EMERGENCY MEDICAL TREATMENT

A Text for EMT-As and EMT-Intermediates

Third Edition

NANCY L. CAROLINE, M.D.
Visiting Professor of Critical Care Medicine
University of Pittsburgh School of Medicine, Pittsburgh

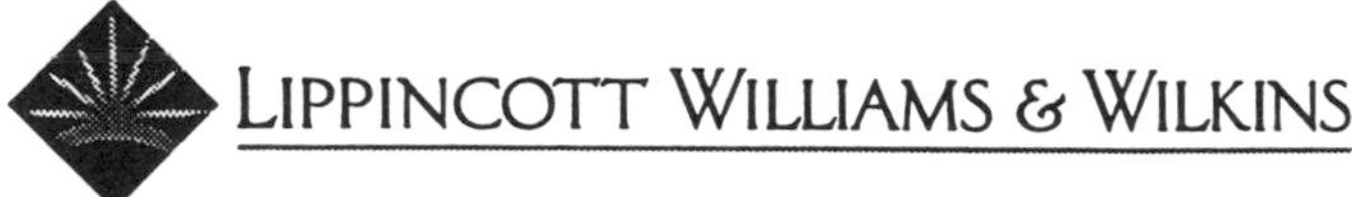

Third Edition

Library of Congress Catalog Card No. 90-63839

ISBN 0-316-12886-4

Printed in the United States of America

MV-NY

Fifth Printing

In memory of

my friend, Asmund Laerdal, whose vision and leadership transformed the field of emergency care;

my uncle, David B. Stearns, M.D., who taught that to care for patients is a privilege that must be earned.

CONTENTS

PREFACE

According to the ancient Greeks, wisdom comes through suffering, a principle that seems to govern the writing of many textbooks. Learning, according to this point of view, must involve a certain amount of tedium to be worthwhile. I do not subscribe to that particular philosophy. One of the underlying assumptions in writing this text, and in writing the workbook that accompanies it, was that learning—especially learning to be an emergency medical technician—ought to be interesting and challenging and sometimes even fun, because ambulance work is interesting and challenging and sometimes even fun. Thus a textbook for EMTs ought to capture some of that excitement and enjoyment.

A textbook ought, furthermore, to be more than just a compilation of facts. It ought to *teach*. That is the aim of this text. **Learning objectives** are clearly defined at the beginning of each chapter to focus the reader's attention on what he or she is expected to master. **Boxed summaries** at the end of each chapter further emphasize important points and permit quick reference during review. Logical processes are summarized in **flowcharts** to help the reader identify key decision points in evaluating and managing various emergencies. New vocabulary is highlighted in boldface type when it is first introduced and summarized in **glossaries** both at the end of each chapter and at the end of the text. **Skill evaluation checklists** are provided to aid in practicing manual skills. **Case histories** are used to illustrate both the classic presentations of various illnesses and the correct format for reporting medical information; and **review questions** accompanying the case histories provide the reader with an opportunity to stop and assess how well he or she has understood the principles covered in the chapter. Finally, a list of **further reading** is included at the end of each chapter for those instructors or students who wish to pursue a given subject in greater depth.

This textbook is designed for use in the United States Department of Transportation (USDOT) course for **EMT-A,** or its equivalent, and thereby it meets the national standard for training emergency medical technicians. In combination with appropriate skill practice and clinical experience, this text provides comprehensive coverage of all the aspects of emergency care that an EMT-A is permitted to render. In addition, more advanced material, indicated in the text with an asterisk, has been included for those taking the **EMT-Intermediate** course.

I received many helpful comments and suggestions regarding the first two editions of this book, and I am grateful to the EMTs and EMT instructors who took the time to let me know what *they* wanted in a textbook. In this third edition, I have tried to incorporate the suggestions I received, in order to make the book more useful to its readers. Thus, **new sec-**

tions have been introduced on "burnout," automated external defibrillators, basic trauma life support (BTLS), cocaine and crack, hazardous materials, and management of violent patients. In addition, many **new illustrations** have been added to help clarify important concepts. Furthermore *all* sections of the book have been updated to reflect current medical opinion and current standards of practice.

Being an EMT is a very special job, and becoming an EMT is a very special process. It is my hope that this text will provide a challenging format for learning the job and a solid foundation for doing the job well.

N. L. C.

ACKNOWLEDGMENTS

Writing a book is not a solitary venture. Especially when the book is a medical textbook, the author is invariably dependent on others for expertise, constructive criticism, and technical and moral support. I am no exception. I would therefore be remiss if I did not acknowledge my gratitude to those whose help has been indispensable in bringing this book, and its new edition, to completion. In particular, I am indebted to:

Dr. Mickey Eisenberg, of the University of Washington in Seattle, who has kept me up to date on advances in emergency medical care while himself contributing prodigiously to those advances.

Dr. William Falk, of Harvard Medical School in Boston, who reviewed the chapter on disturbances of behavior and made enormously helpful recommendations for its improvement.

Dr. Douglas Lindsey, of the University of Arizona in Tucson, who provided invaluable advice regarding the Military Anti-shock Trousers.

Dr. Eugene Nagel, of Winter Haven, Florida, and the University of Florida at Gainesville, who chased down materials that no one else could find and also served as an unfailing source of encouragement.

The EMTs and paramedics of the cities of Boston and Pittsburgh, with whom I "rode rescue" to refresh my own knowledge and whose skill and professionalism were impressive indeed.

The staff of Little, Brown and Company, especially:

Susan Pioli, my editor
Karen Feeney, production editor
Tracey Solon, copy editor
Lou Bruno, production supervisor
Karen Oberheim, the world's most efficient editorial assistant
Mickey Senkarik, medical artist

Finally, I must acknowledge my debt to my students, for it was in the classroom that the material for this book was piloted and refined. A "brilliant" explanation that produced twenty blank stares was eliminated from the text; an explanation that elicited smiles of comprehension was retained. So I am indebted to my students, for, in a very real sense, they are the authors of this book.

N. L. C.

I. THE EMT

Notice
The indications and dosages of all drugs in this book have been recommended in the medical literature and conform to the practices of the general medical community. The medications described do not necessarily have specific approval by the Food and Drug Administration for use in the diseases and dosages for which they are recommended. The package insert for each drug should be consulted for use and dosage as approved by the FDA. Because standards for usage change, it is advisable to keep abreast of revised recommendations, particularly those concerning new drugs. Similarly, the reader is advised to keep abreast of revisions in the standards for cardiopulmonary resuscitation.

1. THE EMT AND THE EMS SYSTEM

OBJECTIVES

In this chapter, we will look at the emergency medical technician (EMT), the EMT's job, and the system in which the EMT operates. What *is* an EMT exactly? What personal qualities are needed for the job? What tasks and responsibilities are involved? What special stresses are imposed by this work? What is the nature of the emergency medical services (EMS) system in which the EMT operates, and what legal constraints govern the EMT's actions?

By the end of this chapter, the reader should be able to

1. Identify the responsibilities of an EMT, given a list of various responsibilities
2. Identify personal qualities desirable in an EMT
3. List the components of an EMS system, and identify weak components, given a description of a hypothetical EMS system
4. Identify those situations in which an EMT may treat a patient without obtaining the patient's consent, given a list of various situations
5. Identify the correct definitions of (a) standard of care, (b) duty to act, (c) consent, (d) abandonment, and (e) negligence, given a list of definitions
6. Identify cases that must be reported to public authorities, given a list of different types of cases

WHAT DOES AN EMT DO?

In the old days of "swoop and scoop" ambulance services, ambulance personnel had one main responsibility: to get the ill or injured patient to a hospital as rapidly as possible. An ambulance was viewed simply as a means of fast horizontal transportation to a medical facility, and the ambulance attendant needed little skill or knowledge except in driving an emergency vehicle.

The strategy of "grab the patient and run" was not an entirely satisfactory one, however. The precipitous ride to the hospital itself often worsened the patient's condition, especially if—as was usually the case—the patient had not received any stabilization before transport and was left unattended, to fend for himself in the back of the ambulance. "Dead-on-arrival" was an all too frequent diagnosis, and in many cases death occurred—preventable death—while the patient was in transit, before he could reach medical treatment. The transportation of critically ill and injured patients to the hospital, in other words, was causing a delay in treatment that frequently resulted in further disability or death.

For that reason, medical professionals began asking, "How can we minimize the delay in treating the seriously ill or injured patient?" The answer was simple yet revolutionary: BRING THE TREATMENT TO THE PATIENT BEFORE BRINGING THE PATIENT TO THE HOSPITAL.

In order to make such a concept work, some very fundamental changes had to occur in ambulance design, equipment, and personnel. The vehicles, to begin with, had to be redesigned to facilitate *care* of the patient, not just transportation (see Chapter 38). Lifesaving equipment had to be added; a stretcher and a few bandages were no longer sufficient. Furthermore, since an unaccompanied ambulance driver could not simultaneously drive and look after a patient, it was necessary to staff ambulances with *at least* two individuals, and these personnel had to acquire a variety of new skills to enable them to take on the additional responsibilities of emergency medical care.

In the mid-1960s, the modern ambulance and the emergency medical technician (EMT) came into existence as a strategy to provide early care, primary stabilization, and safe, supervised transport of the sick and injured. Today's EMT is in another league altogether from yesterday's ambulance driver. The EMT is a *health care professional* with many responsibilities, each requiring a whole set of special skills and knowledge. These responsibilities are listed in Table 1-1 and can be briefly summarized as follows:

What is the EMT's Job?

- To reach the patient as rapidly as possible
- To gain control of the scene, as necessary
- To recognize the nature and seriousness of the patient's illness or injury and provide whatever basic emergency care is needed for sustaining life and reducing further injury
- To move the patient safely and rapidly to a medical facility where definitive care can be given
- To provide the hospital team with a clear and accurate report of findings and treatment in the field

Table 1-1. *EMT's Responsibilities*

EMT's Responsibilities	Necessary Skills and Knowledge
Rapid response to the scene of an emergency	Emergency and defensive driving Knowing traffic laws Knowing the most expeditious route to any given location Knowing special conditions (e.g., roads under repair)
Control of the scene and hazard control (when fire or police officials are not present)	How to handle traffic hazards How to take command of a crowd How to handle environmental hazards (e.g., downed wires, spilled gasoline)
Gaining access to the patient	How to protect oneself from injury Forcible entry
Establishment of priorities for emergency care	Patient evaluation: taking a history, doing a physical assessment Evaluating the relative urgency of different injuries Triage of multiple patients
Administration of prompt and efficient care	Knowing and applying appropriate measures for many medical and traumatic problems, with skills of airway maintenance; CPR; control of bleeding; splinting; bandaging; administering O_2
Extrication and preparation for transport	Basic rescue Use of backboards and various types of stretchers Patient handling and carrying
Supervised transport to the hospital	Monitoring the patient's condition: level of consciousness, vital signs
Orderly transfer of responsibility to the hospital medical team	Communicating medical information
Proper record-keeping	Writing a medical case report
Maintenance of the vehicle and its equipment	Taking inventory How to check the vehicle and each piece of equipment

WHO CAN BECOME AN EMT?

The qualifications for entry into an EMT course vary somewhat from region to region, but most programs require at least the qualifications listed in Table 1-2. These prerequisites for entry into an EMT course are guidelines, and they should be kept flexible. Experience has shown notable exceptions: individuals who did not meet one or more of the requirements who have become first-rate EMTs. Members of disadvantaged minorities, for example, some of whom had not completed even eighth grade, have been trained to very high levels of proficiency as EMTs and paramedics [2]. Petite young ladies, who would not meet the usual height and weight requirements, have shown themselves to be dedicated and effective EMTs [14, 23]. Indeed, the most important requirements for entry into an EMT course have nothing to do with age, sex, height, weight, or years spent in the classroom. What really matters is basic aptitude, motivation, willingness to learn, and emotional maturity.

In addition to the requirements for course entry, which may vary from program to program, there are formal requirements for licensure or registration as an EMT, both at the state and national level. For

Table 1-2. *Qualifications for Entry into an EMT Course*

Requirement	Reason for the Requirement
High school education	An EMT needs to be able to read technical material and write clear reports using technical terminology.
At least 18 years old	The age requirement is to ensure at least a minimum of physical development and emotional maturity.
Good physical health	An EMT must be able to handle hard, stressful work in which exposure to infection is common.
Reasonable strength (able to lift 100 pounds)	An EMT must carry the combined weight of a patient, stretcher, linens, medical equipment, etc., often down several flights of stairs or over difficult terrain.
Good vision, color discrimination, hearing	An EMT needs these senses to make a physical assessment of the patient. Color discrimination is needed for discerning traffic signals and for noting abnormal colorations of the patient's skin (e.g., jaundice, cyanosis).
Manual dexterity	An EMT must be proficient in the use of various devices that require good coordination.
Driver's license	An EMT should be capable of driving an ambulance in case the usual driver becomes disabled.

example, the requirements for registration by the National Registry of Emergency Medical Technicians (NREMT) are as follows:

1. EMT—NONAMBULANCE CATEGORY
   a. Included in the category: health care personnel (e.g., nurses, LPNs, respiratory therapists, x-ray technicians), law enforcement personnel, industrial safety workers, military medical personnel not doing field service
   b. Requirements for registration:
      (1) At least 18 years of age
      (2) Successful completion of an approved EMT training program
      (3) At least 3 months of experience in some health care activity
2. EMT—AMBULANCE CATEGORY
   a. Included in the category: civilians working with emergency ambulance units or rescue units; military medical personnel with field service
   b. Requirements for registration:
      (1) At least 18 years of age
      (2) At least 6 months of emergency ambulance, rescue, or military field experience
      (3) Successful completion of an approved EMT course
      (4) Successful completion of a written and practical examination

THE PERFECT EMT

We have talked so far about the requirements usually used to screen candidates for an EMT course or for certification; but, as noted, these prerequisites do not by themselves necessarily ensure that the student will become an effective EMT. We need to look also at the *personal traits* desirable in an EMT. So let us examine the perfect EMT and see what qualities go into making him so exemplary.

In reality, the perfect EMT has yet to make an appearance, but when he* does show up, it will be possible to recognize him by the following attributes:

- He is highly DEDICATED to his job and to serving other human beings.
- He has HIGH ETHICAL STANDARDS.
- He demands the best of himself and takes PRIDE IN HIS WORK.
- He is FRIENDLY AND PERSONABLE, able to get along well with others in his crew and other members of the health care team.
- He is COURTEOUS AND SYMPATHETIC toward patients and their families. He shows concern for the patient and knows how to give effective, honest reassurance.
- He has a VOICE THAT INSPIRES CONFIDENCE, and his conversation at the scene is appropriate.
- He conveys a PROFESSIONAL APPEARANCE in his grooming, dress, and behavior. His uniform is clean and orderly, his hair is combed, and he has good personal hygiene.
- He does not smoke in the presence of patients. (If he has any sense, he does not smoke at all!)
- He is SELF-CONFIDENT, but not arrogant.
- He has LEADERSHIP ABILITY and can quickly take control of a situation.
- He keeps COOL UNDER PRESSURE, maintaining firm control over his emotions.
- He is DECISIVE.
- He is resourceful and ABLE TO IMPROVISE.
- He is ABLE TO ACCEPT CRITICISM and learn from mistakes.
- He is concerned and involved with PUBLIC EDUCATION and knows that an important part of his job is to teach.

The aspiring EMT may find such a list quite overwhelming, but it is important to realize that no one is

*Bear in mind as you conduct your search for the perfect EMT that "he" may be a "she."

born with the personal qualities listed above. They are qualities that any motivated person can develop, to one degree or another, with time and experience. Probably no one will ever become a truly "perfect EMT," but the EMT who strives to do his or her job as effectively and professionally as possible will come very close.

OBJECTIVES OF THE EMT COURSE

In order to study effectively, students need to know what they are expected to learn in a course. What are the general objectives of a basic EMT training program? Upon successful completion of an EMT course, the student should be able to

- Recognize the nature of a patient's illness or injury, evaluate its seriousness, and assess the need for emergency medical care
- Give the appropriate emergency medical care necessary to stabilize the patient's condition
- Handle and move the patient in such a way as to minimize discomfort and further injury
- Transfer the patient safely to a medical facility and give an accurate account of the patient's problem and status to the health professional who is taking over the patient's care

All of the above sounds very nice, but precisely how will the EMT accomplish these goals? Clearly the student will have to acquire a whole array of new skills. By the conclusion of the course, the student will be expected to demonstrate proficiency in the following:

- PATIENT ASSESSMENT. The student will be able to elicit a relevant history of the patient's illness or injury and to perform a pertinent physical examination. Furthermore, the student will be able to reach appropriate conclusions regarding the implications of clinical findings for treatment at the scene.
- In the MANAGEMENT OF IMMEDIATELY LIFE-THREATENING CONDITIONS, such as cessation of breathing, absence of pulse, or profuse bleeding, the student will be able to
  1. Open and maintain a patient's airway, using manual techniques and adjuncts (e.g., oropharyngeal airway)
  2. Provide effective artificial ventilation to a nonbreathing patient, using mouth-to-mouth, mouth-to-nose, and mouth-to-laryngectomy techniques, and using adjunctive equipment, including
     a. Pocket mask
     b. Bag-valve-mask
     c. Esophageal obturator*
  3. Administer oxygen under appropriate circumstances, using
     a. Face mask
     b. Nasal cannula
     c. Bag-valve-mask
     d. Demand valve and mask
  4. Perform effective cardiopulmonary resuscitation (CPR) on an adult (alone or in conjunction with another rescuer) and infant
  5. Control external bleeding
  6. Treat shock by proper positioning of the patient, application of Military Anti-Shock Trousers, and establishment of an intravenous infusion*
- In the MANAGEMENT OF URGENT CONDITIONS, the student will be able to demonstrate competence in
  1. Dressing and bandaging wounds
  2. Splinting fractures, using commercially available and improvised splints
  3. Immobilizing a spine-injured patient on short and long backboards
  4. Giving obstetric assistance in emergency childbirth
  5. Giving primary emergency care to patients with breathing difficulty, chest pain, seizures, coma, stroke, and a variety of other medical conditions
- The student will have a number of related NON-MEDICAL SKILLS and will be able to demonstrate competence in
  1. Medical reporting and record-keeping
  2. Radio communications
  3. Emergency driving
  4. Vehicle and equipment maintenance
  5. Controlling the scene of an emergency and any hazards therein
  6. Basic rescue

At the beginning of each chapter in this book, we will identify the objectives of the chapter. Where specific manual skills are required, a skill checklist will be supplied at the end of the chapter for the student to use as an aid in practicing.

It must be emphasized that skills are learned by doing, not by reading. No one ever learned to ride a bicycle by reading a book about it, and the same is true of learning cardiopulmonary resuscitation or bandaging or splinting. A textbook can only provide guidelines.

There is a well-known joke about a young music lover who goes to New York City for the first time and loses his way near Rockefeller Plaza. He approaches an elderly man and asks, "Sir, can you tell me how to get to Carnegie Hall?"

The old man smiles kindly and answers, "Practice, son, practice."

*EMT-Intermediate only.

Students who wish to complete their EMT training successfully will do well to heed that advice.

THE EMS SYSTEM

The EMT forms one link in a whole chain of responses, all of which are necessary for an effective emergency medical services (EMS) system. A fully developed EMS system has the following components:

Components of an EMS System

1. RECOGNITION of the emergency and FIRST AID by bystanders
2. INITIATION of the EMS response system by universal emergency telephone number, highway phones, radio, and a communications center
3. TREATMENT AT THE SCENE by members of the system, including firemen, rescuers, and ambulance crews, using mobile intensive care ambulances and, if needed, aircraft ambulances
4. TRANSPORTATION WITH ADVANCED LIFE SUPPORT by members of the system
5. Treatment in the EMERGENCY DEPARTMENT of a hospital or in a separate life support facility
6. Treatment in the OPERATING ROOM
7. Treatment in the INTENSIVE CARE UNIT
8. ORGANIZATION and COMMUNICATION
9. PLANNING, EDUCATION, and EVALUATION
10. RESEARCH

In order to understand how an EMS system works, or breaks down, we need to take a closer look at each of these links in the EMS chain.

RECOGNITION OF THE EMERGENCY AND FIRST AID BY BYSTANDERS

In order to enter the EMS system, the patient or someone in the patient's surroundings must be aware that an emergency exists and thus be motivated to call for help. In general, this is not a problem in the case of injuries, for there are few people who cannot recognize that an injury has occurred. In the case of some medical emergencies, however, there are often significant delays in realizing that an urgent situation exists. Let us consider a case in which this component of the system breaks down:

Marvin Macho is a 45-year-old, hard-driving business executive who lives in a townhouse with his wife, two children (ages 11 and 15), and their Doberman pinscher. Cardiacburgh, the community in which he resides, boasts one of the best ambulance services in the United States. Mobile intensive care units staffed by skilled paramedics are within a 4-minute response time of every location in town. Furthermore, the emergency room of the local hospital is staffed exclusively by doctors and nurses who have been certified in advanced life support, and the hospital's coronary care unit is second to none. All told, Cardiacburgh ought to be about the safest place in America to have a heart attack—if you know you are having one, that is. Take poor Marvin. One night after dinner, he starts feeling a heavy, squeezing pressure in his chest.

"Marvin, dear, you look a little pale," says his wife.

"It's nothing, sweetie," says Marvin, "just a little indigestion. I think I'll just go lie down for a bit."

Two hours later Mrs. Macho finds her husband dead in the bedroom. The best EMS system in the United States could not prevent Marvin's death from heart attack, because Marvin did not know he was having one.

In Marvin's case, the weak link in the EMS chain was LACK OF PUBLIC EDUCATION IN THE SIGNS AND SYMPTOMS OF SERIOUS ILLNESS. All the other links in the chain were strong. The system was poised and ready to respond, but ignorance killed Marvin Macho.

The second aspect of this link in the chain is *first aid by bystanders*. The best ambulance service cannot reach every critically ill patient immediately, and if care is to start immediately—as it must in cases of cardiac arrest—it has to be initiated by people already on the scene. In regions where the lay public has received training in CPR, the rate of successful resuscitation by ambulance teams has increased [5, 7]. Even where lay people have not had prior training in CPR, telephone instruction in CPR by a skilled EMS dispatcher has enabled lay people to perform CPR effectively and save lives [3, 12].

Let us return to the case of Marvin Macho and suppose that the family has seen him collapse:

Mrs. Macho runs over to her husband and shakes him. "Marvin, Marvin, are you all right?" she cries.

Marvin doesn't answer.

"I don't think he's breathing," says Marvin's 11-year-old son.

"We ought to do something," says his 15-year-old son.

"I think you're supposed to bang him on the chest," the 11-year-old volunteers.

"No, stupid, you're supposed to throw cold water on him," says the older brother.

"Maybe we ought to call an ambulance," says the 11-year-old.

"Yeah, that's a good idea. Call an ambulance."

The ambulance is just finishing up a case at the hospital, 15 minutes away. When the ambulance team arrives, they find Marvin cold and lifeless. They attempt CPR, but they cannot revive him.

Here, then, we see another weak link: NO ONE AT THE SCENE KNEW WHAT TO DO. Again, this is a matter of public education. An EMS system does not operate in a vacuum. The lay public form the first link in the EMS chain, and if the average citizen does not know how to recognize an emergency and know what to do until help arrives, the whole system is jeopardized.

INITIATION OF THE EMS RESPONSE SYSTEM

Once an emergency has been recognized, someone has to call for help. That is not always as easy as it sounds. Granted, an increasing number of communities are installing the 911 emergency phone number, but there are still many locations throughout the country where no such universal number exists. The victim of sudden illness or injury may find himself staring at a bewildering array of telephone numbers under the "ambulance" heading in the Yellow Pages and may start phoning those numbers only to discover that he is not in the jurisdiction of any of the services listed. Or the patient may be the victim of an automobile accident on a lonely highway, miles from the nearest phone. An adequate EMS system requires adequate means for notification of emergencies, including

- A universal emergency telephone number (911)
- Public telephones, located at frequent intervals, that do not require a coin for operation of the emergency number
- Linkage between the EMS communications center and other radio systems, especially channel 9 of Citizen's Band (CB) radio

TREATMENT AT THE SCENE BY MEMBERS OF THE SYSTEM

Once the call for help has gone out, it is critical that those who respond to the call be capable of giving the appropriate and necessary treatment at the scene. Take the case of Elsipeth McDwiddle:

Elsipeth is an 80-year-old widow living in Mud Creek, a rural community in the south central part of the country. One day while repairing a leak in the roof, Elsipeth falls and breaks her hip. She finds she cannot move from the spot where she has fallen. Her shouts attract a neighbor, who calls for an ambulance, and about 20 minutes later a sleek, black limousine arrives from Smith's Funeral Home.

"Lord a mercy," says Elsipeth, "what'd you send the hearse for? I'm not dead yet."

"You called for an ambulance, Ma'am?" asks the undertaker, as he pulls a stretcher out of the back of the hearse.

"Lord a mercy," says Elsipeth.

"Now if you'll just step over onto this nice stretcher," says the undertaker. The loud crunch of bones grating together is heard as he helps Elsipeth onto the stretcher.

Elsipeth needed an ambulance, and the arrival of a hearse instead could not have inspired much confidence. Nor was the undertaker properly trained to render emergency care at the scene. Elsipeth's fracture should have been stabilized before any attempt was made to move her. The case is not as farfetched as it seems. In many areas of the United States, there are few minimum standards regarding ambulance vehicles and the personnel who staff them, and much of the ambulance business is still conducted by funeral homes. In Elsipeth's case, the weak link in the chain was the ABSENCE OF AN ADEQUATE AMBULANCE VEHICLE AND OF PROPERLY QUALIFIED RESCUERS.

TRANSPORTATION WITH ADVANCED LIFE SUPPORT BY MEMBERS OF THE SYSTEM

An important component of the EMS system requires that (1) the ambulance or rescue vehicle be equipped to deliver advanced life support, (2) at least some members of the ambulance team be trained to the level of paramedic, and (3) the paramedics be under the command of a physician (usually by radio). Studies have shown that the longer it takes a cardiac arrest victim to receive definitive care (e.g., defibrillation), the less are the chances of successful resuscitation [7, 9, 10]. At this time in many regions, EMTs are not permitted to perform defibrillation, nor are they permitted to administer the drugs necessary to stabilize a patient's cardiac rhythm. Those treatments may be done only by physicians or by paramedics operating under direct physician control. Thus paramedic-staffed mobile intensive care units (MICUs) are a vital component of the EMS system. Unfortunately, a paramedic's training is long and costly, and a fully equipped MICU can cost $50,000 just for the vehicle and its gear. Few communities can afford to supply a paramedic-staffed MICU within a 4-minute response time of every citizen. Furthermore, only a small percentage of emergency calls actually require the services of a paramedic. An EMT is perfectly capable of taking care of routine wounds, splinting fractures, and handling the majority of calls that come in to the emergency dispatcher. Many communities have found that the most cost-effective way to provide emergency medical service is a "tiered system," consisting of several EMT units and a smaller number of paramedic units. The EMTs are expected to respond first to every call and are stationed in such a way as to keep the response times minimal. When the EMTs reach the scene, they make a primary evaluation of the situation, initiate care, and call for paramedic assistance when needed. Without the EMTs, the system would be prohibitively expensive, and the paramedics would often be tied up with minor calls when they are needed for more critical cases. Without the paramedics, the EMTs could not do the most effective job in treating major catastrophes such as cardiac arrest. Thus the two-tiered system benefits all concerned, especially the patient.

In many areas, it simply may not be economically feasible to employ paramedics, and compromise solutions must be sought. One such solution is the intermediate-level EMT (EMT-I), who has all the training of a basic EMT (EMT-A) plus certain advanced life support skills. It has also been suggested that EMTs be given training and authorization in defibrillation, and this strategy has proved successful in early trials [10, 11]. The lesson in all this is that in order for the fourth link in the EMS chain to be strong, the EMS system must be flexible enough to permit alternative solutions to problems when conventional solutions are not feasible.

TREATMENT IN THE EMERGENCY DEPARTMENT

In order for the victim of serious illness or injury to benefit from the EMS system, the care he received at the scene must continue in the emergency department. Not every emergency department is equipped to handle critically ill or injured patients, however. Many emergency departments do not have 24-hour coverage by physicians or do not have x-ray or laboratory facilities available around the clock. Emergency departments that ordinarily do not receive a large volume of patients may have little experience in dealing with major emergencies. Let us look, for example, at the case of Evel Knish:

Evel Knish, age 26, drives a 1,000-cc Honda. One day while he is executing a not-so-controlled skid, Evel upends his bike, which lands on top of him and drags him 50 feet down the highway. The EMT crew arriving first on the scene finds Evel only semiconscious, bleeding from multiple wounds on his arms and legs, and apparently in shock. They call in a paramedic unit, and while the paramedics are on the way, the EMTs control Evel's bleeding, dress his wounds, splint a suspicious looking arm, and ready a backboard. When the paramedics arrive, the team applies Military Anti-Shock Trousers, gets an intravenous line going, and immobilizes Evel to a long backboard. Evel is then loaded into an MICU and transported, with careful attention to his vital signs, to the emergency room of Rosydale Hospital.

Upon arrival at the emergency department, the ambulance team is greeted with the news, "Doc's not in. We'll have to call him at home. Just put the patient over there, in room 2."

Somewhat reluctantly, the EMTs and paramedics do as they are told and leave Evel in the care of a nurse. A few moments later, an orderly comes running out to the ambulance. "You folks won't want to be forgetting these!" he shouts, waving the backboard and the Military Anti-Shock Trousers.

"You mean you took those off the patient!" one of the paramedics says incredulously.

"Sure. Why not?"

By this time, Evel is back in shock. Were he to live, he would be paralyzed from the neck down, due to improper handling in being moved from the backboard to the gurney in room 2. But Evel won't make it, for he will die of internal bleeding before the doctor gets from his house to the hospital.

Another weak link in the chain: THE EMERGENCY DEPARTMENT THAT IS NOT EQUIPPED TO DEAL WITH CRITICALLY ILL AND INJURED PATIENTS. Nothing is more frustrating for the EMT who has done a good job stabilizing a patient in the field than to bring the patient to an emergency room that cannot carry on this same level of care.

TREATMENT IN THE OPERATING ROOM AND INTENSIVE CARE UNIT

Clearly, the same inadequacies that can occur in a hospital emergency department may afflict the surgical and intensive care facilities—deficiencies in coverage, equipment, and training of personnel. When the weak link in the chain is in the operating room or intensive care unit, all the good that has been done can be cancelled out.

ORGANIZATION, COMMUNICATION, PLANNING, EDUCATION, EVALUATION, RESEARCH

The components of organization, communication, planning, education, evaluation, and research may not, at first glance, seem particularly relevant to the day-to-day care of patients in an EMS system. In fact, these links are as vital as any of the others, and they may have enormous impact on the outcome of a patient's illness or injury. Let us look, for example, at evaluation and research:

Collecting data on hundreds of cases of prehospital cardiac arrest, doctors in King County, Washington observe that one of the most critical factors determining whether resuscitation will be successful is the amount of time that elapses between cardiac arrest and defibrillation. The sooner the patient is defibrillated after cardiac arrest, the better his chances for survival [8]. Based on that observation, they postulate that if the first rescuers on the scene —usually EMT-As rather than paramedics—were able to perform defibrillation, more lives could be saved. To test that theory, they train a group of EMT-As in defibrillation and then carry out more studies to compare the survival rates among cardiac arrest victims who did and did not have the benefit of EMT-A defibrillation. Their studies show a clear increase in lives saved where EMT-As are trained and authorized to defibrillate [11]. They are therefore able to make sound recommendations that may save many more lives all across the country.

Evaluation and research mean looking for more effective ways to give emergency medical care. For the EMT, it means critiquing each case and asking, "How could I have done it better?"

It is clear, then, that the total EMS system is only as strong as its weakest link, and for this reason, the EMT needs to be involved not only in his or her own limited phase of the system, but also with the operations of the total system in which the ambulance team works. The EMT needs to examine the EMS services in the community and ask, "Where is the weak link?" and then do whatever is possible to help remedy that weakness. If, for example, the weak link is in public education, the EMT can become involved in programs to teach the public about signs of serious disease, utilization of the EMS system, and basic first aid [20].

The EMT has a vested interest in every link in the EMS chain, for if there is a weak link anywhere, the EMT's efforts—no matter how proficient—may ultimately be for nothing.

MEDICOLEGAL ISSUES

Like all other health care professionals, EMTs can be sued. They can be sued if careless or improper operation of the ambulance results in an accident with injuries to others. EMTs can be sued if their failure to render appropriate care results in further injury to the patient. And this is probably as it should be. In a free society, every citizen has the right to seek legal redress when he feels he has suffered injury through the actions of another, and the courts exist to protect this right.

Whenever a health care professional—doctor, nurse, or EMT—goes to the aid of a patient, he or she automatically accepts certain responsibilities and obligations. It is very important for the EMT to understand what these obligations are, for failure to carry out such obligations can result in a lawsuit. In this section, we will discuss some of the legal concepts relevant to the EMT's work and consider some ways by which the EMT can minimize the risk of being sued.

THE DUTY TO ACT

The duty to act requires that public or municipal ambulance operators respond to the aid of an injured person in their jurisdiction. In general, public ambulance services such as those provided through police or fire departments may not refuse a call. This requirement does not, in many instances, apply to private ambulance services, which are often permitted to select calls at their own discretion. However, local ordinances vary, and it is important for EMTs to know the rules applicable to their own service.

THE STANDARD OF CARE

The standard of care refers to the way an individual is expected to behave; that is, did the EMT provide care according to a given standard or norm? Obviously, the "standard of care" is not one fixed standard; an EMT, for example, would not be expected to give the same level of care as that expected from a physician. The courts consider several factors when examining the standard of care rendered.

The Type of Individual Involved

The courts will compare the behavior of the individual—for example, the EMT—against that of another hypothetical person with similar training and experience. In other words, the court will ask, would another EMT have conducted himself the same way in the same circumstances, with the same equipment and in the same place?

Standards Imposed by Force of Law

In some regions, there may be specific statutes, ordinances, legal precedents, or other rules that require certain standards of care. Such statutes vary considerably from region to region, and it is important for the EMT to be familiar with the legal standards in his or her own state.

Professional or Institutional Standards

Professional standards generally include published recommendations of organizations involved in emergency work, such as the standards of the National Registry of Emergency Medical Technicians governing registration as an EMT. Institutional standards include protocols, standing orders, or other procedural rules of the ambulance service by which the EMT is employed. These standards do not carry the force of law; deviation from these standards does not necessarily imply that any law has been broken. Nonetheless, professional or institutional standards may be introduced as evidence in court to help the jury decide whether the EMT acted appropriately. Thus it is very important for EMTs to be thoroughly familiar with published recommendations pertaining to their work. If the ambulance service has a manual of protocols and standing orders, the EMT should know those procedures and follow them. The EMT should also keep abreast of the standards of the National Registry and similar organizations.

CONSENT

The rendering of emergency medical care requires the *consent*—the concurrence or agreement—of the patient, for every person has the right to be free from interference by another person. Any touching of the patient's body without the patient's consent may be considered technical assault and battery. There are several important aspects of consent.

Informed Consent

Consent must be *informed*. Patients must be told, in a manner they can understand, what is going to be done and for what purpose, what risks are involved, and what alternative treatments are available, if any. After explaining the procedure in this way, the EMT should make sure that the patient understands what has been said and then ask for consent to the procedure. For example, suppose you are attending a conscious, 35-year-old man who fell from a ladder and broke his forearm, and you decide to apply an air splint. You explain to the patient:

It looks like you've got a broken arm, and we want to put it into a splint in order to prevent any more damage and to make you more comfortable. The kind of splint we are using is very safe, but it can interfere with the circulation to your hand if it gets too tight, so you'll have to tell us if you feel any tingling in your fingers. Do you understand what we plan to do?

If the patient has questions, the EMT should answer them as clearly and honestly as possible. For example, the patient might ask, "Will the splint put my bones back in the right position?" The EMT would answer, "No. The splint just holds the broken parts of the bone steady, so that the jagged edges won't damage the tissue around them. In the emergency room, the doctor will realign the bones and put a cast on, if necessary, to hold them in place." Once the patient fully understands, the EMT should ask for consent to splinting.

Informed consent must be obtained from *every* conscious, mentally competent adult.

Implied Consent

In a situation where an adult is unconscious or otherwise unable to give informed consent and is in need of immediate emergency medical care to prevent death or further injury, the law assumes that the individual would consent to receiving emergency care and being transported to the hospital. Such consent is said to be implied, and the EMT may proceed with whatever lifesaving treatment is needed. Even in the situation of an unconscious patient, however, it may be possible to obtain consent from someone other than the patient himself, such as next of kin, a spouse, or a close relative. It is always preferable to obtain consent when possible, and implied consent should be invoked only when the patient is physically incapable of giving consent, when there is an immediate threat to his life or limb, and there is no one else at the scene who can give consent in the patient's behalf.

Consent for the Treatment of Minors

In the case of minors, consent must be obtained from the parent, guardian, or other person legally responsible for the child. In general, a minor is defined as someone less than 18 years of age, but in some states the decision of what constitutes a minor depends on the maturity of the individual. In addition, certain conditions, such as marriage or maintaining a separate household, qualify a minor to be treated as an adult. The consent of a 17-year-old boy who is married, employed, and the head of a household, for example, would probably be considered valid, while the consent of a 6-year-old child would not.

In the situation in which immediate emergency treatment is necessary to save a child's life or prevent further injury and a parent or guardian is not available to give consent, emergency treatment may be undertaken, as consent is considered to be implied.

Consent from a Mentally Disturbed Patient

A person who is mentally disturbed or otherwise mentally incompetent (e.g., a severely retarded adult) is, by definition, incapable of giving informed consent, for he or she is incapable of understanding explanations and of considering those explanations in a rational manner. If the patient's mental disability is well-established and he or she is under the care of a guardian, consent should be sought from the guardian, just as in the case of a minor. Once again, if an immediate threat to life or limb exists and no guardian is present, consent is considered to be implied, and the EMT may proceed with whatever measures are necessary to sustain life and prevent further injury.

The Right to Refuse Treatment

A mentally competent adult has the right to refuse treatment, and this fact can create a very frustrating situation for rescue personnel who feel treatment is necessary. A great deal of tact and judgment is required in dealing with the patient who refuses treatment, and in each case the EMT should try to determine

1. Is the patient truly mentally competent? A severely ill or injured person may be confused or disoriented. In such a circumstance, refusal to accept treatment cannot be assumed to be an informed refusal. If there is substantial doubt regarding the patient's competence, the EMT should probably go ahead with whatever treatment is urgently needed to sustain life. The EMT's task, after all, is to save lives, and the risk of a lawsuit is generally greater for failure to give treatment than for failure to obtain consent. The guideline, then, is that when there is an immediate threat to the patient and doubt exists as to the patient's mental competence, give the necessary treatment.
2. Does the patient understand the possible consequences of refusing treatment? Just as consent

must be informed, refusal to accept treatment must also be informed. The EMT should explain to the patient, in straightforward terms, the possible consequences of refusing care.

Suppose, for example, the patient is a 45-year-old man with severe chest pain who refuses to go to the hospital. The EMT might say to the patient:

"Sir, from the symptoms you're having, it sounds like you may be having a heart attack, and we think it's very important that you get checked out by a doctor. If it's not a heart attack and everything's OK, they'll send you home. But if it is a heart attack, you need to be in a hospital where they can keep a close eye on you, because at home there is a serious risk you would collapse without anyone here to help you."

It is also sometimes useful to try to determine why the patient is refusing treatment or transport to the hospital. In some cases, a person will refuse treatment on religious grounds, and that is certainly within each person's rights. But in other cases, the patient may refuse treatment as a way of denying that he is seriously ill, out of fear of what will happen in the hospital, or out of concern for another family member. An elderly man, for example, may have legitimate concerns about leaving an invalid wife at home alone. By learning the reasons for the patient's refusal, the EMT may be able to provide reassurance or enlist the help of a social service agency where needed.

Consent to Psychiatric Hospitalization
Emergencies involving disturbed behavior present the EMT with complex and difficult problems. On the one hand, the patient's family may be very panicky and demanding ("Take him to the hospital. Can't you see he's crazy and needs to be in the hospital? What are you waiting for?"); on the other hand, the patient himself may refuse to go to the hospital. The EMT cannot invoke the principle of implied consent in such a case, for, although the patient may well be mentally incompetent, there is no immediate threat to the patient's life, such as severe bleeding or choking. Generally speaking, a police officer is the only individual given the authority to restrain or transport a person against his will. An EMT should not do so except at the express request of the police. Each ambulance service should have well-established procedures for this situation, and those procedures should be based on local statutes and preferably be worked out in conjunction with local police authorities. If the patient has a history of emotional problems, consultation with his psychiatrist may facilitate care and transport.

IMMUNITY
Various statutes provide partial immunity from liability to a person who stops at the scene of an accident to help an injured person. The most common statute of this type is a *Good Samaritan Act*, and most states have Good Samaritan laws of one sort or another. The Florida Good Samaritan Law of 1965 (Flor. Stat. Ann. 768.13) is an example of such legislation:

> Any person, including those licensed to practice medicine, who gratuitously and in good faith renders emergency care or treatment at the scene of an emergency outside of a hospital, doctor's office or other place having proper medical equipment, without objection of the injured victim or victims thereof, shall not be held liable for any civil damages as a result of any act or failure to act in providing or arranging further medical treatment where the person acts as an ordinary reasonable prudent man would have acted under the same circumstances.

There are several important things to note about this act:

- The Good Samaritan Law does define a *standard of care* ("where the person acts as an ordinary reasonable prudent man would have acted. . .").
- Most Good Samaritan laws require that the person providing care does not receive payment for doing so ("gratuitously . . . renders emergency care"). Since an EMT who is on duty *is* being paid for his work, the Good Samaritan Law may not offer protection. (An off-duty EMT who helps at the scene of an accident, on the other hand, *would* be protected by such a statute.) Consult the wording of your own state's Good Samaritan Law to determine what protection it offers to an EMT rendering care while on the job.
- The Good Samaritan Law does *not* provide any immunity in cases where negligence or misconduct results in injury to the patient.

NEGLIGENCE
When a person is sued for negligence, he is sued for *neglecting* his responsibility to the patient in such a way that injury was done to the patient. Negligence can apply to any aspect of prehospital care, from dispatch to the selection of the receiving hospital. It can apply when there is faulty or substandard equipment on the ambulance, when the vehicle is not properly maintained, or when the EMT fails to perform his duties properly.

In order to prove negligence, the injured party or his or her survivors must demonstrate all of the following:

- That an injury occurred
- That the person accused of negligence had a *duty to act*
- That the person accused of negligence failed to act as another prudent person with similar train-

ing would have acted under the same circumstances
- That this failure to act appropriately was the cause of the person's injury

Suppose that an EMT employed by the municipality responds to the scene of an automobile accident in his jurisdiction and finds an injured man lying on the road. The EMT thinks the patient looks all right and does not bother to examine him closely, so he does not notice that the patient is bleeding profusely beneath his coat. The EMT loads the patient into the ambulance without treatment and proceeds to the hospital. The patient meanwhile bleeds to death on the way. The EMT is subsequently sued for negligence by the patient's family. It is clear that an injury occurred (1)—the patient died. The EMT accused of negligence had a duty to act (2) because the emergency call was in the jurisdiction of his ambulance service. Furthermore, the EMT failed to act as another prudent EMT would have acted under the same circumstances (3); the hypothetical EMT would have examined the patient carefully and made an attempt to control the patient's bleeding before undertaking transport. Finally, this failure of the EMT to act appropriately, that is, to control the patient's bleeding, was the cause of the patient's death (4). Thus our EMT was clearly negligent, and no Good Samaritan law would protect him in such a case.

Suppose, on the other hand, the EMT had examined the patient carefully, located the bleeding, and used all the measures in which he had been trained to try to stop the bleeding; despite all this, the patient died on the way to the hospital. Once again, the EMT had a duty to act. But in this instance, the EMT *did* act as another prudent person with similar training would have acted; he did the best job he could according to his level of training. In this case, it would be extremely unlikely that a court would find the EMT guilty of negligence.

ABANDONMENT

Abandonment is defined as the termination of contact with a patient without the patient's consent and without giving the patient sufficient time or opportunity to find another health professional who can assume his or her care. The term also implies that the patient had a continuing need for medical care and that the abrupt termination of care was the cause of subsequent injury or death. What this means in practice is that once EMTs have responded to a call for help, they may not leave the patient until there has been an orderly transfer of responsibility to another health professional, such as the doctor or nurse in the emergency room. Let us look at an example of abandonment:

The ambulance is called to the home of a 60-year-old man who is complaining of severe chest pain and difficulty in breathing. The patient says he has had the pain for 2 hours. While the EMT is taking the patient's vital signs (pulse, respirations, and blood pressure), he hears a call on the two-way radio for an auto accident about a mile away. The EMT decides he would like to respond to that call since there might be some serious injuries, so he tells the patient, "Listen, I have to go to an accident. Why don't you just phone a cab and have them take you to the hospital." The EMT leaves and proceeds to the scene of the accident. Meanwhile, the patient with chest pain collapses and dies at home, waiting for a taxi.

This is a clear case of abandonment. The patient was simply left by the EMT without any competent medical professional to take over care, and the patient died as a consequence.

Abandonment may also occur on the threshold of the hospital. The EMT's responsibility is to transfer the patient to another health professional, not to a building, and merely bringing the patient to the emergency room and putting him on a gurney is not sufficient. If the emergency room is crowded and the doctors and nurses are busy with other cases, the patient could lie unnoticed before anyone realizes he is even there. When the EMT arrives at a busy emergency room with a seriously ill or injured patient, therefore, the EMT may have to remain with the patient until emergency department personnel are free to take over.

MEDICAL RECORDS

Even the most skilled, conscientious EMT may eventually have to appear in court as a witness or even as a defendant in a lawsuit. If this happens, the EMT's best protection is a thorough and accurate *medical record* of the case in question. We will learn more about the preparation of medical reports in Chapter 12. For our purposes here, it is sufficient to note that whenever EMTs care for patients, they should make a careful, detailed record of each case and include at least the following information:

Medical Record

1. DATE and TIMES (time call was received, response time, time the patient arrived at a medical facility).
2. Information obtained from the patient and bystanders (HISTORY).
3. Observations of the scene.
4. Findings of the PHYSICAL ASSESSMENT.
5. Any TREATMENT given. Be precise. Do not, for example, write, "Splint," but rather, "An air splint was applied to the right forearm and inflated."
6. Any CHANGES IN THE PATIENT'S STATUS while under the EMT's care.

The EMT should be as precise and detailed as possible. A medical record is a legal document and reflects upon the person who wrote it [17, 18]. A sloppy, incomplete record may suggest to the court that the treatment given the patient was also sloppy and incomplete. Furthermore, a court will often presume that "if it isn't in the record, it wasn't done." If you failed to document that you gave a certain treatment, the burden of proof will be on you to establish that you did indeed give that treatment. So take the time to make your records accurate and thorough. Needless to say, the medical record is not the place for flippant comments about the patient, and the EMT who is tempted to write such comments on the ambulance trip sheet should consider how they might sound if read aloud in a court of law.

AVOIDING LITIGATION

There is no absolute protection against being sued, but the EMT can substantially reduce the risks of a lawsuit by following a few guidelines:

Medicolegal Guidelines

- Always keep the best interests of the *patient* as your first priority.
- When you respond to an emergency, EXPLAIN TO THE PATIENT WHO YOU ARE and WHAT THE PATIENT CAN EXPECT FROM YOU (e.g., "I'm an emergency medical technician, and my job is to get you to the hospital in the best possible shape. I can't fix your fracture, but I can splint it so that it doesn't get any worse before you reach the hospital.").
- EXPLAIN ALL PROCEDURES CAREFULLY to the patient, make certain the patient understands your explanation, and OBTAIN CONSENT.
- Indicate to the patient that you are concerned about his or her well-being, and MAINTAIN A SYMPATHETIC ATTITUDE toward the patient and his family. Most lawsuits stem from poor interpersonal relationships between the health care provider and the patient.
- FOLLOW the ESTABLISHED PROCEDURES and standing orders of your ambulance service.
- DO YOUR BEST, according to your level of training.
- Once you have responded to a call, REMAIN WITH THE PATIENT until there is an orderly transfer of responsibility to another medical professional.
- Maintain DETAILED, ACCURATE, LEGIBLE RECORDS.

In summary, the EMT should be aware of the obligations and responsibilities that one accepts in caring for a patient. The consequences of neglecting these obligations are serious because the obligations are serious—they involve the lives of other human beings. Nonetheless, the EMT should not have an exaggerated fear of being sued. It is very rare that there is a successful lawsuit against an individual who did his job conscientiously and according to the best of his abilities.

REMEMBER, THE FIRST DUTY OF THE EMT IS TO PROVIDE EMERGENCY MEDICAL CARE. UNDER NO CIRCUMSTANCES SHOULD AN EMT WITHHOLD LIFESAVING TREATMENT BECAUSE OF A FEAR OF BEING SUED.

REPORTABLE CASES

In each state, certain types of cases must be reported to the appropriate authorities.

Animal Bites

Animal bites generally are reported to health and public safety officials by hospital personnel. The EMT can provide useful information, however, by giving a description of the precise location of the incident and reporting any information obtained from bystanders about the animal or the circumstances of the attack.

Apparent Suicide or Homicide

If a person is found dead and there is reason to believe that death occurred from suicide, homicide, or other suspicious causes, the death must be reported to police. The EMT should notify the dispatcher about the case and request that the dispatcher contact police officials. Meanwhile, if at all possible, the ambulance team should remain at the scene until the police arrive, being careful not to touch or move anything. Obviously, if the victim is still alive and needs emergency medical care, that care has first priority.

Injury Sustained During the Commission of a Felony

Many states require reporting of any injury likely to have occurred during the performance of a crime—for instance, a person shot while trying to rob a store. Again, bear in mind that an EMT's job is to provide emergency medical care, and your first obligation is to treat the patient.

Child Abuse

If the ambulance team has reason to believe that an injured child in their care is the victim of abuse, the

EMTs are obligated in nearly all states to report their suspicions and the evidence on which they are based to the physician who takes over care of the child in the hospital. Failure to report suspected child abuse may make the EMT liable to prosecution in the event that the child is abused again. EMTs should *not* confront the parents with their suspicions, nor should they discuss their suspicions publicly. Instead, they should wait until they reach the emergency room and confide their suspicions, in private, to the attending doctor.

MUTILATING INJURIES AND DEATH

Much, if not most, of an EMT's work is not pretty. At the scene of an automobile accident, the EMT may encounter patients with an arm or leg torn off, an eye hanging out of its socket, or intestines spilled all over the pavement. A patient rescued from a fire may reek of burning flesh and be charred beyond recognition. An elderly stroke patient may be found lying in a pool of feces and urine, with vomitus all over his face. These examples are intended to be vivid and to produce revulsion. It is only normal to feel sick and repelled by such scenes. With experience, the EMT becomes accustomed to the sight of blood and vomitus; that is part of one's growth as a professional. But even the most hardened veterans of the ambulance service may still become sick at the sight of a mutilating injury. They may become faint or feel an urge to vomit. There is no disgrace in this reaction, but the EMT who wants to be effective must learn how to overcome feelings of revulsion. Perhaps the best method of doing so is to follow a simple rule:

> DON'T STAND THERE GAPING—GET TO WORK!

The very act of doing something constructive—of having a job to do and getting to work at it—is usually sufficient to focus the EMT's attention on the task at hand, rather than dwelling on his or her own reactions to the scene. Getting to work enables the EMT to detach emotionally and thereby gain control of unpleasant feelings. Most EMTs can report the experience of arriving at the scene of an accident and feeling nauseated upon seeing the injuries involved, but then "snapping out of it" as soon as they got busy with the treatment of patients. An experienced EMT will make use of this observation to help out a buddy who looks "a little green around the gills." A decisive command, such as "Get that right leg splinted," is often all that is needed to mobilize an EMT who has become momentarily stunned by the sight of blood and gore.

Emergency medical work will also eventually bring the EMT into contact with death. Inevitably the EMT will now and then be called to care for a patient whose illness or injury is too severe to be reversed, and inevitably some patients will die while in the EMT's care. It is to be expected that an EMT will react to such an experience; indeed it would be very abnormal not to do so. One experienced EMT trainer has reported that "when EMTs have patients die in their care, they may lose sleep, cry, and have bad dreams" [15]. Sadness, guilt, anxiety, frustration, even anger—all of those are normal and frequent reactions to death. What is important is that the EMT realize those reactions *are* normal and expected [13], that everyone has a right to those feelings, and that there is no shame in being touched by death [22].

Often when a patient dies, the EMT must immediately shift attention to the survivors—the patient's family or close friends—and try to give them some kind of comfort [4]. In order to help the survivors, the EMT must first have taken care of his or her own "unfinished business" about death. Each of us has feelings about death, conditioned by our own life experience. If we try to ignore those feelings, they will get in our way. But if we accept our own feelings about death, they can help us deal with the feelings of other people.

When a patient dies, it is also natural for the EMTs to ask themselves, "Could this death have been prevented?" It is a question that causes every health professional to have more than a few sleepless nights. There is only one defense against this kind of insomnia, and that is to be able to say honestly, "I gave it my best."

No one can ask more of the EMT. Nor can the EMT demand any less of himself.

STRESS AND BURNOUT

THE STRESSES OF WORK AS AN EMT

Being an EMT is tough work—tough physically and tough emotionally. The physical stresses, such as carrying a 200-pound patient down four flights of stairs, can be managed by maintaining good physical health. The emotional stresses are sometimes more difficult to handle. Emotional stresses in the EMT's job include the following:

1. *The stress of responsibility.* The EMT may mean the difference between life and death for a patient, and this fact by itself often puts great pressure on EMTs in carrying out their jobs.

2. *The stress of being "alone."* EMTs are out in the field *on their own*, often in very difficult circumstances. No doctor or nurse stands beside them to supervise their work. They must depend solely on their own skills and knowledge and those of their

partners, for no one is there to bail them out if they get into trouble. That is very different from the hospital setting, where a doctor or nurse can in most cases obtain assistance very quickly if the need arises. The EMT does not usually have that option. The patient may be an hour away from a medical facility, perhaps on a lonely stretch of highway where there are not even any bystanders upon whom the EMT can call for assistance.

3. *The stress of working in crowds.* Emergencies often occur in public places, and EMTs may find their work hampered by agitated bystanders or anxious family members. People at the scene may question the EMTs' competence or put pressure on the rescue team to rush the patient to the hospital. Bystanders may demand, "What are you hanging around here for? Why don't you get him to a hospital so he can be seen by a doctor?"

4. *The stress of uncontrolled conditions.* The EMT does not have the luxury of working in a shiny, clean emergency room where all the equipment required is readily accessible and the patient is conveniently placed on a gurney. The EMT may have to do CPR in the stands of a football stadium in the rain; in a tiny bedroom, wedged between the bureau and the wall; or in the aisle of a movie theatre. He or she may have to splint a broken leg in a sewer or crawl into a wrecked car to apply a cervical collar. Such conditions add to the pressure under which the EMT works.

5. *The stresses of other people's stresses.* By the very nature of the scenario in which they work, EMTs will find that many of the people they encounter in their day-to-day activities are also under stress—patients, their families, public safety officials, nurses, doctors. And that stress may be reflected in short tempers, outright hostility, and general unpleasantness. The EMT may feel bombarded from all sides: the patient insisting, "I don't want an EMT, I want a doctor, for heaven's sake"; the police complaining, "Why don't you get him out of here so we can get traffic moving"; the nurse in the emergency room snapping, "Did you have to bring him *here*? Can't you see how busy we are?"

6. *The stress of unrealistic expectations.* EMTs often put unnecessary stress on themselves by subscribing to mistaken beliefs, such as:

- "I have to be right all the time."
- "I am *totally* responsible for what happens to the patient."
- "I am not permitted ever to make a mistake."

Such beliefs are unrealistic and lead very quickly to burnout. Every health professional must try to do the best job he or she can, but rigid perfectionism only produces guilt and stress.

BURNOUT: SIGNS AND SYMPTOMS

The EMT is bound to experience a variety of reactions to the stresses listed above. Many of the reactions are not very pleasant, including sadness, guilt, impatience, anger, anxiety, nausea, and just plain battle fatigue. All of those feelings crop up in the normal course of every EMT's work. If the EMT does not have a strategy for dealing with such stresses, the stresses and the feelings they generate may accumulate over time and produce the syndrome known as "burnout."

As the term implies, burnout occurs when "the fire goes out," when "the spark is gone," or when the EMT no longer feels any interest or enthusiasm for his or her work. Cumulative stress is part of the reason. Inadequate preparation for the job may be another part. Many people are attracted to careers in EMS by the promise of excitement (sirens, flashing red lights) or by fantasies of heroic action. The excitement *is* there, but the fact is that the vast majority of ambulance calls are routine, and the working EMT will usually spend the bulk of his or her time *waiting* for a call. As one EMT wrote:

> The cancelled calls and nursing home runs, the countless hours on the road subsisting on fast food, trying to convince an ER doc that you know how to recognize a PVC all contribute to a sense of frustration. For every call that leaves you pumped and satisfied with your work, there are a hundred others that inspire only tedium. Somehow, in all of your training and preparation, you never imagined how draining the endless waiting could be [1].

All of which—including the stress and the tedium—is a formula for burnout.

How can you tell if burnout is creeping up on you or your colleagues? Here are some of the symptoms and signs of impending burnout:

Warning Symptoms of Burnout

- Chronic fatigue and irritability
- Cynical, negative attitudes
- Lack of desire to report to work
- Emotional lability (crying easily, flying off the handle without provocation, laughing inappropriately)
- Changes in sleep patterns (insomnia or sleeping more than usual), and waking without feeling refreshed
- Loss of interest in hobbies
- Decreased ability to concentrate
- Declining health: many colds, stomach upsets, muscle aches and pains (especially headaches and backaches)
- A feeling of constant tightness in your muscles
- Overeating; smoking; abusing alcohol or drugs

HOW TO PREVENT BURNOUT

The EMT is bound to experience a variety of rections to the stresses listed above, many of them not very pleasant: sadness, guilt, impatience, anger, anxiety, nausea, and just plain battle fatigue. All of those feelings crop up in the normal course of every EMT's work.

First, the EMT who wants to avoid burnout needs to stay physically healthy. That means a good diet (*not* the junk food that is usually wolfed down between calls); regular exercise; sufficient sleep; and avoidance of self-administered poisons (such as cigarettes, drugs, or alcohol in excessive amounts). When you talk to the EMTs who have *not* burned out—the ones who are still on the job and still enjoying it ten or even twenty years after they started out—you find that one thing they all have in common is that they value themselves. People who value themselves take care of themselves.

There is no magic formula for handling stresses that lead to burnout, but there are a few guidelines that can sometimes be helpful. First of all, it is very important to recognize that feelings of anger or fear or sadness *are* perfectly normal. While the EMT on television may be portrayed as a selfless and heroic saint, the EMTs out on the streets are all human. Even very good EMTs get mad, get scared, or feel sick once in a while. What makes them good EMTs is that they have learned how to handle those feelings in order to maintain an outwardly calm and professional manner when with a patient. They have also learned to go easy on themselves, to accept their own limitations.

The second guideline relates to the way in which EMTs deal with their feelings, and one of the most effective ways of dealing with feelings is to talk about them. A rap session with colleagues gives the whole team a chance to "get it off their chests," and it is not unusual for the EMT to discover at such a session that others in the crew have experienced identical emotions. If the stresses arise from a specific interpersonal conflict—for instance, an ongoing feud with a particular emergency room nurse—the EMT may find that talking directly with the person in question (after both parties have cooled down) can resolve many differences, and each person involved can gain a better understanding of the other's viewpoint.

Finally, a more general guideline for the prevention and treatment of burnout. Use your off-duty time for off-duty purposes. Most EMTs are highly motivated individuals who chose their particular line of work because they are genuinely committed to it. Such people often find it hard to go off duty. It is not unusual for off-duty EMTs to hang around the squad in order to help out if there is a difficult call or to carry a two-way radio home so that they can race off to a "big case" on someone else's shift. True, such an EMT has laudable dedication, but that is also the EMT who is going to "burn out" very quickly. No one can work 24 hours a day under the stresses to which EMTs are subjected. The more stressful the job, the more crucial is periodic relief from the job. Some of the best EMTs are part-time volunteers who earn their livings in very mundane occupations; perhaps they are such good EMTs because their lives have a good balance of both stressful and not so stressful activities. The full-time, professional EMT must find that balance in other ways—by pursuing a hobby, by spending time with family and friends. The way one achieves the balance is not important. What is important is spending those off-duty hours in activities different from and unrelated to work.

To sum up, then:

Aids to the Prevention of Burnout

- Recognize your right to have feelings—all kinds of feelings—and your right to be less than perfect.
- Don't be afraid to talk about your feelings.
- Don't be on duty when you are off duty.
- Stay healthy.

CONTINUING EDUCATION

"We've barely started the course, and already we're talking about continuing education! What's going on?" This hypothetical reaction from a hypothetical reader seems at first quite reasonable, but in fact it is based on a serious misconception: that an EMT course has a definite beginning and a definite ending, generally after 81 hours of classroom work and 40 hours of practical experience. It is true that an EMT course has a definite beginning. It is *not* true that it has a definite ending; a good EMT course has no ending at all. Those 81 hours are simply a preparation for a professional lifetime of study and review, for without constant refresher study, EMTs go stale. They lose their skills, and they forget what they have learned. In a study of EMTs conducted in Texas, it was found that by 24 months after the completion of training, only 21 percent of the EMTs remained proficient in CPR. Forty percent of the EMTs could no longer perform traction splinting after this time period, and 30 percent were no longer able to do bandaging and splinting correctly [9]. However, skill retention was considerably better among those EMTs who had participated in some form of continuing education than among those who had not.

Such skill decay translates into poor patient care. Thus the EMT who fails to keep skills sharp and knowledge updated is no less negligent than the EMT who goes out on a call with an empty oxygen tank.

Continuing education, then, is not a separate consideration, to worry about some time in the distant future when recertification becomes mandatory. Continuing education is part of *this* course—the part that begins when the 81 hours end.

If all this sounds rather dreary, it need not be so. Continuing education does not necessarily mean sitting for hours in a classroom listening to lectures. It can take the form of doing a shift now and then in the emergency room, reading the latest EMT journal, or having a workout with Resusci-Anne in the learning lab. For each EMT, the strategies of keeping up professionally will probably be different. What is important is that each EMT take responsibility for his or her own professional competence and find whatever strategy enables maintenance of skills and updating of knowledge.

The moral of the story:

> A PATIENT'S LIFE MAY DEPEND ON THE SKILLS YOU HAVE LOST OR THE KNOWLEDGE YOU HAVE FORGOTTEN. IT IS UP TO YOU TO STAY COMPETENT AND INFORMED.

VOCABULARY

abandonment The abrupt termination of contact with the patient, without the patient's consent and without giving the patient sufficient opportunity to find another health care professional to take over his medical treatment.

advanced life support (ALS) Lifesaving measures that require some "invasive" procedures (e.g., intravenous therapy) that may be performed only by a physician or a specially trained person acting under a physician's supervision.

backboard Any of a variety of long, flat boards used to immobilize patients with suspected spinal injury.

cardiac arrest The sudden and unexpected cessation of cardiac output; for practical purposes, the cessation of pulse.

cardiopumonary resuscitation (CPR) Artificial ventilation and external chest compressions, used to sustain life in cardiac arrest.

consent Agreement, concurrence; in medicine, it usually refers to agreement by the patient to undergo some procedure.

implied consent Assumed agreement to receive emergency lifesaving treatment when the patient is physically or otherwise incapable of giving knowing consent.

informed consent Patient's agreement to accept a given treatment after the nature and risks of the treatment have been fully explained to him.

defibrillation The use of direct current electric shock to terminate ventricular fibrillation and restore an effective cardiac rhythm.

duty to act The obligation of public and certain other ambulance personnel to respond to a call for assistance in their jurisdiction.

EMS Emergency medical services.

EMT Emergency medical technician; an individual specially trained to give basic emergency medical care at the scene of an emergency and in transport to the hospital.

Good Samaritan law One of a variety of statutes that provides limited immunity from prosecution to persons responding voluntarily and in good faith to the aid of an injured person outside the hospital.

intravenous line Tubing inserted inside a vein as a means of supplying fluids or medications directly into the bloodstream.

liability Legal obligation or responsibility.

litigation A lawsuit.

Military Anti-Shock Trousers An inflatable garment applied around the legs and abdomen, used in the treatment of shock.

negligence Failure to exercise the care that circumstances demand; an act of omission or commission that results in injury; carelessness.

paramedic An advanced-level emergency medical technician who is trained to carry out certain invasive procedures under the control of a physician.

response time The time elapsed between receipt of a call for help and arrival of the rescuer at the scene of the emergency.

shock A condition arising when the tissues fail to receive an adequate blood supply because of loss of blood, loss of fluids, damage to the heart, or dilation of blood vessels.

splint Any device used to immobilize a part of the body.

standard of care The norm for providing treatment against which a person's performance is judged.

REFERENCES

Becknell JM. Before you quit, read this. *JEMS* 11(8):46, 1989.

Benson D et al. Mobile intensive care by "unemployable" blacks trained as emergency medical technicians (EMTs). *J Trauma* 12:408, 1971.

Carter WB et al. Development and implementation of emergency CPR instruction via telephone. *Ann Emerg Med* 13:695, 1984.

Costello L. Death and dying. *Emerg Med Serv* 18(8):17, 1989.

Cummings RO, Eisenberg M. Prehospital cardiopulmonary resuscitation: Is it effective? *JAMA* 16:2408, 1985.

Dernocoeur K. Total self-care: Basic stress management—and more. *Emerg Med Serv* 18(2):29, 1989.

Eisenberg M, Bergner R, Hallstrom A. Cardiac resuscitation in the community. *JAMA* 241:1905, 1979.

Eisenberg M et al. Management of out-of-hospital cardiac arrest: Failure of basic emergency medical technician services. *JAMA* 243:1049, 1980.

Eisenberg M et al. Out-of-hospital cardiac arrest: Improved survival with paramedic services. *Lancet* 1:812, 1980.

Eisenberg M et al. Treatment of out-of-hospital cardiac arrest with rapid defibrillation by emergency medical technicians. *N Engl J Med* 302:1379, 1980.

Eisenberg M et al. Treatment of ventricular fibrillation: Emergency medical technician defibrillation and paramedic services. *JAMA* 251:1723, 1984.

Eisenberg M et al. Emergency CPR via telephone. *Am J Public Health* 75:47, 1985.

Floren T. Impact of death and dying on emergency care personnel. *Emerg Med Serv* 13(2):43, 1984.

Foster J, Ramirez-Rude A. Emergency medical technicians: A new career for women. *EMT J* 1:60, 1976.

Gassaway B. Death and the EMT. *Emerg Med Serv* 5(1):66, 1976.

Hinds C. The heat of burnout: How to reduce stress. *Emerg Med Serv* 17(10):52, 1988.

Hirsch H. Legal implications of patient records. *South Med J* 72:726, 1979.

Holder AR. The importance of patient records: Medicolegal rounds. *JAMA* 228:119, 1974.

Latman N, Wooley K. Knowledge and skill retention of emergency care attendants, EMT-As and EMT-Ps. *Ann Emerg Med* 9:183, 1980.

Luterman A et al. Evaluation of prehospital emergency medical service (EMS): Defining areas for improvement. *J Trauma* 23:702, 1983.

McQueen I. Sick and tired. *Emergency* 21(7):40, 1989.

O'Keefe K. Death and dying. *JACEP* 8:275, 1979.

Salvatore N. Females in the field. *Emergency* 11(10):36, 1979.

II. THE HUMAN ORGANISM

2. AN INTRODUCTION TO ANATOMY

OBJECTIVES

Suppose you wanted to be an auto mechanic. One of the first things you would have to learn would be the names of the parts of an automobile engine and roughly where those parts are located. If the instructor started talking about repairing a broken crankshaft, and you couldn't tell a crankshaft from a fan belt, it would be very difficult to understand what the instructor was talking about. The same is true of learning to repair broken or malfunctioning people. First one has to learn the names of the major parts in order to have a basis for talking about the machine in question. In this chapter, we will introduce some basic anatomy and the vocabulary that goes along with it. In later chapters, we will look at various aspects of anatomy and physiology in greater detail; for example, we will examine the lungs and related organs more closely when we discuss respiratory emergencies. This chapter is intended simply to provide the map and the language to help us find our way around the human body. By the end of this chapter, the reader should be able to

1. Describe the location of an injury using correct technical terminology, given a picture of the human body with an injury shown
2. Identify the major regions of the human body, given a diagram of the body
3. Locate the major bones of the human skeleton, given a human skeleton or a picture of a skeleton and a list of bones
4. Locate the major internal organs of the human body, given a diagram of the body
5. Locate the major topographic landmarks of the human body, given another student acting as subject
6. Locate the major arterial pulses of the body, given another student acting as subject

THE VIEW FROM THE OUTSIDE: TOPOGRAPHIC ANATOMY

Before we start taking apart the human body to see what is inside, let us look at what we can observe from the outside. Most patients, after all, do not present themselves to the EMT all neatly dissected, with their internal organs on display. Usually the EMT will be examining the outside of the patient, that is, the patient's *topography*, and drawing inferences from what is seen outside to what is going on inside. A skilled observer can learn a great deal simply by inspection of the patient's exterior, especially if the observer knows the landmarks thoroughly.

DIRECTION AND POSITION

If we want to be able to talk about where things are, we need some terminology. On a map, we refer to north, south, east, and west, but for people we have

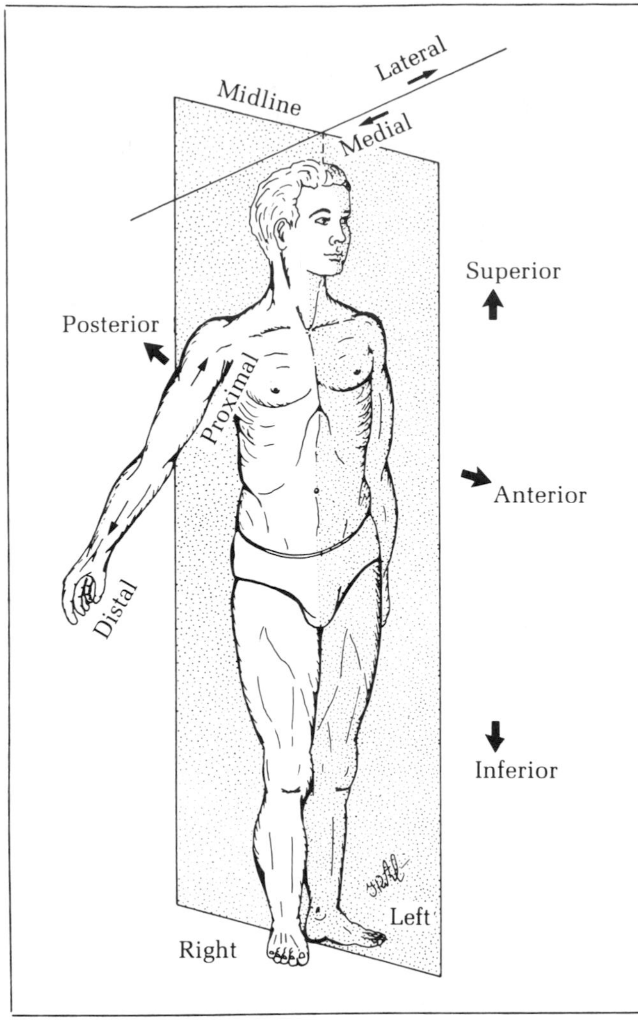

Fig. 2-1. *The east, west, north, and south of the human body.*

other words to indicate direction. In each case, the patient's body, not the examiner's, is the reference point; if we say that the spleen lies in the upper left part of the abdomen, we mean the *patient's* upper left. The words used to describe locations on the human body help indicate whether we are talking about the back or the front, the top or the bottom, the part closer to the center or farther from the center, and so forth (Fig. 2-1).

Front or Back?

When the patient is facing the examiner, the *front* surface of the patient is called the **anterior** surface, and the *back* surface is called the **posterior** surface. (Is the knee anterior or posterior? What about the buttocks?) These terms may also be used in a relative sense, for example, "The nose is *anterior to* the ears" (the nose is more toward the front than are the ears), or "the heel is *posterior to* the toes" (the heel is more toward the back than are the toes). (Which is more anterior, the forehead or the scalp?)

Up or Down?

The part of the patient more *toward the head* is called the **superior** part, while the part more *toward the feet* is called the **inferior** part. Again, these terms are usually used in a relative sense to indicate that a part is above (superior to) or below (inferior to) another part. For instance, the eyes are *superior to* the nose (the eyes are above the nose); the hips are *inferior to* the shoulders (the hips are below the shoulders).

Which is more superior, the neck or the chest? The knee or the belly button (umbilicus)? The chin or the forehead?

Which is more inferior, the nose or the toes? The lips or the hips? The thighs or the eyes?

East or West?

If one were to draw an imaginary line from top to bottom down the middle of the patient's body with the patient facing the examiner, we would call that line the **midline.** Everything east of the midline would be on the patient's **left** side, and everything west would be on the patient's **right** side. We would say that the nose is located *in the midline* of the face. The midline is often used as a reference point to describe the location of injuries; for example, "The patient has a puncture wound of the abdomen at the level of the umbilicus *2 inches to the left of the midline.*" Any medical professional hearing that description would know precisely where the patient's injury was located.

Near the Center or Near the Side?

If we draw our imaginary midline down the front of the patient's body again, locations *nearer the midline* are called **medial,** and locations *farther from the midline* are called **lateral,** irrespective of whether they are on the left or the right. For instance, the eye is *medial to* the ear (the eye is closer to the midline than the ear), while the breast is *lateral to* the sternum or breast bone (the breast is farther from the midline than is the sternum). These terms are also useful in describing the location of an injury. For example, if someone refers to a bruise "1 inch lateral to the left eye," we know that the bruise is toward the side of the face, rather than toward the midline.

Near or Far?

When we talk about the extremities—the arms and the legs—we use terms that give us location with respect to the point of attachment of the extremity to the body. A part that is *nearer to* the point of attachment is called **proximal,** while a part that is *farther* from the point of attachment is called **distal.** Thus the elbow is *proximal to* the wrist (the elbow is closer to the point of attachment of the arm to the body than is the wrist), while the ankle is *distal to* the knee (the ankle is farther from the point of attachment of the leg to the body than is the knee). In general, the proximal part of an arm or a leg is the part nearer the trunk, and the distal part is the part farther from the trunk. If a patient has a burn on the proximal thigh, then, we know that the burn is closer to the hip than to the knee. (Is a burn on the distal forearm closer to the elbow or to the wrist?)

The terms defined above will help get us around the map of the human body with more precision. To summarize:

Words Describing Location

anterior	toward the front
posterior	toward the back
superior	above; toward the head
inferior	below; toward the feet
midline	imaginary vertical line down the middle of the front surface of the body
medial	nearer the midline of the body
lateral	farther from the midline of the body
proximal	nearer the point of attachment to the body
distal	farther from the point of attachment to the body

Position Is Everything in Life

We also need to be able to describe the position in which we find a patient. In addition to commonly used words, such as sitting, standing, and lying down, there are a few more technical words used to indicate the patient's position.

A person who is standing upright is said to be **erect,** while someone who is lying down is **recumbent.** If a person is lying on his back, faceup, he is **supine;** if he is lying facedown, he is **prone.** If our subject chooses to lie on his side, he is said to be in the **lateral recumbent** position ("left lateral recumbent" if he is on his left side, and "right lateral recumbent" if he is on his right side).

Words Describing the Patient's Position

erect	standing upright
recumbent	lying down
supine	lying faceup
prone	lying facedown
lateral recumbent	lying on a side (left or right)

There are also certain positions in which we may want to place a patient, given a specific illness or injury. Again, some of these therapeutic positions are indicated by commonly used words (e.g., sitting, semisitting), while others are named after the person who first suggested their use. In **Fowler's position,** for example, the patient's head is elevated 18 to 20 inches above the rest of the body, usually by elevating the head of the bed or stretcher. It is used for transporting patients with chest pain, for this position minimizes the work of the heart. In the **stable side position** (also called the NATO position), the patient lies on his left side with the left thigh and left knee drawn up toward the waist. This position is used to minimize the danger of inhaling (aspirating) foreign materials into the lungs. We will refer to some of these positions when we discuss the treatment of specific illnesses and injuries.

Finally, we need to be able to describe the position of a given extremity or part of the body—whether it is straight or bent. The act of bending a part of the body, or the condition of being bent, is called **flexion.** When you *flex* your biceps, for example, you are actually bringing the forearm up so that it forms an angle with the upper arm. The arm is then said to be in a state of flexion. The act of straightening the arm out again, on the other hand, is called **extension.** If you crouch, your thighs and legs are in flexion; when you stand up straight, they are in extension. When the head is bent forward so that the chin touches the chest, the head is in flexion; when it is tilted back to normal position, it is in extension, and if you tilt it even farther backward, it is in *hyperextension*.

Words Describing Movement at Joints

flexion	the act of bending a part, or the condition of being bent
extension	the movement that brings the parts of a limb toward a straight condition

THE MAJOR REGIONS OF THE BODY

The human body can be divided into several general regions (Fig. 2-2), the names of which are probably already familiar to most readers: head, neck, trunk (chest and abdomen), and extremities (arms and legs).

The Head

The head (Fig. 2-3) consists of two general regions: (1) the part superior and posterior to (above and behind) the ears, called the **cranium,** and (2) the part containing the ears, eyes, nose, mouth, etc., called the **face.**

The *cranium* contains the brain, which connects with the spinal cord through a hole in the base of the skull. The cranium itself is divided into four regions: the posterior (back) part of the cranium is called the occiput, or **occipital** region, while the anterior part,

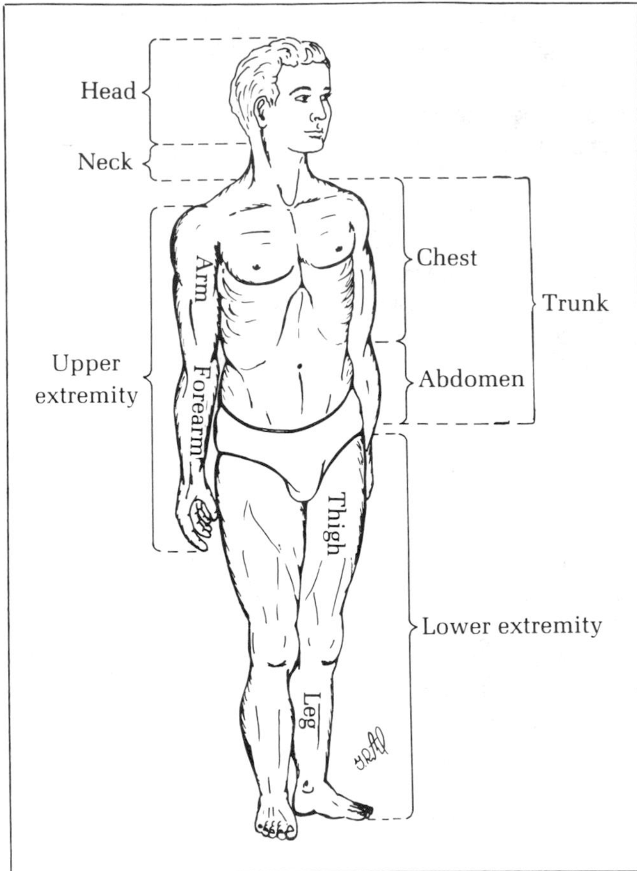

Fig. 2-2. *Major subdivisions of the body.*

just above the forehead, is called the **frontal** region. On each side of the cranium, the more anterior regions (parts nearer the front) are called the **temporal** regions, and the more posterior areas are called the **parietal** regions.

The most obvious landmarks on the *face* are, of course, the eyes, ears, nose, and mouth. Other landmarks that can be easily seen or palpated (felt) are the upper jaw, or **maxilla,** and the lower jaw, or mandible. The chin is located in the center of the **mandible.**

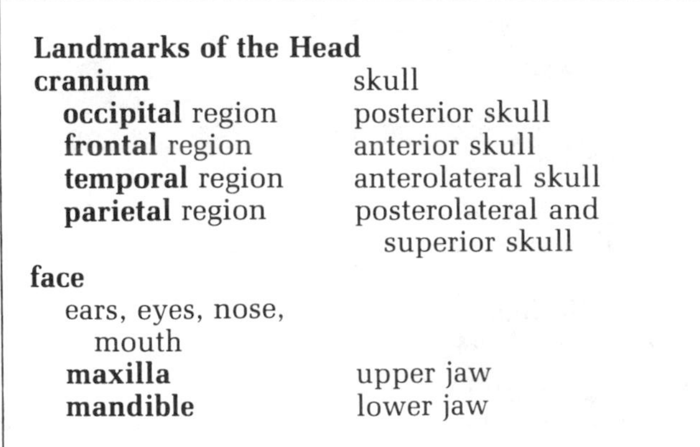

Landmarks of the Head

cranium	skull
occipital region	posterior skull
frontal region	anterior skull
temporal region	anterolateral skull
parietal region	posterolateral and superior skull
face	
ears, eyes, nose, mouth	
maxilla	upper jaw
mandible	lower jaw

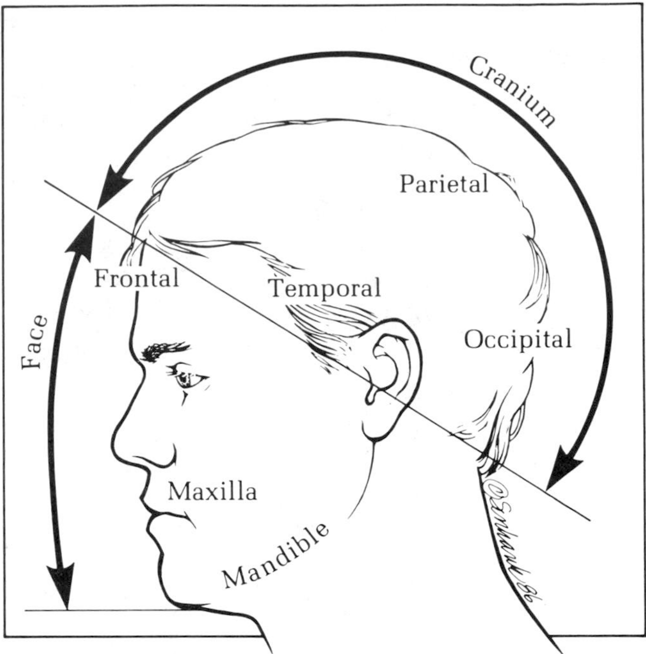

Fig. 2-3. *Regions of the head.*

The Neck

The neck (Fig. 2-4) is inferior to the head and contains many vital structures, including nerves, blood vessels, the windpipe, and the esophagus. If you examine the anterior surface of your own neck in the midline, you will feel a firm prominence or projection that moves up and down as you swallow; this is the thyroid cartilage of the **larynx** (voice box), and it is commonly called the "Adam's apple." If you now tilt your head back and run your finger down the Adam's apple to the base of the neck, you can feel the rings that make up part of the **trachea,** or windpipe. Just posterior to the trachea is the esophagus, but this structure cannot be seen or felt from the outside. An inch or so lateral to the Adam's apple, on the left and the right, the pulsations of the **carotid arteries** can be felt; the carotids are the vital arteries that supply blood to the brain. As we will discuss in Chapter 7, rapid identification of the carotid arteries is critical in carrying out cardiopulmonary resuscitation (CPR) properly. In a recumbent person, or in a person suffering from heart failure, you may also be able to see the major *veins* of the neck, the **external jugular veins,** which appear as prominent cords extending up from the base of the neck about 3 inches lateral to the midline.

On the posterior surface of the neck, there are a series of bony projections, which you can feel if you tilt your head forward and palpate down the midline of the back of your neck. These are the projections of the first seven bones of the spine, or **vertebrae.** These seven vertebrae are called *cervical* vertebrae, because *cervical* is the word that refers to the neck.

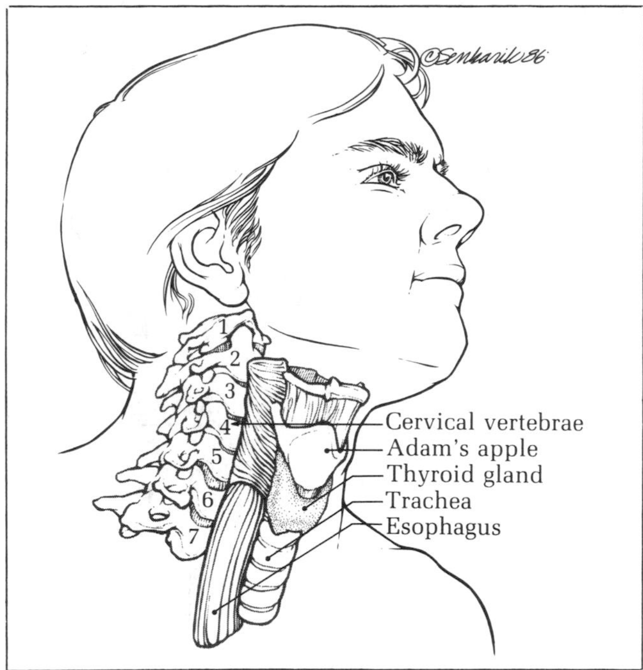

Fig. 2-4. *Major landmarks of the neck.*

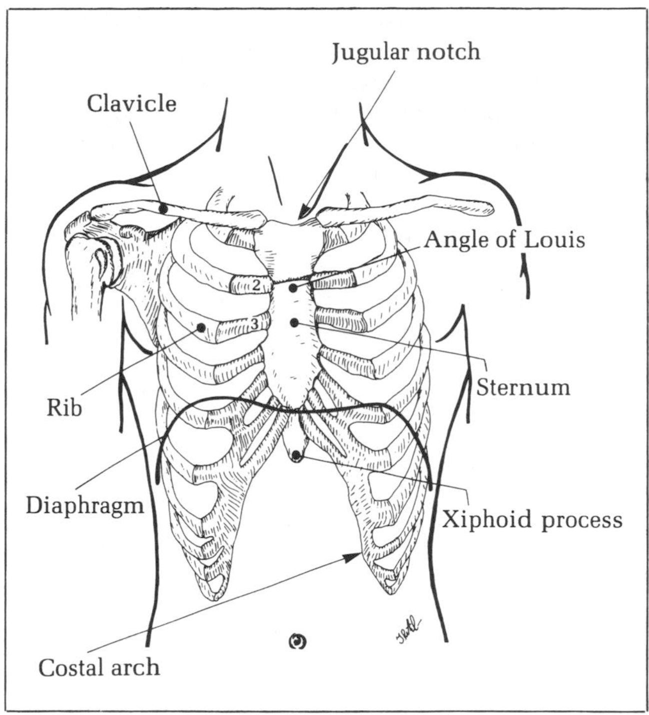

Fig. 2-5. *Major landmarks of the thorax.*

Landmarks of the Neck	
Adam's apple	part of the **larynx** (voice box)
trachea	windpipe
carotid arteries	major arteries of the neck
external jugular veins	major veins of the neck
cervical vertebrae	bones of the spine in the neck

The Trunk

The trunk consists of the **thorax** (chest) and **abdomen**.

The *thorax* (Fig. 2-5) is a cavity containing the heart, lungs, lower part of the esophagus, and great vessels (the aorta, or main artery of the body, and the venae cavae, the main veins of the body).

The collar bones, or **clavicles,** are located on either side of the midline in the superior part of the thorax, and each clavicle can be palpated as a ridge extending from the shoulder toward the base of the neck. Both clavicles attach to the top of the breast bone, or **sternum,** medially. The sternum is a flat bone that lies in the midline of the anterior chest. At its top (superior) border, you can feel a notch, called the **jugular notch.** At its inferior end, the sternum narrows into a small tip, made of flexible cartilage, called the **xiphoid process.** Like the carotid arteries, both the sternum and the xiphoid process are crucial landmarks in doing CPR, and the EMT must be able to locate them rapidly.

The chest is encircled by 12 sets of **ribs.** The upper 10 of these ribs are connected posteriorly to the spine and anteriorly to the sternum or to a cartilage extending from the sternum. The eleventh and twelfth ribs are also connected to the spine in back, but they have no connection in front to the sternum, and for that reason they are called *floating ribs.* The ribs are easy to palpate and they, or the spaces between them **(intercostal spaces),** are often used as landmarks in describing the location of a patient's injury. The first rib is *not* palpable on either side, since it is buried under the collar bone, so the topmost rib one can *feel* is the second rib. One way to check which rib you are dealing with is to palpate the sternum until you find a slight horizontal prominence or elevation; this is located about one-third of the way down the sternum and is called the **angle of Louis** (someone named Louis first described this bump, so it was named after him). The significance of the angle of Louis is that it lies right next to the *second intercostal space* (the space between the second and third ribs). Thus the rib immediately above the angle of Louis is the second rib, and the rib immediately below the angle of Louis is the third rib. (Using the angle of Louis to orient yourself, try to find your seventh left rib anteriorly. Mark it with an X using a ballpoint pen, and have your instructor check to see whether you found the correct rib.) The lower border of the rib cage is called the **costal arch.**

The other obvious landmarks on the anterior chest are the **nipples.** In the male, the nipples are at the level of the fourth intercostal space (the space between the fourth and fifth ribs). In the female, the position of the nipples will vary depending on the size of the breasts, but the center of the breast is still over the fourth intercostal space.

On the posterior portion of the thorax, or back, one can feel the bumps made by the vertebrae of this part of the spine, the **thoracic vertebrae.** On either side of the spine, superiorly, are the **scapulae,** or shoulder blades.

Landmarks of the Chest

clavicle	collar bone
sternum	breast bone
jugular notch	top border of the sternum
angle of Louis	prominence about one-third of the way down the sternum, opposite the second intercostal space
xiphoid process	inferior tip of the sternum
intercostal spaces	spaces between the ribs
costal arch	lower border of the rib cage
nipples	structures overlying the fourth intercostal spaces
thoracic vertebrae	the 12 vertebrae of the thorax, to which the 12 ribs are connected posteriorly
scapula	shoulder blade

The *abdomen* (Fig. 2-6) is the second major body cavity, and it contains the organs of digestion and excretion. The abdomen lies inferior to the thorax. When the abdomen is viewed from the outside, the costal arches form its upper boundary. The region just inferior to the costal arches is referred to as the **epigastrium**.

The most prominent landmark on the abdomen is the **umbilicus,** or navel (belly button), and it is used as a reference point to divide the abdomen into four quarters, or **quadrants:** the right upper quadrant (RUQ), left upper quadrant (LUQ), right lower quadrant (RLQ), and left lower quadrant (LLQ). Once again, these refer to the *patient's* right and left sides. Often a knowledge of the quadrant involved in an injury or giving rise to pain will help the examiner determine what internal organ is involved, and shortly we shall take a look inside the body to see which organs are located in which quadrants.

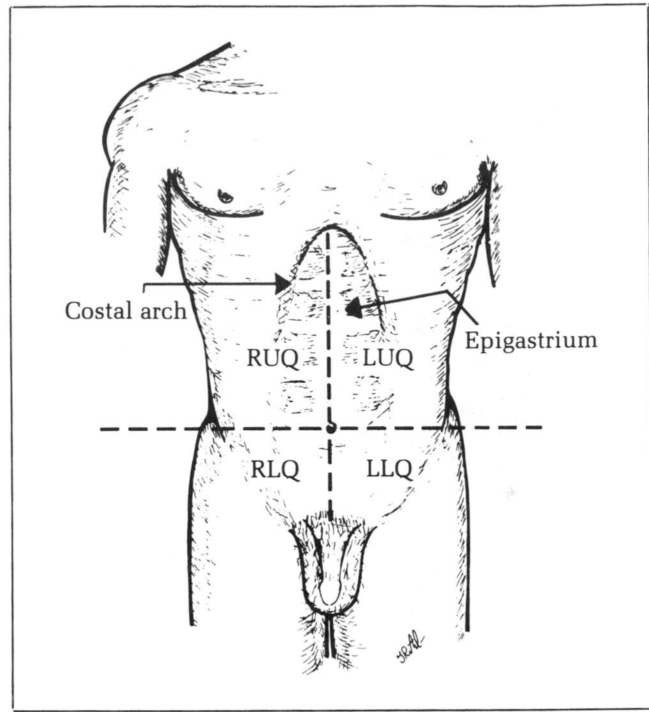

Fig. 2-6. *Quadrants of the abdomen.*

Strictly speaking, the lowest portion of the abdominal cavity is referred to as the **pelvic cavity,** that is, the part of the abdominal cavity bounded by the large hard ring of the pelvic bone. The pelvic cavity contains the urinary bladder, the rectum, and, in females, the reproductive organs (uterus, ovaries).

Landmarks of the Abdomen

costal arches	inferior border of the rib cage, forming the upper boundary of the abdomen
epigastrium	upper portion of the abdomen, just inferior to the costal arches
umbilicus	navel; reference point for dividing the abdomen into quadrants
right upper quadrant (RUQ)	the quarter of the abdomen superior to the umbilicus, on the patient's right
left upper quadrant (LUQ)	the quarter of the abdomen superior to the umbilicus, on the patient's left
right lower quadrant (RLQ)	the quarter of the abdomen inferior to the umbilicus, on the patient's right

left lower quadrant (LLQ)	the quarter of the abdomen inferior to the umbilicus, on the patient's left
pelvic bone	large bony ring that forms the inferior boundary of the abdomen

The Extremities

The *upper extremity* (see Fig. 2-2) extends from the shoulder to the fingertips and consists of the **shoulder, upper arm, forearm,** and **hand**. The **elbow** connects the upper arm to the forearm, and the **wrist** connects the forearm to the hand. The *lower extremity,* which extends from the hip to the toes, comprises the **hip, thigh, leg,** and **foot**. The **knee** connects the thigh to the leg, while the **ankle** connects the leg to the foot.

THE PRINCIPAL PULSES

Each time the heart beats, a bolus of blood is pumped forward through the arteries, creating a pressure wave that is transmitted throughout the whole arterial system. This pressure wave is called the **pulse**, and if the human body were transparent, one could see the pulsation in every artery of the body with each heart beat. In practice, however, people are not transparent, so the only pulses we can readily evaluate are those near the surface of the body, which we can feel. A pulse is most easily felt in those places where an artery is superficial (near the surface) and can be compressed lightly against a fairly rigid structure, such as a bone, muscle, or ligament. Knowing the locations of some of these readily accessible pulses is useful to us for several reasons:

- Palpating any pulse provides information about the rate and quality of the heart beat.
- Palpating the pulse *distal* to an injury on an extremity gives us information about possible damage to the artery in that extremity. For instance, if a person has suffered a severely broken arm and the pulse at the wrist is absent, there is reason to suspect that there has been damage to blood vessels in addition to the damage to bone.
- Firm compression over a pulse that overlies a rigid structure (such as a bone) can help control bleeding from a wound distal to that pulse, for it slows the flow of blood to the site of the injury. In general, direct pressure on a bleeding site is a more effective way to control bleeding, but on occasion, pressure over the supplying artery may be required as well.

Let us look at the major pulses, starting from the head and working our way down (Fig. 2-7).

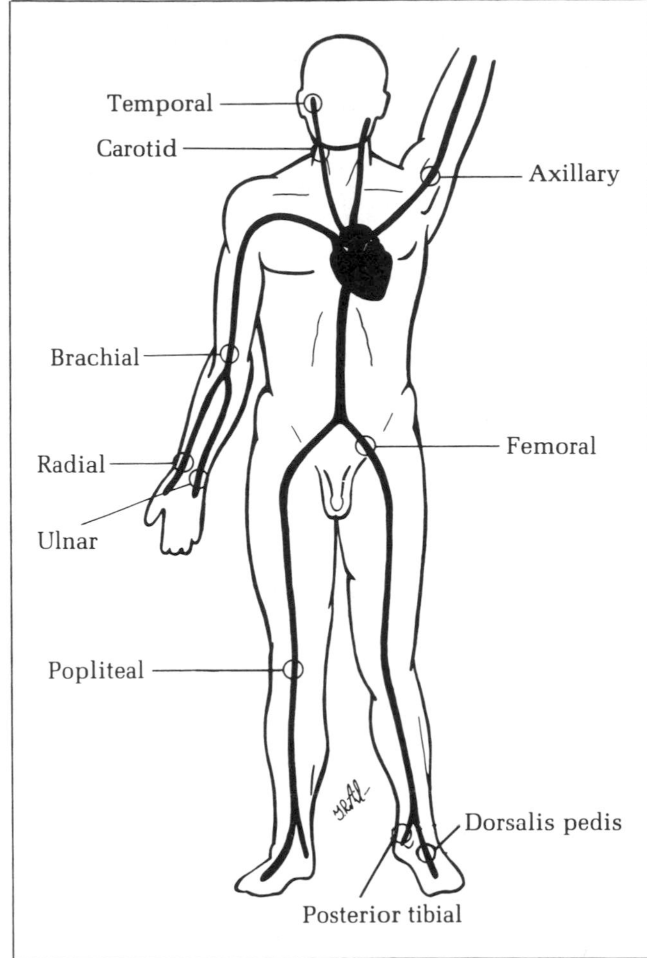

Fig. 2-7. *Locations of the principal pulses.*

The pulse of the **temporal artery** can be palpated just anterior to the upper part of the ear, at a point just above the spot where the lower jaw (mandible) connects with the skull. The temporal arteries supply blood to the *scalp*, and thus firm pressure against the temporal artery on a given side may help control bleeding from that side of the scalp.

The pulsations of the **carotid arteries** are palpable on either side of the neck and are best located by sliding your finger laterally from the Adam's apple. The finger will slip down into a groove beside the Adam's apple, and there the carotid pulse may be felt. The carotid pulse is the one that is usually used to determine whether an unconscious person's heart is beating, for it is ordinarily an easily felt pulse and is readily accessible even in a fully dressed person. The carotids supply blood to the brain, and a carotid artery should be compressed (by pushing it firmly against the vertebra behind it) only when there is severe bleeding from the neck that cannot be controlled by direct pressure over the wound. NEVER compress both carotid arteries at the same time, for this would cut off most of the brain's blood supply and could lead to serious neurologic damage.

The pulse of the **axillary artery** is palpable in the middle of the axilla (armpit). It is not usually used as a pressure point to control bleeding because it is cumbersome to compress and its extensive branching makes it nearly impossible to cut off flow through it.

The pulse of the **brachial artery** can be felt on the inner surface of the arm. The best way to find this artery is to hold the patient's arm out straight (in extension), with the palm up. About an inch or so proximal to the crease of the elbow, and slightly medial, you can feel a small indentation beside the biceps muscle; the brachial artery should be palpable in that indentation. The brachial artery is the artery that is auscultated (listened to) in measuring blood pressure. Firm compression against the brachial artery can be quite effective in controlling bleeding from the forearm.

The pulse of the **radial artery** is felt at the wrist, just proximal to the base of the thumb. This is the pulse usually measured when examining a conscious patient. It is also used to assess the circulation to the hand.

The hand also receives blood from the **ulnar artery,** which is palpated on the little-finger side of the wrist. If the radial artery is firmly compressed and the hand does not become white but remains pink, it can be assumed that the ulnar artery is functional and is supplying blood to the hand.

The pulsations of the **femoral artery** can be felt in the groin, just medial to where the thigh meets the trunk. The femoral artery supplies the entire lower extremity, and very forceful pressure on the femoral artery, applied with the heel of the hand, can help control bleeding from the leg.

The **popliteal artery** lies in the triangular space in the back of the knee, and it can be palpated in the medial part of that space. The popliteal pulse should be sought whenever there is an injury to the upper leg, and its presence or absence should be noted on the patient's record.

The **posterior tibial artery,** as the name implies, lies just posterior to the distal end of the tibia, the main bone of the lower leg. It can be located by putting your finger on the medial malleolus (the inner knob of the ankle) and then sliding your finger back slightly toward the heel. The **dorsalis pedis** pulse is palpable on the anterior surface of the foot, just lateral to the tendon of the big toe. Both the posterior tibial and dorsalis pedis pulses should be checked whenever there is an injury to the leg.

As you review these pulses, try to locate each of them on yourself or a classmate. Or try it on a date—it is a unique way to break the ice!

The Principal Pulses	
temporal	supplies the scalp
carotid	supplies the head, including the brain
axillary	supplies the upper extremity
brachial	supplies the forearm
radial } **ulnar** }	supply the hand
femoral	supplies the lower extremity
popliteal	supplies the leg
posterior tibial } **dorsalis pedis** }	supply the foot

A PEEK INSIDE THE HUMAN BODY

THE INTERNAL ORGANS

We have already mentioned some of the internal organs, and in this section we will learn to locate them on a map of the human interior. We will take a closer look at several of these organs later when we consider injuries to and illnesses of specific body regions or specific organ systems. What is important for our purposes now is simply to "get the lay of the land," that is, to acquire a general idea of where the major internal organs are located.

The major organs of the *chest* (Fig. 2-8) are the heart, lungs, and great vessels. The **heart** is *retrosternal,* that is, it lies *behind* the sternum, a bit to the left of the midline. Into the heart empty the two great *veins* of the body, the **inferior vena cava** carrying blood from the lower part of the body and the **superior vena cava** carrying blood from the upper body regions. The largest *artery* of the body, the

Fig. 2-8. *Organs of the chest.*

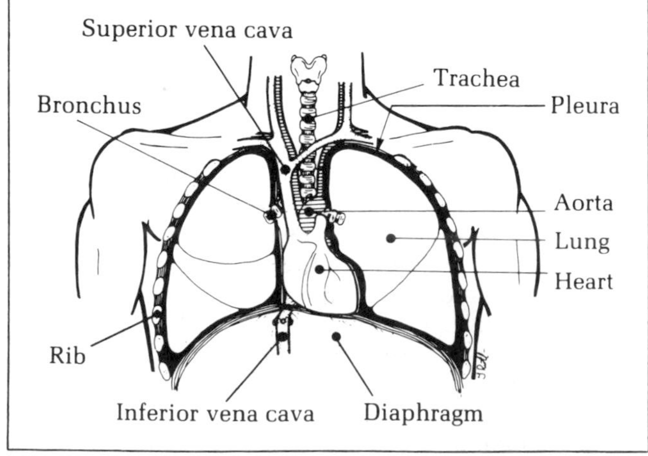

aorta, arises from the heart and arches down behind it. Both the aorta and the inferior vena cava travel down into the abdomen. On either side of the heart are the **lungs,** the principal organs of respiration, which occupy the bulk of the thoracic cavity. At the entrance to the thoracic cavity, the *trachea* (windpipe) divides into two main **bronchi,** which connect with the lungs. The **esophagus** also enters the chest from the neck and extends down to the stomach.

Major Organs of the Chest	
heart	retrosternal, slightly left of midline
aorta	largest artery of the body
venae cavae	largest veins of the body
lungs	organs of respiration
part of **esophagus**	descends to join the stomach in the abdomen

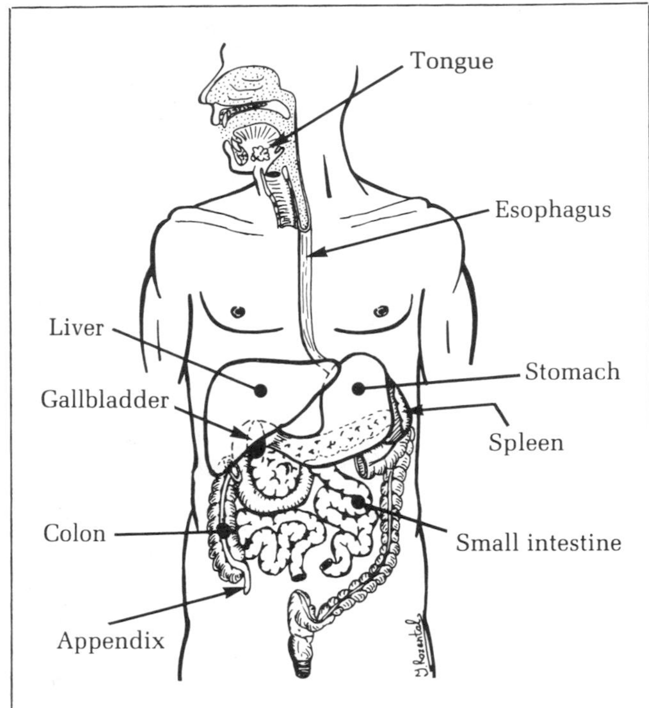

Fig. 2-9. *Organs of the abdomen.*

The *abdomen* (Fig. 2-9) is separated from the chest by a dome-shaped muscle, the **diaphragm.** The abdomen contains the major organs of digestion and excretion. The abdominal wall is lined with a membrane called the *peritoneum*, and the cavity within is known as the **peritoneal cavity.** The contents of the peritoneal cavity can be described according to the four quadrants mentioned earlier.

The *right upper quadrant* (RUQ) contains the **liver**, the **gallbladder**, and a portion of the **colon** (large bowel). Most of the liver lies underneath the rib cage and is thus protected by the ribs, but a strong force applied to the RUQ can still produce considerable injury to the liver. When there is tenderness in the RUQ without a history of injury to the area, the cause is often gallbladder disease.

The *left upper quadrant* (LUQ) contains the **stomach**, the **spleen**, parts of the descending and transverse **colon**, and a bit of the **liver**. The spleen lies laterally, tucked under the eighth to eleventh ribs, and frequently it is injured when any of those ribs are broken.

The major organs in the *right lower quadrant* (RLQ) are the **cecum** (the beginning of the large bowel) and the ascending part of the **colon**. Attached to the cecum is a small, wormlike structure called the **appendix**, and when the appendix becomes inflamed or infected, the patient may experience pain in the RLQ.

The *left lower quadrant* (LLQ) contains the last portions of the large bowel, the descending and sigmoid **colon**.

It is important to bear in mind that some organs lie in more than one quadrant. The urinary **bladder**, for example, sits just behind the pubic bones of the pelvis in the midline of the abdomen; thus it is in both lower quadrants. The **small intestine** winds throughout the abdomen and occupies all four quadrants.

There are some organs that lie *behind* the peritoneal cavity and are thus referred to as *retroperitoneal*. The **pancreas**, the organ that produces digestive enzymes and insulin, lies crosswise in both upper quadrants of the retroperitoneal space. The

Major Organs of the Abdomen by Quadrant	
right upper quadrant (RUQ)	liver gallbladder part of colon
left upper quadrant (LUQ)	stomach spleen transverse colon part of liver
right lower quadrant (RLQ)	cecum appendix ascending colon
left lower quadrant (LLQ)	descending and sigmoid colon
both lower quadrants	urinary bladder uterus and ovaries in the female
all quadrants	small intestine

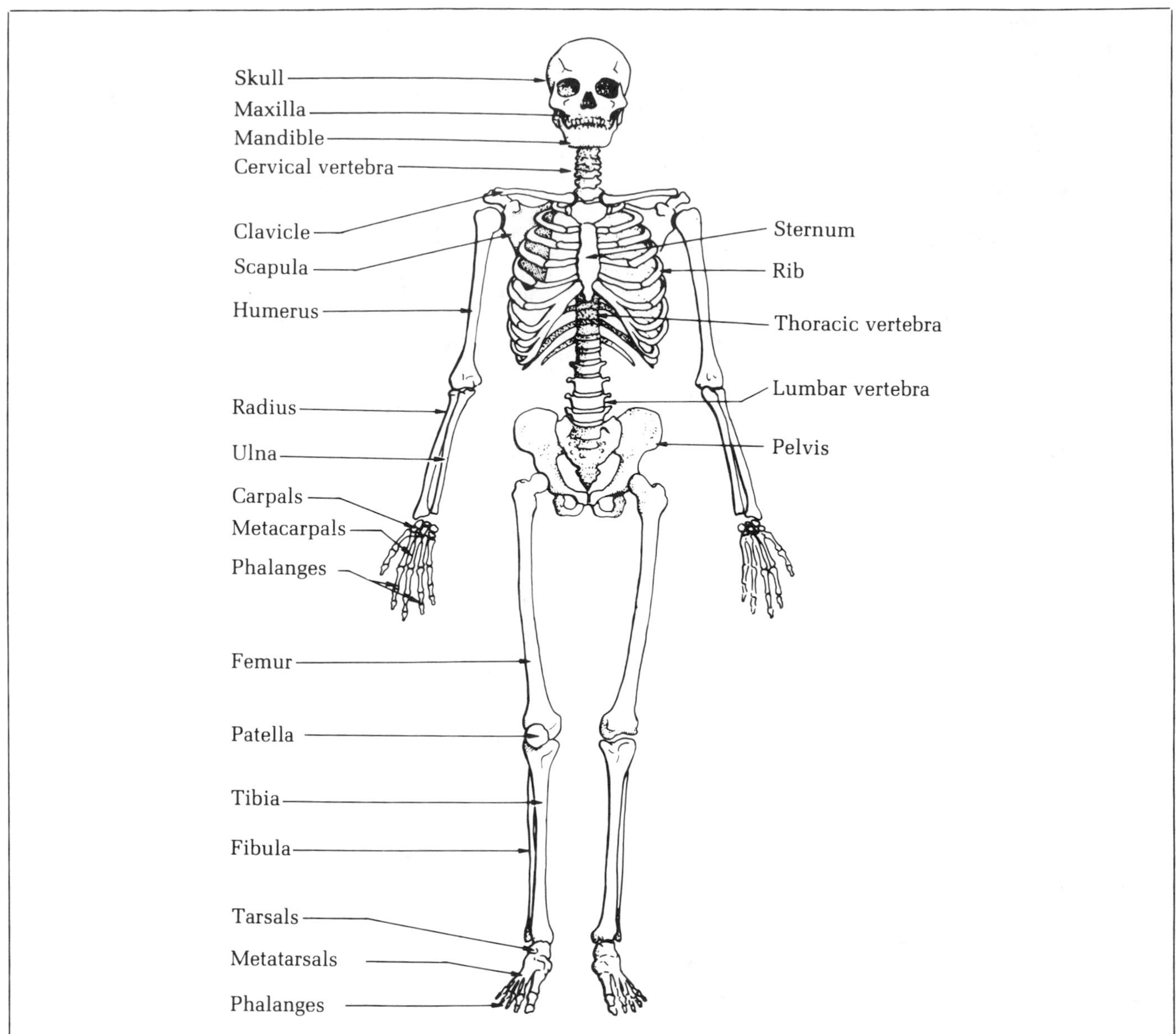

Fig. 2-10. *The human skeleton.*

kidneys also occupy the retroperitoneal space, and they are situated above the level of the umbilicus on either side of the spinal cord.

The internal organs are also classified according to the *system* to which they belong, that is, according to the functions they carry out.

The *skeletal system* consists of the bones, which are the framework of the body.

The *muscular system* consists of specialized tissues (muscles) that are capable of contracting to enable parts of the body to move.

The *nervous system* controls all body activities and is made up of the brain, the spinal cord, and nerves.

The *respiratory system* is in charge of breathing and comprises the upper airways (nose, mouth, throat), lower airways (trachea, bronchi), and the lungs.

The *circulatory system* channels blood throughout the body. It consists of a pump (the heart) and the pipes through which the blood is circulated (arteries, veins, capillaries).

The *digestive system* processes the food we eat, preparing portions of it to be used by the body and eliminating other portions. The main organs of digestion are the mouth, esophagus, stomach, pancreas, gallbladder, liver, small intestine, and large intestine (colon).

The *genitourinary system* is in charge of eliminating liquid wastes and enabling reproduction. It consists of the kidneys, bladder, and male or female reproductive organs.

Major Organ Systems	
skeletal	bones
muscular	muscles
nervous	brain, spinal cord, peripheral nerves
respiratory	upper airway, trachea, bronchi, lungs
circulatory	heart, arteries, veins, capillaries
digestive	mouth, esophagus, stomach, pancreas, gallbladder, liver, small intestine, large intestine
genitourinary	kidney, bladder, reproductive organs

THE CHASSIS: THE HUMAN SKELETON

The human skeleton (Fig. 2-10) consists of 206 bones. The function of the skeleton is to give form and support to the body, to protect the internal organs from injury, and to permit movement. If we look at the human skeleton from top to bottom, we observe the following major bones (indicated in boldface type):

Major Bones of the Human Body	
skull	
cranial bones	frontal, temporal, parietal, occipital
maxilla	upper jaw
mandible	lower jaw
spinal column	**vertebrae**
thorax	
clavicle	collar bone
scapula	shoulder bone
sternum	breast bone
ribs	
pelvis	
upper extremity	
humerus	upper arm bone
radius, **ulna**	forearm bones
carpals	wrist bones
metacarpals, **phalanges**	hand bones
lower extremity	
femur	thigh bone
patella	knee cap
tibia, **fibula**	leg bones
tarsals	ankle bones
metatarsals, **phalanges**	foot bones

Most of these bones are easy to identify and locate on a human skeleton or diagram thereof. The bones that sometimes cause confusion are the radius versus the ulna and the tibia versus the fibula. The distal *radius* attaches to the *thumb side* of the hand, while the distal *ulna* is on the *little-finger side* of the forearm. The proximal end of the ulna forms part of the elbow joint, and it is sometimes referred to as the "funny bone," since a bump on the proximal ulna may hit the ulnar nerve and cause a pins-and-needles feeling in the arm. The *tibia* can be palpated anteriorly down the leg; it is sometimes called the shin bone. At its distal end, where it meets the foot, the tibia forms the inner prominence of the ankle, called the medial malleolus. The *fibula* is much smaller than the tibia and runs posterior to it. The distal end of the fibula forms the outer knob of the ankle, the lateral malleolus.

We will return to the bones and learn more about their structure and function when we consider injuries to the skeletal system in Chapter 17.

VOCABULARY

abdomen The part of the body between the thorax and the pelvis.

angle of Louis A prominence on the sternum that lies opposite the second intercostal space.

anterior Toward the front.

aorta The major artery of the body, which arises from the left ventricle of the heart.

appendix Wormlike structure attached to the cecum; when inflamed, it may cause pain in the right lower quadrant.

axilla Armpit.

axillary artery The artery that supplies blood to the arm; its pulsations can be palpated in the armpit.

bladder Organ of the urinary system, located in the pelvis just behind the pubic bone, that stores urine produced by the kidneys.

brachial artery The artery that supplies blood to the forearm; its pulsations can be felt slightly proximal and medial to the crease of the elbow on the anterior surface of the arm.

bronchi Plural of bronchus, one of the main branches of the trachea that carries air into the lungs.

carotid artery The artery that supplies blood to the head and brain; its pulsations can be felt in the neck, lateral to the Adam's apple.

carpals Bones of the wrist.

cecum The first portion of the large intestine.

cervical Referring to the neck.

clavicle The collar bone.

colon The large intestine.

costal arch The lower border of the ribs.

cranium The part of the head that is superior and posterior to the ears.

distal Farther from the point of attachment to the body.

dorsalis pedis One of the arteries of the foot; its pulsations are palpable on the anterior surface of the foot, lateral to the tendon on the great toe.
epigastrium The upper middle region of the abdomen, just below the costal arches.
erect Standing upright.
esophagus The portion of the digestive tract that lies between the throat and the stomach.
extension The movement that brings the parts of a limb toward a straight condition.
external jugular vein Principal vein that drains blood from the head, sometimes visible in the neck.
femoral artery Artery that supplies the lower extremity; its pulsations may be felt in the groin.
femur Thigh bone.
fibula The smaller bone of the leg; its distal end forms the lateral malleolus of the ankle.
flexion The act of bending a part, or the condition of being bent.
Fowler's position Position in which a patient's head is elevated 18 to 20 inches above the rest of the body.
frontal region The anterior region of the cranium.
gallbladder Sac located just beneath the liver that concentrates and stores bile.
heart The organ, located in the chest behind the sternum, that pumps blood to the rest of the body.
humerus The arm bone.
inferior Below; toward the feet.
intercostal space Space between two ribs.
jugular notch Top border of the sternum.
kidneys Paired organs located in the retroperitoneal space that filter blood and produce urine.
larynx Voice box; lowest portion of the throat.
lateral Farther from the midline of the body.
liver Large organ in the right upper quadrant of the abdomen that secretes bile, produces many essential proteins, and performs other vital functions.
lungs Paired organs in the thorax that supply the blood with oxygen and eliminate carbon dioxide.
mandible Lower jaw.
maxilla Upper jaw.
medial Nearer the midline of the body.
metacarpals Bones of the hand.
metatarsals Bones of the foot.
midline Imaginary vertical line down the center of the anterior surface of the body.
occipital region The posterior region of the cranium.
pancreas Gland that secretes insulin and digestive enzymes.
parietal region Posterolateral and superior region of the cranium.
patella Knee cap.
pelvis The lower bony structure of the trunk.
phalanges Bones of the fingers or toes.
popliteal artery Artery that supplies the leg; its pulsations may be felt in the triangular space behind the knee.
posterior Toward the back; behind.
posterior tibial artery One of the arteries of the foot; its pulsations may be felt posterior to the medial malleolus of the ankle.
prone Lying facedown.
proximal Nearer the point of attachment to the body.
quadrant One of the quarters into which the abdomen is divided by drawing imaginary perpendicular lines that intersect at the umbilicus.
radial artery One of the arteries to the hand; its pulsations can be felt at the wrist, just proximal to the base of the thumb.
radius The larger bone of the forearm.
recumbent Lying down.
rib One of the 12 bones forming the wall of the thoracic cavity.
scapula The shoulder blade.
spleen Organ located in the left upper quadrant of the abdomen that is involved in maintenance of blood cells; because of its fragility, the spleen is easily ruptured by injury.
sternum The breast bone.
stomach The hollow digestive organ in the epigastrium that receives food material through the esophagus.
superior Above; toward the head.
supine Lying faceup.
tarsals Bones of the ankle.
temporal artery Artery that supplies blood to the scalp; its pulsations can be felt just anterior to the upper ear and superior to the temperomandibular joint.
temporal region Anterolateral region of the cranium.
thorax The part of the body between the neck and the diaphragm, encased by the ribs.
tibia The larger bone of the leg; its distal end forms the medial malleolus of the ankle.
trachea The windpipe.
ulna The smaller bone of the forearm; the "funny bone."
ulnar artery One of the arteries supplying the hand; its pulsations can be felt at the wrist on the little-finger side.
umbilicus The navel, or belly button.
vena cava One of the two largest veins of the body.
vertebra One of the bones making up the spinal column.
xiphoid process The cartilaginous lower tip of the sternum.

3. MEDICAL TERMINOLOGY

OBJECTIVES

Medical professionals tend to speak in a secret code that ordinary mortals are apt to find completely unintelligible. Actually the code—the language of medicine—is not all that secret or difficult to crack: It is made up of a fairly limited number of Latin and Greek roots, which are combined in many ways to form medical terms. By learning a relatively few root words, one can unscramble an enormous number of medical terms. In this chapter, we will examine some of those root words, and we will practice putting together and taking apart medical terms.

By the end of this chapter, the reader should be familiar with 75 medical root words and be able to demonstrate the following competencies:

1. Given a medical term composed of two or more of the root words learned in the chapter, the reader will be able to explain the meaning of that medical term.
2. Given a definition of a condition, the reader will be able to form the appropriate medical term for that condition using the roots learned in this chapter.

Why bother with all this Latin and Greek? the reader may wonder. Isn't plain English good enough?

Plain English is very good indeed (and very rare), but it is important to learn some medical terminology for several reasons:

1. Medical terminology permits one to describe medical problems with much greater precision and often more succinctly as well. It is considerably less cumbersome, for example, to say, "The patient has pleuritis," than to say, "The patient has an inflammation of the membrane that surrounds the lungs." Both statements mean exactly the same thing, but the first is much more concise.
2. Medical terminology is the language of health care personnel, and proper use of the medical language identifies the speaker as a professional. Compare two EMTs radioing in the same information about the same patient:

   EMT Melvin McTwiddle: "Doc, I've got a guy here who broke the big bone in his leg, and it's sticking out of the skin."

   EMT Tom Trueblood: "Doctor, we have a 37-year-old man who sustained a compound fracture to the left mid-femur."

   If you were the doctor, which EMT would you be more likely to treat as a professional colleague?
3. A knowledge of medical terminology helps the EMT to communicate effectively with other health professionals, for in order to communicate, people have to speak the same language.

CRACKING THE SECRET MEDICAL CODE

The secret medical code is somewhat like a Lego set: There is a basic set of building blocks that can be linked together in an almost unlimited number of ways to form all sorts of different structures. In the case of medical language, the building blocks are root words, and the structures one forms are medical terms. For example, *cardio-* is a building block meaning "heart"; *peri-* is a building block meaning "around"; *-itis* is the block meaning "inflammation"; *-megaly* means "enlargement."

We have now learned four root words:

cardio-	heart
peri-	around
-itis	inflammation
-megaly	enlargement

Let us put them together in a few ways and see what we get. (Note: When roots are combined, some of the vowels may drop out to make the resulting word easier to pronounce.)

cardio- + -itis	= *carditis* (an inflammation of the heart)
peri- + cardio	= *pericardium* (around the heart; actually this is the name given to the membrane that surrounds the heart)
peri- + cardio- + -itis	= *pericarditis* (an inflammation of the membrane that surrounds the heart)
cardio- + -megaly	= *cardiomegaly* (enlargement of the heart)

Let us take a few more roots:

nephro-	kidney
hepato-	liver
-oma	tumor
-ectomy	surgical removal

Now we have learned eight root words, and our vocabulary of medical terms is growing by leaps and bounds:

nephro- + -itis	= *nephritis* (inflammation of the kidney)
nephro- + -oma	= *nephroma* (tumor of the kidney)
nephro- + -ectomy	= *nephrectomy* (surgical removal of a kidney)
hepato- + -megaly	= *hepatomegaly* (enlargement of the liver)
hepato- + -itis	= *hepatitis* (inflammation of the liver)
hepato- + -oma	= *hepatoma* (tumor of the liver)
peri- + cardio- + -ectomy	= *pericardiectomy* (surgical removal of the pericardium)

(Theoretically, we could also form the words "cardectomy" and "hepatectomy," but in practice the heart and liver are never removed surgically because they are necessary to life.)

Medical root words come in several forms:

1. Root words that tell us *in what direction, how,* or *how much*. These roots are almost invariably *prefixes*, that is, they appear at the beginning of a word.

Common Prefixes (how, in what direction, how much)

a- or **an-**	absence of	**in-, intra-**	inside
ante-	before	**inter-**	between
brady-	slow	**mal-**	bad, disordered
circum-	around		
contra-	against	**oligo-**	few, little
dys-	disordered, painful, difficult	**ortho-**	straight
		para-	beside
		poly-	many, much
endo-	within		
epi-	upon	**post-**	after
extra-	outside of	**pre-**	before
hemi-	half	**quadr-**	four
hyper-	above, excess	**retro-**	behind
		super-, supra-	above
hypo-	below, deficient	**tachy-**	rapid

2. Root words that tell us *what organ* or substance we are talking about, such as *cardio-*, meaning "heart." These roots often appear at the beginning of a word, as in the word "*card*itis." But they may also appear in the middle (as in "peri*card*itis") or even at the end ("dextro*cardia*").

Combining Words (what organ or substance)

angio-	tube, blood vessel	**leuko-**	white
		meningo-	meninges
arthro-	joint	**myo-**	muscle
cardio-	heart	**nephro-**	kidney
cephalo-	head	**neuro-**	nerve
cerebro-	brain	**orchi-**	testicle
chole-	bile	**osteo-**	bone
cyst-	sac	**oto-**	ear
cyt-	cell	**phlebo-**	vein
dermato-	skin	**pneumo-**	air, lung
entero-	gut	**pulmo-**	lung
erythro-	red	**pyo-**	pus
gastro-	stomach	**rhino-**	nose
hem-, hema-, hemato-	blood	**sclero-**	hardness
		uro-	urine, urinary
hepato-	liver	**vaso-**	vessel
hystero-	uterus		

3. Root words that tell us *what is going on* with the organ involved, e.g., *-ectomy* (the organ was cut out surgically) or *-oma* (the organ has a tumor in it). These roots are *suffixes*, i.e., they always appear at the end of a word.

Common Suffixes (what is going on)

-algia	pain in	**-osis**	disease
-asthenia	weakness in	**-ostomy**	opening in
-ectomy	surgical removal of	**-otomy**	incision into
-emia	in the blood	**-paresis**	weakness
-esthesia	sensation	**-pathy**	disease of
-genic	causing	**-plegia**	paralysis
-graph(y)	visualization of	**-pnea**	breathing
-itis	inflammation of	**-rrhea**	profuse flow
-megaly	enlargement of	**-scopy**	to examine, see
-oma	tumor of	**-uria**	urine

Just as in learning French or Spanish, learning the medical language requires practice, and the reader should work at forming and unscrambling medical terms until the roots come easily. For example, what do you think is the meaning of the following?

gastritis
hysterectomy
dysuria

How would you express the following in medical terminology?

inflammation of the meninges (the membranes surrounding the brain)
absence of breathing
rapid heart rate

The lists of root words presented in this chapter are not intended to be exhaustive; rather, they represent some of the roots more commonly used in medical terms. A more comprehensive listing of roots is provided for reference in the Glossary of Common Medical Roots at the end of the book.

In the chapters that follow, we will come upon more new vocabulary, but much of it will seem quite familiar now that we have learned part of the secret code used to construct medical terms.

FURTHER READING

Prendergast A. *Medical Terminology: A Textbook/Workbook*. Reading, Mass.: Addison-Wesley, 1983.
Smith GL, Davis P. *Medical Terminology: A Programmed Text*. New York: Wiley, 1981.

III. IMMEDIATE THREATS TO LIFE

on fire. By the time the rescuers have accomplished their careful extrication with backboards, the patient may have burned to death, and it will be small consolation to a dead patient that his spine was protected from injury. Clearly this is a case in which the usual priorities for managing spine-injured patients must be disregarded, for the *first* priority is always to save the patient's life. This concept is summarized in one of the principles of triage (sorting of patients) that will be discussed later in the book:

> THE SALVAGE OF LIFE TAKES PRECEDENCE OVER THE SALVAGE OF LIMB.

In general, then, we do not like to move a patient until he has been fully assessed and stabilized. But if the patient is in danger, one must get him out of danger—either by taking the danger away from the patient or, if that is not possible, by taking the patient away from the danger.

THE PRIMARY SURVEY

Once the EMT has determined that there is no hazard at the scene (or has eliminated any hazards detected), the primary survey itself can begin. The first thing one must determine is WHETHER THE PATIENT IS CONSCIOUS. If not, the primary survey proceeds through three steps, always in the same sequence—**ABC**—to answer the following questions.

1. Does the patient have an open *AIRWAY* (A)?
2. Is the patient *BREATHING* (B)?
3. Does the patient have an adequate CIRCULATION (C)?
   a. Is there a *pulse*?
   b. Is there profuse *bleeding*?

In some cases, the primary survey may be performed at a glance. If, for example, the patient is alert and talking, it is clear that his airway is open, he is breathing, and he has a pulse; patients in respiratory or cardiac arrest do not talk! On the other hand, if the patient is unconscious, one must proceed step-by-step through the ABCs and correct any problems noted. If the airway is found to be obstructed, one must try to relieve the obstruction. Having accomplished that, one checks whether the patient is breathing; if he is not, artificial ventilation must be started. Then one checks the pulse; if the pulse is absent, one must begin compressions over the sternum, and so forth. There are two important rules relating to the primary survey:

> **Rules of the Primary Survey**
> - The primary survey is the FIRST assessment made of EVERY patient.
> - The primary survey of an unconscious patient is ALWAYS performed in the same sequence: ABC.

Why are these rules important? Suppose, for instance, an EMT comes upon the victim of a hit-and-run accident—a middle-aged man lying unconscious in the road. The most dramatic and obvious thing about the scene is a large pool of blood around the victim's leg. The EMT forgets about the ABCs and starts searching for the source of bleeding. He is so engrossed in this task that he does not notice that the patient has an obstructed airway, and as the EMT is carefully cutting away the patient's trouser leg, the patient stops breathing and quietly goes into cardiac arrest because of the airway obstruction. The EMT finally locates the laceration on the patient's leg, but meanwhile the patient has died of causes the EMT could have easily prevented if he had performed the primary survey systematically, in the correct sequence. THE MOST DRAMATIC INJURY IS NOT ALWAYS THE MOST SERIOUS. The ABCs provide a *list of priorities* and thus help rescuers carry out their jobs in a logical and systematic way. This is particularly important when a patient has multiple injuries and treatment may at first seem overwhelmingly complicated. The ABCs tell us *where to start* and *where to go from there*.

> FIRST THINGS FIRST: KNOW YOUR ABCs.

In this chapter we have presented only an overview of the primary survey (summarized in Fig. 4-1). In the remainder of Section III, we will examine the steps of the primary survey—airway, breathing, and circulation—in greater detail and learn how to manage those conditions that present an immediate threat to life.

VOCABULARY

ABC Airway, breathing, and circulation: the steps of the primary survey.

biologic death Death of the organism, when irreversible brain damage has occurred; also called *brain death*.

cardiac arrest The cessation of effective cardiac action.

clinical death The moment when the heart stops beating, as determined by absence of a pulse.

primary survey The orderly initial assessment of a patient to detect and correct immediately life-threatening conditions.

respiratory arrest The cessation of breathing.

5. AIRWAY OBSTRUCTION

OBJECTIVES

The first letter in the rescue alphabet is *A*, for *Airway*. That vital passage is the body's lifeline to the atmosphere, and if it is blocked, death can occur in minutes. In this chapter, we will examine the airway in detail: its structure, the ways in which it can become obstructed, and the emergency measures one can take to relieve airway obstruction. By the end of this chapter, the reader should be able to

1. Identify the organ in the human body that is most vulnerable to oxygen deprivation, given a list of organs
2. Locate on a diagram the major structures of the respiratory system, given a list of structures
3. Identify the muscles that participate in the breathing process, given a list of muscles
4. Identify the head positions that are most likely to lead to airway obstruction in the adult and in the infant
5. List the major causes of airway obstruction and indicate which of these is most common
6. Describe at least three methods for opening the airway of an unconscious person
7. Identify the maneuver(s) to open the airway in a patient with suspected spine injury, given a list of maneuvers
8. Describe how to remove liquid materials from the mouth and throat of an unconscious person
9. List the signs of choking
10. List in the correct sequence the steps in treating a conscious and an unconscious choking victim, given a list of possible steps in random order
11. List in the correct sequence the steps in treating a choking infant
12. Indicate how to recognize a person with swelling or spasm of the airway and what action to take in such a case

ANATOMY AND FUNCTION OF THE RESPIRATORY TRACT

Every living cell in the body requires oxygen in order to survive. Without oxygen, cells literally suffocate and die. The cells most sensitive to even relatively short periods of oxygen deprivation are those in the *brain*, which begin to undergo irreversible damage within only a few minutes of the oxygen supply being cut off. Cardiac cells can hold out a little longer, but they start to suffer irreparable damage within 20 to 30 minutes of oxygen deprivation, while cells of the skin and nails may continue to reproduce for hours or days, even when the body is already in the grave. In order to ensure an uninterrupted supply of oxygen to the brain and other tissues, the body has a respiratory system, which takes oxygen into the body from the atmosphere, and a circulatory system, which transports the oxygen through the blood to tissues throughout the body. In this chapter, we will look at the first of the two systems, the respiratory system.

Oxygen makes up 21% of the air we breathe, the other 79% being mostly nitrogen. That 21% oxygen is enough, however, for the *healthy* body to get along just fine, and the oxygen taken into the body is exchanged in the lungs for carbon dioxide and other waste gases. In order to reach the lungs, air must pass through several structures.

THE UPPER AIRWAY

Air enters the respiratory system through the **mouth** and **nose** (Fig. 5-1). As it passes through the nose, air is filtered to remove foreign particles, humidified so that it will not dry out the delicate mucous membranes farther down the respiratory tract, and adjusted in temperature to 98.6°F (37°C). The mouth and nasal passages lead to a common passage, the **pharynx** (throat), through which air passes next. The oxygen molecule that has reached the back of the throat now finds itself staring down two tubes. The one in front is the trachea, or windpipe, which leads to the lungs, while the posterior tube is the esophagus, the pipe that carries liquids and solids to the stomach. The lungs do not like liquids and solids; when such foreign matter enters the lungs, pneumonia often follows (aspiration pneumonia), so there is a special trapdoor at the entrance to the trachea whose function is to protect the lower airways and lungs from invasion by food. This trapdoor is called the **epiglottis,** and normally when one swallows, the epiglottis slams shut against the trachea, causing the swallowed material to be directed posteriorly into the esophagus where it belongs. Once in a while, a bit of food or liquid sneaks by the epiglottis (especially if you try to talk and eat at the same time) and "goes down the wrong pipe." When the foreign material touches the sensitive area just beyond the epiglottis, it triggers the *gag reflex* and *cough reflex* by which the airway tries to blow the foreign material back out. In a normal, alert person, these reflexes are very powerful and effective, but in an unconscious person, the cough and gag reflexes may be depressed or even absent; thus an unconscious person is in constant danger of inhaling (aspirating) foreign material into the lungs.

Fig. 5-1. *Components of the respiratory tract.*

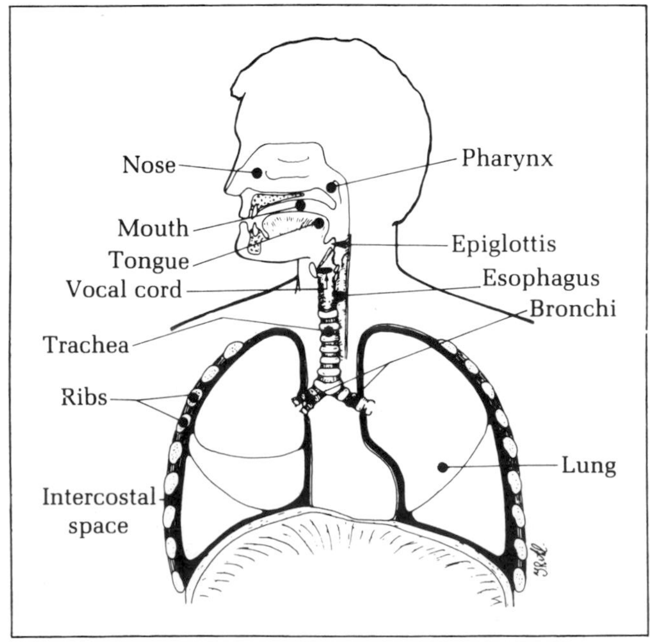

After passing the epiglottis, air journeys on through the lower portion of the throat, called the **larynx,** or "voice box." It is called the voice box because it contains the **vocal cords,** which can produce sound by vibrating as air passes through them. The front part of the larynx, the Adam's apple, can be palpated in the middle of the neck.

THE LOWER AIRWAY

The structures of the airway that lie below the larynx are considered part of the lower airway (Figs. 5-1, 5-2). Leaving the larynx, air whistles down the **trachea,** a tube about 5 inches long that is formed from semirigid rings of cartilage, which prevent the trachea from collapsing during inhalation. You can feel some of these tracheal rings just below the Adam's apple. Where the trachea enters the chest, it divides into two smaller tubes, the **right bronchus** and **left bronchus** (the plural of *bronchus* is *bronchi*). The point at which the trachea divides into the two bronchi is called the **carina**. The right bronchus enters the right lung, and the left bronchus enters the left lung. Within the lungs, the bronchi branch into smaller and smaller tubes that finally end in millions of tiny air sacs, called **alveoli**. Each alveolus sits on top of a **capillary,** a tiny blood vessel, and the exchange of gases takes place here. Oxygen is taken up by the blood from the alveolus to be carried to the rest of the body, while carbon dioxide is given off by the blood into the alveolus to be exhaled into the environment.

Suppose an oxygen molecule came to you and asked for directions on how to get to the circulation. You could now give the following instructions:

1. Enter at the *nose*. Go through a security check in the nasal hairs (to screen out particles), take a shower (humidification), and warm up (temperature adjustment).
2. Proceed down the *pharynx*. Just beyond the *epiglottis,* you will see two tubes. Avoid the posterior tube, for that is the esophagus, which will lead you into the stomach where you will just become part of a burp.

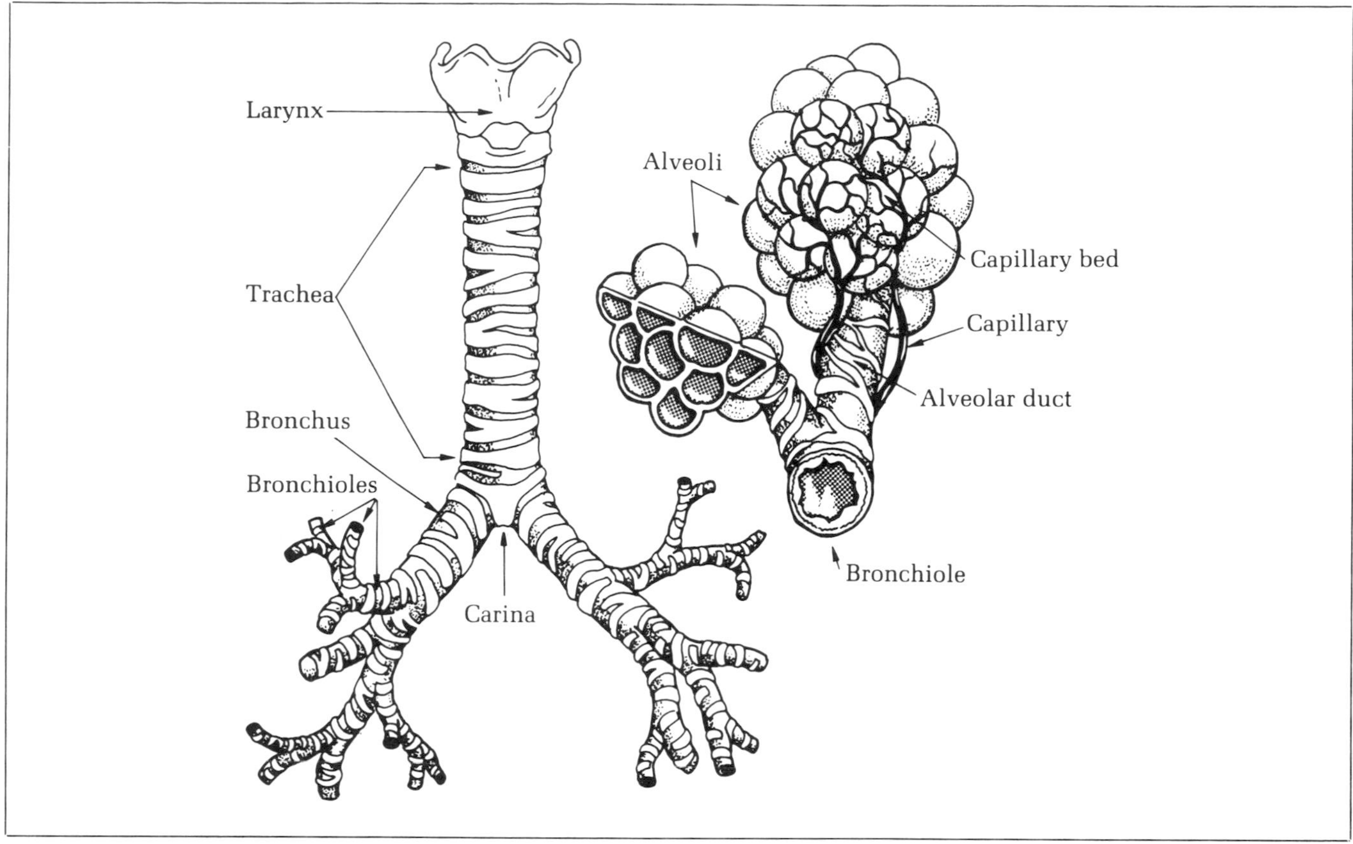

Fig. 5-2. *The lower airway.*

3. Take the tube in front, the *larynx*, and proceed down into the *trachea*.
4. As you enter the chest, make a right or left turn at the *carina* to get to the right or left *bronchus*.
5. Follow the bronchus into smaller and smaller tubes until you get to a sac at the end, an *alveolus*. There, at the capillary border, you will be traded for a molecule of carbon dioxide and permitted to cross into the circulation.

Pathway of Respiration

1. Nose (or mouth)
2. Pharynx
3. Larynx
4. Trachea
5. Bronchus
6. Alveolus

BREATHING

The process of breathing—moving air in and out of the lungs—requires several structures. First of all, we need the lungs themselves, the two big, spongy organs that nearly fill both sides of the thoracic cavity. Each lung is surrounded by a double membrane, called the **pleura.** The inner layer of the pleura is attached to the lung surface, while the outer layer lines the chest cavity. Between the two pleural layers is a potential space—called the **pleural space**—which under normal conditions is hardly a space at all but simply contains a very thin film of fluid lubricant, which permits the lungs to slide smoothly back and forth within the chest. There is a constant vacuum in the pleural space that holds the lungs in expansion, and normal breathing is possible only as long as this vacuum is maintained. If the vacuum should be broken—for example, if a knife penetrates the chest wall and pleura, creating an opening to the outside—the lung will collapse, making breathing impossible.

The lungs are where actual gas exchange takes place between the millions of alveoli and capillaries that make up most of the lung tissue. But in order for gas exchange to occur, we must have a way of getting air in and out of the lungs, the process we call breathing or **respiration.** The most efficient way to do this in a place like the chest is to build a bellows: When the bellows expands, air is drawn in, and when the bellows folds up, air is forced out. To create this bellows, we need a way of expanding the chest to increase its volume. This is accomplished by the **diaphragm,** a tough sheet of muscle that sepa-

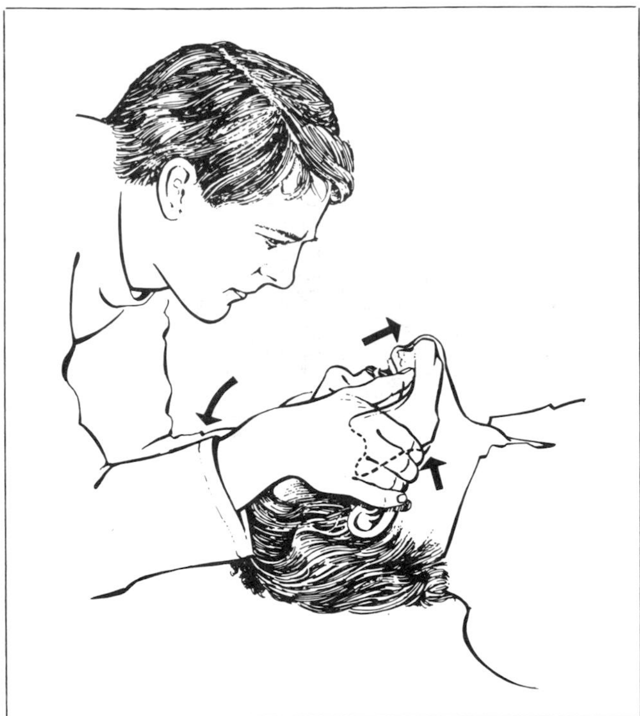

Fig. 5-6. *Triple airway maneuver. (Reproduced courtesy Asmund Laerdal, Stavanger, Norway.)*

placement of the jaw may be needed to open the airway. This can be accomplished by the triple airway maneuver (Fig. 5-6), in which tilting the head back (component 1) is combined with pushing the jaw forward (component 2) and opening the victim's mouth (component 3). This maneuver is easiest to do from the patient's **vertex** (top of the patient's head). Kneel at the vertex and place your fingers behind the angles of the patient's lower jaw, with your thumbs on either side of the lower lip. Then force the mandible forward, tilt the head backward, and push the patient's lower lip open with your thumbs. If the triple airway maneuver has to be performed in conjunction with rescue breathing (artificial ventilation), you will need to be at the patient's side rather than at the vertex. In this situation, it is easiest to perform the triple airway maneuver by resting your elbows on the floor beside the patient to provide some leverage. Then the maneuver is performed just as it was from the vertex. Like other maneuvers involving hyperextension of the head, the triple airway maneuver must not be used in cases where an injury to the cervical spine is suspected.

Jaw Thrust Alone

In cases where there is suspected injury to the cervical spine (see Suspected Spine Injuries, p. 49), the jaw thrust alone is the safest technique for opening the airway. The patient's head is carefully supported, *without* tilting it or turning it in any direction, and the lower jaw is pushed forward by exerting pressure behind the angles of the mandible.

Stable Side Position (NATO Position)

If a patient must be left unattended temporarily—as in a situation where there are many casualties and few rescuers—the patient's airway can be somewhat protected by placing the patient in the stable side position (Fig. 5-7). The patient is turned onto one side, preferably the left side, with the left knee and left thigh flexed beneath him to stabilize him. The head is extended and rests, facing down, on the flexed right arm. This position permits saliva, blood, or vomitus to drain out of the mouth rather than down into the lower respiratory tract. Extension of the head is still required, however, to pull the base of the tongue forward from the back of the throat. Once again, since this maneuver requires movement of the patient and extension of the head, it should not be used when injury to the spine is suspected.

To place a patient in the stable side position, kneel at his left side and flex the left leg at a sharp angle (Fig. 5-7A) so that the foot is near the buttocks. Extend the left arm and put the left hand beneath his hip (Fig. 5-7B). Then pull the right arm toward you,

Fig. 5-7. *Stable side position. See text for details. (Adapted with permission from Asmund Laerdal, Stavanger, Norway.)*

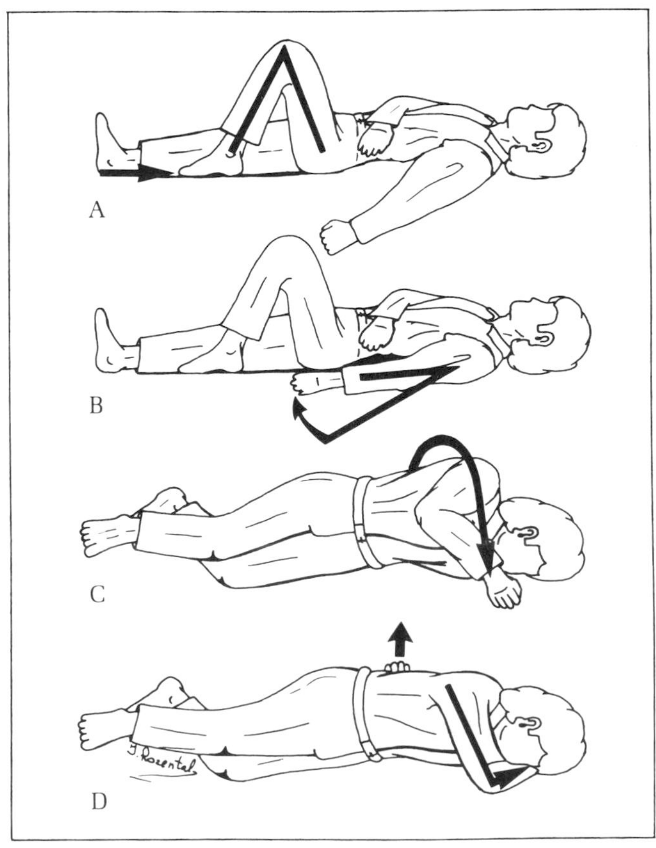

gently rolling the patient onto his left side (Fig. 5-7C). Guide the movement with your hand on the left knee. When he is on his side, tilt the head backward and put his right hand under his cheek to maintain the face in position. Pull the left hand away from the back (Fig. 5-7D).

Techniques for Opening the Airway

head tilt–neck lift*	head tilted back; neck lifted upward; victim supine
head tilt–chin lift*	head tilted back; chin lifted forward; victim supine
triple airway maneuver*	head tilted back; mandible displaced forward; lower lip pushed downward; victim supine
jaw thrust	head in neutral position; mandible displaced forward; victim supine
stable side position*	victim lying on left side with left thigh and leg flexed; head rests on arm, tilted back and turned toward the ground

*Should not be used in suspected cervical spine injury.

Often one of these simple maneuvers for opening the airway is all that is required to enable a nonbreathing patient to start breathing again spontaneously. (These techniques are also effective in correcting the partial airway obstruction that causes **snoring**. Try out one of the maneuvers some time on a snoring companion!)

Suspected Spine Injuries

In any case where there is reason to suspect injury to the cervical spine, *motion of the head and neck*—whether forward, backward, to the left, or to the right—*must be avoided*. Movement may aggravate the injury to the neck and lead to complete paralysis of the trunk and extremities (quadriplegia). Injury to the cervical spine should be suspected in all diving accidents, in any accident involving a fall from a height, and in automobile accidents where the victim shows evidence of injury to the face or head. To be on the safe side, one should use the following guideline:

EVERY ACCIDENT VICTIM HAS A CERVICAL SPINE INJURY UNTIL PROVED OTHERWISE.

If it is necessary to open the airway of an accident victim, the EMT must do so *without* hyperextension of the victim's neck or any movement of the head. The best way to accomplish this is with the JAW THRUST technique. Place your hands on either side of the victim's head, so that it is maintained in a fixed, neutral position. Then use your index fingers to push the mandible forward, *without tilting the head backward* or turning it to either side. If this maneuver does not open the airway, the victim's head may be tilted back very, very slightly and the jaw thrust attempted again. The head, neck, and chest should be kept in alignment throughout. Remember:

IF YOU SUSPECT CERVICAL SPINE INJURY, DO NOT TILT OR TURN THE VICTIM'S HEAD.

Opening the Airway in Infants

The anatomy of a baby's upper airway is a little different from that of an adult, and in addition, the baby's neck is much more pliable. For these reasons, extreme hyperextension of an infant's neck will itself cause airway obstruction. Either the head tilt–neck lift or head tilt–chin lift method may be used to open an infant's airway. (The head tilt–chin lift is the technique favored by the American Heart Association.) In the head tilt–neck lift (Fig. 5-8), the baby is placed supine on a flat surface (e.g., a table top). Place two or three fingers under the baby's neck and your other hand on the baby's forehead; then lift the neck slightly and push the forehead backward with *gentle* pressure. If this maneuver is not sufficient to open the infant's airway, you may try the head tilt–chin lift (Fig. 5-9). Once again, the infant should be supine. With one hand, maintain gentle pressure on the baby's forehead to keep the head in slight exten-

Fig. 5-8. *Head tilt–neck lift for the infant. (Reproduced courtesy American Heart Association.)*

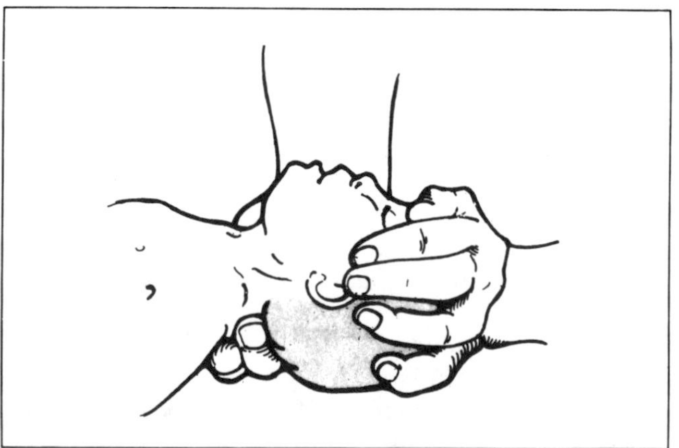

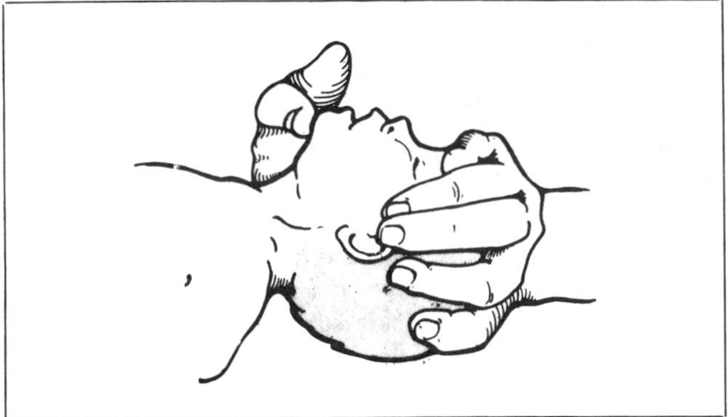

Fig. 5-9. *Head tilt–chin lift for the infant. (Reproduced courtesy American Heart Association.)*

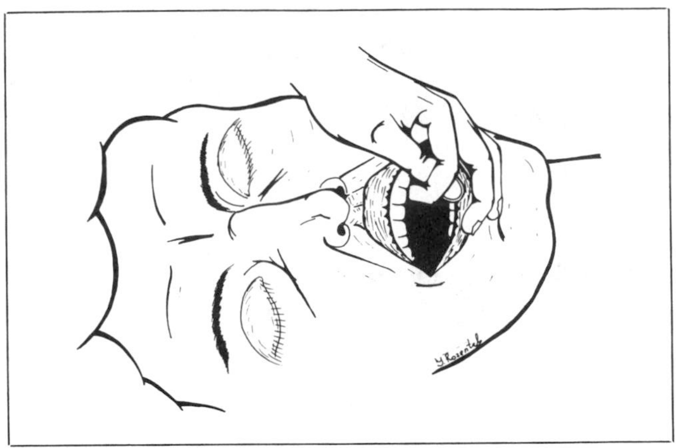

Fig. 5-10. *Crossed-finger maneuver.*

sion; use the tips of the fingers of your other hand to lift the bony part of the baby's jaw, near the chin, forward.

OBSTRUCTION OF THE AIRWAY BY FOREIGN MATERIALS

As noted earlier, by far the most common cause of upper airway obstruction is the tongue. A less common but often more obvious source of airway obstruction is foreign material that gathers in the mouth, throat, or trachea. Such material may be liquid (such as mucus, blood, or vomitus), solid (such as a chunk of meat), or a combination of liquids and solids. Any materials that cannot be removed from the airway by swallowing or coughing may cause airway obstruction and must be removed.

Loose Material

In a patient who is breathing, the presence of liquids or other loose material in the upper airway is suggested by a *gurgling* noise with respiration. The most effective means of removing liquids from the patient's mouth and throat is with the use of a suction device, which will be described in Chapter 9. If there is no equipment available, the EMT must take immediate measures using the equipment he always has with him: his hands. Let us look at two unconscious patients with partial airway obstruction from loose material: (1) the patient without suspected injury to the cervical spine, and (2) the patient with suspected injury to the cervical spine.

In the case where no injury to the cervical spine is suspected, you may turn the patient's head to one side and then sweep your index and middle fingers across the back of the patient's throat to clear out the foreign material. If the patient's mouth is clamped shut, you will have to force it open before you can accomplish this finger sweep. This is done by the **crossed-finger maneuver** (Fig. 5-10): Cross your thumb under your index finger, and apply pressure on the patient's *lower* back molars with your thumb and on the patient's *upper* back molars with your index finger. As you spread your fingers, the patient's jaws will be forced apart. Then, while holding the mouth open in this fashion, use two fingers of the other hand to sweep the mouth and throat clear of debris.

As an alternative to turning the patient's head, you may turn the whole patient. In this case, you need to position yourself beside the patient's shoulder and roll him onto his side, so that he is facing away from you. Keeping your knee against the patient's back to stabilize him, use your fingers to sweep out the patient's mouth. If he is breathing adequately, he may be left on his side (stable side position) to facilitate drainage of fluids from his mouth by gravity.

In a patient with suspected spine injury, the head must *not* be turned. If it becomes critical to remove loose foreign material from the patient's airway without the aid of a suction device, the *whole patient* must be turned onto one side as a unit, with the head, neck, and trunk kept in strict alignment. To do this safely requires at least four rescuers, one of whom maintains the head in traction and guides two of the other rescuers as they roll the patient's shoulders and hips simultaneously. Turning the patient is much safer if he has already been fully immobilized on a long backboard (see Chapter 14). Once the patient is on his side, a fourth rescuer sweeps out the patient's mouth, as described above. The EMT at the patient's head must not release his grip from the head but must continue to hold it in alignment with the neck and trunk at all times. Once the patient's mouth has been swept out, he is rolled back supine—again as a unit, with head, neck, and trunk kept in a straight line.

Impacted Material

Solid foreign materials can become the source of fatal airway obstruction. Foreign body obstruction of the upper airway usually occurs while eating, and in the adult, the most common source of obstruction is a piece of meat, sometimes an astonishingly large piece of meat. Certain factors seem to make a person more susceptible to choking, such as dentures (which may prevent a person from chewing properly), poor chewing habits in general (eating in haste), and consumption of alcohol (which affects a person's judgment regarding the size of a piece of food that can be swallowed). Probably talking while eating is the culprit in some cases, and this fact justifies every mother's warning:

> DON'T TALK WITH YOUR MOUTH FULL!

Choking usually occurs with dramatic suddenness, and perhaps for this reason it is sometimes mistaken for a heart attack—thus the term "cafe coronary" that is sometimes applied to choking incidents. Because meat is often the offending foreign body, choking is also occasionally referred to as the "sirloin strangle." But whatever name one chooses to call it, choking is a dire emergency and will lead to death within minutes if the obstruction is not removed.

RECOGNITION OF UPPER AIRWAY OBSTRUCTION. When a piece of solid food lodges in the airway, the victim becomes suddenly unable to speak, to breathe, to groan, or to cry out. He cannot utter a sound. He may try to get up and walk around, or he may lurch forward and collapse, but all in complete silence. Sometimes the victim will, either instinctively or because he has been taught to do so, give the universal distress signal for choking (Fig. 5-11) by clutching his neck between his thumb and index finger. His skin may become dusky or bluish (**cyanotic**), and he may appear to be making extreme efforts to breathe, although movement of air does not occur with these efforts. Within minutes, he will be unconscious if the obstruction is not relieved.

Fig. 5-11. *Universal distress signal for choking. (Reproduced courtesy American Heart Association.)*

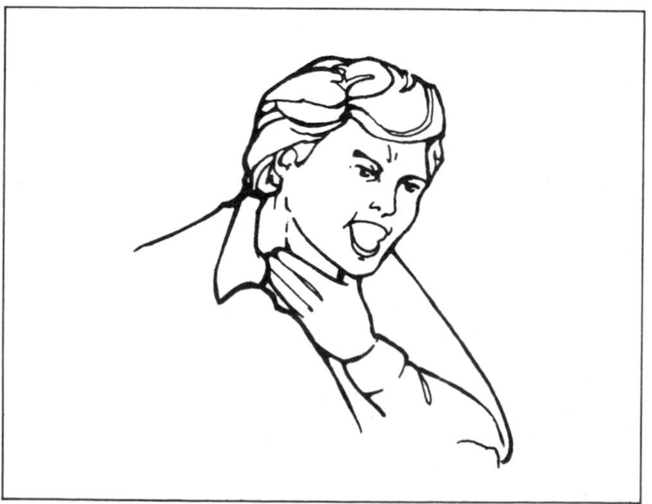

Signs of Choking

- Victim cannot speak or make any sound.
- Universal distress signal for choking: Victim clutches the neck between thumb and index finger.
- Dusky or cyanotic skin.
- Exaggerated but ineffective breathing movements.
- Collapse.

TECHNIQUES FOR RELIEVING UPPER AIRWAY OBSTRUCTION. The techniques of clearing the upper airway of a solid obstructing object are as follows:

1. **Cough.** If a person's airway is only *partially* obstructed and there is still good air exchange, a forceful cough is the most effective means of dislodging the obstruction. The air flow generated by a good cough can be as high as 500 miles per hour (nearly the speed of sound!), and a wind velocity of this magnitude could blow down a large building. Thus, in the partially obstructed airway, a cough can generate more than the necessary force to expel a foreign body. As long as the patient shows good air exchange, the rescuer should not interfere with the patient's own attempts to expel the foreign body but rather should encourage the patient to continue spontaneous coughing.

2. **Back blows.** Back blows produce an instantaneous increase in pressure in the victim's airway. This technique consists of delivering four sharp blows with the heel of your hand between the victim's shoulder blades. *If the victim is sitting or standing* (conscious), you should place yourself beside and slightly behind him (Fig. 5-12). While supporting the victim with one hand in front of his sternum, deliver four sharp blows to the victim's back between the shoulder blades. Needless to say, if the first back blow is successful in dislodging the foreign object, there is no need to proceed with three more. If at all possible (i.e., if you are tall enough), the victim should be leaning over with his head lower than his chest to take advantage of the effects of gravity when the back blows are given. *If the victim is lying down* (unconscious), you need to kneel beside him and roll him onto his side so that he is facing you; his chest should rest against your thigh. Then apply the back blows as described above.

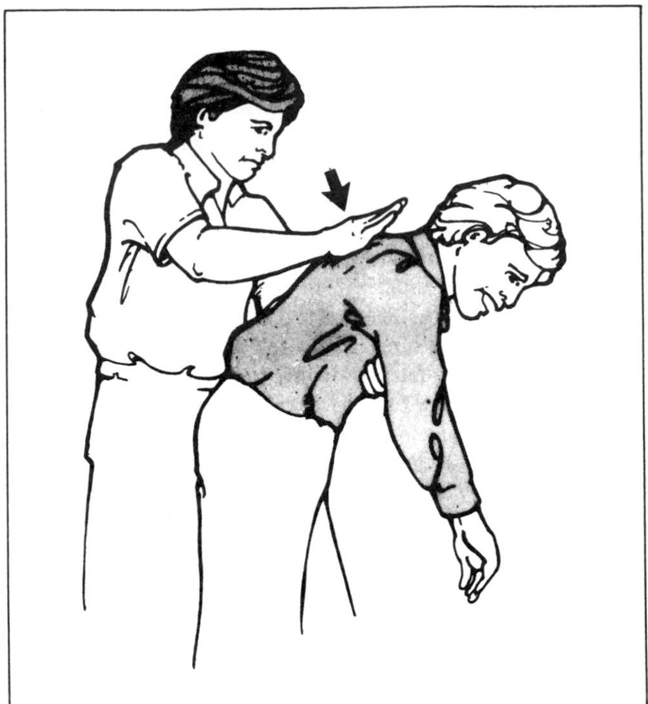

Fig. 5-12. *Back blows, with patient standing. (Reproduced courtesy American Heart Association.)*

3. **Manual thrusts.** The purpose of the manual thrust is to create an *artificial cough* by forcing air out of the victim's lungs by sudden compression either over the upper abdomen (abdominal thrust) or over the chest (chest thrust). Both the abdominal thrust and the chest thrust produce roughly the same flows, pressures, and volumes of air, so there is no particular advantage of one over the other. The chest thrust may be easier to perform than the abdominal thrust on obese or pregnant patients, while the abdominal thrust is probably preferable in elderly patients, whose ribs are brittle and thus more likely to be broken by a chest thrust. At this time, the abdominal thrust is the technique recommended by the American Heart Association. With either maneuver, correct technique is crucial, for improper hand position (e.g., over the xiphoid or costal arches) can cause laceration of internal organs, such as the lungs or liver.

The **abdominal thrust** may be administered with the victim upright or recumbent. *If the victim is sitting or standing* (conscious), stand directly behind him and put your hands around his waist, grasping your fist (thumb side against the victim's abdomen) with your other hand (Fig. 5-13). It is very important that your fist be below the xiphoid to avoid damage to internal organs. Press your fist into the victim's abdomen with a quick inward and upward thrust. You may repeat this three more times as needed. *If the victim is lying down* (unconscious), he should be positioned on his back. You may perform the abdominal thrust either from the victim's side or from an astride position. The position beside the victim enables you to move quickly to his head and chest to recheck the airway and do CPR if needed. For this position, you kneel facing the victim's head, with your knees alongside the hip. Place the heel of the hand closest to the victim in the middle of the abdomen, slightly above the umbilicus, and place your other hand on top of the first. Then rock forward so that your shoulders are directly above the victim's abdomen, and give a quick *upward* thrust toward the diaphragm. Be careful that your thrust does not veer off to the left or right, for that could damage the spleen or liver. Repeat the thrust maneuver three more times as necessary. The position astride the victim is useful when the victim is much larger than you are. It also makes it less likely that your thrust will be misdirected to the left or right side. For the astride position, straddle the victim's hips, and place your fist in the midabdomen just above the victim's umbilicus, with your other hand on top of the fist. Lock your elbows, and give a quick thrust inward and upward.

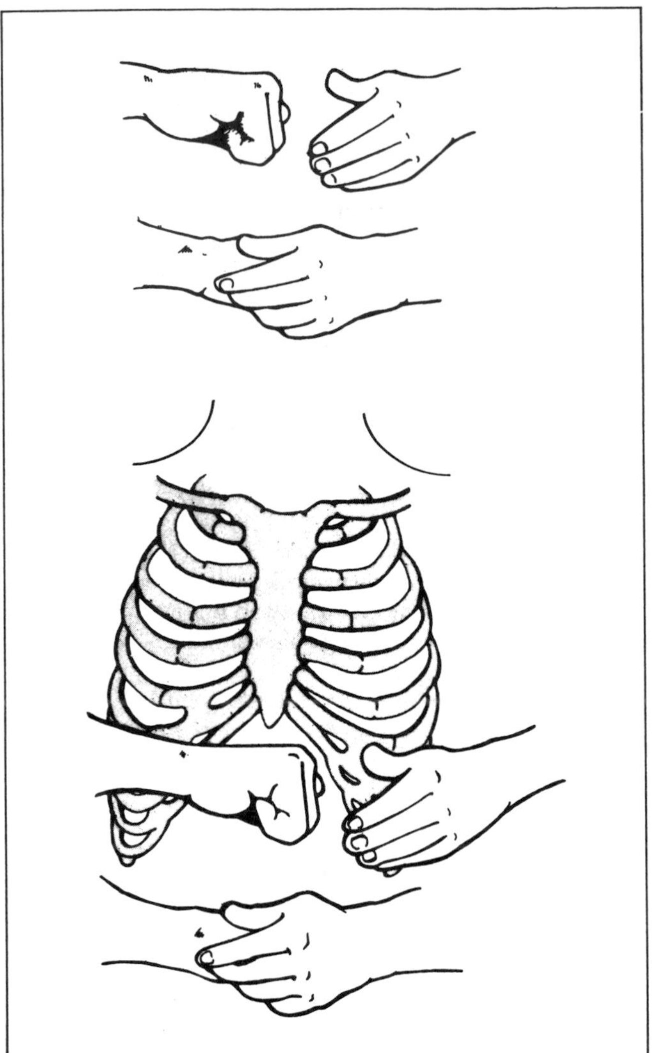

Fig. 5-13. *Hand placement for the abdominal thrust. (Reproduced courtesy American Heart Association.)*

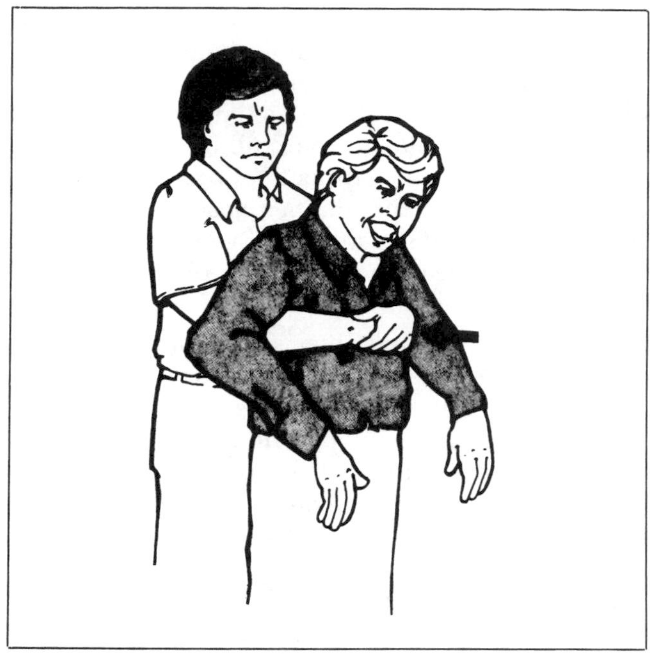

Fig. 5-14. *Chest thrust, with patient standing. (Reproduced courtesy American Heart Association.)*

If you are the victim and there is no one around to help you, you can perform the abdominal thrust on yourself. Just press your fist into your upper abdomen and give a quick thrust upward. Alternatively, you can lean forward and press your abdomen quickly against any firm object, such as a railing or the back of a chair. The life you save may be your own!

The **chest thrust** is an alternative to the abdominal thrust and produces approximately the same air flows and pressures. Like the abdominal thrust, it may be applied to both an erect and a recumbent victim. *If the victim is sitting or standing* (conscious), you should stand directly behind him with your arms encircling his chest just under the armpits (Fig. 5-14). Place the thumb side of your fist (palm down) over the *middle* of the victim's sternum, taking care to stay off the xiphoid and the ribs. Then grasp your fist with your other hand and thrust directly backward (toward you), up to four times. If you are tall enough, it is best to have the victim leaning forward during this maneuver to take advantage of gravity.

If the victim is lying down (unconscious), he should be positioned on his back. Kneel beside him with your knees close to his body, and place the heel of your hand on the lower part of the sternum (about 2 to 3 finger widths above the xiphoid). Place your other hand on top of the first, taking care to keep your fingers off the ribs, and line your shoulders up so they are directly over your hands. Give a quick downward thrust with your arms, and repeat as necessary up to a total of four times.

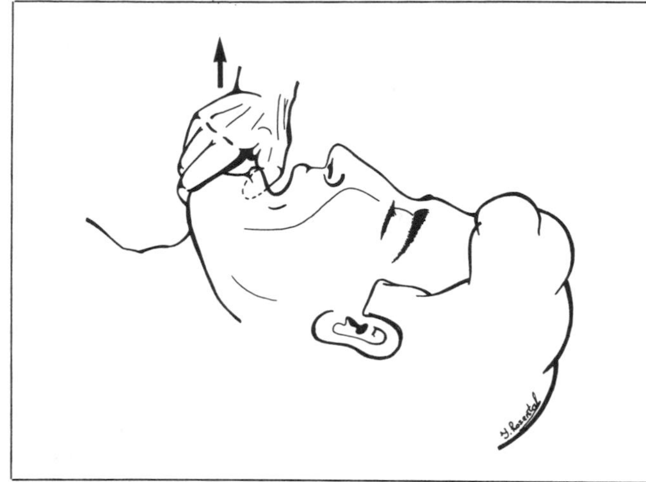

Fig. 5-15. *Jaw lift maneuver.*

4. **Finger sweep.** The finger sweep is an attempt to clear the airway manually of foreign material. With the victim supine, open the mouth by grasping both the tongue and lower jaw between your thumb and fingers and lifting upward (Fig. 5-15). Like the chin lift maneuver, this technique tends to pull the base of the tongue away from the back of the throat and also away from any foreign body that may be lodged there. In some instances, this jaw lift maneuver alone may partially relieve the obstruction. While holding the victim's jaw forward as described, insert the index finger of your other hand along the inside of the victim's cheek and down into the throat to the base of the tongue; try to dislodge the foreign body and hook it into the mouth so you can remove it. Be very careful not to force the foreign body deeper into the airway.

Do *not* place any object other than your fingers in the victim's mouth in an attempt to remove a foreign body. There are several devices marketed today that are purported to be useful in cases of choking, but any device inserted blindly into a person's throat is dangerous and may cause considerable damage. The EMT should not use these devices.

NEVER STICK ANY INSTRUMENT BLINDLY INTO A PATIENT'S THROAT.

In summary, there are four basic techniques for treating the choking victim:

Techniques for Relieving Foreign Body Obstruction

COUGH	If the airway is only partially obstructed and still has good air exchange, do not

	interfere, but encourage the victim to continue spontaneous coughing.
BACK BLOWS	Four sharp blows delivered between the shoulder blades.
MANUAL THRUSTS	Four quick compressions given over either the midabdomen or the sternum.
FINGER SWEEP	Probing the victim's throat with your index finger while holding the victim's jaw and tongue forward.

In the latest standards and guidelines issued by the American Heart Association (AHA), it is recommended that only the abdominal thrust be taught, to minimize the confusion that is apt to arise when a lay rescuer has to confront an emergency situation and remember several techniques. It is the view of this author, however, that *professional* rescuers, such as EMTs, should learn all of the available methods—since none of these methods has been definitively shown to be superior to any of the others—and should therefore have alternative choices should the first method fail. The recommended sequences that follow are based on that view and incorporate several alternative techniques for trying to aid the choking victim. When EMTs are called on to train lay persons, however, they should teach the simpler sequence recommended by the AHA. (See skill evaluation checklists at the end of Chapter 7.)

WHICH TECHNIQUE WHEN? There are several possible scenarios of choking that the EMT may encounter: (1) the conscious choking victim, (2) the choking victim who becomes unconscious in the EMT's presence, and (3) the victim who is found unconscious, and the cause is initially unknown. Each of these situations requires a slightly different approach, utilizing some or all of the maneuvers we learned above.

1. *If the victim is conscious* (Fig. 5-16), first determine whether he has a complete airway obstruction by asking him if he can speak. If he can speak, encourage him to cough. If he cannot speak, however, apply four back blows in rapid succession followed (if the back blows are unsuccessful) by four manual thrusts. Keep repeating the back blows and manual thrusts until they are effective or until the victim loses consciousness.

2. *If the choking victim becomes unconscious* (Fig. 5-17), he should be placed in the supine position. Open the airway (using the head tilt or a similar maneuver), and attempt mouth-to-mouth ventilation (see Chapter 6). If you cannot force any air past the obstruction, quickly roll the victim toward you and deliver four back blows. Then roll him back supine, and give four manual thrusts followed by a finger sweep. Reposition the victim's head, open the airway, and try again to ventilate. If you still cannot get any air in, repeat the sequence of back blows–thrusts–finger sweep.

3. *If the victim is found unconscious and the cause is unknown* (Fig. 5-18), first determine whether the victim is actually unresponsive. If so, it is back to the old ABCs: Open the *airway*, and determine whether the patient is *breathing*. If he is not breathing, attempt to ventilate by the mouth-to-mouth technique. In the event that you cannot ventilate him, reposition his head and try again. If you are still unsuccessful, use the same sequence of back blows–manual thrusts–finger sweep as in the choking victim who becomes unconscious. When first approaching a person who is unconscious from unknown causes, you should not waste time hunting for foreign bodies in the airway unless you have a very good reason to suspect their presence; your first effort to ventilate the lungs will tell you quickly enough whether there is something obstructing the airway.

In addition to the above situations, the EMT needs to know how to manage one other special case: the choking infant or small child. Choking is not uncommon in small children, who have a tendency to put almost anything into their mouths. Small toys, marbles, peanuts, and a variety of other objects are apt to wind up in the child's airway, especially if the child is running or playing while he has something in his mouth. Foreign bodies can cause either partial or complete obstruction of the child's airway. As in the adult, if the obstruction is partial *and* there is good air exchange—that is, the child can still cough forcibly—he should be allowed to cough. If, however, there is poor air exchange (signalled by high-pitched noises on inhalation, ineffective cough, blueness of the lips, nails, or skin), or if there is complete airway obstruction, the rescuer must take immediate action.

If the victim is an infant, straddle him over your arm with the head lower than the trunk (Fig. 5-19), supporting the head with your hand around the jaw and chest. Give four quick back blows with the heel of your hand between the infant's shoulder blades, but be careful: Babies are very little and very delicate, and the back blows should not be as forceful as those given to an adult. As soon as you complete the back blows, place your free hand on the infant's back so that he is sandwiched between your two hands—one supporting the neck, jaw, and chest, the other ready to support the back. Then flip him over and put him on your thigh, with the head still lower than

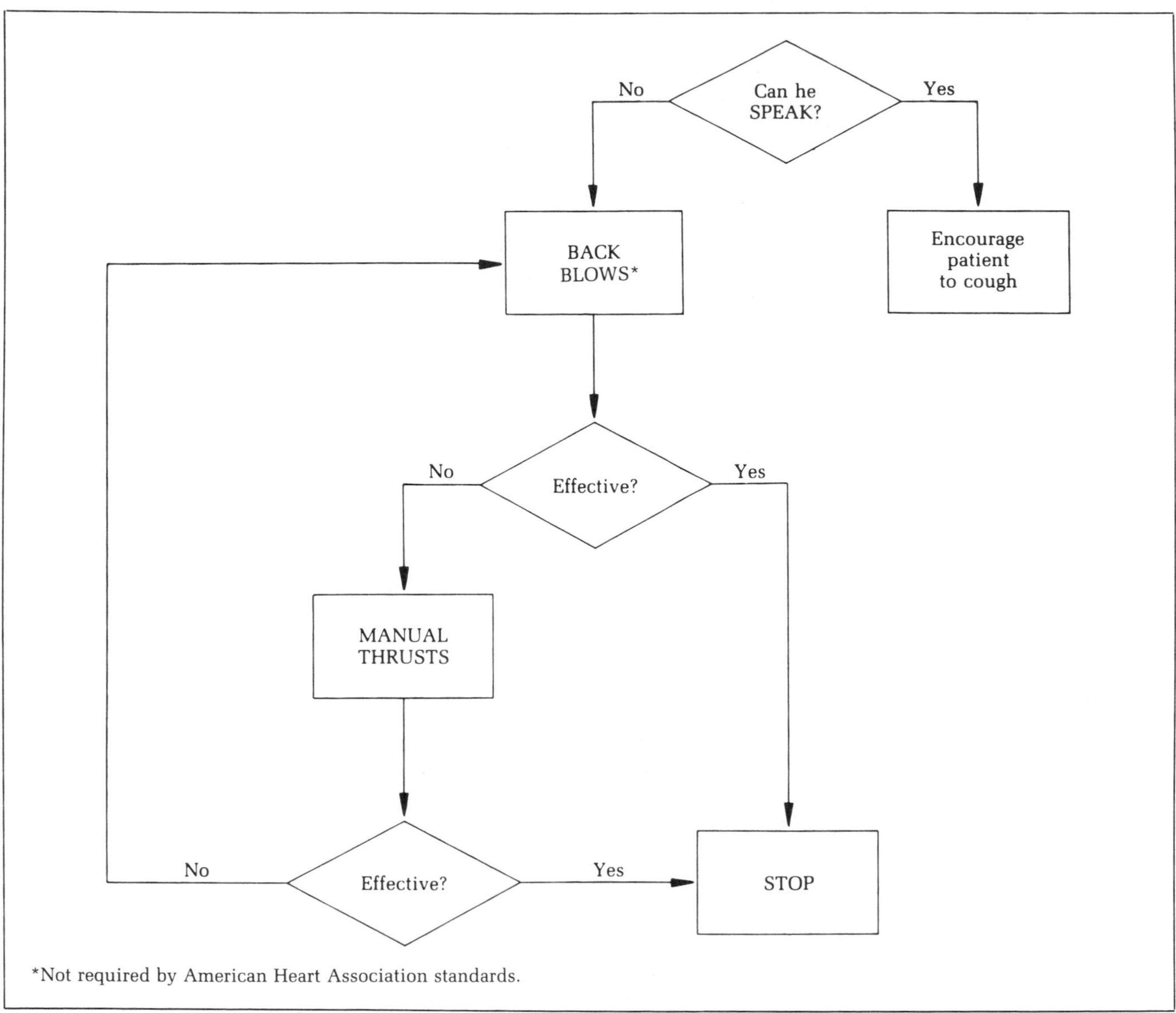

Fig. 5-16. *Management of the conscious choking victim.*

the trunk, and give four quick chest thrusts—using two fingers to push on the midsternum (Fig. 5-20). ABDOMINAL THRUSTS SHOULD NOT BE USED IN INFANTS AND CHILDREN, because abdominal thrusts are more likely in this age group to cause injury to internal organs. *Blind* finger sweeps should also be avoided in infants and children, since the foreign body may be pushed farther back into the child's airway, worsening the obstruction. Pull the child's tongue and jaw forward to open the mouth. If you can *see* the foreign body in the child's mouth, you may remove it with your finger, but do not go poking around for foreign bodies you cannot see. If the child has not started breathing after the back blows and chest thrusts, you should attempt to ventilate. If you cannot do so, the obstruction is still present, and you will have to try the back blows and chest thrusts again.

If the child is too large to straddle over your arm, kneel on the floor and drape him over your thigh so that his head is lower than his trunk. Give four back blows (you can use more force than you would for an infant), then roll him supine onto the floor and give four chest thrusts as you would for an adult, over the lower third of the sternum.

OTHER CAUSES OF AIRWAY OBSTRUCTION

Besides the tongue and foreign bodies, there are other sources of airway obstruction. *Swelling* (edema) or spasm of the structures in the airway itself may narrow the airway to the point that no air exchange can take place. Such swelling or spasm can occur for a variety of reasons—infection, severe allergy, inhalation of noxious gases, and so forth. Whatever the cause, the *sign* of a narrowed airway is **stridor**, a shrill, high-pitched squeak audible when the patient inhales. There is nothing an EMT can do in the field for airway edema or spasm; lifesaving treatment will often require a tracheostomy—a sur-

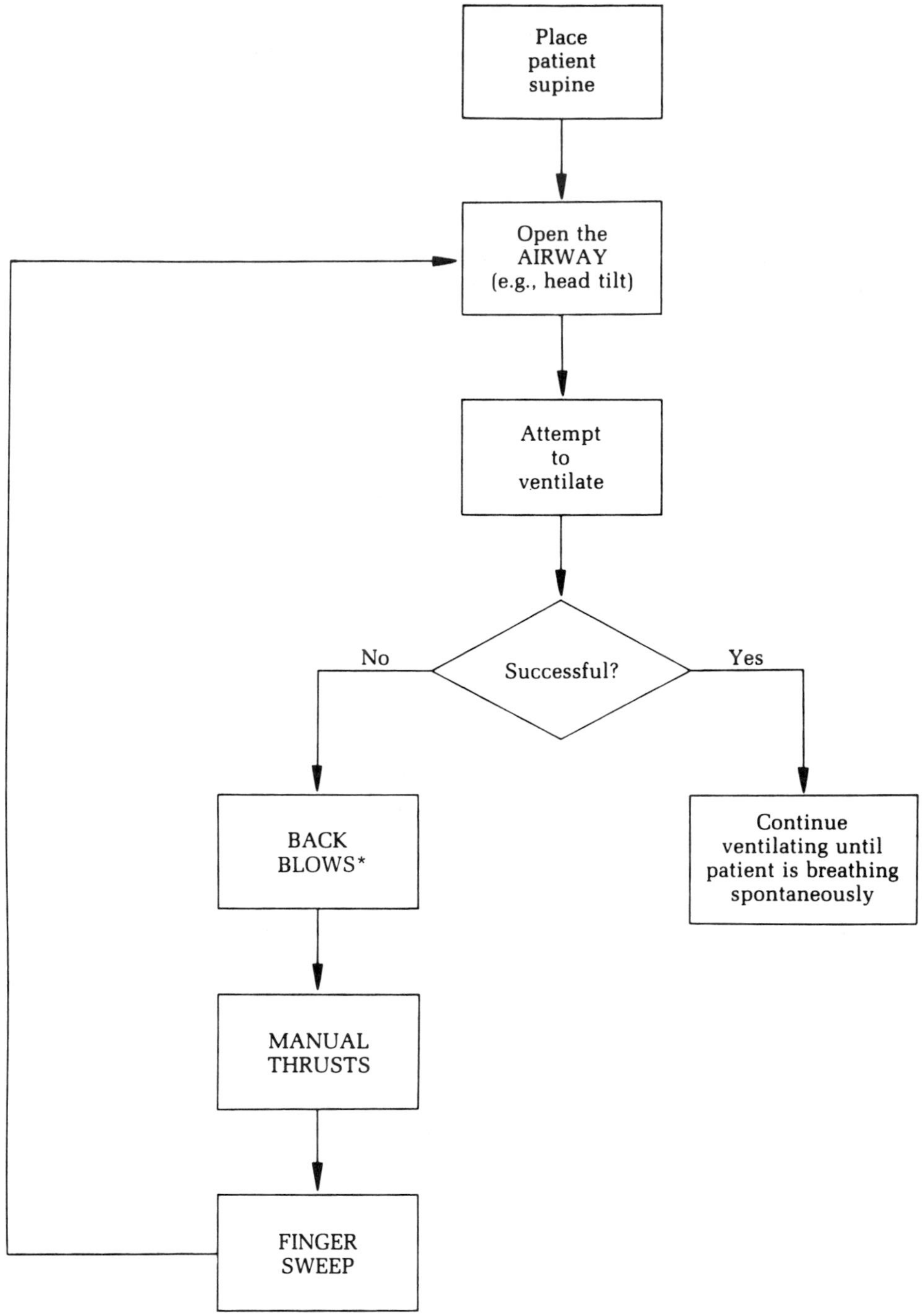

Place patient supine

Open the AIRWAY (e.g., head tilt)

Attempt to ventilate

Successful?

No

BACK BLOWS*

MANUAL THRUSTS

FINGER SWEEP

Yes

Continue ventilating until patient is breathing spontaneously

*Not required by American Heart Association standards.

Fig. 5-17. *Management of the choking victim who becomes unconscious.*

gical opening through the neck into the trachea. Thus the sound of stridor should be a signal to the EMT to GET THE PATIENT TO A MEDICAL FACILITY AS FAST AS POSSIBLE. The EMT should *not* try to insert any object into the patient's mouth or throat, since this may worsen the swelling or spasm and cause sudden, complete obstruction of the airway.

WHEN YOU HEAR STRIDOR, GET A MOVE ON.

Another cause of upper airway obstruction is *collapse of the trachea*, which may occur when there has been severe trauma to the neck (see p. 262). As with airway edema, there is nothing an EMT can do to treat tracheal collapse; the patient must be moved

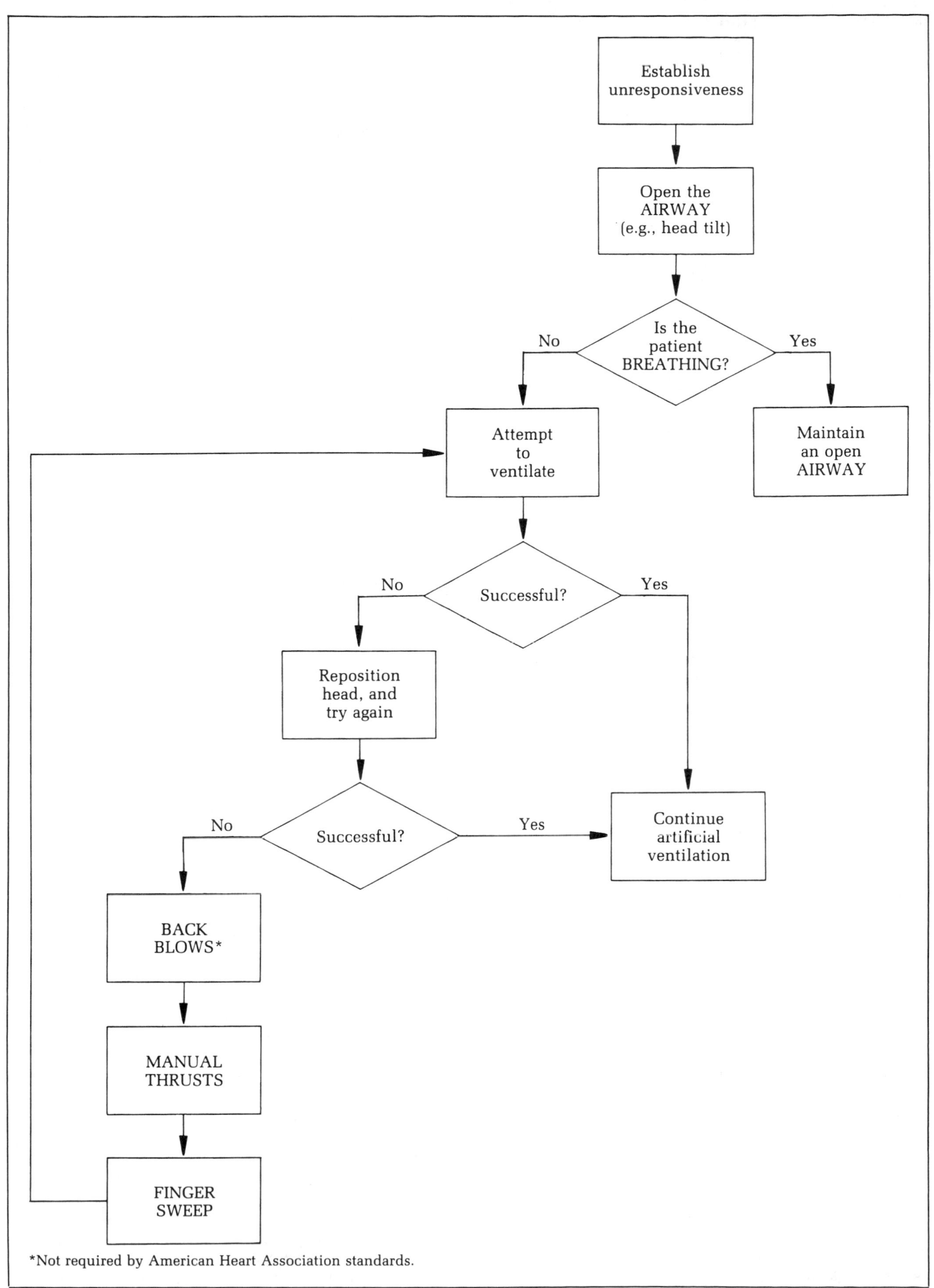

Fig. 5-18. *Management of the victim who is found unconscious and the cause is unknown.*

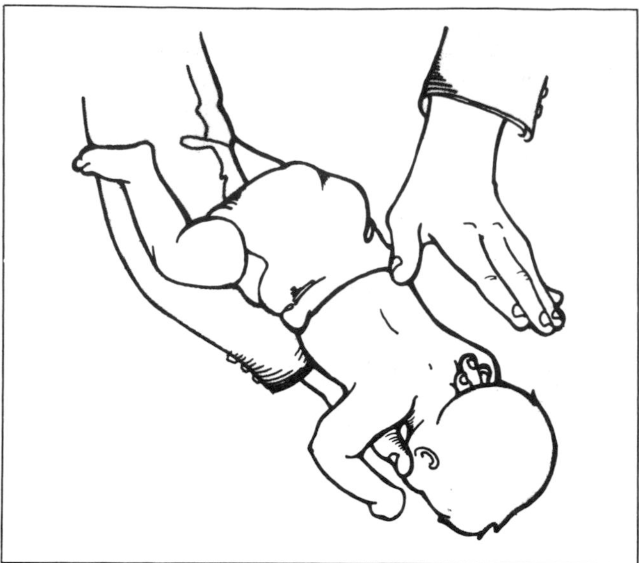

Fig. 5-19. *Back blows for the choking infant. (Reproduced courtesy American Heart Association.)*

to a medical facility with all possible speed, so that appropriate surgical treatment can be instituted.

BEFORE YOU PANIC . . .
The skills presented in this chapter may sound quite complicated on paper, for skills always *sound* complicated if you have to describe them in words. Try writing directions for using a can opener to remove the lid of a soup can, and you will see how complicated a relatively simple manual skill can sound. In reality, these skills are not difficult or complex, but they *do* require practice. So don't panic if you are not an expert on opening the airway after reading this chapter; you are not expected to be. However, it is assumed that the student will spend enough time practicing these skills on manikins to become proficient.

"How do you get to Carnegie Hall?" Remember?

LESSONS OF THE AIRWAY

A cowhand from south Oklahoma
Lapsed quietly one day into coma;
No one checked to see
If his airway was free.
Now he's buried in south Oklahoma.

Moral: EVERY UNCONSCIOUS PERSON HAS AN OBSTRUCTED AIRWAY UNTIL PROVED OTHERWISE.

An unfortunate man named O'Brien
Got a knock on his cervical spine;
Someone let his head loll;
Now he can't move at all,
But his airway is doing just fine.

Moral: NEVER HYPEREXTEND THE HEAD OF A PATIENT WITH A SUSPECTED INJURY TO THE CERVICAL SPINE.

A man with a smile faintly mocking
Bolted up from his steak and stopped talking.
He clutched at his neck
And turned blue as all heck.
He died while the waiter was gawking.

Moral: CHOKING IS A DIRE MEDICAL EMERGENCY AND REQUIRES IMMEDIATE TREATMENT.

A rescuer named Joe McMust
Was uncertain just where he should thrust.
He picked a spot on the chest
And forcefully pressed,
Two ribs and the spleen he did bust.

Moral: CORRECT HAND POSITION IS CRUCIAL FOR MANUAL THRUST MANEUVERS.

There once was a young man named Fred
Who to save a man choking once sped.
He reached in with some pliers
To extract what was mired
And pulled out the tonsils instead.

Moral: NEVER BLINDLY INSERT ANY INSTRUMENT INTO A PATIENT'S THROAT.

VOCABULARY

abdominal thrust Maneuver in which a sharp compression is delivered over the upper abdomen in an attempt to dislodge a foreign body from the airway.

alveolus Terminal air sac in the lung.

back blows Sharp blows delivered with the heel of the hand to the middle of the victim's back, between the shoulder blades, in an attempt to dislodge a foreign body obstructing the airway.

bronchus One of the two subdivisions of the trachea.

cafe coronary A choking incident, so named because its suddenness often leads witnesses to mistake it for a heart attack.

carina The point at which the trachea bifurcates into the right and left bronchus.

chest thrust Maneuver in which a sharp compression is delivered over the sternum in an attempt to dislodge a foreign body from the airway.

chin lift Technique for opening the airway by lifting the chin forward.

cough reflex Automatic, forceful expulsion of air in response to irritation in the back of the throat.

crossed-finger maneuver Technique for forcing a patient's mouth open by pushing on the lower molars with the thumb and on the upper molars with the index finger.

cyanosis Bluish discoloration of the skin, lips, and

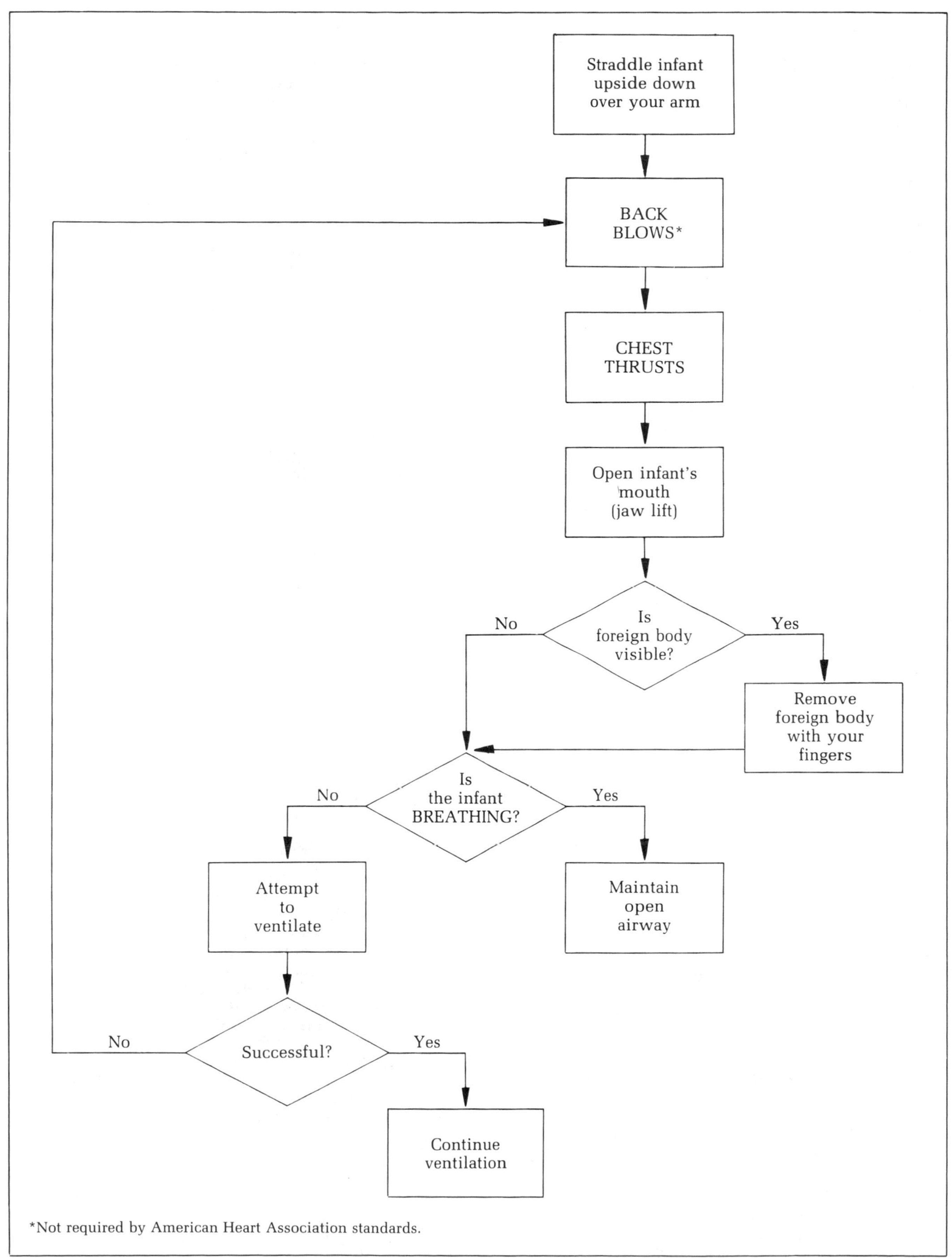

Fig. 5-20. *Management of the choking infant.*

nail beds, suggestive of inadequate oxygen in the blood.

diaphragm Tough sheet of muscle that separates the thoracic cavity from the abdominal cavity; the principal muscle of respiration.

edema Swelling.

epiglottis Small piece of tissue at the entrance to the trachea that acts as a trapdoor to prevent the entry of foreign materials into the lower respiratory tract.

exhalation The passive phase of respiration, during which air is expelled from the lungs.

finger sweep Maneuver to clear the mouth and throat of foreign material by sweeping a finger through them.

gag reflex Automatic spasm of the airway in response to irritation of the throat.

head tilt Maneuver to open the airway by hyperextending the head.

inhalation The active phase of respiration, during which air is drawn into the lungs.

intercostal muscles The muscles between the ribs, which participate in respiration.

jaw thrust Maneuver to open a patient's airway by pushing forward on the angles of the mandible.

jaw-tongue lift Maneuver to open a patient's airway by inserting one's thumb in the patient's mouth over his lower teeth and pulling upward on the tongue and jaw.

larynx Voice box; lower part of the throat.

medulla Area in the base of the brain that controls respiration.

neck lift Maneuver to open the airway by lifting upward on the patient's neck.

oxygen Colorless, odorless gas present in the atmosphere in a concentration of 21% and essential to life.

pharynx The throat.

pleura The double membrane surrounding the lung.

pleural space The potential space between the two layers of the pleural membrane.

snoring Noise made on inhalation when the upper airway is partially obstructed by the base of the tongue.

stable side position Position in which a patient is lying on his left side, with the left thigh and leg flexed, and his head resting on his extended arm.

stridor High-pitched, shrill noise audible on inhalation when there is significant narrowing of the upper airway from edema or spasm.

trachea The windpipe; the tube connecting the throat to the lower airway.

triple airway maneuver Technique for opening the airway by (1) forward displacement of the mandible, (2) backward tilt of the head, and (3) retraction of the lower lip.

vertex Top of the head.

vocal cords Paired structures in the larynx whose vibrations produce sound.

FURTHER READING

Addy DP. The choking child: Back bangers against front pushers. *Br Med J* 286:536, 1983.

American Heart Association. Standards and guidelines for cardiopulmonary resuscitation (CPR) and emergency cardiac care (ECC). *JAMA* 255:2905, 1986.

Baker SP, Fisher RS. Childhood asphyxiation by choking or suffocation. *JAMA* 244:1343, 1980.

Chapman JH, Menapace FJ, Howell RR. Ruptured aortic valve cusp: A complication of the Heimlich maneuver. *Ann Emerg Med* 12:446, 1983.

Day RL. Differing opinions on the emergency treatment of choking. *Pediatrics* 71:976, 1983.

Day RL et al. Choking: The Heimlich abdominal thrust vs. back blows: An approach to the measurement of inertial and aerodynamic forces. *Pediatrics* 70:113, 1982.

Eller WC, Haugen RK. Food asphyxiation: Restaurant rescue. *N Engl J Med.* 289:81, 1973.

Gann DS. Emergency management of the obstructed airway. *JAMA* 243:1141, 1980.

Greensher J, Moffensen D. Emergency treatment of the choking child. *Pediatrics* 70:110, 1982.

Guildner CW. Resuscitation—Opening the airway: A comparative study of the techniques for opening an airway obstructed by the tongue. *JACEP* 5:588, 1976.

Harris CS et al. Childhood asphyxiation by food: A national analysis and overview. *JAMA* 251:2232, 1984.

Haugen RK. The cafe coronary: Sudden deaths in restaurants. *JAMA* 186:142, 1963.

Haynes DE et al. Esophageal rupture complicating Heimlich maneuver. *Am J Emerg Med* 2:507, 1984.

Hoffman JR. Treatment of foreign body obstruction of the upper airway. *West Med J* 136:11, 1982.

Holbrook PR. On opening the airway. *Emerg Med* 14(1): 137, 1982.

Iverson K. Strangulation: A review of ligature, manual and postural neck compression injuries. *Ann Emerg Med* 13: 179, 1984.

Mittleman RE, Wetli CV. The fatal cafe coronary: Foreign body airway obstruction. *JAMA* 247:1285, 1982.

Redding JS. The choking controversy: Critique of evidence on the Heimlich maneuver. *Crit Care Med* 7:475, 1979.

Rund DA. Airway management. *Emerg Med Serv* 19(1):19, 1990.

Safar P, Bircher N. *Cardiopulmonary Cerebral Resuscitation*. Philadelphia: Saunders, 1988.

Safar P. Recognition and management of airway obstruction. *JAMA* 208:1008, 1969.

Safar P. (Ed.). *Advances in Cardiopulmonary Resuscitation*. New York: Springer-Verlag, 1977. Section II: Airway Obstruction and Respiratory Arrest.

Swedish National Food Administration. *The National Food Administration's Ordinance on Foods for Infants and Young Children*. Uppsala, Sweden: Department of Standards, 1978.

Torrey SB. The choking child—a life-threatening emergency: Evaluation of current recommendations. *Clin Pediatr* 22:751, 1983.

Trott A. Recurrent upper airway obstruction. *JACEP* 8:407, 1979.

6. RESPIRATORY ARREST

OBJECTIVES

Breathing is something we do quite spontaneously, without giving it a single thought. But there are many conditions that can interfere with breathing, and in some instances breathing ceases altogether—a situation known as respiratory arrest. In this chapter, we will examine respiratory arrest: how it occurs, how to recognize it, and what to do about it. By the end of this chapter, the reader should be able to

1. Identify the most common cause of respiratory arrest
2. Describe the sequence of events leading to respiratory arrest in (a) an unconscious person, (b) a person who has taken an overdose of narcotics, (c) a victim of electrocution, (d) a victim of head injury, and (e) a person with primary cardiac arrest
3. List the actions to perform and the signs to look for to detect respiratory arrest
4. Identify the most effective method of artificial ventilation, given a list of several methods
5. List in the proper sequence the steps in performing (a) mouth-to-mouth ventilation, (b) mouth-to-nose ventilation, (c) mouth-to-stoma ventilation
6. Indicate the number of breaths per minute that should be given in artificial ventilation of an adult and an infant
7. List the signs that indicate effective artificial ventilation
8. List possible causes of ineffective rescue breathing and indicate the steps that can be taken to correct each
9. Describe the modifications in the technique of artificial ventilation necessary in (a) the patient with suspected injury to the cervical spine, and (b) the infant and small child
10. Explain the danger inherent in gastric distention during rescue breathing and the actions to take if gastric distention occurs

CAUSES OF RESPIRATORY ARREST

Respiratory arrest can occur for several reasons. The most common cause is the one we have already studied: AIRWAY OBSTRUCTION in the unconscious patient. As noted in the previous chapter, when a person loses consciousness, the base of the tongue tends to fall back against the pharynx, thereby closing off the upper airway. Clearly, then, most cases of respiratory arrest are both preventable and easily treatable by simple maneuvers to open the airway.

Less commonly, respiratory arrest may occur because of injury to or depression of the respiratory center in the brain. OVERDOSE OF certain DRUGS, such as narcotics or barbiturates for example, may depress the activity of the medulla to such an extent that the patient breathes very slowly or stops breathing altogether. A high-voltage ELECTRIC SHOCK (e.g., from household current or lightning) can have the same effect, temporarily knocking out the respiratory command center in the brain. Mechanical damage to the brain, such as that occurring from HEAD INJURY, can also affect the respiratory control centers, especially if there is significant swelling of the brain (cerebral edema) that squeezes the medulla against the bones of the skull. Such swelling in the brain can occur even without trauma, as in certain cases of STROKE, and again this may lead to damage to the medulla with resulting respiratory arrest. PRIMARY CARDIAC ARREST—for instance, cardiac arrest caused by massive cardiac damage in a heart attack or by a disturbance of cardiac rhythm—will also lead to respiratory arrest, for once the circulation stops, the brain is cut off from its supply of oxygen and the respiratory center in the brain stops functioning. Thus a person whose heart suddenly stops beating will stop breathing within about 60 seconds thereafter.

Causes of Respiratory Arrest

- AIRWAY OBSTRUCTION
  - Tongue (unconsciousness)
  - Foreign body (choking)
  - Swelling or spasm of the airway
  - Trauma to the airway
- Depressant DRUGS (e.g., narcotics, barbiturates)
- DAMAGE TO THE RESPIRATORY CENTER
  - Electric shock
  - Head injury
  - Stroke
- PRIMARY CARDIAC ARREST

Among these various causes of respiratory arrest, it should be emphasized again that the *most common cause* is unconsciousness followed by airway obstruction by the tongue. This is why the FIRST step in managing EVERY unconscious patient is to open the airway, for this simple maneuver can prevent respiratory arrest from ever occurring.

AN OUNCE OF PREVENTION IS WORTH A POUND OF CURE: IN THE UNCONSCIOUS PATIENT, OPEN THE AIRWAY.

RECOGNITION OF RESPIRATORY ARREST

When a person is breathing spontaneously, his chest rises and falls in a rhythmic fashion, and air can be felt and heard coming out of the mouth and nose. The moment a person stops breathing, these signs are no longer present. Thus to determine whether someone is breathing, the rescuer needs to

LOOK, LISTEN, AND FEEL FOR BREATHING.

First things first though. *A* comes before *B*, and the airway comes before breathing. There is no point in checking for breathing in a person whose airway may be obstructed, for even if the breathing mechanism is quite intact, the obstruction will prevent air from moving in and out of the lungs. Thus the first step in determining whether an unconscious person is breathing is to open the airway, using the head tilt–chin lift or similar technique. Having opened the airway, the rescuer *looks* at the chest and abdomen to see if they are rising and falling in the usual fashion. By itself, however, inspection of the chest and abdomen may be somewhat misleading, for a person may be making breathing efforts (thus showing movement of the chest and abdomen) without succeeding in moving any air. If the rescuer wants to be really sure the patient is breathing, he or she must listen and feel for the movement of air as well. One *listens* by putting one's ear close to the patient's nose. At the same time, this enables the rescuer to *feel* any air exhaled against his or her cheek. If breathing movements are absent and air flow cannot be detected, the patient is in respiratory arrest and requires artificial ventilation.

The steps we have learned so far are summarized in Figure 6-1.

PULMONARY RESUSCITATION

If a person stops breathing, the only way to save his life is to breathe for him. Fortunately, every potential rescuer has a marvelous device with him at all times that can be used to give artificial ventilation to a nonbreathing person: his own lungs. Not all the oxygen we take into our bodies is consumed by the tissues, and consequently our exhaled air contains about 16 to 18% oxygen, enough to sustain life if it is pumped into someone else's lungs. There remains only the small logistic problem of how to get the air from the rescuer's lungs into the victim's lungs, and this problem is solved relatively easily by the techniques of pulmonary resuscitation.

Historically, many techniques have been tried in an attempt to revive people who had stopped breathing. The value of forcing air into the victim's lungs was first recognized by the sixteenth-century physician Paracelsus, who recommended that a bellows, of the type kept beside the household fireplace, be used to ventilate nonbreathing patients. Around the

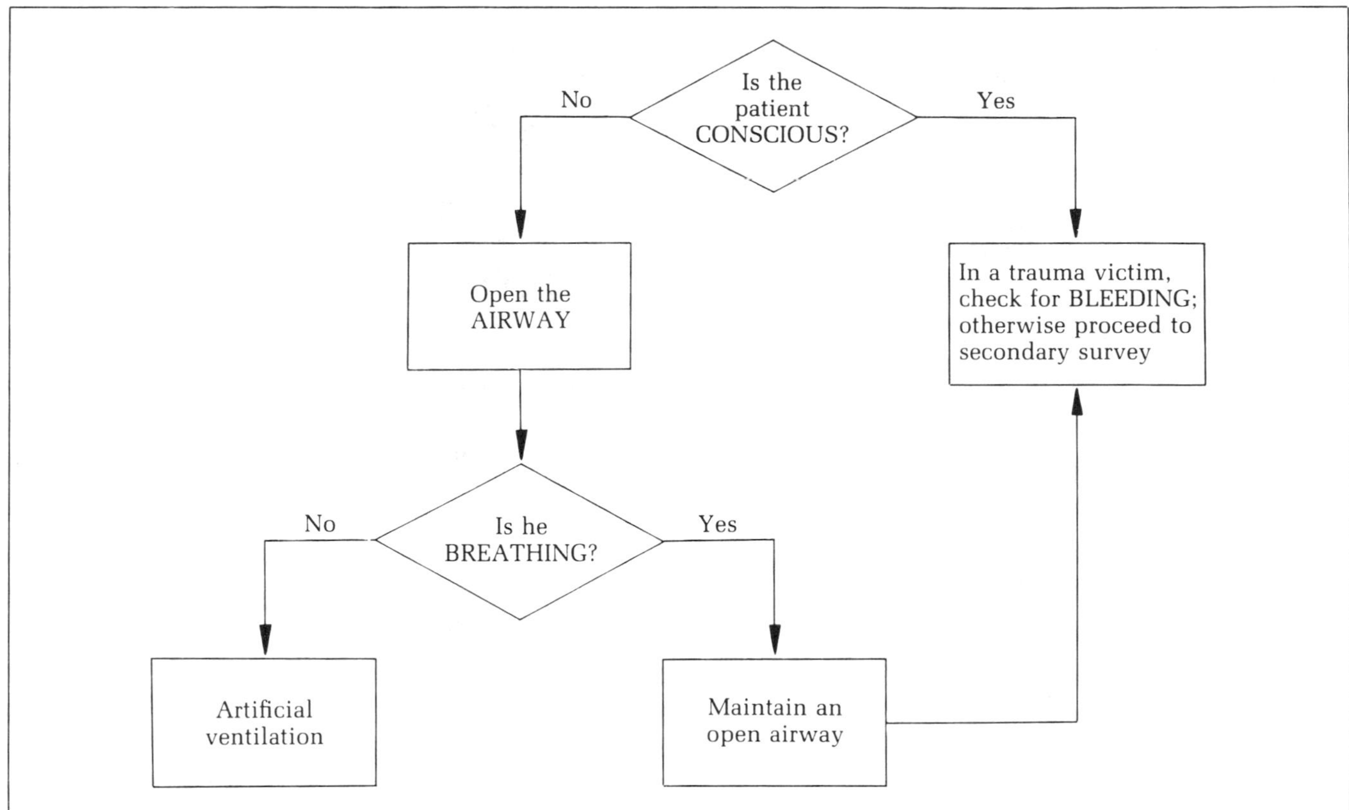

Fig. 6-1. *The airway and breathing.*

same period, midwives were already commonly using mouth-to-mouth ventilation to resuscitate infants who failed to breathe after birth, but physicians apparently considered that technique undignified and paid little attention to it. Nearly 300 years passed before mouth-to-mouth ventilation was rediscovered. Meanwhile, many other methods of resuscitation were tried, including hanging the nonbreathing person by his heels, rolling him over a barrel, and blowing tobacco smoke into his rectum. In the nineteenth century, several methods involving compression over the chest and abdomen became popular. The theory was that pressure over the chest and abdomen would produce movement of the victim's diaphragm and thereby move air in and out of the lungs. During the twentieth century until the early 1960s, two of these compression techniques—Silvester's method (chest pressure–arm lift, with the patient supine) and the Holger Nielsen method (back pressure–arm lift with the victim prone)—were widely accepted and taught as the preferred means of artificial ventilation. In 1958, however, a group of physicians at Baltimore City Hospital reported that the compression techniques were relatively ineffective in moving air in and out of the lungs, partly because it was very difficult to maintain the victim's airway open during these maneuvers. They found that mouth-to-mouth ventilation, on the other hand, could deliver effective volumes of air to the victim's lungs, and thus the instinctive wisdom of the sixteenth-century midwives was confirmed by the medical profession. Since the 1960s, mouth-to-mouth ventilation has been accepted throughout the world as the preferred method of rescue breathing for emergency artificial ventilation.

Rediscovery of the mouth-to-mouth technique opened up a whole new era in saving lives, for the mouth-to-mouth technique has several distinct advantages that make it extraordinarily useful under all sorts of circumstances:

- Mouth-to-mouth ventilation requires *no special equipment* except that supplied with every human being: a pair of hands, a mouth, and a set of lungs.
- Because no special equipment needs to be gathered, the technique *can be applied immediately,* under almost any circumstances. It can be applied by a bystander to a person who has collapsed on the street or by a lifeguard to a drowning victim even while still in the water! In a situation where time is so critical, mouth-to-mouth ventilation permits the rescuer to start treatment right away, without wasting time hunting for special devices or setting up complicated equipment.
- The technique is *easy to learn* and *easy to apply.*

Even children in primary school have been taught to give mouth-to-mouth ventilation effectively. Thus saving lives is no longer the exclusive province of highly trained medical professionals; basic life support is within the capability of nearly every person, and our potential for saving lives is consequently expanded enormously.

- Unlike the pressure–arm lift maneuvers, the mouth-to-mouth technique enables the rescuer to maintain the victim's *airway* open during ventilation.
- Most important, the mouth-to-mouth technique is *effective.*

MOUTH-TO-MOUTH VENTILATION

Once you have determined that a person is unconscious and you have opened the airway, you need to check whether he is breathing. As noted earlier, this is done by looking for chest movement and listening and feeling for the flow of air, while you maintain the airway open (Fig. 6-2). Take at least 5 seconds to make this check, for if the victim is breathing, for example, 12 times a minute, you may miss the respiration if you spend only 1 or 2 seconds checking. If the person is not breathing or if the breathing is inadequate (a few gasping efforts, for instance), you must start artificial ventilation. To do so, use the thumb and index finger of the hand that is maintaining head tilt on the victim's forehead to pinch the victim's nostrils shut (Fig. 6-3). This will prevent air from escaping through the victim's nose when you blow into his mouth. Then take a deep breath, open your own mouth wide, and place it around the victim's mouth, making a tight seal (Fig. 6-4). Exhale forcefully into the victim's mouth, and watch out of the corner of your eye to see whether the victim's chest rises. After delivering the breath, remove your mouth from the victim's mouth so that he can exhale passively, and turn your head slightly to watch the victim's chest fall while you take a breath of fresh air (Fig. 6-5). Then seal your lips over the victim's mouth, give another breath, take your mouth away, and so on.

When *starting* rescue breathing, you should deliver the *first two breaths* in a period of 3 to 5 seconds; that is, give the first breath, lift your mouth away from the victim just enough to permit you to take another breath, and immediately ventilate again. After the first two breaths, the rate of artificial ventilation for an adult is 12 times a minute—that is, one breath every 5 seconds. Rescue breathing should be continued until the patient starts breathing spontaneously.

Let us review the steps of mouth-to-mouth ventilation.

Fig. 6-2. *Look, listen, and feel for breathing.*

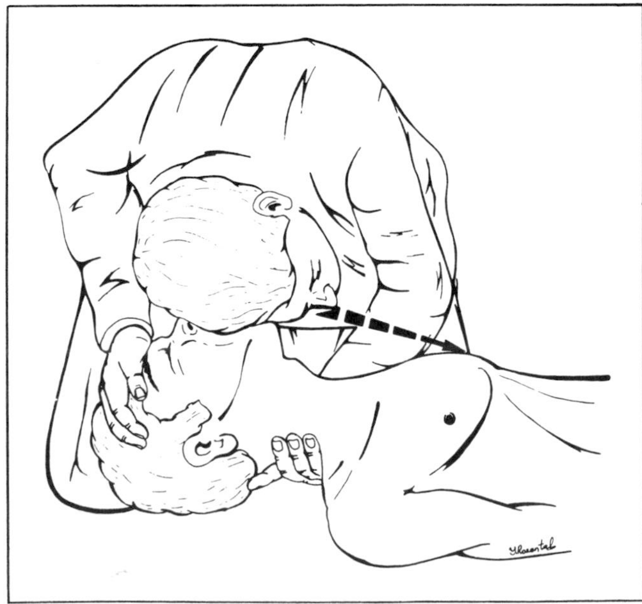

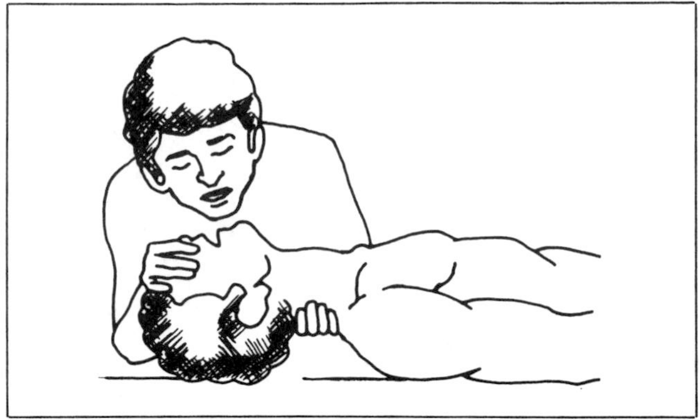

Fig. 6-3. *Position the victim's head, and pinch the victim's nostrils shut. (Reproduced courtesy American Heart Association.)*

Fig. 6-4. *Take a deep breath, open your mouth wide, seal your lips over the victim's lips, and exhale. (Reproduced courtesy American Heart Association.)*

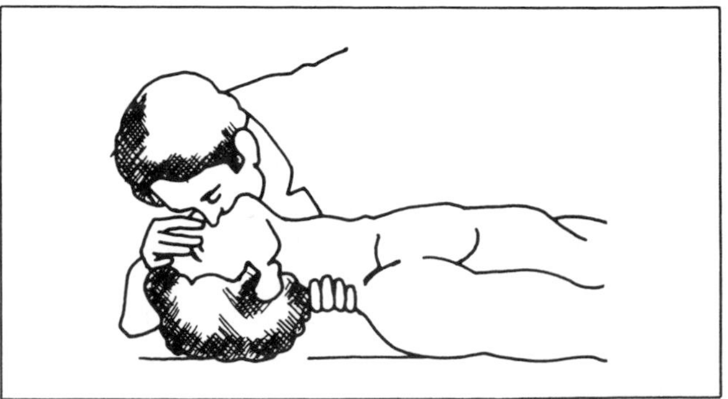

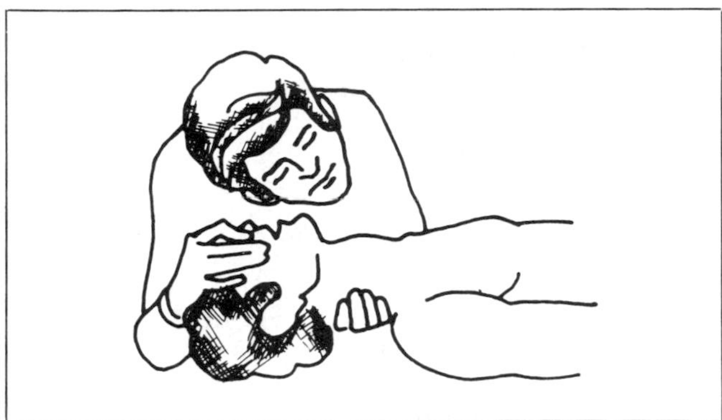

Fig. 6-5. *Remove your mouth from the victim's mouth, and watch the chest fall. (Reproduced courtesy American Heart Association.)*

Mouth-to-Mouth Ventilation

1. Open the victim's airway (head tilt–chin lift), and keep your hands in position.
2. Look, listen, and feel for breathing. If breathing is absent:
3. Pinch the nostrils shut.
4. Take a deep breath.
5. Seal your mouth over the victim's mouth.
6. Exhale forcefully until the victim's chest rises.
7. Turn your head to the side, and take a breath.
8. Repeat steps 5, 6, and 7.
9. Continue steps 5 through 7 at a rate of once every 5 seconds until the patient resumes spontaneous respiration.

Checking the Effectiveness of Artificial Ventilation

How do you know if you are giving *effective* artificial ventilation? You can tell that the patient is being adequately ventilated if (1) you see his chest and abdomen rise and fall with each breath, (2) you can feel in your own airway the resistance of the victim's lungs as they expand (just as you can feel the resistance of a balloon as you inflate it), and (3) you can hear and feel the air escaping from the victim's lungs during exhalation, when his chest falls.

Signs of Effective Artificial Ventilation

- Seeing the chest rise and fall
- Feeling in your own airway the resistance and compliance of the victim's lungs
- Hearing and feeling the escape of air during exhalation

Troubleshooting

What if mouth-to-mouth ventilation does not seem to be working properly? How can you tell what is wrong? For any given situation, you need to check your technique and make sure you are performing each step correctly. Table 6-1 lists some common problems in mouth-to-mouth ventilation and how to deal with them.

What About False Teeth?

What do you do if the victim has false teeth (dentures)? In general, if the dentures are in place, it is best to leave them right where they are. Attempts to

Table 6-1. *Troubleshooting Mouth-to-Mouth Ventilation*

Problem	Possible Cause	Action to Take
Air seems to be going into the victim's mouth, but you do not feel resistance and the chest is not moving.	Probably you are not blowing hard enough. You should be able to feel the resistance of the victim's lungs as you inflate them.	More forceful exhalation.
You feel air resistance as you inflate, and you detect the escape of air as the victim exhales, but you see only slight movement of the victim's chest.	If the victim is fully clothed, it may not be possible to see movement of the chest.	Rely on the feeling of resistance in your own airway and feeling the escape of air when the victim exhales.
You hear air leaking out as you blow into the victim's mouth.	The nose may not be pinched off fully, or your seal over the victim's lips may not be airtight.	Pinch the victim's nose shut; if possible, keep your cheek against the nostrils as you exhale. Make sure your mouth makes an airtight seal over the victim's mouth.
Air does not go in at all; it seems blocked.	The airway may not be open.	Be sure the head is tilted back far enough.
The head is properly tilted back, but air still will not go in.	There may be a foreign body obstructing the airway.	Use procedure for the unconscious choking victim (see Chapter 5).

remove them will only waste time, and the dentures give support to the victim's lips. It is much easier to give mouth-to-mouth ventilation to someone who has teeth (his own or artificial ones) than to someone who does not. If the dentures are in place, be grateful they are there and leave them alone. If dentures are rattling around loose in the victim's mouth, however, you will have to whisk them out before you start rescue breathing, for they will only get in the way and they may obstruct the airway.

MOUTH-TO-NOSE VENTILATION

There are some cases in which effective mouth-to-mouth ventilation is not technically feasible, and ventilation through the patient's nose may be required instead. This may occur, for example, if there is severe injury to the victim's mouth or jaw or if the victim's mouth is clamped shut and the rescuer cannot open it. In patients without teeth it may be difficult to maintain an airtight seal over the mouth, for the lips tend to flop inward between the gums of the victim's upper and lower jaw. Or the rescuer may simply find the mouth-to-nose technique easier to perform, especially when the victim's breath has a very strong, repellent odor.

Indications for Mouth-to-Nose Ventilation

- Victim's mouth cannot be opened.
- Severe trauma to victim's mouth or jaw.
- Victim has no teeth.
- Rescuer preference.

To perform mouth-to-nose ventilation, open the victim's airway using the head tilt–chin lift technique, and keep the head tilted back with one hand maintaining pressure on the forehead. With your other hand, lift the victim's lower jaw farther upward and backward in order to shut his mouth and seal the lips closed. Then take a deep breath, seal your lips around the victim's nose, and blow into the nose until you can feel the victim's lungs expand (Fig. 6-6). Remove your mouth from the victim's nose so that he can exhale passively, and watch to see if his chest falls while you are taking your next breath. It may be necessary to open the victim's mouth or separate his lips so that air can escape through his mouth during exhalation; the soft palate sometimes acts as a one-way valve and obstructs the escape of air through the nose. Just as in mouth-to-mouth ventilation, you need to give two full breaths in the first 5 seconds. Then proceed with one breath every 5 seconds until the victim resumes breathing by himself.

Mouth-to-Nose Ventilation

1. Open the victim's airway, and keep one hand on the forehead to maintain head tilt.
2. Look, listen, and feel for breathing. If breathing is absent:
3. Lift the victim's lower jaw to seal the lips shut.
4. Take a deep breath.
5. Seal your mouth over the victim's nose.
6. Exhale forcefully until the victim's chest rises.
7. Turn your head to the side, and take a breath.
8. Repeat steps 5, 6, and 7.
9. Continue steps 5 through 7 at a rate of once every 5 seconds. If necessary, open the victim's mouth during exhalation.

MOUTH-TO-STOMA VENTILATION

On rare occasions, the EMT may have to give artificial ventilation to a person who has had a **laryngectomy**, a surgical procedure in which the larynx is removed (*laryngo-* + *-ectomy*) and part of the trachea is brought out through a hole (called a **stoma**) on the front or side of the neck (Fig. 6-7). A person who has had this operation is called a **laryngectomee**, or "neck breather," that is, he breathes through the hole in his neck. The stoma may be simply a large round opening in the skin, or the patient may wear a breathing tube in the stoma. Since the larynx has been cut out, there is no longer any connection between the patient's pharynx and lower airway. What this means, practically speaking, is that you cannot ventilate such a patient by the mouth-to-mouth or mouth-to-nose technique, for air blown into the mouth or nose will not reach the lower airway but can only go down the esophagus into the stomach.

To make matters more complicated, there is also another kind of surgery in which only *part* of the larynx is removed. People who have had this operation are called *partial neck breathers* because they breathe through both the stoma and the nose or mouth. A special tube—a so-called speaking tube—is grafted from just within the stoma to the base of the tongue. In practice, it may be impossible to tell initially if an apneic laryngectomee is a neck breather or only a partial neck breather until you attempt artificial ventilation.

Mouth-to-stoma ventilation is actually easier to perform than mouth-to-mouth ventilation, since you do not need any special maneuvers to open the airway: You exhale directly into the patient's trachea. Furthermore, because there is no contact between

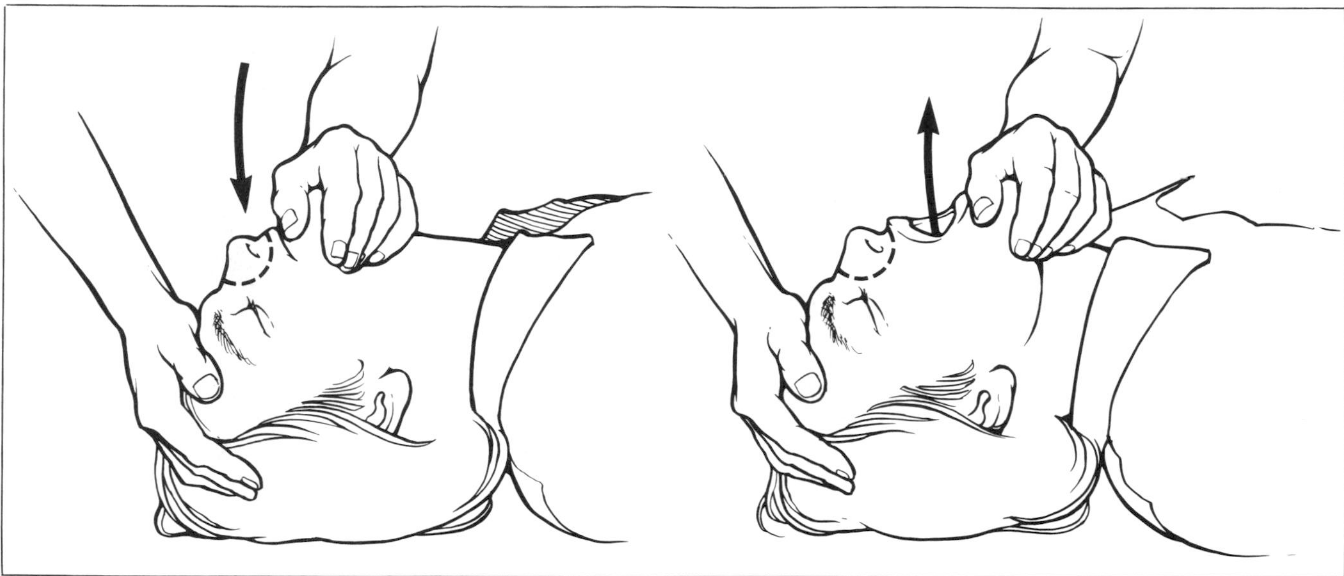

Fig. 6-6. *Mouth-to-nose ventilation, with head tilt–chin lift. Inflation* (left) *and passive exhalation* (right).

the airway and the throat, you do not have to deal with regurgitated stomach contents that sometimes make mouth-to-mouth ventilation a bit unsavory.

To perform mouth-to-stoma ventilation, first remove all coverings (e.g., scarf, tie, necklace) from the stoma area. Then clear the stoma of any foreign material that may have accumulated there. If the patient is wearing a breathing tube, make sure it is not clogged. If the tube is clear, it can be left in place; otherwise it should be removed. Take a deep breath, and make a seal with your mouth over the stoma. Blow into the stoma until you see the victim's chest rise. In general, it will not be necessary to close off the mouth and nose of a laryngectomee, since there is no direct connection between the trachea and the upper airway. However, if the chest does not rise when you ventilate, the patient may be a *partial* neck breather, and you will have to close off the nose and mouth. To do so, pinch the nose closed between your third and fourth finger while you seal the lips with the palm of your hand; then press upward and backward on the jaw with your thumb under the chin.

After you see the chest rise, remove your mouth from the stoma and allow the victim to exhale passively. Use the usual sequence of two full breaths to start mouth-to-stoma ventilation, and continue, as usual, at a rate of one inflation every 5 seconds.

Fig. 6-7. *Laryngectomee.*

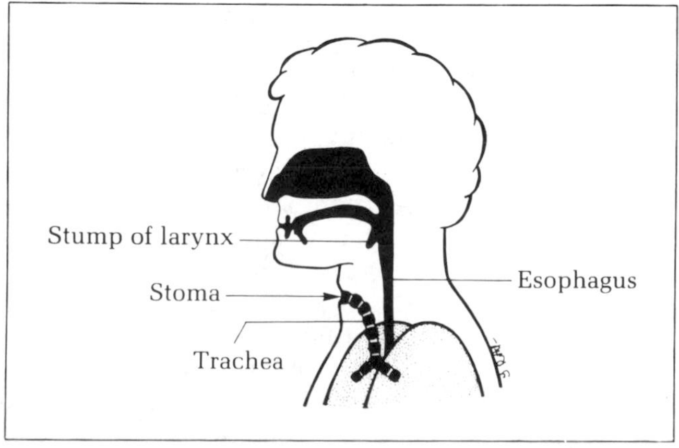

Mouth-to-Stoma Ventilation

1. Identify the patient as a neck breather (obvious stoma or medical identification tag).
2. Remove all coverings from the stoma, and clear the stoma of foreign material.
3. If there is a clogged breathing tube, remove it.
4. Look, listen, and feel for breathing. If breathing is absent:
5. Take a deep breath.
6. Seal your lips over the stoma.
7. Exhale until you see the chest rise.*
8. Turn your head to the side, and take a breath.
9. Repeat steps 6, 7, and 8.
10. Continue steps 6 through 8 at a rate of once every 5 seconds until the patient is breathing spontaneously.

*If the chest does not rise with a full ventilation, close the victim's mouth and nose and try again.

VENTILATING ACCIDENT VICTIMS

Every accident victim, as we recall, has a cervical spine injury until proved otherwise. And maneuvers involving hyperextension of the head, or indeed any forward, backward, or turning movements of the head or neck, must be avoided in patients with suspected cervical spine injury. This does *not* mean, however, that there is no way to give artificial ventilation to an accident victim in respiratory arrest. It simply requires a modified technique and particular care to avoid unnecessary motion.

To ventilate a nonbreathing victim with suspected spine injury, first open the airway using the *jaw thrust* technique. Recall that this is done by placing your hands on either side of the victim's head so that the neck is maintained in a fixed, neutral position *without* extension. Then use your index fingers to move the jaw forward by pushing upward on the angles of the mandible. Take a deep breath, and seal your mouth over the victim's mouth. Since both your hands are tied up holding the head steady and pushing the jaw forward, you will have to use your cheek to seal the victim's nose. Exhale forcefully until you see the victim's chest rise, and continue as you would for mouth-to-mouth ventilation of any other patient. Mouth-to-nose ventilation is also possible for an accident victim and may be somewhat easier, although if you do the mouth-to-nose technique, you will have to use your cheek to seal the patient's *mouth*.

Ventilation of Accident Victims

1. Open the airway by jaw thrust technique, *with the head in neutral position.*
2. Look, listen, and feel for breathing. If breathing is absent:
3. Take a deep breath.
4. Seal your mouth over the victim's mouth; use your cheek to seal the nose.
5. Exhale forcefully until you see the chest rise.
6. Turn your head to the side, and take a breath.
7. Repeat steps 4, 5, and 6.
8. Continue with steps 4 through 6 at a rate of once every 5 seconds until the victim is breathing spontaneously.

VENTILATING INFANTS AND SMALL CHILDREN

The techniques for establishing an airway, recognizing respiratory arrest, and giving artificial ventilation are essentially the same for infants and small children as for adults. Certain modifications in technique are necessary, however, mainly because of the differences in size and normal respiratory rate between infants and adults.

Establishing Unresponsiveness or Respiratory Distress

To examine and treat an infant, it is best to place the infant on a hard surface, like a table top. If you choose to hold the baby, be sure to support the head and neck.

An unconscious infant or child, like an unconscious adult, will not awaken or react when shaken. To determine if an infant or small child is unconscious, tap him or shake him gently. If he begins to move or cry, he is conscious. If he does not respond, he is unconscious.

A conscious infant may also be in serious respiratory trouble and may need to have the airway opened and even need rescue breathing to assist respirations. If the child is gasping or struggling to breathe, he will need treatment even if he is conscious, and the first step of treatment is opening the airway.

Opening the Infant's Airway

Once you have determined that the infant is unconscious or in respiratory distress (gasping, struggling to breathe), open the infant's airway using the techniques described in Chapter 5 (head tilt–chin lift) (Fig. 6-8). Remember to AVOID EXTREME HYPEREXTENSION OF THE BABY'S NECK, as this may itself obstruct the airway.

Recognition of Respiratory Arrest

While maintaining the infant's airway open, the rescuer needs to check whether the infant is breathing. This is done exactly as it is in an adult: look, listen, and feel. Place your ear over the baby's mouth and nose, and (1) *look* to see if the baby's chest and abdomen are rising and falling, (2) *listen* for the sound of air flow, and (3) *feel* for the exhalation of air against your face from the baby's mouth and nose. In many instances, simply opening the airway will be enough to enable the nonbreathing infant to start breathing again. If breathing is absent, however, artificial ventilation will be required.

Artificial ventilation will also be required to *assist* the infant who is not breathing adequately. If the baby is gasping, you should examine the color of the baby's lips. If they are pink, enough oxygen is probably reaching the blood, and you need only maintain an open airway. If the lips are blue (cyanotic), this is a sign of oxygen deficiency, and you should commence rescue breathing.

Artificial Ventilation of Infants

Once you have opened the infant's airway and determined that the infant is not breathing (or not breathing adequately), place your mouth over the baby's

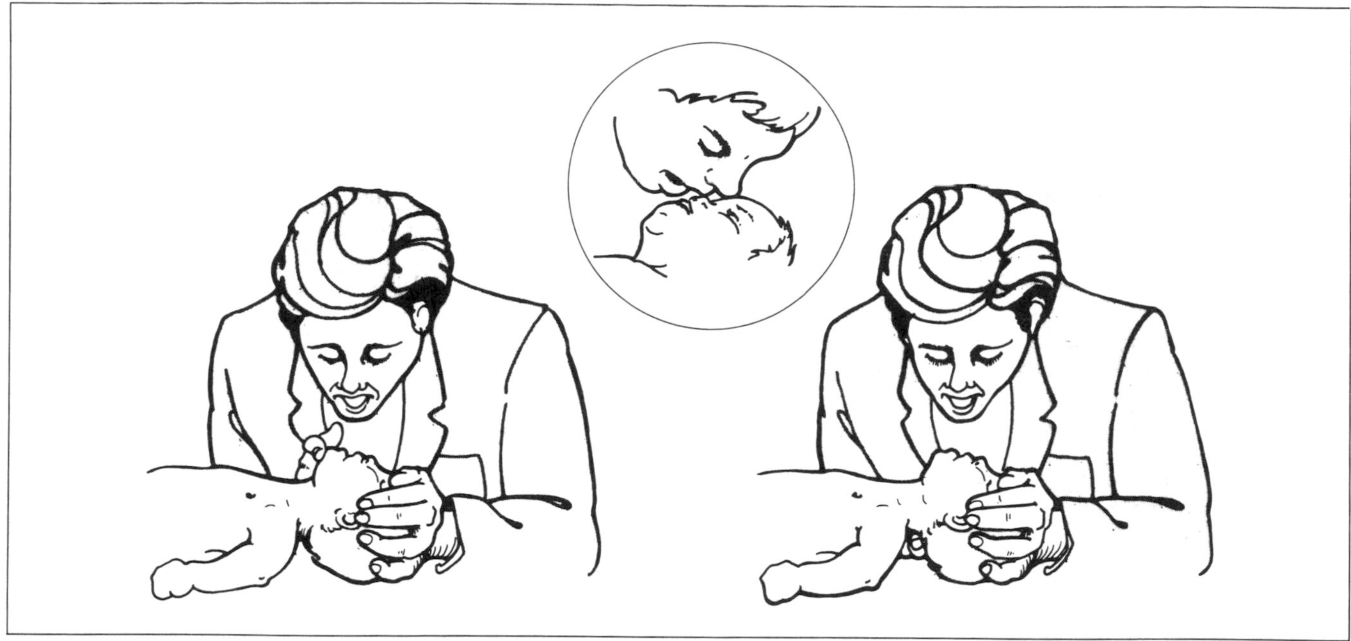

Fig. 6-8. *Artificial ventilation of the infant. (Reproduced courtesy American Heart Association.)*

nose *and* mouth (Fig. 6-8), and make a seal with your lips. Give four quick breaths, just as in the adult, but remember:

BABIES ARE VERY LITTLE!

Babies have much smaller chests than do adults, and they do not need nearly as much air to inflate their lungs. For a small infant, just puffs from your cheeks will usually be sufficient. You can gauge the amount of air needed by watching the baby's chest as you give a breath; give just enough to cause the chest to rise. Then take your mouth away, and watch to see if the chest falls (while you take another breath). If you find you cannot ventilate the infant, the airway may not be fully open, so reposition the head, and try again. If you still cannot ventilate, you should suspect obstruction by a foreign body and follow the procedures learned in Chapter 5 for the choking infant (e.g., back blows, chest thrusts). If ventilation is successful, give two full puffs initially, and continue rescue breathing at a rate of 20 times per minute—that is, *one breath every 3 seconds*—until the baby is breathing spontaneously.

The technique of artificial ventilation for a *child* will depend to some extent on the size of the child. For the child who is sufficiently large that you cannot make a tight seal with your mouth over the child's mouth and nose, use the standard mouth-to-mouth technique as you would for an adult. For any size child, gauge the volume of your ventilations according to the amount of air it takes to make the chest rise.

Ventilation of Infants

1. Open the airway (head tilt–chin lift, but avoid extreme hyperextension of the head).
2. Look, listen, and feel for breathing. If breathing is absent:
3. Make a seal with your mouth over the infant's mouth *and* nose.
4. Give two puffs from your cheeks over 5 seconds, checking to see that the chest rises with each puff.
5. Continue to ventilate once every 3 seconds until the infant resumes spontaneous breathing.

GASTRIC DISTENTION

One problem that can occur with any form of positive pressure ventilation (such as mouth-to-mouth ventilation or ventilation with a bag-mask device) is distention (stretching) of the stomach. This is particularly apt to occur in children. Recall that below the pharynx there are two tubes: the trachea in front and the esophagus in back. Thus when one forces air into the patient's mouth and throat, there are two possible routes the air can take: through the trachea to the lungs or through the esophagus to the stomach. If the head is properly extended to open the airway, most of the air forced into the mouth will take the tracheal route. But some air may still slip into the esophagus and whistle down into the

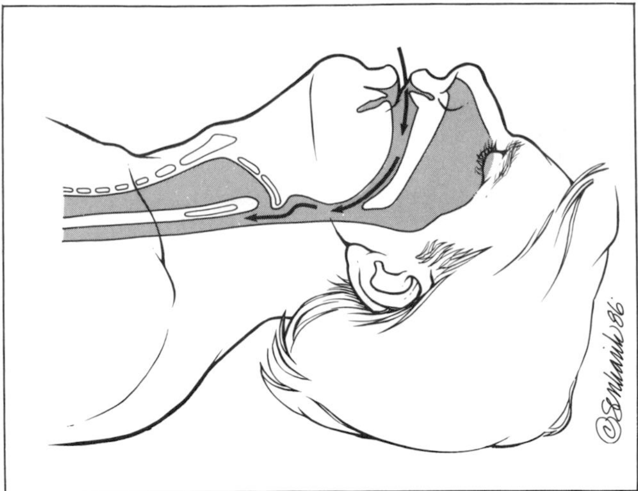

Fig. 6-9. *Partially obstructed airway.*

stomach, causing the stomach to be progressively distended. This is particularly likely to happen when excessive pressure is used for inflation or when the airway is partially obstructed (Fig. 6-9). Gastric distention can therefore be minimized by making sure the airway is fully open (by head tilt–chin lift or similar maneuver) and giving only that volume of air that causes the chest to rise—and no more.

Why bother about gastric distention at all? What difference does it make if the stomach gets filled with air? There are two reasons why gastric distention can be dangerous. First of all, in order to enter the stomach, air must displace whatever is already there. As air enters the stomach, breakfast (or lunch, or whatever) is liable to exit and start creeping up the esophagus toward the mouth. This is called **regurgitation**, the *passive* flow of stomach contents into the throat and mouth. When the patient begins regurgitating and his mouth fills up with semidigested food and gastric juices, life becomes very unpleasant for the rescuer who is trying to do mouth-to-mouth ventilation. But more importantly, regurgitation can lead very quickly to **aspiration**, that is, inhalation of foreign materials into the patient's lungs.

Suppose, for example, you give several forceful ventilations to a victim whose airway is only partially open, and a significant amount of air enters the stomach. And suppose that as air enters, the pieces of the giant cheeseburger that the victim had for lunch begin inching up the esophagus into the throat. Then you open the airway properly and give your next ventilation, and—whoosh!—the giant cheeseburger goes sailing down the trachea. If the pieces are large enough, there will be complete airway obstruction; if they are small enough to enter the lung—and especially if there is a significant amount of liquid material involved—the patient may develop a severe aspiration pneumonia and even die from that pneumonia a few days after he has been saved from his respiratory arrest. Thus the first reason why we want to avoid gastric distention is to prevent subsequent regurgitation and aspiration.

In addition, gastric distention can limit the effectiveness of artificial ventilation. Recall that the stomach sits just under the diaphragm in the abdominal cavity. As the stomach gets bigger and bigger, the diaphragm is pushed upward into the thoracic cavity, so the thoracic cavity gets smaller and smaller. When that happens, the lungs have less and less room in which to expand, so one cannot deliver as effective a volume of air with each ventilation. For both these reasons, then—to avoid regurgitation and to prevent elevation of the diaphragm—every effort should be made to minimize gastric distention during rescue breathing.

Minimizing Gastric Distention

- Make sure the AIRWAY IS FULLY OPEN when you ventilate (proper head position).
- Avoid excessive inflation volumes.

Sometimes the stomach becomes distended during rescue breathing despite proper technique, and the distention is visible as a marked bulging of the victim's abdomen. If you note such bulging, recheck the airway, and make sure you are not giving larger volumes of ventilation than needed to make the chest rise. In general, do *not* attempt to expel the air from the stomach by putting pressure over the victim's abdomen, for experience has shown that this maneuver frequently leads to regurgitation, and the victim may aspirate if suctioning equipment is not available. Only if gastric distention is so severe that it prevents adequate ventilation should you attempt to expel the air—keeping in mind that this is a risky procedure. Roll the victim onto his side, facing away from you, so that his back rests against your knee, and rotate his head slightly so that it is turned toward the floor. Support his head with one hand while you use the flat of your other hand to press firmly over the epigastrium (the part of the abdomen just below the ribs, remember?). Be prepared for regurgitation. If it occurs, keep the victim on his side and use your fingers to sweep the gastric contents out of the victim's mouth and throat. Then roll the victim back supine and continue rescue breathing.

Should regurgitation occur while you are performing artificial ventilation, follow the same procedure as above: Immediately turn the victim onto his side, wipe out his mouth, roll him back to a supine position, and resume artificial ventilation (you may decide to switch to the mouth-to-nose technique).

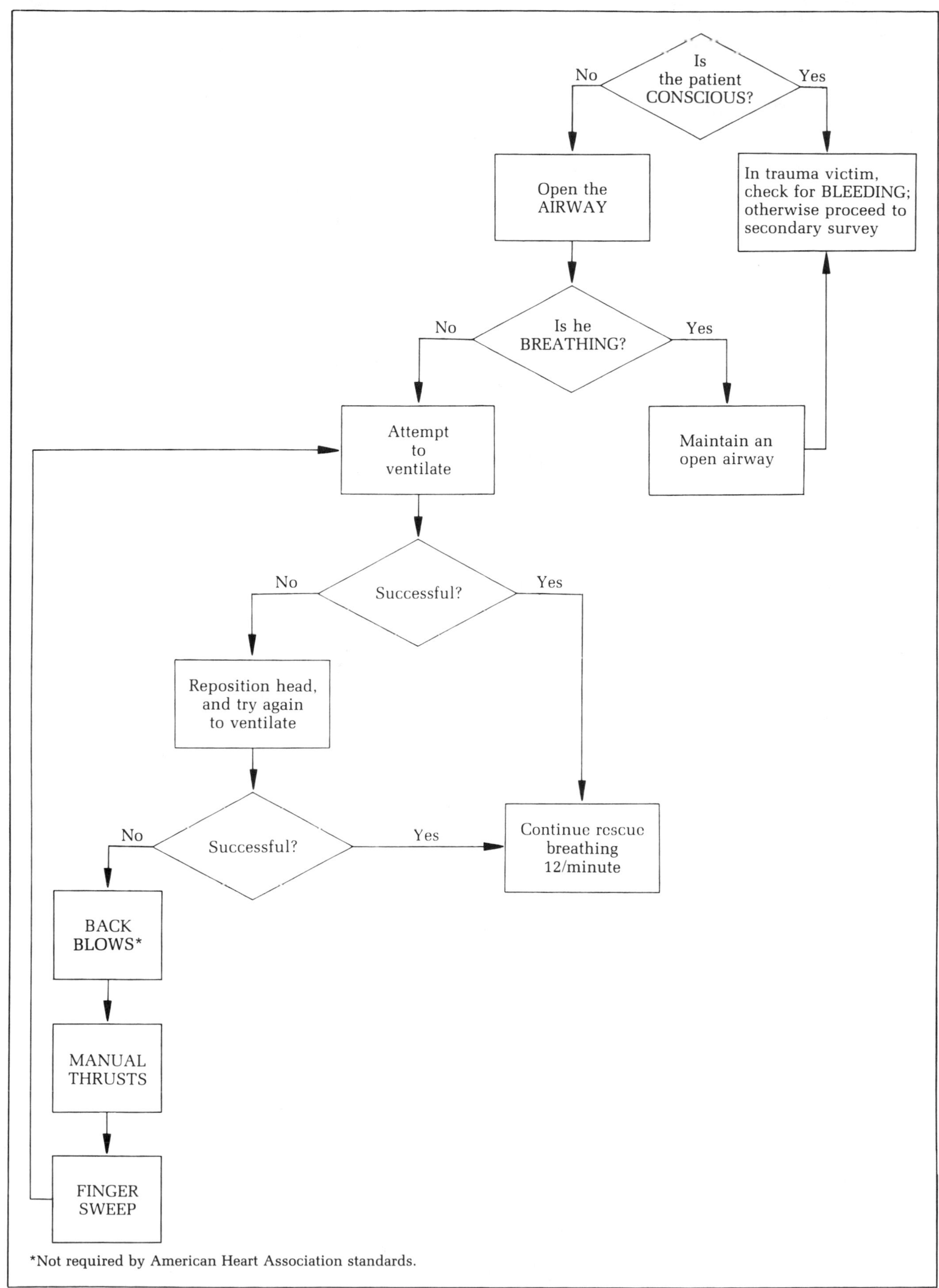

Fig. 6-10. *Management of respiratory arrest.*

PUTTING THE PIECES TOGETHER

In the last two chapters, we have examined the *A* and the *B* of the rescue alphabet: *A*irway and *B*reathing. The steps we have learned are summarized in Figure 6-10. In the next chapter we will move on to *C*—Circulation—and examine the recognition and management of cardiac arrest.

VOCABULARY

apnea Absence of breathing.

artificial ventilation Any means of providing air exchange to a patient who is not breathing or not breathing adequately.

aspiration The inhalation of foreign material into the lungs.

dentures False teeth.

Holger Nielsen method Technique of artificial ventilation involving back pressure–arm lift maneuvers on a prone victim.

laryngectomee Person whose larynx has been removed surgically.

laryngectomy Surgical removal of the larynx.

mouth-to-mouth technique Technique of artificial ventilation wherein air is forced into the victim's mouth from the rescuer's mouth.

mouth-to-nose technique Technique of artificial ventilation wherein air is forced into the victim's nose from the rescuer's mouth.

mouth-to-stoma technique Technique of artificial ventilation wherein air is forced into the stoma of a laryngectomee from the mouth of a rescuer.

neck breather Person who has had a complete laryngectomy.

regurgitation Passive flow of gastric contents from the stomach into the esophagus, throat, and mouth.

rescue breathing Any form of artificial ventilation that utilizes the rescuer's exhaled air to inflate the victim's lungs.

resuscitation The act of reviving an unconscious person or of restoring an apparently dead person to life.

Silvester's method Technique of artificial ventilation involving chest pressure–arm lift maneuvers on a supine patient.

stoma Hole or opening.

FURTHER READING

American Heart Association. Standards and guidelines for cardiopulmonary resuscitation (CPR) and emergency cardiac care (ECC). *JAMA* 255:2905, 1986.

Safar P, Bircher N. *Cardiopulmonary Cerebral Resuscitation.* Philadelphia: Saunders, 1988. Chap. 1B.

Safar P, Escarrago L, Elam J. A comparison of mouth-to-mouth airway methods of artificial respiration with the chest pressure–arm lift methods. *N Engl J Med* 258:671, 1958.

SKILL EVALUATION CHECKLISTS

The following pages contain skill checklists covering the techniques of basic life support we have studied so far. These checklists are intended as a guide for the student in practicing the skills described in this chapter. These skill checklists are reprinted with the kind permission of the American Heart Association. Additional checklists covering the treatment of choking in infants and children appear at the end of Chapter 34.

American Heart Association CPR and ECC Performance Sheet
Obstructed Airway: Conscious Adult

Name ______________________________ Date ______________

Step	Activity	Critical Performance	S	U
1. Assessment	Determine airway obstruction.	Ask "Are you choking?"		
		Determine if victim can cough or speak.		
2. Heimlich Maneuver	Perform abdominal thrusts.	Stand behind the victim.		
		Wrap arms around victim's waist.		
		Make a fist with one hand and place the thumb side against victim's abdomen in the midline slightly above the navel and well below the tip of the xiphoid.		
		Grasp fist with the other hand.		
		Press into the victim's abdomen with quick upward thrusts.		
		Each thrust should be distinct and delivered with the intent of relieving the airway obstruction.		
		Repeat thrusts until either the foreign body is expelled or the victim becomes unconscious (see below).		
Victim with Obstructed Airway Becomes Unconscious (Optional Testing Sequence)				
3. Additional Assessment	Position the victim.	Turn on back as unit.		
		Place face up, arms by side.		
	Call for help.	Call out "Help!" or, if others respond, activate EMS system.		
4. Foreign Body Check	Perform finger sweep.*	Keep victim's face up.		
		Use tongue-jaw lift to open mouth.		
		Sweep deeply into mouth to remove foreign body.		
5. Breathing Attempt	Attempt ventilation (airway is obstructed).	Open airway with head-tilt/chin-lift.		
		Seal mouth and nose properly.		
		Attempt to ventilate.		
6. Heimlich Maneuver	Perform abdominal thrusts.	Straddle victim's thighs.		
		Place heel of one hand against victim's abdomen, in the midline slightly above the navel and well below the tip of the xiphoid.		
		Place second hand directly on top of first hand.		
		Press into the abdomen with quick upward thrusts.		
		Perform 6–10 abdominal thrusts.		
7. Foreign Body Check	Perform finger sweep.*	Keep victim's face up.		
		Use tongue-jaw lift to open mouth.		
		Sweep deeply into mouth to remove foreign body.		
8. Breathing Attempt	Attempt ventilation.	Open airway with head-tilt/chin-lift.		
		Seal mouth and nose properly.		
		Attempt to ventilate.		
9. Sequencing	Repeat sequence.	Repeat Steps 6–8 until successful.†		

* During practice and testing, simulate finger sweeps.
† After airway obstruction is removed, check for pulse and breathing. (a) If pulse is absent, ventilate a second time and start cycles of compressions and ventilations. (b) If pulse is present, open airway and check for spontaneous breathing. (c) If breathing is present, monitor breathing and pulse closely, maintain open airway. (d) If breathing is absent, perform rescue breathing at 12 times/min and monitor pulse.

Instructor ______________________________ Check: Satisfactory __________ Unsatisfactory __________
4/86

American Heart Association CPR and ECC Performance Sheet
Obstructed Airway: Unconscious Adult

Name ______________________________ Date ______________

Step	Activity	Critical Performance	S	U
1. Assessment/ Airway	Determine unresponsiveness.	Tap or gently shake shoulder. Shout "Are you OK?"		
	Call for help.	Call out "Help!"		
	Position the victim.	Turn on back as unit, if necessary, supporting head and neck (4–10 sec).		
	Open the airway.	Use head-tilt/chin-lift maneuver.		
	Determine breathlessness.	Maintain open airway.		
		Ear over mouth, observe chest: look, listen, feel for breathing (3–5 sec).		
2. Breathing Attempt	Attempt ventilation (airway is obstructed).	Maintain open airway.		
		Seal mouth and nose properly.		
		Attempt to ventilate.		
	Reattempt ventilation (airway remains blocked).	Reposition victim's head.		
		Seal mouth and nose properly.		
		Reattempt to ventilate.		
	Activate EMS system.	If someone responded to call for help, send him/her to activate EMS system.		
		Total time, Steps 1 and 2: 15–35 sec.		
3. Heimlich Maneuver	Perform abdominal thrusts.	Straddle victim's thighs.		
		Place heel of one hand against victim's abdomen in the midline slightly above the navel and well below the tip of the xiphoid.		
		Place second hand directly on top of first hand.		
		Press into the abdomen with quick upward thrusts.		
		Each thrust should be distinct and delivered with the intent of relieving the airway obstruction.		
		Perform 6–10 abdominal thrusts.		
4. Foreign Body Check	Perform finger sweep.*	Keep victim's face up.		
		Use tongue-jaw lift to open mouth.		
		Sweep deeply into mouth to remove foreign body.		
5. Breathing Attempt	Attempt ventilation.	Open airway with head-tilt/chin-lift maneuver.		
		Seal mouth and nose properly.		
		Attempt to ventilate.		
6. Sequencing	Repeat sequence.	Repeat Steps 3–5 until successful.†		

* During practice and testing, simulate finger sweeps.
† After airway obstruction is removed, check for pulse and breathing. (a) If pulse is absent, ventilate a second time and start cycles of compressions and ventilations. (b) If pulse is present, open airway and check for spontaneous breathing. (c) If breathing is present, monitor breathing and pulse closely, maintain open airway. (d) If breathing is absent, perform rescue breathing at 12 times/min and monitor pulse.

Instructor ______________________________ Check: Satisfactory __________ Unsatisfactory __________
4/86

7. CARDIAC ARREST

OBJECTIVES

In Chapters 5 and 6 we looked at the threats to life posed by obstruction of the airway and respiratory arrest—the *A* and the *B* of the rescue alphabet. In this chapter we move on to *C*, the circulation, and examine how the circulatory system functions, what happens when it fails, and what the EMT can do about it. By the end of this chapter, the reader should be able to

1. Describe the location of the heart with respect to bones of the thoracic cavity and to other vital organs in the chest and abdomen
2. List the structures through which the blood passes in one circuit through the body
3. Identify the types of cardiac arrest, given a description of the state of the heart in different cardiac arrest situations
4. List the signs of cardiac arrest and indicate which of these signs is the most critical in deciding whether to initiate cardiopulmonary resuscitation
5. Identify the artery that is used to determine pulselessness in the adult and in the infant, and explain why that artery is preferred over others for this purpose in each case
6. Explain what properly performed chest compressions accomplish for the patient in cardiac arrest
7. List the steps of cardiopulmonary resuscitation in the correct sequence for (a) an adult and (b) an infant or small child
8. Identify the correct hand position for external cardiac compressions, and explain the possible consequences of various incorrect hand positions
9. Identify the correct rate of compressions and the correct ratio of compressions to ventilations for (a) one-rescuer CPR, (b) two-rescuer CPR, and (c) CPR of an infant
10. Explain how one can determine whether CPR is being performed effectively
11. List the possible causes of CPR being ineffective
12. List at least three potential complications of CPR and indicate how each can be prevented
13. List the criteria for beginning CPR and for terminating CPR
14. Explain how CPR is carried out in transit (e.g., when the patient is being moved from the scene to the ambulance)
15. Explain the special considerations involved in giving CPR to (a) a victim of near drowning and (b) a victim of electric shock

ANATOMY AND FUNCTION OF THE CIRCULATORY SYSTEM

The circulatory system consists of a pump (the heart) and a network of tubes (blood vessels) through which blood is pumped, and thus it is also known as the *cardiovascular* system (*cardio-* = heart + *vascular* = blood vessels). The function of this system is a very simple one: to deliver a constant supply of oxygen and nourishment through the blood to all the tissues of the body. This simple function is a full-time job, however, for the body does not maintain any emergency depots of oxygen that can be summoned if the supply runs short. All of the oxygen reaching the tissues must be hauled continuously by diligent little **red blood cells** maintaining an endless bucket brigade from the lungs, and the only way for the red blood cells to get from the capillaries in the lungs to the capillaries in the tissues is for the heart to pump them along. The moment the heart stops pumping, the whole bucket brigade lurches to a halt, and the tissues rapidly consume whatever oxygen is left in the blood. Within 2 to 3 minutes, the oxygen supply is depleted, and cells all over the body begin to suffocate. If the red blood cells do not start moving again to fetch more oxygen from the lungs, the organism will die.

What keeps the whole show going is the heart, a muscular organ about the size of a man's fist that sits in the thoracic cavity behind the sternum (Fig. 7-1). Its neighbors to the right and left in the chest are the lungs, while just beneath it lie the spleen (to the left) and the liver (to the right and center). The heart actually consists of *two* pumps (Fig. 7-2), which happen to be right next to one another and are separated only by a thin wall, or **septum.** Each pump has two chambers: an upper chamber (**atrium**) and a lower chamber (**ventricle**).

The *right* side of the heart (right pump) is in charge of pumping oxygen-poor blood through the lungs, where the blood can pick up a fresh supply of oxygen. The right heart receives this oxygen-poor blood from the rest of the body through blood vessels called **veins.** Blood travels through larger and larger veins until it all joins up in the two biggest veins of the body—the **inferior vena cava** and **superior vena cava,** which empty into the upper chamber of the right heart (the **right atrium**). From the right atrium, blood is squirted into the lower chamber of the right heart (**right ventricle**) and then out through the **pulmonary arteries** into the lungs. There the blood distributes through the tiny capillaries that surround the alveoli, and the red cells trade in the carbon dioxide they have picked up in the tissues for a fresh batch of oxygen.

From the lungs, blood travels through the **pulmonary veins** into the *left* side of the heart, emptying first into the **left atrium,** then into the **left ventricle.** The job of the left side of the heart is to pump oxygen-rich blood out to the tissues of the body, so that they can continue to receive the constant supply of oxygen vital to their existence. The blood vessels that carry blood *away* from the heart are called **arteries,** and the biggest artery of all is the **aorta,** which carries blood from the left ventricle to the smaller arteries; from there blood flows into the tiny **capillaries** in the tissues.

Fig. 7-1. *Position of the heart in the chest.*

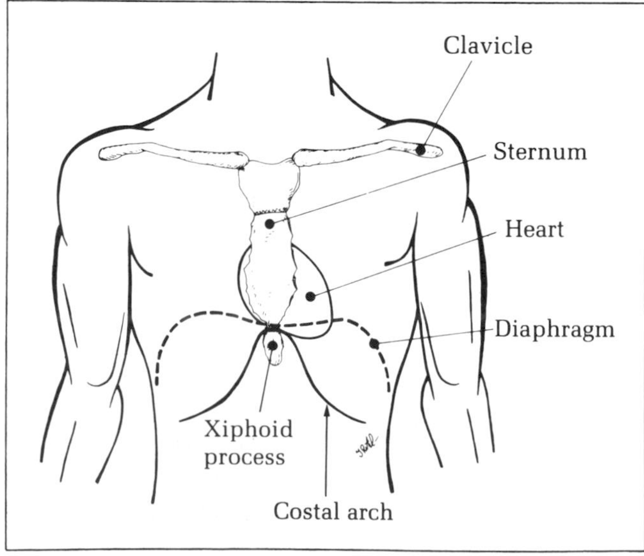

Components of the Cardiovascular System

right heart (right atrium and right ventricle)	receives oxygen-poor blood from the rest of the body and pumps it into the lungs
left heart (left atrium and left ventricle)	receives oxygen-rich blood from the lungs and pumps it into the rest of the body
veins	blood vessels that carry blood *to* the heart; all veins except the pulmonary veins carry blood poor in oxygen
arteries	blood vessels that carry blood *away* from the heart; all arteries except the pulmonary arteries carry blood rich in oxygen
capillaries	tiny vessels that carry blood to the tissues of the lung and other organs so that oxygen exchange can take place

In fact, the two pumps that make up the heart work in parallel. The heart contracts as a unit so that both atria contract at once and then both ventricles con-

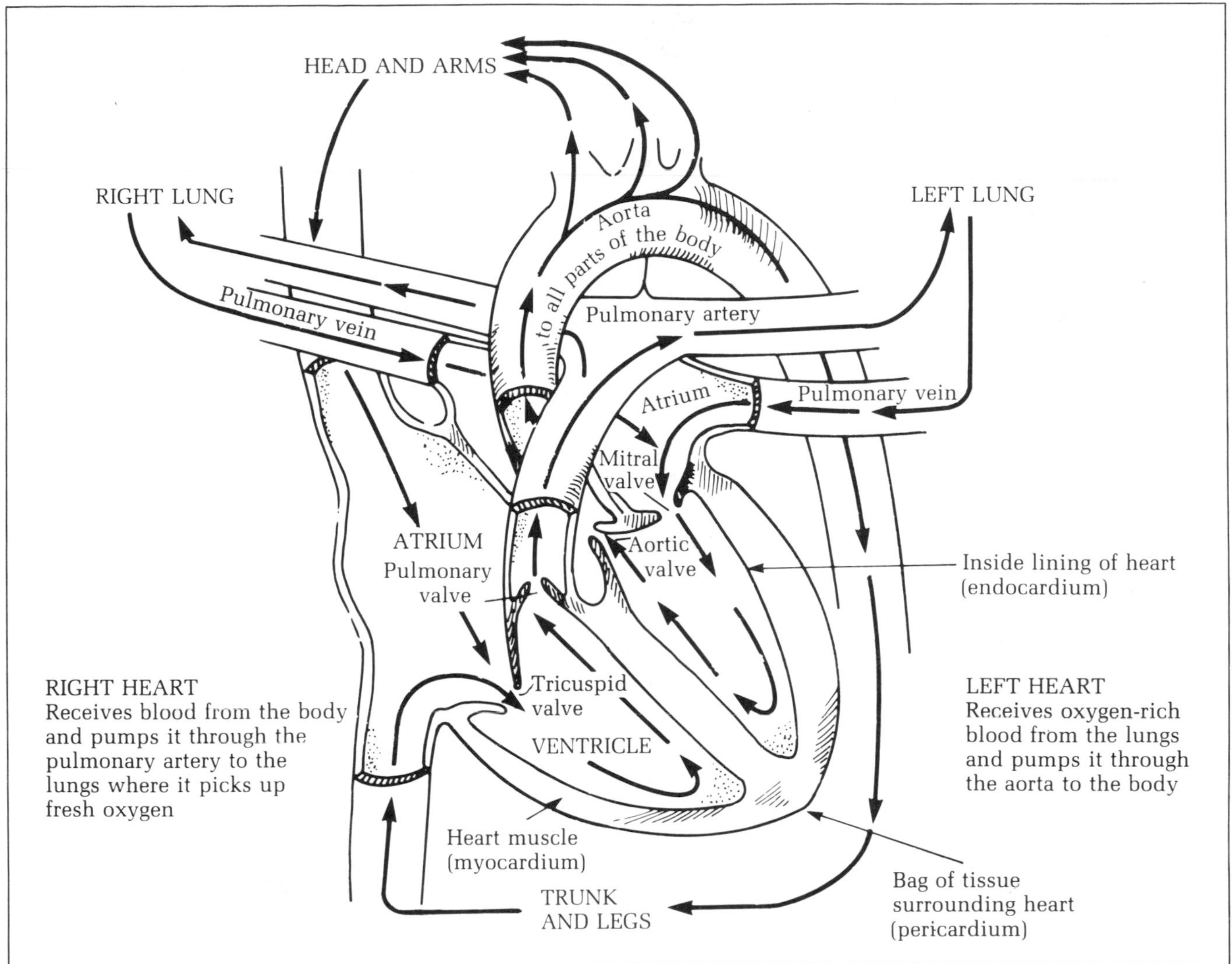

Fig. 7-2. *Function of the heart. (Adapted with permission from American Heart Association.)*

tract at once. What this means is that at the same moment that the right ventricle is squirting its blood into the lungs, the left ventricle is squeezing its blood into the arteries of the rest of the body. A system of one-way valves within the heart keeps blood moving in the right direction and prevents backflow.

In order to get a clearer picture of the cardiovascular system, let us follow Rudolph the Red Cell as he makes a circuit through it. We will join him just as he is leaving the right ear, where he has made an oxygen delivery to the ear lobe.

Rudolph glides out of the ear lobe and makes his way into the jugular vein of the neck, where he meets many of his friends coming from the face and brain. Together they swish into the superior vena cava, the major vein that drains the upper part of the body. The current carries them into the right atrium, and they gurgle past the tricuspid valve into the right ventricle. As the heart makes its next contraction, Rudolph and his friends are catapulted through the pulmonary valve into the pulmonary artery and plummet into the lungs. They begin to split up into smaller and smaller blood vessels, and Rudolph glides into a capillary in the left upper lobe of the lung. Sidling up alongside an alveolus, he dumps the carbon dioxide he picked up in the ear lobe and fills up on oxygen, which makes him turn bright red. Then he is off again, sloshing back into the pulmonary vein to make the trip to the left heart. In no time, he finds himself back with all his bright red friends, being swept into the left atrium, and together they plunge through the mitral valve into the left ventricle. The ventricle gives a mighty squeeze and sends Rudolph and his colleagues gushing through the aorta. Rudolph makes his way quickly to the axillary artery, then takes the turnoff to the biceps. "I thought you'd never make it," the biceps tells him, while greedily taking the oxygen that Rudolph is carrying.

"As long as the heart keeps beating," Rudolph reassures the biceps, "one of us will get through. Don't you worry about that."

Pathway of the Blood

1. Systemic veins	OXYGEN-POOR BLOOD
2. Venae cavae	
3. Right atrium	
4. Right ventricle	
5. Pulmonary artery	
6. Pulmonary capillaries	
7. Pulmonary vein	OXYGEN-RICH BLOOD
8. Left atrium	
9. Left ventricle	
10. Aorta	
11. Systemic arteries	
12. Systemic capillaries	
13. Systemic veins	

CARDIAC ARREST

As Rudolph the Red Cell correctly observed, everything is fine as long as the heart keeps beating. But if the heart stops beating or stops beating effectively, the whole show comes to a halt, and this is the situation called cardiac arrest.

TYPES OF CARDIAC ARREST

Cardiac arrest can be defined as the sudden cessation of effective cardiac functioning, and it can occur in one of several ways. To begin with, the heart can simply stop beating altogether and become perfectly still—a condition called, appropriately enough, **cardiac standstill,** or **asystole.** In other cases, the heart does not stand still, but its component muscle fibers somehow get out of phase with each other and all start contracting separately in a completely uncoordinated fashion. The net effect is that instead of contracting as a unit, the heart just quivers ineffectually. This condition is called **ventricular fibrillation,** and like asystole, it results in the cessation of cardiac output. Finally, cardiac arrest can occur when the heart is still beating, but its contractions are so feeble that it is ineffective in pumping blood through the circulation. This is the condition known as **cardiovascular collapse,** and it occurs with severe bleeding, with severe damage to the heart, or as the result of certain drugs that depress the heart's activity.

Types of Cardiac Arrest

cardiac standstill (asystole)	The heart stops beating altogether.
ventricular fibrillation	The heart quivers as its component muscle fibers contract chaotically.
cardiovascular collapse	The heart continues beating, but its contractions are too weak to maintain the circulation.

In practice, it is impossible to distinguish one type of cardiac arrest from another without an electrocardiograph (ECG machine), a special device that records the electric activity of heart muscle. All three varieties of cardiac arrest have the same clinical signs, all of them are equivalent to clinical death, and all are initially treated in exactly the same fashion.

RECOGNITION OF CARDIAC ARREST

If we observe a person who has collapsed from primary cardiac arrest, we will see that the victim loses consciousness almost immediately (why?); if we check for a pulse, we will not find one. The victim's breathing slows down until there are just a few gasps, sometimes terminating in a crackling sound referred to as a "death rattle," and within about 30 seconds after cardiac arrest, breathing stops altogether. Meanwhile, by about 30 to 60 seconds after cardiac arrest, the victim's pupils begin to dilate (get wider), and they become completely dilated in another minute or two. That sign is variable, however, because there are other factors that can affect the dilation of a person's pupils, such as medications taken. In any case, within about 2 to 3 minutes after cardiac arrest, the victim *looks* dead. Even an observer who has never before seen a dead human being can almost instinctively identify someone in this condition, for the person who is clinically dead lies motionless; his skin may be dusky or bluish; his eyes are lusterless and staring.

Several of these signs of clinical death can, by themselves, be misleading. A person who has fainted, for instance, may lie very still and look very pale but nonetheless will have a good heartbeat. Someone who has taken an overdose of barbiturates may be unconscious with widely dilated pupils and yet not be in cardiac arrest. Anyway, we do not want to spend a lot of time checking out the patient's pupils, skin, or mucous membranes, because time is critical. Thus if we want to be sure we are dealing with cardiac arrest and if we want to make this determination as quickly as possible, we need to look for those signs of cardiac arrest that are consistently reliable and quickly identified. There are two such diagnostic signs of cardiac arrest: (1) UNRESPONSIVENESS and (2) ABSENCE OF A PULSE. Those and only those are the signs we rely on to make a diagnosis of cardiac arrest. An unconscious person in whom a pulse cannot be detected is, by definition, in cardiac arrest and requires immediate treatment.

Diagnostic Signs of Cardiac Arrest
- Victim is UNRESPONSIVE.
- Victim has NO PULSE.

In practice, we use the *carotid* artery in the neck to check whether a pulse is present. Theoretically, any artery would give us the same information, but the carotid has several distinct advantages. First of all, it is *close to the heart* and thus its pulsations are strong and easily felt when the heart is beating. Pulsations in a more peripheral artery, such as the radial, may be more difficult to detect, especially when one is in a hurry. It could be argued that the femoral pulse is also a very strong pulse, but the problem with the femoral is that in most instances one would have to undress the victim to get at it, and this wastes time. Thus the second advantage of the carotid is that it is *easily accessible*. Indeed it is very conveniently located, for the rescuer has to be positioned right near the victim's neck anyway in order to open the airway, so the carotid pulse is already there at the rescuer's fingertips. The third advantage, then, of using the carotid artery to determine pulselessness is that the rescuer need not change position or stop maintaining the airway in order to check for a pulse at the carotid. He or she simply keeps one hand on the victim's forehead to keep the head tilted back and uses the hand that has been maintaining chin lift to feel for the carotid pulse in the groove beside the Adam's apple.

We have now witnessed our hypothetical victim collapse, lose consciousness, and issue a few last, rattling gasps. What are we going to do about it? The answer lies in putting together the *A* (airway) and the *B* (breathing) of the rescue alphabet that we have already learned with a third component, *C* (circulation), to spell out *cardiopulmonary resuscitation*.

CARDIOPULMONARY RESUSCITATION

Cardiopulmonary resuscitation, or CPR for short, is the name given to the technique used to revive a person in cardiac arrest, and it is, as it were, our last stand against death. Recall the pathway from life to death:

Pathway from Life to Death
1. Loss of meaningful communication
2. Loss of consciousness
3. Airway obstruction
4. Respiratory arrest
5. Cardiac arrest (clinical death)
6. Irreversible brain damage (biologic death)

All of our efforts to save lives involve attempts to interrupt that pathway. We have already discussed how to intervene between steps 3 and 4—by opening the airway of an unconscious person to avert respiratory arrest. Similarly we have studied how to interrupt the pathway between steps 4 and 5—by giving prompt artificial ventilation to a person who has stopped breathing. But in CPR, we are dealing with a victim who has already passed the first four way stations on the pathway from life to death, and thus CPR is a last-ditch effort to interrupt the pathway just before the end of the line—between clinical death and biologic death.

As noted, CPR adds the *C* (circulation) to the *A* and *B* we have already studied. Just as in respiratory arrest where we treat the nonbreathing patient by *artificial breathing*, so in cardiac arrest we must also make up for the absence of an effective heart beat by providing an *artificial circulation*. Probably the most effective way to do this is to open the victim's chest and squeeze the heart about 60 times per minute; and indeed, until the early 1960s, this was the only known method of artificial circulation. The technique of open chest cardiac massage has significant limitations, however, for it requires a skilled physician and is practical only in the hospital setting. Fortunately, there is an alternative to open chest cardiac massage. Studies done in the late 1950s showed that intermittent pressure over the sternum, without opening the chest, could also produce a significant cardiac output—only about one-third to one-fourth the output of a normally beating heart, but still enough to sustain life. At first it was thought that *external chest compressions* worked by pressing the heart between the sternum and the spine and thus mechanically squeezing blood out of the heart into the circulation. More recent studies, however, have suggested that external chest compressions raise the pressure in the whole chest cavity, and it is that increase in pressure that results in cardiac output. But whatever the mechanism, it is clear that correctly performed external chest compressions can produce a significant arterial circulation.

Needless to say, artificial *circulation* must ALWAYS be accompanied by artificial *ventilation*. It does the patient little good to circulate blood lacking in oxygen throughout the body, for the whole object of the game in CPR is to GET OXYGEN TO THE TISSUES, especially the brain tissues. Thus artificial ventilation is always required when external chest compressions are applied.

ARTIFICIAL VENTILATION MUST ALWAYS ACCOMPANY EXTERNAL CARDIAC COMPRESSIONS.

THE GENERAL TECHNIQUE OF EXTERNAL CARDIAC COMPRESSIONS

Positioning the Victim

In order for chest compressions to be performed effectively, the patient must be *supine* and lying on a *hard, flat surface.* The amount of blood flow generated by external chest compressions is marginal even with the best technique, and the blood pressure generated is not powerful enough to compete with gravity if the patient's head is higher than the rest of the body. If external chest compressions are applied to a patient who is setting, there will be little if any blood flow to the brain. Thus it is imperative to get the cardiac arrest victim into a horizontal position as quickly as possible. If the victim is sitting in a chair, he should be moved rapidly to the floor; if the victim is a lineman on top of a utility pole, he must be brought down to the ground before external chest compressions are started. Furthermore, the surface on which the victim is placed should be firm and unyielding, such as the floor, a spine board, or a concrete pavement. Effective chest compressions require enough force to depress an adult's sternum 1½ to 2 inches, and that cannot be accomplished if the surface beneath the victim gives every time the rescuer presses on the victim's chest. If the victim is found in bed, a board (such as a spine board) should be placed beneath him. However, if a board is not immediately available, do not waste time running to fetch one, but simply move the patient quickly from the bed to the floor. In the ambulance, it is a good general practice to transport *every* unconscious patient on a spine board, for then the patient will already be on a suitable surface in the event that cardiac arrest occurs in transit.

When possible, the victim's *legs should be raised* (while keeping the trunk horizontal) during external cardiac compressions, for this may assist the return of blood from the lower extremities. Pillows or similar objects can be placed beneath the legs to elevate them, but once again, if pillows are not immediately available, do not waste time hunting for them. Just leave the legs flat and proceed with CPR.

Position of the Patient for CPR

- Supine
- Lying on a hard, flat surface
- Legs elevated, if possible

Technique of External Chest Compressions

To perform external chest compressions, you need to be close to the side of the victim's chest. If the victim is on the floor, kneel facing him so that one knee is about level with his neck and the other is opposite his lower ribs. That position will enable you to perform rescue breathing and chest compressions without having to slide back and forth from the victim's head to the chest. Once you have positioned yourself properly, the next step is to *locate the correct pressure point* on the victim's lower sternum (Fig. 7-3). To do so, use your hand to feel for the lower margin of the victim's rib cage (Fig. 7-4A), and slide your fingers up to the notch where the ribs meet the sternum (this is the point of attachment of the xiphoid process). With your third finger on the notch (Fig. 7-4B), lay your index finger beside it on the lower end of the sternum. Then take the heel of your other hand (the hand closest to the victim's head) and place it on the lower half of the sternum right next to the index finger of the hand you used to locate the notch, so that the heel of the hand is along the long axis of the sternum (Fig. 7-4C). Keeping the heel of your hand aligned along the middle of the sternum will ensure that the line of force is transmitted wholly to the sternum and will decrease the chance of inadvertently fracturing a rib.

Now take the other hand away from the notch, and

Fig. 7-3. *Correct pressure point for external cardiac compression.*

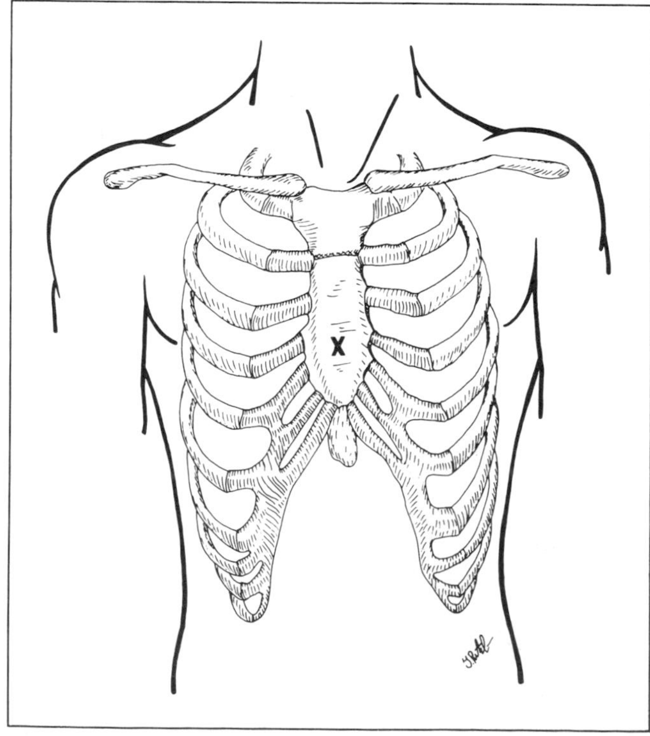

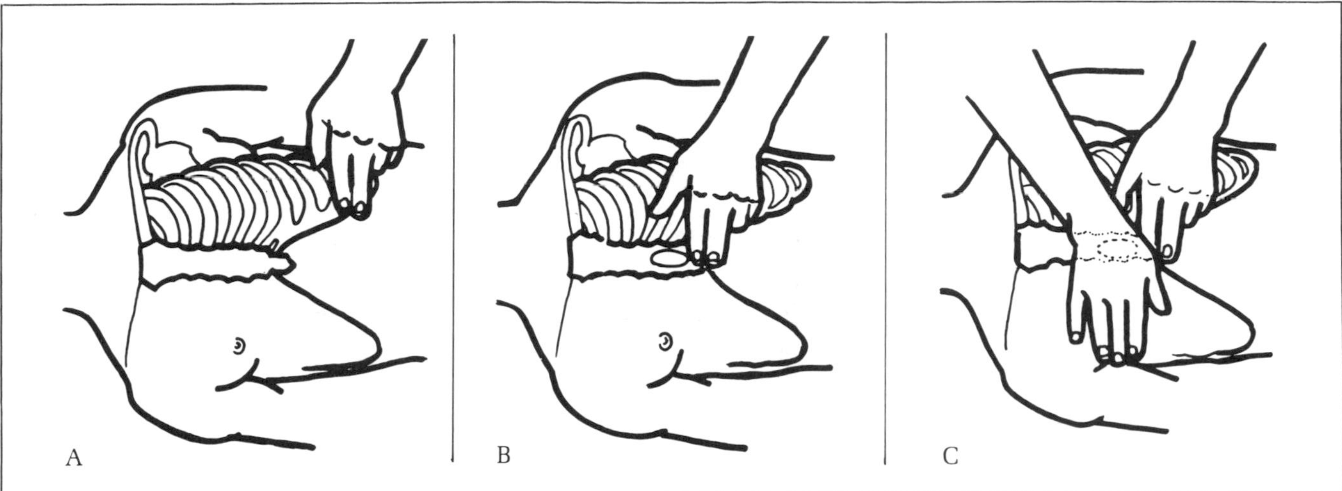

Fig. 7-4. *Locating correct hand position for external cardiac compressions. See text for details. (Reproduced courtesy Asmund Laerdal, Stavanger, Norway.)*

place it directly on top of the hand resting on the sternum, so that the heels of both hands are lined up one on top of the other. The fingers must be kept *off* the chest, so either hold them out straight or interlock them (Fig. 7-5). Alternatively, you can grasp the wrist of the hand that is on the sternum with your other hand if this technique is more comfortable for you.

Straighten your elbows to lock them, and position your shoulders directly over your hands, so that the force of the compression will be delivered straight down and not at an angle (Fig. 7-6). If the thrust is delivered at an angle, the victim's trunk will roll and part of the force will be dissipated, making the compression less effective.

Fig. 7-5. *Keep your fingers off the chest.*

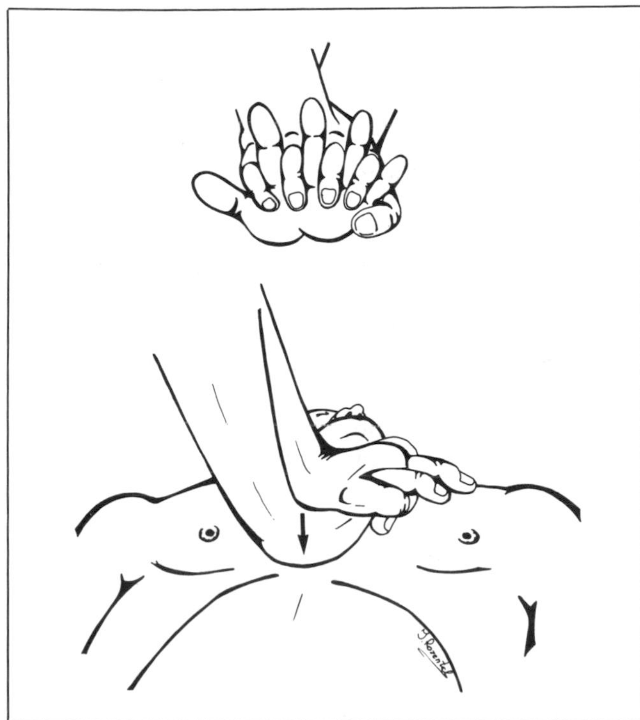

For a normal-sized adult, you will need to apply enough force to depress the sternum 1½ to 2 inches (4–5 cm). This is about as far as it will comfortably go. Depress the sternum by exerting pressure downward from your shoulders as you rock forward on your knees. Then release the pressure completely and allow the chest to return to its normal position, so that the heart can refill with blood. Do not lose your hand position, however; just take the weight off your hands, and leave them resting lightly on the chest. The time allowed for release should be about the same as the time allowed for compression. Compressions should be smooth, regular, and uninterrupted. Avoid bouncing up and down with your compressions, for jerky compressions are less effective and more apt to cause injury.

External Cardiac Compressions: Points to Remember

- The CORRECT PRESSURE POINT is over the midline of the lower third of the sternum, about 1 inch above the lower sternal notch.
- Keep your FINGERS OFF THE CHEST.
- Keep your ELBOWS LOCKED.
- Apply force STRAIGHT DOWN from your shoulders.
- Use the weight of your upper body to exert pressure.
- Depress the sternum 1½ to 2 inches.
- Compression times and relaxation times are of equal duration.
- KEEP YOUR HANDS IN POSITION between compressions.
- AVOID BOUNCING compressions.

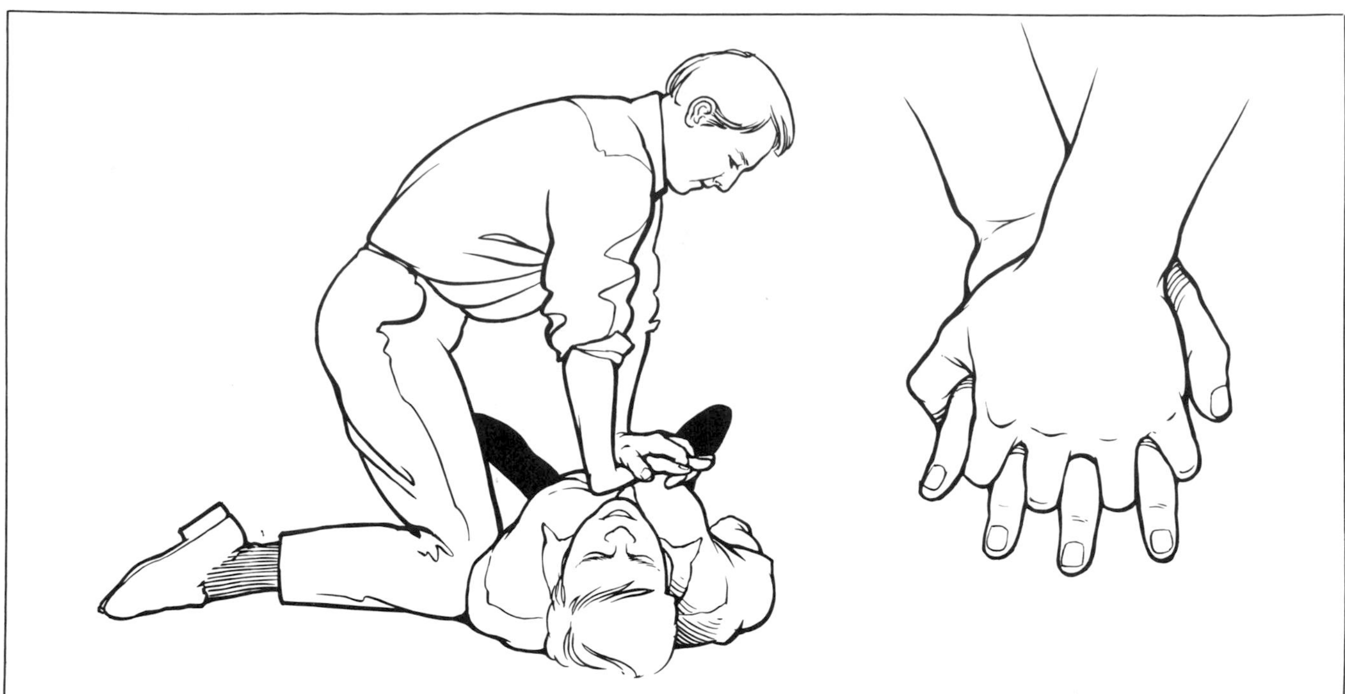

Fig. 7-6. *Line your shoulders up directly over the chest, and deliver your compressions straight down.*

So far we have discussed the general techniques for correct external chest compressions. Now let us put these techniques together with what we have learned about the airway and breathing and learn the correct *sequence* of cardiopulmonary resuscitation. Details of CPR will vary somewhat depending on the number of rescuers and the age of the patient*, so we will examine three different CPR situations: (1) CPR by one rescuer, (2) CPR by two rescuers, and (3) CPR for the infant or small child.

ONE-RESCUER CPR

No matter how many rescuers are available, CPR always follows the same ABC sequence, but when there is only one rescuer, more compressions are performed between ventilations to reduce rescuer fatigue. In any case, the *first* step of CPR is to ESTABLISH UNRESPONSIVENESS, that is, to make certain that the victim is really unconscious. To do so, shake the victim's shoulder gently and shout, "Are you OK?" (a maneuver aptly called the "shake-and-shout technique"). If there is no response, quickly POSITION THE VICTIM so that he is supine on a hard surface, and POSITION YOURSELF beside him. Immediately OPEN THE AIRWAY, using the head tilt–neck lift or head tilt–chin lift method, and —holding the airway open—put your ear close to the victim's nose so that you can LOOK, LISTEN, AND FEEL FOR BREATHING. Take about 5 seconds to determine whether the victim is breathing. If he is not, pinch his nostrils shut, take a deep breath, and give TWO VENTILATIONS OVER 5 SECONDS. The entire process up to this point—from the moment you encounter the victim until you have delivered the first two ventilations—*should not take more than 20 seconds:* 7 to 15 seconds to establish unresponsiveness, open the airway, and check for breathing; and another 5 seconds to deliver the two initial ventilations.

Having given the first two breaths, take the hand you were using to maintain chin lift and CHECK WHETHER THERE IS A PULSE. To do this, put your index finger on the victim's Adam's apple, and then slide your finger *toward* you, into the groove beside the Adam's apple; palpate there for a carotid pulse (Fig. 7-7). Allow 5 to 10 seconds to find the pulse, since it takes a second or two to locate the right spot and another few seconds to detect the pulse, especially if the victim has a very slow heart rate. If the pulse is absent, you must immediately start external chest compressions. You should also send someone to summon an advanced life support

*The new American Heart Association standards recommend that a single technique for CPR, covering all rescue situations, be taught to laypersons. Thus the lay public will be taught to employ a 15:2 ratio of compressions to ventilations irrespective of the age of the patient or the number of rescuers. This change has been made primarily to reduce confusion and simplify training. Professional rescuers, such as EMTs, however, may continue to utilize the 5:1 ratio for infants and for two-rescuer CPR; and certainly the generation that has already been trained in the 5:1 ratio and is accustomed to it need not change their practice.

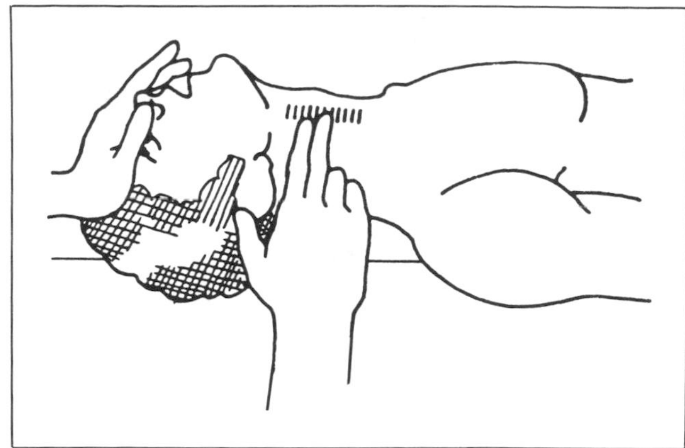

Fig. 7-7. *Palpating for the carotid pulse. (Reproduced courtesy American Heart Association.)*

unit (paramedic unit) if one is available in your community.

Quickly locate the notch at the victim's lower sternum, and place the heel of your other hand on the sternum one fingerbreadth above the notch, as described earlier. Then give 15 COMPRESSIONS at a rate of 80 TO 100 PER MINUTE. If you do not carry a metronome around with you, the easiest way to maintain a rate of 80 compressions per minute is to count out loud: "One and two and three and four and. . ." all the way to fifteen. Keep your compressions smooth and regular. Immediately upon completing the fifteenth compression, return quickly to the patient's head, REOPEN THE AIRWAY (e.g., head tilt–chin lift), and give TWO VENTILATIONS over 3 to 5 seconds (Fig. 7-8). Without pausing, return to the chest, and swiftly locate the correct position on the sternum; give another 15 compressions, and so forth. In this fashion, you should be able to deliver 60 compressions and 8 ventilations in 1 minute.

Fig. 7-8. *Interposing ventilations and compressions. (Reproduced courtesy American Heart Association.)*

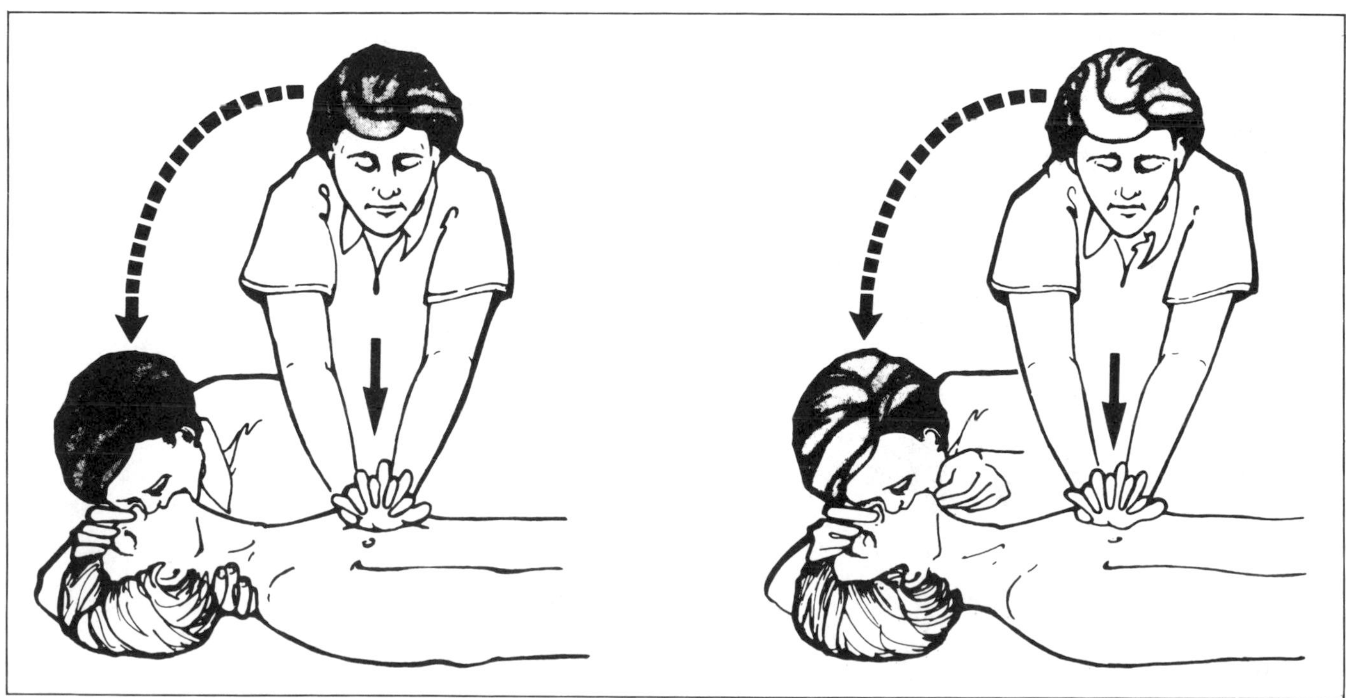

The carotid pulse should be checked periodically during one-rescuer CPR to determine whether there has been a return of an effective, spontaneous heart beat. Check the carotid after the first five cycles of CPR and every few minutes thereafter. If the patient's pulse returns, stop external chest compressions, and continue only with artificial ventilation (once every 5 sec) until there is also a return of spontaneous breathing. It is important to note that checking for the carotid pulse during CPR should not take more than 5 to 10 seconds, nor should CPR be interrupted for more than 5 to 10 seconds for any other purpose.

ONCE YOU HAVE BEGUN, DO NOT INTERRUPT CPR FOR MORE THAN 5 TO 10 SECONDS.

The steps of one-rescuer CPR are summarized in Figure 7-9. The important points to remember are as follows:

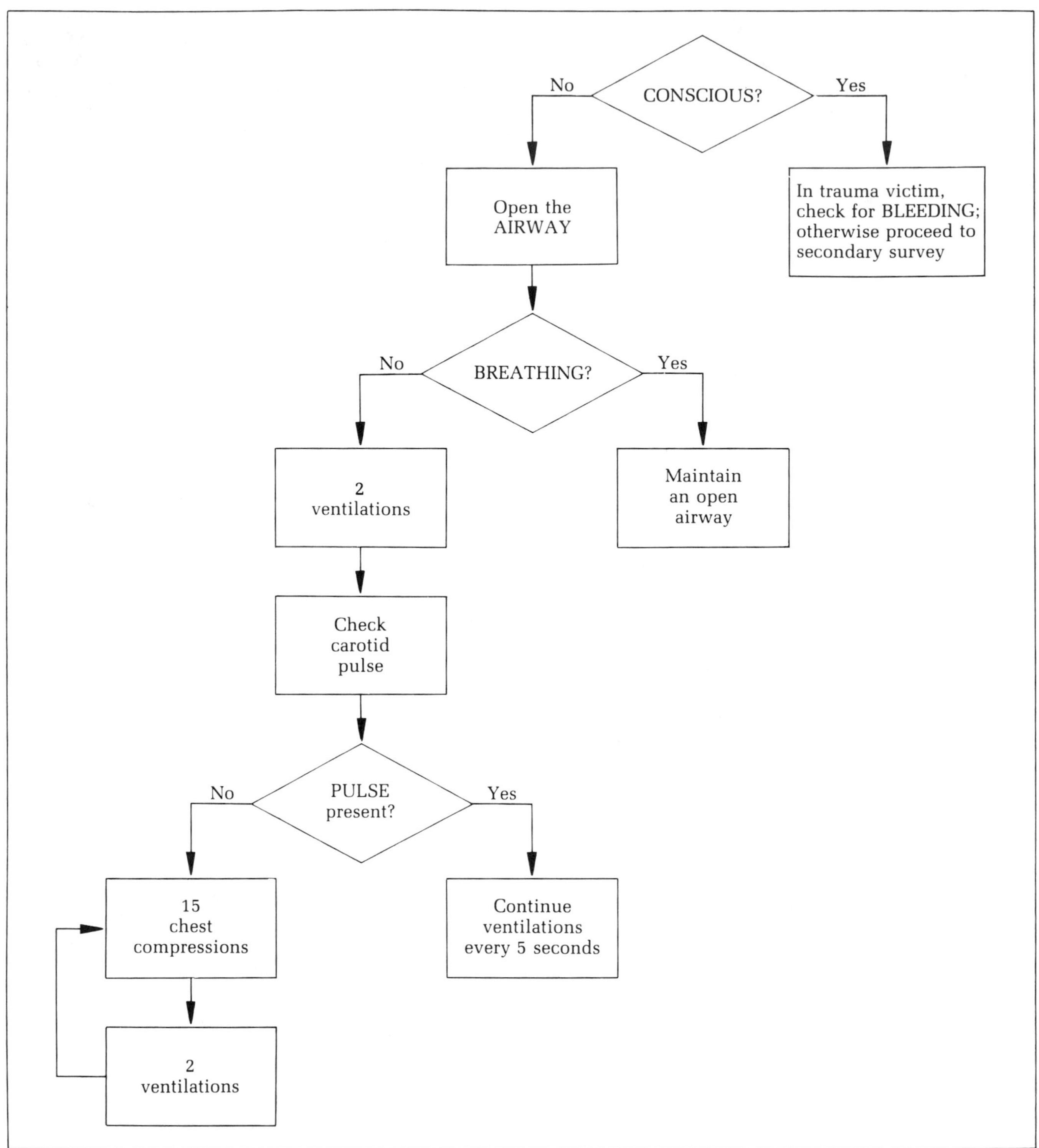

Fig. 7-9. *One-rescuer CPR.*

One-Rescuer CPR: Points to Remember

1. Shake and shout to determine UNRESPONSIVENESS.
2. Open the AIRWAY.
3. Look, listen, and feel for BREATHING.
4. If breathing is absent, give TWO VENTILATIONS over 5 seconds.
5. Check for a CAROTID PULSE.
6. If the pulse is absent, start EXTERNAL CHEST COMPRESSIONS:
   a. The rate of compressions is *80 to 100 per minute.*
   b. The ratio of chest compressions to ventilations is *15:2.*

TWO-RESCUER CPR

Since artificial ventilation must always accompany external chest compressions, it is preferable to have two rescuers to perform CPR, for with two rescuers—one doing chest compressions and the other giving ventilations—chest compressions need not be interrupted to interpose ventilations, and the circulation is more sustained.

The two rescuers should position themselves on *opposite sides* of the victim: the first rescuer in a position to give artificial ventilation and the second rescuer beside the chest, ready to perform chest compressions. The first rescuer goes through the initial steps of CPR as outlined above. He ESTABLISHES UNRESPONSIVENESS, OPENS THE AIRWAY, and CHECKS FOR BREATHING. If breathing is absent, he gives TWO VENTILATIONS over 5 seconds and then CHECKS FOR A CAROTID PULSE. If there is no pulse, he signals the second rescuer to begin EXTERNAL CHEST COMPRESSIONS. In two-rescuer CPR, the rate of compressions is now also 80 to 100 per minute, which can be achieved by having the second rescuer count quickly out loud while compressing: "One-and-two-and-three-and . . . ." As the rescuer doing compressions finishes his fifth compression, he pauses to allow the other rescuer to give a ventilation. (This is a departure from the technique previously recommended, in which no pause was permitted between compressions and ventilations.) It is also permissible according to the new American Heart Association guidelines to use the 15:2 (rather than the 5:1) ratio for two-rescuer CPR. That is, the rescuer giving compressions delivers 15 compressions at a rate of 80 to 100 per minute, then pauses to allow the other rescuer to give 2 breaths over 3 to 5 seconds.

The rescuer doing artificial ventilation should feel for the carotid pulse at frequent intervals to determine whether his partner is giving proper compressions. Effective chest compressions will produce carotid pulsations just as the heart beat does. If these are absent, the rescuer doing compressions should be notified to recheck his or her hand position and to increase the force of compressions. Every 4 to 5 minutes, both ventilations and compressions should be interrupted for 5 seconds to determine whether an effective, spontaneous heart beat has returned.

The important points to remember about two-rescuer CPR are as follows:

Two-Rescuer CPR: Points to Remember

- The two rescuers should position themselves on *opposite sides* of the victim.
- The rate of compressions is 80 to 100 PER MINUTE.
- The ratio of compressions to ventilations is 5:1 or 15:2.
- The rescuer doing ventilations should periodically CHECK THE VICTIM'S CAROTID PULSE to determine the effectiveness of compressions.

Changing Positions

During sustained two-person CPR, one or both of the rescuers may become fatigued and wish to exchange positions. This enables the ventilator to catch his breath and the compressor to give his arms a rest. The important thing about switching positions is that it be done smoothly, *without any interruption in the ongoing rhythm* of CPR. To accomplish this, the rescuer giving compressions signals his intention to switch positions one cycle before the switch is to take place. Then, immediately after giving the next ventilation, the rescuer at the head moves down and positions himself to take over chest compressions. The rescuer at the chest gives his last compression, moves to the head, and gives a ventilation. While he is delivering that ventilation, the rescuer now at the chest locates the landmarks, gets into position, and takes up chest compressions as soon as the ventilation has been delivered. (Note: In *practicing* the switch of positions in two-rescuer CPR, it is probably best that the rescuer taking over ventilations only pretend to ventilate, to reduce the risk of disease transmission during CPR drill.)

CPR FOR INFANTS AND CHILDREN

The basic CPR sequence of ABC is the same whether the victim is 1 month old or 100 years old. The differences in technique relate only to the differences in size and metabolic rate between an adult and an infant or small child.

As in the adult, the first step of CPR for an infant or small child is to ESTABLISH UNRESPONSIVENESS by gently tapping or shaking the victim. If the infant is unresponsive, position him on his back, preferably

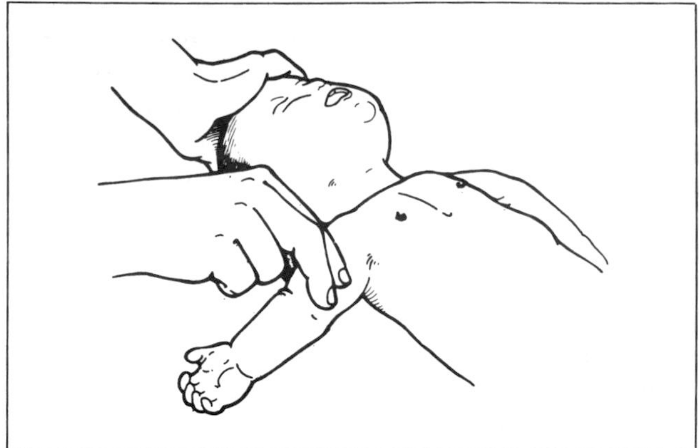

Fig. 7-10. *Locating the brachial pulse of the infant. (Reproduced courtesy American Heart Association.)*

on a hard surface such as a table top. Then OPEN THE AIRWAY by head tilt–neck lift or head tilt–chin lift (but without extreme hyperextension of the head), and maintaining the open airway, LOOK, LISTEN, AND FEEL FOR BREATHING. If the infant is not breathing, give TWO PUFFS FROM THE CHEEKS over 3 to 5 seconds, and FEEL FOR A PULSE. In a *child*, the pulse can be felt over the *carotid* artery in the same fashion as in an adult, but the short and often fat neck of the infant sometimes makes detection of the carotid pulse difficult. Therefore in the *infant*, it may be easier to check for a *brachial* pulse on the inside surface of the arm, midway between the elbow and the shoulder (Fig. 7-10). Steady the outer part of the arm with your thumb, and feel for the brachial pulse with the tips of your index and middle fingers. If the pulse is present, simply continue rescue breathing alone, once every 3 seconds (20 times/min) for an infant, once every 4 seconds (15 times/min) for a small child. These faster rates reflect the fact that the infant's and child's spontaneous rate of breathing is normally faster than that of an adult.

If the infant's pulse is not palpable, then you must start EXTERNAL CHEST COMPRESSIONS. (Remember, just as in the adult, chest compressions are never performed without rescue breathing). The technique of chest compression differs in the infant and child from that used for an adult because the heart sits higher in an infant's chest than it does in the adult. The proper area for compression in the *infant*, therefore, is over the *midsternum* (Fig. 7-11). If you were to draw an imaginary line between the infant's nipples, the correct compression point is right in the center of that line. A child's heart is lower in the chest than that of an infant but not quite as low as that of an adult. To find the correct pressure point on a *child*, locate the notch at the lower

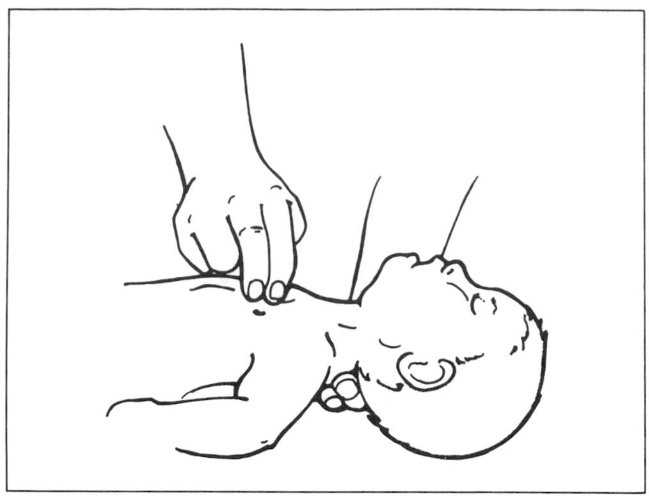

Fig. 7-11. *Chest compressions for the infant—one or two fingers only. (Reproduced courtesy American Heart Association.)*

end of the sternum with your middle finger, and lay your index finger beside it on the sternum. The area just above your index finger is the proper point of compression.

In addition to being smaller than an adult chest, the chest of an infant is much more pliable than that of an adult, and not nearly the same amount of force is needed to achieve proper compressions. In the *infant, two fingers* are more than adequate to exert sufficient force. Place your index and third fingers on the infant's midsternum, and depress ½ to 1 inch (1.3–2.5 cm). In a *child*, more force is required, and if the child is sufficiently large that you cannot depress the sternum with your fingers, use the *heel of one hand*, being careful to keep your fingers off the chest (Fig. 7-12). Increase the depth of your compression to 1 to 1½ inches (2.5–3.8 cm).

The rate of external chest compressions for *infants and children is 80 to 100 per minute*, just as for

Fig. 7-12. *Chest compressions for the child—heel of one hand only.*

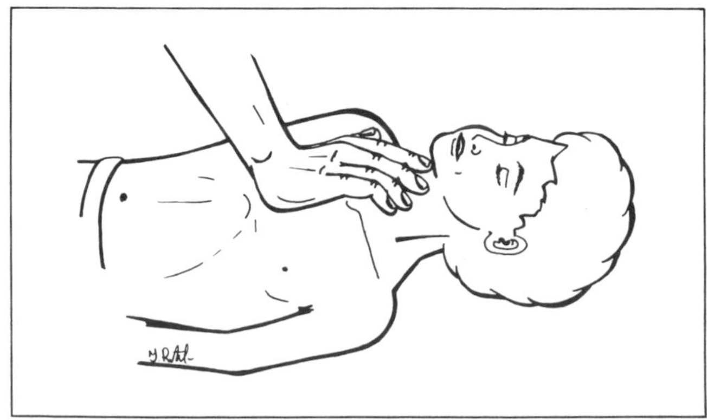

adults, with a ventilation interposed after every fifth compression. Just as in doing CPR on an adult, you must periodically pause for 5 seconds to check the pulse and determine whether an effective, spontaneous heart beat has returned. If so, stop chest compressions, and continue with rescue breathing alone. If not, resume both chest compressions and rescue breathing.

CPR of the Infant and Child: Points to Remember

- The sequence of CPR is the same as for an adult: ABC.
- Differences in INFANTS:
  1. DO NOT HYPEREXTEND THE HEAD in opening the airway.
  2. Ventilate only with PUFFS FROM YOUR CHEEKS.
  3. Use the BRACHIAL ARTERY to check for a pulse.
  4. Pressure point is in the MIDSTERNUM.
  5. Use only TWO FINGERS to depress the sternum.
  6. Depress the sternum only ½ TO 1 INCH.
  7. Ratio of compressions to ventilations: 5:1.
- Differences in CHILDREN:
  1. Use the HEEL OF ONE HAND to depress the sternum.
  2. Depress the sternum 1 to 1½ INCHES.
  3. Ratio of compressions to ventilations: 5:1.

The differences between CPR techniques for adults, infants, and children are summarized in Table 7-1.

SIGNS OF EFFECTIVE CPR

Up to now, we have examined the techniques of CPR and looked at the sequences in which those techniques are employed. But when you are actually *doing* CPR, how do you know whether you are carrying out all the techniques effectively?

There are several signs to look for that indicate CPR is working. First of all, in order for CPR to be effective, A CAROTID PULSE MUST BE PALPABLE with each chest compression. If the pulse is not palpable, the compression is not forceful enough. Needless to say, it is possible to check this only if there are *two* rescuers doing CPR, for a single rescuer cannot simultaneously give chest compressions with two hands and check the carotid pulse. A second sign of effective CPR is improvement in the patient's COLOR; if oxygen is reaching the tissues, they should "pink up." Furthermore, improved oxygenation of the brain is usually reflected by CONSTRICTION OF THE PUPILS when they are exposed to light. If the pupils remain widely dilated and fail to react to light, the brain is probably not being adequately oxygenated. In addition to these signs, there are several other changes that may occur during CPR, all of which may be taken to indicate effective performance. There may, for example, be spontaneous gasping or spontaneous movement of the arms and legs. The victim may try to swallow. In some instances, patients have been known to open their eyes and regain some consciousness while chest compressions were being given, only to lapse back into coma the moment compressions were interrupted. Finally, in some cases the heart may resume beating normally. The presence of any of these signs indicates that CPR is effectively circulating blood and delivering oxygen to the tissues.

Table 7-1. *CPR in Adults, Infants, and Children: A Comparison*

Technique	For the Adult	For the Infant	For the Child
AIRWAY	Head tilt–chin lift	Head tilt–chin lift, but without extreme hyperextension	Head tilt–chin lift
VENTILATION VOLUME	Forceful, until chest rises	Puffs from the cheeks	Intermediate, until chest rises
PULSE CHECKED	Carotid	Brachial	Carotid
PRESSURE POINT	Lower third of sternum	Midsternum	Lower half of sternum
APPLY PRESSURE WITH:	Two hands, one on top of the other	Two fingers	Heel of one hand
DEPRESS STERNUM	1½–2 in.	½–1 in.	1–1½ in.
RATE OF COMPRESSION	80–100/min	80–100/min	80–100/min
RATIO OF COMPRESSIONS TO VENTILATIONS	One rescuer: 15:2 Two rescuers: 5:1 or 15:2	5:1 or 15:2	5:1 or 15:2

Signs of Effective CPR

- Carotid pulsations *must* be palpable with each chest compression.
- Improvement in color: victim "pinks up."
- Pupils constrict in response to light.
- Victim may make spontaneous gasps.
- There may be spontaneous movement of the victim's arms or legs.
- The heart may resume beating on its own.

PITFALLS AND COMPLICATIONS OF CPR

When CPR is performed incorrectly or inadequately, it may be ineffective in supporting life and can lead to unnecessary further damage to the patient. It is important for the EMT to be aware of potential errors in CPR in order to avoid them and the complications they give rise to.

Errors Leading to Ineffective CPR

INTERRUPTIONS. Any time CPR is interrupted, all blood flow ceases entirely for the duration of the interruption. The tissues, particularly brain tissue, cannot tolerate any significant delays in circulation, for they are in a state of very marginal oxygenation even when CPR is in progress (recall that the victim is receiving only 16 to 18% oxygen from the rescuer's exhaled air, and the cardiac output produced by external chest compressions is only about 25 percent of normal). Thus the tissues have no reserve to draw upon, even for very short periods. For this reason, CPR SHOULD NEVER BE INTERRUPTED FOR MORE THAN 5 to 10 SECONDS, except to move the victim (see CPR in Transport, p. 89), in which case the interruption should not exceed 15 to 30 seconds.

BOUNCING OR JERKING COMPRESSIONS. Quick jabs on the chest not only increase the likelihood of injury but also produce only small jets of blood flow. As a result, the cardiac output per compression may be sharply reduced, and blood flow may be inadequate to keep the brain alive. Compressions should be smooth, regular, and uninterrupted—half the cycle being compression and half release.

WEAK COMPRESSIONS. If the rescuer is not positioned so that his or her shoulders are squarely above the victim's sternum, the rescuer is more likely to deliver compressions at an angle rather than straight down. The result is that part of the force of compression is dissipated in rolling the victim's trunk, and the compression itself is ineffective. Improper position will also prompt the rescuer to use wrist or elbow action to produce compressions, which is rapidly fatiguing, and a tired rescuer is less likely to give forceful compressions. The shoulders of the rescuer should be directly over the victim's sternum, and the rescuer's elbows should be locked. To compress the sternum, the rescuer can then rock forward from the knees and use the weight of the upper body, rather than the arm muscles, to produce a compression that is directed straight down.

COMPRESSIONS TOO SLOW OR TOO FAST. Compressions delivered at an incorrect rate can also be ineffective in promoting oxygenation. If compressions are too slow, the rate of oxygen delivery to the tissues may be inadequate. Once again, remember that the blood does not have as much oxygen in it as when the victim is breathing spontaneously and that the cardiac output is considerably reduced from normal. While a spontaneously breathing person with a strong heart beat may be able to tolerate a pulse of 40 or 50, a person being sustained by CPR (and therefore receiving a blood supply with a diminished amount of oxygen) cannot tolerate such a slow rate. On the other hand, compression rates that are too rapid can also be counterproductive. The heart needs time between compressions to refill with blood. If the compressions come one right after another, the ventricles cannot refill completely, and the amount of blood they can eject is accordingly diminished. Therefore, it is important to maintain the appropriate compression rate: 80 to 100 per minute.

ERRORS IN MAINTAINING THE AIRWAY AND IN ARTIFICIAL CIRCULATION. Errors in this category were discussed in Chapters 5 and 6.

Errors Leading to Injury of the Patient

COMPRESSION TOO HIGH ON THE STERNUM. If the rescuer's hands are placed too high on the sternum, external chest compressions can fracture the clavicle or the sternum itself.

COMPRESSION OVER THE XIPHOID. If the rescuer's hands are placed too low on the sternum, pressure may be exerted on the xiphoid rather than on the sternum itself. The xiphoid extends down over the abdomen, and compression over it can drive the xiphoid into the liver, producing laceration of the liver and uncontrollable internal bleeding.

COMPRESSIONS TO THE RIGHT OR LEFT OF CENTER. If the rescuer's hands are placed to the right or left of the midline or if the rescuer's fingers rest on the victim's ribs during compressions, the likelihood of rib fracture is greatly increased. Fractured ribs may in turn lacerate the lung and pleura and thereby cause air to rush into the thoracic cavity, with consequent collapse of the lung—a condition called **pneumothorax** (= *pneumo-*, meaning air + *thorax*, meaning chest).

Pitfalls and Complications of CPR: Points to Remember

- Do not interrupt CPR for more than 5 to 10 seconds.

- Avoid sudden, jerking movements.
- Keep your shoulders directly above the victim's sternum, and keep your elbows locked.
- Maintain correct rates of compressions and ventilations.
- Maintain correct hand position.
- Keep your fingers off the chest.

UNAVOIDABLE INJURY OF THE PATIENT. Sometimes complications occur despite the best possible technique. Elderly patients with brittle bones may suffer broken ribs during CPR even when chest compressions are properly performed. Similarly, fracture of the sternum, bruising of the lungs, and laceration of the liver can all occur despite good CPR technique. These complications can be minimized by scrupulous attention to correct technique, but they cannot be entirely prevented. Concern over injuries that may result from properly performed CPR should *not* inhibit a rescuer from swift initiation of CPR in the cardiac arrest victim. A living patient with a few broken ribs is preferable to a corpse with all the ribs intact. So remember:

FOR THE VICTIM OF CARDIAC ARREST, THE ONLY ALTERNATIVE TO CPR IS DEATH.

BEGINNING AND TERMINATING CPR

When do you begin CPR? Is every person whose heart stops beating a candidate for CPR? Should you try to resuscitate your 107-year-old great-grandmother? And once you have begun CPR, when do you quit? After 5 minutes? After 5 days? CPR is a powerful tool for saving lives, but the EMT needs to have some guidelines about when to apply this tool and how long to persist.

First of all, when do we begin CPR? We know that CPR is most likely to be effective if it can be started immediately after cardiac arrest. The more time that elapses between cardiac arrest and the initiation of CPR, the less the chances of successfully resuscitating the victim. Once cardiac arrest has persisted for more than 10 to 15 minutes, CPR is unlikely to restore the victim to meaningful life (that is, life with an intact brain). The problem is that it is very difficult to document the time of cardiac arrest. EMTs may arrive on the scene 15 minutes after the victim collapsed, but there is no telling whether the victim's heart actually stopped beating immediately when he collapsed or 10 minutes later. Thus the rule of thumb is

WHEN THE DURATION OF CARDIAC ARREST IS UNKNOWN, GIVE THE PATIENT THE BENEFIT OF THE DOUBT, AND START CPR.

Obviously, there are extreme cases where little doubt exists. If, for example, the victim is found cold and stiff in rigor mortis or in various stages of decomposition, there is little to be gained from starting CPR.

CPR is also *not* indicated for a patient known to be in the terminal stages of an incurable condition. The patient who is dying from advanced cancer, for example, should be permitted to die in peace.

What about your 107-year-old great-grandmother? Maybe you had better talk it over with her before the time comes. If she is alert and healthy and says she wants to live to be 150, she has as much right to receive CPR as her 25-year-old great-grandchild. If, on the other hand, she is languishing from a terminal illness, once again she has the right to die in peace.

Once you have started CPR, you should continue until one of the following conditions is met:

- The patient's heart resumes beating, and he begins breathing spontaneously.
- Another person properly trained in CPR takes over resuscitation.
- A physician or other properly trained person (e.g., a paramedic) assumes responsibility for the patient.
- You are exhausted and unable to continue.

In general, once CPR has been started, only a physician is legally entitled to decide that it should be stopped. Thus unless the rescuer is physically incapable of persisting, CPR should continue without interruption all the way to the hospital.

CPR IN TRANSPORT

As a general rule, the victim of cardiac arrest should not be moved until he has been stabilized, that is, until there is a return of spontaneous heart action and respirations. In many if not most instances, this will require advanced life support: the use of intravenous drugs, defibrillation (electric shock to the heart), definitive control of the airway with an endotracheal tube, and so forth. If there is a mobile advanced life support unit readily available, the EMT should remain at the scene and continue CPR until the paramedics arrive. However, if there are no paramedic units in the community or if the arrival of such a unit will be significantly delayed, the EMT must move the patient to a medical facility as quickly as possible. Recent studies have shown that the cardiac arrest victim's chances of survival, even with good basic CPR, decrease rapidly as definitive treatment (defibrillation) is delayed. Thus the main objective after starting CPR must be to get definitive treatment to the patient (by a paramedic unit or EMTs trained in defibrillation) or get the patient to definitive treatment (in the hospital) as fast as possible, *without interrupting CPR* in the meanwhile.

Practically speaking, it is impossible to move a patient without interrupting CPR. Not even an acrobat can perform CPR while carrying a patient on a spine board down a flight of stairs. Some interruptions are inevitable, but they must be kept to a minimum and should not exceed 15 to 30 seconds.

Let us take an example. Suppose a team of three EMTs who work in a community where there are no paramedics respond to a call for a "man down." They find their patient collapsed in the bedroom of his third-floor apartment (winding staircase, no elevator!). Having determined that the patient is in cardiac arrest, one or two of the EMTs start CPR (Fig. 7-13A) while the third EMT returns to the ambulance for a backboard and straps. He places the wheeled stretcher from the ambulance at the foot of the stairs and then returns to the patient's apartment with the backboard. When the third EMT returns, the EMT giving artificial ventilation moves to the same side of the patient as the EMT doing chest compressions, and they continue CPR while the third EMT positions the backboard alongside the victim. As soon as the backboard is lined up next to the victim, CPR is interrupted (for no more than 5 seconds) so the first two EMTs can roll the vicitm toward them. As they do so, the third EMT slides the backboard beneath the patient (Fig. 7-13B), and the first two EMTs roll him back onto the board, immediately resuming CPR. The third EMT secures the straps around the victim's knees and epigastrium.

When the patient is secure, the EMTs—on a signal from the rescuer doing compressions—lift the backboard and move as far as they can toward the door in about 15 seconds. Then they return the backboard to the floor and resume CPR for a minute or two (Fig. 7-13C). In that fashion the team makes its way to the top of the stairs. CPR is interrupted to move down to the first landing (Fig. 7-13D) and is then resumed for 1 to 2 minutes. Then the victim is moved down to the next landing, CPR is resumed again, and so on until the rescuers have reached the stretcher at the bottom of the stairs. The patient and backboard are placed on the wheeled stretcher, and one rescuer pushes the stretcher slowly so that the other rescuers can continue CPR while they are moving (Fig. 7-13E).

If the patient has not resumed spontanous heart action and breathing by the time he is loaded into the ambulance, CPR must be maintained throughout the transport. That will not be feasible if the vehicle is careening wildly around corners and screeching to sudden stops. Therefore the driver must take care to make the trip as smooth as possible. Even so, the EMT doing CPR will have to brace himself in order to avoid lurching as he performs chest compressions.

SPECIAL RESUSCITATION SITUATIONS

Drowning

Approximately 6,500 persons die from drowning in the United States each year, making drowning the fourth leading cause of accidental death. The injury to tissues that occurs in drowning will vary somewhat depending upon whether the victim was submerged in fresh water or salt water, but the initial stages of drowning and the immediate measures for resuscitation are the same in both situations.

When a person is submerged in water, a predictable sequence of events occurs. As the victim first goes under and water begins to enter his mouth and nose, he begins to cough and gasp, and he *swallows* a considerable amount of water. A very small amount of water is aspirated into the larynx and trachea, but this small amount is enough to set off violent spasms of the laryngeal muscles (**laryngospasm**), which effectively seal off the airway and protect it from further aspiration. At this stage, then, the lungs are dry, although there may be a great deal of water in the stomach. Like any other form of airway obstruction, laryngospasm leads to **anoxia** (lack of oxygen in the tissues) and asphyxia, and as a consequence the victim loses consciousness. Soon thereafter, he stops breathing. If the victim is not rescued promptly at this point, the laryngeal muscles will gradually relax, permitting massive amounts of water to enter the lungs. Furthermore, cardiac arrest can be expected to follow promptly on the heels of respiratory arrest, and then the clock starts ticking down toward biologic death.

It should be emphasized that successful resuscitation of drowning victims has been reported even after quite prolonged periods of submersion, especially if the drowning took place in cold water. Indeed, in a recent case in Thunder Bay, Ontario, an 18-month-old child who fell through the ice and was submerged for 30 minutes made a full recovery thanks to prolonged, expert CPR started immediately upon rescue. Thus CPR should be initiated even in cases where the victim was known to be submerged for 20 to 30 minutes or more.

The victim of drowning who is found in a body of water presents several special problems in CPR because of his location and the type of injuries apt to be associated with drowning. Specifically, rescue of a drowning victim poses the following additional dilemmas:

- How to reach the victim
- How to move the victim to a safe location suitable for resuscitation
- How to avoid aggravating possible neck injury

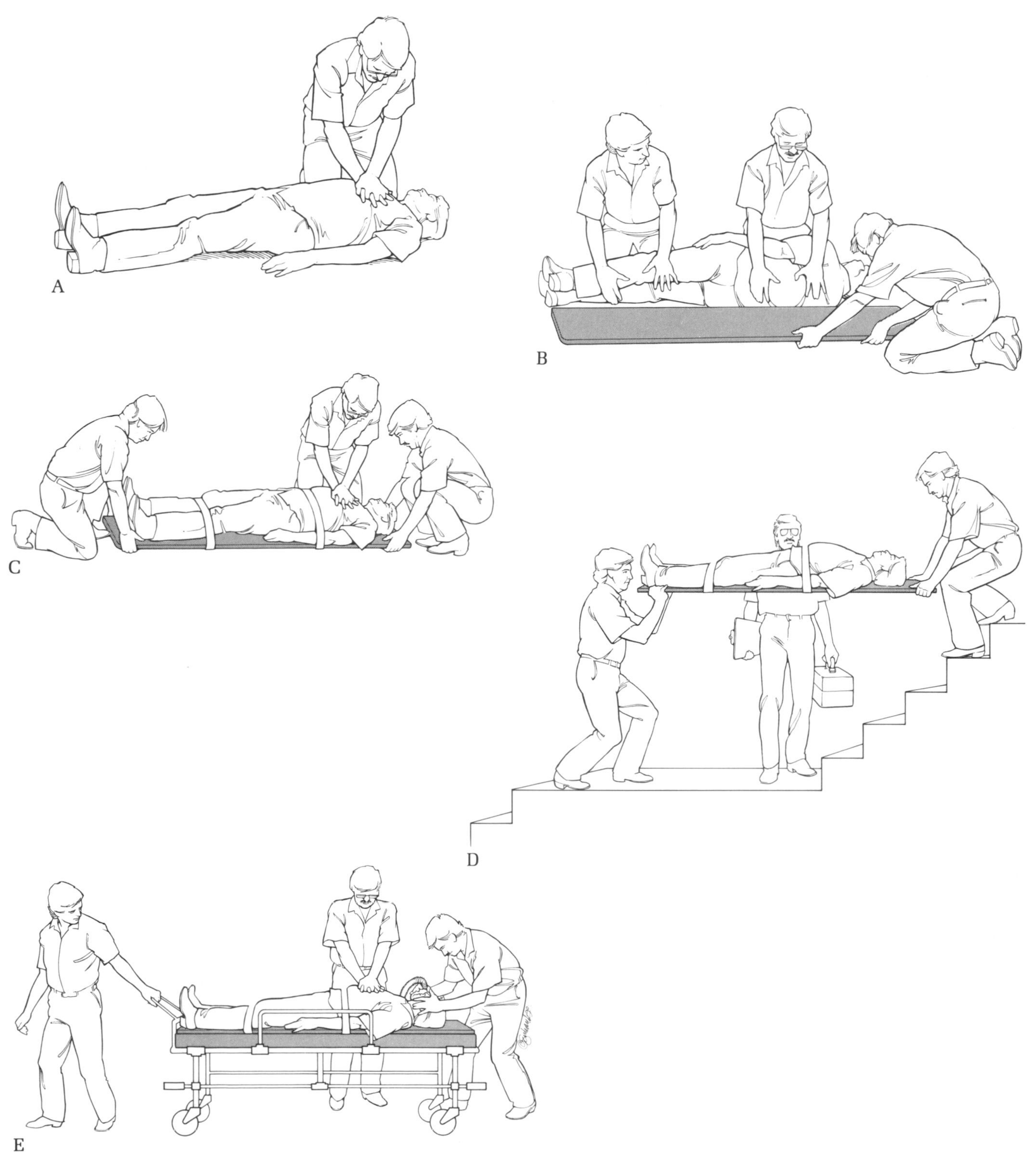

Fig. 7-13. *CPR in transport. A. Start CPR immediately upon reaching the victim. B. Log-roll the victim onto a backboard. C. Move the patient toward the stairs (15 seconds), then resume CPR. D. On signal, descend quickly to the first landing, then put the backboard down and resume CPR. E. Continue CPR as you slowly wheel the stretcher to the ambulance.*

The first problem is getting to the victim. It is of utmost importance that the EMT reach the drowning victim as quickly as possible, preferably with some means of conveyance (e.g., life raft, surfboard, boat) or at least a flotation device. Recall, however, the first rule of rescue: LOOK FIRST TO YOUR OWN SAFETY! An EMT who is not an accomplished swimmer has no business plunging into the water after a drowning victim, for there are likely to be *two* drowning victims as a result.

IF YOU CAN'T SWIM, DON'T PLUNGE IN!

Even if you are a good swimmer, you should not enter deep water without a personal flotation device, and ambulance services that cover regions where drowning is apt to occur should stock such devices in the vehicles.

External chest compressions cannot be performed effectively in the water and should not be attempted until the victim is brought to land or placed in a suitable boat. Mouth-to-mouth or mouth-to-nose ventilation, on the other hand, *can* be performed in the water and should be started at the earliest possible moment after reaching the victim. Usually artificial ventilation is very difficult in deep water, so the victim must be pulled quickly into shallower water. The moment the rescuer can stand in the water, he or she should begin rescue breathing before making any further attempts to pull the victim to dry land.

START ARTIFICIAL VENTILATION AT THE EARLIEST POSSIBLE MOMENT, EVEN BEFORE REMOVING THE VICTIM FROM THE WATER.

If the victim is found lying facedown in the water, approach him from the head. Place one hand down the middle of his back and the other just beneath his armpit, so that his head is sandwiched between your two arms. Then back away, and at the same time gently rotate the victim so that he is supine, with one of your hands still supporting his back. Open the victim's airway (jaw thrust alone!), and start rescue breathing. Remember, drowning accidents are often diving accidents, and any person found in the water must be presumed to have suffered a cervical spine injury. So avoid hyperextension of the head to open the airway, and try to minimize motion of the neck by holding the head steady.

A DIVING ACCIDENT MEANS A BROKEN NECK UNTIL PROVED OTHERWISE.

While you are doing all this, your partner should be fetching the long wooden backboard from the vehicle and floating it out to where you are working. While you support the victim's back, have your partner slip the backboard beneath the victim. Sandbags or wet towels can be placed on either side of the victim's head to prevent lateral motion. Continue rescue breathing as you float the victim to a place where he can be removed from the water on the backboard.

The moment you are on dry land, check for a pulse, and if it is absent, begin external chest compressions. Do not waste time trying to get water out of the victim's lungs or stomach, but be aware that there is a high likelihood of regurgitation (since the stomach is probably full of water), and be prepared to roll the victim quickly to his side, with his head and neck aligned with his body, to sweep out the mouth should any signs of regurgitation appear.

At the earliest possible moment, the victim should be moved to a medical facility, with CPR continuing en route if necessary. Even if the victim regains consciousness at the scene and appears completely recovered, he *must* be evaluated in a hospital, for victims of near drowning very frequently develop serious complications several hours later.

EVERY VICTIM OF NEAR DROWNING MUST BE EVALUATED IN A MEDICAL FACILITY.

Electrocution

The injuries that may follow an electric shock vary depending on the strength of the electric current and the duration of exposure to the current. In later sections, we will study electric burns and injuries that may occur after a fall caused by electric shock. In this section, we are interested in those consequences of electric shock that may require CPR.

When a person comes in contact with a strong electric current, all of his muscles, including the muscles of respiration, go into sustained spasm. Usually this spasm—called **tetany**—is limited to the duration of current exposure, but if the victim remains in contact with the current for any significant period and tetany therefore persists, breathing ceases, and cardiac arrest will follow because of anoxia. In addition, cardiac arrest may occur as a direct result of the electric current itself. Even very small currents can put the heart into fibrillation if they cross through the chest.

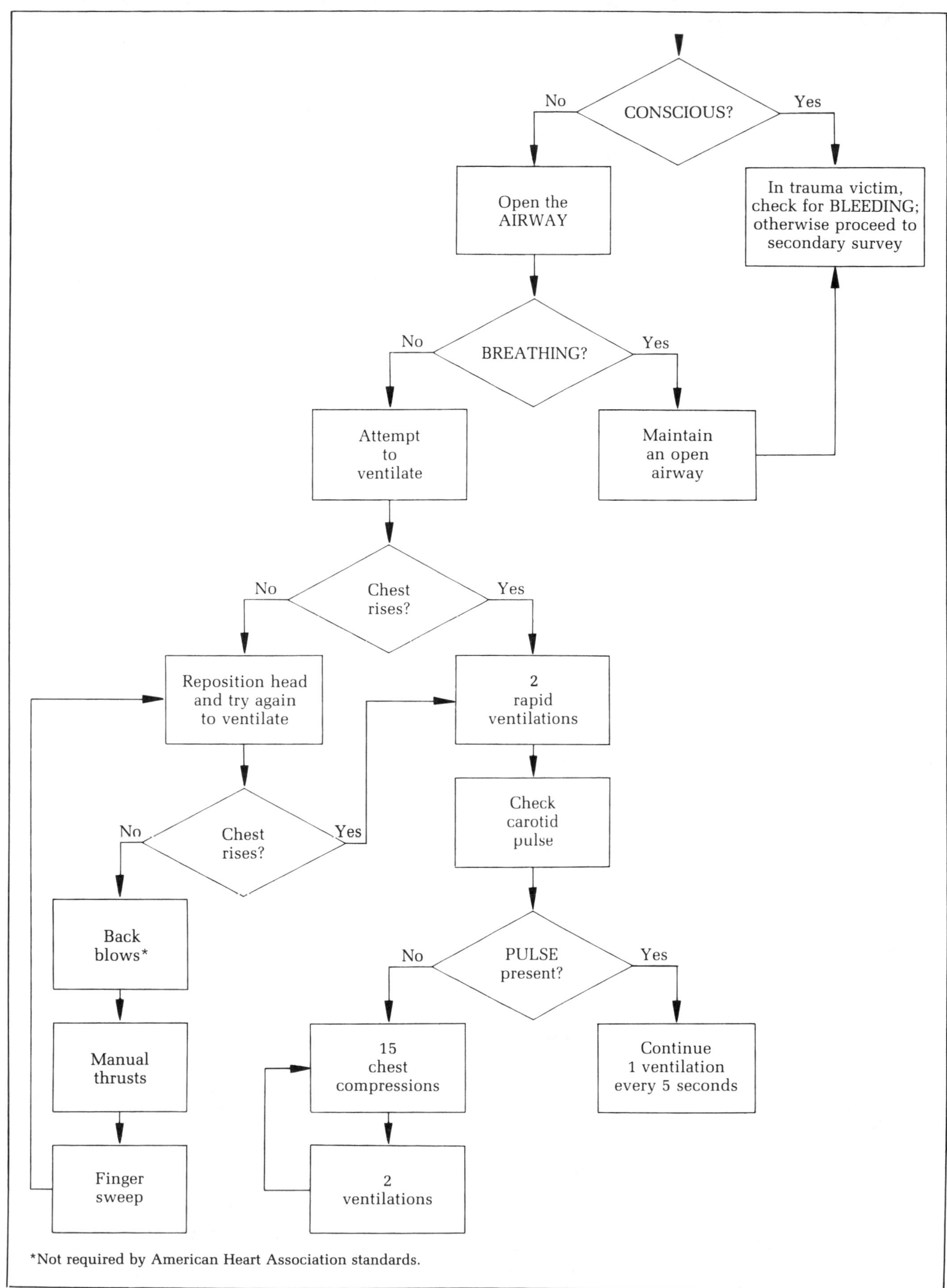

Fig. 7-14. *One-rescuer CPR: Overall summary.*

The treatment of a person who has suffered respiratory or cardiac arrest from electric shock is just like that for any other person in respiratory or cardiac arrest, *with one exception:* First you must make certain the victim is no longer in contact with the current source. If the current can be shut off (e.g., by pulling out a plug or using a circuit breaker in the fuse box), shut it off. If you cannot turn off the current, use some nonconducting item, like a wooden broom handle or a length of rope, to dislodge the victim from the current source. Remember:

> NEVER, NEVER, NEVER TOUCH A VICTIM OF ELECTRIC SHOCK UNTIL YOU ARE ABSOLUTELY CERTAIN HE IS NO LONGER IN CONTACT WITH THE CURRENT SOURCE.

Once the victim has been cleared from the current source, it is back to the old ABCs: Open the airway; look, listen, and feel for breathing, and ventilate if breathing is absent; check for a pulse, and if the pulse is absent, start external cardiac compressions.

In cases where electric shock occurs in a relatively inaccessible location, such as on a utility pole, mouth-to-mouth ventilation should be started as soon as the EMT reaches the victim, while they are both still on the pole. The victim must then be lowered as quickly as possible to the ground, where external chest compressions can be started. As mentioned earlier, CPR is effective only when the victim is horizontal, and thus chest compressions cannot begin until the victim has been brought down from the pole.

PUTTING IT ALL TOGETHER

In the last three chapters, we have examined the threats to life posed by airway obstruction, respiratory arrest, and cardiac arrest. We have studied the various techniques for opening the airway, providing artificial ventilation to a nonbreathing person, and providing artificial circulation to someone whose heart has stopped beating. Figure 7-14 summarizes all of these steps in proper sequence.

In the next chapter, we will look at another major threat to life—profuse bleeding—and find out what to do about it.

DISINFECTION OF TRAINING MANIKINS

With the current widespread anxiety regarding acquired immunodeficiency syndrome (AIDS), there has been renewed concern that CPR training manikins may serve as vehicles for transmitting disease. To date, there have been no recorded cases of *any* communicable diseases—whether bacterial, fungal, or viral—having been transmitted via a CPR manikin. It is, however, considered prudent to maintain a regular schedule for cleaning and disinfecting the manikin surfaces, to minimize whatever risk might exist that the manikin could act as a disease reservoir. The steps described below are sufficient to inactivate harmful microorganisms, including the quite delicate human immunodeficiency virus (HIV) responsible for AIDS.

STEPS IN DISINFECTING A CPR MANIKIN

- At the end of each class or practice session, disassemble the manikin according to the manufacturer's instructions.
- Thoroughly wash all external and internal surfaces with warm soapy water and brushes.
- Rinse all surfaces with fresh tap water.
- Wet all surfaces with a *freshly mixed* sodium hypochlorite solution (¼ cup liquid household bleach per gallon of tap water) for 10 minutes.
- Rinse with fresh water.
- Rinse with alcohol.
- Dry thoroughly.

VOCABULARY

anoxia Lack of oxygen in the tissues.

aorta The largest artery in the body, originating from the left ventricle of the heart.

artery A vessel that carries blood *away* from the heart.

asystole Absence of any ventricular contractions; cardiac standstill.

atrium The upper chamber of the right or left heart.

capillary A tiny blood vessel through which oxygen and carbon dioxide are exchanged in the tissues of the lung and other organs.

cardiac standstill Absence of ventricular contractions; asystole.

cardiopulmonary resuscitation (CPR) Technique to revive a person in cardiac arrest by artificial ventilation and external chest compressions.

cardiovascular collapse Form of cardiac arrest in which the heart continues beating, but its contractions are too weak to sustain the circulation.

CPR Abbreviation for *cardiopulmonary resuscitation.*

external chest compressions Rhythmic pressure exerted over the sternum with the aim of creatingan artificial circulation.

inferior vena cava One of the two largest veins of the body; carries blood from the lower part of the body to the right atrium of the heart.

laryngospasm Violent contractions of the muscles of the larynx, causing partial or complete airway obstruction.

pneumothorax Air in the pleural space.

pulmonary artery Artery that carries blood from the right ventricle to the lungs.

pulmonary vein Vein that carries oxygenated blood from the lungs to the left atrium.

red blood cell Cellular component of blood that carries oxygen from the lungs to the tissues; an erythrocyte.

septum Dividing wall or partition, usually separating two cavities, as the septum that divides the right side of the heart from the left side of the heart.

superior vena cava One of the two largest veins in the body; carries blood from the upper part of the body to the right atrium.

tetany Sustained contraction of a muscle group.

ventricle The lower chamber of the right or left heart.

ventricular fibrillation Form of cardiac arrest in which the individual muscle fibers of the heart contract chaotically, and the heart simply quivers.

FURTHER READING

CARDIAC ARREST

Amey BD, Harrison EE, Straub EJ. Sudden cardiac death: A retrospective and prospective study. *JACEP* 5: 429, 1976.

Barow RC et al. Sudden death among southeast Asian refugees. *JAMA* 250:2947, 1983.

Clinton JE et al. Cardiac arrest under the age of 40: Etiology and prognosis. *Ann Emerg Med* 13:1011, 1984.

Cobb LA. Cardiac arrest during sleep. *N Engl J Med* 311: 1044, 1984.

Crampton R. The problem of cardiac arrest in the community. *Am J Emerg Med* 2:204, 1984.

Goldberg A. Current concepts: Cardiopulmonary arrest. *N Engl J Med* 290:381, 1974.

Raymond JR et al. Nontraumatic prehospital sudden death in young adults. *Arch Int Med* 148:303, 1988.

Singer J. Cardiac arrests in children. *JACEP* 6:198, 1977.

CARDIOPULMONARY RESUSCITATION

Achong MR. Infectious hazards of mouth-to-mouth resuscitation. *Am Heart J* 100:759, 1980.

American Heart Association. Standards and guidelines for cardiopulmonary resuscitation (CPR) and emergency cardiac care (ECC). *JAMA* 255:2905, 1986.

Bieber RM. CPR in transportation: A vital link. *EMT J* 3(3): 59, 1979.

Bircher N et al. A comparison of standard, MAST-augmented, and open-chest CPR in dogs. *Crit Care Med* 8:147, 1980.

Carter WB et al. Development and implementation of emergency CPR instruction via telephone. *Ann Emerg Med* 13:695, 1984.

Chipman C, Adelman R, Sexton G. Criteria for cessation of CPR in the emergency department. *Ann Emerg Med* 10:11, 1981.

CPR—it's come a long way. *Emerg Med* 17(5):77, 1985.

Cummins RO. Infection control guidelines for CPR providers. *JAMA* 262:2732, 1989.

Cummins RO, Eisenberg MS. Prehospital cardiopulmonary resuscitation: Is it effective? *JAMA* 253:2408, 1985.

DeBard ML. The history of cardiopulmonary resuscitation. *Ann Emerg Med* 9:273, 1980.

Eisenberg MS, Bergner L, Hallstrom A. Cardiac resuscitation in the community: Importance of rapid provision and implications for program planning. *JAMA* 241: 1905, 1979.

Eisenberg MS, Bergner L, Hallstrom A. Epidemiology of cardiac arrest and resuscitation in the community. *Ann Emerg Med* 12:672, 1983.

Eisenberg MS et al. Long-term survival after out-of-hospital cardiac arrest. *N Engl J Med* 306:1340, 1982.

Eisenberg MS et al. Survivors of out-of-hospital cardiac arrest: Morbidity and long-term survival. *Am J Emerg Med* 2:189, 1984.

Eisenberg MS et al. Emergency CPR instruction via telephone. *Am J Public Health* 75:47, 1985.

Emergency Cardiac Care Committee, American Heart Association. Risk of infection during CPR training and rescue: Supplemental guidelines. *JAMA* 262:2714, 1989.

Gordon M et al. Cardiopulmonary resuscitation on the elderly. *J Am Geriatr Soc* 32:930, 1984.

Guzy PM, Pearce ML, Greenfield S. The survival benefit of bystander cardiopulmonary resuscitation in a paramedic served metropolitan area. *Am J Public Health* 73: 766, 1983.

Kouwenhoven WB, Jude JR, and Knickerbocker G. Closed chest cardiac massage. *JAMA* 173:1064, 1960.

Lemire JG, and Johnson A. Is cardiac resuscitation worthwhile? A decade of experience. *N Engl J Med* 286:970, 1972.

Lewis JK et al. Outcome of pediatric resuscitation. *Ann Emerg Med* 12:297, 1983.

Lonergan JH, Youngbert JZ, Kaplan JA. Cardiopulmonary resuscitation: Physical stress on the rescuer. *Crit Care Med* 9:793, 1981.

Longstreth WT et al. Neurologic recovery after out-of-hospital cardiac arrest. *Ann Intern Med* 98(Part I):588, 1983.

Luce JM et al. New developments in cardiopulmonary resuscitation. *JAMA* 244:1366, 1980.

Ludwig S et al. Pediatric cardiopulmonary resuscitation: A review of 130 cases. *Clin Pediatr* (Phila.) 23:71, 1984.

Maier GW et al. Optimal techniques of external cardiac massage. *Surg Forum* 33:282, 1982.

Mancini ME et al. The effect of time since training on house officers' retention of CPR skills. *Ann Emerg Med* 3:31, 1985.

Martin WJ et al. CPR skills: Achievement and retention under stringent and relaxed criteria. *Am J Public Health* 73:1310, 1983.

Matthewson Z et al. Mobile coronary care and community mortality from myocardial infarction. *Lancet* 1:441, 1985.

Mayer JD. Emergency medical services: Delays, response times, and survival. *JAMA* 241:1905, 1979.

Melker R et al. One rescuer CPR: A reappraisal of present recommendations for ventilation. *Crit Care Med* 9:423, 1981.

Melker RJ, Banner MJ. Ventilation during CPR: Two-rescuer standards reappraised. *Ann Emerg Med* 14:397, 1985.

Murphy RJ et al. Citizen cardiopulmonary resuscitation training and use in a metropolitan area—the Minnesota heart survey. *Am J Public Health* 74:413, 1984.

Nagel EL. Complications of CPR. *Crit Care Med* 9:242, 1981.

Newton J et al. A physiologic comparison of external cardiac massage techniques. *J Thorac Cardiovasc Surg* 95:892, 1988.

Niemann JT et al. Cough CPR. *Crit Care Med* 8:141, 1980.

Ornato JP et al. Measurement of ventilation during cardiopulmonary resuscitation. *Crit Care Med* 11:79, 1983.

Pergner L et al. Health status of survivors of out-of-hospital cardiac arrest six months later. *Am J Public Health* 74:508, 1984.

Rudikoff MJ et al. Mechanisms of blood flow during cardiopulmonary resuscitation. *Circulation* 6:345, 1980.

Saunders AB, Meislin HW, Ewy G. The physiology of cardiopulmonary resuscitation. *JAMA* 252:3283, 1984.

Safar P, Bircher N. *Cardiopulmonary Cerebral Resuscitation*. Philadelphia: Saunders, 1988. Chap. 1C.

Steen-Hansen JE et al. Pupil size and light reactivity during cardiopulmonary resuscitation: A clinical study. *Crit Care Med* 16:90, 1983.

Taylor GJ et al. Importance of prolonged compression during cardiopulmonary resuscitation in man. *N Engl J Med* 296:1515, 1977.

Torphy DE, Minter MG, Thompson BM. Cardiopulmonary arrest and resuscitation of children. *Am J Dis Child* 138:1099, 1984.

Tresch DD et al. Long-term survival after prehospital sudden cardiac death. *Am Heart J* 108:1, 1984.

Tweed WA et al. Retention of cardiopulmonary resuscitation skills after initial overtraining. *Crit Care Med* 8:651, 1980.

Veatch RM. Deciding against resuscitation: Encouraging signs and potential dangers (editorial). *JAMA* 253:77, 1985.

Vertesi L, Wilson L, Glick N. Cardiac arrest: Comparison of paramedic and conventional ambulance services. *Can Med Assoc J* 128:809, 1983.

Warner LL et al. Prognostic significance of field response in out-of-hospital ventricular fibrillation. *Chest* 87:22, 1985.

Warren ET et al. External cardiopulmonary resuscitation augmented by the military antishock trousers. *Am Surg* 49:651, 1983.

Weaver WD et al. Improved neurologic recovery and survival after early defibrillation. *Circulation* 69:943, 1984.

DROWNING

Harries MG. Drowning in man. *Crit Care Med* 9:407, 1981.

Hooper HA. Near drowning. *Emergency* 12(5):75, 1980.

Knopp R. Near drowning. *JACEP* 7:249, 1978.

Martin TG. Neardrowning and cold water immersion. *Ann Emerg Med* 13:263, 1984.

Orlowski JP. Vomiting as a complication of the Heimlich maneuver. *JAMA* 258:512, 1987.

Pearn J. Secondary drowning in children. *Br Med J* 281:1103, 1980.

Pearn J. Drowning and alcohol. *Med J Aust* 141:6, 1984.

Pluekhahn, V. Alcohol and accidental drowning. *Med J Aust* 141:22, 1984.

Redmond AD et al. Resuscitation from drowning. *Arch Emerg Med* 1:113, 1984.

Schuman SH et al. Risk of drowning: An iceberg phenomenon. *JACEP* 6:139, 1977.

SKILL EVALUATION CHECKLISTS

The following pages contain skill checklists covering the techniques of basic life support we have studied so far. These checklists are intended as a guide for the student in practicing the skills described in this chapter. These skill checklists are reprinted with the kind permission of the American Heart Association. Skill checklists for CPR of infants and children can be found at the end of Chapter 34.

American Heart Association CPR and ECC Performance Sheet
One-Rescuer CPR: Adult

Name ______________________________ Date ______________

Step	Activity	Critical Performance	S	U
1. Airway	Assessment: Determine unresponsiveness.	Tap or gently shake shoulder.		
		Shout "Are you OK?"		
	Call for help.	Call out "Help!"		
	Position the victim.	Turn on back as unit, if necessary, supporting head and neck (4–10 sec).		
	Open the airway.	Use head-tilt/chin-lift maneuver.		
2. Breathing	Assessment: Determine breathlessness	Maintain open airway.		
		Ear over mouth, observe chest: look, listen, feel for breathing (3–5 sec).		
	Ventilate twice.	Maintain open airway.		
		Seal mouth and nose properly.		
		Ventilate 2 times at 1–1.5 sec/inspiration.		
		Observe chest rise (adequate ventilation volume).		
		Allow deflation between breaths.		
3. Circulation	Assessment: Determine pulselessness.	Feel for carotid pulse on near side of victim (5–10 sec).		
		Maintain head-tilt with other hand.		
	Activate EMS system.	If someone responded to call for help, send him/her to activate EMS system.		
		Total time, Step 1—Activate EMS system: 15–35 sec.		
	Begin chest compressions.	Rescuer kneels by victim's shoulders.		
		Landmark check prior to hand placement.		
		Proper hand position throughout.		
		Rescuer's shoulders over victim's sternum.		
		Equal compression–relaxation.		
		Compress 1½ to 2 inches.		
		Keep hands on sternum during upstroke.		
		Complete chest relaxation on upstroke.		
		Say any helpful mnemonic.		
		Compression rate: 80–100/min (15 per 9–11 sec).		
4. Compression/ Ventilation Cycles	Do 4 cycles of 15 compressions and 2 ventilations.	Proper compression/ventilation ratio: 15 compressions to 2 ventilations per cycle.		
		Observe chest rise: 1–1.5 sec/inspiration; 4 cycles/52–73 sec.		
5. Reassessment*	Determine pulselessness. (If no pulse: Step 6.)†	Feel for carotid pulse (5 sec).		
6. Continue CPR	Ventilate twice.	Ventilate 2 times.		
		Observe chest rise; 1–1.5 sec/inspiration.		
	Resume compression/ ventilation cycles.	Feel for carotid pulse every few minutes.		

* 2nd rescuer arrives to replace 1st rescuer: (a) 2nd rescuer identifies self by saying "I know CPR. Can I help?" (b) 2nd rescuer then does pulse check in Step 5 and continues with Step 6. (During practice and testing only one rescuer actually ventilates the manikin. The 2nd rescuer simulates ventilation.) (c) 1st rescuer assesses the adequacy of 2nd rescuer's CPR by observing chest rise during ventilations and by checking the pulse during chest compressions.

† If pulse is present, open airway and check for spontaneous breathing: (a) If breathing is present, maintain open airway and monitor pulse and breathing. (b) If breathing is absent, perform rescue breathing at 12 times/min and monitor pulse.

Instructor ______________________ Check: Satisfactory ________ Unsatisfactory ________

4/86

American Heart Association CPR and ECC Performance Sheet
Two-Rescuer CPR: Adult*

Name ______________________________ Date ______________

Step	Activity	Critical Performance	S	U
1. Airway	One rescuer (ventilator): Assessment: Determines unresponsiveness.	Tap or gently shake shoulder.		
		Shout "Are you OK?"		
	Positions the victim.	Turn on back if necessary (4–10 sec).		
	Opens the airway.	Use a proper technique to open airway.		
2. Breathing	Assessment: Determines breathlessness.	Look, listen and feel (3–5 sec).		
	Ventilator ventilates twice.	Observe chest rise: 1–1.5 sec/inspiration.		
3. Circulation	Assessment: Determines pulselessness.	Palpate carotid pulse (5–10 sec).		
	States assessment results.	Say "No pulse."		
	Other rescuer (compressor): Gets into position for compressions.	Hands, shoulders in correct position.		
	Locates landmark notch.	Landmark check.		
4. Compression/ Ventilation Cycles	Compressor begins chest compressions	Correct ratio compressions/ventilations: 5/1.		
		Compression rate: 80–100/min (5 compressions/3–4 sec).		
		Say any helpful mnemonic.		
		Stop compressing for each ventilation.		
	Ventilator ventilates after every 5th compression and checks compression effectiveness.	Ventilate 1 time (1–1.5 sec). Check pulse to assess compressions.		
	(Minimum of 10 cycles.)	Time for 10 cycles: 40–53 sec.		
5. Call for Switch	Compressor calls for switch when fatigued.	Give clear signal to change.		
		Compressor completes 5th compression.		
		Ventilator completes ventilation after 5th compression.		
6. Switch	Simultaneously switch:			
	Ventilator moves to chest.	Move to chest.		
		Become compressor.		
		Get into position for compressions.		
		Locate landmark notch.		
	Compressor moves to head.	Move to head.		
		Become ventilator.		
		Check carotid pulse (5 sec).		
		Say "No pulse."		
		Ventilate once.†		
7. Continue CPR	Resume compression/ ventilation cycles.	Resume Step 4.		

* (a) If CPR is in progress with one rescuer (lay person), the entrance of the two rescuers occurs after the completion of one rescuer's cycle of 15 compressions and 2 ventilations. The EMS should be activated first. The two new rescuers start with Step 6. (b) If CPR is in progress with one professional rescuer, the entrance of a second professional rescuer is at the end of a cycle after check for pulse by first rescuer. The new cycle starts with one ventilation by the first rescuer, and the second rescuer becomes the compressor.

† During practice and testing only one rescuer actually ventilates the manikin. The other rescuer simulates ventilation.

Instructor ______________________ Check: Satisfactory ________ Unsatisfactory ________

4/86

8. BLEEDING AND SHOCK

OBJECTIVES

Once breathing and circulation are assured, we can turn our attention to another potentially life-threatening condition: profuse bleeding. Just as the absence of breathing or of effective cardiac contractions prevents oxygen from reaching the tissues, so too a serious loss of blood—the medium in which oxygen is carried—jeopardizes tissue survival. In this chapter, we will examine how the normal circulatory system ensures a constant flow of life-giving blood to all parts of the body and what happens when large quantities of blood are lost. On completion of the chapter, the reader should be able to

1. Describe the nature of blood flow and the way in which blood flow is produced
2. Identify the two components of blood pressure and explain their relationship to the phases of the cardiac cycle
3. Describe the differences in blood flow in arteries and in veins
4. List the three major cellular components of blood and describe the function of each
5. Identify the protein responsible for carrying oxygen, given a list of various proteins
6. List two differences between arterial and venous bleeding
7. List three methods of controlling external bleeding and indicate which is the safest and most effective method
8. Identify the location of the pressure points that can be used to help control bleeding from (a) the forearm, (b) the leg, and (c) the neck
9. Describe the dangers in using a tourniquet to control bleeding
10. List the steps in applying a tourniquet correctly and the precautions necessary when a tourniquet is used
11. List two ancillary measures that may help in the control of bleeding
12. Describe what measures should be taken to control a nosebleed in the field, and indicate under what circumstances a nosebleed should *not* be controlled
13. Identify the correct definition of shock, given several definitions
14. List three types of shock and explain the mechanism of each
15. Identify what type of shock is present, given examples of several types of shock
16. Describe how the body attempts to compensate for loss of blood
17. List the symptoms and signs of shock and indicate which of the signs of shock are early signs and which are late signs
18. List in the correct sequence the steps in managing shock

ANOTHER LOOK AT THE CIRCULATORY SYSTEM

As we learned in the previous chapter, the circulatory system has three general components: a pump (the heart), a network of tubing (arteries, capillaries, and veins), and a reservoir of fluid (blood) that is pumped through the tubing. In order for the circulatory system to carry out its job of getting oxygen and nourishment to every cell in the body, all of these components must be intact. In Chapter 7, we focused on the pump and examined what happens when the pump stops working. In this chapter, we will explore the working of the pump a bit more closely and then focus on the other two components of the system: the tubing and the fluid that flows through it.

THE HEART AND BLOOD PRESSURE

As we recall, the heart is the pump that provides the mechanical force to drive blood through the circuit of tubes. With each contraction, the left ventricle ejects 70 to 80 ml of blood. The heart contracts slightly more often than once per second, so in each minute the entire blood volume of 6 liters (about 12 pints) is circulated. This repetitive squeezing action of the heart—squeeze-relax, squeeze-relax—produces a *pulsatile* flow; that is, the blood is pushed along in a somewhat jerky rather than smooth fashion, lurching forward with each ventricular squeeze, then slowing down a bit as the ventricles relax and refill between squeezes. Special names are given to the two phases of the pumping cycle. The time when the ventricles are squeezing, or contracting, is called **systole,** while the period of ventricular relaxation, in between contractions, is called **diastole.** During systole, the forceful ejection of blood from the ventricles causes the pressure throughout the whole network of tubing to rise, especially in the arteries. As the ventricles relax in diastole, the pressure in the system returns to its resting level. If we were to put a probe inside one of the arteries to measure the pressures, the graph we would get would look something like the one in Figure 8-1. Each bump in the graph represents a single contraction of the ventricles and the pressure wave that contraction produces. As each bump is propagated through the arterial circulation, it produces a *pulse beat* (Fig. 8-2).

The pressure that the blood exerts against the walls of the arteries is called the **blood pressure,** and since the cardiac cycle has two phases—systole and diastole—the blood pressure has two components: a *high point,* when the pressure against the arterial wall peaks, called **systolic pressure**; and a *low point,* when the pressure drops to its resting level, called **diastolic pressure.** As the terms imply, systolic pressure corresponds to the period when the ventricles

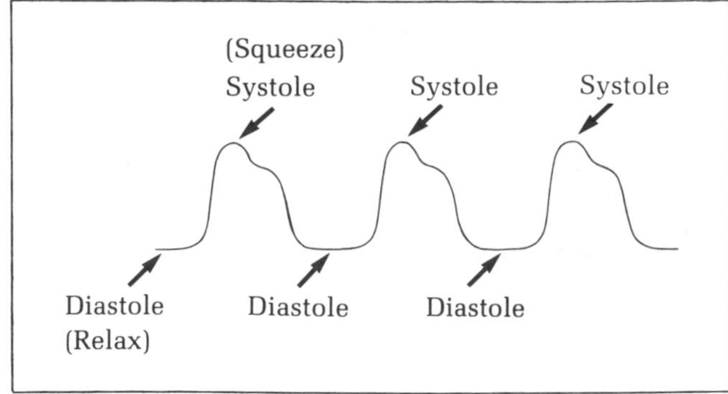

Fig. 8-1. *Arterial pulse pressure.*

are contracting (in systole), while diastolic pressure corresponds to ventricular relaxation (diastole).

The blood pressure can be measured without sticking a probe inside an artery with a device called a **sphygmomanometer,** which consists of an inflatable cuff and a pressure gauge. The cuff is inflated around the arm until it reaches a pressure sufficient to cut off flow through the brachial artery, and this pressure is the systolic pressure; then the cuff is slowly deflated, and the pressure at which blood flow resumes completely through the brachial artery is the diastolic pressure. We could get the same pressure readings in any other artery, but the brachial is the most convenient to use because it is easy to occlude the flow through it. We will learn precisely how to use a sphygmomanometer in Section IV. For our purposes now, it is sufficient to know that the pressures measured with a sphygmomanometer are expressed numerically in millimeters of mercury (abbreviated as **mm Hg**). In normal men, the systolic pressure varies from 100 to about 150 mm Hg (a good general guide is 100 plus the person's age), while the diastolic pressure may be anywhere from 65 to 90 mm Hg. In women, the pressures are normally 8 to 10 mm Hg lower. It is conventional to express blood pressure as a fraction, using the systolic pressure as the numerator and the diastolic pressure as the denominator. Thus if a 20-year-old man has a systolic

Fig. 8-2. *Pulse beat.*

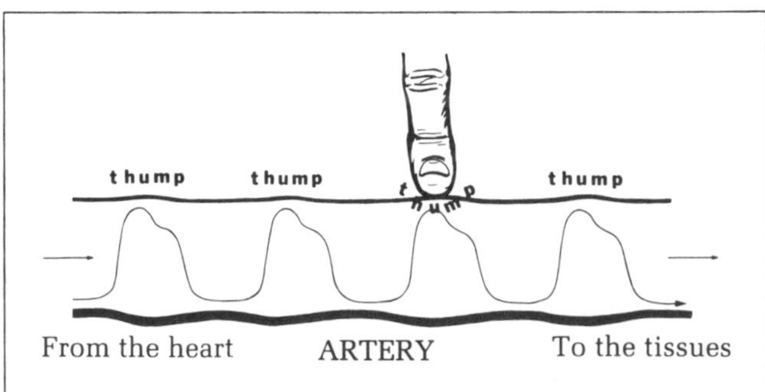

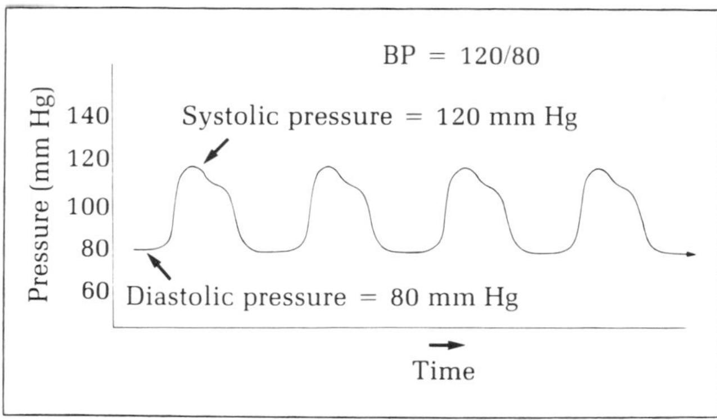

Fig. 8-3. *Blood pressure.*

pressure of 120 mm Hg and a diastolic pressure of 80 mm Hg, one would say that his blood pressure is "120 over 80," and it would be written "120/80" (Fig. 8-3).

Blood pressure is important because it provides the force necessary to drive the circulation. Blood pressure must remain above a certain minimum level in order to keep 6 liters of blood moving through the vast network of tubes. If the blood pressure falls below that minimum level, blood flow becomes sluggish and cannot supply the needs of the peripheral tissues for oxygen.

ARTERIES

The tubes that take the brunt of all this blood pressure are the arteries, for they are the vessels that carry blood *away* from the heart, and thus they are closest to the pumping force. In order to withstand this constant battering from one systolic wave after another, arteries have thick, muscular walls, which also permit the arteries to change their diameter by contracting. The major artery of the body is the *aorta*, which carries freshly oxygenated blood from the left ventricle. The aorta arches back behind the heart and then plunges down all the way to the lower abdomen, where it divides into the two femoral arteries. Other branches extend from the aorta all the way along its course and spread widely to carry oxygenated blood throughout the body. All of the systemic arteries, no matter where they are located, share two important characteristics: (1) blood flow through them is *pulsatile*, reflecting the contraction and relaxation of the ventricles; and (2) the blood moving within them is *oxygenated* and therefore bright red. These two characteristics help us to identify arterial bleeding, for if an artery is cut, *bright red blood* will come out in spurts, each spurt reflecting another squeeze, or systole, of the ventricles.

CAPILLARIES

As the arteries reach the organs of the body, they divide into smaller and smaller branches, finally terminating in the tiniest twigs of the circulatory system, the capillaries. Unlike the thick, muscular arteries, capillaries have very thin walls, which permit oxygen and nutrients to cross out of the blood into the tissues while carbon dioxide and other wastes move in the opposite direction, from the tissues into the blood. Thus the arterial blood that enters the capillaries bright red emerges at the other end of the capillaries a much darker, bluish red, testifying to the fact that the blood has given up its oxygen to the tissues in between. At their distal end, capillaries connect up with tiny veins, and the oxygen-poor blood starts its trek back to the heart.

VEINS

Veins occupy the *low-pressure side* of the circulatory system. Arteries lie in the direct path of the ventricle's force and thus sustain the full impact of each systole; veins experience relatively low pressures, for by the time the blood reaches the veins it is just meandering slowly out of the capillaries. The veins therefore do not have to be nearly as strong and muscular as the arteries. This low pressure in the veins turns out to be quite useful to the circulation, for it aids in returning blood to the heart, since fluids tend naturally to move from an area of higher pressure (like the arteries) to an area of lower pressure (like the veins).

Blood from the whole capillary system returns to the heart through the veins. Capillaries join with very tiny veins, which in turn join to form larger and larger veins, until they all empty into the two venae cavae: the superior vena cava, which receives all the blood returning from the head, neck, shoulders, and upper extremities; and the inferior vena cava, which drains the abdomen, pelvis, and lower extremities. Both venae cavae dump their blood into the right atrium of the heart, and the whole cycle starts over.

All of the systemic veins share two characteristics: (1) the blood flow through them is slow and *steady*, and (2) the blood passing through them is *poor in oxygen* and therefore dark, bluish red. Thus if a vein is cut, dark red blood will ooze or flow in a steady stream from the wound.

The Major Tubes: Arteries and Veins

Arteries	*Veins*
High-pressure side of the system	Low-pressure side of the system
Thick, muscular walls	Thin walls
Pulsatile flow	Steady flow
Bright red blood	Dark, bluish-red blood

BLOOD

The fluid moving through the whole circulatory system is the blood, a red, sticky substance that literally carries life (in the form of oxygen and nourishment) to the remotest frontiers of the body. The blood is actually a very complex fluid, made up of both liquid and cellular elements. The liquid is **plasma**, and in addition to blood cells, the plasma carries all sorts of proteins and mineral elements necessary for proper maintenance of various tissues. Plasma accounts for about half the volume of the blood, the other half being composed of cells. Chief among these are the *red blood cells* (RBCs), or **erythrocytes**, whose sole function is to ferry oxygen from the lungs to the tissues and carbon dioxide from the tissues to the lungs. They are able to carry out this job thanks to a special protein, called **hemoglobin** (*hemo-* = blood + *-globin* = protein), which grabs hold of oxygen in the lungs and then unloads the oxygen in the tissues. Hemoglobin is a pigment, and when it is combined with oxygen it turns bright red, whereas when it releases oxygen it becomes a darker, almost bluish color. Thus it is hemoglobin that gives the red blood cell, and the blood as a whole, its characteristic color.

In addition to red blood cells, the blood contains two other cellular elements: *white blood cells* (WBCs, or **leukocytes**) and *platelets* (**thrombocytes**). Whereas red blood cells are oxygen ferry boats, white blood cells are soldiers whose job it is to defend the body against invasion from foreign forces, such as bacteria. The moment the body's barriers are breached, the white blood cells rush to the spot to fight off enemy bacteria. Thus, for example, if you scrape your knee on the pavement, thousands of bacteria that are everywhere in the environment will immediately attempt to establish a beachhead where the skin is broken. But at the same time, a battalion of white blood cells will speed to the scene and start gulping up the bacteria in an attempt to wipe them out before they can produce an infection. Whenever a person is injured or infected, the body mobilizes the white cell army by calling up the reserves, that is, by increasing the production of leukocytes. If we examine the blood of a person with an injury or infection, we will find the number of white blood cells is increased, and we say that the person has a "high white count," or *leukocytosis*.

The third cellular element of the blood is the platelet. The platelet is a plumber, whose job is to repair leaks in the tubing. If one of the tubes is cut and blood starts to ooze out into the air, the platelets in the area release substances that combine with proteins in the blood to plug up the leak. This is the process we call *clotting*, and under normal circumstances clotting takes about 6 to 10 minutes.

Composition of the Blood

plasma	clear, yellowish fluid that carries the cells and also contains many proteins and minerals
red blood cell	ferry boat: carries oxygen
white blood cell	soldier: fights infection
platelet	plumber: repairs leaks by promoting clotting

BLEEDING

Since every organ in the body depends on a continuous stream of blood to furnish oxygen and nutrients, virtually any hole in the vascular system through which blood can escape the circulation is potentially dangerous. When blood escapes from the tubing of the vascular system, we call it bleeding, or **hemorrhage** (*hemo-* = blood + *-rrhagia* = profuse flow), and the seriousness of the hemorrhage depends on how much blood is lost, how rapidly it is lost, and how much there is to begin with. An adult man, for instance, who normally has 6 liters (12 pints) of blood in his circulation, can comfortably tolerate a loss of 500 ml of blood, especially if this loss occurs over more than 10 to 15 minutes—as is the situation in donating a pint of blood. However, if the same person loses a larger quantity of blood, or even if he loses only a pint of blood but the loss occurs very rapidly, he may develop signs and symptoms of shock. Now take a newborn infant, whose *total* blood volume is only in the neighborhood of 300 ml. Clearly it would take very little bleeding to have serious consequences in someone that small.

Bleeding may be *external*, visible from a wound on the surface of the body, or *internal*, within the body. Both external and internal bleeding, if profuse, are potentially fatal within minutes to hours, and the EMT must be aware of the measures that can be taken to control bleeding.

EXTERNAL BLEEDING

External bleeding is a hemorrhage that can be seen coming from the surface of a wound. Theoretically, external bleeding can be classified according to its source—arterial, venous, or capillary. *Arterial bleeding*, as described earlier, is characterized by the rhythmic spurting of bright red blood from the wound, and because the blood on the arterial side of the circuit is under high pressure, a great deal of blood can gush out of an artery in a very short time.

Furthermore, the force with which the blood spurts through a significant cut in an artery makes it very difficult for the platelets to do their job of plugging up the leak, for each time they start to glue a clot in place, another jet of blood comes along and blows the clot right out of the hole. Thus, unless the hole in the artery is a very small one or the artery itself is quite small, arterial bleeding is not likely to stop by itself. *Venous bleeding,* on the other hand, is characteristically a slow and steady flow of dark, bluish-red blood. Because the blood is under less pressure on the venous side of the circulation, venous bleeding is somewhat easier to control and is more apt to stop by itself as the clotting process takes effect. Nonetheless, a person *can* bleed to death from a significant opening in a vein—it will just take a little longer—so venous bleeding must also be controlled. *Capillary bleeding* is that which occurs from superficial wounds, such as a scraped elbow, and is characterized by slow oozing of blood that usually clots off by itself. Capillary bleeding alone does not pose a significant danger in terms of blood loss, and usually the main concern in wounds that involve only capillary bleeding is to prevent contamination by bacteria.

In practice, one usually sees a combination of arterial, venous, and capillary bleeding, especially in serious wounds where there has been a major disruption of tissue. Furthermore, significant bleeding requires treatment no matter what its source, so there is no point spending a lot of time scrutinizing the color of the blood and the characteristics of its flow. What *is* important is to realize that when you do see bright red blood spurting from a wound, this is a situation of extreme urgency and demands prompt treatment.

There are three principal methods to control external bleeding: (1) direct pressure, (2) pressure point control, and (3) tourniquet.

Direct Pressure

By far the most effective, not to mention the simplest, means of controlling external hemorrhage is to apply steady, direct pressure over the wound. Such pressure physically prevents any more blood from escaping the artery or vein, which gives the platelets a chance to glue a clot firmly in place over the hole.

Initially, direct pressure should be applied over the wound with whatever means you have immediately available. Ideally, you should place a sterile gauze pad over the wound and press down firmly on the pad with your fingers or the heel of your hand (Fig. 8-4). However, if you do not have a sterile pad handy, use any available means—a clean handkerchief, a sanitary napkin, a clean cloth, or even your bare hand.

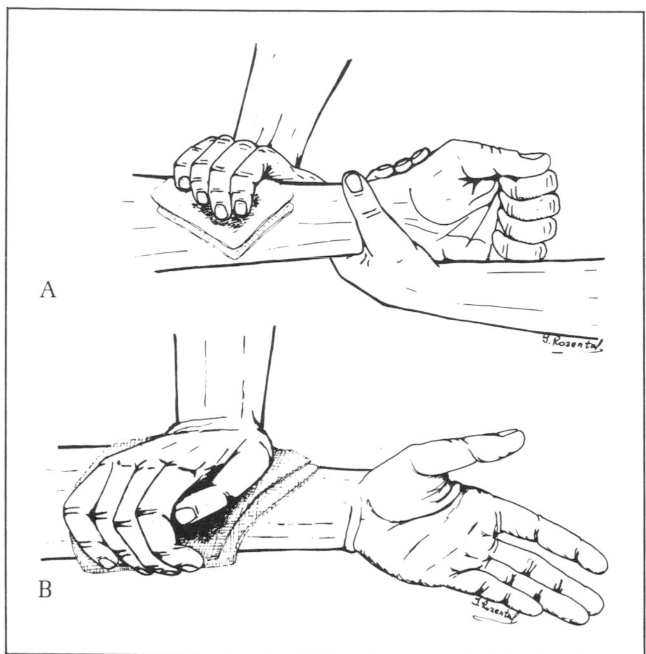

Fig. 8-4. *Manual control of bleeding by direct pressure on the wound. A. Pressure with the fingers. B. Pressure with the heel of the hand.*

Since you cannot tend to any of the victim's other injuries as long as you are holding pressure on the wound, you will want to replace direct manual pressure with a *pressure dressing* as soon as possible. To do this, remove your hand from the sterile pad over the wound, and apply a universal dressing (a bulky dressing, 9 × 36 in., or something similar) on top of the gauze pad. To apply the necessary pressure, wrap the wound circumferentially and firmly with a clean, self-adhering roller bandage. The bandage should cover the entire dressing, from above the wound to below the wound, and should be tight enough to stop the hemorrhage. However, if it is on an extremity, the bandage should not be so tight that it cuts off all circulation to the limb. To make sure, check a pulse distal to your pressure dressing (e.g., if the dressing is on the arm, check the radial pulse). If the pulse is absent, loosen the bandage just enough so that the pulse reappears. If the bleeding does not stop when the pressure dressing is in place, you will have to apply additional manual pressure over the dressing.

Needless to say, there are certain areas of the body where a pressure dressing is not practical, such as the neck (think about why). In these instances, pressure over the wound must be maintained manually.

Once a dressing has been put on a wound, it should not be taken off until the patient is examined by a doctor in the emergency room. Removing the dressing releases the pressure over the wound and disrupts the clotting process. Furthermore, taking the dressing off increases the risk of contaminating the wound. Should the dressing become soaked, do *not* change it, but simply add another clean dressing on top of it.

Direct pressure may also be applied to a wound with inflatable pressure splints or, if the wound is on the lower extremities, an inflatable garment known as the Military Anti-Shock Trousers (MAST). The use of the latter device will be described in detail in Chapter 9.

Remember:

DIRECT PRESSURE ON THE WOUND IS THE FASTEST, EASIEST, SAFEST, AND MOST EFFECTIVE WAY TO STOP BLEEDING.

Pressure Point Control

If bleeding persists despite direct pressure, compression over the supplying artery can sometimes control the bleeding. In general, pressure point control is not as effective in controlling hemorrhage as direct pressure over the wound, for it is rare that the bleeding vessel is supplied only by the artery you are compressing. Compression over the supplying artery is unlikely to stop bleeding altogether, but it may slow the bleeding down to the point where direct pressure over the wound is more effective.

The location of the arterial pressure points was discussed in Chapter 2. Among the several pressure points mentioned in that chapter, the ones that can be most effectively used to control bleeding are the *femoral,* for bleeding from the leg (Fig. 8-5A); the *brachial,* for bleeding from the arm (Fig. 8-5B); and the *carotid,* for bleeding from the neck. When pressure point control is used, the pressure must be strong enough to squeeze the artery shut against the bone behind it.

It must be emphasized that pressure point control should *never* be the first method applied to control bleeding. Pressure points may be difficult to locate, especially in a heavy person, and critical time can be wasted searching for an elusive pressure point while the victim's blood drains away unchecked by direct compression over the wound. Thus pressure point control should be regarded only as an adjunct to direct pressure, to be used together with direct pressure when the latter has been ineffective in controlling hemorrhage by itself.

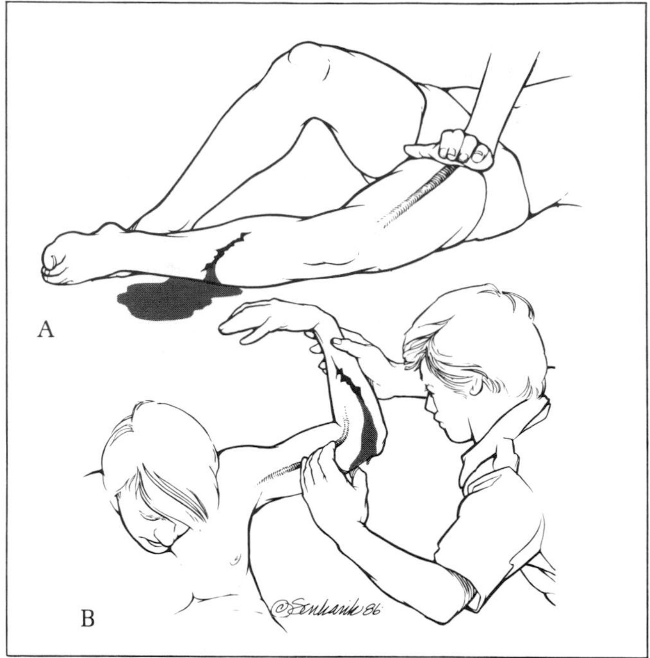

Fig. 8-5. *Pressure point control of bleeding. A. On the femoral artery. B. On the brachial artery.*

Tourniquet

The use of a tourniquet to control bleeding must be considered a *last resort.* It is very rare indeed that external bleeding cannot be effectively controlled with the techniques described above, and a tourniquet may itself lead to significant injury. A tourniquet crushes the tissues beneath it and thereby can cause permanent damage to nerves and blood vessels. Furthermore, by its very nature, a tourniquet cuts of the *whole blood supply* to the limb distal to it. We know that tissues do not like being cut off from their blood supply; as we learned in earlier chapters, tissues deprived of circulation, and the oxygen carried therein, soon die. For this reason, if a tourniquet is left on for any significant period of time, the whole extremity distal to the tourniquet may die and have to be amputated (cut off). When you apply a tourniquet, then, you must accept the risk that you may be sacrificing the extremity involved.

Nevertheless, a properly applied tourniquet can in some instances save the life of a person whose bleeding is uncontrollable by any other means. In such a case, the risk of losing the extremity is acceptable, for as the rule of triage states: *the salvage of life takes precedence over the salvage of limb.* Such a case may occur, for example, in a patient whose arm or leg has been partially amputated in an accident and in whom direct pressure over the wound and pressure point control have not succeeded in slowing the hemorrhage from major arteries.

If a tourniquet is used, it must be applied correctly. A tourniquet applied too loosely may actually *increase* bleeding because it permits blood to keep flowing into the extremity through the arteries but shuts off the exit of blood from the extremity through

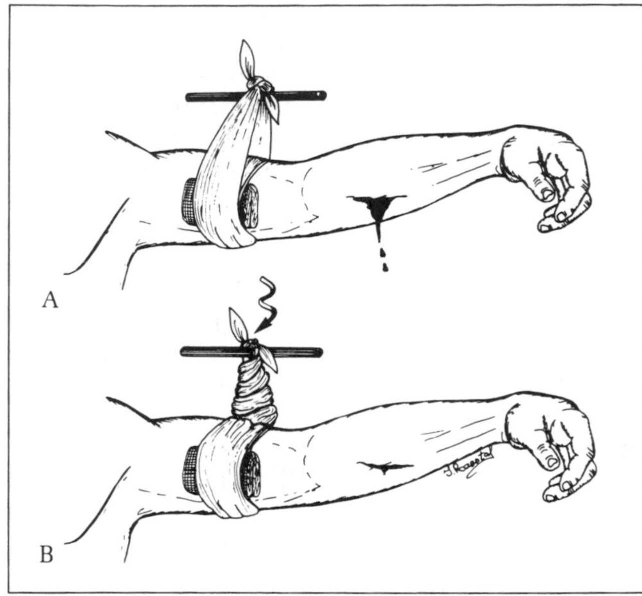

Fig. 8-6. *Use of a tourniquet. A. Cravat is wrapped twice around arm over padded artery. B. Cravat is twisted with a stick until bleeding slows and can be controlled thereafter by direct pressure.*

the veins. A tourniquet fashioned from inappropriate materials may cut into the skin and injure tissues beneath. Thus strict attention to technique is required whenever a tourniquet is used.

To apply a tourniquet, use a wide, flat material of sufficient length. A triangular bandage folded 3 or 4 times so that it is about 3 or 4 inches wide is ideal. If a triangular bandage is not available, a scarf, handkerchief, or wide belt may be used. Do *not* use narrow materials such as a wire or rope, for these may cut into the skin and damage underlying tissue. Choose a spot proximal to the bleeding but as far distal on the arm or thigh as possible, and wrap the tourniquet *twice* around the spot. Do not place a tourniquet below the knee or elbow because of the possibility of injuring nerves that lie close to the skin in the leg and forearm. If the site for the tourniquet happens to coincide with an arterial pressure point (e.g., over the brachial pulsation), apply a pad over the artery before wrapping the extremity (Fig. 8-6A). Tie the ends of the bandage with half a square knot; place a stick, pencil, or similar object on top of the half-knot; and tie the ends of the bandage over the stick to complete the square knot. Then twist the stick to tighten the bandage *until the bleeding slows and no further* (Fig. 8-6B). Secure the stick in that position, and leave it there. Do not loosen the tourniquet once it is in place. When an appropriate bandage cannot be found to make a tourniquet, a blood pressure cuff can be used instead. The cuff is wrapped proximal to the wound and inflated just to the point where bleeding slows and no further. To minimize leakage of air from the cuff, the tubing can be clamped off with a hemostat.

Whatever you use as a tourniquet, do *not* cover the tourniquet with any sort of bandage, but leave it in full view so that it will not escape notice by medical personnel at the receiving hospital. As an added precaution, use a grease pencil or indelible marker to write "TK" on the patient's forehead, and attach a tag to the patient in a conspicuous place. The tag should indicate the location of the tourniquet and the exact time it was applied. Even with all these labels, it is still vital for the EMT to notify the receiving doctor or nurse that the victim has a tourniquet in place.

Tourniquets: Points to Remember

- Use a tourniquet ONLY AS A LAST RESORT, when all other methods to control bleeding have failed.
- Use WIDE, FLAT MATERIALS ONLY. Never use rope, wire, or anything else that can cut into the skin.
- Never place a tourniquet below the knee or elbow.
- TIGHTEN a tourniquet UNTIL THE BLEEDING SLOWS AND NO FURTHER.
- Once the tourniquet has been properly tightened, DO NOT LOOSEN IT or remove it.
- NEVER CONCEAL A TOURNIQUET lest it escape notice by hospital personnel.
- Be triply sure that the medical team receiving the patient knows a tourniquet is in place:
  1. Write "TK" on the patient's forehead.
  2. Attach a TAG to the patient, indicating the LOCATION of the tourniquet and the TIME it was APPLIED.
  3. TELL the doctor that a tourniquet was applied.

Ancillary Measures

When hemorrhage is from an extremity, there are two additional measures that may assist in the control of bleeding: (1) elevation of the extremity and (2) splinting.

ELEVATION OF THE EXTREMITY. If an injured arm or leg is raised above the level of the rest of the body, the amount of blood reaching the limb will be diminished for simple hydraulic reasons, for the pressure driving the blood has to overcome gravity. A wounded leg may be raised on pillows, while an injured arm can be held above the victim's head. If, however, there is any reason to suspect a fracture of the extremity, it should not be elevated or subjected to any other motion unless it has been immobilized in a splint.

SPLINTING. In many cases, bleeding from an injured extremity occurs because the sharp ends of broken bones pierce the surrounding tissues or because the blood vessels in the bones themselves continue to bleed. As long as the fracture remains unstable, the broken bone ends can continue to tear into muscle, and the clotting process in blood vessels already lacerated is constantly disrupted. Often putting a splint on a fractured, bleeding extremity is all that is required to permit very rapid control of bleeding that was otherwise profuse. Even in instances where no fracture has occurred, motion of an extremity promotes blood flow into the limb and thereby increases bleeding. Thus it is a good general rule to splint *any* extremity in which there is significant bleeding.

> SPLINT A WOUNDED EXTREMITY.

The management of severe external bleeding is summarized in Figure 8-7.

NOSEBLEED: A SPECIAL CASE

A nosebleed (**epistaxis**) is a common emergency and often regarded as trivial. But a person can lose substantial amounts of blood from a nosebleed, sometimes enough even to cause shock. The blood seen coming from the nose may be only a fraction of the total blood lost, for usually much of the blood flows down the throat and is swallowed. If the patient swallows enough blood, often he will become sick to his stomach and vomit dark clots.

Most nosebleeds result from injury to the blood vessels in the anterior part of the nose, after a direct blow to the face, and these are usually controlled without too much difficulty. Nosebleeds may also be caused by infection in the nasal passages or sinuses, by high blood pressure, by bleeding disorders in which the ability of the blood to clot is impaired, and by a fractured skull. The extent to which a nosebleed can or should be controlled will depend very much on what caused it.

> **Causes of Epistaxis**
> - Facial injury
> - Nasal infection or sinusitis
> - High blood pressure
> - Bleeding disorders
> - Skull fracture

To begin with, it is important for the EMT to know when *not* to try to stop a nosebleed. When there has been a serious head injury, bleeding from the nose (or ears) may indicate that the skull has been fractured. If this is the case, an attempt to stop the nosebleed can be dangerous, for if blood is prevented from escaping through the nose, it can accumulate within the skull, causing a rise in the pressure inside the skull (increased *intracranial* pressure) and consequent damage to the brain. For this reason, if you have any reason to suspect skull fracture (see Chapter 14), do *not* attempt to stop any flow of blood from the patient's nose or ears.

> WHEN YOU SUSPECT SKULL FRACTURE, DO NOT TRY TO DAM UP THE FLOW OF BLOOD FROM THE NOSE OR EARS.

Nosebleeds from causes other than skull fracture *should* be given initial treatment at the scene. The patient should be kept in a sitting position (unless there are signs of shock, in which case he must be recumbent), preferably leaning slightly forward (Fig. 8-8A). He should be kept calm and quiet, especially if he suffers from high blood pressure, for agitation and anxiety will increase the blood pressure and promote further hemorrhage. Excited or hysterical bystanders should be kept at a distance, and the patient himself should be given quiet reassurance.

Apply pressure either by pinching the victim's nostrils (Fig. 8-8B) or by placing a rolled gauze pad betweeen his upper lip and gum and pressing over the upper lip. The patient may be able to apply enough pressure himself if he can stretch his upper lip tightly over the gauze pad. If ice is available, it is often helpful to apply an ice pack to the nose as well. Wrap the ice in a towel or similar material, and hold it firmly over the patient's nose.

> **Treatment of Simple Epistaxis**
> - Keep the patient SITTING UP, unless there are signs of shock.
> - Keep the patient quiet.
> - Pinch the patient's nostrils, or
> - Place a rolled dressing between the patient's upper lip and gum, and press.
> - Apply an ICE PACK, if available, over the nose.

Most nosebleeds arising from the anterior part of the nose can be controlled by the methods outlined above. Some nosebleeds, however, arise in the *posterior* portion of the nasopharynx, especially in older patients suffering from high blood pressure, and epistaxis of this type cannot be readily controlled in the field. The only way to stop this kind of epistaxis is to pack both the anterior and posterior nasal passages with dressings, and this has to be done by a doctor in a medical facility. Thus any patient whose nosebleed

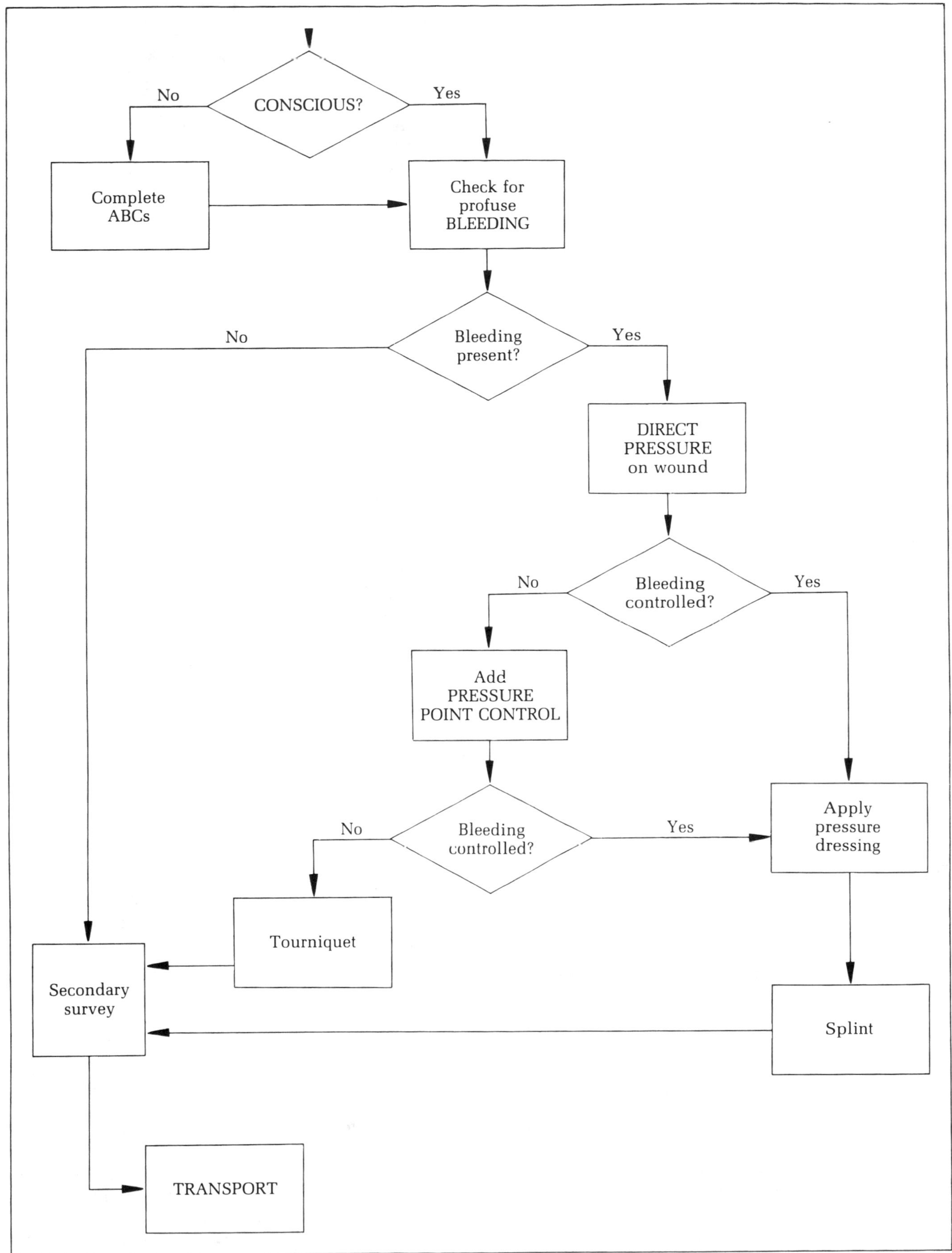

Fig. 8-7. *Control of external hemorrhage.*

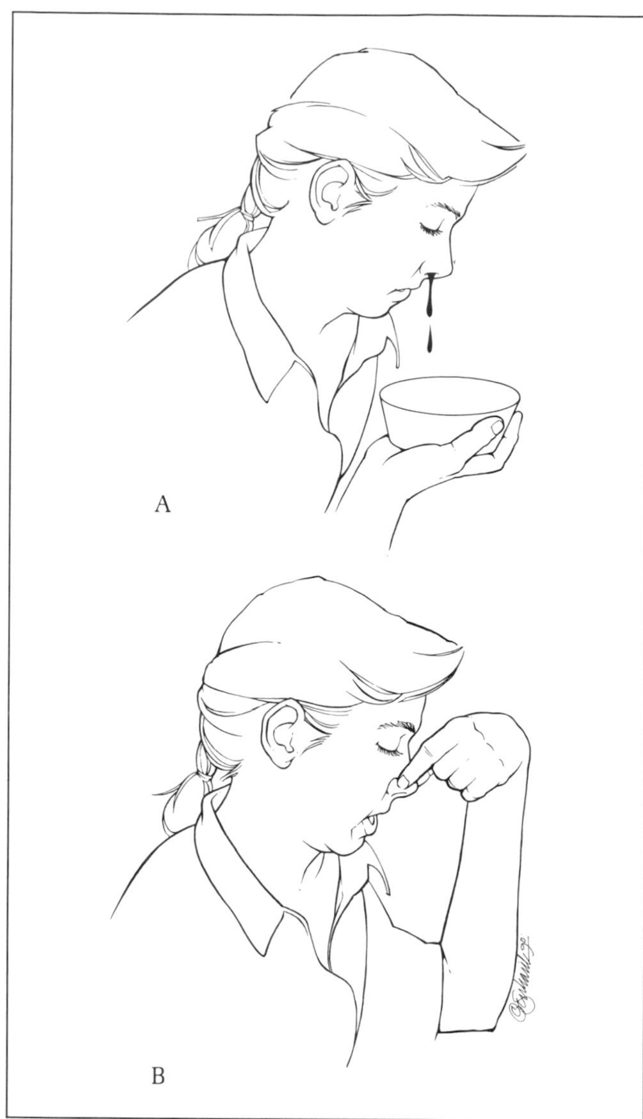

Fig. 8-8. *Control of epistaxis. A. Have the patient sit up, leaning slightly forward, and instruct her to breathe through her mouth. B. Pinch the nostrils shut.*

is not rapidly controlled by pressure, or whose nosebleed recurs after stopping, must be taken to the hospital and seen by a physician.

THE PATIENT WHOSE NOSEBLEED IS DIFFICULT TO STOP MUST BE BROUGHT TO THE HOSPITAL.

INTERNAL BLEEDING

Internal bleeding is not visible on the surface of the body, although in some instances blood may emerge through one of the body orifices. A patient bleeding internally from a stomach ulcer, for example, may vomit blood or pass blood through the rectum. Blood may appear in the urine of a person who has suffered injury to the kidneys or bladder, or a woman may pass blood from her vagina at a time when she is not having her menstrual period. All of these are signs of internal bleeding and must be regarded as serious. In many cases, however, especially in victims of trauma, there may be massive internal bleeding without any external signs of blood at all. This is probably the most dangerous kind of bleeding, for it is apt to be overlooked if the EMT is not very alert to the mechanisms of the injury and signs of shock (see Shock, next). A person who suffers a closed fracture of the femur (a fracture without any break in the skin) can lose as much as 3 units of blood into the surrounding tissues. Blunt trauma to the abdomen with rupture of the spleen or liver can cause the loss of the entire blood volume into the abdominal cavity. Thus a person can literally bleed to death (**exsanguinate**) internally without spilling a single drop of blood outside the body.

There is very little an EMT can do in the field, without equipment, for internal bleeding, and when internal bleeding is suspected, the emphasis must be on moving the patient to the hospital as rapidly as possible. If the bleeding is within an extremity, such as in the thigh after a fractured femur, the extremity should be splinted prior to transport. If the bleeding is in a major body cavity, such as the abdomen, the victim should be treated for shock, as described below.

SHOCK

As we learned earlier, the circulatory system requires three intact components in order to function properly: a working pump (the heart), a closed network of tubing (arteries, capillaries, and veins), and an adequate volume of fluid (blood) within the tubing. If any one of these components is damaged, the circulation of blood within the tissues (called **perfusion** of the tissues) will be jeopardized, and a condition called **shock** will occur.

The word *shock* has many meanings. To lay people, it usually means an unpleasant surprise or the feeling you get when you stick your finger into a light socket. In medicine, shock has a different and very specific meaning. Most simply stated, shock exists when there is *inadequate perfusion of the tissues by the blood.* An organ is perfused if there is blood entering it through the arteries and blood leaving it through the veins, and every organ in the body depends on constant perfusion to bring food and oxygen and to take away waste products. The moment perfusion slows down below a critical minimum rate or stops altogether, the organs involved begin to suffocate and die.

Shock can occur if there is a malfunction of any one of the three components of the circulatory system—the pump, the tubing, or the fluid—and the *type* of shock involved is classified according to which component has failed. Let us look at these types of shock one at a time.

To begin with, shock can occur because of a breakdown of the *pump*, that is, severe damage to the heart. If a person suffers a major heart attack, for example, the injury to heart muscle may be so extensive that the heart simply cannot squeeze effectively and therefore it cannot push the blood along through the circulation. As a result, blood flow becomes more and more sluggish, and the other organs of the body are not perfused at a rate sufficient to supply their needs for oxygen and nutrients. When shock is due to damage to the heart, it is called **cardiogenic shock** (*cardio-* = heart + *-genic* = caused by).

Shock can also occur because of malfunctioning in the *tubing*. Normally, the diameter of arteries and veins is controlled by the nervous system and is constantly readjusted according to the amount of blood available. Recall that the 6 liters of blood normally present in an adult exerts a certain pressure (blood pressure) within the vascular system, and it is this pressure that keeps the blood moving. Now if the arteries and veins were just ordinary tubes and you lost a pint of fluid from the system, the pressure inside the tubes would drop and might no longer be adequate to maintain the circulation. Fortunately, arteries and veins are *not* ordinary tubes at all, and when a person loses a small amount of blood, the blood vessels *constrict* to provide a smaller bed for the reduced volume of blood. Thus the blood pressure is maintained, for even though the volume of blood becomes smaller, the container (blood vessels) becomes smaller as well, so the pressure inside the container stays at the same level.

Under normal circumstances, the nervous system is constantly readjusting the diameter of the blood vessels to compensate for changes in posture (e.g., going from a lying to a standing position) and for variations in fluid volume within the body. But suppose something were to happen to this control system and the blood vessels could not contract—that instead the muscles in the blood vessel walls relaxed completely. As the diameters of all the vessels increased, we would suddenly have a much larger container, far too large for the amount of blood available. The blood pressure would plummet, and there would consequently be insufficient pressure to maintain the circulation. Once again, we would have a state of shock—of inadequate tissue perfusion—but this time because of a malfunction in the tubing. When shock occurs for this reason, it is called **neurogenic shock** (*neuro-* = *nerve* + *-genic* = caused by), that is, shock caused by loss of vascular control by the nervous system. Neurogenic shock can occur when there is direct damage to the nervous system itself, as in a spinal cord injury, or it can follow overdose of certain drugs, such as barbiturates. Some episodes of fainting are also examples of a temporary state of neurogenic shock.

Finally, shock can occur when there is significant loss of *fluid* from the system, a condition called **hypovolemic shock** (hypo- = deficient + *-volemic* = volume). The most obvious type of hypovolemic shock is **hemorrhagic shock,** which occurs when the fluid lost from the body is *whole blood*. However, people can lose massive amounts of other fluids in other ways. In severe burns, for example, there are often considerable losses of *plasma* across the damaged skin. People with significant vomiting or diarrhea can lose large volumes of fluid through the gastrointestinal tract. Profuse sweating can result in dangerous fluid loss if not compensated by an increased intake of water. One can even "lose" fluids within the body itself, as when there is an inflammation in the abdomen and fluids ooze out of blood vessels to pour into the abdominal cavity. In all of these situations, if the loss of fluids is significant enough, hypovolemic shock will result.

In some instances, more than one component of the circulatory system can be affected by illness or injury, and the resulting state of shock will be a combination of two or more of the above general types. This is the case, for example, in **septic shock,** which sometimes occurs in patients with severe bacterial infections. Septic shock combines elements of neurogenic shock (widespread dilation of blood vessels) and hypovolemic shock (leakage of large amounts of plasma from the capillaries). Similarly, **anaphylactic shock,** a kind of shock that occurs with a violent allergic reaction, has features of neurogenic shock and cardiogenic shock.

Types of Shock

- **Cardiogenic shock** (*pump* failure)
- **Neurogenic shock** (failure of the *tubing* to constrict)
- **Hypovolemic shock** (inadequate volume of *fluid*)
  1. Loss of BLOOD (hemorrhagic shock)
  2. Loss of PLASMA (burns)
  3. Loss of GASTROINTESTINAL FLUIDS (vomiting, diarrhea)
  4. Loss of SWEAT
  5. Internal losses (peritonitis)
- Mixed types
  1. Septic shock (from severe infection)
  2. Anaphylactic shock (severe allergic reaction)

In all of the above types of shock, the net result is the same: The perfusion of blood through the tissues of the body is inadequate to provide the oxygen that the tissues require for survival. And if the condition

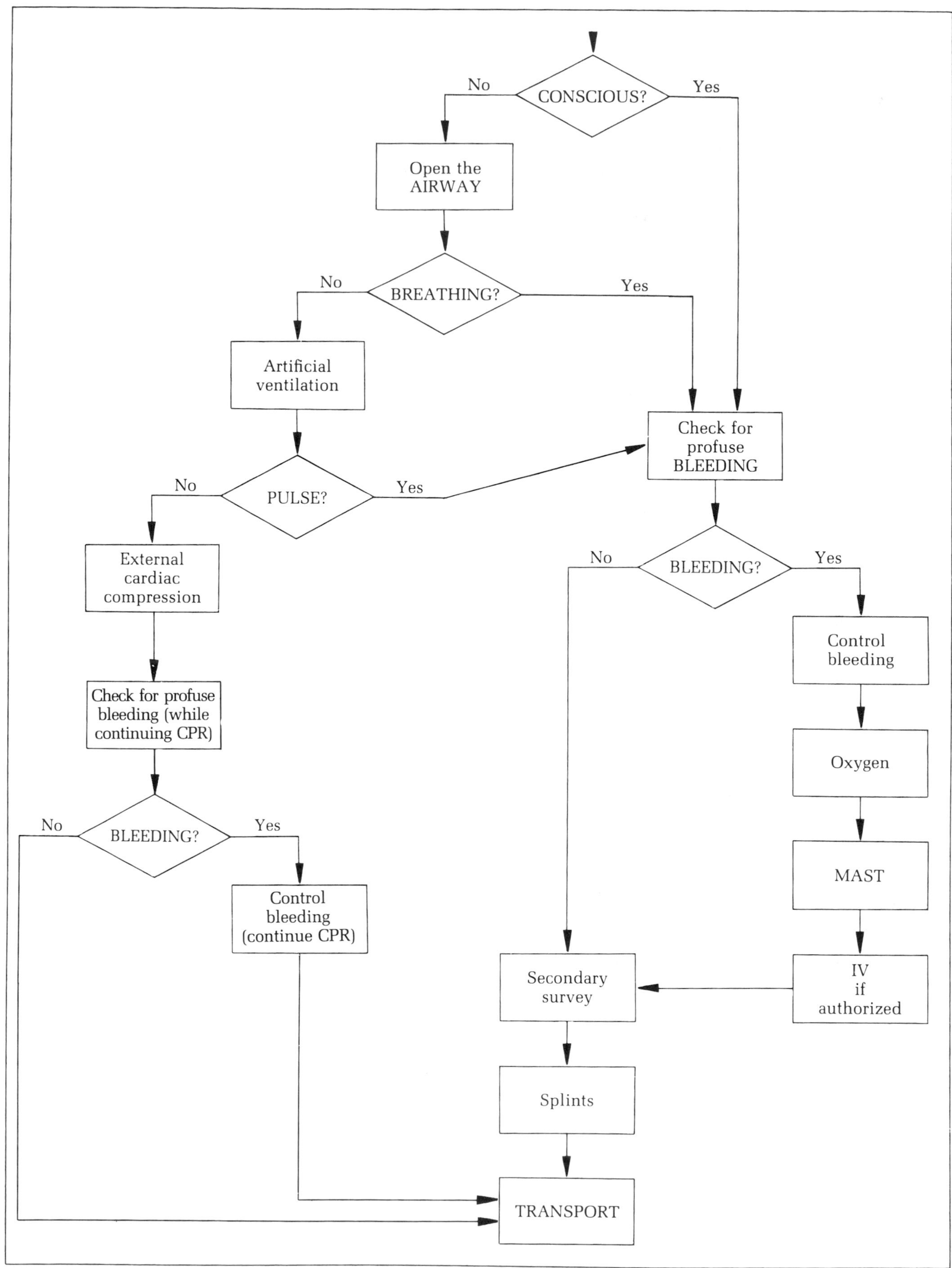

Fig. 8-9. *Treatment of hemorrhagic shock.*

if we decreased the number of people carrying buckets from 10 to 5, then each of the remaining bucket carriers had to run twice as fast and make two trips per minute, rather than one, to keep up the same supply of water (10 buckets/min) at the fire. At this rate, sooner or later our bucket carriers are going to run out of energy and be unable to maintain the water supply. But suppose each of our 5 remaining bucket carriers could take *two buckets of water at a time*. Then they could slow down and make only one trip per minute between the well and the fire. This is just what happens when we give oxygen to the patient in hemorrhagic shock. Each red cell now finds much more oxygen available in the alveoli, so each red cell can grab two or three times its normal oxygen load and carry it to the tissues. Thus the red cells do not have to rush so fast between the lungs and the tissues, and the heart does not have to work so hard to keep them speeding along.

As soon as you get a chance, SPLINT any obvious FRACTURES. Splinting will often help control bleeding and will also decrease the pain in a fractured extremity. Alleviating pain is very important in shock, not just for reasons of compassion, but because pain itself can aggravate shock.

Keep the victim at normal body temperature. Usually this means covering the victim with a BLANKET to prevent heat loss from the body. Extreme warmth should be avoided, however, so do not turn the heaters in the ambulance on full blast unless the weather is cold or the victim is clearly shivering.

Do not give the patient anything to eat or drink. If you are trained and authorized to do so, give fluid by the intravenous route but NOTHING BY MOUTH. If the patient complains of intense thirst, as is often the case in shock, his discomfort may be somewhat relieved by allowing him to such on a moistened gauze pad.

When you have finished treating the victim's major problems, make a RECORD of HIS VITAL SIGNS (pulse, blood pressure, and rate of respirations), and continue to check and record those signs at 5-minute intervals thereafter. Then prepare the victim for transport, and move him to the hospital as expeditiously as possible.

The importance of getting a severely injured patient promptly to the hospital cannot be overemphasized. This does not mean that you should return to the "swoop and scoop" tactics of the old days. What it does mean is that the EMT must rapidly determine what has to be done at the scene and do what has to be done as efficiently as possible. In other words, DO THE JOB RIGHT, BUT DON'T DAWDLE!

Treatment of Hemorrhagic Shock

1. Secure and maintain a clear AIRWAY.
2. Give ventilatory assistance as needed (BREATHING)
3. If there is cardiac arrest, start external cardiac compressions (CIRCULATION).
4. Control all obvious BLEEDING.
5. Administer OXYGEN as soon as possible.
6. If you are more than 20 minutes from the hospital, apply Military Anti-Shock Trousers (MAST); if MAST is not available, elevate the victim's legs.
7. If you are trained and authorized to do so, start an INTRAVENOUS INFUSION with Ringer's solution or normal saline.
8. Give NOTHING BY MOUTH.
9. SPLINT fractures.
10. Cover the victim with a BLANKET.
11. Record the victim's VITAL SIGNS, and recheck every few minutes.
12. Transfer the patient to the HOSPITAL promptly.

VOCABULARY

anaphylactic shock Form of shock occurring as a result of a violent allergic reaction.

cardiogenic shock Failure of perfusion caused by damage to the pump, the heart.

diastole The period of the cardiac cycle when the ventricles are relaxing and refilling with blood.

diastolic pressure The low point of the blood pressure.

epistaxis Nosebleed.

erythrocyte Red blood cell.

exsanguination Bleeding to death.

hemoglobin Pigmented protein in the red blood cell that carries oxygen and is responsible for the characteristic color of blood.

hemorrhage Profuse bleeding.

hemorrhagic shock Failure of tissue perfusion caused by loss of blood.

hypotension Low blood pressure, or deficient blood pressure.

hypovolemic shock Failure of tissue perfusion caused by a deficiency of the fluid volume in the body.

leukocyte White blood cell.

mm Hg Abbreviation for millimeters of mercury, the units in which blood pressure is measured.

neurogenic shock Failure of tissue perfusion caused by massive dilation of blood vessels, due to failure of nervous system control.

perfusion The flow of blood through tissues.

platelet Thrombocyte; the cellular element of the blood responsible for repairing leaks in blood vessels and promoting clotting.

pulsatile Characterized by throbbing or rhythmic motion.

septic shock Failure of tissue perfusion caused by changes in the circulation that occur as a result of severe infection.

shock A state of inadequate tissue perfusion.

sphygmomanometer Device used to measure the blood pressure.

systole The phase of the cardiac cycle in which the ventricles are contracting.

systolic pressure The high point of the blood pressure.

tachycardia Rapid heart rate.

tachypnea Rapid breathing.

thrombocyte Platelet.

tourniquet Any device placed circumferentially on a limb to exclude the flow of blood into the limb.

FURTHER READING

Barber JM. EMT checkpoint: Early detection of hypovolemic states. *EMT J* 2(2):72, 1978.

Bennet BR. Shock: An approach to teaching EMTs normal physiology before pathophysiology. *EMT J* 2(1):41, 1978.

Carveth S, Olson D, Bechtel J. Emergency medical care system. *Arch Surg* 108:528, 1974.

Garvin JM. Keeping shock simple. *Emerg Med Serv* 9(5):49, 1980.

Geelhoed GW. Shock and its management. *Emerg Med Serv* 5(6):42, 1976.

Gervin AS, Fischer RP. The importance of prompt transport in salvage of patients with penetrating heart wounds. *J Trauma* 32:443, 1982.

Pedowitz R, Shackford S. Noncavitary hemorrhage producing shock in trauma patients: Incidence and severity. *J Trauma* 29:219, 1989.

Shock. *Emerg Med* 12(19):47, 1980.

9. MECHANICAL AIDS TO LIFE SUPPORT

OBJECTIVES

Up to this point, we have discussed those lifesaving techniques that can be performed without the use of any equipment. We started that way intentionally to emphasize that the EMT should never delay basic life support procedures in order to secure equipment. Every EMT has on his or her body all the equipment needed to open an airway, start rescue breathing, perform external cardiac compressions, and control bleeding. Critical time should never be wasted securing mechanical devices before initiating the ABCs of basic life support.

There is no doubt, however, that certain devices can make the ABCs more effective once begun, and in this chapter we will examine the use of equipment that can help in maintaining an airway, giving artificial ventilation, providing oxygen to the tissues, doing chest compressions, controlling hemorrhage, and treating shock. By the end of this chapter, the reader should be able to

1. List the indications and contraindications for use of (a) an oropharyngeal airway and (b) a nasopharyngeal airway
2. List the steps in inserting (a) an oropharyngeal airway and (b) a nasopharyngeal airway
3. List the equipment necessary to carry out suctioning of the patient's mouth and pharynx
4. List the steps in suctioning (a) through the mouth, (b) through the nose, and (c) through a laryngectomy stoma; and indicate the safety precautions necessary in suctioning a patient

*5. List the steps in suctioning the lower airway through an endotracheal tube, and indicate how the intubated patient should be prepared for suctioning

6. Identify which patients should receive oxygen, given a description of several patients with various conditions
7. Identify which patients are showing signs and symptoms of acute respiratory insufficiency, given a description of several patients with different signs and symptoms
8. List at least 10 causes of acute respiratory insufficiency
9. Explain the function of (a) the reducing valve, (b) the flow meter, and (c) the humidifier on the oxygen cylinder
10. Calculate the amount of oxygen remaining in a cylinder (in terms of duration of flow), given the size of the cylinder and the reading on the pressure gauge
11. List at least six safety precautions in the handling of oxygen cylinders
12. Identify situations in which oxygen cylinders have been improperly or unsafely handled,

*Not required of the EMT-A. Included here for students taking the EMT-Intermediate course.

given a description of several situations involving the use of oxygen

13. List in the proper sequence the steps in operating an oxygen cylinder
14. Indicate which device can deliver the highest oxygen concentration to a spontaneously breathing patient, given a list of various oxygen cannulas and masks
15. Indicate which device for providing oxygen to a nonbreathing patient is the preferred device if the patient does not have an esophageal obturator airway (EOA) or endotracheal tube in place, and list the reasons it is the preferred device
16. Identify the device(s) for providing controlled ventilation that (a) give the highest oxygen concentration, and (b) can also be used to assist ventilation
17. Indicate which device is most suited to providing oxygen to a patient, given a description of several patients with different medical problems

*18. Indicate under what circumstances an EOA should be used and in what circumstances it is contraindicated
*19. List in the correct sequence the steps of inserting an EOA
*20. Identify errors in the use of an EOA, given a description of incorrect uses, and indicate what complications may result from the errors in question
*21. Indicate under what circumstances the EOA may be removed, and describe the steps in removing it
*22. List at least three advantages of endotracheal intubation over other means of airway control
*23. Describe the steps in preparing for endotracheal intubation, and list the equipment that must be assembled
*24. Describe, or demonstrate on a manikin or fellow student, the correct position of a patient for endotracheal intubation
*25. List at least three ways of confirming that an endotracheal tube has been inserted in the right place
*26. Describe the appropriate action to take if (a) breath sounds are absent on one side of the chest after intubation and (b) breath sounds are absent on both sides of the chest after intubation
*27. State the maximum permissible time for an intubation attempt
*28. List the steps in carrying out suction through an endotracheal tube
*29. State the hazard involved in suctioning through an endotracheal tube, and describe what actions can be taken to minimize that hazard

30. List in the correct sequence the steps in using (a) a cardiac press and (b) a gas-powered chest compressor

*31. Calculate the heart rate, given a 6-second electrocardiogram (ECG) strip
*32. Identify which ECG rhythm requires defibrillation, given pictures of several ECG rhythms
*33. List three possible causes of artifacts in the ECG
*34. Identify which patients an EMT should monitor, given a description of several patients with various conditions
*35. List in the correct sequence the steps in managing (a) unwitnessed cardiac arrest and (b) witnessed cardiac arrest
*36. List in the correct sequence the steps of defibrillation
*37. Identify the correct (a) placement of defibrillator paddles and (b) energy levels for defibrillation, given several alternatives

38. Identify which patients should be treated with the MAST, given a description of several patients with different conditions
39. Identify which patients should *not* be treated with the MAST, given a description of several patients with different conditions
40. Identify for which patients only the leg sections of the MAST should be inflated, given a description of several patients
41. List in the correct sequence the steps in applying and inflating the MAST
42. Indicate under what conditions the MAST may be deflated, and describe the steps in so doing

*43. Identify which patients should receive intravenous therapy in the field, given a description of several patients
*44. Identify which intravenous solution should be used in the field to treat a patient in shock, given a list of different intravenous solutions
*45. Identify the signs and symptoms of a transfusion reaction, given a list of signs and symptoms of various conditions
*46. Describe the action to take if a patient develops a transfusion reaction
*47. List in the correct sequence the steps in establishing an intravenous (IV) infusion
*48. Indicate at what point in the overall care of a trauma patient the IV should be started
*49. List at least four potential complications of intravenous therapy, and indicate (a) how each of these complications can be prevented, (b) how each is recognized, and (c) how each is treated.

*Not required of the EMT-A. Included here for students taking the EMT-Intermediate course.

ARTIFICIAL AIRWAYS

The first step in treating any unconscious patient is to open the airway, and initially this is always done by manual methods (e.g, head tilt–neck lift, head tilt–chin lift). After the airway has been opened by manual methods, however, it may be desirable to use an artificial airway to keep the victim's airway unobstructed, especially if the rescuer needs to free his hands for other tasks. An artificial airway is particu-

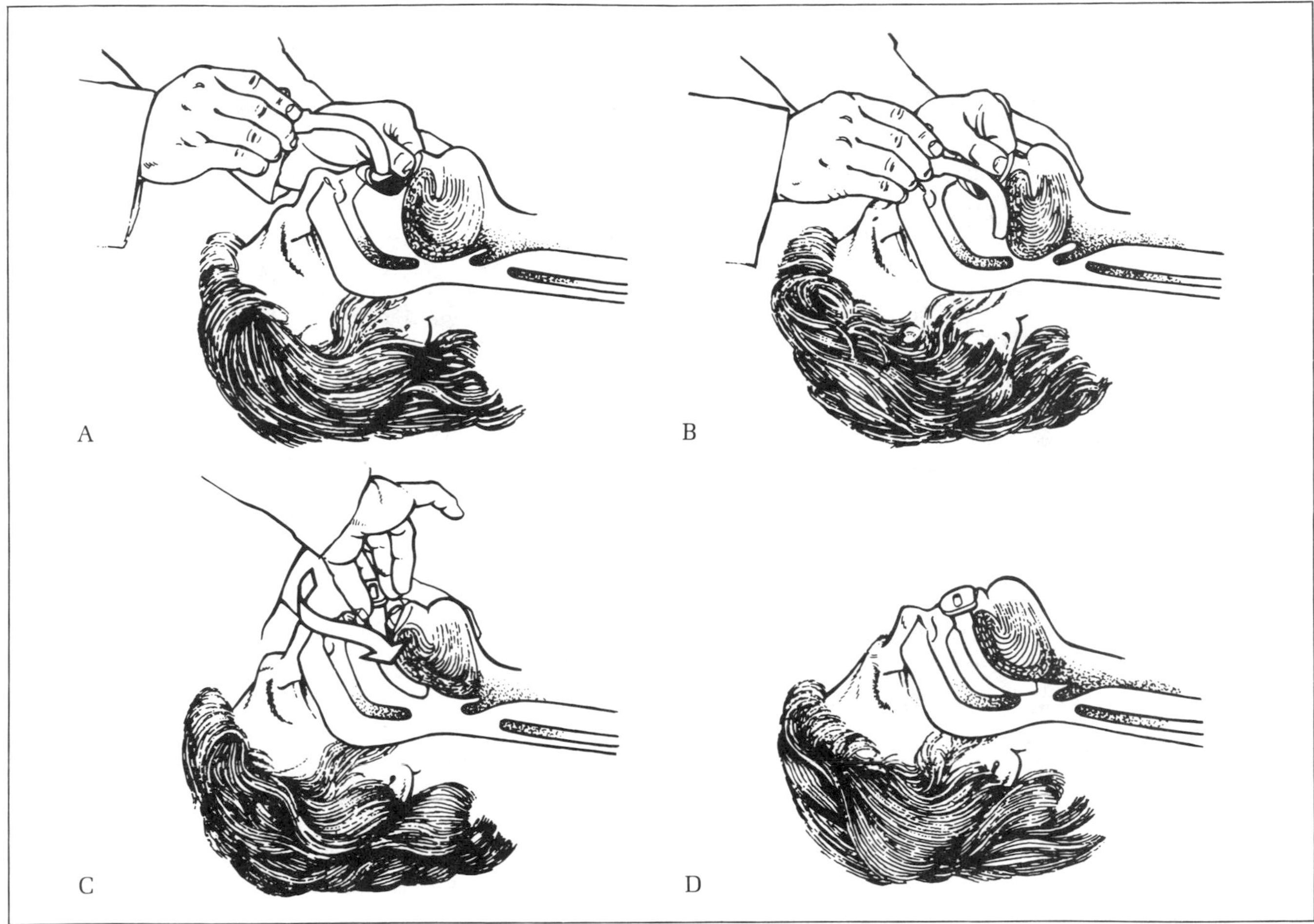

Fig. 9-1. *Insertion of oropharyngeal airway. (Reproduced courtesy Asmund Laerdal, Stavanger, Norway.)*

larly useful if the victim is breathing spontaneously or if rescue breathing is applied by a bag-mask device rather than by mouth-to-mouth or mouth-to-nose.

There are two types of artificial airway that an EMT may use in the field: the oropharyngeal airway and the nasopharyngeal airway.

THE OROPHARYNGEAL AIRWAY

As the name implies, the oropharyngeal airway extends from the mouth (*oro-*) into the back of the throat (*-pharyngeal*). The oropharyngeal airway is a curved, plastic or hard rubber device designed to fit over the back of the tongue and thereby hold the tongue away from the posterior part of the throat. Its curvature is such that it fits the natural curvature of the tongue.

The oropharyngeal airway is useful in deeply unconscious patients who are breathing spontaneously or who are being ventilated by a mask. It should NOT be used in conscious or semiconscious patients because their reflexes are still intact, and the presence of a hard piece of plastic against the back of the throat will cause gagging and sometimes vomiting and laryngospasm as well.

To insert an oropharyngeal airway (Fig. 9-1), first select an airway of the appropriate size for the patient. Oropharyngeal airways come in a range of sizes, to fit infants, children, and adults, and you need to choose the one that conforms best to the patient's dimensions. Hold the airway against the patient's face; if it is the right size, it will extend from the mouth to the angle of the jaw.

Having chosen an appropriate airway, hyperextend the patient's head, open the mouth using the crossed-finger technique, and begin to insert the airway *with the tip facing upward* (toward the roof of the patient's mouth). When the airway is about halfway in, rotate it 180 degrees so that the curvature follows that of the tongue, and continue to insert it until the flange rests against the patient's lips or teeth. The reason for rotating the airway as you insert it is to avoid pushing the tongue backward into the pharynx, which would cause airway obstruction. Another way to accomplish the same thing is to use a tongue blade to depress the tongue while you insert the airway. If the patient should begin to gag while you are putting in the oropharyngeal airway, remove

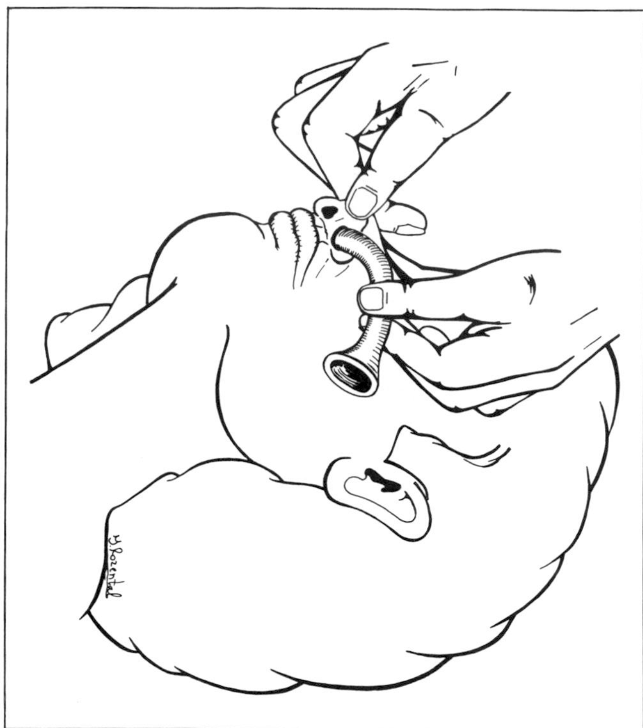

Fig. 9-2. *Insertion of nasopharyngeal airway.*

it immediately and do not make any further attempt to insert it.

> **Oropharyngeal Airway: Points to Remember**
> - Use ONLY in UNCONSCIOUS PATIENTS.
> - Avoid pushing the tongue backward as you insert the airway.
> - If the patient begins to gag, remove the airway at once.

THE NASOPHARYNGEAL AIRWAY

The nasopharyngeal airway is a soft rubber tube that is inserted through the nose (*naso-*) and extends down into the back of the pharynx, behind the tongue, thereby allowing free passage of air from the nose to the lower airways. This type of airway is better tolerated by semiconscious patients than is the oropharyngeal airway. The nasopharyngeal airway is useful in situations where (1) the patient's mouth cannot be opened, (2) there is trauma to the mouth or lower jaw, or (3) the patient is sufficiently awake that he will not tolerate an oropharyngeal airway but is not sufficiently conscious to maintain an open airway by himself. Since the nasopharyngeal airway comes in only one size, it can be used only in adults. The airway should NOT be used where there is trauma to the nose or bleeding from the nose suspected to be caused by skull fracture.

To insert the nasopharyngeal airway (Fig. 9-2), first lubricate it thoroughly with a water-soluble jelly, and then insert it gently into one nostril, following the natural curvature of the nasal passage (tip downward), until the flange rests against the nostril. Make sure you use a nasopharyngeal airway made of very soft, compressible rubber; the hard, plastic varieties cause unnecessary trauma to the nasal passages.

> **Nasopharyngeal Airway: Points to Remember**
> - Better tolerated than the oropharyngeal airway in semiconscious patients.
> - Do NOT use when there is trauma to the nose or suspected skull fracture.
> - Use only a nasopharyngeal airway made from SOFT RUBBER.
> - LUBRICATE the nasopharyngeal airway well before inserting.

ADVANCED AIRWAY CONTROL*

In many programs, EMT-Intermediates are trained in more invasive procedures for airway control and ventilation—the use of either the esophageal obturator airway (EOA) or the endotracheal tube. At the time of this writing, there is some controversy regarding the safety and efficacy of the EOA (see references on the subject cited under Further Reading). It is, furthermore, the view of this author that endotracheal intubation provides more definitive airway control and is therefore the preferred method. Because both techniques are currently taught in EMT-Intermediate programs, however, both are presented here. Instructors should decide which technique to teach according to local practice and the recommendations of national advisory boards.

ESOPHAGEAL OBTURATOR AIRWAY

The esophageal obturator airway (EOA) is a long tube, open at the proximal end and closed at the distal end, with numerous side holes in between (Fig. 9-3). As the name implies, the tube is designed to be inserted into the *esophagus*, and it attaches to a mask at its proximal end. When the tube is in place in the esophagus and the mask is sealed against the patient's face, air or oxygen forced into the tube will flow out through the side holes of the tube into the patient's pharynx. Since the esophagus is closed off, air will tend to go down the trachea into the lungs (Fig. 9-4). Thus the EOA is helpful in preventing gastric distention during artificial ventilation, and it thereby minimizes the incidence of regurgitation.

*The sections on the esophageal obturator airway and endotracheal intubation are intended for the EMT-Intermediate. These skills are not required of the EMT-A.

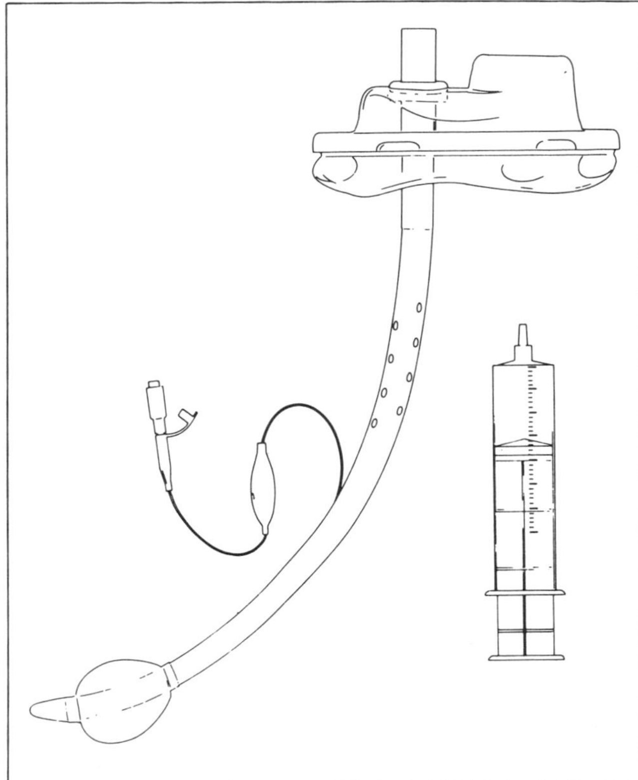

Fig. 9-3. *Esophageal obturator airway. (Reproduced courtesy Cavitron, Anaheim, California.)*

The name *esophageal obturator "airway"* is a bit misleading, for strictly speaking it is not an airway. While it does to some extent keep the tongue off the back of the throat by passing behind the tongue into the esophagus, it does not by itself maintain an adequately open airway. Thus the EOA is *not* a substitute for proper head position. It is simply a type of mask that happens to provide a means for minimizing regurgitation during artificial ventilation.

The primary indication for using the EOA is the situation of full CARDIOPULMONARY ARREST, for the device can be used only in deeply unconscious patients. In conscious or semiconscious patients, insertion of a rigid tube into the esophagus will cause gagging and vomiting. The EOA also should *not* be used in children under 16 years old (the obturator may be too large for the esophagus) or in any patient known to have swallowed a corrosive substance (the obturator may perforate the damaged wall of the esophagus).

Do Not Use the Esophageal Obturator Airway in

- Conscious or semiconscious patients
- Children under 16 years old
- Patients known to have swallowed corrosive substances

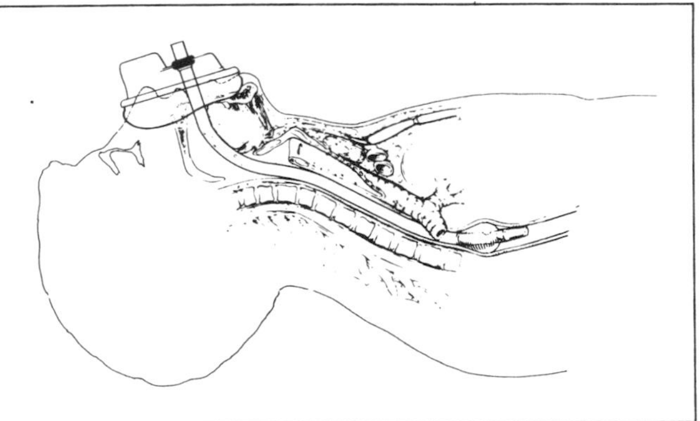

Fig. 9-4. *EOA in position in the esophagus. (Reproduced courtesy Cavitron, Anaheim, California.)*

Insertion of the EOA

Insertion of the EOA requires at least two rescuers, for one or more rescuers must initiate and continue CPR while another prepares the EOA. Furthermore, it is preferable that the patient be well oxygenated before any attempt is made to insert the EOA, so CPR must be initiated with mouth-to-mouth methods and then continued with a pocket mask and oxygen or bag-valve-mask and oxygen while one rescuer sets up for EOA insertion. The steps in inserting the EOA are as follows:

1. PREPARE THE EQUIPMENT
   a. While your partner maintains CPR, check to make sure that all the components of the EOA are present, including the OBTURATOR, the MASK, and a 35-ml SYRINGE. You will also need a water-soluble LUBRICANT.
   b. Prepare the MASK by injecting air through the one-way valve until the mask cushion is firm enough to provide a good seal against the patient's face. The mask will give a better fit if it is not inflated too hard, but it should be sufficiently firm that it will not collapse when pressed against the patient's face.
   c. Check the CUFF on the obturator for leaks by injecting 35 ml of air through its one-way valve (Fig. 9-5). Once you are satisfied that there is no leak in the cuff, withdraw the air back into the syringe and leave the syringe attached to the tubing of the obturator.
   d. Snap the obturator into the mask so they form a single unit.
   e. Lubricate the distal end of the obturator generously with water-soluble jelly, but take care not to put lubricant in the area of the side holes.

2. INSERT THE EOA
   a. Hold the tube in one hand, just below the face mask, and position yourself at the patient's vertex. The tip of the tube should be pointing toward the patient's feet, and the upper part of

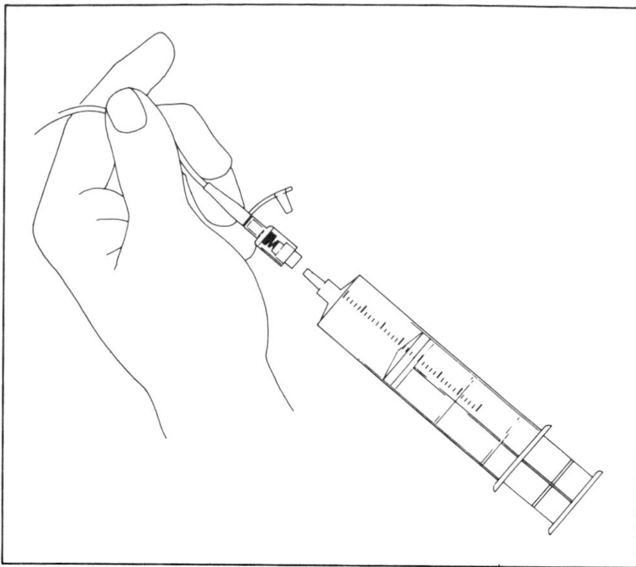

Fig. 9-5. *Check the cuff for leaks. (Reproduced courtesy Cavitron, Anaheim, California.)*

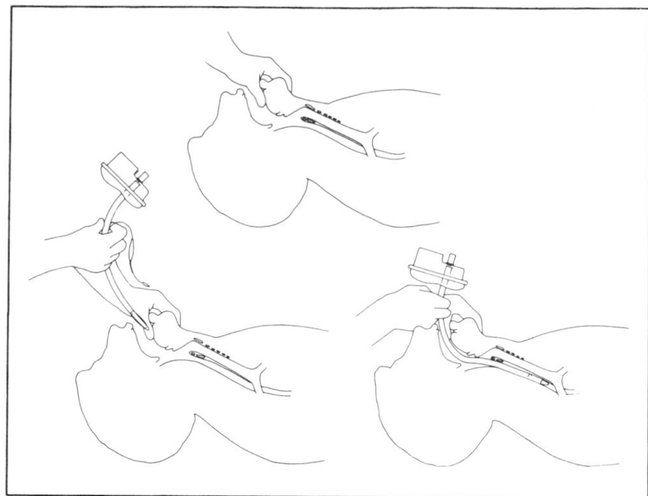

Fig. 9-6. *Steps in inserting the EOA. (Reproduced courtesy Cavitron, Anaheim, California.)*

the mask (the part that fits over the patient's nose) should be pointing toward you.

b. Notify your partner (who has been doing CPR all this time) that you are ready.

c. As soon as your partner completes two ventilations and moves to the patient's chest, tilt the patient's head slightly *forward*. Insert the thumb of one hand into the patient's mouth, with your index finger under the chin, and grasp his tongue and lower jaw between your thumb and index finger (Fig. 9-6). Lift straight up without hyperextending the neck, and insert the tip of the obturator into the patient's mouth.

d. While continuing to hold the jaw upward, SLOWLY and GENTLY advance the obturator behind the patient's tongue, through the pharynx, and into the esophagus, until the mask fits flush against the patient's face. DO NOT TRY TO FORCE THE TUBE DOWN. If you meet resistance, withdraw the obturator part way and try again to ease it into place.

NEVER JAM THE EOA INTO THE ESOPHAGUS.

e. Insertion of the EOA should not take more than about 10 to 12 seconds; that is, it should be in place in time for the next two ventilations. If you have not succeeded in inserting the EOA by the time your partner has finished 15 chest compressions, withdraw the obturator, and let your partner ventilate the patient on schedule before you try again.

3. TESTING FOR CORRECT POSITION. Once the obturator has been inserted and the mask is seated on the patient's face, it will be necessary to make sure the obturator is indeed in the esophagus and has not found its way into the trachea instead. Since the EOA is inserted blindly, one cannot be absolutely certain that it is entering the esophagus. One attempts to minimize accidental tracheal intubation by keeping the patient's head tilted slightly forward during EOA insertion, but nonetheless, in about 5 to 10 percent of insertion attempts, the EOA is accidently placed in the trachea. Clearly, if the EOA remains in the trachea it will be lethal to the patient, for all of the air or oxygen forced into the patient's pharynx will be blown into the stomach, the trachea being sealed off. The fact that no air can reach the lungs is by itself quite enough to kill the patient; but to make matters worse, the stomach will be inflated to the point where it ruptures, causing air to spread throughout the abdomen, chest, and subcutaneous tissues. Thus it is crucial to be absolutely certain the EOA is in the right place. To do so:

a. Hold the mask firmly against the patient's face as you would hold a pocket mask—that is, with your index fingers pressing the mask down against the face while your fourth and fifth fingers pull up on the jaw to establish backward head tilt. Remember:

THE EOA DOES NOT ELIMINATE THE NEED TO MAINTAIN HEAD TILT.

b. Take a deep breath, and blow into the mouthpiece of the EOA (Fig. 9-7). If the patient's *chest* rises with your ventilation, the obturator is probably in the esophagus as it should be.

c. To be doubly sure, have your partner listen with a stethoscope over both sides of the chest,

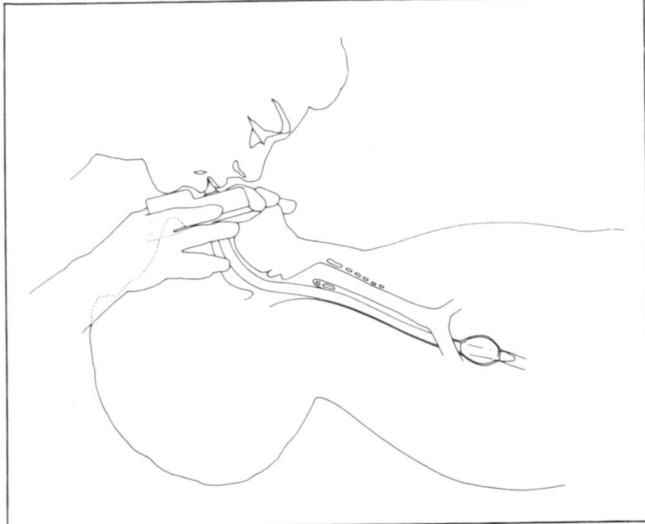

Fig. 9-7. *Ventilating through the EOA. (Reproduced courtesy Cavitron, Anaheim, California.)*

near the clavicles, and over the epigastrium as you ventilate through the mouthpiece on the mask. If the obturator is in the right place, your partner should be able to hear air entering the patient's lungs each time you blow into the EOA. If the obturator is in the trachea, on the other hand, breath sounds will not be audible in the lungs, but air may be heard entering the stomach (or gurgling through the stomach contents).

d. If the chest does *not* rise when you ventilate through the EOA or if your partner does not hear air entering the lungs with each of your ventilations, then the obturator is in the trachea and must be removed IMMEDIATELY. Withdraw the obturator smoothly, and have your partner resume CPR until you are ready to try again to insert the EOA.

4. INFLATION OF THE CUFF. Once the EOA is in place and its position has been verified, the cuff must be inflated to close off any leaks between the obturator and the wall of the esophagus. Squeeze the plunger of the 35-ml syringe (which should still be attached to the EOA) until you have injected 20 to 30 ml of air into the cuff. Then detach the syringe from the one-way valve. If by chance the one-way valve has been lost, the tubing may be clamped off with a hemostat before you detach the syringe.

Ventilation with an EOA

Once the EOA is properly positioned, it is used like any other mask for mouth-to-mask, bag-valve-mask, or demand valve–mask ventilation (see pp. 139–144). As mentioned, proper head tilt must be maintained.

USE THE EOA LIKE ANY OTHER MASK.

Removal of the EOA

In general, the rule to remember about removing an EOA is DON'T! Under most circumstances, the EOA should not be removed until the patient reaches the hospital and an endotracheal tube has been inserted to protect the trachea from aspiration. The only exception to this rule is when the patient resumes spontaneous breathing in the field and seems to be regaining consciousness; a patient with intact reflexes will not tolerate having a big, thick tube down his esophagus, and if you do not remove it, he will.

It is important to be aware that removal of an EOA is often accompanied by massive regurgitation, and you should have a good strong suction close at hand, preferably with a rigid (tonsil tip) suction catheter. The steps in removing the EOA are as follows:

1. Check your suction apparatus, and place the suction catheter where you can reach it in a hurry.
2. Roll the patient onto his side.
3. Snap the mask off the EOA. Insert the syringe into the one-way valve of the EOA, and slowly withdraw the air from the cuff until the cuff is fully deflated.
4. Hold the suction catheter ready in one hand while you remove the EOA smoothly with the other hand. If the stomach contents follow the obturator, suction the mouth and pharynx thoroughly before returning the patient to the supine position.

When you remove the EOA, then, remember the words of Louis XIV:

"APRÈS MOI LE DELUGE."*

Complications of the EOA

While the EOA is in general a safe and simple device to use, improper technique can result in serious and even fatal complications. Attempts to jam the tube past resistance, for example, have resulted in perforation of the esophagus, with subsequent leakage of air into the chest, abdomen, and beneath the skin. A second, relatively more common complication is unrecognized accidental intubation of the trachea, which, as noted, results in sealing off the lower airway and thus asphyxiates the patient. Both of these complications are ENTIRELY PREVENTABLE. The EOA should never be forced into the

*"After me, the flood."

esophagus, and proper checking of the EOA after insertion will ensure that it is not left in the trachea if it has been accidently placed there. Remember:

> WITH PROPER TECHNIQUE, *NO* COMPLICATIONS RESULT FROM USING AN EOA.

Like any other skill, use of the EOA requires constant practice, both to learn the skill and to maintain it. So visit your local manikin periodically to keep up your proficiency on the EOA.

> **Esophageal Obturator Airway: Points to Remember**
>
> - Use the EOA ONLY IN DEEPLY UNCONSCIOUS PATIENTS. In practice, this usually means patients in cardiac arrest.
> - DO NOT USE THE EOA IN
>   1. Conscious or semiconscious patients.
>   2. Children under 16 years old.
>   3. Patients known to have swallowed corrosive materials.
> - Do not interrupt artificial ventilation for more than 15 to 20 seconds to insert the EOA.
> - PREOXYGENATE the patient before attempting EOA insertion.
> - NEVER USE FORCE to insert the EOA.
> - ALWAYS CHECK THE POSITION OF THE EOA after it has been inserted.
> - Maintain proper HEAD TILT to ventilate through the EOA.
> - DO NOT REMOVE THE EOA in the field unless the patient begins breathing spontaneously.
> - If you do remove the EOA, be prepared for massive regurgitation, and have suction readily available.

ENDOTRACHEAL INTUBATION

Endotracheal intubation provides the most definitive control over a patient's airway. Not only does intubation with a cuffed endotracheal tube ensure that the airway remains open, but it also seals off the airway from foreign materials, thereby preventing aspiration. Once an endotracheal tube is properly placed within the trachea, furthermore, it is then possible to provide controlled ventilation with 100% oxygen, without the danger of causing gastric distention. The endotracheal tube also provides direct access to the lower airway for suctioning of secretions. For all these reasons, many EMT and paramedic programs that teach advanced airway skills regard endotracheal intubation as the method of choice to be taught to emergency medical personnel.

Endotracheal intubation does have its hazards. The two complications most likely to occur in the emergency setting are accidental intubation of the esophagus and accidental intubation of a main bronchus (usually the right main bronchus). Both of those potential complications are avoidable, however, with careful attention to correct technique.

Probably the most common error made by those inexperienced in endotracheal intubation is trying to intubate a patient too early, before either the patient or the operator is fully ready. Indeed, most intubation failures occur before the operator has even picked up the laryngoscope—from inadequate preparation of the patient or inadequate preparation of the equipment. There is nothing to be gained by haste in endotracheal intubation. Quite the contrary. So the first rule to remember is:

> START ARTIFICIAL VENTILATION WITH A POCKET MASK OR BAG-VALVE-MASK, AND MAKE SURE THE PATIENT IS FULLY OXYGENATED *BEFORE* YOU ATTEMPT TO INTUBATE.

During the 15 to 20 seconds it will take you to place an endotracheal tube between the patient's vocal cords, he will be without oxygen altogether. So he will need a good oxygen reserve on board to tide him over your intubation attempt.

Preparing the Equipment

The first step in endotracheal intubation is to MAKE CAREFUL PREPARATIONS FOR INTUBATION. This means that while your partners initiate and continue CPR, with supplemental oxygen for ventilation, you begin assembling and checking all your equipment. Ideally, you should have an intubation kit in which everything you need is collected in one place. The things you will need to check are as follows:

- You will need two or three cuffed ENDOTRACHEAL TUBES in different sizes. The average adult takes about a (French) size 8 tube, but some people are bigger and some people are smaller. So you need to have several alternative sizes close at hand, in order to choose the appropriate size tube once you have gotten a look at the size of the opening between the patient's vocal cords. Endotracheal tubes are usually longer than necessary when received from the manufacturer, and a tube that is too long easily passes beyond the trachea into the main bronchus. So the tube should be cut to a more manageable size before you insert the plastic connector. Table 9-1 shows approximately what length a tube should be for a patient of a given age. But one way to make a good estimate of

Table 9-1. *Dimensions of Endotracheal Tubes*

Age	Weight (lb)	Internal Diameter (mm)	Optimal Length (cm)
Newborn	to 8	2.5	10
1–6 months	8–12	3.5	11.5
6–12 months	12–20	4.0	12
1 year	20	4.5	13
2 years	25	5.0	14
3–4 years	30–35	5.5	15
5–6 years	40–45	6.0	15
6–8 years	45–60	6.5	17
9–11 years	65–80	7.0	18–19
12–13 years	80–100	7.5	20
14 years–adult	100+	8.0	20–24
Adult female	100+	7.5–8.0	20–24
Adult male	100+	8.0–9.0	20–24

the length is to lay the tube alongside the patient's face and neck; the tube should be long enough to reach from the angle of Louis (remember where that is?) to the teeth.

1. Once the excess length has been cut from the top of the tube, INSERT A CONNECTOR (standard 15 mm/22 mm fitting) of the appropriate size. The connector should fit very snugly into the endotracheal tube, preferably distending the end a bit as it is pushed into place. If the connector slips into the endotracheal tube very easily, it will also slip out very easily, and that is something you would like to avoid.
2. Next, TEST THE CUFF of the endotracheal tube by injecting 10 to 20 ml of air into the cuff through the inflation tubing. Clamp off the inflation tube with a hemostat, and make sure there are no leaks in the cuff. Then unclamp the tubing, and let the cuff deflate. Test every endotracheal tube you think you might use (e.g., one size 7.5, one size 8, one size 8.5). The time to discover that a cuff is not working is *before* you insert the tube into a patient's trachea.
3. Most people find an endotracheal tube easier to insert if a flexible metal stylet is placed within the tube. The stylet makes the tube a bit more rigid and also allows you to bend the tube into a convenient shape. The most effective shape for an endotracheal tube is like a hockey stick, that is, with the last few inches bent at an angle to the rest of the tube.
4. To PLACE A STYLET INTO THE ENDOTRACHEAL TUBE, first lubricate the stylet with water-soluble jelly, so that it will be easier to remove the stylet from the tube when the time comes. Then insert the stylet into the endotracheal tube so that the end of the stylet is about an inch short of the end of the tube. Bend the other end of the stylet over the tube connector, so that the stylet cannot slip farther into the tube. Do NOT allow the distal end of the stylet to protrude beyond the end of the endotracheal tube, for it could tear or otherwise damage delicate structures in the throat.
5. Finally, LUBRICATE THE OUTSIDE OF THE ENDOTRACHEAL TUBE with water-soluble jelly, to make it easier to pass across mucous membranes.

- ASSEMBLE AND TEST THE LARYNGOSCOPE. A laryngoscope consists of two parts: a handle, which contains the batteries, and a lighted blade. You should have two or three blades available, to allow for differences in size and anatomy among different patients. For adults, one size 3 straight (Miller) blade and size 3 and size 4 curved (MacIntosh) blades are usually sufficient. The curved blade is the easier for most people to use and will work for the majority of intubations. But sometimes, especially when the patient is very muscular or has a short, thick neck, a straight blade gives better visualization. So it is a good idea to have at least one of each. Snap each blade, one after the other, onto the laryngoscope handle, and CHECK THE LIGHT. It should be bright white and steady. If it is flickering, try tightening up the bulb in its socket. If it is yellow or dim, you need fresh batteries or a new bulb. (You *should* have checked the bulb and batteries at the beginning of your shift!) Keep one blade—the one you think will be the right size for the patient—snapped onto the laryngoscope handle, but folded down in the "off" position until you are ready to use it.
- CHECK YOUR SUCTION APPARATUS. Turn on the suction, clamp the tubing, and make sure that the pressure gauge goes right up to 300 mm Hg. Then ATTACH A RIGID (TONSIL-TIP) CATHETER TO THE TUBING, for that is the catheter you will need first. But make sure you also have one or two STERILE SUCTION CATHETERS nearby; you will need these later, once the patient is intubated, to suction through the endotracheal tube.
- Now assemble the last few odds and ends: a BITE-BLOCK, which you will use once the patient is intubated, to prevent him from biting down on the endotracheal tube (an oropharyngeal airway will do fine); a MAGILL FORCEPS, which you may need to help steer the distal end of the endotracheal tube through the patient's vocal cords; and some ADHESIVE TAPE OR UMBILICAL TAPE (or both) to tape or tie the endotracheal tube in place once it has been properly inserted.

If you are well organized, it should not take very long to carry out the above steps (especially if you have been keeping your equipment in good condition and checking it at the beginning of every shift). But no matter how long it takes, DO NOT TRY TO MAKE ANY SHORTCUTS. Your chances of performing a successful intubation depend critically on the thoroughness of your preparations; so do not start with a handicap. And if it takes you an extra minute or two to get ready, no problem; that simply means that the patient is getting another minute or two of oxygenation, as your partners continue CPR—and that is all to the good.

Equipment for Endotracheal Intubation
2–3 endotracheal tubes, different sizes
20-ml syringe
Hemostat
Bandage scissors (to cut tube to right length)
Plastic connectors for endotracheal tubes
Malleable stylet
Water-soluble lubricating jelly
Laryngoscope handle
1–2 curved (MacIntosh) blades
1–2 straight (Miller) blades
Spare batteries for laryngoscope
Magill forceps
Suction unit
Rigid (tonsil-tip) suction catheter
Several flexible suction catheters (sterile)
Bite-block (or oropharyngeal airway)
Adhesive tape or umbilical tape (preferred)

Intubating the Patient

Once you have all your equipment set up, preferably on a tray that you can place at your right side, the next step is to POSITION THE PATIENT. The patient's position will determine whether you locate the vocal cords quickly or waste precious seconds groping around unfamiliar anatomy. So it is worth taking care to make sure the patient is positioned correctly.

The optimal position of a patient for endotracheal intubation is called the "sniffing position," because the patient's nose is pointing up, as if he were sniffing the air. To place a patient in the sniffing position, you need to FLEX HIS NECK FORWARD AND EXTEND HIS HEAD BACKWARD. If the patient is on a bed or stretcher, this is best accomplished by placing one or two pillows under his head (to flex the neck forward) and then extending the head back. If however, as is all too often the case, the patient is on the floor, it is better to rest the patient's head on your lap (otherwise, you will have to perform the intubation from a prone position on the floor). Kneel at the patient's vertex—with your buttocks supported on your heels and your knees to the left of the patient's head—but leave enough room for your partner to continue artificial ventilation until you are ready to begin. Arrange your equipment to the right of the patient's head, for your right hand will be reaching for the suction, the endotracheal tube, and so on. (Your left hand will be holding the laryngoscope.) When you are ready to begin your intubation attempt, lift the patient's head and quickly slide your knees beneath it, so that his head is resting on your thighs. Extend the head backward, and you are ready to begin.

It is a good idea before you insert the laryngoscope to check the patient's mouth for dentures or loose bridgework; remove them if present, and put them in a safe place. Also use the opportunity to suction out any vomitus or other secretions readily visible in the mouth. Then let your partner ventilate the patient with oxygen again for a minute or so.

Now you need to work swiftly but deliberately. As soon as your partner takes the ventilating mask away from the patient's face, use the fingers of your right hand to open the patient's jaws wide and spread his lips apart, so that they will not become trapped underneath the laryngoscope blade. Now, take the laryngoscope in your *left* hand. Place your hand low on the laryngoscope handle, so that the junction of the blade and the handle rests against the heel of your hand. Holding the laryngoscope in that fashion gives you maximum control over the angle of the blade while enabling you to lift the patient's jaw with minimum force. Don't clench your fist around the laryngoscope handle—that decreases control over the blade and leads to fatigue. Slip the laryngoscope blade into the *right* corner of the patient's mouth (Fig. 9-8). Keep the rigid, tonsil-tip suction in your right hand, in case you need to clear vomitus or secretions out of your line of vision. If you are using a curved blade, use the flange on the blade to displace the patient's tongue to the left. Slowly advance the blade forward and and toward the center, holding your wrist rigid. Keep advancing the blade until its tip reaches the epiglottis (Fig. 9-9). What you do when you see the epiglottis will depend on which type of blade you are using. If you are using a *straight blade,* you need to advance it just slightly beneath the tip of the epiglottis. If you are using a *curved blade,* the tip of the blade should come to rest in the little pocket, called the **vallecula,** between the epiglottis and the base of the tongue.

Now, holding your left wrist rigid, lift the laryngoscope forward and upward at a 45-degree angle to the patient's face. If you do this properly, you will find you are lifting the patient's mandible and head. DO NOT USE THE TEETH AS A FULCRUM! As you lift forward and upward with the laryngoscope, the **glottis,** that is, the space between the vocal cords, should come into view, as shown in Fig. 9-10. When you see the vocal cords, pick up your endotracheal tube in your right hand, holding it as you would hold a pencil, and pass it, with its curve facing forward, into the patient's mouth to the right of the tongue and laryngoscope. Advance the tube slowly through the glottic opening until the cuff just disappears from sight beyond the vocal cords. YOU MUST SEE THE TIP OF THE TUBE PASS THROUGH THE GLOTTIS! If you just shove the tube in blindly, the chances are very good that you will deftly intubate the esopha-

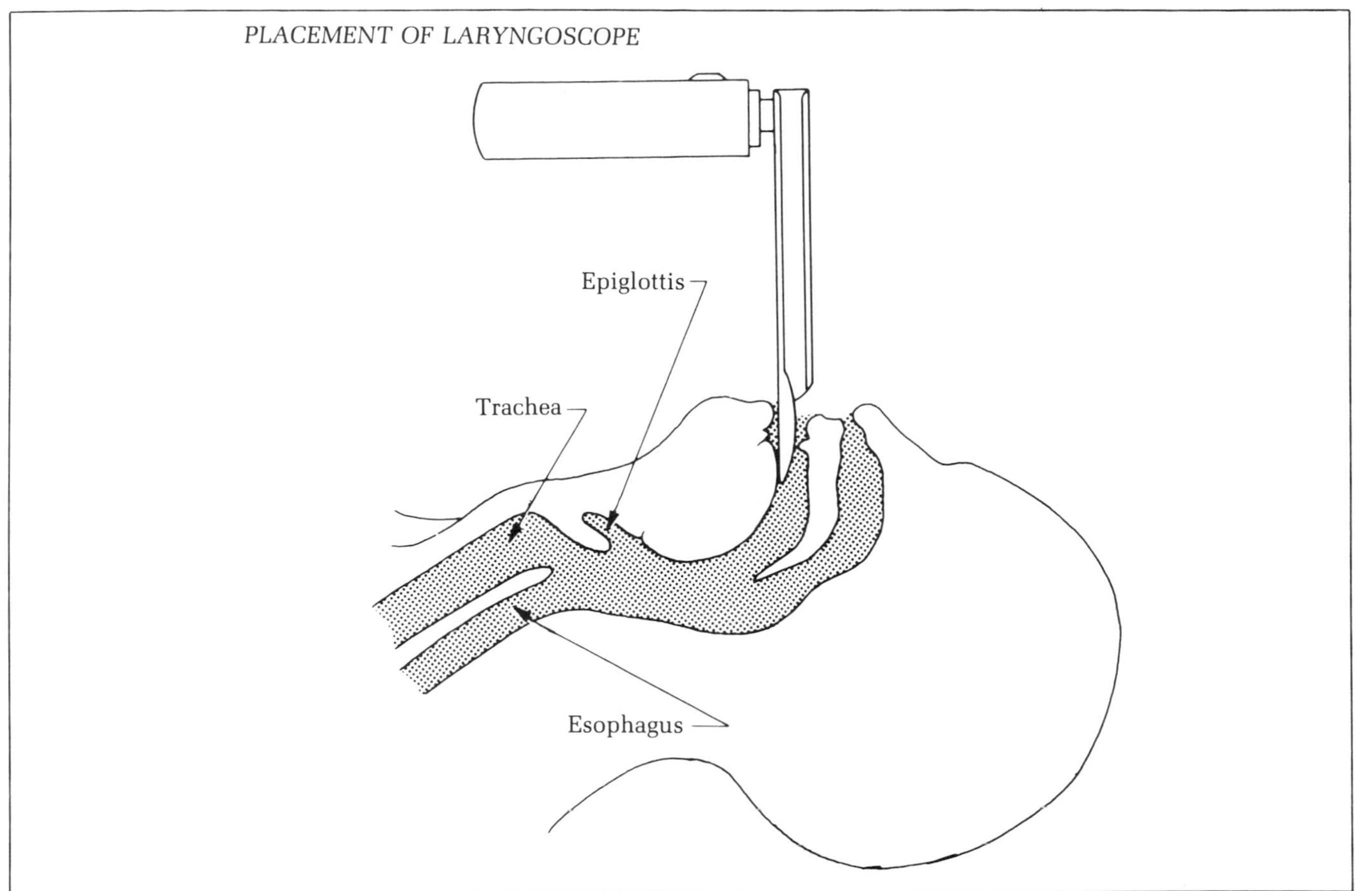

Fig. 9-8. *The laryngoscope is inserted into the right side of the patient's mouth.*

gus. The only way to be absolutely sure that the endotracheal tube is where it should be—in the trachea—is to *see* it enter the trachea.

Once you have gotten the tube into the trachea, hold it firmly in place with your left hand, pull out the stylet, and attach a ventilating bag to the plastic connector. Then, as you ventilate the patient, have your partner inflate the cuff of the endotracheal tube. Keep one finger on the patient's neck, just above the upper border of the sternum, as the cuff is being inflated. If the tip of the endotracheal tube is in the right place, you should be able to feel the cuff in the trachea. The cuff should be inflated with only enough air to seal off any leaks between the tube and the wall of the trachea. You can usually hear those leaks as you ventilate. So have your partner slowly inflate the cuff until you do not hear any more leakage around the cuff. Then clamp off the inflating tube with a hemostat.

The whole process of inserting the endotracheal tube—from the time your partner takes the bag-valve-mask away from the patient's face to the moment you give the first ventilation through the tube—should not take more than about 20 seconds. Since it is difficult to count aloud or keep looking at your watch during an intubation attempt, the best way to keep track of the time elapsed is to HOLD YOUR OWN BREATH. When *you* start getting uncomfortable from hypoxia and accumulation of carbon dioxide, it is a good bet that the patient's cells are at least as uncomfortable. So if you have not gotten the tube in by then, stop the attempt, reoxygenate the patient for a few minutes, and get your own breath back. Then try again.

Once the tube is placed in the trachea, but before you get the tube all taped and trussed down, you want to CHECK AGAIN THAT IT IS IN THE RIGHT PLACE. So as you continue to ventilate, holding the tube firmly in place, LOOK to make sure the chest is rising with each ventilation. At the same time, have your partner listen to at least six sites on the patient's chest:

Listen over the right and left sides of the upper chest.
Listen over the right and left mid-axillary line (a few inches below the armpits).
Listen over the sternal notch.
Listen over the epigastrium.

Breath sounds should be clear and equal on both sides of the chest. If they are not, SOMETHING IS WRONG.

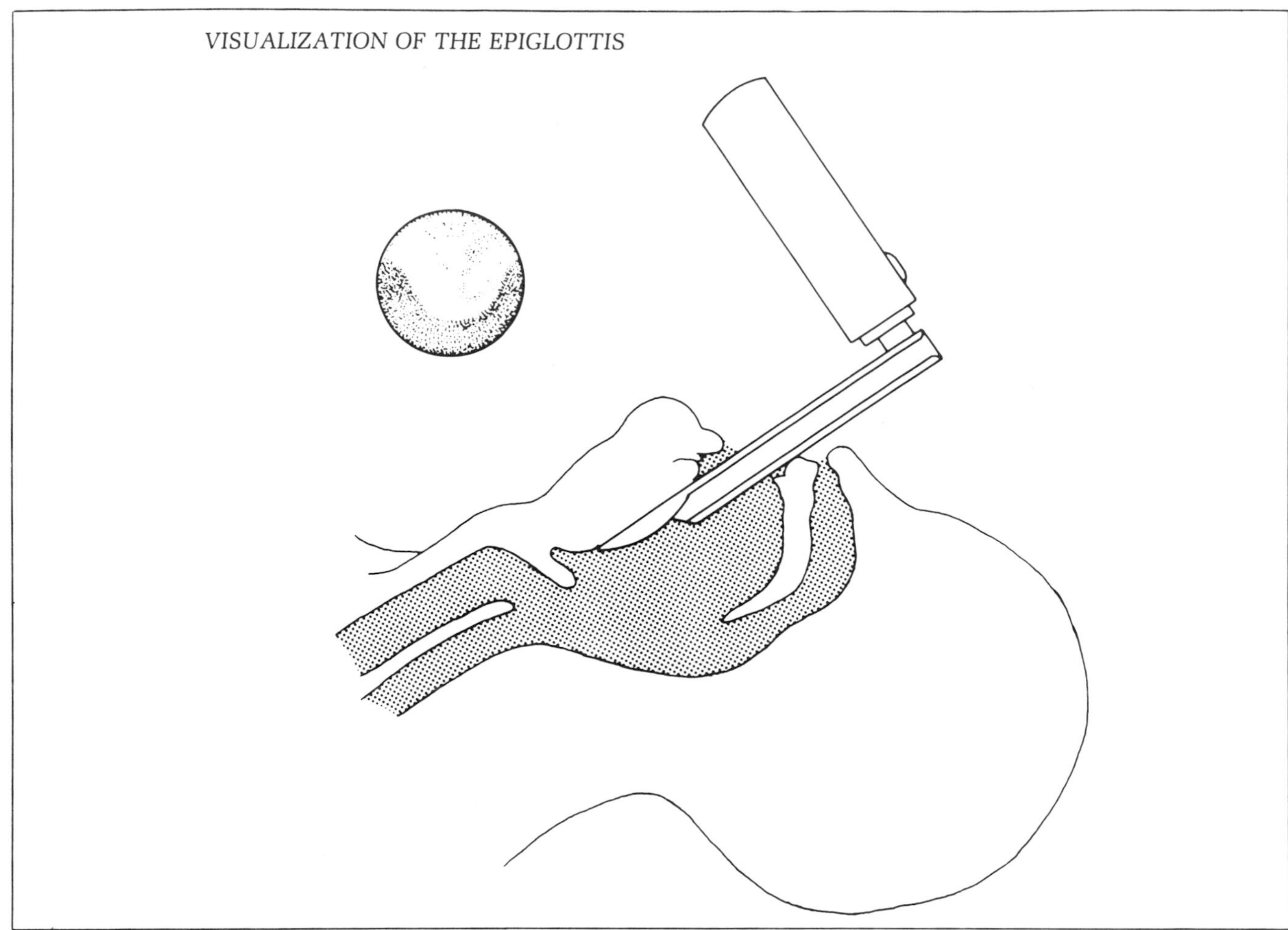

Fig. 9-9. *As the blade is advanced, the epiglottis comes into view.*

If you hear breath sounds on only one side of the chest (usually the right), you have inserted the endotracheal tube too far and it has come to rest in a main bronchus. What you need to do is deflate the cuff on the tube and pull back *very slightly* on the tube, while you continue to ventilate and your partner continues to listen over the silent chest. As soon as your partner can hear breath sounds on that side, stop pulling back on the tube, for the tip is now in the trachea.

If you do not hear breath sounds on *either* side of the chest (or if you hear whistling or gurgling over the epigastrium with each ventilation), you have most likely intubated the esophagus, not the trachea. What you must do is deflate the cuff, withdraw the endotracheal tube, and immediately resume ventilating the patient with the bag-valve-mask for several minutes before you make another intubation attempt.

Let us assume that you have inserted the endotracheal tube, inflated the cuff, and confirmed that the tube is in the right place. The next step is to SECURE THE TUBE IN PLACE. In the field, the best way to secure an endotracheal tube is to tie it in place with umbilical tape, for adhesive tape often pulls loose under field conditions. And the last thing you want is for the tube to slip out, necessitating another intubation, for you may be sure that the second attempt is going to be much more difficult than the first. So make sure the tube is anchored securely.

First, holding firmly to the tube, insert an oropharyngeal airway into the patient's mouth, to serve as a bite-block. Next, mark the tube at the point at which it emerges from the patient's mouth. This mark will help you determine later if the tube has slipped out or farther into the trachea. Then take a generous length of umbilical tape—at least 2 feet long—and wind it once around the tube, once around the oropharyngeal airway, and then behind the patient's neck, where it should be securely tied. Even when the endotracheal tube is well secured, the prudent EMT holds the tube in place as he ventilates the patient. A sudden jarring of the patient (e.g., in a moving vehicle) can wrench loose even the most sturdily tied tube.

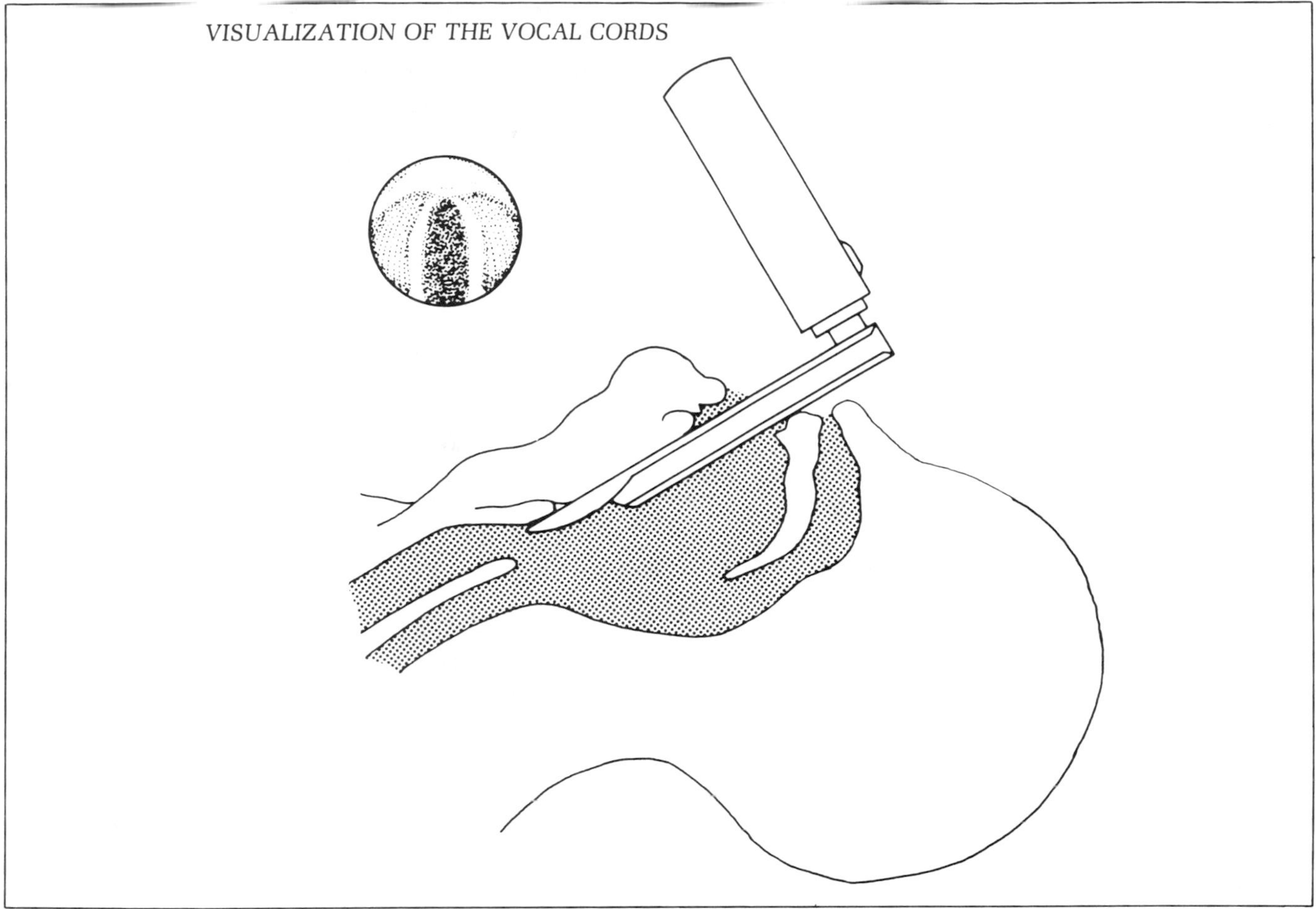

Fig. 9-10. *As the epiglottis is lifted upward, the vocal cords become visible.*

Endotracheal Intubation: Points to Remember

- Never attempt endotracheal intubation before the patient has been thoroughly preoxygenated.
- Assemble and check all your equipment before you start.
- Position the patient properly: neck flexed forward, head extended back.
- DO NOT RUSH. Work with *deliberate* speed.
- Hold your breath during an intubation attempt. When *you* get hypoxic, it is time to reoxygenate the patient!
- Get it right the first time; the second try will be much more difficult.
- Verify that the tube is in the right place. Take nothing for granted.
- Secure the endotracheal tube well. You do not want to have to try to insert it a second time.
- Even when the tube is tied in place, stabilize it with one hand as you ventilate the patient.

SUCTION

When the mouth or throat is filled with blood, vomitus, or other semiliquid material, the use of a suction device allows rapid and efficient removal of the foreign material. Every ambulance should be equipped with both a fixed suction unit that operates off the engine manifold and a portable suction that can be carried from the vehicle to the patient.

DESIGN OF SUCTION DEVICES

Fixed Suction Unit

A fixed suction unit is permanently installed in the vehicle and is usually powered by vacuum from the engine manifold or by an electric vacuum pump. In either case, the unit should be capable of generating a VACUUM of 300 mm Hg within 4 seconds after the collection tube is clamped off, and it should be able to provide a constant air flow of at least 30 liters per minute. One should check the vacuum on the suction apparatus at the beginning of each shift and before each use by switching on the suction, clamping the tubing, and examining the pressure gauge to make sure it registers at least 300 mm Hg.

In addition to a strong vacuum source, the suction unit should have a nonbreakable COLLECTION BOTTLE; a stiff, transparent COLLECTION TUBE long enough to reach comfortably to the patient's head regardless of what position he is in; and a variety of sterile, disposable SUCTION CATHETERS. The catheters come in two general types. The first type, the *flexible rubber catheter*, is used for suctioning the nose, mouth, pharynx, and in laryngectomees, the stoma. The second type is the rigid plastic or metal suction tip—called a *tonsil suction tip*, or Yankauer suction tip—and is very useful for suctioning the pharynx of an unconscious patient, since it is easier to direct the tip where you want it to go. Whichever type of catheter you use, you will need a supply of WATER for rinsing the system after suctioning. There must also be some means of controlling the suction, that is, of shutting the flow off and turning it back on without having to keep turning the whole system on and off. This is most easily accomplished by placing a Y TUBE in the line—a small piece of plastic shaped like a Y and inserted between the collection tubing and the catheter. Two arms of the Y are connected into the system, while the third arm is left open. So long as this third arm is open, air will be pulled in through it, and the suction at the end of the catheter will be minimal. When you need to use the suction, you simply cover the open end of the Y with your fingertip, and air will be drawn in through the suction catheter.

All the components of the suction system should be cleaned or disposed of after each use.

Portable Suction Units

Portable suction units are of several types, depending on the power source used to create the necessary vacuum. *Electrically powered units* operate off either a rechargeable battery or a 110-volt outlet and overall are the most satisfactory type of portable suction for everyday field use. Electrically powered units are compact, relatively lightweight, and capable of generating vacuums well above the 300 mm Hg standard. The *oxygen-powered suction* operates off an oxygen-powered resuscitator (see under Aids to Breathing). It does not generate as strong a vacuum as an electrically powered suction. Furthermore, it quickly uses up the oxygen in a cylinder, and oxygen is a gas too valuable to waste on suctioning. *Air-powered suction units* do not have this disadvantage, and they tend to be more effective besides, although they are generally heavier and more cumbersome than the electrically powered models. Suction units powered by compressed *freon* in disposable cans are also available. These generate powerful suction, but occasional freezing of the valves and the necessity to maintain an inventory of freon cans limits their usefulness for day-to-day ambulance work; they are, however, a good ancillary device to stock in disaster kits. Finally, there are *manually powered suction units*, operated by squeezing a rubber bulb or stepping on a foot pump. Manual units of this type are ineffective and unsatisfactory for emergency work.

TECHNIQUE OF SUCTIONING

Suctioning removes not only liquids from the airway but air as well. Thus it is preferable to *preoxygenate* the patient for at least 3 minutes before suctioning by providing him with supplemental oxygen to breathe. This will give him a small oxygen reserve in his tissues, which he can draw upon while you are suctioning. This reserve is very limited, however, so each suctioning attempt must be kept brief (less than 15 sec), with adequate oxygenation, and, if necessary, artificial ventilation in between.

To suction a patient's mouth and throat, first inspect the suction unit to make certain all parts are properly assembled. Switch on the suction, clamp the tubing, and check that the pressure gauge reaches 300 mm Hg. Once you have made sure the equipment is functioning properly, attach a flexible catheter or tonsil suction tip to the tubing, and recheck the suction by placing the catheter tip in the rinse water, with the Y tube closed. Position yourself at the patient's head, and turn his head to the side. Then open his mouth by the crossed-finger technique, and use your fingers to clear the mouth of any solid debris or large collections of fluid. If you are using a flexible catheter, measure off the distance from the patient's mouth to his ear lobe with the catheter, and insert the catheter into the patient's pharynx just this distance, with the suction OFF (i.e., without occluding the opening in the Y tube). Once the catheter is in place, apply suction by putting your finger over the Y tube to close the hole, and move the suction catheter around so that it will not attach itself to any soft tissues. If you are using a rigid tonsil suction, insert it so that the convex side goes along the roof of the patient's mouth until the tip of the catheter reaches the pharynx. Once again, keep the vacuum off until the suction tip is in place. Then occlude the Y tube, and move the rigid suction catheter around the pharynx to "vacuum clean" it out. Bear in mind that a semiconscious patient may gag or vomit if a hard object touches the back of his throat. Apply suction for NO MORE THAN 15 SECONDS AT A TIME. Then take your finger off the Y tube to release the suction, remove the catheter from the pharynx, quickly suction the patient's mouth, and rinse the catheter and collection tubing through with water—while you reoxygenate the patient—before suctioning again.

If a patient's mouth is clamped shut and you cannot open it by the crossed-finger maneuver, you can use a *flexible* rubber catheter to suction the back of the throat through the nose. To do this, moisten the catheter in water, and insert it *gently* through one of the nostrils, with the suction OFF. When the tip of the catheter is in place in the back of the throat, apply intermittent suction (by occluding and releasing the Y tube) as you slowly draw the catheter out of the patient's nose. Once again, the suction attempt should not exceed 15 seconds, and the patient should be permitted to breathe oxygen for a minute or two before another attempt is made.

If suctioning is carried out during CPR, it must be done swiftly, between ventilations. Do not interrupt artificial ventilation for more than 5 seconds at a time to carry out suctioning, and resume ventilations, preferably with oxygen, immediately after each suctioning procedure.

Suctioning the Mouth and Pharynx: Points to Remember

- PREOXYGENATE the patient for 2 to 3 minutes before *every* suctioning attempt.
- CHECK YOUR EQUIPMENT *before* you insert a suction catheter.
- Do not use a rigid (tonsil) suction tip to suction the throat in a conscious or semiconscious patient.
- Keep the suction OFF as you are inserting the suction catheter.
- Do not suction for more than 15 SECONDS at a time in any patient. REOXYGENATE immediately after suctioning.
- Do not interrupt artificial ventilation for more than 5 seconds for a suctioning attempt.

Suctioning the Laryngectomee

To suction a "neck breather," first preoxygenate the patient and clean the area around the stoma or breathing tube of any encrusted mucus. Then moisten a flexible catheter in sterile water, and insert it 2 to 3 inches through the stoma or breathing tube, with the suction OFF. Once the catheter tip is in place, apply intermittent suction as you slowly withdraw the catheter. Once again, do not suction for more than 15 seconds, and allow the patient to breathe oxygen in between suctioning attempts.

If the patient is conscious, he may wish to suction out his trachea by himself, and you should let him do so. Laryngectomees receive training in this procedure and are usually more comfortable carrying it out for themselves, if able.

*SUCTIONING THROUGH AN ENDOTRACHEAL TUBE**

The first rule to remember about suctioning through an endotracheal tube is DON'T DO IT IF YOU DON'T HAVE TO. Tracheal suctioning requires, first of all, strict attention to sterile technique, which is very difficult to achieve under field conditions. In the second place, suctioning the trachea carries a constant danger of causing disturbances in the cardiac rhythm. Ideally, a patient should be hooked up to a cardiac monitor while being suctioned, so that any irregularities in the heart beat can be detected right away. If you do not carry a monitor in your vehicle and therefore cannot monitor the patient during tracheal suctioning, the hazards of inducing an unrecognized cardiac dysrhythmia are considerable. So suction the trachea in the field *only* if the patient has a lot of secretions in the lower airway that are interfering with ventilation.

A suction catheter removes more than secretions from the airway. It removes oxygen as well. For this reason, a patient must be thoroughly preoxygenated before any attempt is made to suction his trachea, for you want the patient to have a good reserve of oxygen on board when you start. Our second rule about tracheal suctioning, then, is

PREOXYGENATE THE PATIENT WITH 100% OXYGEN FOR AT LEAST THREE MINUTES BEFORE EACH TIME YOU SUCTION.

While your partner is ventilating the patient with 100% oxygen, you need to get set up. You will need the following equipment:

Equipment Required for Endotracheal Suctioning

Functioning suction apparatus
2–3 sterile suction catheters
Sterile gloves
Sterile water
A sterile cloth on which to lay out the equipment

Once you have gathered these supplies together, proceed as follows:

1. Set up and TEST THE SUCTION APPARATUS. Make sure it has a good vacuum (when the tubing is kinked, the vacuum should reach 300 mm Hg). Make sure as well that all the connections are snug and that there are no leaks. If you can set the vacuum level on your suction machine, set it to between 80 and 120 mm Hg.
2. Unfold and SPREAD OUT THE STERILE CLOTH, being careful not to touch the upper surface, on which you will be laying out your sterile equipment.
3. CHOOSE ONE OR TWO STERILE CATHETERS.

*This section intended for EMT-Intermediates trained in endotracheal intubation; not required for EMT-As.

A suction catheter should have at least one or two side holes or a ring tip with multiple holes to prevent it from catching on the respiratory mucosa. It should also have a large side hole near the end that attaches to your suction apparatus, to enable you to control the suction (when you cover the hole with your thumb, the suction is on; when you uncover the hole, the suction is effectively off). The catheter SIZE is also very important. The diameter of the catheter should never be greater than one-third to one-half the diameter of the endotracheal tube, for a suction catheter that nearly fills the endotracheal tube will pull out too much gas (hence oxygen) from the airway. A No. 12 or 14 (French) suction catheter is usually a good choice for most adults.

4. LAY THE STERILE EQUIPMENT OUT ON THE STERILE CLOTH. To do so, handle only the *outside* of the sterile packages as you open them, and let their contents fall out onto the sterile cloth. You should have one or two sterile suction catheters and a sterile container for water also laying on the cloth.
5. Open a bottle of sterile water, and pour it into your sterile container.
6. Touching only the proximal tip of the suction catheter (the end opposite to the end that you will insert in the endotracheal tube), connect the suction catheter to the tubing of the suction apparatus.
7. DON STERILE GLOVES. Once you have these gloves on, do not touch anything unsterile.
8. Dip the end of your suction catheter in sterile water to lubricate the catheter, and occlude the side vent with your thumb to test the suction. The water should be rapidly drawn up the catheter.
9. Have your partner disconnect the ventilating bag from the endotracheal tube.
10. Insert the catheter into the endotracheal tube with the SUCTION OFF (i.e., with the side hole open), taking care that the suction catheter does not touch anything outside the endotracheal tube. Advance the catheter until you meet an obstruction. Then pull back a bit and apply suction intermittently (by covering and uncovering the side hole) as you slowly withdraw the catheter.
11. DO NOT SUCTION FOR MORE THAN 10 SECONDS AT A TIME! If there are still secretions that need to be removed after your first 10 seconds of suctioning, have your partner reoxygenate the patient—by ventilating him with 100% oxygen for 3 minutes—before you try again. Meanwhile, flush the catheter with sterile water. Take care, between suctioning attempts, not to let the catheter touch anything that is unsterile.
12. When you have finished suctioning through the endotracheal tube, you may use the same catheter to suction out the mouth and back of the throat, if necessary. But once the catheter has been used in the mouth, DO NOT USE IT AGAIN INSIDE THE ENDOTRACHEAL TUBE. The human mouth is full of nasty germs, and you do not want to introduce any of them into the patient's lungs.

Endotracheal Suctioning: Points to Remember

- Do not try endotracheal suctioning in the field unless it is really necessary.
- Always preoxygenate the patient (ventilate with 100% oxygen) for 3 minutes before *every* suctioning attempt.
- Maintain strict sterile technique.
- Never suction the trachea for more than 10 seconds at a time.
- Reoxygenate the patient immediately when you finish suctioning.
- Do not put the suction catheter back into the endotracheal tube after it has been in the patient's mouth or has touched any other unsterile object.

AIDS TO BREATHING

There are several devices in every properly equipped ambulance whose function is to make ventilation more efficient in delivering oxygen to the tissues or to provide mechanical assistance to ventilation. In the first category is oxygen itself, probably the most vital life support equipment carried in the ambulance. In the second category are several ventilation assist devices, ranging from a simple mask to an oxygen-powered resuscitator. In this section, we will examine the different means of improving ventilation and look at the circumstances in which each is most appropriately used.

OXYGEN

Oxygen (abbreviated as O_2, pronounced "Oh-two") is a colorless, odorless gas present in a concentration of 21% in our atmosphere. In a healthy person, this concentration of oxygen available in the air is more than adequate to furnish the needs of all body tissues, at least so long as the supply of air is constant and uninterrupted. In severe illness or injury, however, 21% oxygen may not be sufficient, either because of an isolated oxygen deficiency in one or more body organs or because of widespread oxygen deficiency throughout the body. In such circumstances, survival of the organism may depend upon receiving extra oxygen—above the usual 21%—to boost the concentration of oxygen in the lungs and thereby permit delivery of a higher oxygen concentration to the tissues.

What kind of situations produce a need for supplementary oxygen? Probably the most obvious and dramatic is full CARDIOPULMONARY ARREST (absence of breathing and pulse). We have already learned that even effective CPR produces a flow of blood only 25 to 30 percent of normal; that is, the red blood cells manning the bucket brigade from the lungs to the tissues are plodding along at one-third to one-fourth their usual speed. Thus the tissues are receiving oxygen at only one-third to one-fourth the usual rate. To make matters worse, the tissues are receiving a lower concentration of oxygen than usual, for the exhaled air used for mouth-to-mouth ventilation contains only 16% oxygen, rather than 21%. Clearly, the only way to increase the delivery of oxygen to the tissues under these circumstances is to give each red blood cell a bigger bucket (a higher concentration of oxygen) to carry on each trip. If we do that, the tissues will receive a larger net supply of oxygen every minute despite the fact that the red blood cells are not moving any faster. The rule to remember, then, is

> START OXYGEN AS SOON AS POSSIBLE AFTER BEGINNING CPR.

Cardiac arrest is one member of a larger category of disorders that we have termed SHOCK, that is, disorders in which there is a failure of adequate tissue perfusion. Cardiac arrest simply represents the most extreme form of cardiogenic shock. But the tissues face the same problems of oxygenation in other forms of shock. We have already seen, for example, how in hemorrhagic shock there are fewer red blood cells traveling through the circulation, so each red blood cell needs to carry much more oxygen in order to keep up the supply to the tissues. Thus extra oxygen is needed in all cases of shock.

> ANY PATIENT IN SHOCK NEEDS OXYGEN.

The need for supplementary oxygen in cardiac arrest and in shock in general is clear. But what about the patient with AIRWAY OBSTRUCTION or RESPIRATORY ARREST only? Does he need extra oxygen? At first glance, the answer would seem to be no, for as long as the patient's heart continues to beat, the red blood cells are moving along at a proper rate. The problem is, however, that the red blood cells are making the trip from the lungs to the tissues *empty-handed*. The moment a person stops breathing, the oxygen in the lungs is rapidly depleted by the red cells, and the oxygen carried by the red cells is just as rapidly gobbled up by the tissues. Within a minute or two after airway obstruction or respiratory arrest, the red blood cells find themselves trekking back and forth through the circulation with empty oxygen buckets, and even though they continue for a short while (until cardiac arrest occurs) to visit the tissues, they have no oxygen to leave there. Oxygen levels throughout the body fall lower and lower as a consequence. If at this point the person starts breathing again, or if someone starts breathing for him, and the red cells find they have a little oxygen to put in their buckets, the tissues—now starved for oxygen—will wolf down the oxygen as fast as the red cells can bring it, and they will barely be able to manage. But suppose the patient is given a higher concentration of oxygen—say 100%. Now each red cell can carry a much larger load of oxygen on each trip to the tissues, and the deficits can be remedied more quickly. Giving 100% oxygen in this situation is like sending a large relief shipment into an area devastated by natural disaster: The relief shipment of oxygen feeds the hungry tissues and keeps them going until normal breathing is restored.

> ANY PATIENT WHOSE AIRWAY HAS BEEN OBSTRUCTED OR WHO NEEDS ARTIFICIAL VENTILATION NEEDS OXYGEN.

Please note that this category includes patients who may be reasonably *suspected* of having had an airway obstruction, such as unconscious patients or patients who have had seizures.

We have seen that any person who is not breathing—with or without a pulse—needs supplementary oxygen. But what about ill or injured people who *are* breathing spontaneously? Do they need extra oxygen too?

In many cases, yes. There are a variety of conditions that can interfere with the normal transfer of oxygen from the alveoli into the blood, all of which are grouped together under the general heading of **acute respiratory insufficiency.** In such circumstances, it is necessary to supply extra oxygen to the lungs in order to ensure a sufficient reservoir of oxygen for the red blood cells to pick up. For example, if some of the alveoli get filled with *fluid*, red blood cells coming to these alveoli will not find any oxygen at all, and they will leave the lungs empty-handed. In order to compensate for this, the red blood cells that visit normal alveoli will have to carry bigger buckets of oxygen (higher oxygen concentration), and the only way they can do so is if we give the patient more oxygen to breathe. Examples of situations in whicn some of the alveoli are filled with fluid include PULMONARY EDEMA (plasma in the alveoli), PNEUMONIA (pus in the alveoli), and TRAUMA TO THE CHEST (blood in some alveoli). Similarly, there are circumstances in which alveoli may *collapse*, such as in patients with RIB FRAC-

TURE or patients who for any reason are not breathing deeply enough, and once again the red cells passing by the collapsed alveoli will not find any oxygen. Thus once again it will be up to their buddies, the red cells that circulate past normally open alveoli, to pick up a bigger oxygen load in order to compensate. Finally, alveoli may become full of *other gases* that displace oxygen. A victim of SMOKE INHALATION or one who has been exposed to TOXIC FUMES may have very little oxygen in his lungs, and the fastest way to get oxygen back into the lungs—and from there into the circulation—is to supply it to the patient in high concentrations.

Causes of Acute Respiratory Insufficiency

- FLUID IN THE ALVEOLI
  1. Pulmonary edema (plasma)
  2. Pneumonia (pus)
  3. Near drowning (salt water)
  4. Chest trauma (blood)
- COLLAPSE OF ALVEOLI
  1. Airway obstruction
  2. Failure to take deep breaths
     a. Pain (e.g., broken ribs)
     b. Paralysis of the respiratory muscles (spine injury)
     c. Depression of the respiratory center (head injury, drug overdose)
     d. Collapse of an entire lung (pneumothorax)
- OTHER GASES IN THE ALVEOLI
  1. Smoke inhalation
  2. Carbon monoxide poisoning
  3. Inhalation of toxic fumes

In all of the above conditions, the amount of oxygen in the air may be insufficient to furnish an adequate supply of oxygen to the blood, and supplementary oxygen will be required.

In many cases, the patient or his body will *tell* us that he needs more oxygen by certain signs and symptoms. When a person is suffering from acute respiratory insufficiency—that is, when, for whatever reason, not enough oxygen is reaching the tissues—the body responds with certain characteristic signs that it needs more oxygen. If the patient is alert and conscious, he will usually be aware of the difficulty and will report that he has SHORTNESS OF BREATH (**dyspnea**). His body, meanwhile, will be showing various reactions to hypoxia. In an attempt to bring more air into the lungs, the respiratory muscles will start working faster, and the patient will be seen to be breathing faster (**tachypnea**) and more deeply (**hyperpnea**). In order to do this, the patient may have to use additional muscles besides the diaphragm and the intercostals: *accessory muscles of respiration* in the neck, above the clavicles, and in the abdomen. As a result, when a person is in respiratory distress, one may be able to see RETRACTION OF THE NECK MUSCLES or upward motion of the Adam's apple (**"tracheal tugging"**) during inhalation and pushing with the abdominal muscles during exhalation. Often there will be FLARING OF THE NOSTRILS as they open wide to permit freer air flow. This kind of breathing is very tiring, and as the patient becomes fatigued, his breathing may grow more and more labored, until it consists mainly of GASPS.

An unconscious person with respiratory insufficiency, on the other hand, may show his inadequate respiration in other ways, especially if the respiratory depression is due to drugs or head trauma. In these instances, the RESPIRATIONS may be very SLOW AND SHALLOW and thus inadequate to move sufficient quantities of air in and out of the lungs.

If any patient, conscious or unconscious, is suffering from severe oxygen deficiency, he *may* have CYANOSIS of the skin, nail beds, and mucous membranes. When present, cyanosis is a reliable sign of hypoxia, but its absence is no guarantee that the patient is well oxygenated.

Signs and Symptoms of Acute Respiratory Insufficiency

- Dyspnea (shortness of breath)
- Tachypnea (rapid breathing) and hyperpnea (deep breathing)
- Labored or gasping respirations, or
- Slow, shallow respirations (unconscious patient)
- Use of accessory muscles in the neck and abdomen to assist respirations
- Nasal flaring
- Cyanosis

Whenever a patient displays any one of these symptoms or signs, he is telling us in no uncertain terms that he NEEDS OXYGEN, and the EMT's *first* action, before asking any further questions or conducting any further examination, should be to GIVE HIM OXYGEN. No ifs, ands, or buts.

EVERY PATIENT COMPLAINING OF SHORTNESS OF BREATH AND EVERY PATIENT DISPLAYING SIGNS OF RESPIRATORY INSUFFICIENCY SHOULD RECEIVE OXYGEN IMMEDIATELY.

Up to now, we have discussed those patients whose total body supply of oxygen is somehow compromised: patients in respiratory or cardiac arrest, patients whose respiratory function is impaired by illness or injury, and patients showing clear signs of respiratory distress. In all of these situations, we have seen that extra oxygen is clearly needed. But what about a patient who is breathing spontaneously, whose lungs are perfectly normal, and who shows no signs whatsoever of respiratory distress? Are there any circumstances in which such a patient might need extra oxygen?

Once again, the answer is yes. There are some conditions in which *part* of the patient's body may not be receiving enough oxygen, even though the oxygen supply to the body as a whole is adequate. Take for example the case of a HEART ATTACK, or myocardial infarction. A heart attack occurs when part of the cardiac muscle does not get the blood supply it needs. There may be a partial or complete blockage in the artery that supplies that portion of the cardiac muscle, and as a result the flow of oxygenated blood to the area is reduced to a tiny trickle or stops altogether. The rest of the body is doing fine, for oxygenated blood is flowing normally through all the other arteries in the body. But the heart, or a portion of the heart, is suffocating, for not enough blood is reaching it to furnish the oxygen it needs. Once again, the only way to increase the oxygen supply to the heart is to give *all* the red blood cells a bigger bucket of oxygen; then the red blood cells that do reach the heart can make up for the fact that fewer of them are getting through. A similar situation exists in a patient who has suffered a STROKE. In this case, it is part of the brain whose circulation has been interrupted. A clot may have formed inside one of the arteries supplying the brain tissue, and as a consequence, that part of the brain has a markedly reduced blood flow. Once again, the way to approach this problem is to increase the amount of oxygen each red blood cell is carrying—by giving the patient extra oxygen to breathe. Thus the patient with a possible heart attack (which means, practically speaking, any adult patient with chest pain) and the patient with a possible stroke NEED OXYGEN, *even though their lungs may be perfectly normal and they show so signs of respiratory distress.*

To return, then, to our original question: Who needs oxygen?

Patients Who Need Oxygen

- Any patient at risk of AIRWAY OBSTRUCTION
  1. Any patient who is UNCONSCIOUS
  2. Any patient who is having SEIZURES
- Any patient who requires ARTIFICIAL VENTILATION
- Any patient in CARDIAC ARREST
- Any patient in SHOCK
- Any patient complaining of SHORTNESS OF BREATH
- Any patient with signs of RESPIRATORY DISTRESS (tachypnea, hyperpnea, gasping, use of accessory muscles to breathe)
- Any patient BREATHING LESS THAN 10 TIMES PER MINUTE
- Any patient rescued from DROWNING
- Any patient with TRAUMA TO THE CHEST
- Any patient exposed to SMOKE, TOXIC FUMES, or CARBON MONOXIDE
- Any patient complaining of CHEST PAIN
- Any patient with suspected STROKE

We have already dealt with airway obstruction, respiratory arrest, cardiac arrest, and shock in previous chapters. We will consider the other conditions listed above in more detail later in the book. What is important to remember now is that there are many circumstances in which a patient needs oxygen, even when he appears to be breathing normally and has no apparent impairment of his respiratory system. Oxygen is a life-giving gas. Do not be afraid to use it!

WHEN IN DOUBT, GIVE OXYGEN.

OXYGEN CYLINDERS AND REGULATORS

Pure or 100% oxygen is usually supplied as a compressed gas in steel or aluminum cylinders. These cylinders are given letter descriptions according to their size. For example, an E cylinder is 4.5 inches by 30 inches and contains about 625 liters of oxygen. A D cylinder is somewhat smaller and contains 350 liters of oxygen, while the larger M cylinder contains 3,000 liters of oxygen. In all of these cylinders, large or small, gas is stored under very high pressures—2,000 *pounds per square inch* (2,000 **psi**)—much too much pressure to deliver directly into a patient's airway; a blast of oxygen or any gas at 2,000 psi would literally send the patient into orbit. For this reason, the gas flow from an oxygen cylinder is controlled by a **pressure regulator,** or *reducing valve,* which (as the name implies) reduces the pressure of gas coming out of the cylinder from 2,000 psi to levels more suitable for administration to patients, that is, about 40 to 70 psi. Cylinders of E size or smaller have special outlet valves to which the pressure regulator attaches by means of a *yoke* containing one or more pins. Each yoke is designed so that its pins will fit only the cylinder for one type of gas (e.g., oxygen or helium); thus the pressure regulator for oxygen cannot be accidently attached to a cylinder containing a different gas. As an additional safety measure, all gas

the flow rate to the duration of flow. Since cylinders of different sizes hold different quantities of oxygen, we also have to take into account the cylinder size in our equation. We do this with a "cylinder constant," that is, a factor that is constant for any given cylinder size. Our equation looks like this:

Calculating Duration of Remaining Oxygen Flow

$$\text{Duration of flow (min)} = \frac{(\text{gauge pressure} - 200 \text{ psi}) \times \text{cylinder constant}}{\text{flow rate (L/min)}}$$

Cylinder Constants

D cylinder = 0.16 liter/psi
E cylinder = 0.28 liter/psi
G cylinder = 2.41 liters/psi
M cylinder = 1.56 liters/psi

If we look closely at this equation, it is clear that the higher the gauge pressure, the more oxygen is left in the cylinder (the longer the duration of oxygen flow). On the other hand, the faster the flow, the more quickly the oxygen will be used up. This can be understood intuitively.

Let us take a couple of examples to see how this equation works.

1. Suppose the ambulance carries a fixed M cylinder for the piped-in oxygen supply of the vehicle. The reading on the pressure gauge of the M cylinder is 500 psi, and you are presently running the oxygen at a flow rate of 4 liters per minute (i.e., this is the reading on the flow meter). How long can you expect the oxygen to last before you reach the safe residual of 200 psi and must replace the cylinder?

$$\text{Duration of flow} = \frac{(\text{gauge pressure} - 200 \text{ psi}) \times \text{cylinder constant}}{\text{flow rate (L/min)}}$$
$$= \frac{(500 \text{ psi} - 200 \text{ psi}) \times 1.56 \text{ L/psi}}{4 \text{ L/min}}$$
$$= \frac{300 \text{ psi} \times 1.56 \text{ L/psi}}{4 \text{ L/min}}$$
$$= \frac{468 \text{ L}}{4 \text{ L/min}}$$
$$= 117 \text{ min} = 1 \text{ hr and } 57 \text{ min}$$

2. Suppose you carry a portable oxygen unit utilizing an E cylinder. The pressure gauge on the E cylinder reads 1,200 psi, and you are administering oxygen during CPR at a rate of 10 liters per minute. How long can you continue before the pressure reaches the safe residual of 200 psi and you have to switch to a new cylinder?

$$\text{Duration of flow} = \frac{(\text{gauge pressure} - 200 \text{ psi}) \times \text{cylinder constant}}{\text{flow rate (L/min)}}$$
$$= \frac{(1{,}200 \text{ psi} - 200 \text{ psi}) \times 0.28 \text{ L/psi}}{10 \text{ L/min}}$$
$$= \frac{280 \text{ L}}{10 \text{ L/min}}$$
$$= 28 \text{ min}$$

Thus, even though the pressure in the cylinder is relatively high, the cylinder will not last very long because it is not very large and is being emptied rapidly.

It should be part of the EMT's daily routine to check the pressure remaining both in the main cylinder of the vehicle's oxygen supply and in the cylinders of all the portable units on board, so that they can be replaced when the supply of oxygen runs low. Wherever possible, a backup main cylinder should be carried on the vehicle, while backup portable cylinders should always be available. Remember:

IT IS GROSS NEGLIGENCE TO RESPOND TO A CALL WITH AN EMPTY OXYGEN CYLINDER.

Safety Precautions

As mentioned previously, oxygen cylinders contain gas under very high pressure, and improper handling of an oxygen cylinder can convert it into an unguided missile with enormous destructive power. Furthermore, while oxygen is not an explosive gas, it does *support combustion;* a small spark becomes a flame in an oxygen-enriched atmosphere, and the glowing end of a cigarette can become a small torch. For these reasons, certain safety rules must be followed in the handling of oxygen cylinders.

- Combustible materials, such as oil or grease, must never be permitted to come in contact with the cylinders, regulators, fittings, valves, or hoses. NEVER USE OIL OR GREASE to lubricate any part of the oxygen assembly, and do not manipulate any part of the oxygen assembly if your hands are greasy.
- NEVER PERMIT SMOKING in any area where oxygen cylinders are in use or on standby. The interior of the ambulance and any oxygen storage areas should be clearly marked with large signs reading "OXYGEN—NO SMOKING."
- The oxygen cylinder should never be subjected to temperatures above 125°F (about 50°C). Store reserve cylinders in a COOL, WELL-VENTILATED AREA.

- An oxygen cylinder should never be used without a safe, PROPERLY FITTING REGULATOR VALVE. Regulator valves for one gas should never be modified for use with another gas. Use only those regulator valves intended for attachment to an oxygen cylinder.
- The PRESSURE REGULATOR and FLOW METER should be CLOSED when the oxygen cylinder is not in use, even if the cylinder is empty.
- Oxygen cylinders should be SECURED to prevent toppling over. In transit, they should be in a proper carrier or rack or strapped onto the stretcher with the patient.
- When attaching the pressure regulator or turning on the valves, ALWAYS POSITION YOURSELF TO THE SIDE OF THE CYLINDER. NEVER PLACE YOUR FACE OR ANY PART OF YOUR BODY OVER THE PRESSURE REGULATOR. A loose regulator can be blown off the cylinder with sufficient force to amputate a head or demolish any other object in its path.
- Oxygen cylinders must be retested every 10 years to ensure that they can still sustain the high pressures required. The original test date is stamped onto every oxygen cylinder, together with its serial number and other information.

Cylinder Safety in Brief

- No grease
- No smoking
- No heat
- Appropriate regulator valve
- All valves closed when not in use
- Firmly secured
- Face and body to the side of the cylinder
- Periodic testing

Operating the Oxygen Cylinder

With the above precautions in mind, let us go through the steps in operating the oxygen cylinder:

1. Place the cylinder securely UPRIGHT, and position yourself TO THE SIDE.
2. "CRACK" THE TANK with the wrench supplied; that is, slowly open and rapidly close the cylinder valve to clear it of any dust or debris.
3. Inspect the PRESSURE REGULATOR (reducing valve) to make sure it is the right type for an oxygen cylinder and that is has an intact washer (rubber ring).
4. Apply the pressure regulator to the cylinder and tighten it securely.
5. Open the MAIN CYLINDER VALVE slowly to about one-half a turn beyond the point where the reducing valve becomes pressurized.
6. Open the FLOW METER CONTROL VALVE to the desired liter flow.
7. When you are ready to terminate oxygen therapy, shut off the flow meter control until the liter flow is zero.
8. Shut off the main cylinder valve.
9. Bleed the valves of any residual pressure by reopening the flow meter control and leaving it open until the needle or ball indicator returns to zero.
10. Shut off the flow meter control.

DELIVERY OF OXYGEN TO PATIENTS WHO ARE BREATHING SPONTANEOUSLY

There are a variety of devices available for delivering oxygen to spontaneously breathing patients, from simple face masks to oxygen tents. Some of these devices are more practical for work outside the hospital than others, and in this section, we will look at those oxygen delivery devices that have applicability to field situations (Fig. 9-13).

Nasal Catheter

The nasal catheter (Fig. 9-13A) is a soft rubber or plastic tube with several holes at the end and is designed to be inserted through the patient's nostril so that it comes to rest in the posterior nasopharynx. At a flow rate of 6 to 8 liters per minute, the nasal catheter can deliver concentrations of oxygen of 30 to 50%. Higher flow rates should not be used, for they will simply cause drying of the mucous membranes without any appreciable gain in oxygen concentration. The nasal catheter should NOT be used in unconscious or debilitated patients, for such patients have impaired reflexes, and large quantities of oxygen may flow into their stomachs, causing gastric distention. The steps in inserting a nasal catheter are as follows:

1. Explain to the patient what you are about to do.
2. Place the tip of the catheter at the patient's ear lobe, and measure the distance to the tip of the patient's nose. Mark this distance off on the catheter.
3. Lubricate the end of the catheter with water-soluble jelly.
4. Gently insert the catheter into one nostril, and advance it slowly until its tip is visible in the back of the throat. If you encounter resistance, try the other nostril.
5. Pull the catheter back very slightly, just until its tip is no longer visible in the back of the throat.
6. Tape the catheter securely to the patient's nose and cheek.
7. Attach the catheter to the oxygen tubing, and turn on the oxygen to the desired flow rate.

Be very careful not to advance the nasal catheter beyond the mark you have placed on it; if the catheter descends too far, it can enter the esophagus and quite literally inflate the stomach like a balloon.

In general, nasal catheters are NOT the best means of administering oxygen, for they are not particularly comfortable for the patient, and there is the constant risk of the catheter's slipping into the esophagus. This means of oxygen delivery should not be used unless more suitable equipment is unavailable.

It is worthwhile to note one rather unusual but effective use of the nasal catheter, which justifies stashing one or two of the devices in the vehicle, and that is to provide supplementary oxygen to the patient during mouth-to-mouth ventilation. What makes this application of the catheter unusual is the fact that the catheter is inserted into the *rescuer's* nasopharynx, not the patient's. This fills the rescuer's airway with a moderately high concentration of oxygen, and when the rescuer exhales into the victim's mouth, he can deliver up to about 40% oxygen, instead of the 16% oxygen normally present in exhaled air.

Nasal Cannula

Far more desirable for use in the field when moderate oxygen concentrations are needed is the two-pronged nasal cannula (Fig. 9-13B). This is a circle or semicircle of plastic tubing with two plastic tips that fit into the patient's nostrils. A nasal cannula will deliver an oxygen concentration of 25 to 40% with a flow rate of 4 to 6 liters per minute (higher flow rates will not increase the delivered oxygen concentration and will only dry the mucous membranes). The nasal cannula is probably the most comfortable oxygen delivery device for the patient, and its only drawback is that it cannot deliver high oxygen concentrations.

> THE TWO-PRONGED NASAL CANNULA IS THE PREFERRED MEANS OF DELIVERING OXYGEN TO A SPONTANEOUSLY BREATHING PATIENT WHEN ONLY MODERATE OXYGEN CONCENTRATIONS ARE REQUIRED.

Simple Face Mask

The simple face mask (Fig. 9-13C) is just a piece of clear plastic molded to fit over the face, with an inlet tube for oxygen to enter and multiple holes to allow the escape of excess oxygen and exhaled air. It is held in place by an elastic strap. At high flow rates (8–12 liters/min), the simple face mask can deliver 50 to 60% oxygen, although if the mask is not tightly applied or if the patient is breathing deeply, air may be drawn into the mask and dilute the oxygen concentration. The simple face mask in general delivers only a slightly higher oxygen concentration than the nasal cannula, and it is usually not as well tolerated as the cannula, for many patients feel "suffocated" wearing a mask. Thus the simple face mask usually offers no particular advantage over the nasal cannula in situations where moderate oxygen concentrations are required.

Venturi Mask

The Venturi mask (Fig. 9-13D) is designed in such a way that the flow of oxygen into the mask pulls air into the mask with it in a fixed combination, thereby permitting the delivery of accurate, relatively low oxygen concentrations. Masks are available that can deliver 24, 28, 35, and 40% oxygen. Venturi masks are especially useful for the long-term treatment in the hospital of patients with chronic lung disease, for some of these patients do not tolerate high oxygen concentrations. These masks offer no particular advantage in the field, except for the long-range transport of patients with chronic lung disease who are in relatively stable condition.

Partial Rebreathing Mask

A partial rebreathing mask (Fig. 9-13E) is a face mask with a reservoir bag attached to it, and it enables the patient to rebreathe about one-third of his own exhaled air. Since this air is primarily from the patient's "dead space" (i.e., the part of the respiratory tract where oxygen exchange does *not* take place: the larynx, trachea, bronchi, etc.), it contains mostly oxygen inspired during the previous inhalation. At flow rates of 6 to 10 liters per minute, a partial rebreathing mask will provide oxygen concentrations of 35 to 60%.

Nonrebreathing Mask

The nonrebreathing mask (Fig. 9-13F) resembles a partial rebreathing mask in that it also has an oxygen reservoir bag, but in this case the reservoir bag is equipped with a one-way valve that permits inhalation of oxygen from the reservoir but prevents exhaled air from entering the reservoir. During inhalation the patient breathes 100% oxygen from the reservoir bag, while during exhalation the bag refills with oxygen from the oxygen source and the patient's exhaled air is vented out of the mask. The oxygen flow rate is adjusted to prevent collapse of the bag during inhalation, usually about 10 to 12 liters per minute. If the mask is fitted tightly to the patient's face, the nonrebreathing mask can deliver oxygen concentrations approaching 100%. Thus this mask is ideally suited to situations in which there is a need to deliver high oxygen concentrations to a spontaneously breathing patient.

> THE NONREBREATHING MASK IS THE PREFERRED MEANS OF DELIVERING *HIGH* OXYGEN CONCENTRATIONS TO A SPONTANEOUSLY BREATHING PATIENT.

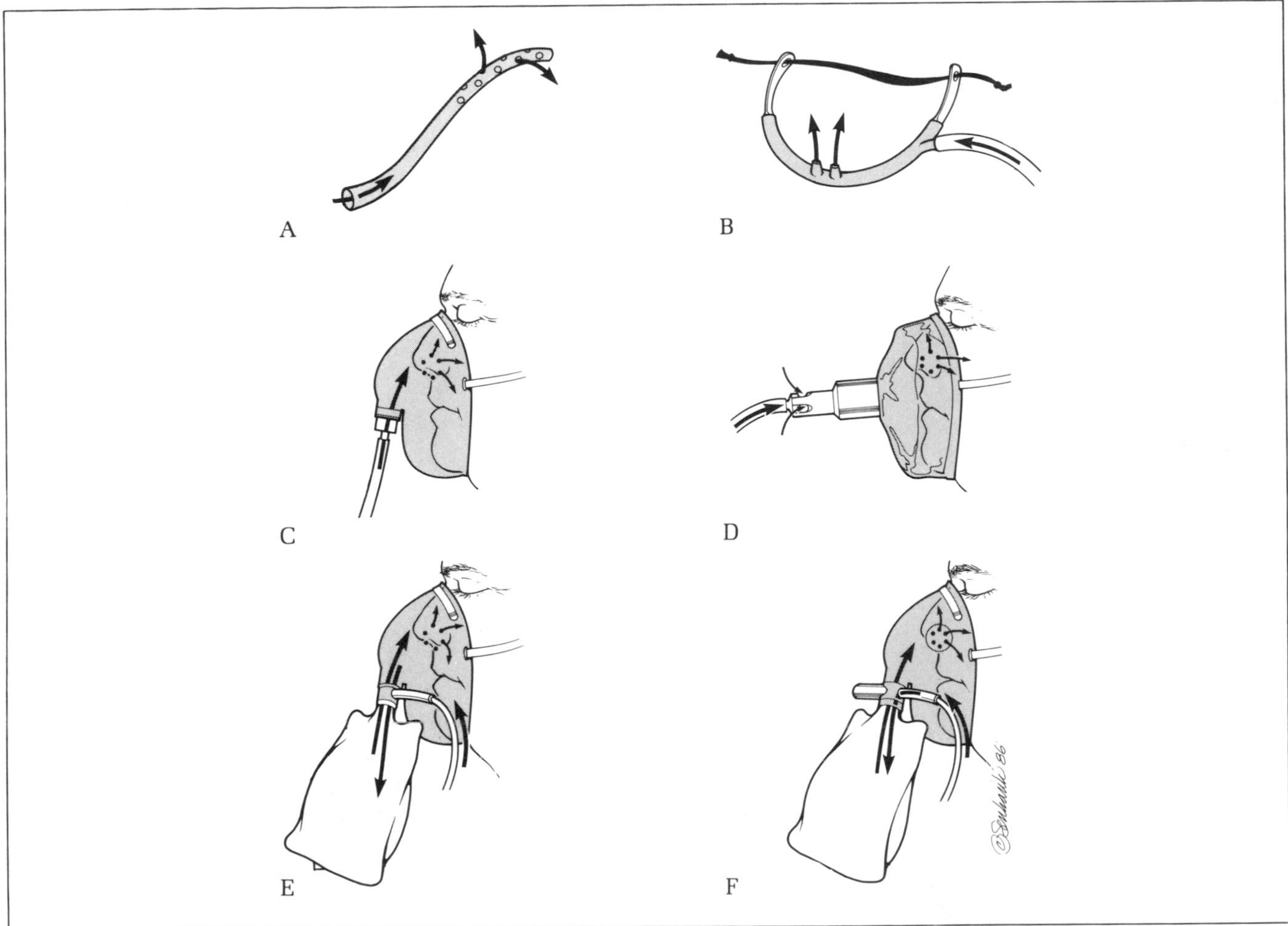

Fig. 9-13. *Oxygen administration devices. A. Nasal catheter. B. Two-pronged nasal cannula. C. Simple face mask. D. Venturi mask. E. Partial rebreathing mask. F. Nonrebreathing mask.*

As noted earlier, some patients—indeed, often the very patients who need oxygen most desperately—simply will not tolerate any sort of face mask because the mask makes them feel as if they are suffocating. This is often the case, for example, in patients with pulmonary edema (a condition where the lungs literally fill up with fluid, which may even bubble out of the mouth—see Chapter 19). These patients are apt to be frantic from **hypoxia** (oxygen deficiency), and often they will rip the mask off as fast as you can put it on. In such a situation, you may have to switch to the nasal cannula, even though the patient needs 100% oxygen and would be much better off with a nonrebreathing mask; but the 30 or 40% oxygen delivered by the nasal prongs is better than the 21% he would get without any supplementary oxygen at all. In a calmer patient, an explanation may enable the patient to tolerate the mask better. If you forewarn the patient that the mask may feel confining, but that in fact it is providing "more air" than breathing without it, he may be able to overcome his anxiety about having something over his face.

The properties of different types of cannulas and masks are summarized in Table 9-2.

DELIVERY OF OXYGEN TO PATIENTS WHO ARE NOT BREATHING

The cannulas and masks described in the previous section do not deliver oxygen with sufficient pressure to inflate a person's lungs, and thus they cannot be used to provide oxygen to a nonbreathing patient. If by now you have had a chance to practice mouth-to-mouth ventilation, you are aware that it takes considerable force to overcome the resistance of a patient's lungs and drive air into them. In artificial ventilation, then, one needs a *power source* to generate the pressure required for lung inflation. This power source can be the rescuer's lungs, a bag that is squeezed by hand, or a direct line off the pressure regulator of the oxygen cylinder.

Table 9-2. *Oxygen Delivery Systems for Spontaneously Breathing Patients*

Device	Flow Rate Used	Oxygen Delivered (%)	Comments
Nasal catheter	6–8 L/min	30–50	Do NOT use in unconscious patients. Be careful not to insert too far. Use chiefly for giving supplementary oxygen during mouth-to-mouth ventilation (inserted into rescuer's nasopharynx).
Nasal cannula	4–6 L/min	25–40	Recommended device for delivering moderate oxygen concentrations in the field; well-tolerated. Do not exceed 6 L/min flow rate.
Simple face mask	8–12 L/min	50–60	Minimum advantage over nasal cannula.
Venturi mask	4–8 L/min	24, 28, 35, 40	Useful in long-term treatment in the hospital of patients with chronic obstructive lung disease; limited value in the field.
Partial rebreathing mask	6–10 L/min	35–60	
Nonrebreathing mask	10–12 L/min	90	Recommended device for delivering high oxygen concentrations to spontaneously breathing patients. Must have good mask fit to achieve high oxygen concentrations.

Mouth-to-Mask Ventilation

In mouth-to-mask ventilation, the power source for artificial ventilation is the rescuer's lungs, but the ventilations are delivered to the patient through a mask, rather than directly to the patient's mouth. Since, as we have already learned, it is desirable to administer oxygen to *every* patient who requires artificial ventilation, the ideal mask for mouth-to-mask ventilation is one that will permit oxygen to be piped in to supplement the rescuer's exhaled air. Such a device is the POCKET MASK with oxygen inlet valve, which can provide oxygen concentrations of up to 50% in mouth-to-mask ventilation when used with an oxygen flow rate of 10 liters per minute. The pocket mask is clear plastic and collapses to fit in a small case easily carried in one's pocket (hence the name). If you have the mask with you, it can be used to initiate artificial ventilation simply with exhaled air, and then an oxygen line can be hooked to it as soon as oxygen is available. For those who are somewhat squeamish about mouth-to-mouth ventilation, the pocket mask is an ideal device to carry on one's person.

To use the pocket mask with oxygen, perform a triple airway maneuver from the patient's vertex, and apply the lower rim of the pocket mask between the patient's lower lip and chin to pull the lip down and hold the mouth open (Fig. 9-14). Clamp the remainder of the mask to the face with both thumbs along the sides of the mask. The fingers grasp the jaw just beneath the angles and pull upward, to maintain backward tilt of the head. Then exhale intermittently into the mask, forcing your own breath—now enriched with oxygen—into the patient's lungs. After each breath, remove your mouth from the mask to permit the patient to exhale. As with any means of artificial ventilation, when ventilating with a pocket mask it is still necessary to look for the rise and fall of the chest as a sign of effective ventilation.

If the oxygen flow rate into the mask is high enough (15 liters/min or more), you can simply occlude the opening of the mask periodically with your tongue and allow the oxygen flow to ventilate the patient. With this method, oxygen concentrations considerably higher than 50% can be delivered, but you must make certain that the chest rises with each ventilation. If it does not, you must add your own ventilation to the oxygen flow.

The pocket mask is an excellent device for artificial ventilation, and it has several significant advantages over the other devices to be described:

- It has the same advantage as mouth-to-mouth ventilation; that is, it permits the rescuer to deliver *higher volumes* of air than can be delivered with a bag-valve-mask device.
- *Both* hands can be used to hold the mask on the patient's face, thus ensuring a tight seal and also facilitating head tilt.
- The rescuer can *feel the resistance* of the patient's lungs in his own lungs and thus gauge the efficacy of inflations more accurately.
- If the pocket mask is indeed carried in the rescuer's pocket, artificial ventilation can be initiated and continued with the same method.
- Should the patient resume spontaneous ventilation, the pocket mask may be strapped to his face and used, with high flows, as a simple face mask.

For the above reasons, it is this author's view that a pocket mask should be carried by every EMT and

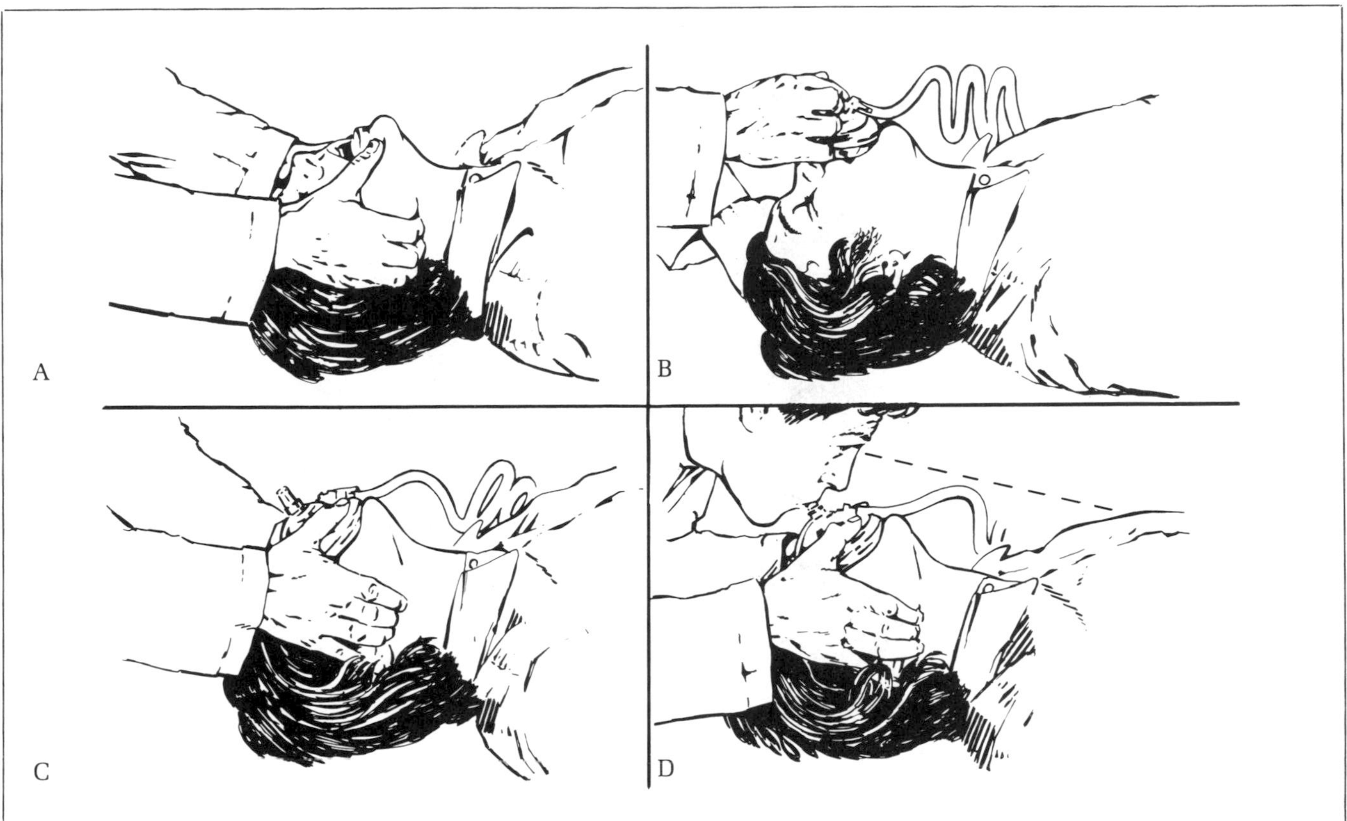

Fig. 9-14. *Application of pocket mask. A. Perform triple airway maneuver from the vertex. B. Fit mask over nose and mouth. C. Clamp mask to face, maintaining head tilt. D. Exhale into mask until the chest rises. (Reproduced courtesy Asmund Laerdal, Stavanger, Norway.)*

should be regarded as the *preferred method of administering artificial ventilation* until an esophageal obturator airway or endotracheal tube is in place.

Bag-Valve-Mask Ventilation

The second principal power source for artificial ventilation is the rescuer's hand, used to squeeze the contents of a bag of air or oxygen into the patient's lungs. A bag used for this purpose is called a BAG-VALVE-MASK UNIT, after its three main components: a rubber or plastic bag that serves as a reservoir of air, a one-way valve that prevents exhalation back into the bag, and a mask to fit the unit to the patient's face. The mask is usually detachable so that the bag-valve unit can be fitted to an endotracheal tube (a tube placed directly into the patient's trachea) or an esophageal obturator airway (see Esophageal Obturator Airway).

The operational principle of the bag-valve-mask is quite simple. When the bag is squeezed, air leaves the bag through the nonrebreathing valve in front and is delivered to the patient. Another one-way valve prevents air from escaping through the air inlet. When the bag is released and it reexpands, air is pulled into the bag through the inlet valve. At the same time, the air being passively exhaled from the patient's lungs passes through the mask and out into the atmosphere through the nonrebreathing valve. If an oxygen supply is connected to the bag, both air and oxygen are pulled into the bag each time it reexpands, and depending on the oxygen flow rate, the oxygen concentration in the bag can reach about 40%. If, in addition, one attaches a long, wide tube (Fig. 9-15A) or a reservoir bag (Fig. 9-15B) to the air inlet valve, then oxygen will be pulled in from *both* the oxygen source and the air inlet valve as the bag reexpands. With this system, the oxygen concentration in the bag can approach 100%. This setup—with an oxygen reservoir—is the ideal way of using the bag-valve-mask unit, for it enables delivery of the high oxygen concentrations that are needed in artificial ventilation.

The American Heart Association has proposed the following minimum design standards for the bag-valve-mask unit:

- The bag should be self-refilling, but without any sponge rubber inside. Sponge rubber filling makes the interior of the bag difficult to clean and disinfect, and the sponge rubber also tends to break apart with use.
- The valve system should work freely, without jamming, at an oxygen flow of 15 liters per minute. The valve should be a true nonrebreathing valve and should be designed in such a way that it

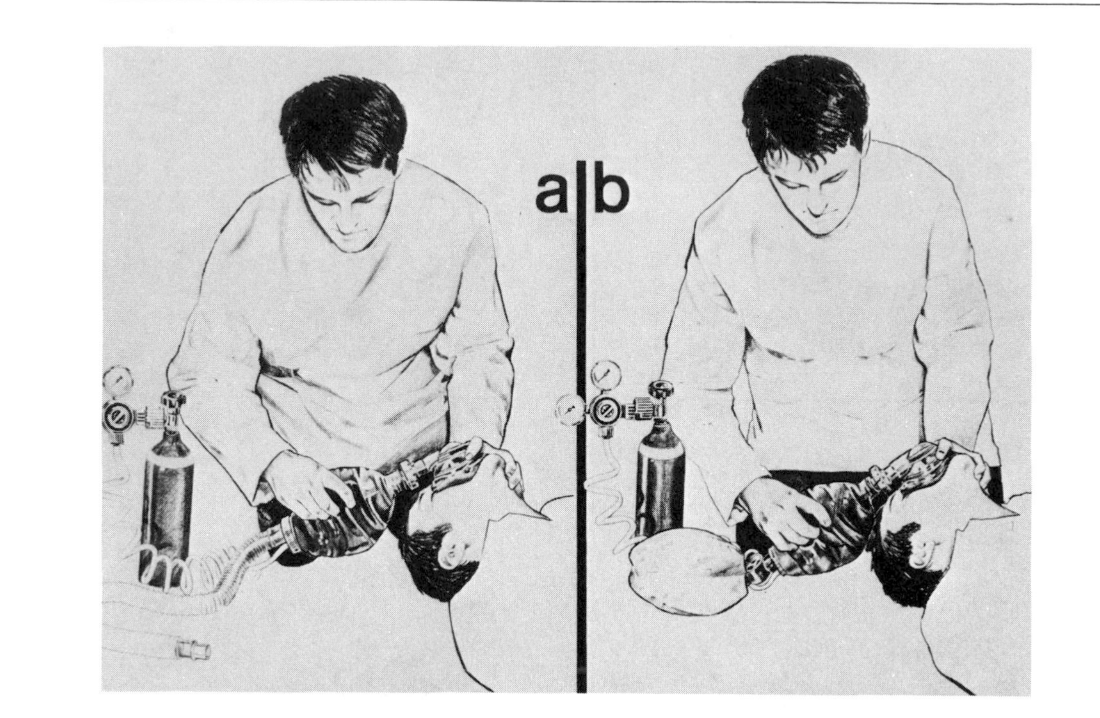

Fig. 9-15. *Bag-valve-mask unit with oxygen. A. With reservoir tube. B. With reservoir bag. (Reproduced courtesy Asmund Laerdal, Stavanger, Norway.)*

cannot be incorrectly assembled (e.g., inserted in the bag backward).

- The valve should fit not only the mask, but should have a standard 15 mm/22 fitting so that it can also be attached to an endotracheal tube or esophageal obturator airway.
- There should be no pop-off valve (a valve that opens at a certain pressure to vent the system).
- The face mask should be of transparent plastic to enable the rescuer to observe the victim's mouth for vomitus or secretions, and it should have a resilient cuff that molds tightly to form a seal around the patient's nose and mouth.
- There should be a system for delivering high concentrations of oxygen, through an inlet at the back of the bag or through an oxygen reservoir.
- The unit should be available in both adult and pediatric sizes.
- The unit should function properly under all environmental conditions and extremes of temperature.

The bag-valve-mask is more difficult to use than the pocket mask, and it requires considerable practice to perform ventilations with the bag-valve-mask properly. The device usually provides less volume for ventilation than the mouth-to-mouth or mouth-to-mask technique, partly because of the difficulty in maintaining a leakproof seal between the mask and the face using only one hand. (To check this for yourself, try both mouth-to-mouth and bag-valve-mask ventilation on a recording manikin and see which method delivers more air with each breath.) For these reasons, the pocket mask with oxygen supplementation is preferable to the bag-valve-mask for giving artificial ventilation to a patient who has not yet been intubated with an endotracheal tube or esophageal obturator airway.

To operate the bag-valve-mask, it is first of all desirable to insert an oropharyngeal airway into the patient's mouth, for you will find it difficult otherwise to maintain an open airway by manual methods when one of your hands is tied up squeezing the bag. Once the oropharyngeal airway is in place, position yourself at the patient's vertex; tilt the patient's head back (Fig. 9-16A), and place your thumb and index finger on the mask—the thumb above and the index finger below the valve connection. Use your other fingers to grip the mandible and hold a tight seal to the mask (Fig. 9-16B). Then compress the bag at the proper rate, observing for the rise and fall of the chest with each ventilation. If the chest does not rise, recheck the patient's head position and the seal of the mask against his face.

Some people—especially those with small hands—find it more comfortable to place the palm of the hand over the mask and lock the mask in place with their fingers curled under the patient's chin (Fig. 9-16C). This method is also acceptable, but one must take care not to flex the patient's head forward as one pushes down on the mask. The fingers grasping the

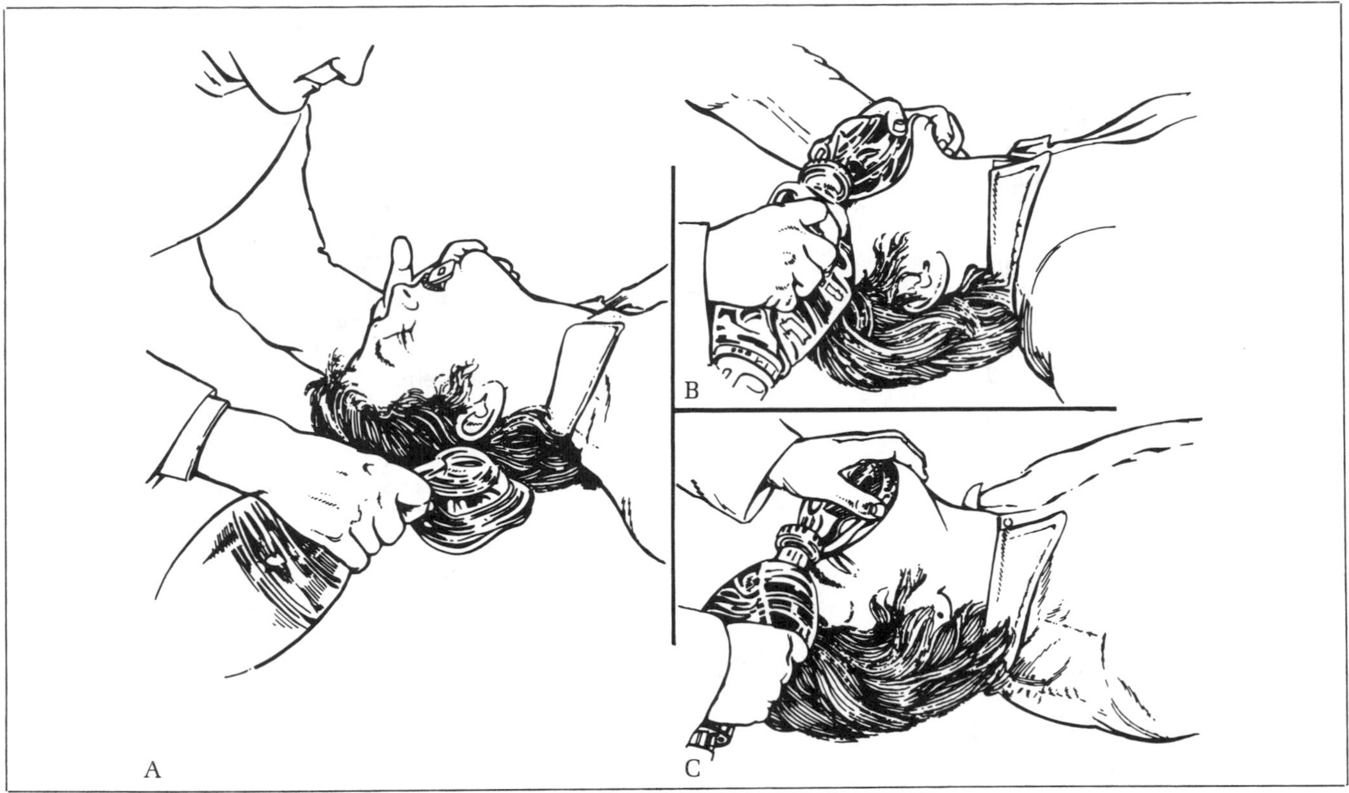

Fig. 9-16. *Use of bag-valve-mask. A. Patient's head tilted back, oropharyngeal airway in place. B. "C-clamp" grip to hold mask to face. C. Use of palm to hold mask to face. (Reproduced courtesy Asmund Laerdal, Stavanger, Norway.)*

chin should be used to pull backward and thereby maintain hyperextension of the head.

The bag-valve-mask device with oxygen can also be used to *assist* the ventilations of a patient who is breathing spontaneously but not breathing adequately. The mask is applied to the patient's face as described, and the bag is *gently* squeezed each time the patient begins to inhale. By this technique, one can increase the volume of each breath the patient takes.

Manually Triggered, Oxygen-powered Resuscitator (Demand Valve)

The third potential source of power for artificial ventilation is the pressure from the oxygen cylinder, and the device that utilizes this power source is the manually triggered, oxygen-powered resuscitator, more commonly called a **demand valve.**

The demand valve is connected by a reinforced rubber hose to the pressure regulator of the oxygen cylinder and is inserted into a face mask (which should, like any face mask, be transparent plastic). On top of the valve unit, there is a push button that controls oxygen flow; when the push button is depressed, oxygen streams out at very high flow rates (in the range of 100–150 liters/min) until the operator takes his finger off the push button *or* until a preset pressure (40–50 mm Hg) is reached, at which point the oxygen flow immediately stops. This pressure limit is a safety feature to prevent the rescuer from literally blowing out a hole in the patient's lung. Thus as the lungs inflate and the pressure within them increases, the oxygen flow automatically shuts off. When the push button is depressed periodically to provide ventilation to a nonbreathing patient in this fashion, it is called **controlled ventilation,** for the rescuer has control over the patient's breathing.

The demand valve also has a second mode of operation designed to augment the ventilations of a patient who is breathing spontaneously. When the face mask is sealed against the patient's face, the negative pressure created by the patient's inhalation will open the valve, without the rescuer depressing the push button, and oxygen will flow into the patient's lungs until the cutoff pressure is reached, at which point the oxygen flow shuts off automatically. This serves to increase the volume of each breath the patient takes and to enrich each breath with oxygen. This mode of operation is the reason for the name *demand valve,* for the patient receives a breath "on demand." When the device is used in this fashion—triggered by the inhalations of the patient rather than by the rescuer—the process is called **assisted ventilation.**

Table 9-3. *Devices for Delivering Oxygen to Nonbreathing Patients*

Device	Mode of Use	Oxygen Delivered (%)	Comments
Pocket mask	Exhaled air 10 L/min O_2 flow 15 L/min O_2 flow	16 50 90	Preferred method of giving artificial ventilation to a patient who does not have an endotracheal tube or EOA in place. Can be used as a simple face mask to give oxygen to a patient who resumes spontaneous breathing.
Bag-valve-mask	Room air 10–12 L/min O_2 flow 10–12 L/min O_2 flow with reservoir	21 40 90	Does not provide as much volume as mouth-to-mouth or mouth-to-mask ventilation. Best to restrict its use to patients who have an endotracheal tube or EOA in place.
Demand valve	Any mode	100	Very dry gas delivered; causes gastric distention if used with mask; do not use in children under 12. Best to restrict its use to patients who have an endotracheal tube or EOA in place. Can be used to assist ventilations.

Since the demand value is oxygen-powered, it delivers 100% oxygen to the patient. The oxygen delivered is very dry because it comes directly from the oxygen cylinder without passing through a humidifier. For this reason, prolonged use of the demand valve can cause drying of the patient's mucous membranes.

The American Heart Association has recommended the following minimum design standards for the demand valve:

- The device should provide instantaneous oxygen flow rates of at least 100 liters per minute and should have a safety release valve that opens at approximately 50 cm H_2O (about 32 mm Hg) pressure in order to prevent damage to the lung.
- It should provide 100% oxygen.
- It should operate satisfactorily under varying environmental conditions and extremes of temperature.
- It should have a standard 15 mm/22 coupling for attachment to an endotracheal tube or esophageal obturator airway.
- It should be rugged, compact, and easy to hold.
- It should have a trigger attached to the push button positioned in such a way that the rescuer can depress the valve while keeping both hands on the mask to hold it in position and maintain head tilt (i.e., so that the rescuer can hold the mask as he would hold a pocket mask).

The demand valve is most useful for (1) spontaneously breathing patients who require high concentrations of oxygen under pressure (e.g., patients in pulmonary edema) or (2) nonbreathing patients who have an endotracheal tube or esophageal obturator airway in place. When the demand valve is used for any length of time with a standard mask, the high air flows almost invariably cause gastric distention; for this reason, demand valve–*mask* ventilation is NOT recommended for controlled ventilation of nonbreathing patients. Because of the relatively high cutoff pressure, the demand valve also should NOT be used to ventilate children under 12 years old.

Controlled ventilation with a demand valve does *not* eliminate the need to maintain proper backward tilt of the head or to observe the chest for a rise and fall with each ventilation.

The devices for delivering oxygen to a nonbreathing patient are summarized in Table 9-3.

AIDS TO CIRCULATION

Up to now, we have examined adjunctive equipment that can help maintain an open *airway* and that can provide effective artificial *breathing*. Moving on through the ABCs, we come next to those devices designed to assist in providing artificial or spontaneous *circulation*. In this discussion, we will cover two types of equipment that aid in maintaining or restoring the circulation: (1) mechanical devices for chest compression and (2) defibrillators. The latter topic, defibrillation, is included for EMT-Intermediates who work under physician control in a system where specially trained EMTs are authorized to carry out this procedure.

MECHANICAL DEVICES FOR CHEST COMPRESSION

There are several devices available that can depress the patient's sternum and thus maintain external chest compressions. Those devices are used to (1) reduce the rescuers' fatigue, especially in prolonged resuscitation efforts, (2) increase the effectiveness of CPR by providing more uniform compressions, and (3) reduce the number of rescuers required to perform CPR.

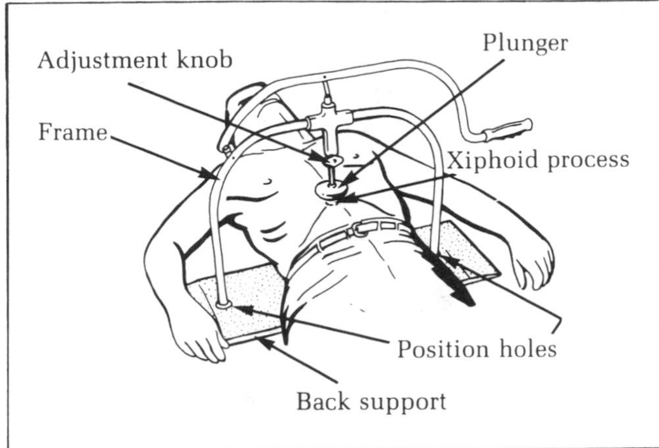

Fig. 9-17. *Cardiac press.*

Certain general guidelines apply to the use of any mechanical CPR device:

1. Use of these devices requires EXTENSIVE TRAINING and FREQUENT TEAM DRILL to ensure correct application, smooth coordination of team action, and rapid assembly time.
2. A mechanical CPR device should NEVER BE USED TO INITIATE CPR. Resuscitation should always be started manually and continued by manual techniques until the mechanical compressor is fully assembled and ready to be deployed. CPR should not be interrupted for more than 15 to 20 seconds to position a mechanical compressor.
3. Mechanical CPR devices should NOT BE USED ON INFANTS AND CHILDREN.

Mechanical CPR devices are best suited for use in the ambulance when a long transport with ongoing CPR is required, for manual CPR is very difficult to perform effectively in a moving vehicle. These devices also provide an excellent means for applying uninterrupted, uniform chest compressions while moving a patient down stairs or from any other location to the vehicle.

Mechanical chest compressors fall into two general categories: (1) manually operated cardiac presses and (2) automatic, gas-powered compressors.

Cardiac Press

The cardiac press (Fig. 9-17) is a hinged, manually operated chest compressor, which usually provides an adjustable stroke of 1.5 to 2.0 inches (3.8–5.1 cm). The advantages of this unit are its relatively low cost, ease of storage and assembly, light weight, and minimal possibility of mechanical breakdown. The steps in using the cardiac press are as follows:

1. INITIATE CPR BY MANUAL METHODS. One rescuer continues CPR while the second rescuer assembles the cardiac press.

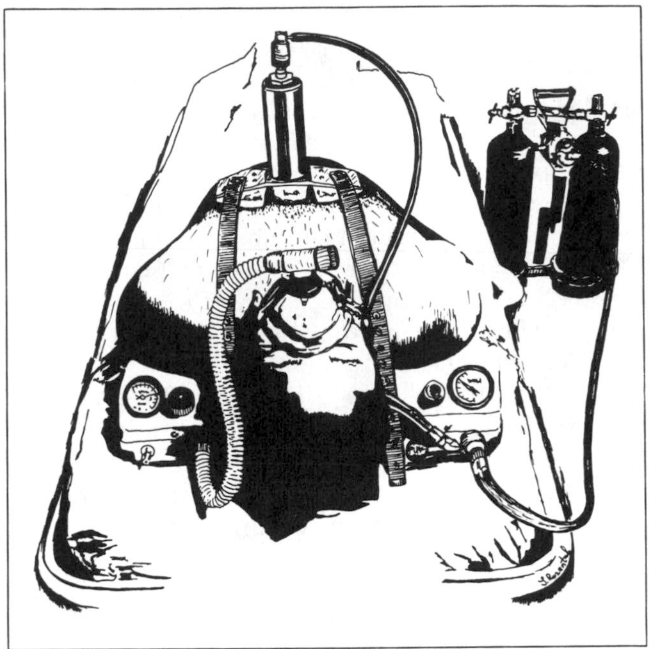

Fig. 9-18. *Automatic, gas-powered chest compressor.*

2. The second rescuer slides the BACK SUPPORT of the cardiac press beneath the victim's back and places the FRAME of the press into the position holes.
3. While the first rescuer is doing ventilations, the second rescuer loosens the adjustment knob of the press and POSITIONS THE PLUNGER centrally over the lower half of the sternum. Then the adjustment knob is retightened.
4. The second rescuer can now start external cardiac compressions by pushing down the handle of the press with a brisk stroke, then releasing the handle to allow the plunger to return to its up position. As with manual chest compressions, compressions with the cardiac press should be smooth; jerky, bouncing compressions must be avoided.
5. The first rescuer should CHECK periodically for the EFFECTIVENESS OF COMPRESSIONS by feeling for a carotid pulse with each compression. If compressions do not produce a palpable carotid pulse, readjust the length of the plunger shaft to give a deeper thrust and retighten the adjustment knob.

In using the cardiac press, you need to keep a sharp eye on the plunger to make sure that it does not shift position and inadvertently apply force over the ribs or abdomen. The adjustment knob should also be checked periodically, for if it becomes loose, the plunger will not deliver an adequate compression.

Automatic, Gas-powered Compressors

The automatic, gas-powered compressor (Fig. 9-18) delivers its compressions by a plunger that is mounted on a back support and driven by compressed oxygen; the same oxygen source may be used to provide artificial ventilation (in a manner similar to a demand valve) with an oxygen concentration of about 80%. The gas-powered compressor is very popular among ambulance personnel, for it enables them to give consistently effective compressions with a minimum of fatigue, even while moving the patient down stairs or out of difficult terrain. The device also permits delivery of more sustained compressions, which are believed to result in more effective artificial circulation. Its major disadvantage is that it consumes a lot of oxygen—41 liters per minute. Thus it will empty a D cylinder in about 7½ minutes of use, so one must either carry larger cylinders or bring a good supply of full D cylinders. A further disadvantage of the unit is that it is relatively expensive and also relatively heavy.

The ventilator unit of the gas-powered compressor is best used with an endotracheal tube or EOA in place, for—like a demand valve—it tends to cause gastric distention in the nonintubated patient because of the high oxygen flow rates. If the ventilator is used with a mask only, the rescuer must be highly skilled in maintaining an open airway.

The use of the gas-powered compressor requires at least two rescuers: one to initiate and maintain CPR, the other to secure and set up the equipment (Table 9-4).

Just as in using a cardiac press, one must keep a close watch on the plunger of the gas-powered compressor to make sure it does not shift position. Compressions over the ribs or xiphoid process are just as dangerous (if not more so) when applied by the plunger as when applied with the rescuer's hands.

Table 9-4. *Steps in Using the Gas-Powered Compressor*

First Rescuer	Second Rescuer
Initiates CPR by manual methods.	Secures the equipment.
Rolls patient onto side (5 sec)	Positions base plate under the patient so that the lower part of the patient's sternum is lined up over the center of the plate.
Rolls patient back supine.	
Resumes CPR.	Mounts and positions automatic chest compressor so that the plunger is over the lower third of the sternum in the midline.
	Turns on chest compressor.
Interposes a ventilation after every fifth compression.	Sets up ventilation equipment.
Switches to powered ventilator; maintains head tilt.	Checks for carotid pulsation with each compression.
Checks that chest rises with each ventilation.	
	Straps unit in place.

*DEFIBRILLATION**

Recent studies have suggested that the most critical factor in determining whether a patient who suffers ventricular fibrillation outside the hospital will be successfully resuscitated is the amount of time between the onset of ventricular fibrillation and the administration of definitive treatment, that is, defibrillation. The longer it takes to apply defibrillation, the less the chances of successful resuscitation. In regions with full advanced life support systems—that is, mobile intensive care units staffed by paramedics—defibrillation can be performed within minutes of starting CPR, and in such systems, successful resuscitation rates (= percent of patients in cardiac arrest who survive to be discharged from the hospital) of more than 40 percent have been reported. On the other hand, in communities that do not have paramedic services, defibrillation usually must be postponed until the patient reaches the hospital; reported rates of successful resuscitation in communities having only basic EMT services are in the range of 4 to 6 percent. While the solution to this problem would seem to be the establishment of paramedic units in every region, the very high cost of setting up and maintaining such services puts them out of the reach of many communities. For this reason, it has been proposed to train basic- or intermediate-level EMTs to perform defibrillation in those communities whose EMS resources are limited to basic life support units. The rationale for training EMTs in defibrillation is simple:

- The majority of cardiac arrests occurring outside the hospital are ventricular fibrillation (VF).
- The sooner a defibrillating shock can be delivered to a patient in VF, the greater the patient's chance of survival.
- Defibrillation, if delivered soon enough after the onset of cardiac arrest, is sufficient treatment for VF.
- Most communities are served by EMTs, either as sole providers of prehospital emergency care or as first responders in systems with paramedic backup.

*Not required of the EMT-A. This discussion is intended for EMT-Intermediates who work under physician control in a system where EMTs are authorized to perform defibrillation.

The first trial of this proposal in an area of King County, Washington, showed promising results. EMTs serving a suburban and semirural community of 79,000 people were given a 10-hour course in recognition of cardiac arrhythmias and defibrillation, and they were provided with detailed standing orders regarding when and how to perform defibrillation. In the 2 years prior to the course, when the EMTs gave standard basic life support only, 4 of 100 patients (4%) suffering cardiac arrest outside the hospital were resuscitated and discharged alive from the hospital. By contrast, during the year following the course, when EMTs were permitted to defibrillate according to standing orders, 10 of 54 patients (19%) found in cardiac arrest were successfully resuscitated. These findings suggested that EMTs could be considerably more effective in CPR if trained and equipped to perform defibrillation at the scene.

Since that first study in King County, several additional studies have amply confirmed the original findings. Furthermore, subsequent controlled trials have shown that even in regions where paramedic services are available, the provision of defibrillation skills to basic-level EMTs, who are the first responders, increases the number of lives saved. As a consequence of this research, programs authorizing EMT defibrillation are now operative in 18 states, and many other states are currently considering enabling legislation.

The encouraging results of EMT defibrillation need to be weighed in terms of the practical requirements and possibilities of a given community. In a suburban area with a relatively high population density, defibrillation by EMTs may indeed have considerable lifesaving potential and may represent an acceptable compromise between a basic and an advanced life support system. In rural areas, on the other hand, where the population is widely dispersed and response times are apt to be prolonged, the addition of a $7,000 defibrillator to a basic life support unit may not be a reasonable expense. Furthermore, in such areas, where the ambulance service as a whole may be called upon to respond to fewer than one cardiac arrest a year, it is very difficult for the EMT to maintain the high level of skill required to recognize and treat ventricular fibrillation. Thus the medical authorities in each community need to determine whether defibrillation by EMTs is a practical, safe, and cost-effective option.

In any system where defibrillation is performed by nonphysicians—be they EMTs or paramedics—there must be STRONG MEDICAL CONTROL. What this means in practice is (1) direct radio communications between the ambulance personnel and the responsible physician, ideally with the possibility of telemetry (a system for sending the patient's ECG to the physician by radio), (2) frequent case reviews involving the ambulance personnel and their medical director, and (3) periodic in-hospital refresher training. Case reviews and evaluation are greatly facilitated if the defibrillator unit is equipped with a dual-channel cassette recorder that can simultaneously record the patient's ECG and the conversation of the rescue team.

What Is Defibrillation?

Probably the first thing an EMT needs to know in learning how to perform defibrillation is what precisely defibrillation is and does. We have already learned that when the heart is in fibrillation all of its muscle fibers contract chaotically, completely out of phase with one another. The result is that the heart, instead of squeezing rhythmically as a single unit, simply quivers; if you were to look at a heart in fibrillation, its motion would resemble that of a plastic bag full of energetic worms. A heart that is quivering instead of beating cannot squeeze blood out into the circulation, so when we examine a patient in ventricular fibrillation, we cannot detect any pulse; that is, the patient is in cardiac arrest.

A defibrillator is a machine designed to deliver a precisely measured electric shock to the fibrillating heart, and what the shock does is momentarily paralyze all the muscle fibers in the heart so that they stop contracting altogether. The paralysis is only temporary, however, and within a few seconds, the muscle fibers resume their contractions. But what is important is that, if the defibrillation has been successful, all the muscle fibers resume contracting *at the same time*. If this happens, then the heart muscle is once again contracting and relaxing as a single unit, and it starts pumping again the way it is supposed to.

Defibrillation is effective *only* in treating ventricular fibrillation. It cannot restore the pulse of a patient whose cardiac arrest is due to asystole (cardiac standstill) or cardiovascular collapse. The problem is that it is impossible to distinguish from clinical signs alone which patients in cardiac arrest have ventricular fibrillation, which have asystole, and which have cardiovascular collapse, for all three of these conditions have exactly the same clinical sign: absence of a pulse. The only way to tell them apart is with an electrocardiogram.

The Electrocardiogram

As the heart contracts and relaxes, it generates tiny electric currents, and these currents can be measured by electrodes placed on the surface of the body. The machine that records these currents is called an **electrocardiograph,** and the record it produces is called an **electrocardiogram** (ECG). The ECG consists of a

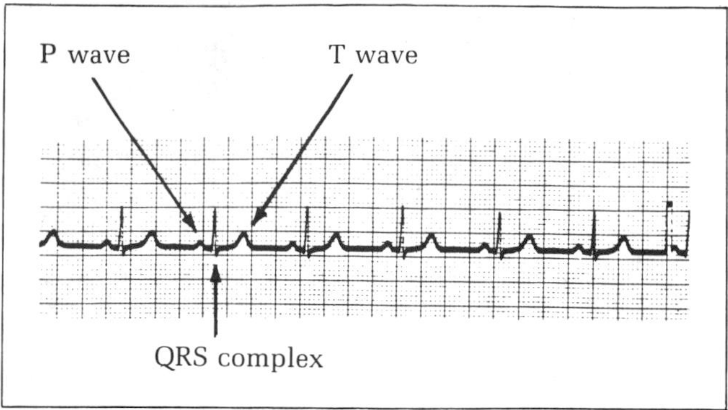

Fig. 9-19. *Normal electrocardiogram.*

series of waves and complexes that tell us what electric events are going on in the heart at any given time. Each of these waves and complexes has a name, and each corresponds to a specific electric event in the heart.

The main features of the *normal* ECG (Fig. 9-19) are the P wave, QRS complex, and T wave. The rounded hump called the **P wave** corresponds to depolarization of the two atria, which in general means the contraction of the atria. After a small fraction of a second, the P wave is followed by the spiked **QRS complex,** which represents depolarization of the ventricles—the time the ventricles are contracting. The next bump in the ECG, after the up-and-down spikes of the QRS complex, is the **T wave,** and it reflects the electric activity involved in gearing up for the next cardiac contraction. Thus a single cardiac cycle is represented by one P-QRS-T series: First the atria contract, then the ventricles contract, then the heart muscle recharges itself for the next contraction.

If you look closely at the paper on which the ECG is recorded, you will notice that it consists of a kind of grid, formed from horizontal and vertical lines. Since the ECG paper is run at a known speed, a given distance on the ECG paper is equivalent to a given time. This fact is very helpful, for it enables us to use the ECG to calculate the patient's heart rate. The simplest and often the most accurate way to do this is to count the number of ventricular contractions (QRS complexes) in a 6-second length of the ECG and multiply by 10 to determine how many times the ventricle is contracting in 60 seconds (1 min). Most ECG paper has markings along the top to indicate 3-second intervals, and you need to count the number of QRS complexes in two successive 3-second intervals to determine the number of contractions in 6 seconds (Fig. 9-20). Then multiply this figure by 10 to get the heart rate per minute.

NUMBER OF QRS COMPLEXES IN 6 SECONDS × 10 = HEART RATE PER MINUTE

It is very important to realize that an ECG provides information only about the *electric* events in the heart, *not* about the mechanical events. That is, the ECG measures only the travels of little electric currents through the heart muscle; it gives us no information whatsoever about how strongly the heart is pumping or indeed whether it is pumping effectively at all. For that information, one must feel the patient's pulse.

The ECG in Cardiac Arrest

Each of the three forms of cardiac arrest has a different ECG associated with it, and it is crucial for the EMT performing defibrillation to be able to recognize rapidly the characteristic ECG of ventricular fibrillation, for it is in this condition—AND THIS CONDITION ONLY—that defibrillation is permissible.

The ECG in VENTRICULAR FIBRILLATION (VF) is just like the movement of the heart muscle fibers in fibrillation—chaotic. Instead of a regular sequence of clearly defined waves and complexes, one sees merely a completely irregular, wavy line (Fig. 9-21), reflecting the fact that all the muscle fibers are

Fig. 9-20. *Calculation of heart rate: 8 complexes × 10 = 80/min.*

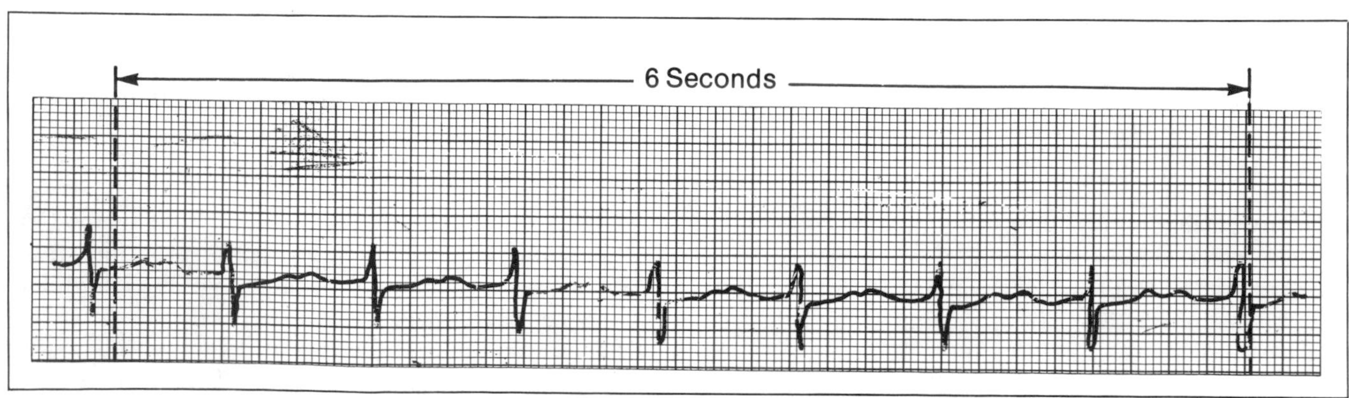

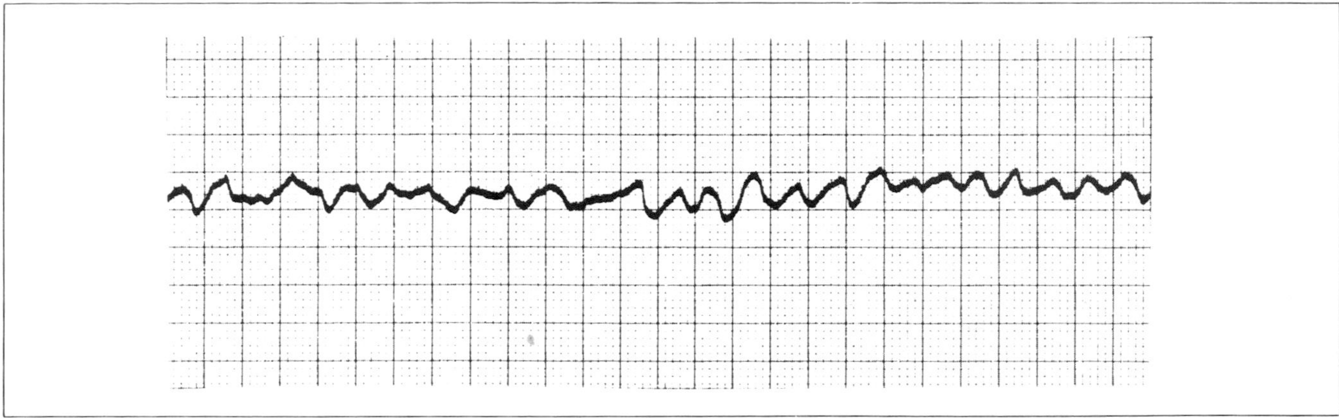

Fig. 9-21. *Ventricular fibrillation.*

firing off at different times, completely out of phase with one another.

In ASYSTOLE, by contrast, the heart is perfectly still. There are no muscle fibers contracting at all, so the heart is electrically "silent"—reflected in the ECG by a relatively flat, straight line (Fig. 9-22).

In CARDIOVASCULAR COLLAPSE, the heart is still beating, but it is beating too weakly to pump blood effectively. The ECG in cardiovascular collapse is variable. Because the heart is still contracting, the ECG may closely resemble a normal ECG, with a regular sequence of clearly defined waves and complexes. For this reason, the diagnosis of cardiovascular collapse is not made by the ECG per se, but by the fact that *despite* the complexes visible on the ECG, the patient has no pulse.

It cannot be overemphasized that what you see on the ECG *must* be correlated with the patient's clinical findings. If the ECG shows a wavy line and the patient is alert and talking, he is NOT in ventricular fibrillation, and you had better check your equipment.

Imposters in the ECG

There are several circumstances in which the ECG may look alarmingly like ventricular fibrillation or asystole when in fact neither VF nor asystole is present at all, and the cardiac rhythm may be perfectly normal. These ECG "rhythms" are called **artifacts,** that is, they are due to various technical problems in the equipment that produce disturbances in the electrocardiographic record. Artifacts are potentially dangerous "rhythms" because they may look a lot like VF and thus prompt the unwary EMT into giving a blast of electric current to a patient who has a perfectly normal heart beat. If the EMT does "defibrillate" someone with a normal rhythm, the patient *will* go into ventricular fibrillation in short order, and this is, in effect, a form of homicide. Thus it is crucial for the EMT to be able to distinguish VF from various imposters.

Who are these evil imposters? First of all, there is **Louie the Loose Lead.** If the ECG electrodes are applied too loosely, they are apt to flop back and forth, intermittently losing contact with the skin. If this happens, the electric activity of the heart will be picked up only intermittently, and the result can be a very wavy ECG that looks much like VF.

Two other dangerous imposters are **Trevor the Tremor** and his cousin **Mavis the Moving Patient.** When a patient is trembling or shivering, all sorts of electric currents from his skeletal muscles will be detected by the ECG electrodes and recorded on the ECG together with the electric impulses from the heart. Similarly, if the patient is shifting about, with the ECG cables flopping all over the stretcher, all

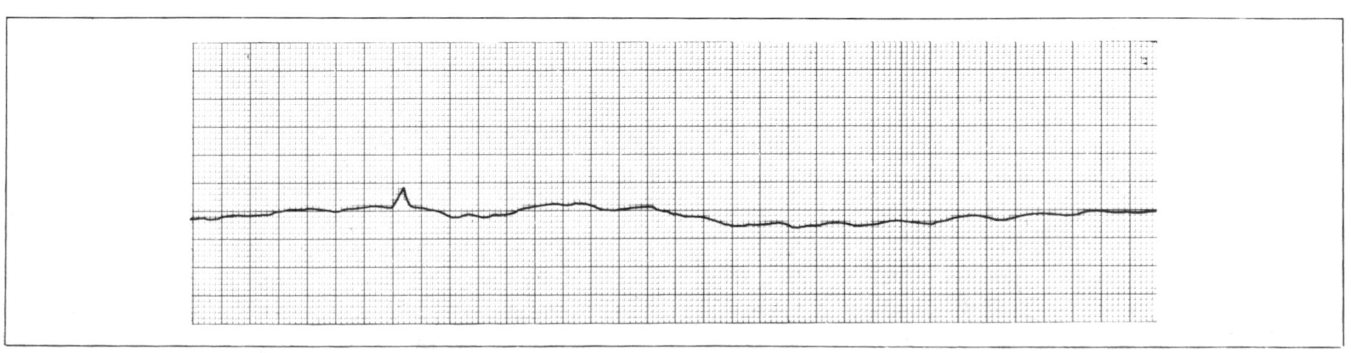

Fig. 9-22. *Asystole.*

kinds of strange bumps and blips may find their way onto the ECG. Both Trevor the Tremor and Mavis the Moving Patient can thus produce an ECG picture alarmingly similar to VF.

Bugsy the Broken Cable can also mimic VF. Rough handling of ECG cables may eventually break some of the wires running through the cable, leading to faulty transmission of the ECG signal.

Finally there is **Dietrich the Detached Lead,** who prefers to impersonate asystole. If an electrode being used for monitoring should fall off the patient, the ECG will record a flat line and be virtually indistinguishable from the ECG of asystole.

Louie, Trevor, Mavis, and Dietrich are always skulking around nearby whenever ECG monitoring equipment is in use, and the EMT must keep a constant eye out for them, lest they lure him into giving "the juice" to the wrong patient. Fortunately, there is one very powerful weapon against which the ECG imposters are defenseless: examination of the patient. The moment you see something funny happening on the ECG, the first thing to do is LOOK AT THE PATIENT! If he is sitting up, perfectly alert and cheerful, the problem is in your equipment and not in the patient. Remember:

> IF THE PATIENT HAS A PULSE, HE IS NOT IN VENTRICULAR FIBRILLATION, NO MATTER WHAT YOU SEE ON THE ECG.

Thus, when there is a discrepancy between what you see on the ECG and the patient's clinical condition, check to make sure that none of the ECG imposters have sneaked into your ambulance, and correct any problems you find with the equipment.

> **Causes of ECG Artifacts**
> - Loose lead(s)
> - Muscle tremor
> - Patient or cable movement
> - Broken cable
> - Detached lead(s)

The Defibrillator-Monitor

There are at least a dozen portable defibrillator-monitor units on the market, each of which has a somewhat different design. All of them, however, have certain basic components in common (Fig. 9-23). To begin with, there is the DEFIBRILLATOR component. This consists of a large, rechargeable battery; a capacitor capable of storing energy; and two big paddles with large metal plates, through which the energy is delivered to the patient. The second component of the unit is a MONITOR, which consists of a screen (oscilloscope) on which the ECG is constantly displayed. Defibrillators for use by EMTs in the field should also have a write-out device, that is, a means for recording on paper the ECG seen on the monitor, so there will be a permanent record of the patient's cardiac rhythms. Some monitor units have a small cassette recorder, which enables one to tape-record the entire ECG from the time the monitoring leads are attached to the patient until the patient reaches the hospital. This feature provides an excellent tool for reviewing cases later with the medical director; when the tape is played back, the entire course of the patient's cardiac rhythm can be reviewed.

In order for the monitor to work, it must be connected to the patient, and this is done by placing **electrodes**—devices that can detect small electric currents—on the patient's skin and connecting these electrodes by wires to the monitoring unit. The types of electrodes most commonly in use are silver plate, or CLAMP ELECTRODES, which are fastened onto the patient's extremities, and stick-on DISC ELECTRODES, which are applied to the patient's chest. The stick-on electrodes are somewhat faster and easier to apply, but because they are disposable, the long-term expense associated with stocking them is higher. Both the clamp-on extremity electrodes and the stick-on disc electrodes are used when there is a need for continuous monitoring of the patient's rhythm (see below). In urgent situations, however, such as when you first come upon a patient in cardiac arrest, it is desirable to have a way of checking the patient's ECG rhythm immediately, without having to spend the minute or two it takes to get all the electrodes hooked up. In such situations, the PADDLES of most defibrillator-monitor units can be used as monitoring electrodes simply by positioning them correctly on the chest. Paddles designed for both delivery of electric energy and monitoring are called "quick-look" paddles, for they enable the rescuer to get a quick look at the patient's ECG rhythm without having to hook up conventional leads.

Who Should Be Monitored, and How Is It Done?

In general, a patient is monitored when he is considered to be at risk of developing a dangerous disturbance in his cardiac rhythm that might require treatment. For the EMT, this means chiefly a patient who might develop ventricular fibrillation, since the EMT is not trained to recognize other rhythm disturbances or authorized to give the appropriate drug treatment. Patients in danger of developing VF include (1) all patients complaining of chest pain, (2) all patients who have been successfully resuscitated from cardiac arrest, (3) all patients who have suffered significant periods of hypoxia (e.g., airway obstruc-

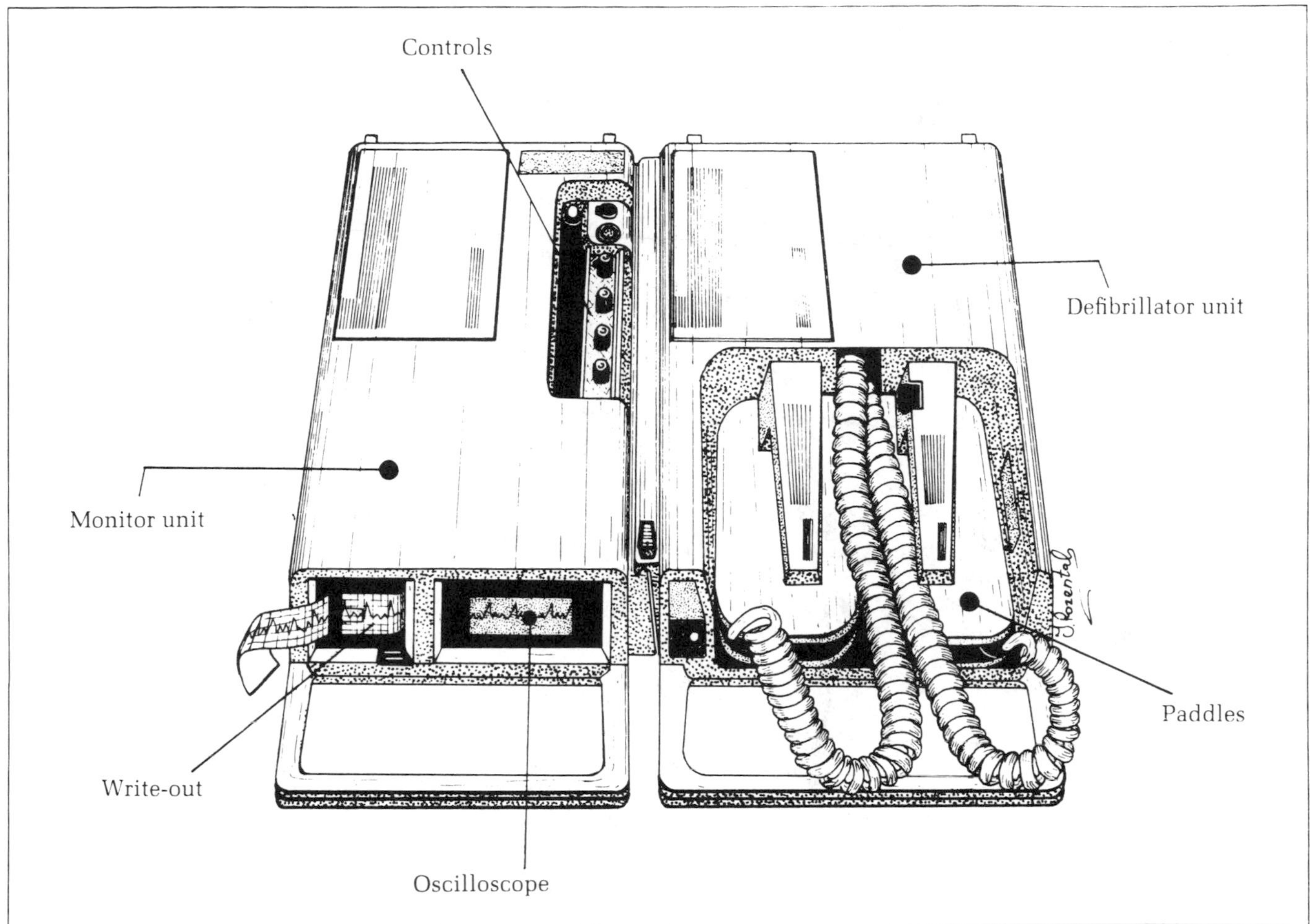

Fig. 9-23. *Defibrillator-monitor.*

tion, respiratory arrest), and (4) all patients who have sustained major trauma to the chest in which the heart may have been bruised. We will examine these categories in greater detail in other sections of the book as we discuss specific emergency situations. As a general rule, though, if you have any doubts at all about the status of a critically ill or injured patient, it is best to be on the safe side and monitor his ECG rhythm.

To apply electrodes for *continuous* monitoring, first sort out the lead wires, which are color-coded and labeled LA (left arm), LL (left leg), RA (right arm), and RL (right leg). If you are using clamp-on electrodes for the extremities, they should be placed on the *inner* surfaces of the arms and legs, because there is less hair in these areas and hair can interfere with the contact between the electrode and the skin. Also try to place clamp-on electrodes as high (proximal) on the arms and legs as possible, so that motion of the patient's extremities will cause minimal movement of the electrodes. If you are using stick-on disc electrodes for the chest, you may have to shave some of the hair from the chest to allow the discs to stick properly. The stick-on electrode for the right arm lead may be placed over the right clavicle, for the left arm lead over the left clavicle, for the right leg lead over the lowest right rib, and the left leg lead over the lowest left rib (Fig. 9-24).

Whether you use clamp-on or stick-on electrodes, you must first prepare the electrode site to promote optimal contact between the electrode and the skin. Oil or dirt on the skin will interfere with that contact and weaken or distort the ECG signal. Vigorously rub with alcohol the spot where you intend to put the electrode in order to remove oil and dead tissue from the skin, and wait a minute for the skin to dry. Then apply special electrode paste or jelly to the electrode, and attach it firmly to the spot you have cleaned. The electrode jelly serves to improve the contact between the electrode and the skin. Now attach the cables from the monitor, making sure that the appropriate cable is attached to each electrode (e.g., RA cable to the electrode on the right arm or right shoulder). Turn on the monitor, and switch the dial to a lead where you get a good clear ECG picture.

For *emergency* monitoring (e.g., in cardiac arrest), the paddles of the defibrillator are initially used as electrodes until there is time (after getting CPR well

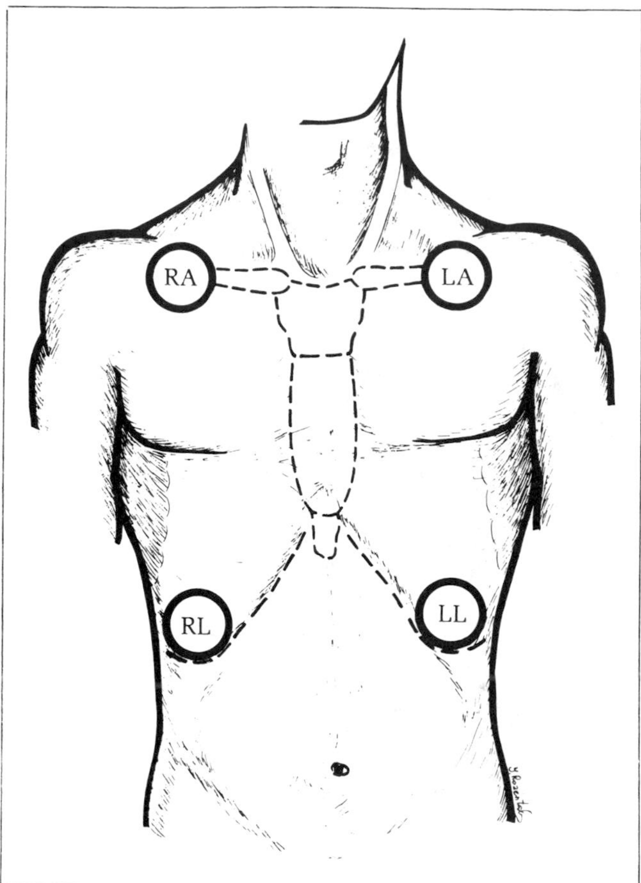

Fig. 9-24. *Position of chest leads for monitoring.*

under way) to hook up the standard electrodes. To use the defibrillator paddles in this fashion, you must first quickly turn on the monitor and bare the patient's chest. Electrode jelly is applied to each of the paddles, and then the positive (red) paddle is pressed firmly below the patient's left nipple while the negative (black) paddle is applied to the upper right chest where the clavicle meets the sternum. Hold the paddles firmly in place, and check the rhythm on the oscilloscope.

When to Defibrillate

There are two possible scenarios in which defibrillation may be necessary. First of all, the EMT may arrive at the scene and find the victim already in cardiac arrest, having been without a pulse for an undetermined period of time. This is the situation of so-called *unwitnessed* cardiac arrest, that is, cardiac arrest that occurred without your observing it, usually before you arrived. On the other hand, the patient may still have a pulse and may even still be conscious when the EMT arrives but may go into VF while under the EMT's care, a situation termed *witnessed* cardiac arrest, that is, cardiac arrest that you saw occur. These two situations require slightly different approaches, for the patient who has had an unwitnessed cardiac arrest may be in a quite different physical condition when you find him from the patient whose arrest occurs in your presence.

UNWITNESSED CARDIAC ARREST. By definition, the patient who has had an unwitnessed cardiac arrest became pulseless at an indeterminate time before your arrival. Information from bystanders regarding when the patient *lost consciousness* is helpful in establishing the *maximum* possible duration of the arrest, but it tells you very little about when the arrest actually occurred. For instance, bystanders may report that the patient collapsed 20 minutes before you arrived, so you know that the patient could not have been in cardiac arrest much *longer* than 20 minutes. But you have no way of knowing whether the arrest occurred immediately after the patient collapsed or 10 minutes later. For purposes of treatment, you have to assume the worst, and in the case of our hypothetical patient, you must assume that he has been without breathing or circulation for the whole 20 minutes and thus is severely hypoxic. In general, defibrillation is unlikely to be successful when there is extreme tissue hypoxia and accumulation of carbon dioxide in the body. So before you can even consider defibrillation, you have to try to clear some of the carbon dioxide out of the patient's system and deliver some oxygen to the tissues. In other words, you have to get CPR started, preferably with oxygen for ventilation as quickly as the oxygen can be secured. Only after good CPR has been in progress for a minute or two should you take time to check the patient's ECG rhythm (with the quick-look paddles). If the rhythm is *not* VF, continue CPR and ready the patient for transport, with CPR all the way to the hospital. If you do see VF on the monitor, that is the cue to defibrillate.

Immediately after you have delivered the shock, resume artificial ventilation. Meanwhile keep an eye on the monitor for about 5 seconds to see if a rhythm returns; if it does, check immediately for a pulse. If there is no pulse despite the monitor rhythm, resume external cardiac compressions. Should the pulse return, however, you may cease external cardiac compressions and continue only with artificial ventilation as needed. At this point, the patient should be hooked up to the monitor with regular leads so that you can watch constantly for a return of VF. You also need to keep a finger on the patient's pulse, for if the pulse disappears, you will have to resume external cardiac compressions, even if the monitor shows regular complexes.

If the defibrillation attempt is not successful, you must immediately resume CPR and continue for another minute or so before trying again to defibrillate. Remember:

IN UNWITNESSED CARDIAC ARREST, START CPR FIRST, CHECK THE MONITOR LATER.

The management of unwitnessed cardiac arrest is summarized in Figure 9-25.

WITNESSED CARDIAC ARREST. The patient who has had a witnessed cardiac arrest is in a somewhat different situation. While he is just as clinically dead as the patient who arrested before your arrival, his tissues are still relatively well oxygenated. After all, only moments before he was still breathing oxygen. So he is a much better candidate for successful defibrillation, and the sooner the shock can be given the better. Let us take two hypothetical cases. In the first case, you have responded to a call from a 52-year-old man with chest pain. You find him alert and conscious, and since he says he has chest pain, the FIRST thing you do is give him some supplementary oxygen to breathe through a nasal cannula. As he is telling you his story, his eyes suddenly roll backward, and he pitches over to the side. What do you do? The answer is that first you must VERIFY THAT HE IS IN CARDIAC ARREST. Just because he keeled over does not mean that his heart has stopped beating. So you must take 15 seconds to open the airway, check for breathing, and determine whether there is a pulse. If the pulse is absent, immediately use the quick-look paddles to determine if the rhythm is VF. If so, keep the paddles in place and deliver the defibrillating shock. If the rhythm is other than VF (e.g., asystole), put away the paddles and start CPR immediately.

What if you left the defibrillator in the ambulance, which is down three flights of stairs and around the corner? In that case, you will have to start CPR and continue it while your partner goes down to the vehicle and fetches the equipment. The moment he gets back, interrupt CPR to apply the quick-look paddles, and defibrillate immediately if the rhythm on the monitor is VF.

Now let us look at another case of chest pain: a 42-year-old man who called for an ambulance because of "squeezing" in his chest for 3 hours. The case is pretty uneventful: The patient is fully alert, so you give him oxygen, get him hooked up to the monitor (every patient with chest pain should be monitored), and load him into the ambulance. As you are jouncing along to the hospital, you suddenly notice VF on the monitor. What should you do?

If you said, "Defibrillate," or even "Open the airway," you are wrong! The FIRST thing you should do is LOOK AT THE PATIENT, remember? If he is wide awake, this is *not* a witnessed cardiac arrest; it is a witnessed loose lead or cable movement or some other ECG artifact. It cannot be overstressed that a witnessed cardiac arrest, even in a monitored patient, MUST be verified by checking for pulselessness. Not every unconscious patient is without a pulse, and not every wavy line on the monitor is VF.

WHETHER THE PATIENT IS MONITORED OR NOT, YOU *MUST* VERIFY CARDIAC ARREST BY CLINICAL SIGNS. **NEVER** "DEFIBRILLATE" A PATIENT BEFORE YOU HAVE CHECKED FOR A PULSE.

The steps in treating witnessed cardiac arrest are summarized in Figure 9-26.

How to Defibrillate

Now that we know *when* to defibrillate, we have to learn exactly *how* to do it. A defibrillator is a potentially lethal machine, and an EMT can wipe out his partner or himself with an incorrectly applied shock. For this reason, it is vital for the EMT to know precisely what he or she is doing and to observe all the necessary safety precautions. The use of a defibrillator is a skill, and like any other skill it requires frequent practice.

There are two types of defibrillators in use nowadays. The first is a standard defibrillator, like that described earlier in this section, which requires the rescuer to activate it. The second type of defibrillator is an automated external defibrillator (AED), which makes its own assessment of the patient's cardiac rhythm and delivers a shock automatically if the rhythm is found to be ventricular defibrillation.

HOW TO USE A STANDARD DEFIBRILLATOR. To perform defibrillation with a standard defibrillator, you must first turn the SYNCHRONIZE SWITCH OFF and the MAIN POWER SWITCH ON. The synchronize switch is a control used for treating certain rhythms *other than* VF, and if it is left on during defibrillation, the shock may not be delivered.

SET THE ENERGY LEVEL on the defibrillator initially to a charge of 200 JOULES, and CHARGE THE PADDLES by pushing the "charge" button.

It is then necessary to LUBRICATE THE PADDLES to reduce the electric resistance of the patient's skin; otherwise the electric energy put out by the defibrillator will be delivered to the surface of the skin itself, resulting in burns to the skin and ineffective energy delivery to the heart. The skin resistance can be overcome with either 4- × 4-inch pads soaked in

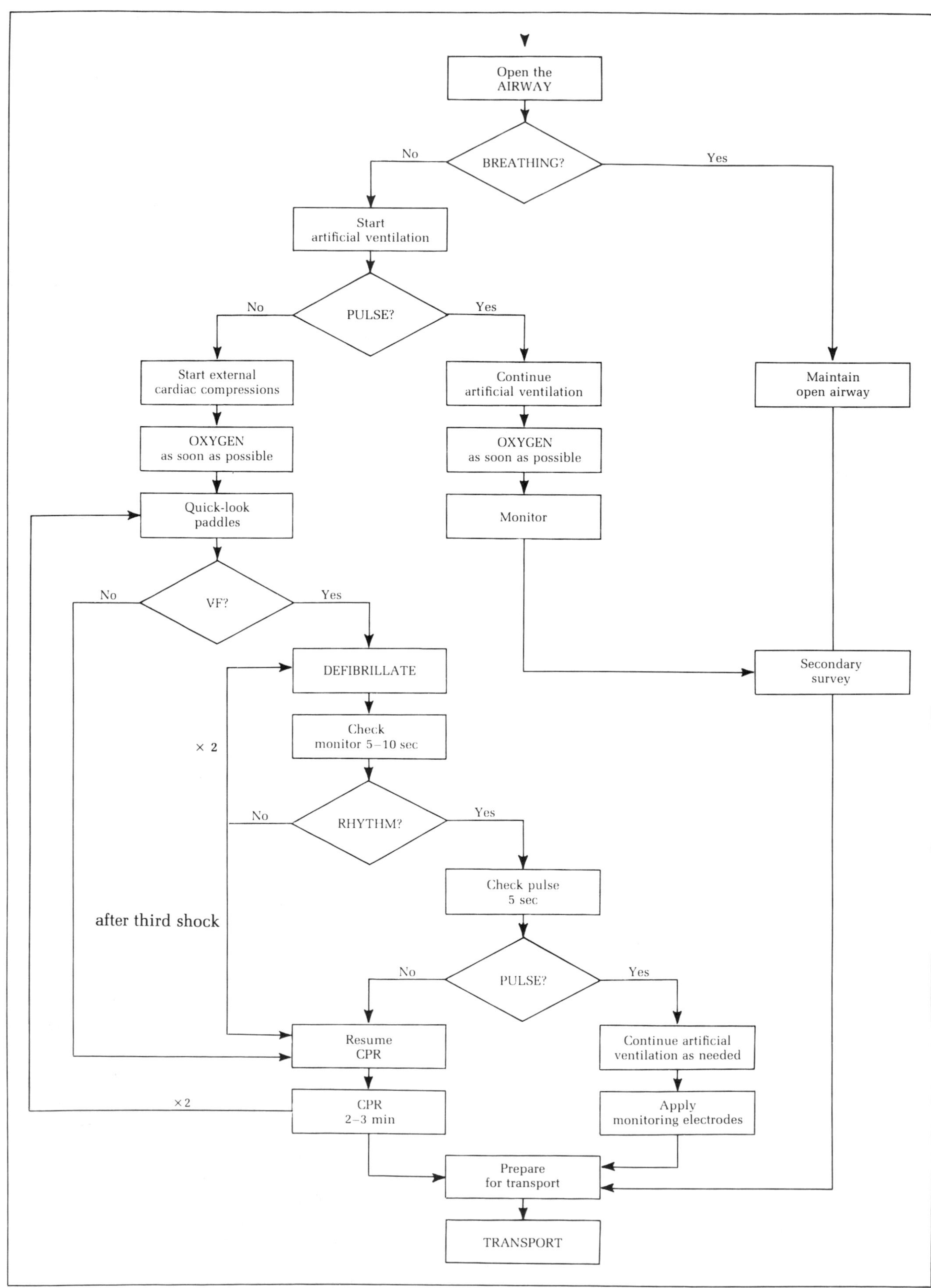

Fig. 9-25. *Management of unwitnessed cardiac arrest.*

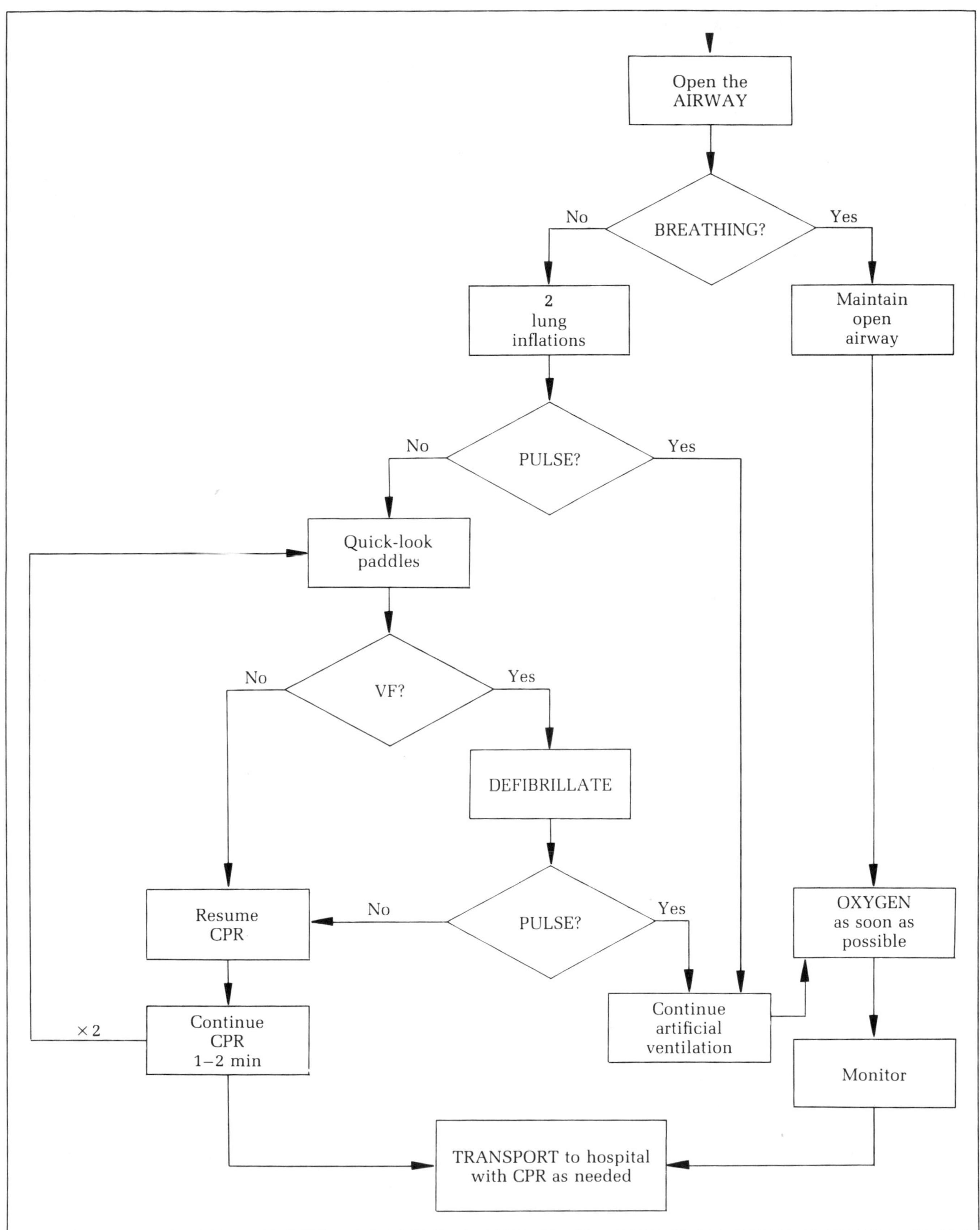

Fig. 9-26. *Management of witnessed cardiac arrest.*

saline (one under each paddle) or electrode jelly. The saline pads have the advantage that they do not leave a slippery residue on the chest; so if you have to resume CPR after the defibrillation attempt, your hands will not be skidding all over the chest with each compression. If saline pads are used, they must be thoroughly soaked but not so wet that they ooze saline all over the skin. Do NOT use any fluid other than saline to soak the pads. ALCOHOL-SOAKED PADS SHOULD NEVER BE USED, for they may ignite into flames when the electric energy passes through them. If electrode jelly is used for lubrication, it should be squeezed generously onto the paddles and rubbed into the patient's skin with the paddles. Whichever method of lubrication you choose—saline pads or electrode jelly—you must take care not to allow contact (bridging) between the two paddles, which will occur if the saline or jelly from one paddle oozes along the chest and comes into contact with the other paddle. If this happens, all of the electric energy will simply cross the skin from one paddle to the other; the skin will be burned, and the shock will not reach the heart. Also be very careful that saline does not dribble off the chest and form a puddle where you are kneeling, for in that instance you will be the recipient of the 200-joule shock.

Once the paddles have been lubricated with jelly or saline pads have been placed on the chest, POSITION THE PADDLES so that the positive (red) paddle is just below the patient's left nipple and the negative (black) paddle is to the right of the sternum, just where the right clavicle meets the sternum (Fig. 9-27). Exert FIRM PRESSURE downward on the paddles to ensure good skin contact. Ineffective contact is another cause of burns and unsuccessful shock.

When the paddles are in place, CLEAR THE AREA, so that no one, including yourself, is in contact with the patient or the stretcher. Give a loud command, "Everybody off!" and look around quickly to make sure no one is touching the patient. Then FIRE THE DEFIBRILLATOR by pushing simultaneously on the two paddle buttons. If the defibrillator is of the type where the discharge button is on the main console rather than on the paddles, instruct your partner to fire the defibrillator by commanding, "Hit it!" when you are ready to deliver the shock. If the current has reached the patient, marked contractions of the patient's chest and extremity muscles will be evident. He may even appear to rise an inch or so off the floor. If you do not see these muscle contractions, check the defibrillator to be certain that the synchronize switch is off, the main power switch is on, and the battery is fully charged.

Immediately after delivering the shock, observe the monitor (leave the quick-look paddles in place on the chest for that purpose if monitoring leads have not already been attached). If the patient is still in VF, RECHARGE THE PADDLES to 200–300 joules and GIVE A SECOND SHOCK IMMEDIATELY. If VF persists, GIVE A THIRD SHOCK up to 360 joules. If still unsuccessful, resume CPR for 15–30 seconds and then reassess the rhythm. If *still* VF, you may give three more shocks of up to 360 joules. If at any point a regular rhythm is present, palpate for a carotid pulse to determine whether rhythm is associated with an effective heart beat. Remember:

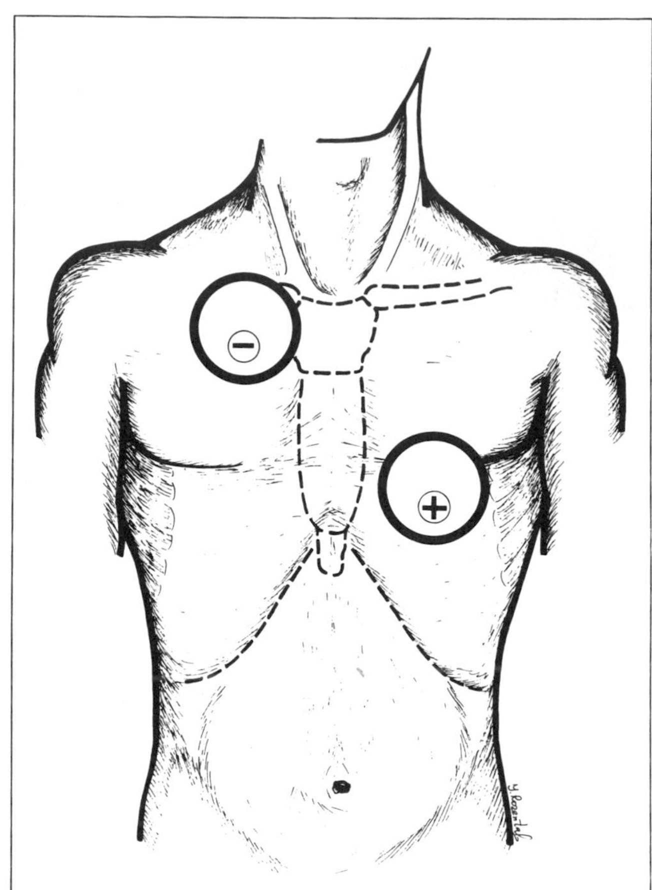

Fig. 9-27. *Position of paddles for defibrillation.*

IF THE PULSE IS ABSENT, RESUME CPR NO MATTER WHAT THE MONITOR SHOWS.

No more than 10 seconds should be taken to check the monitor and the pulse after a defibrillation attempt, and the whole sequence—application of the paddles, shock, checking the monitor, checking the pulse—should not interrupt CPR for more than 15 to 20 seconds. You should have practiced defibrillation on the manikin enough times to be able to accomplish all the steps within this 15- to 20-second time limit.

Steps of Defibrillation
1. Turn the SYNCHRONIZE SWITCH OFF and the MAIN POWER SWITCH ON.
2. Set the energy level at 200–300 JOULES.
3. CHARGE the paddles.
4. LUBRICATE the paddles, and POSITION them on the chest.
5. CLEAR the area.
6. FIRE the defibrillator.
7. CHECK the MONITOR and the PULSE.

The Automated External Defibrillator
The automated external defibrillator (AED) is a "smart defibrillator" that can—thanks to sophisticated computer chips—analyze the patient's ECG rhythm and determine whether a defibrillating shock is needed. AEDs may be either fully automatic or semi-automatic. The **fully automatic** versions assess the patient's rhythm and, if VF is present, charge the paddles and deliver countershocks, without any intervention by the rescuer. The **semi-automatic** AEDs, on the other hand, require decisions by the rescuer. That is, the semi-automatic AED identifies the rhythm and then instructs the rescuer what to do about it! If, for example, the AED detects ventricular fibrillation, a message may appear on the liquid crystal display (LCD) screen saying, "SHOCK ADVISED. PRESS TO SHOCK." The rescuer must then depress the "shock" button in order to defibrillate the patient.

Whether the AED is fully automatic or semi-automatic, the basic sequence of steps in using an AED are the same:

1. The patient's chest is exposed.
2. Two self-adhesive electrode pads are attached firmly to the patient's chest—one (the *sternal pad*) at the junction of the right clavicle and upper border of the sternum; the other (the *apex pad*) along the left lower rib margin at the anterior axillary line (see Fig. 9-27).
3. The AED is turned on.
4. CPR is stopped and everyone gets clear of the patient.
5. The AED assesses the rhythm (for about 6–20 seconds) and determines whether it is "shockable" (i.e., whether the rhythm is one that will respond to defibrillation).
6. If the AED does detect a "shockable" rhythm, it automatically starts charging up the paddles, which takes about 5–10 seconds.
7. Defibrillating shocks of 200–300 joules are then delivered, either automatically or by the rescuer, depending on the type of AED.

We shall not present here the details of operating the currently available automated external defibrillators. New AEDs are coming on the market all the time, and each model is furnished with its own operational manual. EMTs who will be using an AED should train with the specific apparatus carried by their service, according to the manufacturer's instructions for that machine.

Care and Maintenance of the Equipment
A broken defibrillator or one with a dead battery is worse than no defibrillator at all. It is the EMT's responsibility to check the equipment at the beginning of each shift to be certain that (1) the battery is fully charged, (2) the defibrillator charges properly, and (3) all ancillary equipment (e.g., leads, electrodes, jelly) is present. Follow to the letter the maintenance instructions supplied with your particular defibrillator-monitor, and have it checked on a regular basis by the local service representative. Remember:

A DEAD DEFIBRILLATOR CANNOT HELP A DEAD PATIENT.

AIDS TO THE TREATMENT OF BLEEDING AND SHOCK

MILITARY ANTI-SHOCK TROUSERS
The idea behind shock trousers has been around since 1909, when Crile first used a pneumatic rubber suit to treat a patient in hemorrhagic shock. The idea of a pressurized suit, or G suit, did not come into its own until World War II, however, when it was used by fliers to combat the loss of consciousness produced by centrifugal force. Interest in using the suit for the treatment of *shock* revived in the late 1950s. At that time, researchers reported successful use of a modified aviation G suit to treat abdominal bleeding. But the real impetus for the development of an antishock garment came during the Vietnam War, where the pneumatic antishock devices were used for the first time to treat victims of trauma. This was also the first *prehospital* application of this sort of equipment, and it set the stage for the introduction of the military anti-shock trousers (MAST) into civilian prehospital use. In the early 1970s, the MAST was tested for civilian use by the Miami paramedics, and during the first 6 months that the MAST was used in the Miami system, 47 of 53 patients with otherwise fatal shock were saved—a salvage rate of 89 percent. The MAST subsequently came into widespread use in both basic and advanced life support ambulances, and since 1977 antishock trousers have been listed by the American College of Surgeons as essential equipment for *every* ambulance.

During the mid-1980s, questions were raised regarding the real effectiveness of anti-shock trousers, and the MAST became a subject of controversy: Are anti-shock garments useful or not? Many paramedics and physicians (including the present author) can cite extensive field experience in which the MAST produced favorable and sometimes dramatic responses, and such experience should not be dismissed out of hand. Nonetheless, some very careful studies carried out at Baylor College of Medicine in Houston, Texas, have failed to document any benefit from use of anti-shock garments and, indeed, suggest that use of the MAST may even be harmful. The final word on the subject has not yet been spoken; therefore, EMTs and their medical advisors need to keep abreast of new findings on anti-shock trousers as they are reported in the emergency medicine journals.

There are several types of anti-shock trousers on the market today. For convenience, we shall refer in our discussion to the military anti-shock trousers (MAST), since those were the prototype for all others. (In the medical literature, you may also find anti-shock trousers referred to as pneumatic anti-shock garments, or PASG.) The principles involved in using the MAST are the same for all anti-shock garments, which differ from one another only in details of design.

What is the MAST, and What Does it Do?

The MAST is an inflatable garment that is wrapped around the patient's legs and abdomen and can generate up to about 100 mm Hg of pressure. The question is, what does that uniform blanket of pressure actually do? As noted, ideas about the MAST are in the midst of considerable revision, but the current evidence would seem to support at least the following statements:

1. When inflated to pressures between 30 and 40 mm Hg, the MAST probably HELPS CONTROL BLEEDING from the lower extremities. Recall that the most effective means to control hemorrhage is to apply *direct* pressure over the bleeding site, and that is just what the MAST does if there is bleeding from injury to the legs or pelvis. The pressure exerted by the inflated MAST is uniform and sustained. Unlike the EMT, the MAST does not get tired; it can maintain pressure for hours if necessary. Furthermore, it can maintain pressure over an extensive area, which is useful if there are multiple sources of bleeding or if bleeding is internal and its source therefore cannot be accurately pinpointed. Because it can keep sustained pressure on the bleeding site, the MAST is also believed to PROMOTE HEMOSTASIS (the cessation of bleeding), for it gives the patient's platelets time to do their job of plugging up holes in blood vessels.

2. The MAST provides an effective SPLINT for a fractured pelvis and a good partial splint for lower extremity fractures. The function of a splint is to prevent motion of an injured extremity, and that is just what happens when you surround an extremity with an air-filled bag.

3. The MAST RAISES THE BLOOD PRESSURE of a patient in shock. It remains to be determined whether the rise in blood pressure is, in fact, good for the patient; but there is no doubt that it is good for the *EMT* trying to find a vein in which to start an intravenous line!

What the MAST Does

- CONTROLS BLEEDING in the lower extremities
- SPLINTS fractures of the pelvis and femur
- RAISES THE BLOOD PRESSURE in a patient in shock

What remains to be determined beyond doubt is whether the MAST improves (or worsens!) the ultimate outcome for a seriously injured patient.

Most versions of the MAST have three separate compartments—one for each leg and one for the abdomen—that can be inflated and deflated as a unit or individually. The MAST is transparent to x-rays, so it does not have to be removed to x-ray the patient. An opening in the groin area also permits insertion of a urinary catheter without removal of the MAST.

When Do You Use the MAST?

In view of the current controversy about the MAST, the indications for its use have been narrow (some EMS systems have stopped using anti-shock garments altogether). The data available at the time of this writing would support the following guidelines:

When to Use the MAST (Indications)

- To control DIFFUSE BLEEDING OF THE LOWER EXTREMITIES (inflate to 30–40 mm Hg)
- To stabilize PELVIC FRACTURES
- For cases of NEUROGENIC SHOCK with systolic blood pressure below 80–90 mm Hg and signs of poor perfusion
- For cases of HYPOVOLEMIC SHOCK with systolic blood pressure below 80–90 mm Hg and signs of poor perfusion
- For HEMORRHAGIC SHOCK when not contraindicated

When NOT to Use the Abdominal Section of the MAST

- PREGNANCY
- EVISCERATION
- IMPALED OBJECT in the abdomen

When NOT to Use the MAST at All
(Contraindications)

- For patients with CHEST INJURY or ANY INJURY ABOVE THE MAST
- For patients with HEAD INJURY
- For patients in heart failure with PULMONARY EDEMA

Application of the MAST

Application of the MAST is shown in Figure 9-28. The method described here is one for use in patients with suspected spinal injury, for any patient with multiple trauma severe enough to cause shock should be handled as if he has a spinal injury. A well-trained EMT team should be able to apply and inflate the MAST, even with these precautions, in about 60 seconds.

While one EMT stays with the patient, a second EMT fetches the MAST and a long backboard from the vehicle. The backboard is placed alongside the patient, and the MAST is unfolded and laid flat on top of the backboard (Fig. 9-28A). The patient is then rolled onto his side, facing away from the backboard—a maneuver that will require three rescuers in order to keep the body straight and the head and neck aligned with the trunk. As the patient is brought onto his side, a fourth rescuer slides the backboard beneath him so that the top of the MAST is lined up with the bottom of the patient's rib cage. The patient is carefully rolled back to the supine position so that he is lying on the MAST (Fig. 9-28B). Check to make sure the patient's trouser pockets are empty. Then one EMT can begin fastening the three MAST sections. The left leg of the MAST is wrapped snugly around the patient's left leg and secured with velcro fasteners (Fig. 9-28C); next the right leg is secured (Fig. 9-28D); and lastly the abdominal section is fastened (Fig. 9-28E). Once the garment has been secured, the MAST is inflated, using a foot pump, to a pressure of 30 to 40 mm Hg. Then close the stopcock valves to all three segments. It is a good idea to leave the foot pump attached in case you need to inflate the MAST further later on. If the patient has an angulated fracture of the leg, be sure to hold the leg in traction until the MAST is inflated.

It is important to be aware that changes in temperature or atmospheric pressure can alter the pressure within the MAST. If you move the patient from a very cold environment into your toasty warm ambulance, for example, the air inside the MAST will expand and thus increase the pressure exerted by the garment. Similarly, if the patient is evacuated by helicopter or airplane, the lower atmospheric pressures at high altitudes will permit the air inside the MAST to expand and increase the pressure of the suit. Should you have to let some of the air out of the MAST during air transport, do not forget to reinflate the garment as you prepare for landing! Otherwise

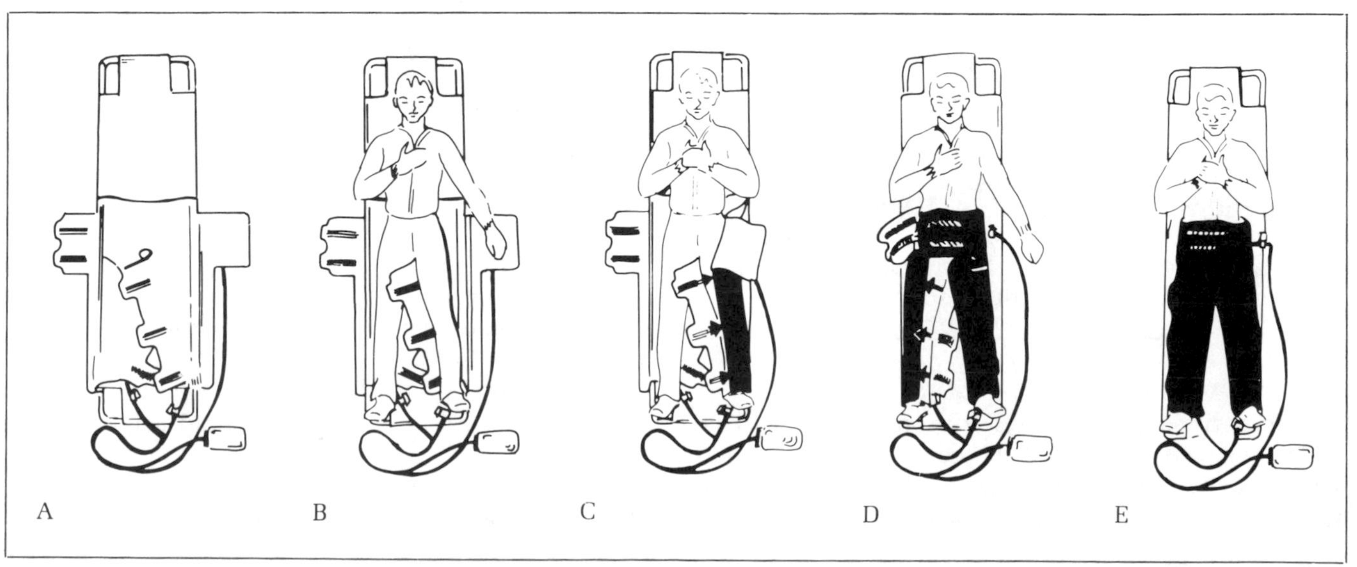

Fig. 9-28. *Application of the Military Anti-Shock Trousers (MAST). A. Unfold the MAST and lay flat (if stretcher is to be used lay MAST on it). Attach foot pump and open stopcock valves. B. Put the patient on the MAST face up (supine), so that the top of the garment will be just below the lowest rib. C. The left leg of garment is wrapped around the patient's left leg and secured with velcro strips. D. The right leg of garment is wrapped around the patient's right leg and secured with velcro strips. E. The material corresponding to the abdominal area is then put into place and secured with velcro strips.*

Using the foot pump, inflate the trousers until air exhausts through the relief valves, the patient's vital signs become stable, or both. Close the stopcock valves. (Reproduced courtesy Armstrong Industries, Northbrook, Illinois.)

you may find that your patient, who was perfectly stable at 10,000 feet, is back in shock down on the ground.

Deflation of the MAST

The rule regarding deflation of the MAST is quite simple:

DO NOT DEFLATE THE MAST IN THE FIELD.

Whatever salutory effects the MAST might have, they will be reversed immediately upon its deflation. Ideally, therefore, fluid replacement should be well under way, through at least two large-bore intravenous lines, and arrangements for definitive control of bleeding (usually in the operating room) should have been completed before any attempt is made to deflate the MAST. In any case, the decision to deflate the device should be made by a physician.

When the MAST *is* deflated, the steps for doing so are as follows:

Steps in Deflation of the MAST

1. Record the patient's pulse and blood pressure.
2. Obtain permission to begin deflation from attending physician knowledgeable in the use of this equipment.
3. SLOWLY DEFLATE ABDOMINAL SECTION ONLY.
4. RECHECK PATIENT'S VITAL SIGNS over a 5- to 10-minute period. If the blood pressure drops by 5 mm Hg or more, infuse 100 to 200 ml of volume over 10 minutes or until the blood pressure stabilizes again.
5. When the patient's vital signs are again stable, SLOWLY DEFLATE ONE LEG SECTION.
6. Again, RECHECK THE PATIENT'S VITAL SIGNS over a 5- to 10-minute period. If there is a blood pressure drop or the pulse starts to rise, infuse volume until the vital signs stabilize.
7. If the vital signs are stable, DEFLATE THE OTHER LEG SECTION, again slowly, with careful monitoring of the pulse and blood pressure at 2- to 3-minute intervals.

Care and Maintenance of the MAST

By the very nature of the conditions in which it is used, the MAST often gets covered with blood, vomitus, and various excreta, and thus it is essential that it be cleaned after use. Fortunately, most antishock garments can be easily cleaned with warm water and soap, and after cleaning they should be hung out to dry with all the valves open. Follow the manufacturer's instructions for precise cleaning methods.

In storing the MAST, take care that the rubber tubing does not kink inside the bag or plastic case, for this will shorten the life of the tubing and make it more difficult to pump air through it. Wind the tubing around a cardboard cylinder or similar device to keep it free of kinks, and store the MAST in a relatively cool place when not in use.

*INTRAVENOUS THERAPY**

Up to this point, we have considered two methods to try to improve the circulating blood volume of a person who has lost fluids and is in, or approaching, shock. The first method requires no special equipment, and that is to elevate the victim's legs. This maneuver permits blood to drain by gravity out of the veins of the legs, where it has pooled, and makes this blood available to perfuse more vital organs, such as the brain. Elevation of the legs can be very effective for this purpose, but the technique has limitations if there has been injury to the lower extremities that precludes raising them. The second method we have learned for increasing the effective blood volume utilizes the MAST garment, which may improve blood flow to vital organs, perhaps by shunting blood away from the legs. Nonetheless, the MAST does not bring about any actual *replacement* of lost fluid or blood. At best, it merely transfers blood from one part of the circulation to another, and sooner or later (preferably sooner), one has to give the patient back the fluid volume he has lost. That is the objective of intravenous (IV) therapy. Fluid of one sort or another is piped directly back into the patient's circulation to replace the fluid or blood that has been lost. Every patient in hypovolemic shock will require extensive intravenous fluid replacement, and the sooner this replacement can be started the better, for the body does not tolerate long periods of poor perfusion. Thus it is all to the good if intravenous fluids can be started before the patient reaches the hospital.

Who Needs Intravenous Therapy?

In general, the EMT's use of intravenous therapy in the field will be confined to patients in hypovolemic shock, the vast majority of whom will be in hemorrhagic shock, but shock from other fluid losses (e.g., plasma losses in burns) also requires treatment. Needless to say, it is preferable if you can get the intravenous therapy going *before* the patient actually goes

*Not required of the EMT-A. This discussion is intended for students taking the EMT-Intermediate course.

into shock—not only to spare the patient's body the extreme stress of shock, but also for the very practical reason that veins collapse in shock. Once the patient's blood pressure begins to fall significantly, you will have a very tough time finding a vein in which to insert the IV catheter. Thus intravenous therapy should be started as soon as possible in any patient who is a *good candidate for shock,* without waiting for shock to develop. Such candidates include patients who have significant external bleeding; patients who report having vomited blood or passed blood through the rectum; patients who have had excessive vaginal bleeding; patients who have sustained blunt trauma to the abdomen; patients with severe fracture of one or both femurs; patients with severe or extensive burns; patients who have collapsed from heat exposure; and any other patients whose illness or injury is likely to produce hypovolemic shock or who show signs of impending shock (e.g., tachycardia; cool, clammy skin).

WHEN THE MECHANISMS OF INJURY SUGGEST THAT SHOCK MAY OCCUR, START INTRAVENOUS THERAPY *BEFORE* SHOCK DEVELOPS.

If the patient is already in shock by the time you find him (systolic blood pressure below 90 mm Hg) and requires the MAST, then there is a definite need for intravenous therapy. The MAST can often be very helpful in this situation, for addition to the several nice things the MAST does for the patient in shock, it does one very nice thing for the *EMT*: It refills collapsed veins. Inflation of the MAST commonly causes veins magically to pop up all over in a patient whose veins were entirely undetectable just moments before. This makes the job of putting a catheter into one of those veins immeasurably easier. The MAST, then, goes hand in hand with intravenous therapy, and it is a safe general rule that

ANY PATIENT WHO NEEDS THE MAST NEEDS AN IV.

To summarize, the patients for whom the EMT-I should provide intravenous therapy are as follows:

Patients Who Need IVs

- All patients in HYPOVOLEMIC SHOCK
- Patients who are LIKELY TO DEVELOP HYPOVOLEMIC SHOCK from
  1. Profuse external bleeding
  2. Internal bleeding
     a. Ulcer (vomiting blood, or blood in the stool)
     b. Vaginal bleeding
     c. Blunt trauma to the abdomen
     d. Femoral fracture(s)
  3. Severe or widespread burns
  4. Heat exhaustion

Certain restrictions apply to the above categories. In most regions, EMTs will not be permitted to start an IV on a child under 14 years old. Furthermore, because an IV is an "invasive" procedure—that is, a procedure that penetrates the patient's body—it requires the direct order of a physician. In some ambulance services, the order for intravenous therapy is part of a set of standing orders for shock, while in others a voice order from the physician by radio is required. Under no circumstances, however, is an EMT permitted to initiate intravenous therapy *without* a physician's order, whether written or spoken.

Which Intravenous Fluid?

The EMT-I will be using only one intravenous fluid in the field, and that is either normal saline or Ringer's solution, for these are the fluids used in the prehospital situation to treat hypovolemic shock. However, the EMT may be called upon to transport a patient who is already receiving intravenous therapy with another fluid, and for this reason the EMT should be aware of what those fluids are and what complications they may cause.

There are two general categories of fluids that are given intravenously to patients. In the first category are whole blood and blood products, such as plasma or packed red blood cells. The term for administering blood or blood products intravenously is **transfusion.** EMTs will not be called upon to start a transfusion on a patient, but they may have to transport a patient who has a transfusion running and should be alert for any sign of a **transfusion reaction.**

Transfusion reactions can occur because of improperly matched blood, contamination of the intravenous equipment, or hypersensitivity of the patient to some element in the donor's blood. Such reactions are more likely when whole blood is given than when plasma is transfused. The signs and symptoms of a transfusion reaction may be quite mild or catastrophic. The most common symptom is FEVER, sometimes accompanied by PRURITUS (itching) and URTICARIA (hives). In more serious reactions, usually of the type caused by improper matching of the blood, the patient's face may become flushed, then cyanotic. If he is conscious, he will complain of severe LOW BACK PAIN, THROBBING HEAD-

ACHE, SUBSTERNAL PAIN, and DIFFICULTY IN BREATHING; he will appear very ANXIOUS and RESTLESS. The SKIN becomes COLD and CLAMMY, as in shock, and sometimes the BLOOD PRESSURE FALLS, again presenting a picture similar to shock.

Signs and Symptoms of Transfusion Reaction

- Fever
- Pruritus (itching)
- Urticaria (hives)
- Throbbing headache
- Severe pain in the lower back and/or chest
- Dyspnea
- Anxiety and restlessness
- Shocklike picture
    1. Cold, clammy skin
    2. Falling blood pressure

If you should note ANY of these signs or symptoms in a patient who is receiving a blood transfusion, you should take the following steps:

1. STOP THE TRANSFUSION IMMEDIATELY. Shut the clamp on the IV tubing, and detach the entire transfusion set (blood bag plus tubing) from the IV catheter. Hook up a bag of normal saline, and run it at the same rate the blood was running. However, if the patient is showing signs of shock, you may have to infuse saline very rapidly and even apply the MAST. Radio your physician for instructions.
2. SAVE THE DONOR BLOOD AND ALL THE TUBING, so that it can be tested after you reach the hospital.
3. MAKE A CAREFUL RECORD of the TIME you noted the transfusion reaction and all of the patient's SIGNS AND SYMPTOMS. Also record his VITAL SIGNS (pulse, blood pressure, respirations), and recheck (and record) the vital signs every 5 minutes until you reach the hospital.

The second major category of intravenous fluids includes all those fluids that are NOT whole blood or blood products, and when such fluids are administered intravenously, the term used to describe the process is **infusion.** Nonblood fluids may be further subdivided into sugar solutions, salt solutions, and blood substitutes. **Sugar solutions** contain the simple sugar dextrose dissolved in water and labelled according to the amount of dextrose in the solution. For example, 5% dextrose in water (usually called "D5 and W" for short) contains 5 gm of dextrose in every 100 ml of solution. In emergency medicine, sugar solutions are used primarily in situations where one does NOT want to give a large volume of fluid but merely to "keep the vein open," so that there will be a route for administering drugs directly into the circulation. Thus sugar solutions are usually given at very slow flow rates with a special infusion set ("microdrip") that delivers very small drops of fluid at a time.

Salt solutions, on the other hand, are used when there is a need to give large volumes of fluid, as in shock. They are better suited to this purpose than sugar solutions because they tend to remain inside the blood vessels longer, while sugar solutions quickly seep out of the blood vessels to equilibrate between the blood and the body tissues. The most commonly used salt solutions are normal saline and Ringer's solution. **Normal saline** is simply ordinary salt (sodium plus chloride, or NaCl) dissolved in water in the same concentration that sodium and chloride are normally present in the blood. **Ringer's solution** also contains sodium and chloride, but in addition it has other elements present in the blood: potassium and calcium. These elements—sodium, chloride, potassium, and calcium—are called **electrolytes,** and in the healthy body, the concentration of each of these electrolytes in the blood is regulated very precisely. If one were to infuse suddenly a liter of pure water into a vein, the electrolytes in the blood would be considerably diluted, and vital organs could not function properly. For this reason, salt solutions are made in such a way that they closely approximate the plasma concentrations of the most important electrolytes (sodium and chloride), so as not to disturb the concentration of these elements in the blood.

The third category of nonblood solutions are **blood substitutes.** These are solutions that remain in the blood vessels even longer than salt solutions because they contain very large molecules that cannot squeeze out of the capillaries easily. One such solution is dextran, which contains very large sugar molecules and is sometimes used for patients in hemorrhagic shock when blood or plasma is not immediately available. It is generally NOT used in the field because its use may be associated with various complications and thus usually requires the supervision of a physician.

Intravenous Solutions

- Blood and blood products (transfusion)
- Nonblood solutions (infusion)
    1. Sugar solutions (to keep the vein open)
    2. Salt solutions (to give volume)
    3. Blood substitutes (to give volume)

Steps in Establishing an Intravenous Infusion

Once you have determined that a patient needs intravenous fluids and you have received a physician's order to start the infusion, you need to follow a systematic routine for establishing the IV line. If the IV is inserted in an orderly way, the procedure is much less stressful for both the EMT and the patient. The following are the steps in establishing the intravenous infusion:

1. EXPLAIN THE PROCEDURE TO THE PATIENT, AND OBTAIN CONSENT. Nobody likes needles, and no one—especially a person who is already anxious and in pain—is going to be particularly thrilled when you come marching up with a 5-inch needle, an enormous bag, and all sorts of tubes. After you have gained some experience in the field, starting an IV may seem pretty routine to you; but remember, it is NOT routine to the patient. Thus you need to explain carefully (a) why the IV line is necessary and (b) what is involved in the procedure. An unhurried, informative, and confident attitude on the part of the EMT will do a great deal to allay the patient's fears.
2. ASSEMBLE ALL THE NECESSARY EQUIPMENT. The well-organized EMT will have all the equipment he needs for the IV procedure neatly laid out beside him and will never find himself in the awkward situation of inserting an IV needle only to discover that there is no infusion set to which to hook it up. Check and double-check before you start that everything you will need is close at hand:
   a. INTRAVENOUS FLUID. Take a 1-liter bag of normal saline or Ringer's solution, and check it carefully for leakage, contamination, cloudiness, and the manufacturer's expiration date. NEVER USE ANY FLUID THAT IS CLOUDY, OUTDATED, OR SUSPECT IN ANY OTHER WAY. For field use, intravenous fluids should be stocked in plastic bags rather than bottles, since bottles are apt to break under field conditions.
   b. INFUSION SET. For administering large volumes of fluids, you will want a standard infusion set (i.e., *not* a microdrip), which usually delivers 0.1 ml in each drop. Attach the infusion set to the IV bag (Fig. 9-29). Clamp the tubing shut, and squeeze the drip chamber until it is about half full. Then open the flow control clamp, and flush the tubing through so that it is completely filled with fluid and all the air has been expelled.
   c. IV CATHETER. For giving significant volumes of fluid, you will need an IV catheter with a relatively wide diameter, or bore. The diameter of an IV needle or catheter is expressed in a *gauge number*, and the lower the gauge number, the wider the diameter of the needle. Thus an 18-gauge needle, for example, has a wider diameter than a 21-gauge needle. For the patient in shock, the larger the needle you can insert the better—fluids move faster through a wider needle—and a 16- or 18-gauge IV needle or catheter is probably ideal.

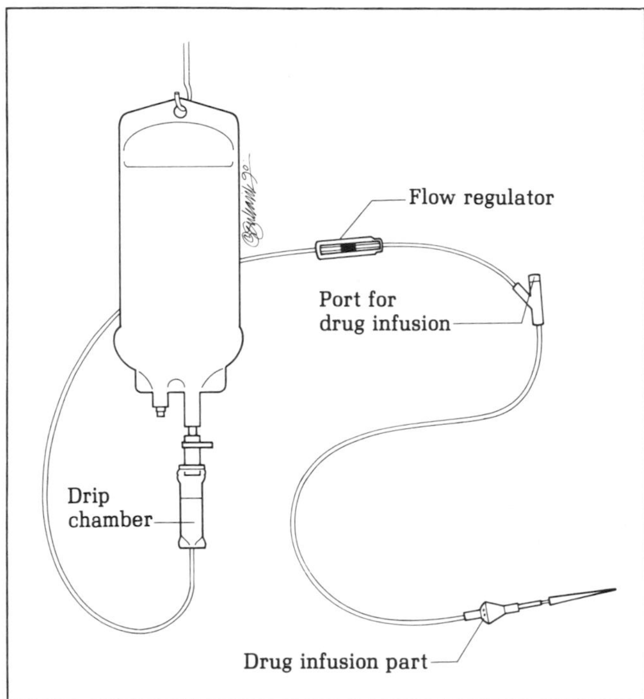

Fig. 9-29. *Intravenous infusion set.*

   IV needles and catheters come in several types. The preferred type for field use is the over-the-needle catheter. This consists of a plastic catheter threaded over a sharp, hollow needle. The catheter and needle are inserted into the vein as a unit, and then the needle is withdrawn, leaving the plastic catheter in the vein. A somewhat less desirable alternative is the "butterfly" needle, which consists of a hollow needle with two plastic "wings" to facilitate gripping it. The butterfly is easier to insert, but it is also easier to dislodge, and its steel needle is more likely to perforate the vein than is the flexible plastic catheter. If neither an over-the-needle catheter nor a butterfly needle is available in an emergency, one can use a standard 16- or 18-gauge hypodermic needle.
   d. ANTISEPTIC CLEANING SOLUTION, for preparing the site for the IV. Povidone-iodine swabs and alcohol swabs, used in succession, are the best means for disinfecting the skin.
   e. ANTISEPTIC OINTMENT, for placing over the puncture site. Povidone-iodine ointment is preferable; antibiotic ointments should be avoided if possible.
   f. STERILE DRESSING, to cover the puncture site. A 4 × 4–inch sterile gauze pad will do fine.
   g. ADHESIVE TAPE, CUT INTO STRIPS of 4 to 6 inches in length, to secure the IV. After you have inserted the IV needle is no time to start tearing adhesive tape, for you need two free hands to tear adhesive tape and at least one hand will be holding the needle in place. Some EMTs regularly walk around with several doz-

en strips of adhesive tape stuck to their trousers, just to have tape handy when it is needed. Usually, however, there is enough time before inserting the IV to prepare a few lengths of tape.

h. TOURNIQUET. This may be a length of soft rubber tubing, a commercial tourniquet, or a blood pressure cuff. The last often helps one find a vein when other methods have been unsuccessful. To use a blood pressure cuff as a tourniquet, determine the patient's systolic blood pressure, and then reinflate the blood pressure cuff to about 20 mm Hg *below* the systolic pressure. Clamp the tubing on the blood pressure cuff so it will not slowly deflate as you are working. When you are ready to release the pressure around the arm, simply unclamp the tubing.

i. PEN AND LABELS. The IV bag should be labelled with the time and date it was started and the initials of the person who started it.

j. ARMBOARD. It is often desirable to immobilize the extremity in which you have placed the IV, for undue movement can dislodge the IV needle. A short length of heavy cardboard or a padded arm splint can be used as an armboard.

3. SELECT A SUITABLE VEIN. Let the patient's arm hang dependent for a few minutes so that blood will pool by gravity in the veins of the forearm and hand. Then attach a tourniquet to the arm, midway between the elbow and the armpit. Take care not to make the tourniquet so tight that it cuts off arterial flow into the arm; check the radial pulse to make sure, and if you cannot feel a pulse, loosen the tourniquet until you can. Inspect the back of the hand and the forearm for a vein that looks fairly straight and lies on a flat surface. Ideally it should be well fixed to the surrounding tissues so that it does not roll off to one side, and it should feel springy to the touch. AVOID the following:
   a. VEINS THAT LIE OVER JOINTS. IVs in such veins are easily dislodged and require firm immobilization of the joint, which is uncomfortable for the patient.
   b. VEINS THAT LIE CLOSE TO ARTERIAL PULSATIONS. If the vein is very close to an artery, you may accidently puncture the artery when you insert the needle through the skin.
   c. VEINS NEAR INJURED AREAS.
   d. VEINS OF THE LOWER EXTREMITIES. The leg veins are much more prone to develop phlebitis (inflammation of the vein) and should be avoided, except in cases where there are no options (e.g., severe burns of both arms).

   In general, the preferred site for inserting an IV catheter is the forearm (Fig. 9-30), with the back of the hand the second choice (Fig. 9-31).
4. PREPARE THE SITE. Scrub the spot you have chosen with several povidone-iodine swabs. Start from the spot where you plan to insert the needle, right over the vein, and wipe in widening circles around it, giving yourself a broad margin around the site to be punctured. Then give a final wipe with an alcohol swab to remove the povidone-iodine from the skin (some patients develop a rash from iodine left on the skin).
5. INSERT THE IV CATHETER. Stabilize the vein so it will not roll by applying pressure to it with your thumb distal to the spot you intend to puncture. Do not push down too hard though, or the vein will empty and collapse. With the needle lined up in the same direction as the vein and the bevel of the needle pointing upward, insert the needle firmly through the skin. Avoid jamming it in, for you may jam it right through the vein as well. Once the needle has penetrated the skin, angle it so that it is almost parallel with the vein, and advance it toward the vein. You can enter the vein from the side or from above, but in either case you should be able to feel a small "pop," or give, as the needle pierces the wall of the vein. Once the needle is in the vein, blood will flow back and appear in the needle hub. If you are using an over-the-needle catheter, advance the needle just a millimeter or so more, so it is securely in the vein, and then slide the catheter smoothly over the needle into the vein. When the catheter is in all the way to its hilt, hold it steady against the arm and withdraw the needle from it. An important precaution: Once you have advanced a plastic catheter over a needle into a vein, NEVER PULL IT BACK. Doing so can cause a piece of the catheter to be sheared off against the sharp edge of the needle, and the piece of catheter then becomes a very dangerous foreign body in the bloodstream, which may ultimately lodge in the lungs and cause serious damage.
6. ATTACH THE IV TUBING. While continuing to hold the catheter steady, release the tourniquet, and attach the tubing from the solution bag to the catheter hub. Open the flow control clamp on the tubing wide to flush the catheter and check its position. If the catheter is indeed in the vein, the fluid should flow into the drip chamber in a brisk, steady stream. If the flow is feeble with the flow control wide open—just a few slow drops—the tip of the catheter may be up against the wall of the vein. Pull back *very slightly* on the catheter, and recheck the flow. If the flow is still feeble, and meanwhile you notice a lump developing over the puncture site, the catheter has probably slipped out of the vein. In this case, you must clamp the IV shut, withdraw the catheter, and hold firm pressure over the puncture site for several minutes before trying again at some other spot.
7. SECURE THE IV CATHETER. Once good flow has been established, squeeze a dab of povidone-iodine ointment over the skin at the point where the catheter emerges, and cover the site with a

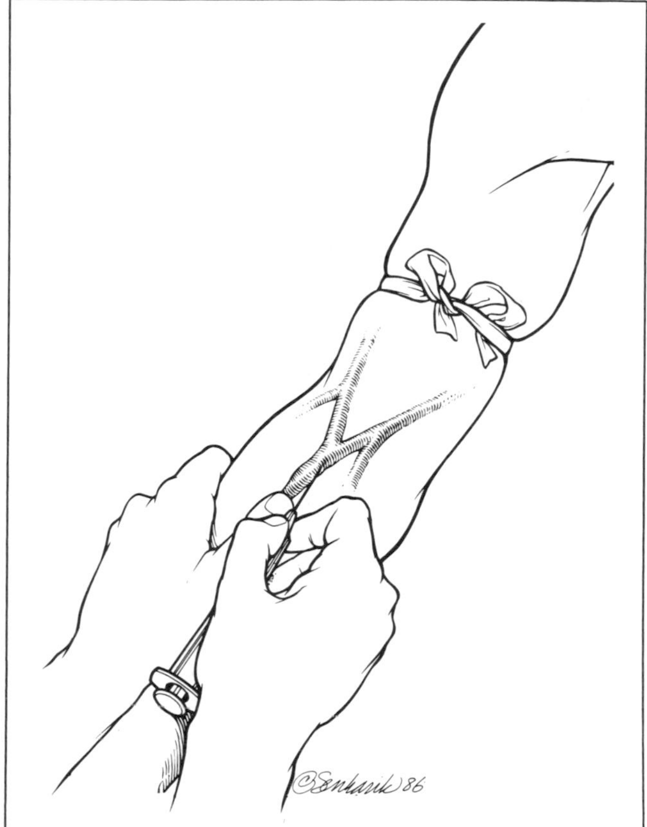

Fig. 9-30. *Starting an intravenous infusion in an antecubital vein.*

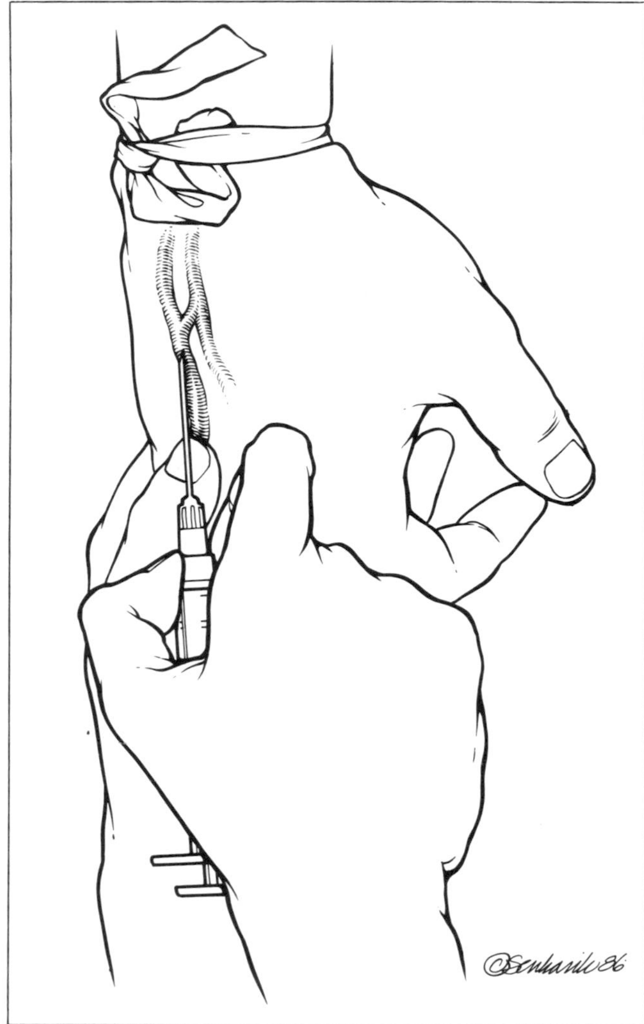

Fig. 9-31. *Starting an intravenous infusion in a hand vein.*

sterile dressing. Tape down the dressing and the catheter. Put a loop in the IV tubing, and tape its distal segment to the arm. The loop will serve to protect the catheter from receiving the direct force of any sudden jerk on the tubing and will thereby help prevent the catheter from being accidently pulled out. If the IV is on the back of the hand, stabilize it further by securing the patient's arm and forearm to an armboard.

8. ADJUST THE FLOW RATE. The flow rate is calculated according to a simple equation that relates the number of drops per milliliter (a characteristic of the infusion set) to the time over which the infusion is to be given, and it tells you how fast you have to run the infusion (in drops/min) to deliver a given volume (in ml/hr). In order to calculate the flow rate, you need to know (a) how many drops = 1 ml in the infusion set you are using and (b) how fast (in ml/hr) you want the infusion to run.

The rate is easiest to calculate in two steps:

a. Determine how many milliliters you have to give per minute:

$$\text{ml/min} = \frac{\text{ml/hr}}{\text{60 min/hr}}$$

b. Determine how many drops you have to give to provide this volume per minute:

$$\text{drops/min} = \text{ml/min} \times \text{drops/ml}$$

Let us take an example. Suppose the physician orders you to give an infusion of normal saline at a rate of 180 ml per hour. You have an infusion set that delivers 10 drops per milliliter. How many *drops per minute* will you have to infuse in order to give the patient the desired volume of 180 ml per hour?

a. How many milliliters per minute must you infuse?

$$\text{ml/min} = \frac{\text{180 ml/hr}}{\text{60 min/hr}}$$
$$= \text{3 ml/min}$$

b. How many drops per minute are equivalent to this volume?

$$\text{drops/min} = 3\ \text{ml/min} \times 10\ \text{drops/ml} = 30\ \text{drops/min}$$

Thus, in order to deliver 180 ml per hour to the patient with the infusion set you are using, you must run the IV at 30 drops per minute, and you will have to adjust the flow clamp until the drops are falling at this rate.

Let us practice with one more example. The physician decides that he does not want the patient to have much fluid after all, and he instructs you to start the IV with a microdrip infusion set, which delivers 60 drops per milliliter, and to maintain the IV at 30 ml per hour (a "keep-open" rate—i.e., just enough to keep the line from clotting off). How many drops per minute should the patient receive?

a. $\text{ml/min} = \dfrac{30\ \text{ml/hr}}{60\ \text{min/hr}} = 0.5\ \text{ml/min}$

b. $\text{drops/min} = 0.5\ \text{ml/min} \times 60\ \text{drops/ml} = 30\ \text{drops/min}$

Thus, using this infusion set, you will have to adjust the rate to 30 drops per minute in order for the patient to receive the desired volume of 30 ml per hour.

9. LABEL THE IV BAG with the date, time, and your initials.

Steps in Establishing an Intravenous Infusion: Summary

1. EXPLAIN the procedure to the patient, and OBTAIN CONSENT.
2. ASSEMBLE all the necessary EQUIPMENT:
   a. Intravenous fluid bag.
   b. Infusion set.
   c. IV catheter.
   d. Antiseptic swabs.
   e. Antiseptic ointment.
   f. Sterile 4 × 4–inch dressing.
   g. Strips of adhesive tape.
   h. Tourniquet.
   i. Pen and label.
   j. Armboard.
3. APPLY TOURNIQUET, and select a suitable vein.
4. DISINFECT THE SKIN.
5. INSERT the IV CATHETER.
6. ATTACH the IV TUBING to the catheter, and release tourniquet.
7. SECURE the CATHETER.
8. ADJUST the FLOW RATE.
9. LABEL the bag.

In the Greater Scheme of Things

Suppose you are called upon to treat a man who has been run over by a truck, and you find him lying unconscious in the street, with a pool of blood around him. At what point in his care do you pause to start the IV?

Recall the ABCs. Airway. Breathing. Circulation (= pulse, bleeding). Thus the IV is quite a way down the road. First things first.

1. Open the AIRWAY.
2. Make sure the patient is BREATHING. (If not, start rescue breathing.) As soon as possible, start OXYGEN.
3. Make sure the patient has an effective CIRCULATION (pulse). (If not, start external cardiac compressions.)
4. Control any obvious BLEEDING, first by manual methods.
5. Apply the MAST.
6. Start the INTRAVENOUS INFUSION.
7. Dress WOUNDS.
8. Splint FRACTURES.

Experienced EMT-intermediates and paramedics often wait until they have the patient in the vehicle and are en route to the hospital before they start the IV in order not to spend any more time at the scene than absolutely necessary (see Chap. 18 for a discussion of the "golden hour" in trauma victims). It takes considerable skill to start an IV in a moving vehicle—more skill than the average *doctor* possesses—but experienced EMTs carry it off with finesse.

Potential Complications of Intravenous Therapy

Every invasive medical procedure has its potential complications, and intravenous therapy is no exception. Most of the potential complications of intravenous therapy, however, can be avoided with proper attention to technique.

LOCAL INFILTRATION. Local infiltration of intravenous solution into the subcutaneous tissues (tissues just beneath the skin) happens quite commonly. It occurs when a catheter or needle tip is dislodged from the vein, and the intravenous solution infuses into the tissues rather than into the circulation. When this happens, the patient develops edema (swelling) and pain at the site of the IV catheter. The infusion slows down or stops altogether, and if you lower the IV bag below the level of the patient's arm, there will be no blood return through the tubing, which you *would* see if the catheter were in the patient's vein. If local infiltration occurs, you must STOP THE INFUSION IMMEDIATELY AND REMOVE THE IV CATHETER. Cold compresses applied over the infusion site will help reduce the swelling and diminish the pain.

PYROGENIC REACTIONS. Pyrogenic reactions are caused by the presence of contaminants in the intravenous solution, and they are more apt to occur when the patient is given an intravenous solution that is cloudy or that is packaged in a leaking bag. The reaction is characterized by a very sudden onset of high fever, severe chills, backache, headache, nausea, vomiting, and sometimes cardiovascular collapse. Such a reaction will usually occur (if it is going to occur at all) within 20 to 30 minutes of the time the infusion with the IV bag in question was started. A pyrogenic reaction can be life-threatening, and if it occurs, you must take the following steps:

1. STOP THE INFUSION IMMEDIATELY, AND REMOVE THE IV CATHETER.
2. Start ANOTHER INFUSION in the other arm, using a fresh IV catheter, a new bag of IV solution, and a new infusion set.
3. If signs of shock are present, treat as any other case of shock.

The best treatment of all is prevention, so be sure to check every bag of intravenous solution carefully for cloudiness and evidence of leaks. If the bag does not look quite right, *do not use it*!

INFECTION OF THE INFUSION SITE. Infection of the infusion site is almost always the result of poor sterile technique on the part of the person who inserted the IV. Infection may take a day or two to develop, so you will not know whether your IVs are getting infected unless you stop back at the hospital periodically to check up on patients you have transported there. Infection can be almost entirely prevented by strict adherence to sterile procedures when establishing an intravenous infusion.

THROMBOPHLEBITIS. Thrombophlebitis, or inflammation and clotting within the vein, is a relatively common complication of intravenous therapy. It is generally *not* a problem in the field because thrombophlebitis takes a few days to develop. It may be due to mechanical factors, such as excessive motion of the IV catheter, or it may be caused by the intravenous solution itself. Certain intravenous solutions are more irritating to veins than others: 5% dextrose solution, for instance, is quite acid, and prolonged infusion can cause significant inflammation of the vein in which the IV catheter has been placed. The signs and symptoms of thrombophlebitis are *pain* along the course of the vein, which may be tender to palpation, and *redness* and *swelling* at the puncture site. You probably will not see thrombophlebitis unless you are transferring from one hospital to another a patient who has had an IV running for a few days. If you should note signs of thrombophlebitis, stop the infusion, and remove the IV catheter. Apply cold compresses to the puncture site.

CIRCULATORY OVERLOAD. Circulatory overload can occur if the patient is given an excessive volume of intravenous fluid—either because of a miscalculation of the patient's volume needs, a miscalculation of the IV rate, or a "runaway IV" (an IV that starts flowing faster than the original rate because the control clamp has loosened). Circulatory overload is more apt to occur in older patients, especially patients with preexisting heart disease, for they are less able to adapt to sudden changes in blood volume. When the circulation has become overloaded with fluid, the result is often pulmonary edema, that is, fluid in the alveoli, and the chief manifestations are increasing DYSPNEA and TACHYPNEA.

If a patient receiving intravenous therapy begins showing signs of circulatory overload, slow the IV to the lowest possible flow rate. SIT THE PATIENT UP with his feet dangling (unless he is still in shock, in which case you should raise the head of the stretcher to about 45 degrees)—a maneuver that will help blood and fluid to drain out of the lungs by gravity. If the patient is not already receiving OXYGEN, provide it in high concentration. (Why?)

AIR EMBOLISM. An embolism is a kind of plug that is swept through the circulation until it reaches a blood vessel small enough to trap it, and then it lodges in that blood vessel and obstructs the flow of blood. Generally one thinks of an embolism as being formed from a blood clot, but—strange as it seems—air introduced into the bloodstream can also serve as an embolism and can plug up a blood vessel just as effectively as a blood clot can. A healthy adult can probably tolerate as much as 100 ml of air being introduced into a peripheral vein, but in a critically ill or injured patient, as little as 10 ml of air in a vein can be fatal. Once again, the best treatment is prevention, and air embolism can be prevented by taking the following precautions:

- Inspect the tubing of the infusion set for any defects before you hook it up to the IV bag.
- Make sure all connections (e.g., between the IV catheter and the infusion set) are *fitted tightly*, so no air can seep in.
- *Avoid* circumstances that will increase the negative pressure in the IV tubing, such as
    1. Elevation of the extremity receiving the IV above the level of the patient's heart.
    2. Placement of the flow control clamp too high on the tubing (it should be at the level of the patient's heart).

If air embolism does occur, you will know about it, for the signs are very dramatic: sudden shock, with cyanosis, hypotension, tachycardia, and a decreasing level of consciousness. If these signs occur, immediately CLAMP THE IV TUBING OFF, and TURN THE PATIENT ONTO HIS *LEFT* SIDE WITH THE STRETCHER TILTED HEAD DOWN. This position makes the air bubble in the circulation rise into the

Table 9-5. *Potential Complications of Intravenous Therapy*

Complication	Prevention	Signs and Symptoms	Treatment
Local infiltration	Secure IV catheter firmly.	Pain and swelling at puncture site; IV slows down or stops; no blood return.	1. Stop the infusion, and remove IV catheter. 2. Cold compresses.
Pyrogenic reaction	Inspect bag for leaks, cloudiness, expiration date.	Sudden fever, chills, headache, backache, nausea, vomiting, shock.	1. Stop the infusion, and remove IV catheter. 2. Start a new IV in the other arm (fresh bag, fresh infusion set). 3. Treat for shock.
Infection	Strict sterile technique.	Pain, redness, and swelling at puncture site; possible fever.	1. Stop the infusion, and remove IV catheter. 2. Antibiotics.
Thrombophlebitis	Secure IV firmly. Do not leave IV in more than 24–36 hr.	Pain and tenderness along the vein; redness and swelling at puncture site.	1. Stop the infusion, and remove IV catheter. 2. Cold compresses, then warm compresses.
Circulatory overload	Check flow rate often.	Dyspnea, tachypnea, tachycardia.	1. Slow IV. 2. Sit patient up with legs dangling. 3. Oxygen (high concentration).
Air embolism	Check tubing for defects; all connections fitted tightly; arm with IV below heart level.	Sudden cyanosis, hypotension, tachycardia, decreasing consciousness.	1. Clamp off infusion. 2. Roll patient to left side, head down.
Catheter shear	Never pull back on a plastic catheter being advanced over a needle.	May be absent; may not be detected until catheter is removed.	None in the field; report to physician.
Arterial puncture	Do not try to cannulate a vein that lies close to an artery.	Bright red blood spurts back through IV catheter.	1. Remove IV catheter. 2. Hold firm pressure over puncture site at least 5 min.

right atrium and keeps it from moving into the lungs. The patient should be kept in this position until he reaches the hospital, where a long IV catheter may have to be snaked into the right atrium to "snare" the air bubble and draw it out of the circulation.

If you should ever notice a bubble of air wending its way through the IV tubing, immediately shut the flow control clamp, disconnect the tubing from the IV catheter, and then open the control clamp to flush the air out of the tubing before you reconnect it to the catheter.

CATHETER SHEAR. As noted earlier, an IV catheter that is threaded over or through a needle may get partially sheared off if it is pulled back against the sharp edge of the needle. For this reason, once a catheter is advanced over or through a needle, it must NEVER, NEVER, NEVER be pulled back. If it is necessary to remove the catheter, *first* withdraw the needle, then withdraw the catheter.

INADVERTENT ARTERIAL PUNCTURE. Inadvertent arterial puncture can occur if the vein you have chosen for the IV lies right next to an artery, for if your aim is a little off or your needle slips, the IV catheter can pierce the artery rather than the target vein. You will know if the catheter has accidently entered an artery, for bright red blood will come spurting back through the catheter. If that happens, immediately withdraw the needle and catheter, and hold firm pressure over the puncture site for at least 5 minutes, or until the bleeding stops.

The potential complications of intravenous therapy are summarized in Table 9-5.

SUMMARY

The following verses summarize some of the important points of this chapter.

An EMT named Ollie O'Blake
Shoved an airway into a man quite awake.
An uppercut to the jaw
And a left hook to the craw
Convinced O'Blake that he'd made a mistake.

MORAL: A CONSCIOUS PATIENT WILL NOT TOLERATE AN OROPHARYNGEAL AIRWAY.

A man who'd been bleeding most swiftly
Appeared to be breathing just niftily.

The EMT thus saw no need
To give O_2 for a bleed.
And death came both quickly and thriftily.

MORAL: EVERY PATIENT IN SHOCK NEEDS OXYGEN.

An incautious man named Decatur
Leaned over the O_2 regulator.
He failed to peruse
That the valve had come loose.
They'll find his head sooner or later.

MORAL: NEVER PLACE ANY PART OF YOUR BODY OVER THE REDUCING VALVE OF A COMPRESSED GAS CYLINDER.

With sirens and great falderal,
An EMT took his first call—
A respiratory arrest;
So imagine his distress
To find he'd no oxygen at all.

MORAL: IT IS GROSS NEGLIGENCE TO RESPOND TO A CALL WITH AN EMPTY OXYGEN CYLINDER.

McGrew was a good sort of bloke
Who thought he'd just have a quick smoke.
While rings he was blowing,
The oxygen was flowing.
In the hospital burn unit he woke.

MORAL: NEVER SMOKE IN AN AREA WHERE OXYGEN IS IN USE OR BEING STORED.

VOCABULARY

acute respiratory insufficiency Condition in which breathing is inadequate to supply oxygen to and remove carbon dioxide from the tissues.
assisted ventilation Use of adjunctive equipment, such as a demand valve, to increase the volume of each breath in a spontaneously breathing patient.
controlled ventilation Artificial ventilation of a patient who is not breathing spontaneously.
demand valve Oxygen-powered resuscitator.
dyspnea The sensation of being short of breath.
evisceration Condition in which internal organs, such as the intestines, protrude through a wound in the abdomen.
flow meter Device that controls the flow rate of oxygen from an oxygen source.
hyperpnea Abnormally deep respirations.
impaled object Foreign body that remains in a wound and protrudes from it.
nasopharyngeal airway Soft rubber tube that is inserted through the nose so that its distal tip lies in the pharynx.
O_2 Abbreviation for *oxygen*.
oropharyngeal airway Curved plastic device that is inserted through the mouth and passes behind the tongue to hold the tongue away from the back of the throat.
psi Abbreviation for *pounds per square inch*.
pulmonary edema Condition in which the lungs fill with fluid.
reducing valve Pressure regulator that reduces the pressure of gas inside the oxygen cylinder so that it emerges at workable pressure levels.
safe residual Minimum permissible pressure in an oxygen cylinder, defined as 200 psi.
tachypnea Abnormally rapid respirations.
tonsil tip Type of rigid suction catheter; also called Yankauer suction catheter.
tracheal tugging Upward motion of the trachea on inhalation—a sign of respiratory distress.
yoke The part of the reducing valve that connects the regulator assembly to the oxygen cylinder.

ADDITIONAL VOCABULARY FOR EMT-INTERMEDIATES

air embolism Bubble of air that enters the circulation and acts as an obstruction when it becomes trapped in a blood vessel.
artifact Interference in the ECG signal.
defibrillation Use of unsynchronized electric shock to terminate ventricular fibrillation.
ECG Abbreviation for *electrocardiogram*.
electrocardiogram Written record of the electric activity of the heart.
electrocardiograph Machine used to record the electric activity of the heart.
electrode Probe used to sense electric activity.
electrolyte Substance whose molecules dissociate into charged components when placed in water (e.g., sodium, chloride).
infusion Intravenous therapy with nonblood products.
gauge Diameter of a needle or catheter.
glottis Opening between the vocal cords.
normal saline Intravenous salt solution used to replace volume.
pruritus Itching.
P wave First component of the ECG, reflecting depolarization of the atria.
QRS complex Spiking lines that follow the P wave and reflect depolarization of the ventricles.
Ringer's solution Intravenous salt solution used to replace volume.
thrombophlebitis Inflammation and clotting within a vein.
transfusion Intravenous therapy with blood or blood products.
T wave Third component of the ECG, reflecting recharging of the ventricles.
urticaria Hives.
vallecula Groove between the epiglottis and the back of the throat.

FURTHER READING

GENERAL

American Heart Association. Standards and guidelines for cardiopulmonary resuscitation (CPR) and emergency cardiac care (ECC). *JAMA* 255:2905, 1986.

ESOPHAGEAL OBTURATOR AIRWAY

Auerbach PS, Geehr EC. Inadequate oxygenation and ventilation using the esophageal obturator gastric tube airway in the prehospital setting. *JAMA* 250:3067, 1983.

Bass R, Allison E, Hunt R. The esophageal obturator airway: A reassessment of use by paramedics. *Ann Emerg Med* 11:358, 1982.

Brain A. The laryngeal mask—a new concept in airway management. *Br J Anaesth* 55:801, 1983.

Don Michael T. Comparison of the esophageal obturator airway and endotracheal intubation in prehospital ventilation during CPR. *Chest* 87:814, 1985.

Don Michael T. Mouth-to-lung airway for cardiac resuscitation. *Lancet* 2:1329, 1968.

Donen N et al. The esophageal obturator airway: An appraisal. *Canad Anaesth Soc J* 30:194, 1983.

Goldenberg I et al. Morbidity and mortality in patients receiving the esophageal obturator airway and the endotracheal tube in prehospital cardiac arrest. *Minnesota Med* 69:707, 1986.

Greenbaum DM, Poggi J, Grace WM. Esophageal obstruction during oxygen administration: A new method for use in resuscitation. *Chest* 65:188, 1974.

Hammargren Y et al. A standard comparison of esophageal obturator airway and endotracheal tube ventilation in cardiac arrest. *Ann Emerg Med* 14:933, 1985.

Harrison E et al. Esophageal perforation following use of the esophageal obturator airway. *Ann Emerg Med* 9:21, 1980.

Johnson KR, Genovesi MG, Lassar KH. Esophageal obturator airway: Use and complications. *JACEP* 5:36, 1976.

Kassels SJ, Robinson WA, O'Bara KJ. Esophageal perforation associated with the esophageal obturator airway. *Crit Care Med* 8:386, 1980.

Meislin HW. The esophageal obturator airway: A study of respiratory effectiveness. *Ann Emerg Med* 9:54, 1980.

Shea SR et al. Prehospital endotracheal tube airway or esophageal gastric tube airway: A critical comparison. *Ann Emerg Med* 14:102, 1985.

Smith JP et al. The esophageal obturator airway. *JAMA* 250:1081, 1982.

Smith JP et al. A field evaluation of the esophageal obturator airway. *J Trauma* 23:317, 1983.

ENDOTRACHEAL INTUBATION

Bishop MJ. Endotracheal tube lumen compromise from cuff overinflation. *Chest* 80:100, 1981.

Bissinger U. Unrecognized endobronchial intubation of emergency patients. *Ann Emerg Med* 18:853, 1989.

Chander S et al. Correct placement of endotracheal tubes. *NY State J Med* 79:1843, 1979.

DeLeo BC. Endotracheal intubation by rescue squad personnel. *Heart & Lung* 6:851, 1977.

Dick T. Tubular tricks. Foolproofing your field intubations. *JEMS* 14(5):26, 1989.

Hardwick WC et al. Digital intubation. *J Emerg Med* 1:317, 1984.

Jacobs LM et al. Endotracheal intubation in the prehospital phase of emergency medical care. *JAMA* 250:2175, 1983.

Natanson C, Shelhamer J, Perrillo J. Intubation of the trachea in the critical care setting. *JAMA* 253:1160, 1985.

Owen RL, Cheney FW. Endobronchial intubation: A preventable complication. *Anesthesiology* 67:255, 1987.

Stanford TM. ET: A different approach. *Emergency* 20(12):34, 1988.

Stein JM. Difficult adult intubation. *Emerg Med* 17(3):121, 1985.

Stein JM. Endotracheal intubation in a hurry. *Emerg Med* 14(15):129, 1982.

Stein JM. Nasotracheal intubation. *Emerg Med* 16(13):183, 1984.

Stewart RD et al. Effect of varied training techniques on field endotrachial intubation success rates. *Ann Emerg Med* 13:1032, 1984.

Stewart RD et al. Field endotracheal intubation by paramedical personnel: Success rates and complications. *Chest* 85:341, 1984.

Stewart RD, Paris PM. Signs of endotracheal intubation in the field setting (Letter). *Ann Emerg Med* 14:276, 1985.

Whitten CE. Common errors and how to avoid them. *Emerg Med* 21(15):91, 1989.

Whitten CE. Difficult intubations: Tricks to remember. *Emerg Med* 22(1):85, 1990.

Whitten CE. Endotracheal anatomy. *Emerg Med* 21(8):171, 1989.

Whitten CE. Equipment for airway management. *Emerg Med* 21(12):91, 1989.

Whitten CE. Oral intubation in adults. *Emerg Med* 21(14):81, 1989.

Whitten CE. Tests for tube placement. *Emerg Med* 21(17):93, 1989.

AIDS TO BREATHING

Barnes TA, Watson ME. Oxygen delivery performance of four adult resuscitation bags. *Disaster Med* 1:204, 1983.

Bourne S. You can breathe easy. *JEMS* 14(5):59, 1989.

Campbell EJ et al. Subjective effects of humidification of oxygen for delivery by nasal cannula: A prospective study. *Chest* 93:289, 1988.

Committee on Trauma, American College of Surgeons. Essential equipment for ambulances. *Bull Am Coll Surg*, September, 1977.

Elling R, Politis J. An evaluation of emergency medical technicians' ability to use manual ventilation devices. *Ann Emerg Med* 12:765, 1983.

Harrison R et al. Mouth-to-mask ventilation: A superior method of rescue breathing. *Ann Emerg Med* 11:74, 1982.

Jesudian M et al. Bag-valve-mask ventilation: Two rescuers are better than one: Preliminary report. *Crit Care Med* 13:122, 1985.

Lawrence PJ. Ventilation during cardiopulmonary resuscitation: Which method? *Med J Austral* 143:433, 1985.

Safar P. Pocket mask for emergency artificial ventilation and oxygen administration. *Crit Care Med* 2:273, 1974.

Stewart RD et al. Influence of mask design on bag-mask ventilation. *Ann Emerg Med* 14:403, 1985.

Tinits P. Oxygen therapy and oxygen toxicity. *Ann Emerg Med* 12:321, 1983.

Tendrup TE et al. A comparison of infant ventilation methods performed by prehospital personnel. *Ann Emerg Med* 18:707, 1989.

Waxman K. Oxygen delivery and resuscitation. *Ann Emerg Med* 15:1420, 1986.

Whelan G. Ensuring ventilation. *Emerg Med* 16(15):109, 1985.

MECHANICAL CPR

Barkalow CE. Mechanical cardiopulmonary resuscitation: Past, present, and future. *Am J Emerg Med* 2:262, 1984.

Little K, Auchinloss JM, Reaves CS. A mechanical cardiopulmonary life-support system. *Resuscitation* 3:63, 1974.

Roberts BG. Dallas EMS system advocates mechanical CPR. *Emerg Med Serv* 7(4):39, 1978.

Taylor GJ et al. External cardiac compression: A randomized comparison of mechanical and manual techniques. *JAMA* 240:644, 1978.

DEFIBRILLATION

American College of Emergency Physicians. Prehospital defibrillation by basic level emergency medical technicians. *Ann Emerg Med* 13:974, 1984.

Bocka JJ. Automatic external defibrillators. *Ann Emerg Med* 18:1264, 1989.

Copass MK, Eisenberg MS, Damon SK. *EMT Defibrillation*. Westport, CT: Emergency Training, 1984.

Cummins RO et al. Automatic external defibrillation: Evaluation of its role in the home and in emergency medical services. *Ann Emerg Med* 13:798, 1984.

Cummins RO. Defibrillation. *Emerg Med Clin North Am* 6(2):217, 1988.

Cummins RO. From concept to standard of care? Review of the clinical experience with automated external defibrillators. *Ann Emerg Med* 18:1269, 1989.

Cummins RO et al. An innovative approach to medical control: Semiautomatic defibrillators with solid-state memory modules for recording cardiac arrest events. *Ann Emerg Med* 17:818, 1988.

Cummins RO et al. Sensitivity, accuracy, and safety of an automatic external defibrillator. *Lancet* 2:318, 1984.

Cummins RO et al. Training of lay persons to use automatic external defibrillators: Success of initial training and one-year retention of skills. *Am J Emerg Med* 7:143, 1989.

Eisenberg MS et al. Management of out-of-hospital cardiac arrest. Failure of basic emergency medical technician services. *JAMA* 243:1049, 1980.

Eisenberg MS et al. Treatment of out-of-hospital cardiac arrest with rapid defibrillation by emergency medical technicians. *NEJM* 302:1379, 1980.

Eisenberg MS et al. Treatment of ventricular fibrillation. Emergency medical technician defibrillation and paramedic services. *JAMA* 251:1723, 1984.

Eisenberg MS et al. Use of the automatic external defibrillator in homes of survivors of out-of-hospital ventricular fibrillation. *Am J Cardiol* 63:443, 1989.

Fotre TV. Automated defibrillators: Their history and utilization. *Emerg Med Serv* 18(4):33, 1989.

Graves JR, Austin D, Cummins RO. *Rapid Zap: Automated Defibrillation*. Englewood Cliffs, NJ: Prentice-Hall, 1989.

Heath RL, Pendergrast R. Controlling defibrillation attempts. *Emergency* 12(4):44, 1980.

Heath RL, Pendergrast R. Current problems in defibrillation. *Emergency* 12(1):33, 1980.

Heath RL, Pendergrast R. Difibrillation: Long term vs. short term survival. *Emergency* 12(5):70, 1980.

Heath RL, Pendergrast R. Misconceptions in defibrillation. *Emergency* 12(3):69, 1980.

Hunt RC et al. Influence of emergency medical services systems and prehospital defibrillation on survival of sudden cardiac death victims. *Am J Emerg Med* 7:68, 1989.

Iversen WR et al. AICDs spark hope for cardiac care. *JEMS* 14(9):37, 1989.

Kerber RE et al. Determinants of defibrillation: Prospective analysis of 183 patients. *Am. J Cardiol* 52:739, 1983.

Olsen DW et al. EMT-defibrillation: The Wisconsin experience. *Ann Emerg Med* 18:806, 1989.

Pulley SA, Ferko JG, Defibrillation—EMT style. *Emergency* 21(7):36, 1989.

Stults K. *EMT-D Prehospital Defibrillation*. Englewood Cliffs, NJ: Prentice-Hall, 1986.

Vukov LR et al. New perspectives on rural EMT defibrillation. *Ann Emerg Med* 17:318, 1988.

Weaver WD et al. Cardiac arrest treated with a new automatic external defibrillator by out-of-hospital first responders. *Am J Cardiol* 57:1017, 1986.

Weaver D et al. Use of the automatic external defibrillator in the management of out-of-hospital cardiac arrest. *N Engl J Med* 219:661, 1988.

Weigel A, Atkins JM, Taylor J. *Automated Defibrillation*. Englewood, CO: Morton, 1988.

MILITARY ANTISHOCK TROUSERS

Abraham E et al. Effect of pneumatic trousers on pulmonary function. *Crit Care Med* 10:754, 1982.

Aprahamian C et al. Effect of circumferential pneumatic compression devices on digital flow. *Ann Emerg Med* 13:1092, 1984.

Bass RR et al. Thigh compartment syndrome without lower extremity trauma following application of pneumatic antishock trousers. *Ann Emerg Med* 12:382, 1983.

Bickell WH et al. Effect of antishock trousers on the trauma score: A prospective analysis in the urban setting. *Ann Emerg Med* 14:218, 1985.

Bickell WH, Dice WH. Military antishock trousers in a patient with adrenergic-resistant anaphylaxis. *Ann Emerg Med* 13:189, 1984.

Bickell WH et al. Randomized trial of pneumatic antishock garments in the prehospital management of penetrating abdominal injuries. *Ann Emerg Med* 16:653, 1987.

Bircher N, Safar P, Stewart RD. A comparison of standard, MAST augmented, and open chest CPR in dogs. *Crit Care Med* 8:147, 1980.

Bivens HG et al. Blood volume displacement with inflation of antishock trousers. *Ann Emerg Med* 11:409, 1982.

Brotman S, Browder B, Cox E. MAS trousers improperly applied causing a compartment syndrome in lower extremity trauma. *J Trauma* 22:598, 1982.

Chipman CD. The MAST controversy. *Emerg Med* 15(3):206, 1983.

Chisholm CD, Clark DE. Effect of pneumatic antishock garment on intramuscular pressure. *Ann Emerg Med* 13:581, 1984.

Christiansen KS. Pneumatic antishock garments (PASG): Do they precipitate lower-extremity compartment syndromes? *J Trauma* 26:1102, 1986.

Civetta JM et al. Prehospital use of the military antishock trouser (MAST). *JACEP* 5:581, 1976.

Cogbill TH et al. Pulmonary function after military antishock trouser inflation. *Surg Forum* 32:302, 1981.

Cram AE. Effects of pneumatic antishock trousers on canine intracranial pressure. *Ann Emerg Med* 10:28, 1981.

Crile GW. *Hemorrhage and Transfusion: An Experimental and Clinical Research*. New York: Appleton, 1909. P. 139.

Davis JW, McKone TK, Cram AE. Hemodynamic effects of military antishock trousers (MAST) in experimental cardiac tamponade. *Ann Emerg Med* 10:185, 1981.

Flint LM et al. Definite control of bleeding from severe pelvic fracture. *Ann Surg* 189:709, 1979.

Gaffney FA et al. Hemodynamic effects of medical antishock trousers (MAST garment). *J Trauma* 21:931, 1981.

Gilbert RD. Depression of respiratory function by pneumatic antishock trousers in traumatic quadriplegia. *Ann Emerg Med* 12:378, 1983.

Goldsmith SR. Comparative hemodynamic effects of antishock suit and volume expansion in normal human beings. *Ann Emerg Med* 12:348, 1983.

Gustafson RA et al. The use of the MAST suit in ruptured abdominal aortic aneurysms. *Am Surg* 49:454, 1983.

Lee HR et al. MAST augmentation of external cardiac compression: Role of changing intrapleural pressure. *Ann Emerg Med* 10:560, 1981.

Lee HR et al. Venous return in hemorrhagic shock after application of military anti-shock trousers. *Amer J Emerg Med* 1:7, 1983.

Lilja GP, Long RS, Ruiz E. Augmentation of systolic blood pressure during external cardiac compression by the use of the MAST suit. *Ann Emerg Med* 10:182, 1981.

Lilja GP et al. MAST usage in cardiopulmonary resuscitation. *Ann Emerg Med* 13:833, 1984.

Ludewig RM, Wangensteen SL. Effect of external counterpressure on venous bleeding. *Surgery* 65:515, 1969.

Mahoney BD, Mirick MJ. Efficacy of pneumatic trousers in refractory prehospital cardiopulmonary arrest. *Ann Emerg Med* 12:8, 1983.

Mannering D et al. Application of the medical anti-shock trouser (MAST) increases cardiac output and tissue perfusion in simulated, mild hypovolaemia. *Intens Care Med* 12:143, 1986.

Mattox K. Blind faith, poor judgment, and patient jeopardy. *Prehosp Disaster Med* 4:39, 1989.

Mattox K et al. Prospective randomized evaluation of antishock MAST in post-traumatic hypotension. *J Trauma* 26:779, 1986.

McBride G. One caution in pneumatic anti-shock garment use. *JAMA* 247:112, 1982.

McCabe JB, Seidel DR, Jagger JA. Antishock trouser inflation and pulmonary vital capacity. *Ann Emerg Med* 12:290, 1983.

McSwain NE. Pneumatic anti-shock garment: Does it work? *Prehosp Disaster Med* 4:42, 1989.

McSwain NE. Pneumatic anti-shock garment: State of the art 1988. *Ann Emerg Med* 17:506, 1988.

Niemann JT et al. Hemodynamic effects of pneumatic external counterpressure in canine hemorrhagic shock. *Ann Emerg Med* 12:661, 1983.

Oertel T, Loehr M. Bee-sting anaphylaxis: The use of medical antishock trousers. *Ann Emerg Med* 13:459, 1984.

Palafox BA et al. ICP changes following application of the MAST suit. *J Trauma* 21:55, 1981.

Pepe P, Bass R, Mattox K. Clinical trials of the pneumatic antishock garment in the urban prehospital setting. *Ann Emerg Med* 15:1407, 1986.

Ransom KJ, McSwain NE. Physiologic changes of antishock trousers in relationship to external pressure. *Surg Gynecol Obstet* 158:488, 1984.

Rockwell DD et al. An improved design of the pneumatic counter pressure trousers. *Am J Surg* 143:377, 1982.

Sanders AB, Meislin HW. Alterations in MAST suit pressure with changes in ambient temperature. *J Emerg Med* 1:37, 1983.

Sanders AB, Meislin HW. Effect of altitude change on MAST suit pressure. *Ann Emerg Med* 12:140, 1983.

Savino J et al. Overinflation of pneumatic antishock garments in the elderly. *Am J Surg* 155:572, 1988.

Wangensteen SL et al. The effect of external counterpressure on arterial bleeding. *Surgery* 64:922, 1968.

Wayne, MA MacDonald SC. Clinical evaluation of the antishock trouser: Prospective study of low-pressure inflation. *Ann Emerg Med* 12:285, 1983.

Wayne, MA MacDonald SC. Clinical evaluation of the antishock trouser: Retrospective analysis of five years of experience. *Ann Emerg Med* 12:342, 1983.

Williams TM, Knopp R, Ellyson JH. Compartment syndrome after antishock trouser use without lower extremity trauma. *J Trauma* 22:595, 1982.

INTRAVENOUS THERAPY

Jones S, Nesper T, Alcouloumre E. Prehospital intravenous line placement: A prospective study. *Ann Emerg Med* 18:244, 1989.

Lawrence DW et al. Complications from IV therapy: Results from field-started and emergency department-started IVs compared. *Ann Emerg Med* 17:314, 1988.

Lawrence DM. Prehospital IV therapy: Are we contributing to patient complications? *JEMS* 15(1):51, 1990.

Lewis FR. Controversy: Prehospital fluid administration. Ineffective therapy and delayed transport. *Prehosp Disaster Med* 4:129, 1989.

O'Gorman M, Trabulsy P, Pilcher D. Zero-time prehospital IV. *J Trauma*, 29:84, 1989.

Pons PT et al. Prehospital venous access in an urban paramedic system: Prospective on-scene analysis. *J Trauma* 28:1460, 1988.

Rottman SJ. Controversy: Prehospital fluid administration. Prehospital fluid administration in trauma. *Prehosp Disaster Med* 4:127, 1989.

SKILL EVALUATION CHECKLISTS

The following pages contain checklists for correct performance of some of the skills described in this chapter. The checklists can be used as a review and as a guide for practicing the respective skills.

Performance Test
Pocket Mask

Student ____________________________ Date ______________

Instructor: Place an "X" in the Fail column beside any step that is done incorrectly, out of sequence, or omitted.

Maximum Time (sec)	Activity	Critical Performance*	Fail
10	Positioning mask	Pointed end of mask over bridge of nose	
		Rescuer at patient's vertex	
		Triple airway maneuver to clamp mask to face	
	Proper head position	Hyperextends patient's head	
	Ventilates	Blows into mask until chest rises	
		Removes mouth from mask; observes chest fall	
		Records volume of at least 500 ml/breath	
10	Addition of oxygen	Attaches tubing to O_2 cylinder	
		Attaches other end of tubing to mask	
		Sets flow rate to 10 L/min	
		Resumes ventilations through the mask	
	Interposition of ventilations	Interposes ventilation between every 5 compressions	
		No pause for ventilations	

*CPR is in progress; second student doing compressions.

Instructor ____________________________

Performance Test
Oropharyngeal Airway and Bag-Valve-Mask Ventilation

Student ______________________ Date ______________

Instructor: Place an "X" in the Fail column beside any element that is done incorrectly, out of sequence, or omitted.

Maximum Time (sec)	Activity	Critical Performance*	Fail
10	Airway selection	Measures airway against face, from lips to angle of jaw	
		Selects appropriate airway	
	Opening victim's mouth	Crossed-finger maneuver	
	Airway insertion	Tip of airway faces roof of patient's mouth	
		Rotates airway 180 degrees when halfway in	
		Tongue not pushed back into throat	
		Flange against patient's lips or teeth	
10	Positioning mask	Pointed end of mask over bridge of nose	
		Clamps mask to face with "C" clamp or palm	
		Tight seal	
	Proper head position	Hyperextends patient's head	
	Ventilation (4 times)	Squeezes bag until chest rises	
		Releases bag and observes for chest falling	
		Records volume of at least 500 ml for each breath	
10	Addition of oxygen	Attaches oxygen tubing to O_2 cylinder	
		Attaches other end of tubing to bag-valve-mask	
		Opens oxygen tank	
		Turns on flow to 10–12 L/min	
		Resumes ventilations	
	Interposition of ventilations	Interposes ventilation between every 5 compressions	
		No pause for ventilations	

*CPR is in progress; second student doing compressions.

Instructor ______________________

Performance Test
Oropharyngeal Airway and Demand Valve

Student ______________________ Date ______________

Instructor: Place an "X" in the Fail column beside any element that is done incorrectly, out of sequence, or omitted.

Maximum Time (sec)	Activity	Critical Performance[a]	Fail
10	Airway selection	Measures airway against face, from lips to angle of jaw	
		Selects appropriate airway	
	Opening victim's mouth	Crossed-finger maneuver	
	Airway insertion	Tip of airway faces roof of patient's mouth	
		Rotates airway 180 degrees when halfway in	
		Tongue not pushed back into throat	
		Flange against patient's lips or teeth	
10	Opening oxygen tank	Face and body not over pressure regulator	
		Regulator fully pressurized	
	Positioning mask	Pointed end of mask over bridge of nose	
		Mask clamped over face correctly	
		Tight seal	
	Proper head position	Hyperextends patient's head	
	Ventilation (4 times)	Depresses button until chest rises[b]	
		Releases button and observes for chest falling	
		Records volume of at least 1,000 ml for each breath	
	Interposition of ventilations	Interposes ventilation between every 5 compressions	
		No pause for ventilations	

[a]CPR is in progress; second student doing compressions.
[b]Care must be taken when using a demand valve unit with a manikin, lest the lungs of the manikin be blown out. Depress button on demand valve only until gauge or signal light indicates adequate inflation.

Instructor ______________________

Performance Test
Suctioning the Mouth and Pharynx

Student ______________________________ Date ________________

Instructor: Place an "X" in the Fail column beside any element that is done incorrectly, out of sequence, or omitted.

Maximum Time (sec)	Activity	Critical Performance*	Fail
	Preoxygenation	Patient given oxygen while student prepares equipment	
		Oxygen administered for at least 3 min before suction	
	Equipment assembly	Checks that collection bottle is screwed tight	
		Connects collection tubing to suction	
		Connects catheter or suction tip to collection tubing	
		Turns on suction unit	
	Equipment check	Kinks collection tubing to block flow	
		Checks that pressure gauge reaches 300 mm Hg	
		Unkinks tubing	
		Places catheter tip in rinse water and flushes through	
	Catheter measurement	Measures off catheter from patient's mouth to ear lobe	
	Opening victim's mouth	Removes oxygen mask from patient's face	
		Turns patient's head to side	
		Crossed-finger maneuver to open mouth	
		Uses fingers of other hand to sweep mouth of debris	
	Catheter insertion	Suction OFF (Y tube open) during insertion	
		Inserts catheter correct distance	
		If tonsil suction, inserts convex side up	
15	Suction	Occludes Y tube	
		Moves catheter tip around	
		Pulls catheter tip back into mouth	
		Suctions mouth	
	Catheter removal	Suction OFF (Y tube open)	
		Replaces oxygen mask on patient's face	
		Flushes system with water	

*Assume spontaneously breathing, unconscious patient.

Instructor ______________________

Performance Test
Use of an Oxygen Cylinder

Student ______________________________ Date ________________

Instructor: Place an "X" in the Fail column beside any element that is done incorrectly, out of sequence, or omitted.

Activity	Critical Performance	Fail
Proper position	Oxygen cylinder securely upright	
	Rescuer to side of cylinder; no part of body over cylinder valve	
Cracking tank	Slowly opens main cylinder valve until rush of air is audible	
	Rapidly closes main cylinder valve	
Application of pressure regulator	Checks that pressure regulator is correct one for cylinder	
	Checks for intact washer	
	Checks that humidifier bottle contains sterile water	
	Checks that humidifier bottle is tightly closed	
	Applies pressure regulator to cylinder in correct position	
	Tightens regulator securely to cylinder	
Opening cylinder	Opens main cylinder valve slowly to pressurize regulator	
	Turns cylinder valve one-half turn more	
Connection of equipment	Selects oxygen delivery device to be used	
	Connects tubing from cylinder to device	
Flow adjustment	Opens flow regulator	
	Adjusts flow to rate ordered by instructor	
Termination of O_2 therapy	Shuts flow meter to zero	
	Closes main cylinder valve	
	Opens flow meter to bleed system, until indicator is at zero	
	Closes flow meter securely	

Instructor ______________________

Performance Test
Endotracheal Intubation[a]

Student ______________________ Date ______________

Instructor: Place an "X" in the Fail column beside each item that is performed incorrectly, out of sequence, or omitted.

Maximum Time (sec)	Activity	Critical Performance[b]	Fail
	Preparation of equipment	Chooses endotracheal tube	
		Measures length against patient	
		Cuts tube to correct length	
		Inserts tight-fitting connector	
		Tests cuff; leaves syringe attached	
		Lubricates stylet	
		Inserts stylet into endotracheal tube	
		Stylet distal end not protruding	
		Bends proximal stylet over connector	
		Bends endotracheal tube to hockey-stick shape	
		Lubricates endotracheal tube	
		Assembles laryngoscope	
		Checks light for brightness, constancy	
		Leaves laryngoscope in "off" position	
		Turns on suction	
		Tests vacuum	
		Attaches tonsil-tip catheter to suction	
		Places within easy reach: Bite-block (or oropharyngeal airway)	
		Magill forceps	
		Umbilical tape	
		Hemostat	
20	Positioning the patient	Neck flexed on pillow	
		Head extended	
	Intubation	All equipment accessible at right hand	
		Grasps laryngoscope in left hand	
		Snaps blade into "on" position	
		Opens patient's jaws with right hand	
		Patient's lips spread apart	

Maximum Time (sec)	Activity	Critical Performance[b]	Fail
		Inserts blade into right corner of mouth	
		Suctions mouth/pharynx as needed	
		Advances blade to vallecula	
		Lifts mandible/head with laryngoscope	
		Blade not touching teeth	
		Visualizes vocal cords	
		Passes tip of endotracheal tube through cords under direct vision	
		Removes laryngoscope from patient's mouth	
		Removes stylet from endotracheal tube	
		One hand stabilizing tube at all times	
		Attaches bag-valve to endotracheal tube	
		Ventilating, inflates cuff until no leak	
	Testing position	Instructs assistant to listen to six areas on chest during ventilations	
		Watches for rise and fall of chest	
		Palpates sternal notch for cuff	
	Securing tube	Asks assistant to ventilate and hold tube	
		Inserts bite-block (or oropharyngeal airway)	
		Marks endotracheal tube where it emerges from mouth	
		Ties tube/bite-block securely in place	
		Resumes ventilations, holding tube with one hand to stabilize it	

[a]EMT-Intermediates only.
[b]It is assumed that someone else is ventilating the patient (or manikin) while the student prepares for intubation.

Instructor ______________________________

Performance Test
Esophageal Obturator Airway[a]

Student ______________________________ Date ______________

Instructor: Place an "X" in the Fail column beside any element that is performed incorrectly, out of sequence, or omitted.

Maximum Time (sec)	Activity	Critical Performance[b]	Fail
	Preparation of equipment	Checks to see there is a mask, obturator, and syringe	
		Inflates cuff of mask until firm	
		Inflates cuff of obturator to check for leaks	
		Deflates cuff of obturator and leaves syringe attached	
		Snaps obturator into mask	
		Lubricates obturator	
12	Obturator insertion	Moves to patient's head	
		Tells rescuer doing CPR, "Ready."	
		Tilts patient's head slightly forward	
		Uses thumb and forefinger to pull jaw forward	
		Does not hyperextend neck	
		Slowly advances obturator until mask is flush with face	
10	Testing position	Performs triple airway maneuver from vertex; mask tight	
		Takes deep breath	
		Exhales into mask	
		Observes to see if chest rises	
		Records volume of at least 1,000 ml for each breath	
5	Cuff inflation	Inflates cuff with 20–30 ml of air	
		Detaches syringe	
		Resumes ventilations	
	Interposition of ventilations	Interposes ventilation between every 5 compressions	
		No pause for ventilation	
		Adequate volumes (at least 1,000 ml)	
	Use of adjunct	Attaches bag-valve with O_2 to EOA	
		Interposes ventilation between every 5 compressions	
		No pause for ventilations	
	EOA removal	Instructor says, "The patient is breathing spontaneously." Assembles and tests suction (tonsil tip)	
		Turns patient's head to side	
		Snaps mask off obturator	
		Deflates cuff	
		Smoothly withdraws obturator, with suction in other hand	
		Suctions pharynx and mouth	
		Places oxygen mask or cannula on patient	

[a]For EMT-Intermediates only.
[b]CPR is in progress; second student doing compressions.

Instructor ______________________

Performance Test
Military Anti-Shock Trousers (MAST)

Students ______________________________ Date ______________

____

____

____

Instructor: Place an "X" in the Fail column beside each item that is performed incorrectly, out of sequence, or omitted.

Maximum Time (sec)	Activity	Critical Performance	Fail
	Positioning MAST	MAST unfolded on long backboard, right side up	
		Backboard lined up beside patient; top edge of MAST level with patient's lowest ribs	
	Positioning the patient	3 rescuers roll patient to side, facing away from board	
		Head and neck kept in alignment with trunk	
		One rescuer slides backboard under patient	
		Other rescuers roll patient back supine; head and neck kept in alignment with trunk	
60	Fastening MAST	Left leg snugly wrapped and secured with velcro fasteners	
		Right leg snugly wrapped and secured with velcro fasteners	
		Abdomen snugly wrapped and secured with velcro fasteners	
	Inflation of MAST	Tubing attached to each compartment	
		Stopcocks opened	
		MAST inflated with foot pump	
		Stopcocks shut	

Instructor ______________________

Performance Test
Defibrillation*

Student ______________________ Date ______________

Instructor: Place an "X" in the Fail column beside any item that is performed incorrectly, out of sequence, or omitted.

Maximum Time (sec)	Activity	Critical Performance	Fail
	CPR and oxygen therapy	Assistant starts CPR	
		Brings assistant pocket mask with oxygen	
	Preparation of defibrillator	Turns synchronize switch OFF	
		Turns main switch ON	
		Turns monitor switch ON	
		Sets energy level to 200–300 joules	
		Charges paddles	
		Lubricates paddles	
15–20	Checking rhythm	Informs assistant, "Ready."	
		Positions paddles correctly on patient's chest	
		No bridging by saline or electrode jelly	
		Holds firm pressure on paddles	
		Checks rhythm on monitor	
	Defibrillation	Instructor says, "Rhythm is VF." Shouts, "Everybody off!"	
		Checks that no one is touching patient or stretcher	
		Depresses buttons on paddles simultaneously	
	Checking result	Leaves paddles in position	
		Checks rhythm on monitor (instructor says, "Regular rhythm.")	
		Checks pulse (instructor says, "No pulse.")	
	CPR	Assistant resumes CPR for at least 1 min	
15–20	Repeat attempt	Repeats rhythm check, defibrillation, pulse check Instructor says, "Pulse present."	
	Preparation to transport	Assistant continues artificial ventilation	
		Hooks up monitor leads	

*For EMT-Intermediates working under physician control in a system where defibrillation by EMTs is authorized.

Instructor ______________________

Performance Test
Intravenous Therapy[a]

Student ______________________________ Date ______________

Instructor: Place an "X" in the Fail column beside any item that is performed incorrectly, out of sequence, or omitted.

Activity	Critical Performance[b]	Fail
Explaining procedure	Explains need for IV to patient	
	Explains what procedure involves	
	Obtains consent	
Assembling equipment	Checks IV fluid bag for cloudiness, leaks, date of expiration	
	Attaches infusion set with sterile technique	
	Fills drip chamber halfway	
	Flushes tubing through	
	Closes clamp and covers tip of tubing	
	Selects IV cannula	
	Assembles in a convenient place: Antiseptic swabs	
	Antiseptic ointment	
	Sterile dressing	
	Strips of adhesive tape	
	Tourniquet	
	Pen and label	
	Armboard and roller bandage	
Selecting vein	Lets arm hang dependent	
	Secures tourniquet (radial pulse not obliterated)	
	Selects straight vein on forearm (not over joint)	
Disinfecting the skin	Uses povidine-iodine swabs to clean skin	
	Cleans in widening circles around the puncture site	
	Final wipe with alcohol swab	
IV insertion	Stabilizes vein	
	Inserts needle through skin	
	Advances needle into vein (blood return seen)	
	Slides catheter over needle into vein; does not pull catheter back	
	Withdraws needle from catheter	
	Releases tourniquet	
Attachment of tubing	Holds catheter steady	
	Attaches IV tubing with sterile technique	
	Opens flow control clamp wide to test catheter position	
Securing catheter	Places antiseptic ointment on puncture site	
	Covers puncture site with sterile dressing	
	Secures dressing and catheter in place	
Adjustment of flow rate	Instructor orders flow rate in ml/min Adjusts flow rate to correct drops/min	

[a]For EMT-Intermediates only.
[b]Second student serves as patient.

Instructor ______________________

IV. THE SECONDARY SURVEY

Up to this point we have considered only the ***primary survey****, that is, the initial assessment of the patient to determine whether there is any immediate threat to life and the initial steps to correct any life-threatening conditions detected. We have seen that for a conscious, alert patient, the primary survey may be conducted at a glance, while for an unconscious patient, one must proceed systematically through the ABCs, treating each problem as it is encountered.*

Once the primary survey has been completed—whether it was accomplished at a glance or after several therapeutic steps—the EMT can move on to the ***secondary survey****, the purpose of which is to detect those problems that do not pose an immediate threat to life but that can become more serious or even life-threatening if they are not promptly managed. Such problems may be medical, such as chest pain, or due to injury, such as an open fracture of the leg. In either case, the EMT must discover these problems and initiate treatment in order to prevent the condition of the patient from deteriorating.*

The secondary survey consists of two parts: information gathering and physical assessment. In the INFORMATION-GATHERING PHASE, one seeks to determine the nature of the patient's problem by asking questions of the patient and witnesses and by noting the surroundings. If the patient was injured, when and how did it happen? Where does it hurt? If the patient has a medical problem, what precisely is bothering him? When did it start? And so forth. The PHASE OF PHYSICAL ASSESSMENT is a rapid but complete, hands-on evaluation of the patient to determine vital signs and detect injuries or signs of illness. Unlike the primary survey, in which no special equipment is needed, the secondary survey requires the use of several diagnostic aids, such as a stethoscope, blood pressure cuff, and flashlight.

Steps in Patient Assessment

1. PRIMARY SURVEY: To detect and correct immediately life-threatening problems
   a. Airway
   b. Breathing
   c. Circulation
      (1) Pulse
      (2) Profuse bleeding
2. SECONDARY SURVEY: To detect problems that do not pose an immediate threat to life but that can become more serious or life-threatening if not treated
   a. Medical history
   b. Physical assessment

In practice, the information-gathering phase of the secondary survey may be performed together with the physical assessment or even after some treatment has begun, depending on the circumstances. For instance, if the patient is a middle-aged man with chest pain, the first step the EMT should take is to administer oxygen (treatment). Then the EMT will want to keep a finger on the patient's pulse (physical assessment), while asking questions about the patient's symptoms (information gathering). For purposes of discussion, we shall present the secondary survey in the traditional sequence: information gathering (history taking) first, physical assessment next. In the field, however, this sequence may have to be altered.

We will conclude this section with a chapter on reporting medical information. The EMT has access to a great deal of information that might otherwise be unavailable to the medical personnel at the hospital, such as the condition of an accident scene, the condition of the patient when first observed, and so forth. Such information can be of enormous value to the emergency room physician, but it can be useful only if it is reported accurately and systematically. Thus we will learn the standard format for reporting the findings of the patient survey and the information necessary for a complete medical record.

10. OBTAINING THE MEDICAL HISTORY

OBJECTIVES

The initial phase of the secondary survey is the phase of information gathering, or obtaining the medical history: What happened to the patient that turned his everyday existence into an emergency? In the phase of gathering information, the EMT becomes a detective—scrutinizing the scene and questioning witnesses in a search for clues that will help define the patient's problem. By the end of this chapter, the reader should be able to

1. List three potential sources of information about what happened to a patient
2. List the kinds of information that can be obtained from observations of the scene
3. Indicate where medical identification materials should be sought and what kind of information they can provide
4. Identify questions about the patient's medical history that are improperly phrased, given a list of questions
5. List the preliminary steps that should be taken before eliciting the history from a conscious patient
6. Define the chief complaint
7. Differentiate between signs and symptoms, given a list that contains both signs and symptoms
8. List the kind of questions one asks to gain more information about the patient's chief complaint, given an example of a chief complaint
9. List the kinds of information one needs to obtain in the field regarding the patient's past medical history
10. Identify the chief complaint, elements of the present illness, and elements of the past medical history, given the medical history of a patient.

PURPOSE OF TAKING THE MEDICAL HISTORY

What exactly are we trying to find out when we start looking around and asking questions? To begin with, we want to know WHAT HAPPENED to the patient. If he has been injured, how did the injury occur? What parts of his body were affected? How badly does it hurt? If he is ill, when did it all start? What is bothering him? In addition, it is useful to know what OTHER PROBLEMS the patient has that might have some bearing on his present condition or on the treatment he will need. For instance, an asthmatic is likely to have a much more severe reaction to smoke inhalation than a person with normal lungs, so it is important to know, when dealing with someone rescued from a fire, whether that person has any preexisting respiratory problems. Finally, in our information gathering, we would like to obtain PERTINENT DATA NOT OTHERWISE AVAILABLE TO THE HOSPITAL PERSONNEL. The EMT has a unique opportunity to learn a great deal about the patient and his problem. An unconscious patient simply left at the doorstep of a hospital presents a complete mystery to the medical staff. But if the EMT brings in the unconscious patient and also brings three empty medication bottles found by the patient's side, the emergency room doctor already has a valuable lead in treating the patient. Similarly, the unconscious victim of an automobile accident presents an unknown collection of injuries to the emergency room staff. But if the EMT can report that the steering column of the patient's car was bent, the doctors immediately know they must be extra alert for chest injury. Thus the EMT gives the doctor an extra set of eyes and ears, and the additional information the EMT can provide may literally save a patient's life.

SOURCES OF INFORMATION

Like any good detective, the EMT may have to get information from several sources. The most obvious source is THE PATIENT; and in most cases where the patient is conscious, he or she will serve as the principal source of information, for no one is better qualified than the patient to tell you where it hurts. Furthermore, questioning the patient directly establishes the fact that he or she is the center of your attention, which helps create an atmosphere of confidence and trust. It is very irritating to any person—sick or well—to be talked about as if he were not there ("When did he start having pain?"), for it makes a person feel as if his opinions are not considered significant. Thus, whenever possible, you should question the patient directly; his information is usually the most accurate, and he needs to feel that you respect him and his ability to tell you what is wrong.

> THE PATIENT IS THE MOST IMPORTANT PERSON AT THE SCENE OF AN EMERGENCY.

There may be circumstances, however, in which the patient cannot give you any information or his information is of unknown reliability. The most obvious example is an *unconscious patient* who, by definition, cannot communicate at all. But even some conscious patients can present difficulties in responding to questions. A *very small child*, especially one who cannot yet talk, is unlikely to be able to provide much information. Similarly, a person who is very *confused or disturbed* may be unable to give reliable answers. Some patients, such as those with chest pain, may minimize their symptoms or neglect to mention certain symptoms in an attempt to deny to themselves that they may be suffering a serious illness. A patient with a *stroke* may have his speech impaired to such a degree that he cannot understand your words or cannot formulate words with which to answer your questions. In all of these instances, it is very helpful to try to obtain information from BYSTANDERS—friends, family, or anyone else who may have witnessed what happened to the patient. Bystanders can provide valuable information about how an accident happened or when a patient collapsed. Bystanders trained in first aid may already have started treatment, and they can tell you what they did and how the patient responded. Family members or friends may be able to provide important details about the patient's other medical conditions—for example, that the patient had three heart attacks in the past or suffers from diabetes. Sometimes they can also fill in parts of the story that the patient omitted. Our hypothetical man with chest pain, for instance, may tell you he "just had a little indigestion—it was nothing," while his wife informs you that her husband was up all night with the pain and "looked pale as a ghost."

It should be emphasized that bystanders represent a *secondary* source of information. If the patient is conscious, you should always try to talk first with the patient himself, even if he appears confused or uncommunicative. The disturbed patient may calm down considerably if you address him in an assured, respectful manner. A child who has reached the age of speaking may be able to tell you a great deal about where and how it hurts. Even a person who has been robbed of speech by a stroke may be able to nod or shake his head in response to specific questions. So always start your interviewing with the patient, and use bystanders to help fill in missing information. On some occasions, it may be useful for one EMT to talk with the patient while his or her partner interviews a family member or bystander in another room. But in any case, remember:

> NEVER ASSUME THAT IT IS IMPOSSIBLE TO TALK WITH A PATIENT UNTIL YOU HAVE TRIED.

Besides the patient and bystanders, there is a third very valuable source of information, and that is THE SCENE ITSELF (Fig. 10-1). The place where the patient is found—whether the patient is the victim of an accident or suffering from a medical condition—can provide valuable clues to the nature of the patient's problem. Take the unconscious victim of an automobile accident, for example. He cannot tell you anything about what happened, but a keen observer may be able to piece together a lot of the story just by looking around. Are there skid marks on the road

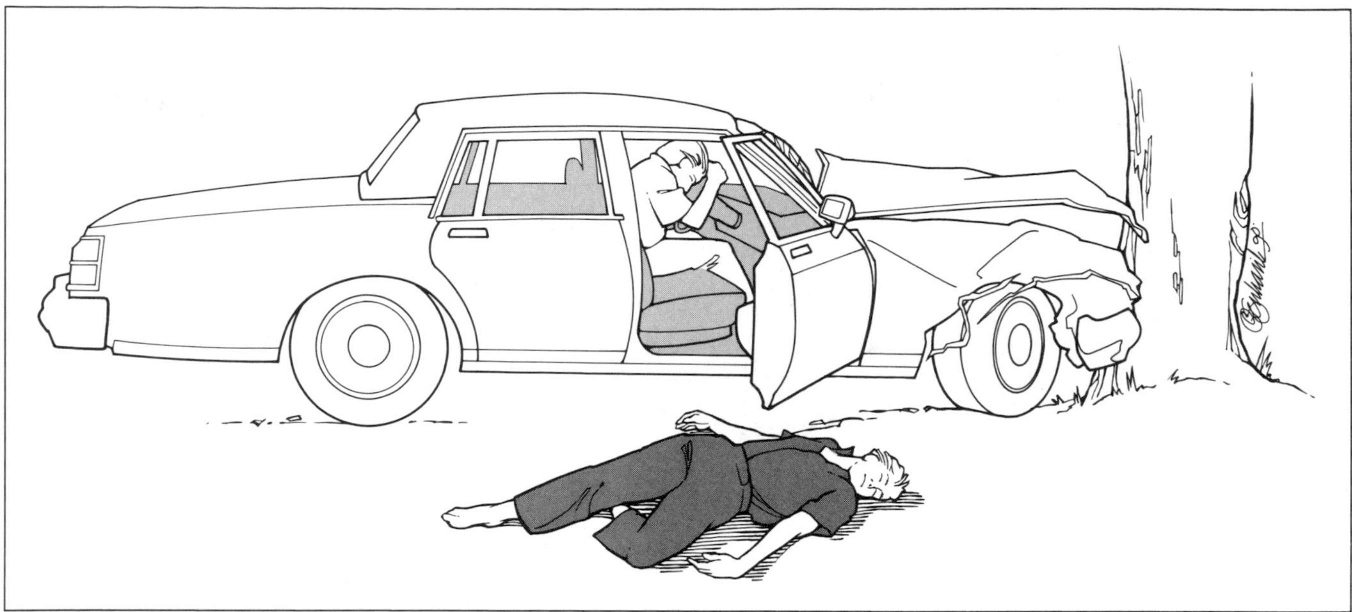

Fig. 10-1. *Mechanisms of injury. Observe the accident scene for clues to the nature of the victims' injuries.*

that suggest the victim had to apply the brakes suddenly? Or is there no apparent reason for the accident, suggesting that it may have been a medical problem, such as a blackout, that caused the victim to lose control of the car. And what about the condition of the car? A smashed windshield suggests a severe blow to the head and alerts you to the possibility of scalp or facial lacerations or even a fractured skull. A bent steering column or broken steering wheel tells you that the victim was hurled forward with considerable force against the wheel and points to the possibility of serious chest injury. A fastened lap belt may have produced abdominal trauma, while a shoulder harness could have caused a fractured clavicle if the patient was hurled forward against it. All of these observations point to the **mechanisms of injury**, that is, the way in which the injury took place. And the more one knows about *how the injury occurred*—and the forces involved—the more accurately one can predict the types of injury sustained.

The accident scene can also provide clues to the *seriousness* of the injury. A large pool of blood around the patient, for example, immediately suggests the possibility of hemorrhagic shock, and you should try to form an estimate of the amount of blood involved. Is it just a few teaspoons? A cup? A quart? Such information can be helpful to the emergency room physician in estimating the patient's need for transfusion. In addition, the place where you find the patient can be informative. Is he still in the car, suggesting that he lost consciousness around the time of the accident? Or is he 300 feet down the road, suggesting that he was conscious immediately after the accident and only lost consciousness later, after wandering out of the car? Information of this sort can help the neurosurgeon decide whether to rush the patient to the operating room or whether there is time to wait and watch the patient's condition.

Thus the scene of an accident has much to tell about the mechanisms of injury and the potential seriousness of the patient's problem. But what about the scene in which an unconscious patient with a *medical* problem is found? What clues can you detect there? Once again, a keen observer can learn a great deal from looking around. Are there empty bottles of sleeping pills, suggesting a drug overdose? Is there an improperly vented space heater that could have caused carbon monoxide poisoning? Is there a smell of gas? Are there medications by the patient's bedside or in the bathroom medicine cabinet that give clues to illnesses for which he is receiving treatment? Is a doctor's name printed on the medication bottle? Are there any cards in the patient's purse or wallet that indicate regular attendance at a certain clinic?

With regard to the last question, it is important to note that you should be circumspect about going through someone's belongings, since bystanders may misinterpret your intentions. Wherever possible, it is preferable to search a patient's purse or wallet in the presence of a police officer or some other reliable witness, so that there can be no accusations of theft afterward.

A fourth valuable source of information about the patient is a MEDICAL IDENTIFICATION DEVICE. One of the most commonly used of these in the United States is the MEDIC ALERT TAG (Fig. 10-2) that is worn as a necklace, bracelet, or anklet. The tag is engraved on the front with the caduceus (the snake

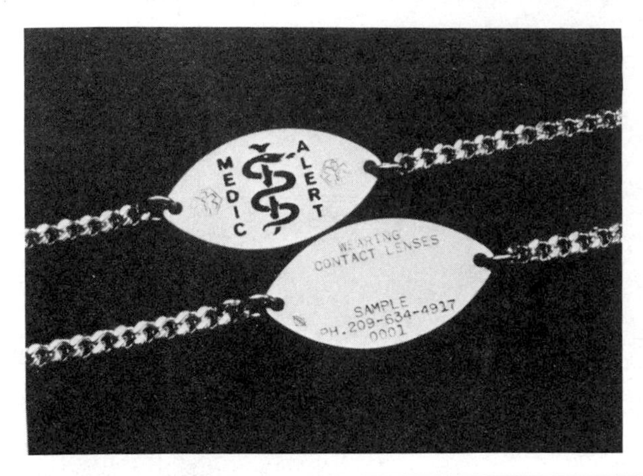

Fig. 10-2. *Medic Alert bracelet. (Reproduced courtesy Medic Alert Foundation, Turlock, California.)*

and staff, which is the symbol of the medical profession) and the words "Medic Alert." On the back of the tag is engraved a brief statement of the patient's chief medical problem (e.g., "epileptic" or "allergic to penicillin"), together with the patient's membership number and the Medic Alert telephone number. A similar bracelet, which is somewhat more common in Europe than in the United States, is issued by an organization called SOS. The SOS BRACELET has a small compartment that can be unscrewed, and inside is a long strip of paper containing information about the wearer's identity, medical problems, immunizations, whom to notify in an emergency, and so forth. In addition to medical identification devices that are worn as jewelry on the patient's body, there are others that are carried in the wallet or even stored in the home. The VIAL OF LIFE, for example, is a small cylinder containing information about the patient and is usually kept in the refrigerator, with a label on the refrigerator door to indicate that the Vial of Life is inside.

If you should find a Medic Alert tag on an unconscious person, it is a good idea to radio the wearer's membership number and the Medic Alert telephone number to the hospital to which you will be transporting the patient, so that they can start getting the detailed information about the patient from Medic Alert's answering service while you are en route. If you have no way of contacting the hospital directly, radio your dispatchers and have them relay the information to the hospital or call Medic Alert themselves. You should not call Medic Alert yourself, since your primary responsibility at the scene is to care for the patient, and you cannot afford to delay treatment by engaging in a lengthy phone conversation, especially if the patient is unconscious.

Sources of Information

- The PATIENT
- OTHERS: Bystanders, friends, family members
- The SCENE:
  1. Mechanisms of injury
  2. Clues to the patient's underlying illness(es)
- MEDICAL IDENTIFICATION DEVICES

TAKING THE MEDICAL HISTORY IN THE FIELD

Eliciting information about the patient from the report of the patient himself or from others is called taking the medical history. The "history" may be very recent, for instance a twisted ankle suffered 5 minutes before you arrived, but it may also include information about the patient's past medical problems that have possible relevance to the patient's present condition. The medical history one elicits in the field is much more abbreviated than the medical history a doctor would take in his office in the course of a routine examination, for its purpose is a very limited one: to identify the patient's immediate problems and any other factors that may have a bearing on those problems. Thus one does not, for example, go into a lengthy inquiry about past illnesses in the patient's family or the case of measles the patient had 30 years ago, for such information is unlikely to be useful in defining or treating the patient's current, urgent condition. Interviewing in the field under emergency conditions must be as efficient as possible and thus requires the use of direct questions. Nonetheless, the questions should not be phrased in such a way that they put words into the patient's mouth. In particular, one should avoid asking questions that can be answered with a "yes" or "no." For instance, it is better to ask, "What makes the pain worse?" than to suggest an answer to the patient by asking, "Does the pain get worse when you climb up the stairs?" To direct the questions, you can provide the patient with alternatives, for example, "Does the pain come and go, or is it there all the time?"

AVOID ASKING QUESTIONS THAT CAN BE ANSWERED WITH A "YES" OR "NO."

If circumstances are such that you must question the patient at the same time you are examining him, it is a good practice to ask your questions about a given part of the body *before* you examine it, for otherwise the patient is likely to get the impression that you have found something terribly wrong, and this creates needless anxiety. For instance, if you listen to a patient's chest and then pipe up, "Tell me, sir, have you ever had a heart attack?" the patient is liable to conclude that in your examination of his chest you found some telltale sign of heart disease.

The information one elicits in the field consists of three components: (1) the chief complaint, (2) the history of the present illness, and (3) the past medical history.

THE CHIEF COMPLAINT

The chief complaint (CC) is the problem that prompted the patient or bystanders to call for help. In the case of an accident victim, the chief complaint may seem obvious without asking, as for example when you find the patient lying on the street bleeding after having been struck by an automobile. Even in such situations, however, it is worthwhile finding out what is bothering the *patient*, for *his* chief complaint may lead to unexpected findings. Our accident victim, for instance, may have a very dramatic laceration of the leg, but his chief complaint may be "I can't breathe"—leading you to discover an unsuspected chest injury much more dangerous than the leg laceration. The chief complaint is elicited by asking the patient, "What seems to be the trouble?" or, if there is an obvious injury, "What is bothering you the most?" The chief complaint is usually stated in a word or phrase, preferably in the patient's own words, such as "difficulty breathing" or "squeezing in my chest" or "twisted ankle." Some patients may have a whole catalogue of complaints, and in such cases it is useful to ask, "Which of those things is bothering you the most?" in order to define the *chief* complaint.

It is very helpful if the dispatcher can elicit the chief complaint on the telephone when the patient or bystander calls for the ambulance, for this information enables the rescue team to plan while en route to the scene what equipment they will need to take with them from the vehicle. If the chief complaint given to the dispatcher is "chest pain" or "shortness of breath," for example, the rescue team knows in advance that they should take a portable oxygen unit with them when they leave the vehicle to seek out the patient. Similarly, if the chief complaint is "I'm having a baby," the EMTs know they will need the obstetric kit and they can leave the traction splint in the ambulance. Knowing the chief complaint in advance also enables the EMTs to anticipate what backup units may be required, such as police for a shooting victim or an engine company when the emergency involves a fire.

Whatever the chief complaint given to the dispatcher, the EMT will want to ascertain firsthand what is bothering the patient. If the patient is not in critical condition, a few preliminaries are necessary for purposes of establishing a good relationship with the patient and recording some basic identifying information. First of all, you need to INTRODUCE YOURSELF and indicate what organization you represent; for instance, "I'm Tom Trueheart. I'm an EMT with the Doonsburgh Fire Department, and I understand you need some help." After the patient has acknowledged your presence, you will want to learn his or her NAME AND AGE, and once you have elicited this information, you should address the patient by name thereafter. For a patient over 18 years of age, this means "Mr. Smith," "Mrs. Smith," or "Miss Smith"—*not* "Tom," "Sadie," or "Mary." Unless you are considerably older than the patient, the use of the patient's first name implies disrespect, so stick to formal terms of address for adults.

It is a good idea to initiate some form of physical contact with the patient as soon as possible after your arrival. This can consist simply of placing your hand on the patient's arm or holding your fingers over the pulse, but even this minimal contact can in itself give considerable reassurance to someone who is anxious or in pain.

Meanwhile, one elicits the chief complaint, and from this initial brief statement of the patient's main problem, one proceeds to develop a line of questioning to learn more about the chief complaint: when, where, how, how much, and so forth. This amplification of the chief complaint is called the history of the present illness.

HISTORY OF THE PRESENT ILLNESS

The "present illness" may be a medical problem (e.g., heart attack) or an injury (e.g., broken leg), but in either case, one needs to learn more about how it occurred and what it feels like. In performing this part of the secondary survey, it is important to know the distinction between symptoms and signs. A *symptom* is something the PATIENT FEELS and that therefore only he can tell you about—for instance, pain, nausea, dizziness, weakness. A *sign* is something YOU CAN SEE, whether the patient tells you about it or not—such as bleeding, a bruise, cyanosis, dilated pupils. When you take a medical *history*, you are gathering information about symptoms—the things the patient has felt. Signs are discovered only when you do the *physical assessment*.

The kind of information that makes up the history of the present illness (HPI) includes the following:

- LOCATION: *Where* in the body is the problem? If the problem is pain, is it in one place only? Does it radiate to any other place?
- QUALITY: If the problem is pain, *what is it like*? Dull? Sharp? Throbbing? Steady? Intermittent?
- INTENSITY: *How bad* is the problem? If the patient's complaint is shortness of breath, for in-

stance, is it so bad he can barely talk to you, or is it just noticeable when he has walked up a flight of stairs? If the problem is pain, how severe is it?
- QUANTITY: How many? How often? How much? How big?
- CHRONOLOGY: If the chief complaint relates to an injury, *when* did the injury occur? If the problem is a medical one, *when* did it start? *How long* has it been going on? If there is more than one symptom, which one came first?
- SETTING: In trauma, one wants to know *how* the injury took place. What exactly occurred? Were there any medical problems that contributed to the injury (e.g., a fainting spell in which someone fell down a flight of stairs). If the problem is a medical one, under what circumstances did the symptoms occur (e.g., dyspnea that woke the patient from sleep versus dyspnea after running to catch a bus).
- AGGRAVATION AND ALLEVIATION: Does anything make the symptom worse? Does anything make it better? Has the patient done anything or taken anything to try to relieve the symptoms? If so, did it help?
- ASSOCIATED COMPLAINTS: Are there any other *related symptoms*? Has the patient noted any other abnormal feelings or changes in body function in association with this illness or injury?

In order to illustrate these categories of information, let us look at a middle-aged man with a fairly classic story of a heart attack. The history of this man's present illness might be as follows:

CHIEF COMPLAINT: Chest pain.
- LOCATION: Retrosternal, radiating into the left arm.
- QUALITY: "Squeezing."
- INTENSITY: Very severe; patient feels as if he is being "choked in the chest."
- QUANTITY: The patient had just this one attack of pain. He has never had pain like it before.
- CHRONOLOGY: The present attack of chest pain started about an hour ago and has not let up since.
- SETTING: The patient was changing the tire on his car when the pain came on.
- AGGRAVATION AND ALLEVIATION: The patient took some antacid and lay down after he got the pain, but it did not help. Nothing seems to relieve the pain; neither does anything make it worse.
- ASSOCIATED COMPLAINTS: The patient feels very weak and somewhat sick to his stomach.

Now let us consider a victim of trauma, a 52-year-old farmer who was injured when he fell off a ladder.

CHIEF COMPLAINT: "I fell off a ladder and hurt my leg."
- LOCATION: Mid-thigh of right leg.
- QUALITY: Throbbing pain.
- INTENSITY: Severe.
- QUANTITY: Pain is limited to the right leg.
- CHRONOLOGY: The patient felt dizzy and lost his balance, then fell off the ladder.
- SETTING: The patient was picking apples, and he turned to reach some apples behind him.
- AGGRAVATION AND ALLEVIATION: The leg feels better if he keeps it still, but the moment he tries to move it, the pain gets more severe.
- ASSOCIATED COMPLAINTS: The patient has some pins-and-needles sensations in his right foot.

Thus by asking relatively few questions, we have been able to form a clear picture of what happened to each of our two patients. As we learn more about specific illnesses and injuries, we will learn other questions that can be asked to clarify a given problem. For example, we would want to ask our patient with chest pain whether he has had any difficulty breathing, dizziness, or sweating, for these symptoms sometimes go along with a heart attack. But even without knowing anything about specific diseases, we can learn a great deal about the patient's problem just by obtaining the details mentioned above.

History of the Present Illness
- Location: WHERE is the pain or discomfort?
- Quality: WHAT IS THE PAIN LIKE?
- Intensity: HOW BAD is it?
- Quantity: HOW MANY times? HOW BIG an injury?
- Chronology: WHEN did it occur?
- Setting: WHERE did it occur? WHAT happened? HOW did it happen? What was the patient doing when it happened?
- Aggravation and alleviation: What makes the symptom WORSE? What makes it BETTER?
- Associated complaints: WHAT ELSE is the patient experiencing?

PAST MEDICAL HISTORY

After we have completed our inquiry into the patient's present problem, we want to obtain *pertinent* information about his past medical history (PMH) and other medical problems. The word *pertinent* is stressed, for there is no time in the field to ask a lot of questions about the patient's childhood illnesses or the wart he had removed from his toe 10 years ago. Nor would such information be useful to us even if we did have the time to elicit it. In emergency care, the purpose of asking about the past medical history is to find out if the patient has any other problems that may relate to his present problem or the treatment of it. For example, in a patient who suffered multiple lacerations in an accident, it is very important to know that he has a history of clotting disorders, for this will affect our ability to control his bleeding. On the other hand, it is of no use to us to know that he had chicken pox at the age of three. Similarly, in a patient with a large, contaminated wound, it is crucial to know that he is allergic to penicillin, for the doctor may want to give him an antibiotic to try to prevent infection; but it is not particularly helpful to know that he is also allergic to rhubarb.

The term "*past*" *medical history* is a bit misleading, for the category in fact includes all the patient's medical problems—past and present—that are *not* directly related to his chief complaint. Furthermore, to make matters even more confusing, those problems that the patient had in the past but that *are* related to his chief complaint are considered part of the history of the *present* illness, not part of the past medical history. For instance, if the patient's chief complaint is "vomiting blood," then the fact that he suffered from an ulcer 2 years ago would be considered part of the history of the present illness because it is probably directly related to his present symptoms. On the other hand, the fact that he is currently under treatment for high blood pressure would be considered part of the "past" medical history—even though it is not past—because it is not directly connected with the chief complaint. Probably "*other*" *medical problems* would be a better term than *past medical history*, but *past medical history* has come to be the accepted name for this category of information.

> THE HISTORY OF THE PRESENT ILLNESS INCLUDES ALL THE DETAILS ABOUT THE PATIENT'S *CHIEF COMPLAINT*. THE PAST MEDICAL HISTORY IS ABOUT *OTHER* MEDICAL PROBLEMS.

In the field, the information one needs about the patient's past medical history is as follows:

- Is the patient currently UNDER A DOCTOR'S CARE for any medical condition(s)? If so, WHAT CONDITIONS? (Ask specifically if there is any history of heart problems, lung problems, or diabetes.) What is the name of the doctor? (Radioing ahead will permit the hospital to contact the patient's doctor and learn more about the patient's medical background. It will also give the doctor time to get to the hospital, if he or she chooses to meet the patient there.)
- Has the patient ever been HOSPITALIZED for a serious medical or surgical problem? If so, when? What was the problem? At what hospital? (Where practical, it is preferable to transport a patient to a hospital where the patient has been treated before and where his medical records are on file, providing that the hospital is close enough and has the facilities to deal with the patient's current problem.)
- Is the patient taking any MEDICATIONS? What are the names of the medications? (If possible, bring the bottles with you to the hospital.) Did he take any medications *today*?
- Does the patient have any known ALLERGIES to medications?
- In trauma victims, find out when they ate their LAST MEAL, since that information will be important to the anesthesiologist if the patient must undergo surgery.

If the patient is unconscious, do not forget to check for a medical identification bracelet or necklace, which may be able to provide information about the patient's other medical problems.

> **Past Medical History**
> - OTHER MEDICAL CONDITIONS for which the patient is being treated and the name of the DOCTOR who is treating him
> - HOSPITALIZATIONS for major illness or injury, and the name of the hospital(s)
> - MEDICATIONS the patient takes regularly
> - ALLERGIES to medications
> - In trauma victims, time of LAST MEAL

THE HISTORY AS A WHOLE

Let us look at an interview between a skilled EMT and a patient to see how the elements of the history are obtained in practice. We will suppose that EMT Tom Trueheart has responded to a call for a "man down" in a shopping center. Tom and his partner arrive at the scene, grab a portable oxygen unit and a "jump kit" from the vehicle, and head for the store where the patient is said to be located. In the store, they find a man who appears to be about 70 years old sitting on the floor, looking a bit dazed, surrounded by a group of very anxious people. Tom notices that one of the bystanders is kneeling down beside the patient, and he addresses her:

TOM: What seems to have happened?

BYSTANDER: He passed out about 15 minutes ago.

TOM: How long was he out?

BYSTANDER: I'd say 10 minutes.

TOM: I'd like to examine him. Could you stay around for a few minutes so that I can ask you some more questions when I finish?

The bystander agrees, for Tom has made it clear by his attitude that he regards her information as significant. Meanwhile, Tom kneels beside the patient and takes the patient's wrist. His partner readies the oxygen and also prepares to make some notes on the history.

TOM: Hello, sir. I'm Tom Trueheart, an EMT from the Doonsburgh Fire Department. It seems you passed out, and we've come to help you out. First of all, we'd like to give you a little oxygen to breathe. Here, I'll just put this around your face, and you can feel the extra oxygen going into your nose.

The patient nods. He seems to be looking a bit more alert.

TOM: Can you tell me your name, sir?

PATIENT: Uh, James Patterson.

TOM: And how old are you, Mr. Patterson?

PATIENT: Seventy-two.

TOM: Can you remember what happened?

PATIENT: No. I just remember coming in the store to look at some shoes. That's all I remember.

TOM: How do you feel now?

PATIENT: I feel very dizzy.

TOM: Has anything like this ever happened before?

PATIENT: Yes, I passed out twice last week. It was at home both times. I didn't think much about it. I thought I had the flu or something.

TOM: This dizziness—does anything seem to make it better or worse?

PATIENT: It gets worse if I try to stand up.

TOM: Is anything else bothering you? Are you having any pain or any trouble breathing?

PATIENT: No, no pain. But I feel as if my heart is going 90 miles an hour.

TOM: Are you under a doctor's care for any problems?

PATIENT: Yes, Dr. Cassidy. He takes care of my high blood pressure.

TOM: Besides the high blood pressure, do you have any other medical problems—with your heart or lungs? Or any diabetes?

PATIENT: No. I have a cough—smoking you know. But no other problems.

TOM: Were you ever in the hospital?

PATIENT: Two years ago. I was in the hospital—Lakewood Medical Center, right down the street—for the prostate. Plumbing trouble, don't you know.

TOM: Tell me, Mr. Patterson, do you take any medicine regularly?

PATIENT: Just the blood pressure pills. And some other little white pills.

TOM: Do you know the name of the pills?

PATIENT: No, but I've got 'em right here in my pocket.

TOM: Did you take your medicines today?

PATIENT: Well, I took the blood pressure pills, but I ran out of the little white pills a few weeks ago. I keep meaning to get some more, but you know how you forget things.

TOM: Are you allergic to any medicines?

PATIENT: Not so's I know of. Only strawberries. I break out in a rash if I even see a strawberry.

While keeping his hand on the patient's wrist, Tom turns back to the bystander and asks her to fill in details about what she saw happen. Did the patient give any warning that he was going to fall? Did he strike any part of his body as he fell? Did he have a seizure? Did he stop breathing at any point? Then he turns back to the patient.

TOM: OK, Mr. Patterson, I'd like to have a quick look at you, just to make sure you didn't hurt yourself when you fell, and then I think we'd better have you checked out at the hospital.

If you read through the above dialogue out loud and clock yourself, you will find that it took only about 3 minutes to gather all of this information about Mr. Patterson. The main reason it was accomplished so quickly was that Tom had a very systematic approach to the history. He knew what kind of information he wanted, and he knew as well what order he wanted to follow in asking the questions. This systematic approach also helped Tom not to forget any of the questions he needed to ask.

The Medical History

1. CHIEF COMPLAINT	The reason the patient or bystanders called for an ambulance
2. HISTORY OF THE PRESENT ILLNESS	An elaboration of the chief complaint
3. PAST MEDICAL HISTORY	Other pertinent medical problems of the patient

As we left Tom Trueheart, he was just about to begin the physical assessment of the patient, which is precisely what we shall do in the next chapter.

VOCABULARY

chief complaint (CC) The problem that prompted the patient or bystanders to call for an ambulance.

history of the present illness (HPI) An elaboration of the chief complaint.

mechanism of injury The way in which an injury occurred and the forces involved in producing the injury.

past medical history (PMH) All of the patient's medical problems that are not directly related to his chief complaint.

secondary survey Assessment of the patient undertaken to detect problems that are not immediately life-threatening but that can become more serious or life-threatening if not treated.

sign An indication of illness or injury that the *examiner* can see, hear, feel, smell, etc.

symptom A pain, discomfort, or other abnormality in bodily function that the *patient* feels.

FURTHER READING

Caroline NL. Hidden at the scene: Clues to social emergencies. *Emerg Med Serv* 11(4):83, 1982.

11. PHYSICAL ASSESSMENT

OBJECTIVES

While we were interested in symptoms when taking the patient's medical history, the physical assessment is a search for signs—signs of illness or injury. In the physical assessment, we try to define more precisely the nature and seriousness of the patient's problem by checking the body for clues. In this chapter, we will learn how the physical assessment is conducted: what signs we look for and what those signs mean. On completion of the chapter, the reader should be able to

1. List the equipment needed to perform the secondary survey
2. List the observations that should be made in evaluating the patient's general appearance
3. Explain how the state of consciousness is assessed and how it should be described
4. Identify behavior that should alert the EMT to the possibility of hypoxia or impending shock, given a description of patients with different behaviors
5. Explain the reason for making a quick check for obvious injuries before beginning the head-to-toe survey
6. Indicate the possible significance of skin condition (color, temperature, moisture), given a description of a patient's skin condition
7. List the aspects of the pulse that should be assessed and indicate how the pulse is described
8. Describe the method of measuring the respiratory rate
9. List the aspects of respiration that should be assessed and indicate how the respirations should be described
10. Indicate the significance of abnormal respiratory sounds, given a list of abnormal sounds
11. Describe the usual method of measuring the arterial blood pressure and indicate what alternative method can be used under noisy field conditions
12. Identify the normal vital signs for an adult, given a list of various sets of vital signs
13. Identify the significance of various abnormal physical signs in an injured patient, given a list of signs
14. Identify the significance of various abnormal physical signs in a medical patient, given a list of signs
15. Indicate the differences between the examination of an injured patient and a patient with a medical problem, with respect to examination of (a) the head, (b) the neck, (c) the chest, (d) the abdomen, and (e) the extremities and back.

TOOLS OF THE TRADE

Unlike the primary survey, which is carried out without any equipment, the secondary survey requires a few basic tools to aid in the detailed examination of the patient. Perhaps the most useful of these tools is a **stethoscope**, which is used both to check the blood pressure and to listen to the patient's chest and abdomen for abnormal sounds. In acquiring a stethoscope, the EMT should choose one that fits comfortably in the ears (the stethoscope is worn with the earpieces pointing forward), that is easily carried, and that has long enough tubing to reach from the patient's vertex, where the EMT will be seated in the ambulance, to the chest and arm.

In addition to the stethoscope, the EMT will need a **watch** with a sweep second hand, to measure the pulse and respiratory rate, and a **flashlight**, preferably pocket-size, with a good, focussed beam, to examine the patient's pupils, ears, and mouth. A heavy-duty **scissors** is also sometimes necessary for cutting away a sleeve or pant leg in order to expose a wound or an injured extremity. The EMT should carry a **pen** with waterproof ink and a small **pad of paper**, on which to make notes of vital signs and other observations until the data can be recorded on the trip sheet. Most EMTs find it convenient to carry the above equipment on their person, often in some sort of holster attached to the belt.

Finally, the secondary survey requires a **sphygmomanometer**—a blood pressure cuff and pressure gauge. If there is a blood pressure apparatus permanently installed in the vehicle, it is preferable that there be a second, portable unit that the EMT can carry to the patient so that a complete set of vital signs can be recorded immediately and need not be postponed until the patient is brought to the ambulance.

Equipment Needed for the Secondary Survey

- Stethoscope
- Watch
- Sphygmomanometer
- Penlight
- Pen and paper
- Heavy-duty scissors

OVERVIEW OF PHYSICAL ASSESSMENT

The physical assessment must be carried out systematically, for otherwise it is easy to leave out a step here and there, especially when working under pressure or caring for a patient with multiple injuries. For this reason, the PHYSICAL ASSESSMENT SHOULD ALWAYS BE CONDUCTED IN THE SAME ORDER. Needless to say, circumstances will dictate what particular signs one looks for in any given patient. It does not make much sense, for example, to make a painstaking search for fractures in a patient whose chief complaint is chest pain. Nonetheless, the examination of the patient with a medical problem will follow the same general *sequence* as the examination of the injured patient, and the difference between the two examinations will be one of emphasis.

The sequence of physical assessment, then, should always be the same, and the first step is an evaluation of the patient's GENERAL APPEARANCE. This is followed by the taking of VITAL SIGNS (pulse, blood pressure, respiratory rate, and occasionally temperature) and then the HEAD-TO-TOE SURVEY. It is in the head-to-toe survey that the differences in emphasis for the injured patient and the patient with a medical problem are apparent.

After dealing with the first two steps of the secondary survey, we will discuss the head-to-toe examination of an injured patient and then start all over at the beginning with the examination of a medical patient.

GENERAL APPEARANCE

The physical assessment begins by spending a moment or two to take a careful look at the patient and make note of (1) his position, (2) his level of consciousness, (3) his behavior and degree of distress, (4) any obvious wounds or deformities, and (5) the condition of his skin. A trained observer can derive a great deal of information from this preliminary survey, and making early note of possible areas of injury minimizes the chances of aggravating an unsuspected injury as you proceed through the examination.

POSITION

The position in which the patient is found can in itself be very informative. If the patient is the victim of trauma, his position often suggests the mechanism of injury or the type of injury sustained. The patient who lies supine with his hands stretched out above his head, for instance, may have an injury of the lumbar spine, while the patient who walks toward you holding his wrist with the other hand usually has a fracture of the distal radius and ulna.

In a medical patient, the position in which the patient is found often gives clues to the nature of the patient's problem. A person with difficulty breathing, for example, will usually sit bolt upright (Fig. 11-1) or may even get up and pace around, but he will not voluntarily assume a recumbent position. A person with peritonitis (an inflammation of the adbominal lining) will lie very still and avoid any movement, while a person with a kidney stone will thrash around trying to find a position in which the pain is less severe. In general, a conscious patient—whether ill or injured—will assume the position that is most comfortable for him, and it is best not to move him unless his remaining in that position is likely to aggravate his condition.

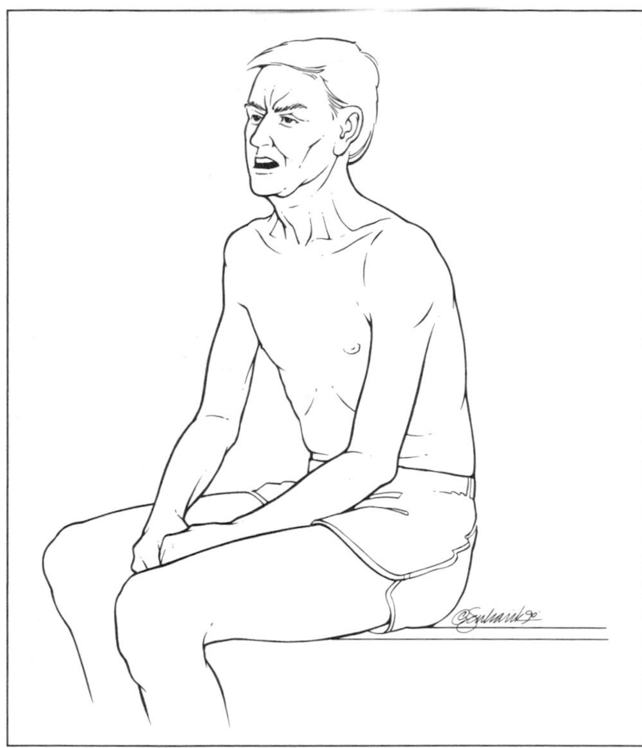

Fig. 11-1. *The patient's position. A person in respiratory distress will usually sit bolt upright or leaning slightly forward.*

STATE OF CONSCIOUSNESS

It is very important to determine the level of the patient's consciousness when you first encounter him and at periodic intervals thereafter. A healthy person is alert; he knows who he is, where he is, and usually what day it is; and he responds when you talk to him. But illness or injury can alter a person's state of consciousness in a variety of ways. There are many terms to describe altered states of consciousness—confusion, disorientation, stupor, coma, semicoma, obtundation—but the trouble with these terms is that they are not precise, and they mean different things to different people. What you consider "stupor," the emergency room doctor may call "semicoma," and the doctor may therefore conclude that the patient's condition has deteriorated when in fact there has been no change at all in his condition—only a difference in terminology. Thus you should test and describe the patient's state of consciousness in terms of SPECIFIC RESPONSES TO SPECIFIC STIMULI. This type of report provides the doctor with information that can be rechecked very precisely later to determine if there has been any change in the patient's status. For example, you might find that the patient does not respond to your voice, even when you shout, but that he does pull his arm away if you pinch it. Later, in the emergency room, the doctor may find that the patient does not even withdraw his arm in response to pain, so the doctor immediately knows there has been a deterioration in the patient's condition (which often means a need for urgent surgery). On the other hand, you may find in the field that the patient is very confused and can barely recall his name, but by the time you reach the emergency room, he can tell the doctor his address, the date, and his social security number—a clear indication of improvement in the patient's status.

If the patient is *conscious*, try to determine his degree of ALERTNESS AND ORIENTATION. Does he give appropriate answers to your questions, or does his mind seem to wander? Does he know his name? His address? The day of the week? The date? His social security number? Estimate the alertness of small children or infants by noting whether they seem to take an interest in their surroundings and how much they move about. Do they make eye contact in response to your voice?

If the patient is *unconscious*, determine what kind of stimulation is required to get some response. Does the patient waken or move in response to a shout? If not, does he move in response to a painful stimulus (e.g., a pinch or a pinprick)? Is the movement purposeful? Does he withdraw his arm or try to push your hand away, or does he simply go into a generalized spasm? Does he have any reaction at all? Make a detailed note of precisely what stimulus you applied, what response you observed, and the time of your observation (e.g., "9:21 A.M.—patient withdraws right arm in response to pinprick of right palm").

BEHAVIOR AND DEGREE OF DISTRESS

If the patient is conscious, his behavior, facial expression, movements, and apparent degree of distress can tell you a good deal about the seriousness of his problem. Is the patient sitting quietly, in no apparent distress? Is his face contorted with pain? Is he struggling for breath? Does he look scared?

Be particularly alert for signs of restlessness. RESTLESSNESS IS A DANGER SIGNAL, for it often indicates impending shock or an inadequate state of oxygenation, and in some patients it may be the *only* sign of serious internal injury. Never dismiss restlessness as insignificant.

RESTLESSNESS IS OFTEN THE EARLIEST SIGN OF HYPOXIA OR INTERNAL BLEEDING.

OBVIOUS WOUNDS OR DEFORMITIES

As you do your preliminary inspection, make a quick note of any areas of clothing soaked with blood or any extremities that seem to be positioned at an unusual angle. This quick survey will help guide your more thorough head-to-toe survey later and will also alert you to areas of the body that should not be moved pending closer examination.

SKIN

The patient's skin should be examined for color, temperature, and degree of moisture. In lightly pigmented people, the SKIN COLOR gives considerable information about peripheral perfusion. Under normal circumstances, the skin of a lightly pigmented person is pink, reflecting good blood flow to the skin and moderate dilation of the blood vessels beneath the skin surface. If the blood vessels *dilate* more widely, or if the blood flow to the skin increases, the skin becomes flushed or RED. This may occur, for example, in fever, in which the body tries to dissipate its extra heat by dilation of blood vessels just beneath the skin surface. Through this mechanism, more blood is brought to the surface of the body, where it can be cooled. Very red skin is also seen in some allergic reactions. In poisoning with carbon monoxide, the skin sometimes takes on a "cherry red" appearance, which is a classic sign of this kind of poisoning.

On the other hand, if the blood vessels just beneath the skin surface *constrict*, the skin becomes WHITE—a condition called **pallor**. This is the case, for example, in fright; when a person is frightened, the body releases adrenalin, a chemical that causes the heart to beat faster and the blood vessels to narrow. Pallor is also seen in shock or in fainting, because of the widespread arterial constriction that the body uses in an attempt to maintain blood pressure. Constriction of blood vessels beneath the skin can also produce blotchy or MOTTLED skin, which is again sometimes seen in shock. Furthermore, any time the circulation to the periphery is reduced or the level of oxygen in the blood falls, the skin is apt to take on a BLUE color (**cyanosis**). Bluish skin is seen in patients exposed to cold because the blood vessels of the skin constrict in order to shunt blood away from the body surface and conserve heat. It is also seen in hypoxia. In darkly pigmented people, cyanosis can be detected in the mucous membranes of the mouth and eyes and beneath the fingernails. Finally, certain diseases can cause changes in skin color. When there is disease involving the liver or gallbladder, for instance, the skin may turn YELLOW, a condition called **jaundice.**

Changes in Skin Color

RED	Fever; allergic reactions; blushing; exposure to heat; carbon monoxide poisoning
WHITE (pallor)	Fright; blood loss; fainting; shock
BLUE (cyanosis)	Hypoxia; cold exposure; poor skin perfusion
MOTTLED	Shock
YELLOW (jaundice)	Liver or gallbladder disease

The TEMPERATURE AND MOISTURE of the skin is estimated by placing the back of your hand on the patient's skin. In a healthy person, the skin is warm and relatively dry. The skin temperature rises as the blood vessels beneath the skin dilate, as in fever; the skin temperature drops when there is constriction of the subcutaneous blood vessels, as in shock. The degree of moisture on the skin reflects the amount of sweating, which is a mechanism the body uses to cool itself by evaporation of water from the skin. Sweating is also a reflex reaction to stress, and most people have had the experience of going into a "cold sweat" under stressful conditions or feeling their palms get sweaty during moments of anxiety.

Changes in Skin Temperature and Moisture

HOT, DRY SKIN	Excessive body heat (heat stroke; early phase of fever)
HOT, WET SKIN	Reaction to increased internal or external temperature
COOL, DRY SKIN	Exposure to cold
COOL, CLAMMY SKIN	Shock or other extreme stress

At the outset of the patient assessment, then, we have already acquired a good overall impression of the seriousness of the patient's condition simply by taking a few moments to observe the patient's general appearance. To summarize this phase of physical assessment:

General Appearance

- Position
- State of consciousness
- Behavior and degree of distress
- Obvious wounds and deformities
- Skin condition

VITAL SIGNS

Having completed the initial overview of the patient, we move on to the patient's vital signs: pulse, respirations, blood pressure, and sometimes temperature.

These signs are called "vital" signs because they measure the patient's vital functions: heart beat, breathing, and the state of the vascular system. Changes in vital signs are a very sensitive indicator of illness or injury, and in a critically ill or injured patient, such changes can occur in minutes or even seconds. Thus when caring for a patient in serious condition, the EMT should check and record the vital signs frequently to detect changes in the patient's status.

PULSE

The pulse, as we learned earlier, is the pressure wave generated by the heart beat and transmitted through the arteries, and thus the PULSE RATE is a measure of how many times the heart is beating each minute. The normal pulse rate for an adult at rest can be anywhere from about 60 to 80 per minute. In a well-trained athlete, the normal resting pulse may be somewhat lower—in the range of 50—while poor physical fitness tends to increase the resting pulse toward 90. In children, the normal pulse is 80 to 100, while in infants, it averages 120 (range 80–160).

The pulse is most conveniently measured in the radial or carotid artery (Fig. 11-2). Use the tips of your index and middle fingers (*not* your thumb) to palpate lightly over the patient's pulse. If you press on the artery too firmly, you may interfere with the blood flow through it. Using the sweep second hand of your watch to indicate the time elapsed, count the number of beats you feel in 15 seconds, and then multiply by 4 to obtain the pulse rate per minute. If the pulse is very slow, you will get a more accurate measurement of the rate by palpating for 30 seconds (and multiplying by 2).

In addition to the rate, you should note the RHYTHM AND FORCE of the pulse. The *rhythm* is an estimate of the regularity of the pulse. A normal pulse is regular; each beat follows the next at precise intervals, like the ticking of a clock. If one or more beats come early or late, the pulse is considered irregular. The *force* of the pulse refers to the degree of pressure you feel against your fingertips with each pulse beat. A normal pulse is "**full**"; that is, it produces a feeling that a strong wave has passed beneath the fingertips. If the heart is beating more forcefully than usual (as after strenuous exercise), the pulse will be "**bounding**"; that is, it will feel stronger than usual. If, on the other hand, the heart is beating less forcefully or the fluid inside the tubing is reduced in volume (as in shock), the pulse will feel weak, or "**thready**." When you describe the pulse, you should always indicate the rate, force, and rhythm; for example, "The patient's pulse was 70, full, and regular."

Evaluation of the Pulse

- RATE — Number of beats per minute
- FORCE — Full, bounding, or thready
- RHYTHM — Regular or irregular

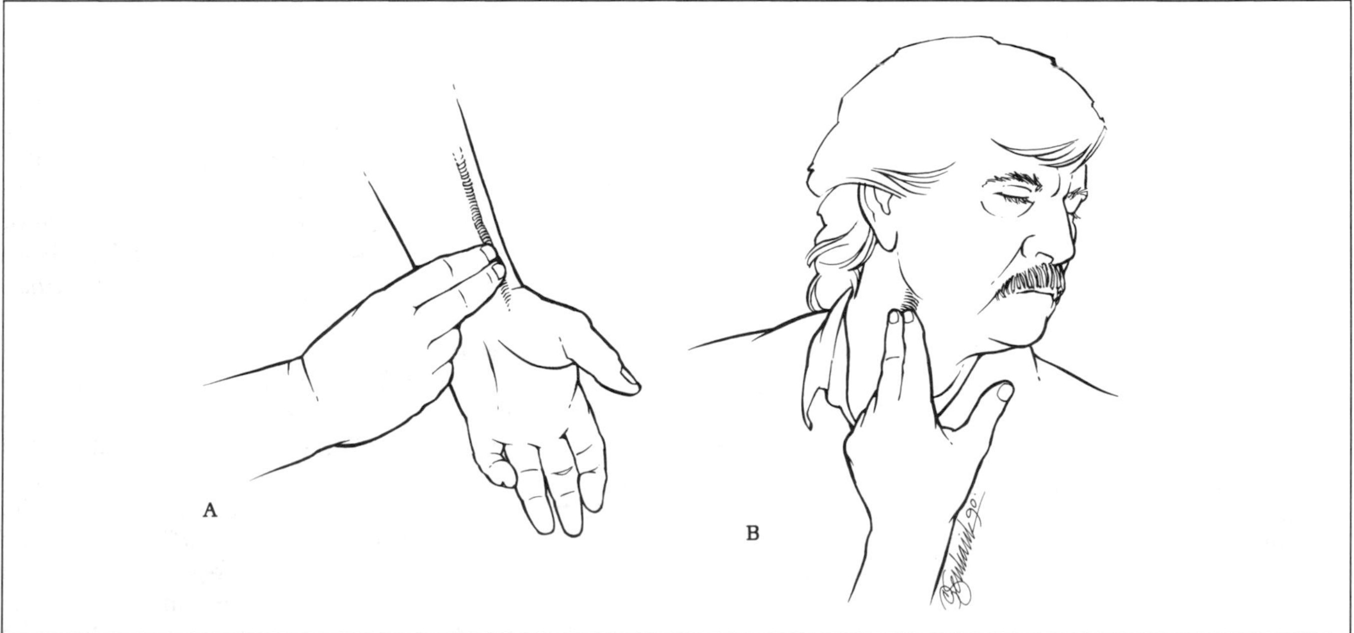

Fig. 11-2. *Checking the pulse. The pulse is most conveniently measured in the radial artery (A) or the carotid artery (B).*

RESPIRATIONS

Without taking your fingers off the patient's pulse, you should immediately proceed to measuring the RATE OF RESPIRATIONS. Again, use the sweep second hand of your watch to indicate the time elapsed, and count the number of times you see the chest rise and fall in 30 seconds; then multiply by 2 to get the number of respirations per minute. The reason for keeping your fingers on the patient's pulse all this time is to give the impression that you are still measuring the pulse. When a person is aware that his breathing is under scrutiny, the respiratory rate will often change (try thinking about your own breathing for a minute, and see what happens). Thus when you finish measuring the pulse, you should simply keep your fingers on the pulse but surreptitiously shift your gaze to the patient's chest and abdomen to count the breaths. The normal respiratory rate is somewhat variable, but it is usually between 12 and 20 per minute in an adult, somewhat slower for a trained athlete, and faster in a child.

In addition to counting the respiratory rate, note the RHYTHM of respirations. Breathing is normally fairly regular, but some illnesses and injuries can produce irregular respiratory rhythms. For example, a patient with head injury may show a pattern of breathing called **Cheyne-Stokes respiration**, in which the breathing gets deeper and deeper, then shallower and shallower, and then stops for a second or two before resuming another series of shallow-deep-shallow breathing.

Note also the EASE AND DEPTH of respirations. In a healthy person, breathing is relatively effortless, while a person in respiratory distress may have labored or gasping respirations. Broken ribs or inflammation of the pleura can produce pain on breathing. The depth of respiration refers to the volume of air the patient takes in with each breath. Normally this is about 500 ml, but a person with severe hypoxia ("air hunger") may take very *deep* breaths, while someone who has taken an overdose of narcotics may have *shallow* respirations.

Listen for ABNORMAL RESPIRATORY NOISES. A healthy person breathes quietly at rest. **Snoring** indicates partial obstruction of the upper airway, usually by the tongue, which can be corrected by head tilt. **Gurgling** noises suggest fluid in the upper airway, while **stridor**—a high-pitched, squeaking noise heard on inhalation—indicates narrowing of the airway, usually caused by swelling (laryngeal edema).

Finally, note any ABNORMAL ODORS ON THE BREATH, such as the smell of alcohol. In diabetic acidosis, the patient often has a sweet, fruity odor to his breath. Bowel obstruction can give the breath the odor of feces. In cyanide poisoning, the breath is said to smell like "bitter almonds," an observation useful to those who know what bitter almonds smell like.

When reporting on the respirations, include all the information mentioned above. For instance, "The patient's respirations are regular, deep, and labored at 24 per minute. There is slight stridor on inhalation, and the patient's breath smells of alcohol."

Evaluation of Respirations

• RATE	Number of breaths per minute
• RHYTHM	Regularity of respirations
• EASE	Labored? Painful?
• DEPTH	Deep? Shallow?
• ABNORMAL NOISES	Snoring; gurgling; stridor
• ABNORMAL ODOR	Alcohol; fruity odor; fecal odor

BLOOD PRESSURE

The blood pressure (BP) is the pressure that circulating blood exerts against the walls of arteries. As we learned in Chapter 8, the blood pressure has two components: a high point, the systolic pressure, which reflects the contraction of the heart (ventricular systole); and a low point, the diastolic pressure, which reflects the relaxation of the heart (ventricular diastole) and represents the minimum pressure constantly present in the arteries.

Normal blood pressure varies with age and sex. In a healthy adult man, the *systolic* pressure is usually between about 120 and 150 mm Hg (you can make a rough estimate by adding 100 to the patient's age, up to a total of 150). The *diastolic* pressure is normally 65 to 90 mm Hg. Both pressures are usually about 8 to 10 mm Hg lower in a woman of the same age. Disease or stress can elevate a person's blood pressure (*hypertension*), and the blood pressure that gets too high can damage or rupture arteries, particularly in the brain. Abnormally low blood pressure (*hypotension*), on the other hand, leads to inadequate perfusion of vital organs and results from failure of the heart to pump forcefully, from loss of fluid from the circuit (e.g., hemorrhage), or from widespread dilation of blood vessels (e.g., neurogenic shock).

To measure the blood pressure, first explain to the patient what you are planning to do, for some people may be unfamiliar with the procedure and fearful when they see the equipment. Wrap the cuff of the sphygmomanometer snugly around the patient's arm with its lower border about an inch or two above the elbow. It is preferable to use the LEFT ARM if this arm is uninjured, for it will be more accessible to you for rechecking the blood pressure when the patient is lying on the stretcher in the ambulance. Once the blood pressure cuff is in place, palpate to find the pulsation of the brachial artery, and place the diaphragm (flat part) of your stethoscope over the brachial pulsation (Fig. 11-3). While holding the stethoscope in position, rapidly inflate the cuff by squeezing the rubber bulb until the needle on the pressure gauge stops bouncing with each pulse beat—usually somewhere between 150 and 200 mm Hg. Then, while you keep an eye on the pressure gauge, SLOWLY release the air from the cuff by opening the adjustable valve on the rubber bulb. The pressure in the cuff should be allowed to drop at a rate of about 2 to 3 mm Hg per second. As the pressure in the cuff falls and blood resumes flowing through the brachial artery, you will start to hear the thumping of the pulse, and the point at which you hear the *first* thump is the *systolic* pressure. Continue to listen as you let the cuff deflate further, and at the point where the thumping grows very soft or disappears altogether, you have reached the *diastolic* pressure. Deflate the cuff completely when you finish measuring the blood pressure, but leave it in position on the arm so that you can recheck the pressure at frequent intervals without having to reapply the cuff each time.

As noted in Chapter 8, the blood pressure is expressed as a fraction, with the systolic pressure as the numerator and the diastolic pressure as the denominator. Thus if you measured a systolic pressure of 120 mm Hg and a diastolic pressure of 80 mm Hg, you would write it "120/80" and say it as "120 over 80."

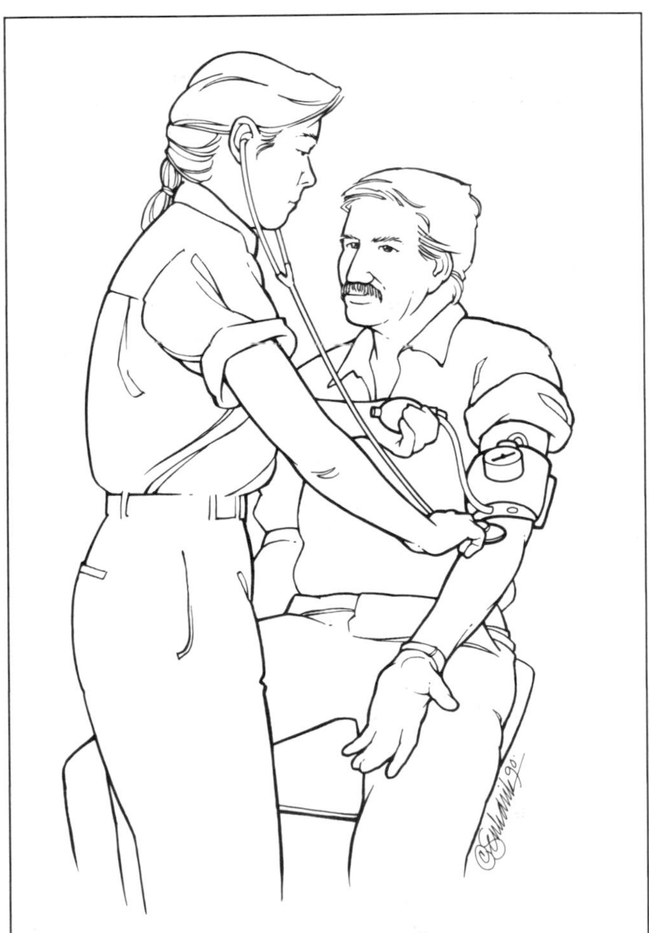

Fig. 11-3. *Measuring the blood pressure. Hold the diaphragm of the stethoscope over the pulsation of the brachial artery.*

Sometimes field conditions or noises in the ambulance make it impossible to hear the blood pressure sounds. In such circumstances, you can measure the *systolic* pressure by palpation. Apply the blood pressure cuff in the usual fashion, but before you inflate it, locate the radial artery on the same arm, and keep your finger on the radial pulse. Then inflate the cuff to a point about 20 mm Hg higher than the point at which the radial pulse disappears. Deflate the cuff slowly while continuing to palpate the radial artery and keeping an eye on the blood pressure gauge. The point at which you first feel the pulse beat return is the systolic pressure. At that point, the needle on the dial will usually begin to bounce slightly with each pulse beat, and this serves to confirm the reading you got by palpation.

It should be stressed that a single measurement of blood pressure is of minimal value, especially when the individual's usual blood pressure is not known. What is important is the *trend* of the blood pressure, and in order to determine this, you must make several measurements during the time the patient is under your care. Each time you measure the blood pressure (or any other vital signs), immediately record the values together with the time the measurements were made. Do not leave it to memory.

Sometimes a patient will want to know what reading you obtained for his blood pressure and may become alarmed if your measurement is significantly different from one obtained in his doctor's office. It is important to explain to the patient that a single measurement of blood pressure may not be significant, for anxiety, excitement, or stress can cause temporary blood pressure elevations in an otherwise perfectly healthy person. If the reading you obtain is abnormally high, you should suggest to the patient that he have his blood pressure rechecked some time after his acute illness or injury is over, under less stressful circumstances.

TEMPERATURE

In the hospital, it is standard practice to measure the patient's temperature as part of the routine assessment of vital signs. In the field, this is not usually practical, and the temperature is measured only when it is relevant to the patient's problem—for example, in fever or heat stroke. Otherwise it is simply estimated by feeling the patient's skin with the back of your hand.

The temperature is measured in the field by placing the mercury bulb of a standard oral thermometer under the patient's tongue for at least 3 minutes. This should not be done in a moving ambulance or in any other circumstances in which the patient is apt to bite down through the thermometer. In the hospital, temperatures are also taken in the axilla or rectum; but the axillary temperature tends to be inaccurate in the field, and measurement of rectal temperature is not practical under field conditions.

Normal body temperature is 98.6°F (37°C). When you report the temperature, indicate the reading and how the temperature was taken; for instance, "The patient's temperature is 100°F orally."

Vital Signs: Normal Values at Rest

PULSE	Adults: 60 to 80 per minute Children: 80 to 100 per minute Infants: 80 to 160 per minute (average = 120)
RESPIRATIONS	Adults: 12 to 20 per minute Children: 18 to 26 per minute Infants: 25 to 36 per minute
BLOOD PRESSURE	Adult man Systolic: 100 mm Hg + age (up to 150) Diastolic: 65 to 90 mm Hg Adult woman: systolic and diastolic 8 to 10 mm Hg lower than in man of the same age
TEMPERATURE	98.6°F (37°C)

Whenever you measure vital signs in the field, be sure to observe these guidelines:

- Measure vital signs FREQUENTLY in any seriously ill or injured patient.
- RECORD THE TIME each set of vital signs was taken.
- RECORD the vital signs IMMEDIATELY as you take them: do not trust them to memory.

HEAD-TO-TOE SURVEY

Once the vital signs have been measured and recorded, we proceed to a systematic examination of the patient's body, literally from head to toe. By starting at the head and working down in this fashion, one is less likely to forget part of the examination and thereby miss a significant finding. The head-to-toe survey requires the examiner to use his or her senses of sight, hearing, and touch in a search for abnormalities—the process of LOOK, LISTEN, AND FEEL that we already learned when checking for breathing. These three techniques of the physical examination are given special names:

- **Inspection** is the process of LOOKING at a part of the body for visible abnormalities. In order for an area of the body to be properly inspected, it must be visible—which means good lighting and proper exposure. You cannot inspect a wound that is covered with clothing, so clothing must be removed or cut away from the area to be inspected. Remember, though, to safeguard the patient's privacy, try to carry out your inspection so that the patient is shielded from the stares of bystanders.
- **Auscultation** is LISTENING with a stethoscope for sounds made by the passage of air through the patient's lungs, by the beating of the heart, or by the passage of air and fluids through the intestines. The diaphragm of the stethoscope is designed to detect sounds of relatively high frequency, such as those of the lungs, while the bell (the concave part) of the stethoscope conducts low-frequency sounds, such as certain heart sounds.
- **Palpation** is FEELING with the hands for contours, textures, temperature, and so forth. The fingertips are best suited to detecting differences in texture and consistency, while the back of the hand is more sensitive to elevated or lowered temperatures.

In describing the head-to-toe survey, we will proceed first through the survey of an injured patient and then repeat the survey for a patient with a medical problem. As noted earlier, the *sequence* in which the two surveys are conducted is the same; the difference is in emphasis.

THE INJURED PATIENT

Throughout the head-to-toe survey of the injured patient, extreme care must be taken not to move the patient's head, neck, or the rest of the spine any more than absolutely necessary. Unless the injury is clearly confined to a limited area (e.g., a twisted ankle), you must assume the possibility of spinal injury and handle the patient accordingly.

Examination of the Head

Begin your examination of the head by checking the SCALP for lacerations. When the patient is lying on his back, check the posterior scalp by placing your fingers behind the patient's neck and sliding them gently upward along the back of the head, taking care not to move the head as you do so. If you see or feel blood on the scalp, try to separate the hair to determine exactly where the blood is coming from. Also palpate the SKULL gently, and make note of any unusual lumps or depressions. Be careful not to press too hard, however, lest you push a fragment of broken bone into the brain.

Examine both EARS for evidence of external trauma, such as bruising, swelling, or laceration of the ear lobe. Shine your penlight into the ear canals to check for blood or clear fluid. If clear fluid is seen coming from an ear, it is likely to be **cerebrospinal fluid (CSF)**, a watery substance that bathes the brain and spinal cord and whose presence in the ear canals is a sign of skull fracture. Blood coming from the ears usually has the same significance. If you see either blood or clear fluid emerging from an ear, DO NOT ATTEMPT TO STOP THE FLOW, for this can cause dangerous increases in the pressure within the skull. Also examine the area just behind the ear, over the mastoid bone of the skull, for the bluish discoloration (**ecchymosis**) that is a sign of blood beneath the skin. Bluish discoloration over the mastoid bone is called **Battle's sign** (Fig. 11-4A) and indicates a fracture of the base of the skull.

Inspect the NOSE for swelling, bruises, or deformity. Here too, note the presence of blood or clear fluid draining from the nose, but do not attempt to stop the flow.

Observe the patient's EYES for evidence of trauma. Check for swelling of the area around the eyes (**periorbital** area). Ecchymoses around the eyes (Fig. 11-4B, "coon's eyes") without evidence of a direct blow to the face suggest skull fracture. Gently open the patient's eyes and examine the PUPILS (Fig. 11-5). Normal pupils are equal in size and constrict (get smaller) when a light is shone into them. In an injured patient, *widely dilated pupils*—especially if they do not constrict in response to light—suggest hypoxia or brain injury. *Narrowly constricted pupils* suggest the patient may have taken some narcotic drug. *Unequal pupils* occur normally in 2 to 4 percent of the population, but in the context of head trauma, unequal pupils should always be assumed to be a sign of serious brain injury.

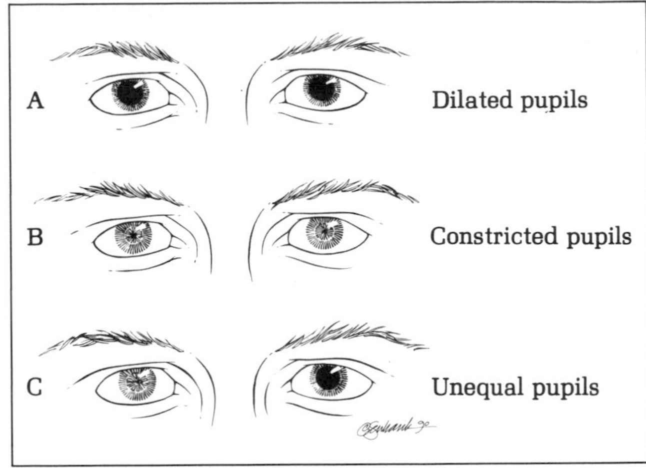

Fig. 11-5. *Examination of the pupils. A. Dilated pupils. B. Constricted pupils. C. Unequal pupils.*

Also observe the MOTIONS OF THE EYES. Normally the two eyes move together in the same direction, but in head injury or direct trauma to the eyes, the eyes may turn in different directions. If the pa-

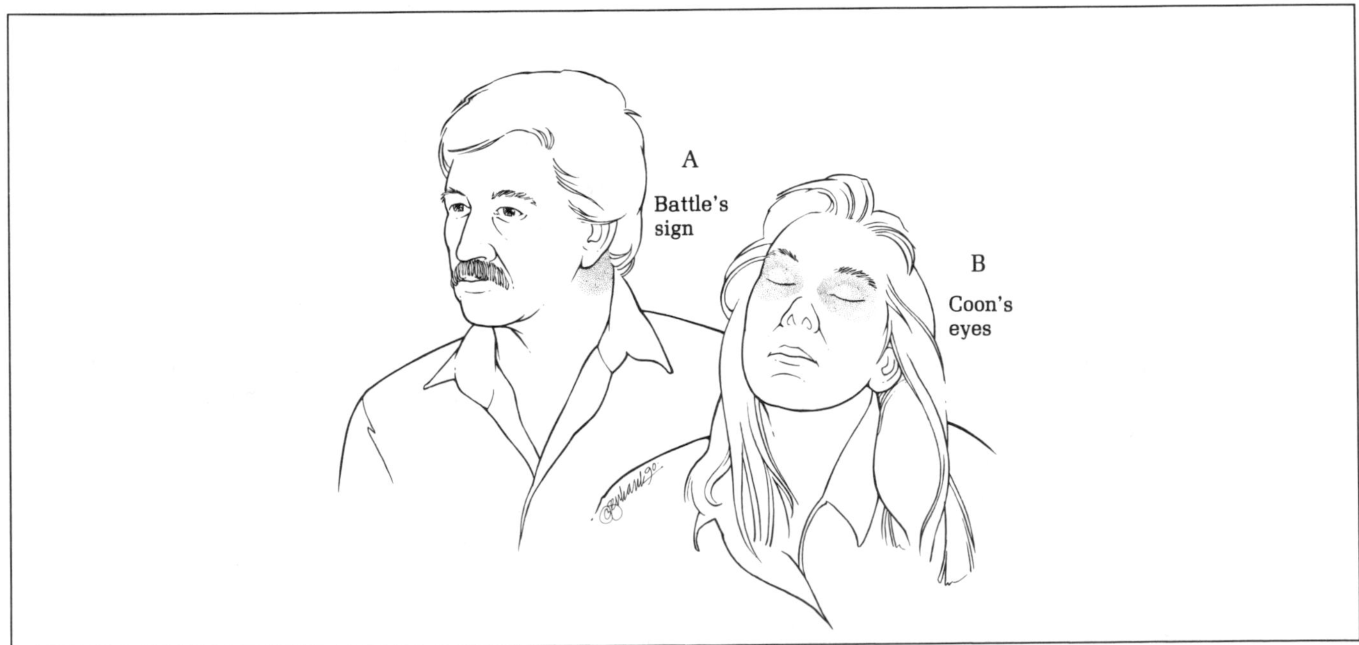

Fig. 11-4. *Signs of basilar skull fracture. A. Ecchymosis over the mastoid bone, behind the ear (Battle's sign). B. Periorbital ecchymosis ("coon's eyes," or raccoon sign).*

tient is conscious, ask him to follow your finger with his gaze as you move your finger 90 degrees up, down, left, and right, and note whether the eyes move fully in each direction.

Palpate the patient's JAW for instability. If there is no evidence of fracture, gently open his MOUTH, and shine your penlight inside to inspect for blood, vomitus, or foreign bodies, such as broken dentures. Remove any easily accessible foreign objects, and suction the mouth if there is considerable blood, vomitus, or other liquid material. Observe the LIPS AND MUCOUS MEMBRANES for cyanosis.

Examination of the Head

• SCALP	Lacerations; lumps; depressions
• EARS	External trauma; blood or clear fluid in canals; ecchymoses over mastoid
• NOSE	Swelling; deformity; bruising; blood or clear fluid coming from nostrils
• EYES	Trauma to lid or eye; periorbital swelling or ecchymosis Pupils: equality and reaction to light Eye movements
• JAW	Stability
• MOUTH	Foreign materials; blood; vomitus
• LIPS	Cyanosis

Examination of the Neck

Expose the neck for inspection by unbuttoning any collar or removing any tie or scarf—but once again, DO NOT MOVE THE NECK to do so. Look first at the *front* of the neck to determine whether there is a stoma or breathing tube; if so, it must be kept unobstructed. Observe and palpate the trachea to see whether it is in the midline or whether it appears to be pulled to one side. Look lateral to the trachea for distended jugular veins, which may be a sign of trauma within the chest. Check for open wounds of the neck, which must be covered immediately. Then slide your fingers behind the neck, and gently feel for any deformities. If the patient is conscious, ask him to report any tenderness he feels as you palpate. Detection of either tenderness or deformity in the victim's neck should prompt you to interrupt the survey at that point and temporarily stablize the victim's head with sandbags or some other device before continuing with the examination.

Examination of the Neck

- LOOK:
  1. For a stoma or breathing tube
  2. For trachea out of the midline
  3. For open wounds (close immediately)
  4. For distended jugular veins
- FEEL for tenderness or deformity

Examination of the Chest

Expose the chest by opening the patient's shirt all the way, and observe the patient as he breathes, noting whether the two sides of the chest seem to expand equally with each inhalation. (If the patient is female and you are male, explain why you must examine the chest, and if at all possible, have a woman EMT or woman bystander present with you.) Inspect the chest for bruises, open wounds, or objects impaled in the chest wall. If you see an open wound of the chest, place your ear over it to listen for air being drawn into the pleural cavity; a penetrating wound of this kind must be closed immediately with an occlusive dressing before you proceed further with the survey.

Spread your hands lightly on the chest with your thumbs at the xiphoid process, and note whether both hands move equally with respiration. Palpate the ribs for tenderness, and compress the sides of the rib cage to check for instability of the chest wall. Also feel for air crackling beneath the surface of the skin—a sign of pneumothorax. Feel the trachea during inhalation, and note whether it remains in the midline or is pulled to one side.

Listen to the BREATH SOUNDS with your stethoscope—just below the left clavicle and then just below the right clavicle; below the left axilla and then below the right axilla—and compare the breath sounds on the two sides. In a normal person, the breath sounds should be equal in intensity on the right and left, but collapse of a lung or blood in one side of the chest can alter the breath sounds on the affected side. Also listen over the left chest for HEART SOUNDS, which should be clear and regular. Muffled heart sounds suggest blood in the sac that surrounds the heart (pericardium).

Examination of the Chest

- LOOK
  1. For symmetry of breathing
  2. For bruises; lacerations; impaled objects
- LISTEN
  1. For air being sucked into a wound
  2. For equal breath sounds on both sides of the chest
  3. For a clear heart beat

- FEEL
  1. For symmetry of breathing
  2. For instability of the rib cage
  3. For air crackling beneath the skin

Examination of the Abdomen
Expose the abdomen, and inspect it for distention, ecchymoses, or any penetration of the skin surface. If circumstances permit, listen with your stethoscope for bowel sounds. In a normal person, one can usually hear at least a gurgle or two from the intestines by listening for 60 seconds with the diaphragm of the stethoscope lying lightly on the abdominal wall. If there has been significant internal injury to the abdomen, however, bowel sounds may be absent, for the intestine goes into a state resembling paralysis. Do not take time to listen for bowel sounds in noisy conditions or if the patient is badly injured. Lightly palpate the abdomen for tenderness. If the victim is complaining of abdominal pain, palpate the part that hurts *last*. Note whether tenderness is localized to a single spot or is widespread throughout the abdomen. If the abdomen is tender *and* distended, it is probably full of blood, and you can expect hemorrhagic shock to become evident very soon. Also note the *consistency* of the abdomen: Is it soft and compliant, as in a healthy person, or is it rigid and boardlike, suggesting internal injury?

Examination of the Abdomen
- LOOK
  1. For ecchymoses
  2. For penetration of the skin
- LISTEN for the presence of bowel sounds
- FEEL
  1. For consistency (soft vs. rigid)
  2. For tenderness

Examination of the Back
Without moving the patient, gently slide your hands beneath him, and palpate the lower spine for tenderness or deformity. Feel for any blood and for localized bumps.

Examination of the Pelvis
Place your hands on either ilium (the wide bones of the patient's hips), and compress the pelvis. Pain on compression or instability of the pelvis suggests a fracture to the pelvic bone.

Examination of the Genital Region
If there is blood on the patient's clothing suggesting injury to the genital region, you should expose the area and examine it. You must shield the patient from onlookers during this procedure, and if the patient is female and you are male, you must have a woman EMT or woman bystander present during the examination. Note the source of bleeding and any associated bruises or swelling. In the male, check for **priapism** (sustained erection of the penis), which is a sign of injury to the spinal cord.

Examination of the Extremities
Start with the lower extremities, and check each extremity separately. It may be necessary to cut away a trouser leg or a shirt sleeve to get a better look at an extremity that seems injured. Do not try to pull clothes off or rip them loose, for this can cause unnecessary jarring of the limb. Use your heavy-duty scissors to cut along the seam of the pant leg or shirt sleeve. Once you have exposed the extremity, look for bleeding, ecchymosis, swelling, or deformity. Observe the position of the extremity, and take note of any ABNORMAL POSITION suggesting fracture or dislocation (compare the injured extremity to the uninjured extremity). Feel for a DISTAL PULSE in each extremity (i.e., the dorsalis pedis in each foot and the radial in each wrist) to check the arterial supply to the limb. An absent pulse suggests that the artery may have been damaged or pinched off by a broken bone end at a more proximal location in the extremity.

If the pulse is present, test for the ABILITY TO MOVE by asking the patient to flex and extend each foot (Fig. 11-6A) (when you are examining the upper extremity, ask the patient to squeeze your hand with each of his hands). Check for SENSATION by asking the patient to tell you when he feels you touching his toe (Fig. 11-6B) (or finger). If sensation is absent in the toes, keep moving up the leg, and make a note of the point at which the patient begins to have some feeling. If movement and sensation are absent in both legs but intact in the arms (**paraplegia**), there is an injury to the spinal cord somewhere in the back; if movement and sensation are absent in both legs *and* the arms (**quadriplegia**), an injury has occurred to the cervical spine. If the patient is unconscious, test for movement by applying a painful stimulus (e.g., a pinprick) to the sole of each foot and the palm of each hand, and note whether the patient withdraws the extremity in response to pain.

Examination of the Extremities
- Inspect for BLEEDING, BRUISES, DEFORMITY, abnormal POSITION.
- Distal PULSES: present or absent.
- Ability to MOVE feet and hands.
- SENSATION in feet and hands.

Cheyne-Stokes respiration Abnormal breathing pattern in which periods of hyperpnea are interspersed with periods of apnea.
conjunctiva Pink membrane on the inside of the eyelid.
ecchymosis Bluish discoloration of part of the skin caused by injury; a "black-and-blue mark."
edema Swelling.
hemiparesis Weakness of one side of the body.
hemiplegia Paralysis of one side of the body.
hemoptysis Coughing up blood.
inspection Examination of a part of the body by looking at it for visible signs of injury or illness.
jaundice Yellow discoloration of the skin, usually caused by disease of the liver or gallbladder.
mastoid bone Part of the skull just behind the ear.
pallor Whiteness or paleness of the skin.
palpation Examination of part of the body by feeling for abnormal textures, contours, masses, etc.
paraplegia Paralysis of the lower extremities.
periorbital Pertaining to the region around the eyes.
priapism Sustained erection of the penis, often a sign of spinal injury.
quadriplegia Paralysis of the arms and the legs.
rales Abnormal respiratory sounds with a crackling or bubbling quality that indicate the presence of fluid in the alveoli.
rhonchi Abnormal respiratory sounds with a rattling quality that indicate the presence of mucus or other material in the bronchi or bronchioles.
sclera The white of the eye.
wheezes Abnormal respiratory sounds with a whistling quality that indicate narrowing of the lower airways.

SKILL EVALUATION CHECKLISTS

The following pages contain checklists for testing the mastery of skills learned in association with this chapter. The student may find these checklists useful as a guide to practicing the skills involved.

Performance Test
Vital Signs

Student ______________________________ Date ______________

Instructor: Place an "X" in the Fail column beside any element that is performed incorrectly, out of sequence, or omitted.

Minimum Time (sec)	Activity	Critical Performance	Fail
15	Pulse measurement	Correctly locates artery (radial or carotid)	
		Palpates with fingertips, not thumb	
		Times pulse for at least 15 sec	
		Reports pulse rate, rhythm, and strength	
		Assessment is accurate (instructor checks)	
30	Measurement of respirations	Keeps fingers on pulse	
		Shifts gaze to patient's chest	
		Times respirations for at least 30 sec	
		Reports rate, depth, rhythm, and ease of respirations	
		Assessment is accurate (instructor checks)	
60	Measurement of blood pressure	Explains procedure to the patient	
		Attaches cuff snugly in correct position	
		Palpates brachial artery	
		Places stethoscope over brachial pulsation	
		Inflates cuff to sufficient pressure	
		Deflates cuff 2–3 mm Hg/sec	
		Obtains accurate reading (instructor checks)	
		Indicates whether reading is normal, high, or low for patient of this age	

Instructor ______________________________

Performance Test
Examination of the Injured Patient (Unconscious)

Student ______________________ Date ____________

Instructor: Place an "X" in the Fail column beside any element that is performed incorrectly, out of sequence, or omitted.

Maximum Time (sec)	Activity	Critical Performance	Fail
30	Primary survey	Opens the airway correctly (jaw thrust without head tilt)	
		Checks for breathing (Instructor says, "Breathing present.")	
		Checks for pulse (Instructor says, "Pulse present.")	
		Checks for exsanguinating hemorrhage	
60	Assessment of general appearance	Inspects patient and reports on State of consciousness	
		Position	
		Degree of distress	
		Obvious wounds and deformities	
		Skin color, temperature, moisture	
60	Vital signs	See performance test for vital signs	
	Head-to-toe survey	No motion of head or neck	
	Head	Examines scalp; feels back of scalp	
		Inspects external ears and ear canals	
		Looks behind ears for ecchymoses	
		Inspects nose for deformity, bleeding, discharge	
		Inspects eyes for injury, eye movements	
		Checks pupils for equality, reactivity, size	
		Checks jaw for stability	
		Opens mouth; checks for foreign material	
	Neck	Checks for wounds in neck, midline trachea	
		Feels back of neck for deformity	
	Chest	Observes for symmetry, penetrating wounds	
		Listens to both sides of chest for equal breath sounds	
		Palpates ribs for instability	
	Abdomen	Observes abdomen for ecchymoses, wounds	
		Listens for bowel sounds (at least 60 sec)	
		Palpates for rigidity	
	Pelvis	Checks for instability	
	Back	Slides hand behind lower back to feel for deformity	
	Extremities	Checks each extremity for Distal pulse	
		Withdrawal from painful stimulus	
		Medical identification tag	

Instructor ______________________

Performance Test
Examination of a Medical Patient (Unconscious)

Student ______________________ Date ______________

Instructor: Place an "X" in the Fail column beside any element that is performed incorrectly, out of sequence, or omitted.

Maximum Time (sec)	Activity	Critical Performance	Fail
30	Primary survey	Opens the airway (head tilt–neck lift or head tilt–chin lift)	
		Checks for breathing (Instructor says, "Breathing present.")	
		Checks for pulse (Instructor says, "Pulse present.")	
60	Assessment of general appearance	Observes patient and reports on: State of consciousness	
		Position	
		Degree of distress	
		Skin color, temperature, moisture	
90	Vital signs	See performance test for vital signs	
	Head-to-toe survey	Checks face for symmetry	
		Examines pupils for size, equality, reactivity	
	Head	Checks conjunctivae for pallor, cyanosis	
	Neck	Checks for distention of jugular veins	
	Chest	Observes respiratory movements	
		Listens to four quadrants of chest, anterior and posterior, for abnormal breath sounds	
	Abdomen	Inspects for distention	
		Listens for presence of bowel sounds	
		Palpates for rigidity	
	Extremities	Inspects arms for needle marks	
		Checks for medical identification tag	
		Checks for withdrawal of each extremity from painful stimulus	
		Checks ankles for edema	
	Back	Rolls patient to side, and checks back for edema	

Instructor ______________________

12. MEDICAL REPORTING AND RECORD-KEEPING

OBJECTIVES

In taking the patient's history and conducting the physical assessment, we have acquired a great deal of information about the patient and his problem. If this information is to be useful to others—specifically to the medical team that will be taking over care of the patient in the emergency room—it must be well organized and concise. In emergency situations, no one has the time or patience to listen to a long, rambling recital and try to pick out the important details. In this chapter, we will learn how to organize the information gathered in the field and how to communicate this information to other medical professionals in an orderly, concise, and accurate fashion. By the end of the chapter, the reader should be able to

1. Indicate what information belongs in the patient's history and what information belongs in the report of the patient's physical assessment, given a list of information about a patient
2. Identify the elements of the chief complaint, history of the present illness, past medical history, and physical examination, given a list of statements from a report on a patient
3. Present the report of a patient in the correct sequence, given the information about the patient in random order
4. Indicate what additional information, besides the patient's history and physical findings, should be recorded on every trip sheet
5. State two reasons for making certain that medical reports are accurate and complete

MEDICAL REPORTING

When the EMT calls in information over the radio, reports to the doctor in the emergency room, or writes up the record of the case, he or she must do so in an *orderly* fashion, so that all the information will be received and understood. In order to facilitate this process, the EMT should use the standard format for presenting medical information. In this format, INFORMATION IS *ALWAYS* PRESENTED IN THE SAME SEQUENCE, even if the steps of assessment and treatment were carried out in a different sequence. For instance, it is customary when presenting medical information to mention the treatment *last*, no matter when the treatment was given. Thus, even if you administered oxygen as one of the first steps upon reaching a patient with chest pain, you would not mention the oxygen administration until the end of your report.

The reason for sticking to a single sequence in presenting information is twofold. First of all, you are less likely to forget details of the report if you run down a standard list of items as you proceed through the report. In the second place, doctors are used to hearing medical information presented in a certain order. When you finish reporting on the patient's general appearance, for instance, the doctor will be waiting to hear the vital signs. If you give him some other information, such as how the lungs sounded, that information may not register, for the doctor's mind is "programmed" to process medical information in a certain way. Thus the standard reporting format helps both the EMT to remember all the details of the case and the doctor to "hear" all the information.

The purpose of presenting medical information is to paint a vivid and accurate picture of the patient. This is especially true when you are reporting by radio, for the doctor at the other end of the radio has only your words to provide a picture of the patient. The format of presenting the information helps the doctor build this picture in a logical way.

The traditional format for medical reporting is divided into four parts: (1) the patient's history, (2) the physical findings, (3) the treatment given, and (4) the patient's condition during transport.

THE HISTORY

The patient's history consists of all the information you picked up from talking to the patient and bystanders. It reports who the patient is, what happened to him, how it happened, and what he is *feeling* (his SYMPTOMS). You will not confuse the information belonging in the history with that belonging in the report of the physical assessment if you bear in mind that you can take a complete history over the telephone, without ever seeing or touching the patient. On the other hand, you can perform a complete physical assessment on an uncommunicative patient (e.g., someone who is unconscious) without his telling you anything, for the physical assessment requires only direct observation.

In reporting the history, it is customary to proceed in the following order.

Age and Sex of the Patient

The first information to report is the age and sex of the patient. This information immediately gives the doctor a frame of reference, especially if the patient has a medical problem. If you say, for example, "The patient is an 18-year-old man," the doctor already knows there is a whole group of illnesses that can be excluded from further consideration because those illnesses (e.g., heart attack, stroke) would be very unlikely in a young person. The fact that the patient is male also tells the doctor that this is unlikely to be a case involving pregnancy, vaginal bleeding, and so forth. The age and sex of the patient thus give the first broad outlines of the portrait you are painting and enable the doctor to begin to form a mental picture of the patient as, for example, a young man, an old woman, or a small child. If the patient is unconscious or for some other reason cannot tell you his or her age, try to make an estimate, for instance, "The patient is a man who appears to be in his 50s. . . ."

Chief Complaint

As we learned in Chapter 10, the chief complaint is the reason the patient or bystanders called for help. It is stated in a word or two, such as "chest pain," "vomiting blood," "twisted ankle," or "went into labor." The chief complaint is usually reported in the same sentence as the age and sex of the patient:

"The patient is a 48-year-old man who called for an ambulance because of chest pain."

"The patient is an elderly man who was found unconscious in an alley."

"The patient is a 12-year-old girl who fell from a horse."

Present Illness

The present illness is an elaboration of the chief complaint, and it answers questions such as how, how much, when, where, and how long. The present illness includes all the information you have gathered from the patient or bystanders regarding the patient's present problem (including any information from the patient's past that may be *directly connected* to the present problem). Take, for instance, the 48-year-old man with chest pain; his present illness might be reported like this:

The pain began 2 hours ago when the patient was watching television. It is squeezing in nature and radiates into his jaw. It is accompanied by nausea and dizziness, but there is no shortness of breath. The patient took two aspirin shortly after the pain started but got no relief. He was hospitalized 2 years ago at Lakeview Hospital for a heart attack, but he hasn't had any further heart symptoms until today.

There are two important features to note about the above presentation of the present illness. First of all, it INCLUDES INFORMATION FROM THE PATIENT'S PAST, that is, his previous hospitalization for a heart attack. The EMT has placed this information here, rather than in the past medical history, because the EMT has a hunch that the patient may be having another heart attack and thus feels there is a connection between that past hospitalization and the patient's current chief complaint.

Secondly, note that the EMT said, "There is no shortness of breath." This is a type of observation known as a PERTINENT NEGATIVE; that is, it is a symptom that a patient with this chief complaint might be expected to have but DOES NOT have. The EMT knows that in some cases of heart attack there is also heart failure, which causes dyspnea. So he specifically asked the patient, "Have you had any trouble breathing" and the patient apparently answered, "No."

Why bother to mention symptoms that the patient *does not* have? If you do not mention the pertinent negatives, the doctor has no way of knowing whether you bothered to check that particular detail. If you say nothing, for example, about whether the patient felt sick to his stomach, the doctor is faced with two possibilities: (1) the patient was not sick to his stomach, or (2) you neglected to ask the patient whether he was sick to his stomach. Mentioning the pertinent negatives clarifies this confusion.

The trick is, of course, to know what is *pertinent*. Clearly, there could be an endless list of symptoms the patient *does not* have (e.g., "His teeth do not itch," "He has no pain in his toenails"). Learning the pertinent negatives for a given chief complaint comes with learning more about specific illnesses and injuries. As we progress through this book, you will acquire much more information about specific conditions, which will help you determine what questions to ask in any given case.

Past Medical History

In reporting the patient's past medical history, you should include

- Any other SIGNIFICANT MEDICAL CONDITIONS the patient has that are *not* directly related to the chief complaint, and the doctor who is treating the patient for these conditions
- The patient's past HOSPITALIZATIONS that are not directly related to his chief complaint
- The MEDICATIONS the patient takes regularly, and whether he took his medications today
- Any known ALLERGIES, especially to medications
- In a trauma victim, the time of the patient's LAST MEAL

Let us return to our man with chest pain. His past medical history might sound like this:

The patient is treated by Dr. Koff for chronic bronchitis. Besides his hospitalization for a heart attack, he was hospitalized in 1972 for a kidney stone. He takes tetracycline and Tedrol regularly and has no known allergies.

With the past medical history, we have completed the first part of the report—the part that is basically hearsay, that is, what other people *told* you. We then move on to the objective part of the report—the physical assessment, which tells the doctor what you saw and touched and auscultated.

THE PHYSICAL ASSESSMENT

General Appearance

The first thing the doctor wants to hear is what the patient *looks* like. Is he conscious? Is he in pain? Is he struggling to breathe? Once again, this information gives the doctor a framework in which to form a mental picture of the patient. As we learned in Chapter 11, the description of the general appearance should include

- The patient's POSITION when found
- The patient's STATE OF CONSCIOUSNESS
- The patient's DEGREE OF DISTRESS
- The condition of the patient's SKIN

Obvious wounds and deformities may be mentioned at this point if they are part of the patient's principal problem. For example, in a patient whose main problem derives from having been stabbed in the chest, it is relevant to mention an obvious wound, and you might say, "The patient is conscious, lying on his left side, with a knife protruding from his right chest. He is in moderate distress, and his skin is cold and clammy." If, on the other hand, obvious deformities are not the main problem—for instance, a broken wrist in a patient who is in shock from massive external bleeding—they can wait until you reach the report on the part of the body involved.

We return to our patient with chest pain for an example of how one describes the general appearance:

The patient was alert and sitting upright in a chair. His skin was pale, cold, and damp, and he appeared to be in moderate distress.

Vital Signs

Next, we report the vital signs in the manner we learned in Chapter 11, starting with the pulse, then respirations and blood pressure. For instance:

"The patient's pulse was 110, thready, and regular. His respirations were 18 and slightly labored. His BP was 110 over 60."

Head-to-Toe Survey

Having reported the vital signs, we proceed next through the findings of the physical examination in head-to-toe order. Once again, as in the present illness, it is important to mention pertinent negatives so that the doctor will know you checked for certain findings and that those findings were indeed absent. The report on the head-to-toe survey of our man with chest pain might sound as follows:

The patient's pupils were round, regular, midposition, and reactive to light. There was no cyanosis of the conjunctivae or lips. The jugular veins were distended with the patient at 45 degrees. The chest was clear; no rales were heard. The abdomen was soft. There was no edema of the back or lower extremities.

We have now completed the second part of the report, the part dealing with direct observations. The next thing we have to tell the doctor is what we did for the patient.

TREATMENT
The treatment section of the report includes any measures taken to relieve the patient's distress or stabilize his condition. Treatment may consist of nothing more than placing the patient in a recumbent position, or it may involve dressings, bandages, splints, backboards, and a whole host of other equipment. In either case, the treatment should be spelled out *in detail*. For our 48-year-old man with chest pain, for example, we might report:

The patient was kept in a semisitting position and given oxygen at 6 liters per minute by nasal cannula.

CONDITION DURING TRANSPORT
Finally, we need to report on the transport of the patient—the position in which he was transported and any changes that may have occurred in his condition en route. The latter information will help the doctor determine whether the patient's status has been improving or deteriorating during the time you were observing him, and it thus gives an indication of the urgency and seriousness of the patient's underlying condition. So we finish the report on our man with chest pain as follows:

The patient was transported in a semisitting position. His color improved during transport, but otherwise there was no change in his condition. Vital signs were rechecked twice and remained unchanged.

Now let us take it from the top and listen to the EMT's whole report:

The patient is a 48-year-old man who called for an ambulance because of chest pain. The pain began 2 hours ago when the patient was watching television. It is squeezing in nature and radiates into his jaw. It is accompanied by nausea and dizziness, but there is no shortness of breath. The patient took two aspirin shortly after the pain started but got no relief. He was hospitalized 2 years ago at Lakeview Hospital for a heart attack, but he hasn't had any further heart symptoms until today. The patient is treated by Dr. Koff for chronic bronchitis. Besides his hospitalization for a heart attack, he was hospitalized in 1972 for a kidney stone. He takes tetracycline and Tedrol regularly and has no known allergies. On physical exam, the patient was alert and sitting upright in a chair. His skin was pale, cold, and damp, and he appeared to be in moderate distress. His pulse was 110, thready, and regular; respirations were 18 and slightly labored; BP was 110 over 60. The patient's pupils were round, regular, midposition, and reactive to light. There was no cyanosis of the conjunctivae or lips. The jugular veins were distended with the patient at 45 degrees. The chest was clear; no rales were heard. The abdomen was soft. There was no edema of the back or lower extremities. The patient was kept in a semisitting position and given oxygen at 6 liters per minute by nasal cannula. He was transported in a semisitting position. His color improved during transport, but otherwise there was no change in his condition. Vital signs were rechecked twice and remained unchanged.

The EMT making this report has managed to present all the information collected during 15 or 20 minutes of history-taking and physical assessment in the space of less than 90 seconds. In addition, the material has been presented in such a way that it is easily grasped by any medical person listening, for the information proceeds in a logical sequence.

Compare the above report to the report on the same patient given by an EMT who is not very well organized:

"We have a man here with chest pain, and we're giving him some oxygen. He looks pretty bad. He's 48. He had a heart attack a couple of years ago. His pulse is 110, thready, and regular; his BP is 110 over 60, and his respirations are 18. He says the pain started 2 hours ago. He takes tetracycline and Tedrol for chronic bronchitis. His skin is very pale and cold. He says the pain is squeezing and goes into his jaw. He was in the hospital for a kidney stone in 1972. Uh, his pupils are equal. Let's see, what else? He's not allergic to anything. Oh yeah, and his lungs are clear. Uh, did I mention that he feels dizzy and sick to his stomach? There's no edema. Oh yeah, and he's conscious, by the way."

Which version of the report gives you a clearer picture of the patient and his problem? Which version gives you more confidence in the EMT who is making the report?

Presenting Medical Information

1. AGE and SEX of the patient 2. CHIEF COMPLAINT 3. History of the PRESENT ILLNESS 4. PAST MEDICAL HISTORY	INFORMATION FROM THE PATIENT OR BYSTANDERS

5. PHYSICAL EXAMINATION a. General appearance b. Vital signs c. Head-to-toe survey	DIRECT OBSERVATIONS
6. TREATMENT GIVEN IN THE FIELD	
7. CONDITION during transport	

MEDICAL RECORDS

Ideally, the report you write up in your trip sheet would follow the same format as the report you give orally in the emergency room. This is not usually very practical, however, for writing out the history and physical findings in the format for medical reporting is quite time-consuming, and an EMT who works a busy shift simply will not be able to keep up with the paperwork. For this reason, most ambulance forms are constructed in such a way that the EMT simply checks off boxes and fills in blank spaces. What is important is that the trip sheet be designed so that the EMT can record *all* the pertinent information about the call. This includes not only the information about the patient's history, physical findings, and treatment mentioned earlier, but also information pertaining to time, mileage, personnel, and so forth. There should also be ample space for drawing small diagrams—for example, a sketch of the accident scene to illustrate the position of a victim with respect to a damaged vehicle, or a body diagram to show the location of specific injuries on the patient.

DATE AND TIMES

The ambulance trip sheet should contain a record of the following times:

a. Time call was received
b. Time ambulance left for the call
c. Time ambulance reached the scene
d. Time ambulance left the scene
e. Time ambulance reached the hospital
f. Time ambulance back in service

These times are important for both legal and management purposes. The times listed above enable calculation of the duration of various aspects of the call. For example:

RESPONSE TIME = (c) − (a)
TIME SPENT AT THE SCENE = (d) − (c)
TIME UNTIL DEFINITIVE TREATMENT = (e) − (c)
TOTAL "DOWN" TIME = (f) − (b)

Accurate information about RESPONSE TIME enables the service to handle complaints regarding how long it took the ambulance to reach the patient. For a critically ill person, or his family, minutes can seem like hours, and it may seem as if the ambulance took forever to arrive when in fact the response time was only 5 minutes. Complete time data on the trip sheet can resolve such questions definitively.

The TIME SPENT AT THE SCENE and the TIME UNTIL DEFINITIVE TREATMENT are of concern to the medical advisor to the service. In reviewing the trip sheets, he or she will want to evaluate whether the EMTs are taking enough time to stabilize the patient properly or, on the other hand, whether they are spending too much time at the scene, thereby causing needless delay in the patient's receiving definitive care in the hospital.

The TOTAL "DOWN" TIME, that is, the time the ambulance was tied up with the call, is of interest to the manager of the service, who has to figure out how many ambulances are needed to cover the region. This is a matter not only of the number of calls but also of the amount of time each call keeps an ambulance occupied.

If the EMTs find it cumbersome to keep track of the times during a call, they should radio in to their dispatcher at each time indicated (e.g., "Arrived at the scene" or "Leaving for the hospital"). The dispatcher can make a note of each time, and the EMTs can get the information from dispatch later, when they write up their trip sheet.

MILEAGE

The mileage of the run is important for two reasons. First, it can be compared against the response time to determine whether the response was appropriate to the distance that had to be covered. If the distance to the call is 15 miles, for instance, it is unreasonable to expect a response time of 5 minutes. On the other hand, if the distance is half a mile and your response time was 20 minutes, you had better have some note in your trip sheet explaining why (e.g., "heavy traffic," "heavy snow on the road").

The second reason for noting the mileage is that these data, totalled up over a month or so, help the manager of the service plan the fuel and maintenance budget.

Ideally, the ambulance should be fitted with an odometer that can be reset to zero at the beginning of each run. Such a device makes it much easier to note the mileage for a given call.

CODE NO. | AMB. NO. | MO. | DAY | YEAR | TRIP NUMBER | PTS. TRN | GEOGRAPHICAL SITE CODE

E.D./FAMILY/PHYSICIAN AT SCENE SIGNATURE

E.D. NO.

PATIENT'S NAME — PHONE

TIMES: CALL RECEIVED · ENROUTE · ARRIVED AT SCENE · ENROUTE W/PAT. · ARRIVED AT DEST. · BACK IN SERVICE

MILEAGE TO SCENE · TO DEST. · TO BASE

SEX: 1 M 2 F — AGE — MOS.

PATIENT'S ADDRESS — ZIP

LOCATION PATIENT PICKED UP

NATURE OF CALL (AT SCENE)

MEDICAL COMMAND

1 BY TELEPHONE
2 WRITTEN STAND. ORDERS
3 VERBAL STAND. ORDERS
4 PHYSICIAN AT SITE
5 RADIO
6 NOT AVAILABLE
7 NONE REQUESTED

✓ IF COMMUN. DIFFICULTY ☐

NATURE OF CALL

1 EMERGENCY
2 URGENT
3 TRANSPORT
4 ASSIST
5 STAND BY

INCIDENT LOCATION

1 MOTOR VEHICLE
2 HOME
3 COMMERCIAL
4 FACTORY/INDUSTRY
5 MINE
6 STREET
7 FARM

✓ IF ACCIDENT ☐

CASE SEVERITY

1 MINOR
2 MODERATE
3 SEVERE
4 LIFE THREAT
5 D.O.A

PATIENT STATUS DURING TREATMENT

1 IMPROVED
2 UNCHG'D. STABLE
3 UNCHG'D. UNSTABLE
4 WORSENED
5 EXPIRED ENROUTE

COMMAND MD

COMMAND HOSPITAL

A-SYMPTOMS/INJURY TYPE

B-ANATOMICAL INJURY SITE

CREW — NO. — RTG.

INSURANCE COVERAGE

1 MEMBERSHIP PLAN
2 MEDICARE
3 DPA
4 UMWA
5 BLUE CROSS
6 TAX BASE
7 NONE
8 OTHER (write in)
9 UNKNOWN

INSURANCE COVERAGE NO.

PATIENT PICK'D UP — IF HSP

1 HOSPITAL
2 MORGUE/FUNERAL HOME
3 LONG TERM CARE FACILITY
4 RESIDENCE
5 DR.'S OFFICE/CLINIC
6 OTHER

PATIENT TAKEN TO — IF HSP

CPR IN PROGRESS ON ARRIVAL

1 GENERAL PUBLIC
2 1ST RESPONDER (inc. police/fire)
3 QRS
4 OTHER MEDICAL PERS.

☐ ✓ ADEQUATE
☐ ✓ INADEQUATE

CHECK IF APPLICABLE

1 ☐ NO PATIENT TRANSPORTED
2 ☐ CALLED OFF ENROUTE

PATIENT DECLINED: 3 ☐ TREATMENT 4 ☐ TRANSPORT

NONE DEEMED NECESSARY: 5 ☐ TREATMENT 6 ☐ TRANSPORT

7 ☐ TRANSPORTED BY OTHER MEANS

NARRATIVE

INITIAL — TIME — C-LUNG (S, L) — D-SKIN (C, T) — E-PUPILS (S, R, P)

FINAL — TIME — C-LUNG (S, L) — D-SKIN (C, T) — E-PUPILS (S, R, P)

PAIN

1 MINOR
2 MODERATE
3 SEVERE
4 VERY SEVERE

ALLERGIES

T ALS ARRIVED: I M E

MILITARY TIME	F	G-PULSE S R W I	H-RESP. R N I D S	B.P. SYST. / DIAST.	I-CARDIAC MONITOR (write-in)	CODE	RATE	J-DRUG/FLUID	K-ROUTE	L-AIDS GIVEN	AIDS & DRUG/FLUIDS GIVEN (write-in - incl. dosage)	M-IV S U D	BY EMT
	LEVEL OF CONSCIOUSNESS												

HEALTH OPERATIONS RESEARCH GROUP, UNIVERSITY OF PITTSBURGH/EMERGENCY MEDICAL SERVICE INSTITUTE

PAGE ____ OF ____ DRIVER ____________ ATTENDANT ____________

AMBULANCE COPY

Fig. 12-1. *Pittsburgh ambulance form. (Reproduced courtesy Professor Harvey Wolfe, University of Pittsburgh.)*

A - SYMPTOM INJURY CODES

01 Abrasion
02 Amputation
03 Asphyxiation
04 Avulsion
43 Bite - poisonous
44 Bite - non-poisonous
05 Burn - incl. thermal, chem., elect.
06 Cardiac Symptoms
39 Cardiac Arrest
07 Chills
08 Contagious disease
09 Contusion/bruise - minor trauma
10 Convulsions/seizure
unspec., petit mal, focal - site 00
systemic, grand mal - site 26
11 Crushing
42 Dehydration
12 Diabetic
13 Difficulty breathing/shortness of breath
14 Dislocation
41 Disorientation
15 Dizziness/fainting - weakness
16 Drowning
17 Electrical Shock
18 Fever
46 Foreign body - obstruction
19 Fracture
A - closed
B - open
20 Hemorrhaging
45 Hypersensitivity - incl. allergic rxn. to meds.
21 Impairment - similar to that caused by alcohol
47 Insect bite/sting
22 Internal trauma (closed blunt) - major
23 Laceration - cut
24 Mental disorder
25 Nausea
26 Obstetrics - delivery
27 Pain
28 Paralysis
48 Paresthesia (incl. numbness)
29 Penetrating/puncture wound (incl. stab)
30 Poison (incl. drug overdose)
31 Poison (other)
32 Projectile wound - high velocity (incl. gunshot)
40 Respiratory arrest
33 Shock
34 Sprain - strain
35 Stroke
49 Swelling
36 Unconscious
38 Vomiting

B - ANATOMICAL SITE CODE

01 Head
02 Face
03 Eye
04 Ear
05 Neck
06 Shoulder
07 Arm (upper)
08 Elbow
09 Forearm
10 Wrist
11 Hand
12 Fingers
13 Back
14 Chest
15 Abdomen - GI
16 Pelvis
17 Buttocks - perineum
18 Hip
19 Thigh
20 Knee
21 Leg (lower)
22 Ankle
23 Foot
24 Toes
25 Genito-urinary
26 Systemic
27 Upper respiratory tract/airway

C - LUNG CODES

SOUNDS
1 Clear
2 Stridor
3 Rales - incl. wheeze, ronchi
4 Diminished
5 Absent

LOCATION
1 Bilaterally Equal
2 Right
3 Left

D - SKIN CODES

COLOR
1 Normal
2 Cyanotic
3 Pale, ashen
4 Flush

TEMPERATURE
1 Normal
2 Hot, dry
3 Hot, wet
4 Cool, dry
5 Cool, wet

E - PUPIL CODES

SIZE
1 Equal
2 Unequal
3 Med./surg anomaly

REACTIVITY
1 Reactive
2 Not reactive

POSITION
1 Midposition
2 Dilated
3 Constricted

F - CONSCIOUSNESS LEVEL

1 Alert & oriented
2 Disoriented
3 Response to verbal stimuli
4 Response to pain stimuli w. purpose
5 Response to pain stimuli w/o purpose
6 Decorticate/decerebrate (rigid)
7 Flaccid/unresponsive

G - PULSE CODES

Include both Character and Regularity with Rate.

CHARACTER
S - Strong
W - Weak

REGULARITY
R - Regular
I - Irregular

H - RESPIRATORY CODES

Include both Rhythm and Depth with Rate.

RHYTHM
R - Regular, smooth
I - Irregular

DEPTH
N - Normal
D - Deep
S - Shallow

I - MONITOR CODES

01 N.S.R.
02 Sinus tach
03 Sinus brad
04 Sinus arrhythmia
05 S. A. arrest
06 Wandering pacemaker
07 P.A.C.'s
08 P.A.T.
09 Atrial flutter
10 Atrial fibrillation
11 P.N.C.'s
12 AV nodal tach
13 Nodal rhythm/junctional
14 SVT
16 1st° A.V. block
17 2nd° A.V. block T-1
18 2nd° A.V. block T-2
19 3rd° A.V. block
20 PVC-5 or less per min.
21 PVC-6 or more per min.
22 PVC on T-wave
23 PVC - Bigeminy
24 PVC - Trigeminy
25 V. tach
26 V. fibrillation
27 Asystole
31 Idioventricular rhythm
32 EMD - electro.mech. dissoc.
98 Other (explain on form)

J - DRUG/FLUID CODES

03 Atropine
09 Calcium chloride or gluconate
20 Corticosteroids
10 Dextrose in water - D_5W
19 Dextrose in water - $D_{50}W$/Glucose
11 Dextrose in saline
12 Dextrose in ringers lactate
21 Diazepam (Valium)
22 Diphenhydramine HCL (Benadryl)
16 Dopamine
05 Epinephrine
18 Furosemide (Lasix)
23 Ipecac
07 Isoproterenol
01 Lidocaine HCL
06 Metaraminol (Aramine)
15 Naloxone (Narcan)
08 Narcotic (incl. M.S.)
24 Nitroglycerine (NTG)
25 Nitrous Oxide (NO_2)
26 Oxygen
17 Plasmanate
13 Ringers Lactate (RL)
14 Saline (NSS)
04 Sodium bicarbonate
98 Other

K - MEDICATION ROUTE

50 Endotracheal
51 Intramuscular
52 Subcutaneous
53 Oral
54 Sublingual
55 Suppository
56 IV bolus (push)
57 IV infusion (drip)
58 Inhalation
59 Topical
98 Other

M - IV

S - Successful
U - Unsuccessful
D - Discontinued

L - AIDS GIVEN

03 Aspirate (suction)
37 Blood drawn
06 CPR
07 Cervical collar
08 Control bleeding
09 Defibrillation
10 Demand Valve
11 Dress wound
29 EKG transmitted
12 Esophageal Obturator Airway
13 Extricate patient
34 Ice pack
39 Irrigate with water/saline
15 MAST trousers
17 OB delivery
18 Oropharyngeal airway
19 Orthopedic stretcher
04 Positive Pres. Ventilation (excl. demand valve)
38 Precordial thump
22 Psychiatric intervention
23 Restrain patient
24 Rotating tourniquet
25 Sand bags
26 Sling
27 Spine board (3 ft.)
28 Spine board (6 ft.)
36 Splint - incl. air, board, other
42 Stairchair
35 Stretcher
40 Thrust - abd./chest
30 Tourniquet
31 Tracheal intubation
32 Traction splint
41 Valsalva maneuver
98 Other

TRI-COUNTY EMS COUNCIL

CLINTON · EATON · INGHAM

Standard Ambulance Report Form

1.

AGENCY NAME: ______________________ DATE ________

YOUR RUN NUMBER ________ YOUR UNIT NUMBER ________ TOTAL MILES TRAVELED ________

2.

TIMES (No Military): CIRCLE

Call Received	________	AM PM
Ambulance Enroute	________	AM PM
Arrived Location	________	AM PM
Departed Location	________	AM PM
Arrived Hospital	________	AM PM
Available for Next Call	________	AM PM

3. PATIENT INFORMATION:

NAME ______________________ ☐ M ☐ F AGE ______

HOME ADDRESS ______________________

PICKUP LOCATION ______________________
Street Address City Village Township County

AREA: ☐ Urban ☐ Model city ☐ Suburban ☐ Rural

LOCATION TYPE: ☐ Street-Highway ☐ Home ☐ Public Bldg. ☐ Business ☐ Industrial ☐ Recreation area ☐ Hospital ☐ Dr. Office ☐ Other ________

4. NATURE OF CALL WHEN RECEIVED: ☐ Emergency ☐ Urgent Transfer

5. AID PROVIDED BEFORE AMBULANCE ARRIVED:

☐ None ☐ Yes—Helpful ☐ Yes—Harmful ☐ CPR ☐ Splinting ☐ Controlled Bleeding ☐ Extrication ☐ Shock Treatment

BY WHOM? ☐ City Police ☐ County Sheriff ☐ State Police ☐ Fire Dept. ☐ Citizen ______________________

6. STATUS OF PATIENT:

	1	2	3	4
Appearance:	☐ Good	☐ Fair	☐ Poor	☐ Critical
Consciousness:	☐ Normal	☐ Dazed	☐ Disoriented	☐ Unconscious
Breathing:	☐ Normal	☐ Rapid	☐ Labored	☐ Absent
Bleeding:	☐ None	☐ Minimum	☐ Moderate	☐ Severe
Pain:	☐ None	☐ Minimum	☐ Moderate	☐ Severe
Pulse:	☐ Normal	☐ Slow	☐ Rapid	☐ Absent
Pupils:	☐ Equal	☐ Unequal __ side larger	☐ Constricted	☐ Dilated
Range of Motion:	☐ Normal (full)	☐ None below the waist	☐ One side only	☐ None below neck
Skin:	☐ Normal	☐ Warm and wet	☐ Hot and dry	☐ Cold and clammy

7. CAUSE OF INJURY: ________ INJURY (TYPE CODE) ________

ILLNESS (TYPE CODE) ________ INJURY (SITE CODE) ________

OTHER ILLNESS OR INJURY ______________________

8. AID PROVIDED BY AMBULANCE CREW:

☐ DRY RUN (CODE ________)
☐ AID GIVEN, NOT TRANSPORTED
☐ TRANSPORTED, NO AID GIVEN
☐ CPR
☐ AIRWAY CLEARED
☐ SUCTION
☐ ESOPHAGEAL AIRWAY
☐ RESPIRATORY ASSIST
☐ OXYGEN
☐ CONTROLLED HEMORRHAGE
☐ BANDAGING
☐ ANTI-SHOCK
☐ IV FLUIDS (SPECIFY IN #9)
☐ MAST TROUSERS
☐ LIMB SPLINTS
☐ EXTRICATION
☐ SHORT BACKBOARD
☐ LONG BACKBOARD
☐ PSYCHOLOGICAL AID
☐ RESTRAINTS
☐ OB ASSIST/DELIVERY

9. COMMENTS AND DETAIL AID: ______________________

10. VITAL SIGNS

	1	2
BLOOD PRESSURE	____	____
PULSE	____	____
RESPIRATION	____	____

11. COMMUNICATIONS WITH HOSPITAL

☐ YES — HEAR
☐ YES — TELEPHONE
☐ NO

12. RUN CONDITIONS

	TO SCENE	TO DEST.
LIGHTS	☐	☐
SIREN	☐	☐
SEVERE TRAFFIC	☐	☐
SEVERE WEATHER	☐	☐
MECHANICAL TROUBLE	☐	☐
COMMUNICATION TROUBLE	☐	☐

13. DESTINATION: HOSPITAL CODE

OTHER ________

14. AMBULANCE CREW INFORMATION: circle number in crew 1 2 3 4

DRIVER ________ EMT ☐ Yes ☐ No ATTENDANT ________ EMT ☐ Yes ☐ No

ATTENDANT ________ EMT ☐ Yes ☐ No ATTENDANT ________ EMT ☐ Yes ☐ No

AMBULANCE COPY

Fig. 12-2. *Tri-county ambulance form, Lansing, Michigan. (Reproduced courtesy Garry Briese.)*

SUSPECTED ILLNESS CODES

Code	
ABP	— Abdominal Pain
ABM	— Abortion-Miscarriage
AST	— Asthma
CRD	— Cardiac Problems
CHL	— Chills
CMM	— Communicable Disease
CNV	— Convulsions (Describe on Form)
DIA	— Diabetic Coma
SOB	— Difficulty in Breathing—Shortness of Breath
DIZ	— Dizziness—Fainting—Weakness
EMP	— Emphysema
FVR	— Fever
STM	— Stomach Problems
GEN	— Genitourinary Problems
HEX	— Heat Exhaustion
HES	— Heat Stroke (Sunstroke)
HMN	— Hemorrhaging (Nasal)
HMV	— Hemorrhaging (Vaginal)
HMO	— Hemorrhaging (Other—Describe on Form)
DNK	— Impairment Similar To That Caused By Alcohol
INS	— Insulin Shock
MEN	— Mental Disorder(s)
NAU	— Nausea
OBS	— Obstetric
PAR	— Paralysis (Describe on Form)
PSN	— Poison (State Type, Amount and Route Taken in Section 9) (Includes Drug Overdose)
SHK	— Shock
CVA	— Stroke—CVA
TRM	— Terminal Illness
VOM	— Vomiting
UNK	— Unknown
OTH	— Other (Describe on Form)

SUSPECTED INJURY CODES

Code	Site
HED	— Head
FAC	— Face
EYE	— Eye
NEK	— Neck
UAS	— Upper Arm—Shoulder
LAE	— Lower Arm—Elbow
HWR	— Hand—Wrist
FGR	— Fingers
BCK	— Back
CHT	— Chest
ABD	— Abdomen
PLV	— Pelvis
BUT	— Buttocks—Perineum
ULH	— Upper Leg—Hip
LLK	— Lower Leg—Knee
FTA	— Foot—Ankle
TOE	— Toes
MLT	— Multiple
OTH	— Other (Explain on Report Form)

Code	Type
ABS	— Abrasion
AMP	— Amputation
AVL	— Avulsion
BRN	— Burn
CNC	— Concussion
CNT	— Contusion—Bruise
CRU	— Crushing
DSL	— Dislocation
FXR	— Fracture
INT	— Internal
LAC	— Laceration—Cut
PUN	— Puncture
SPR	— Sprain—Strain
APH	— Asphyxiation
DWN	— Drowning
ELC	— Electrocution (Electrical Shock)
OTH	— Other (Explain on Report Form)

DRY RUN CODES

(Explain Circumstances Under Comments)

Code	
5	— No Emergency Health Care Needed
10	— Cancelled By Requester
15	— Patient Needed But Refused Care
20	— Patient Went By Other Means (Explain Under Comments)
25	— Prank
30	— Victim DOA—Not Moved
35	— Unable To Locate
40	— Other (Explain Under Comments)

(A Dry Run Is Any Run In Which Patient Is Not Transported)

PATIENT INFORMATION
Some identifying information about the patient is necessary, both for billing purposes in areas that charge for ambulance service and to enable follow-up of selected cases. At the least, one should record the patient's name, age, sex, and address.

DESTINATION
The trip sheet should indicate to what hospital the patient was taken and, when possible, the name of the physician who received the EMT's report. This information permits follow-up of selected cases and also establishes the transfer of responsibility for the patient's care.

CREW
The names of all crew members should be recorded on each trip sheet, together with the unit number of the ambulance. If anyone other than the ambulance team participated in the care of the patient in the field (e.g., a nurse or physician bystander), his or her name should also be recorded. Any orders received by radio from a physician should be noted as well, with the name of the physician who issued the orders. All of this information is necessary for legal purposes in the event that the case should ever go to court.

ADDITIONAL INFORMATION
Depending on local needs and research interests, the ambulance service in any given area may wish to include additional types of information on the trip sheet. There may be an interest, for example, in tabulating the locations of patients: what percentage of calls came from the home versus the place of work, and so forth. Or it may be of interest to know how often the call came from the patient himself versus how often a family member or bystander initiated the call. These and many other types of information can be built into the trip sheet, but extra information should be kept within reasonable bounds so that the trip sheet does not become too complicated to fill out accurately.

The ambulance record should always be filled out in at least TWO COPIES, and the original should be left with the patient in the emergency room. The EMT's record of the patient's condition in the field provides crucial baseline information for the emergency room staff, and probably the most important function of the trip sheet is to *communicate* information, in a permanent form, to those who will take over responsibility for the patient.

Sample trip sheets are shown in Figures 12-1 and 12-2—one from the greater Pittsburgh area and the other from Lansing, Michigan. Each reflects the specific needs and concerns of the ambulance services involved, but both contain the fundamental information listed in this chapter.

Always keep in mind when filling out an ambulance form that it is a LEGAL DOCUMENT and can be introduced as evidence in court. For that reason, the trip sheet should be as accurate and complete as possible and should be free of flippant comments. So take time as soon as possible after the call to record all the details of the case thoroughly and legibly.

> THE MEDICAL RECORD IS A LEGAL DOCUMENT. MAKE SURE YOUR RECORDS ARE ACCURATE, LEGIBLE, AND COMPLETE.

Once you have completed your record, do not alter it. If you have made a mistake, draw a single line through the error, make a note that it was an error, and explain. Do not erase any part of the record or use correction fluid to cover anything you've written.

SAMPLE CASE PRESENTATION

To summarize the material presented in this chapter, we conclude with a sample patient report, with the various components labelled. In the chapters that follow, we shall present more such sample cases—dealing with specific illnesses or injuries—in order to depict typical examples of various conditions and also to refresh our memories about the way medical information is presented.

SEX — AGE — CHIEF COMPLAINT — PERTINENT NEGATIVE — PRESENT ILLNESS — PAST MEDICAL HISTORY

The patient is an 18-year-old [AGE] woman [SEX] who called for an ambulance because of shortness of breath. [CHIEF COMPLAINT] The patient is a known asthmatic and regularly takes Tedrol for her asthma. During the past few days, however, her symptoms have been getting worse despite the medications, and she has begun coughing a lot and bringing up yellow sputum. She denies having had any fever. [PERTINENT NEGATIVE] Presently she is so short of breath that she says she can't even sleep. [PRESENT ILLNESS] She's used her inhaler, but it hasn't helped. The patient has no other known medical problems. She was hospitalized for an appendectomy last year. She takes no medications other than those for her asthma. She is allergic to ragweed, pollen, dust, and aspirin. [PAST MEDICAL HISTORY] On physical exam, she was sitting bolt upright, struggling to breathe, obviously in acute distress. Skin was warm and moist. Pupils were equal and reactive to

PERTINENT NEGATIVES	light. There was no cyanosis of the lips or nail beds. Neck veins were flat. There were very tight wheezes audible all over the chest on inhalation, and the chest appeared hyperinflated. There was no edema.	PHYSICAL EXAM
	The patient was given oxygen at 6 liters per minute by nasal cannula and was transported in a sitting position to the hospital.	TREATMENT
	There was no change in her condition during transport.	CONDITION DURING TRANSPORT

VOCABULARY

down time The total amount of time an ambulance is tied up on a call, from the time the ambulance leaves for the call until the ambulance goes back into service, ready for another call.

pertinent negative A symptom or sign that the patient does *not* have but might be expected to have, given his or her chief complaint.

response time The total time elapsed from the moment the ambulance service receives a call for help to the moment the ambulance team reaches the patient.

trip sheet The written record of an ambulance call.

FURTHER READING

Briese G. SIFRA—A standard information reporting form for ambulances. *Emerg Med Serv* 5(2):58, 1976.

Editorial. The ultimate run sheet. *Emerg Med Serv* 13(10): 152, 1984.

Griffin PM. An audit method for ambulance calls. *Emergency* 11(2):9, 1979.

Henry GL (Ed.). Legal rounds: About the medical record. *Emerg Med* 22(2):47, 1990.

Hirsch HL. Legal implications of patient records. *South Med J* 72:726, 1979.

V. TRAUMA

It was the publication by the National Academy of Sciences in 1966 of a pamphlet called Accidental Death and Disability: The Neglected Disease of Modern Society *that spurred the modernization of ambulance services in the United States. That landmark study reported that, in 1965, 52 million accidental injuries killed 107,000 Americans, temporarily disabled another 10 million, and caused permanent disability to another 400,000—at a cost to the nation of $18 billion. The report further pointed out that, as of that time, "most ambulances used in this country are unsuitable, have incomplete fixed equipment, carry inadequate supplies, and are manned by untrained attendants." There was clearly a need to upgrade the care given to injured people before they reached the hospital.*

The EMT was born of this necessity. During the 20 years since publication of the National Academy of Sciences report, the EMT has come into his own and become a vital link in the EMS chain. And although the EMT has acquired skills in managing many types of emergencies outside the hospital, it is in the management of trauma—the "neglected disease" that gave impetus to the creation of the EMT—that the EMT can have the greatest potential impact.

Today, there are about 165,000 deaths from trauma each year in the United States, and for each death there are at least two cases of permanent disability. Furthermore, trauma is primarily a disease of the young and of people in their prime. It is the leading cause of death and disability among Americans under the age of 38. Thus the cost in lost productivity is very high. According to recent statistics, the total annual cost in the United States of accidental trauma—including medical expenses, lost wages, and indirect work losses—comes to around $50 billion. And this cost is rising as the death rate from trauma continues to rise—by about 1 percent a year. Thus, now even more than 20 years ago, trauma is one of the most urgent health problems in the United States and most other countries.

Like the word shock, *the word* trauma *has several meanings. When a lay person speaks of trauma, often he is referring to a shattering emotional experience; for instance, "It was very traumatic for me when my son died." In medicine, the word* trauma *means "injury," and it implies that the injury was sustained rapidly or violently. Cuts, bruises, fractures, and burns are all considered trauma, for they involve destructive forces and occur within minutes or seconds. The injury that a smoker does to his or her lungs, on the other hand, is not trauma, strictly speaking, for it occurs gradually, over several years.*

In this section, we will look at various forms of trauma: trauma to the skin, to the nervous system, to bones, and to other specific parts of the body. In each case, we will consider the normal function of the system involved, the mechanisms and signs of injury, and the method of treatment in the field. Then, having reviewed the various types of trauma, we will conclude the section with a consideration of triage—the sorting of patients according to the severity of their injuries.

While the chapters on trauma that follow focus on the assessment and treatment of injured people, it is important for the EMT to be aware that trauma is, by and large, a preventable disease. Studies have shown beyond any doubt, for example, that the reduction of speed limits, the use of seat belts by motorists, and the wearing of helmets by motorcyclists can drastically reduce the incidence of serious injury and death on our highways. We have mentioned earlier that one important role of an EMT is that of health educator. Perhaps nowhere is health education more critical today than in the area of accident prevention. Emergency medical personnel should be in the forefront of this health education effort—campaigning for enforcement of drunk driving penalties, for mandatory use of seat belts and motorcycle helmets, for industrial safety programs, and so forth. And remember: Accident prevention begins at home. So when you get into your ambulance (or your family car), buckle up for safety. The life you save may be your own.

FURTHER READING

Alexander RH et al. The effect of advanced life support and sophisticated hospital systems on motor vehicle mortality. *J Trauma* 24:486, 1984.

Alyono D, Perry J. Impact of speed limit. I. Chest injuries: Review of 966 cases. *J Thorac Cardiovasc Surg* 83:519, 1982.

Avery JG. The overall assessment of the medical effects of seat belt legislation in the United Kingdom. *Arch Emerg Med* 2:232, 1985.

Bachulis BL et al. Patterns of injury in helmeted and nonhelmeted motorcyclists. *Am J Surg* 155:708, 1988.

Berger LR et al. Promoting the use of car safety devices for infants—an intensive health education approach. *Pediatrics* 74:16, 1984.

Cales R, Trunkey D. Preventable trauma deaths: A review of trauma care systems development. *JAMA* 254:1059, 1985.

Carr WP et al. Injury patterns and helmet effectiveness among hospitalized motorcyclists. *Minn Med* 64:521, 1981.

Decker MD et al. The use and efficacy of child restraint devices. *JAMA* 252:2571, 1984.

Dreghorn C. The effect of seat belt legislation on a district general hospital. *Injury* 16:415, 1985.

Freedman LS. Initial assessment of the effect of compulsory use of seat belts on car occupants' injuries and the trauma department workload. *Injury* 16:60, 1984.

Goldbaum GM et al. Failure to use seat belts in the United States: The 1981–1983 behavioral risk factor surveys. *JAMA* 255:2459, 1986.

Guerrin D, MacKinnon P. An assessment of the California child passenger restraint requirements. *Am J Pub Health* 75:142, 1985.

Heilman D et al. Motorcycle-related trauma and helmet usage in North Dakota. *Ann Emerg Med* 11:659, 1982.

Hicks TC et al. Resuscitation and transfer of trauma patients: A prospective study. *Ann Emerg Med* 11:296, 1982.

Krantz KPG. Head and neck injuries to motorcycle and moped riders with special regard to the effect of protective helmets. *Injury* 16:253, 1985.

Lowe DK et al. Patterns of death, complication, and error in the management of motor vehicle accident victims: Implications for a regional system of trauma care. *J Trauma* 23:503, 1983.

Lowenfels A, Miller T. Alcohol and trauma. *Ann Emerg Med* 13:1056, 1984.

Luna GK et al. The influence of ethanol intoxication on outcome of injured motorcyclists. *J Trauma* 24:695, 1984.

Luna GK et al. The role of helmets in reducing head injuries from motorcycle accidents. *West J Med* 135:89, 1981.

Maull K. Alcohol abuse: Its implications in trauma care. *South Med J* 75:794, 1982.

McSwain N, Petrucelli E. Medical consequence of motorcycle helmet nonusage. *J Trauma* 24:233, 1984.

Munoz E. Economic cost of trauma, United States, 1982. *J Trauma* 24:237, 1984.

National Academy of Science, National Research Council. Accidental Death and Disability: The Neglected Disease of Modern Society. *U.S. Department of Health, Education and Welfare, Emergency Medical Services No. A-13.* Washington DC: Government Printing Office, 1966.

Ornato JP et al. Impact of improved emergency medical services and emergency trauma care on the reduction in mortality from trauma. *J Trauma* 25:575, 1985.

Orsay EM et al. Prospective study of the effect of safety belts on morbidity and health care costs in motor-vehicle accidents. *JAMA* 260:3598, 1988.

Polen MR, Friedman GD. Automobile injury—selected risk factors and prevention in the health care setting. *JAMA* 259:77, 1988.

Pye G et al. Effect of seat belt legislation on injuries in road traffic accidents in Nottingham. *Br Med J* 288:756, 1984.

Rivara FP et al. The public cost of motorcycle trauma. *JAMA* 260:221, 1988.

Sanders RS et al. Bless the seats and the children: The physician and the legislative process. *JAMA* 252:2613, 1984.

Trunkey D. Trauma. *Sci Amer* 249:28, 1983.

13. WOUNDS AND BURNS

OBJECTIVES

In this chapter, we shall look at one of the most vital and also the most visible of human organs: the skin. We will examine the structure of normal skin and the tasks it carries out, and we will look at a variety of injuries that produce damage to the skin and underlying soft tissues. On completion of this chapter, the reader should be able to

1. List at least three functions of normal skin
2. Identify the layers of skin, given a description of various layers
3. Identify the following soft tissue injuries, given a description of their signs and symptoms: (a) contusion, (b) abrasion, (c) laceration, (d) avulsion, and (e) puncture wound
4. List the measures in treating (a) a closed soft tissue injury and (b) an open soft tissue injury
5. List the special measures that should be taken in the case of (a) an amputated part and (b) an impaled object
6. List the information that should be obtained in taking the history of a burned patient
7. Indicate in the correct sequence the steps in evaluating a burned patient
8. Identify the correct techniques of extinguishing the flames of a burning person, given a list of various techniques
9. Identify the signs of impending airway edema in a burned patient, given a list of various signs
10. Identify those burn victims who should receive oxygen, given a description of several victims
11. Identify first-, second-, and third-degree burns, given a description of several types of burns
12. Calculate the extent of a burn using the rule of nines, given a description of the parts of the body involved in the burn
13. Identify those patients who have critical burns, given a description of several patients with various burn injuries
14. List the items of particular emphasis in the secondary survey of the burned patient
15. Identify the correct methods of treatment for first-, second-, and third-degree burns, given a list of various treatments
16. List the steps in treating a chemical burn (a) to the skin and (b) to the eye
17. Indicate what differentiates an electric burn from a thermal burn
18. Identify the FIRST step in treating a victim of electric burns, given a list of steps
19. Indicate what items should be given particular emphasis in the secondary survey of the electric burn victim
20. Identify the kind of injuries one should anticipate in (a) an electric burn victim and (b) a lightning victim, given a list of various injuries
21. Identify those situations in which one is more likely to be struck by lightning, given a list of situations
22. Indicate which victim(s) of lightning injury

should be treated first, given a description of several casualties found at the scene of a lightning strike
23. List the items of particular emphasis in the secondary survey of a lightning victim
24. Indicate what materials are suitable for (a) dressings and (b) bandages, given a list of materials
25. Identify improperly applied bandages, given a description of the bandaging techniques

STRUCTURE AND FUNCTION OF THE SKIN

The skin is one of the most important and most remarkable of human organs, and it does much more than simply keep the rest of the body neatly packaged. The skin is a tough, resilient tissue that forms the interface between our bodies and the environment, protecting what is inside from what is outside.

FUNCTIONS OF THE SKIN

The skin serves several crucial functions in adapting the human animal to its environment. To begin with, the skin has a PROTECTIVE function, for it acts as a fortress to seal the body off from harmful elements in the environment. Bacteria, for example, are everywhere around us, but unless the skin is broken, bacteria cannot gain access to the body through it. Bacteria are found on the skin surface but not in its deeper layers, for the skin effectively restricts them from passing into the tissues beneath. The skin also protects by cushioning the structures within it from bumps and bruises, thereby blunting the impact of blows.

In the second place, the skin is the principal organ of TEMPERATURE REGULATION. In order to survive, the body must maintain a nearly constant internal temperature around 98.6°F (37°C), regardless of whether the body is out shovelling snow in subzero temperatures or sunbathing in 100°F heat. It is the skin that helps the body maintain its internal temperature at a constant level, despite enormous variations in the environmental temperature, and it does so through several mechanisms. When the body is exposed to *high* temperatures, the blood vessels of the skin dilate, allowing more blood to reach the body surface and excess heat to radiate into the atmosphere. Furthermore, the skin cools the body through evaporation of water from its surface—the process we call sweating. In a *cold* environment, the blood vessels of the skin constrict, thereby shunting blood away from the cold temperatures outside. The layer of fat just beneath the skin also serves as good winter insulation, minimizing heat loss to the outside.

A third function of the skin is to PREVENT EXCESSIVE WATER LOSS from the body. Over 70 percent of the human body is composed of water, and without skin to enclose it, this water would simply evaporate and we would all look like prunes on the first warm day of spring. Fortunately for us, however, the skin forms a watertight seal around the human body and thereby keeps our internal fluids intact.

Finally, the skin serves as a SENSE ORGAN, providing us with all kinds of vital information about our environment. Through a vast network of nerve endings, the skin is constantly relaying messages to the brain: "Hot—don't touch!" "Ouch—danger!" "Someone's pushing!" or "That feels nice." The skin thus sends us information about heat, cold, pressure, pain, and pleasant stimuli, and it thereby helps the brain decide what situations to avoid.

If there is significant damage to the skin, it is clear that all of the above functions may be jeopardized. Bacterial invaders will come charging into the body through any breach in the skin, even a small cut. When there is widespread damage to the skin, as in burns, the ability to regulate body temperature may be impaired, and massive fluid loss—enough to cause shock—can also occur across the skin surface. Deep burns can even destroy the nerve endings in the skin, rendering the victim incapable of feeling heat, cold, or even pain in the damaged area and thus incapable of preventing further damage to the area. For these reasons, the skin is as necessary to life as the heart and lungs.

Functions of the Skin
- PROTECTION
- TEMPERATURE REGULATION
- PREVENTION OF WATER LOSS
- SENSATION

STRUCTURE OF THE SKIN

The skin comprises two principal layers, called the epidermis and the dermis (Fig. 13-1). The **epidermis,** or outermost layer, is the body's first line of defense against bacterial or chemical invaders and is particularly tough and resilient. The outer cells of the epidermis are hardened, dead cells that are constantly being rubbed off and replaced by new cells. The deeper layers of the epidermis contain cells that are constantly duplicating to give rise to the cells of the upper layer. In addition, the deeper epidermal layers contain special cells with granules of **melanin**; it is these melanin-containing cells, together with capillary blood flow in the skin, that determine the skin color. A person with only a small amount of melanin will have relatively light skin that visibly reflects changes in blood flow, while large amounts of melanin make the skin brown or black.

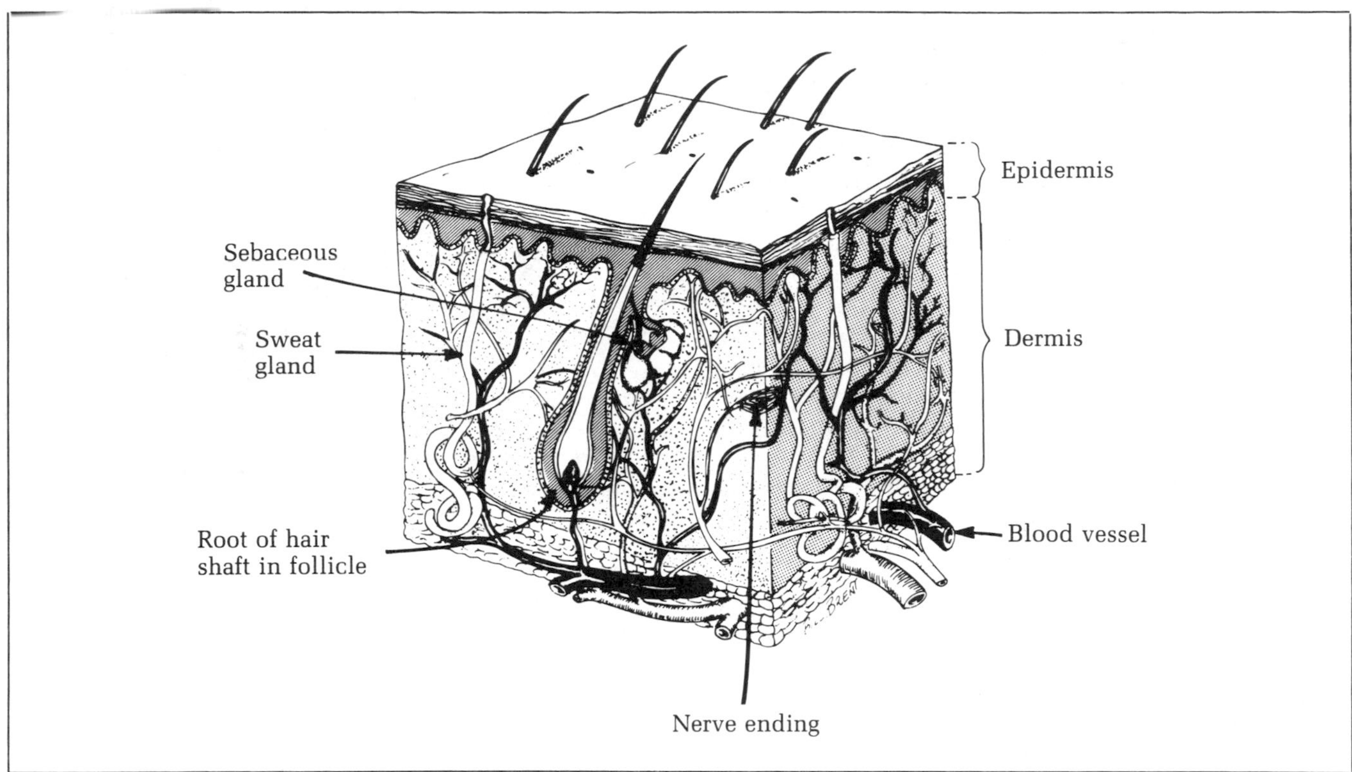

Fig. 13-1. *Structure of the skin.*

Beneath the epidermis is a tough, elastic layer of connective tissue called the **dermis,** which contains several specialized structures:

- NERVE ENDINGS located in the dermis are of several types, allowing one to perceive temperature, touch, pressure, and pain.
- BLOOD VESSELS in the dermis carry oxygen and nutrients to the skin.
- SWEAT GLANDS in the dermis produce sweat, which consists of water and salt and which is discharged from the sweat glands through a duct that leads to the outer surface of the body. Each sweat gland connects with a single pore. Normally, the body secretes about 500 to 1,000 ml (1 pint–1 quart) of sweat in a 24-hour period, but during strenuous activity, the sweat glands are capable of increasing their output to as much as 1 liter per hour.
- HAIR FOLLICLES are structures that produce hair and enclose the hair roots. Each follicle contains a single hair, and attached to each hair follicle is a tiny muscle that makes the follicle stand up vertically when it contracts. Cold or fright can cause contraction of these tiny muscles, and the result is an appearance of the skin known as "goose flesh."
- SEBACEOUS GLANDS are located beside hair follicles and produce an oily substance called **sebum,** which is discharged to the skin surface along the hair shafts. Sebum gives the hair and skin their natural oiliness, and it is important in both waterproofing the skin and keeping the skin soft, so that it does not crack.

Just beneath the surface lies the **subcutaneous tissue,** which is composed mainly of fat. This subcutaneous layer serves as insulation for the body and also gives the body some of its characteristic curves.

The skin and soft tissues beneath it can be injured in a variety of ways: by blunt impact, by penetration, by extremes of temperature, or by corrosive chemicals. In the following discussions, we will look at three types of soft tissue injury: blunt (closed) injury, open injury, and burns.

CLOSED SOFT TISSUE INJURIES

A blunt or closed wound is one in which there is damage to tissues beneath the skin but no break in the skin surface itself. If a blunt object, such as a baseball bat, strikes the skin with sufficient force, it crushes the tissues beneath the skin and causes disruption of small blood vessels. Blood and plasma leak out of the damaged blood vessels, causing SWELLING AND PAIN, and as the blood migrates toward the skin surface, it becomes visible as a black-and-blue mark (ECCHYMOSIS). This kind of injury is called a bruise, or **contusion.** If large blood vessels are torn at the site of the contusion, or if there is extensive tissue damage, blood may pool and form a lump beneath the skin surface called a **hematoma.** A hematoma represents the most serious form of contusion, and hematomas associated with fractures can contain as much as a pint of blood.

The treatment of a contusion depends upon its size. A small bruise requires no special treatment, although the application of cold compresses may provide some pain relief and also lessen swelling. More extensive or severe soft tissue injuries do require treatment, for subcutaneous bleeding and leakage of plasma can be of such volume as to cause shock. Thus the following measures should be taken:

1. Apply COUNTERPRESSURE to the injured area to control bleeding. If the contusion is on an extremity, an air splint is an excellent means of providing uniform pressure to the extremity, and it also stabilizes any fractures that might be associated with the injury. If the contusion is on the trunk, use a pressure dressing to control subcutaneous bleeding.
2. Apply COLD PACKS to the injured area to reduce swelling. If cold packs are used, they must be kept in place for at least 30 minutes to be effective, for it takes at least that long for the cold temperature to be conducted to the subcutaneous tissues. Placing the cold pack in a moistened towel makes it conduct cold more effectively.
3. If the contusion is on an extremity, ELEVATE THE EXTREMITY after it has been placed in an air splint. A badly contused arm or leg can be elevated on a pillow, for example, which encourages drainage of excess fluid from the limb by gravity.

OPEN WOUNDS

An open wound, as the name implies, is one in which there is a break in the skin, thus rendering the body vulnerable to invasion by bacteria and subsequent infection.

TYPES OF OPEN WOUNDS

Open wounds are of four general types: (1) abrasions, (2) lacerations, (3) avulsions, and (4) puncture wounds.

Abrasion

An abrasion is a superficial wound in which rubbing or scraping causes loss of part of the skin surface, as in a "brush burn" or "mat burn" (Fig. 13-2). Abrasions tend to be quite painful and are often embedded with dirt, gravel, or other foreign materials. Usually bleeding is minimal—just a little oozing here and there from broken capillaries at the skin surface.

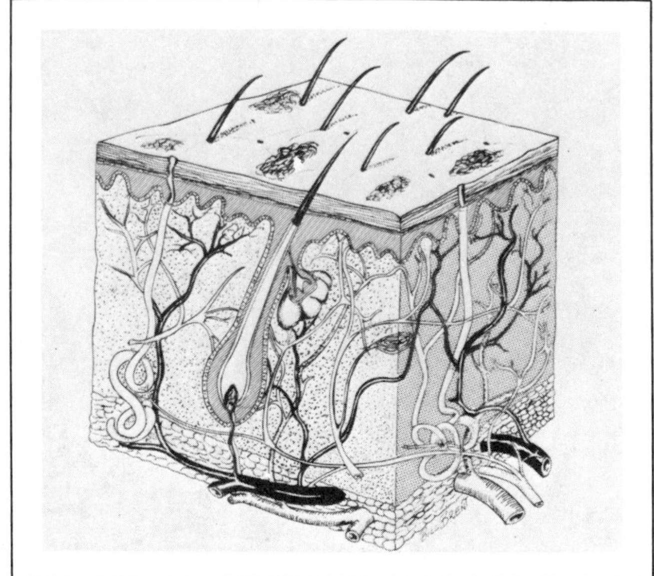

Fig. 13-2. *Abrasion.*

Laceration

A laceration is a cut made with a sharp instrument, such as a knife or fragment of glass (Fig. 13-3). Sometimes the word *laceration* is used specifically to refer to a jagged cut (like the ragged tear that comes from being mauled by a dog), while a clean, smooth cut (like one made by a sharp knife) is called an *incision*. A laceration can be superficial, involving only the skin itself, or it can be very deep, cutting through skin, subcutaneous tissue, nerves, blood vessels, muscle, and even internal organs. Significant external bleeding is apt to be present with a laceration, especially if the sharp instrument that made the cut also disrupted the wall of a large blood vessel.

Avulsion

In an avulsion, a piece of skin, with or without various underlying tissues, is torn loose from the body

Fig. 13-3. *Laceration.*

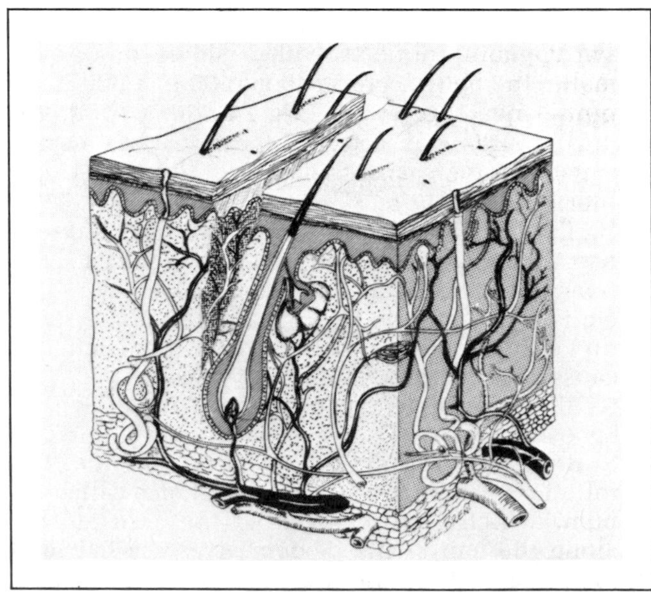

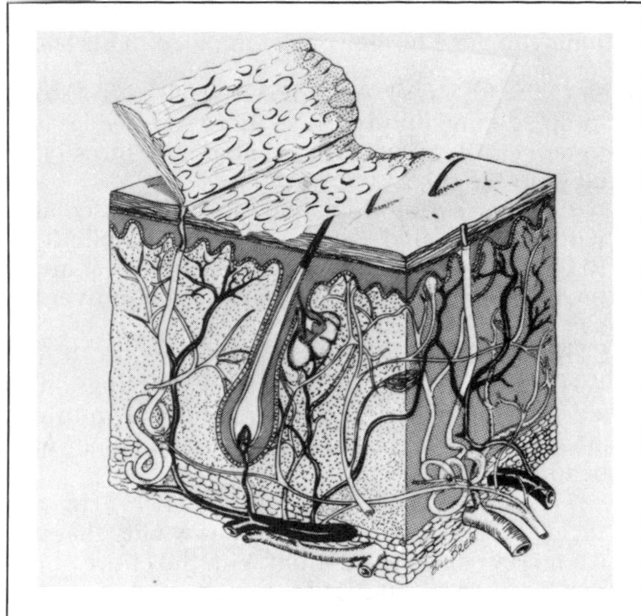

Fig. 13-4. *Avulsion.*

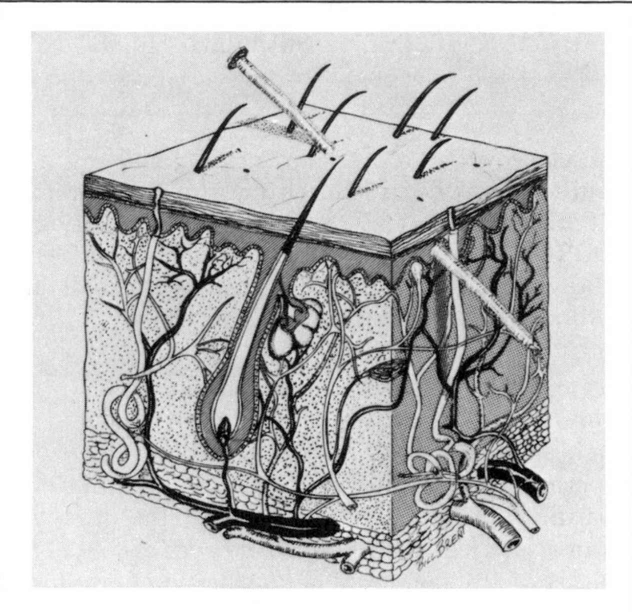

Fig. 13-5. *Impaled object.*

and hangs as a flap (Fig. 13-4). So long as part of the tissue remains attached to the patient, it is regarded as an avulsion; parts of the body that are entirely torn away are said to be amputated. Amputated tissues—such as part of a finger or leg—should always be collected and brought with the patient to the emergency room, for frequently prompt surgery can successfully reimplant the amputated part.

Puncture Wound

A puncture wound is a stab made by a pointed object, such as a knife, scissors blade, nail, or sliver of wood; a puncture wound can also be caused by an object travelling at high velocity, such as a bullet. If the instrument that caused the injury remains embedded in the wound, it is referred to as an **impaled object** (Fig. 13-5). Puncture wounds can be very deceptive, for the injury visible at the skin surface is apt to be minimal or even nearly undetectable, but there may be devastating damage to organs and blood vessels within. A classic example is a bullet wound, which may be so small that it causes little, if any, external bleeding, yet there may be exsanguinating hemorrhage within the chest or abdomen. There is no way that an EMT can assess the damage from a puncture wound, so one must always assume the worst.

Some puncture wounds, especially on the extremities, may penetrate the whole depth of the body and come out the opposite side. This is particularly apt to be the case with bullet wounds. The path taken by the bullet or other instrument can provide clues to the internal structures likely to have been injured. For this reason, the EMT should always look for both an **entrance wound** and an **exit wound** when examining a patient who has sustained a puncture wound, especially if the offending agent was a bullet.

MANAGEMENT OF OPEN WOUNDS

The management of open wounds has three general objectives: (1) to control bleeding, (2) to prevent further contamination of the wound, and (3) to prevent further damage to the injured part.

Control of Bleeding

The methods for the control of bleeding were discussed in detail in Chapter 8, and we shall review them only briefly here. By far the most effective method of hemorrhage control is the application of DIRECT PRESSURE over the wound. Pressure is initially applied manually, but as soon as possible, manual pressure is replaced with a PRESSURE DRESSING. The dressing can be held in place either by a pressure bandage or—if the wound is on an extremity—by an air splint. The MAST garment can also be used to apply pressure if the wound is on the leg, hip, or abdomen. A seriously bleeding extremity should *always* be SPLINTED, whether or not there is an associated fracture, for motion of an extremity increases the blood flow into it. Splinting therefore, by preventing motion, reduces the amount of blood that is pumped into the extremity and out through the wound. The *air splint* is the preferred type of splint for this purpose, because it serves a dual role of maintaining pressure on the wound and immobilizing the extremity.

ALWAYS SPLINT A SEVERELY BLEEDING EXTREMITY.

In cases where a pressure dressing and splint are insufficient to control bleeding from an extremity, PRESSURE POINT CONTROL should be tried. A TOURNIQUET is used ONLY AS A LAST RESORT, to prevent death from exsanguination when all other methods to control bleeding have failed.

Prevention of Further Contamination

Every wound is contaminated, for the moment there is a break in the skin, all the bacteria that have been congregating hopefully on the skin surface go swarming through the barricades into the underlying tissues. Nonetheless, there are degrees of contamination. A minimal amount of contamination from skin bacteria may not necessarily lead to infection, for the body's defenses—the white blood cells and other mechanisms—may be able to beat back a small invasion. But the more massive the contamination by foreign materials, the more likely is the possibility of infection, for at a certain point the body's defenses simply become overwhelmed. For this reason, the EMT should try to KEEP THE WOUND AS CLEAN AS POSSIBLE, by observing the following guidelines:

- CUT AWAY any CLOTHING covering the wound.
- If the surface of the wound is covered with dirt, FLUSH THE WOUND by pouring sterile water over it or placing it under a brisk stream of tap water. Do not try to pick out foreign material embedded in the wound, for this simply wastes time and can in fact increase the degree of contamination.
- Wherever possible, USE STERILE MATERIALS for the initial dressing. While it is true that severe external bleeding must be controlled immediately with whatever materials are at hand, a good EMT will *have* sterile dressings at hand, for he or she will have grabbed a "jump kit" upon leaving the vehicle to seek out the patient.

Prevention of Further Injury

Prevention of further injury in general means IMMOBILIZATION OF THE INJURED PART. This requires not only the use of splints, but also the *verbal* immobilization of the patient; that is, the EMT must try to keep the patient quiet and still, for a splint on a leg will not do very much good if the patient is hopping up and down.

A very special kind of immobilization is required in the case of an IMPALED OBJECT, for any motion of the impaled object can cause additional damage to the tissues in which it is embedded. There are several guidelines the EMT should follow in treating a patient who has a foreign object impaled in his body:

- DO NOT REMOVE AN IMPALED OBJECT. Efforts to do so may simply cause more serious damage to nerves, blood vessels, or other structures lying close to the object.
- If there is serious external bleeding associated with an impaled object, CONTROL HEMORRHAGE BY DIRECT PRESSURE, but do *not* apply pressure over the impaled object itself or over tissue that lies beside its cutting edge.
- STABILIZE THE IMPALED OBJECT IN PLACE WITH A BULKY DRESSING. Pack dressings on all sides of the object so that its motion is minimal after the dressings have been secured in place with bandages (Fig. 13-6).
- DO NOT ATTEMPT TO SHORTEN THE IMPALED OBJECT, unless it is so unwieldy that you cannot transport the patient with the entire object in place (e.g., a 10-foot fence post sticking out of the chest). If you must shorten an impaled object, stabilize it in place as securely as possible before doing so, for any motion caused by sawing the object will otherwise be transmitted to the patient and is likely to cause further injury.
- TRANSPORT THE PATIENT WITHOUT DELAY TO THE HOSPITAL. An impaled object will usually necessitate immediate surgery, so wherever possible, try to notify the receiving hospital of the nature of the case and your estimated time of arrival, so that they can summon the necessary personnel.

Amputated Parts

As noted earlier, amputated parts should always be searched for at the accident scene and brought with the patient to the emergency room. Any amputated part (e.g., a finger, a hand, part of an ear) should be rinsed free of gross dirt with sterile saline and then wrapped gently in a bulky sterile dressing, which in turn should be soaked with cool saline or Ringer's solution. The wrapped part is then sealed in a plastic bag, which may be placed on ice. Do NOT place amputated parts directly in ice or in dry dressings. Do NOT use any solution other than a sterile salt solution to moisten the dressing. Be sure to notify the hospital of the type of case you are bringing in so that a surgeon specializing in reimplantation can be summoned.

Management of Open Wounds

- CONTROL BLEEDING.
  1. Manual pressure.
  2. Pressure dressing held in place with bandage or air splint.
- PREVENT FURTHER CONTAMINATION.
  1. Cut away clothing from the wound.
  2. Flush gross contaminants from the wound.
  3. Use sterile materials for dressings.

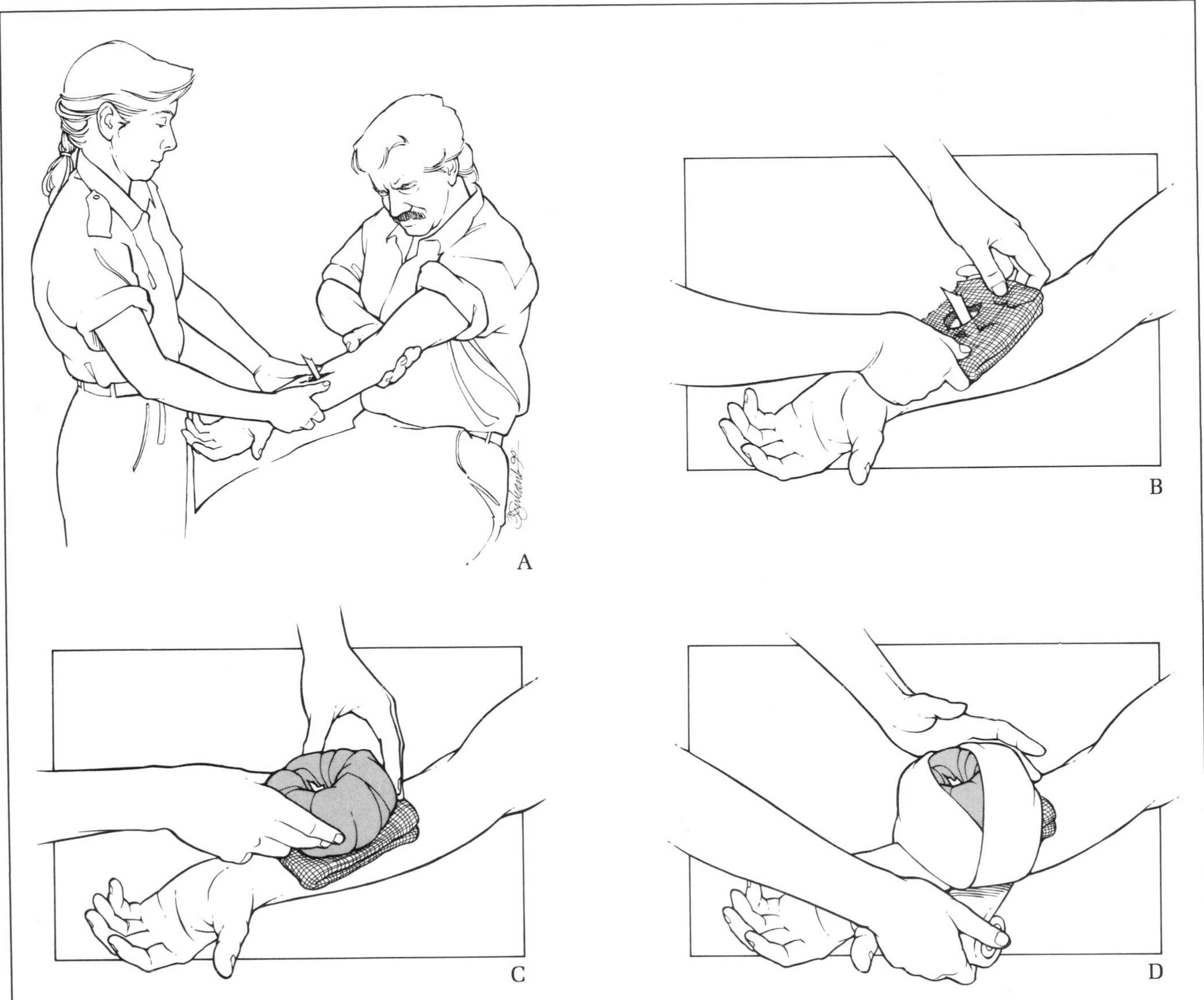

Fig. 13-6. *Stabilizing an impaled object. A. to control bleeding, apply direct pressure at the wound edges. B. Cut a hole in the center of several layers of gauze pads, then gently slip the pads over the impaled object. C. Make a "doughnut" out of a triangular bandage and place it around the impaled object. If is is not higher than the object, add another "doughnut" on top of the first. D. Secure the "doughnuts" and gauze pads with diagonally applied bandage (do not bandage over the impaled object).*

- PREVENT FURTHER INJURY.
  1. Immobilize any injured extremity; keep the patient still.
  2. Stabilize an impaled object in place.
- PRESERVE AMPUTATED PARTS.

BURNS

A burn is an injury in which the skin—and sometimes underlying tissues as well—is damaged by extremes of temperature, caustic chemicals, electric current, or radiation. In this chapter, we will look at the first three types of burns. Radiation injuries, which require very special precautions, will be discussed in Chapter 31.

THERMAL BURNS

Thermal burns are caused by open flame, hot liquids, or other extremely hot objects. In the United States, approximately 2 million people suffer some kind of thermal injury each year, of whom more than 100,000 are hospitalized and 12,000 die. The most common victims are small children and the elderly.

Taking the History

One of the most important contributions an EMT can make to the care of a burned patient is to provide a thorough and accurate history, complete with observations of the scene. Obviously, if the patient is in critical condition when you arrive, you will have to tend first to any life-threatening problems and ask questions later. But sometime during your time at the scene, you should try to find out at least the following:

- HOW LONG before the ambulance arrived did the burn occur? If the burn occurred 5 minutes ago, it is still worthwhile to treat it with cold applications. A burn that is several hours old, on the other hand, is unlikely to benefit from cold compresses or immersion in cold water.
- Was the patient in a CLOSED SPACE with smoke, steam, or other products of combustion? If so, for how long? DID HE LOSE CONSCIOUSNESS? Respiratory injuries are much more likely in patients who were confined in a closed, smoky area or who lost consciousness in a smoke-filled environment.
- WHAT WAS BURNING? The products of combustion from certain materials—such as wood, cloth, paint, upholstery, and plastics—are highly toxic to the respiratory tract. A fire in a closed car, for example, may give rise to the very dangerous fumes of polyvinyl bromide, the plastic used in automobile seat covers. The more precisely you can determine the nature of the fire, the more accurately the emergency room doctor will be able to gauge the possibility of lung damage in the victim.
- WHAT EXACTLY HAPPENED? What were the mechanisms of injury? Was the patient found unconscious in a smoke-filled room, or did he jump three stories out of a window—the latter circumstance suggesting that there are probably significant associated injuries.
- WITH WHAT WAS THE PATIENT BURNED? Open flame? Hot liquids? Scald burns from hot liquids are not likely to be as deep as burns caused by flame or electric burns.
- Does the victim have any UNDERLYING MEDICAL CONDITIONS, such as heart disease, respiratory problems, diabetes, or other serious underlying illness, that could complicate his condition? Is he taking any MEDICATIONS?

Steps in Evaluation and Management of the Thermal Burn Victim

1. PUT OUT THE FIRE! The most important first step in the treatment of any burned victim is to extinguish any fire in the patient's clothes, hair, and so forth. While this may seem obvious, it is remarkable how many burned patients arrive in the emergency room with their clothes still smoldering. One of the most critical factors in the depth of a burn is the amount of time the patient's skin is in contact with the heat source; thus the first priority in treatment must be to terminate the contact between the patient and the agent that is burning. If the patient's clothes are on fire, he should be prevented from running, since this will only fan the flames. Similarly, he must not be allowed to stand, for he is more likely to ignite his hair or to inhale flames in the erect position. Instead, the victim should be placed on the ground and instructed to roll to extinguish the flames. Residual flames can be smothered by covering the victim briefly with a blanket. Smoldering clothes should be extinguished with fire blankets, a Water-Jel blanket, or cool water.

If the burn victim cannot be moved (e.g., if he is trapped inside a flaming car), the fire should be extinguished using a DRY CHEMICAL MULTIPURPOSE (ABC) EXTINGUISHER. The dry chemical extinguisher can put out a broad range of fires without damaging the patient's skin or soft tissues. Avoid water extinguishers, which can react adversely on class B (flammable liquid) fires, causing the fire to flame up and spread. Water extinguishers are also a potential hazard in class C (electric) fires, for the water stream may conduct electric current back to the rescuer and cause fatal shock. Also avoid sodium bicarbonate and potassium bicarbonate (Purple K) dry chemical extinguishers (used for class B and C fires), for these may damage the victim's skin.

Learn how to use your fire extinguisher *before* the call comes in which you need it. There is no time to practice when you are faced with an incinerating patient, for once activated, a 10-pound multipurpose extinguisher has a discharge time of between 8 and 12 seconds—and you had better be aiming it in the right direction. Hold the extinguisher upright, and discharge it at a distance of 5 to 10 feet from the flaming victim, aiming it just below the flames and using a sweeping motion to spray the chemical from side to side along the entire width of flames.

Once you have put out the fire, move the patient upwind from the area where you discharged the fire extinguisher, for the chemicals in a multipurpose extinguisher are irritating to the mucous membranes if inhaled in high concentration.

As soon as the fire is out and the patient is in a safe place, quickly REMOVE ALL BURNED CLOTHING from the victim's body, since such clothing can continue to be a source of heat even after the flames have been extinguished. Do not attempt to pull away any fabric that is stuck to the patient's skin, however, as this may aggravate a burn wound and lead to further contamination. Simply cut around the areas where clothing adheres to the skin, and remove the rest.

A special case of "putting out the fire" involves hot tar burns; for so long as hot tar or asphalt remains hot, the burning process will continue. Thus the first measure you should take in managing a patient who has been spattered by hot tar is to try to cool the tar to room temperature as fast as possible. If the tar burn is on an arm or leg, immerse the affected extremity in cold water to dissipate the heat and speed up the hardening process. Do *not* attempt to remove the tar in the field. Safe removal of tar from burned skin will require the use of special solvents in the emergency room. (If you get a *minor* tar burn at home, a little margarine or mayonnaise will remove the cooled tar from the skin.)

2. ENSURE AN ADEQUATE AIRWAY. Remove any dentures or foreign materials from the patient's mouth, and examine the face, mouth, and neck carefully for signs of burns that can cause respiratory problems. BURNS OF THE FACE AND NECK, SINGED NASAL HAIR, HOARSENESS, STRIDOR, AND SOOTY SPUTUM ARE ALL DANGER SIGNALS, indicating probable damage to the airway. Laryngeal edema can develop within minutes in such patients, completely sealing off the airway; if that happens, the only way to save the patient's life will be a tracheostomy (a surgical opening through the neck into the trachea) performed in the emergency room. Thus if you note any signs suggesting a respiratory burn, GET THE PATIENT TO THE HOSPITAL WITHOUT DELAY!

Signs and Circumstances Suggesting Respiratory Injury

- Burns of the FACE or NECK
- SINGED NASAL HAIRS
- STRIDOR
- BRASSY COUGH
- SOOT IN SPUTUM
- Burn occurred in a CLOSED SPACE
- Patient FOUND UNCONSCIOUS in a smoky environment

3. ENSURE ADEQUATE BREATHING. It is a good rule of thumb to assume that all victims of fire have some degree of injury to their lungs or some other impairment to respiration, such as high carbon monoxide levels in the blood. This includes fire fighters who have been overcome by smoke. In general, the signs of pulmonary injury from smoke or toxic fumes do not appear for 8 to 24 hours after exposure. For this reason, any person exposed to significant amounts of smoke—especially if the victim was unconscious or in a closed space—MUST be evaluated in the hospital, even if the patient has no present symptoms of respiratory difficulty.

If the patient is not breathing, he should of course be ventilated artificially. Do not use a demand valve, since the very dry gas delivered by a demand valve will aggravate respiratory damage. If the victim is breathing spontaneously, he should be given OXYGEN, preferably by nonrebreathing mask at 10 to 12 liters per minute. Do not wait for the patient to show signs of hypoxia. If he has been in a fire, give him oxygen.

4. ENSURE ADEQUATE CIRCULATION. As always in the primary survey, the next step after breathing is circulation. If a pulse is absent, you must start external cardiac compressions. If there is exsanguinating hemorrhage associated with the burn, you will need to control the bleeding. Should you note a rapid, thready pulse or other signs of *shock*, begin treatment for shock by elevating the patient's legs. If shock is severe and the victim will not reach the hospital within 20 minutes, the EMT-Intermediate should request orders for an intravenous infusion. Burned patients should receive lactated Ringer's solution (without glucose) through a wide-bore IV catheter placed in an unburned extremity.

5. NOTE THE GENERAL APPEARANCE of the patient. If the patient has jumped from a window or done anything else likely to result in injury, be alert for the possibility of spinal damage, and handle the patient accordingly.

6. CHECK AND RECORD THE VITAL SIGNS.

7. GAUGE THE DEPTH OF THE BURN. Burns are traditionally classified according to the depth of tissue damage they produce (Table 13-1). (Note that until now we have not given any attention to the burn itself. This is because a burn is NOT an immediately life-threatening injury; airway obstruction, apnea, cardiac arrest, and profuse bleeding are.

Table 13-1. *Depth of a Burn*

Type	Layer of Skin Involved	Signs and Symptoms
First degree	Epidermis	Redness and pain Slight tenderness Edema Blanching on pressure
Second degree	Epidermis and part of dermis	Redness or mottling and pain Hypersensitive to pinprick Blisters Blanching on pressure
Third degree	Full thickness: epidermis, dermis, and subcutaneous tissue	Leathery, charred, or pearly gray Burn odor Painless Impaired sensation to pinprick No blanching

It is only when we get to the head-to-toe survey that we begin to look at the burns.)

A **first-degree burn** (Fig. 13-7A), or superficial burn, the mildest type of burn, is limited to the most superficial layers of skin, and it is characterized by REDNESS AND PAIN. A moderate scald or sunburn is an example of a first-degree burn. First-degree burns are initially very painful, but because they involve only the outer epidermal layers of the skin, they usually heal without complication in about a week.

Second-degree burns (partial-thickness burns) (Fig. 13-7B) penetrate the skin more deeply than do first-degree burns, causing damage to *both* the epidermis and the underlying dermis. A second-degree burn looks mottled or red, swollen, and somewhat wet. It is also characterized by BLISTER FORMATION, although blisters may not become apparent until several hours after the burn was sustained. Second-degree burns are also very painful, unless there has been extensive damage to the nerve endings in the dermis. The burn is tender to the touch and blanches on pressure, but the red color returns as soon as you take your finger off the burn. Second-degree burns are most commonly caused by contact with boiling liquids, such as the classic "tea burn" seen in toddlers who upset a cup of boiling tea from a table or counter above them. If a second-degree burn is kept clean and free of infection, healing usually occurs in 2 to 3 weeks.

Third-degree burns (Fig. 13-7C) are also called full-thickness burns because they involve damage to or destruction of the full thickness of the skin, from the epidermis down into the subcutaneous fat and sometimes underlying muscle as well. When muscle or bone is involved, the burn is sometimes categorized as fourth, fifth, or sixth degree, but for field purposes, any burn deeper than a second-degree burn should be considered third degree. The skin in a third-degree burn looks charred, leathery, or pearly gray. Usually redness is not present, and if it is (from coagulation of blood near the burn surface), it does not blanch on pressure. The skin often has a "burn smell," that is, it has the odor of burning flesh. Unlike first- and second-degree burns, third-degree burns are INSENSITIVE TO PAINFUL STIMULI because of destruction of the nerve endings for pain in the dermis. For this reason, a patient usually will not be able to feel a pinprick over an area where there are third-degree burns, whereas a pinprick will be perceived as unusually painful over a second- or first-degree burn.

In practice, most patients will be found to have varying combinations of burns—for example, a small area of second-degree burn in the center of a larger first-degree burn, or varying areas of all three degrees of burn. In the field, one can make only a rough estimate of what degrees of burn are present and which predominate.

8. GAUGE THE EXTENT OF THE BURN. In addition to determining how deep the burns are, one must also make an estimate of their extent—that is, how wide an area of the body is covered by the burns. The extent of a burn is also a measure of its seriousness, for a first-degree burn that covers 50 percent of the body is clearly more serious than one that covers only 2 percent of the body, and it can even be more serious than some third-degree burns of smaller area. It is customary to gauge the extent of a burn in terms of the percentage of the body surface involved, and to determine this, one uses a rough guide known as the RULE OF NINES (Fig. 13-8). That system assigns a percentage value to each part of the body. For ex-

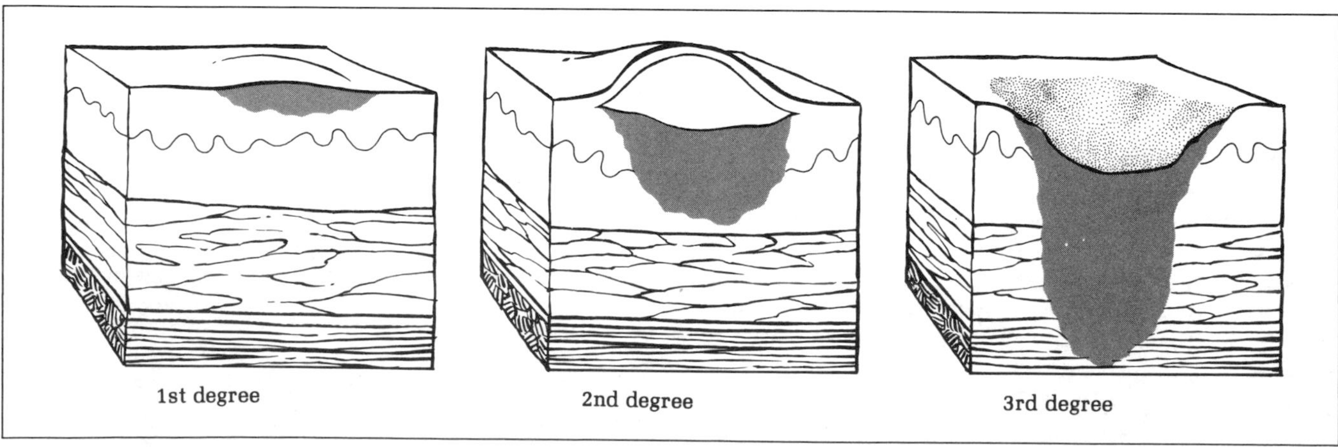

Fig. 13-7. *Assess the depth of the burn. A. First degree (epidermis only). B. Second degree (epidermis and part of dermis). C. Third degree (epidermis, dermis, and subcutaneous tissues).*

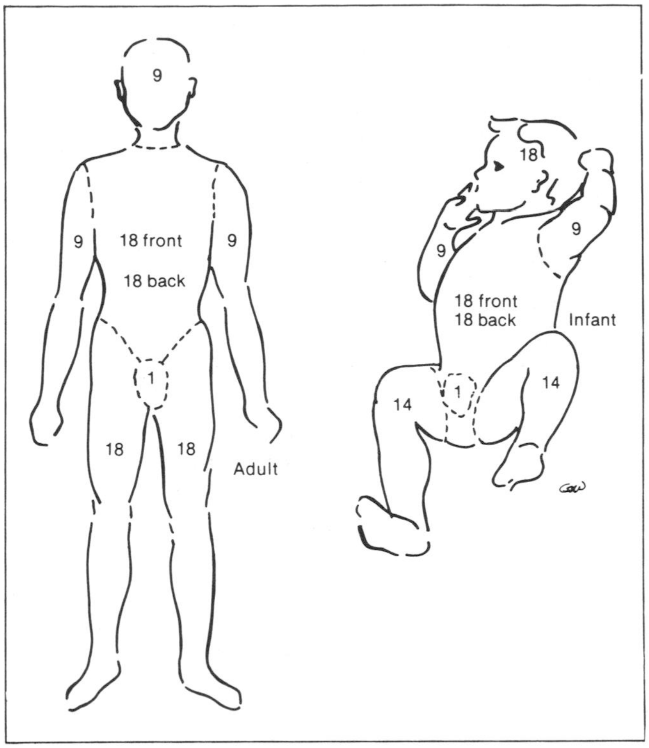

9
18 front
18 back
9
9
1
18
18
Adult
18
9
9
18 front
18 back
Infant
1
14
14

Fig. 13-8. *Rule of nines.*

ample, an arm (front and back) represents 9 percent of the body surface, while a leg (front and back) is 18 percent. Suppose then that a patient had burns covering his entire right arm and the anterior surface of the right leg. According to the rule of nines, the patient would have an 18-percent burn (whole arm = 9% + anterior leg = 9%). In children, the chart looks a little different because a child's head is much larger than an adult's in proportion to the rest of the body. For gauging the extent of small or scattered burns, some authorities use the "rule of the palm"; that is, the palm of the victim's hand represents about 1 percent of his body surface. So if he has scattered burns of the body covering about the area of both of his palms, he has a 2 percent burn.

9. DETERMINE WHETHER A CRITICAL BURN IS PRESENT. A burn is considered critical if it involves any of the following:

- Burns complicated by RESPIRATORY INJURY
- Burns (any degree) involving MORE THAN 30 PERCENT OF BODY SURFACE
- THIRD-DEGREE BURNS OF MORE THAN 10 PERCENT OF BODY SURFACE
- Nearly all burns of the FACE, HANDS, FEET, OR GENITALIA
- Burns complicated by FRACTURE or MAJOR SOFT TISSUE INJURY
- Deep ACID or ELECTRIC BURNS (see discussions below)
- Burns occurring in PATIENTS WITH SERIOUS UNDERLYING DISEASE (e.g., heart disease or emphysema)

Wherever possible, patients having burns regarded as critical according to the above criteria should be transported to a regional burn center, if such a center is within reasonable travel time.

10. EXAMINE THE PATIENT FOR OTHER INJURIES. One must examine the burned patient with particular care, for associated injuries are apt to be obscured by the burn. In checking the HEAD, be alert for eye injuries, which must be covered with moist, sterile pads. If there has been a jump or fall from a height, check the NECK for tenderness or deformity. Also look closely to determine whether there are *circumferential burns* on the neck, for such burns can act as a tourniquet and literally strangle a patient as they swell and tighten around the throat. A similar situation can arise from burns that cover the whole CHEST, for such burns can restrict movement of the chest during respiration. In both circumstances, the patient will require urgent treatment in the emergency room, where an incision will have to be made through the burned skin to release the tourniquet effect of the burn. Observe the ABDOMEN for distention, which is very common in burned patients and which will need to be relieved with a nasogastric tube as soon as the patient reaches the hospital. When examining the EXTREMITIES, first remove all rings, bracelets, and other potentially constricting items from burned extremities, for swelling of the hands and fingers can occur very rapidly after a burn; and once swelling does occur, the only way to get this jewelry off will be to cut it off. Check each burned extremity carefully for PULSES, MOVEMENT, AND SENSATION. Like circumferential burns on the neck or chest, circumferential burns on an extremity may act as a tourniquet and completely cut off circulation to the extremity. IF A PULSE IS ABSENT IN A BURNED EXTREMITY, THE PATIENT NEEDS URGENT SURGICAL TREATMENT AND MUST REACH THE HOSPITAL WITHOUT DELAY! Be sure to check for fractures, which should be stabilized before the patient is moved. Swelling from a burn can distort the appearance of an extremity, so fractures may be hard to detect. Thus you have to maintain a high index of suspicion when a burned extremity just "doesn't look right" or when the mechanisms of injury (e.g., a fall from a high place) suggest that fractures *might* be present.

Assessment and Management of the Burned Patient

1. PUT OUT THE FIRE!
2. AIRWAY:
   a. Maintain an open airway.
   b. Remove dentures, foreign materials.
   c. Check for signs of airway damage.
3. BREATHING: Give humidified oxygen.
4. CIRCULATION:
   a. Control bleeding.
   b. Elevate legs.
5. GENERAL APPEARANCE.
6. VITAL SIGNS.
7. BURN ASSESSMENT:
   a. Depth.
   b. Extent (rule of nines).
   c. Presence of critical burns.
8. SEARCH FOR OTHER INJURIES:
   a. EYE injury.
   b. SPINE injury.
   c. CIRCUMFERENTIAL BURNS on neck or chest.
   d. Absence of distal PULSES.
   e. FRACTURES.

Treatment of Thermal Burns

FIRST-DEGREE BURNS. The major consideration in the treatment of first-degree burns is RELIEF OF PAIN, for unless first-degree burns cover very large areas of the body, they pose no particular threat to the patient. If you reach the patient within about 15 minutes of the injury, immerse the burned area in cold water or apply towels that have been soaked in ice water to the burn. Do not apply cold compresses to more than 10 percent of the body surface, however, because widespread cooling can cause a dangerous drop in the patient's core body temperature. Furthermore, never apply ice directly to the burn, for this can cause a burn of another type—called frostbite.

DO NOT UNDER ANY CIRCUMSTANCES APPLY SALVES, OINTMENTS, BUTTER, CREAM, SPRAYS, OR ANY OTHER COATING ON ANY TYPE OF BURN. These home remedies will simply have to be scrubbed off in the emergency room, a procedure that will cause unnecessary additional pain to the patient. So remember:

NEVER, NEVER, NEVER PUT GOO ON A BURN!

SECOND-DEGREE BURNS. The treatment of second-degree burns is similar to that of first-degree burns, although one needs to take greater care to avoid contamination of the burn. Once again, significant pain relief and some reduction of swelling can be achieved by application of towels that have been soaked in ice water, but with the same provisos as before: Do not cool more than 10 percent of the body surface, and do not place ice in direct contact with the burn. If the burn is on an arm, be sure to remove all rings, bracelets, and similar pieces of jewelry before the extremity becomes so swollen that these items begin to act as tourniquets. Keep a burned leg or arm elevated on pillows to promote drainage of edema fluid out of the extremity by gravity.

If the patient has blisters, DO NOT RUPTURE THEM, for this is simply an open invitation to bacteria to invade the burn. Blister fluid is sterile so long as the blister remains intact, and blisters are an excellent burn dressing—so do not disturb them. If a blister *has* been inadvertently ruptured, cover it with a *dry*, sterile dressing. Once again, do NOT use goo, and do NOT use dressings that have been impregnated with goo (e.g., petrolatum gauze, Xeroform). Extensive burns should be covered with a sterile burn sheet, on top of which is placed a clean blanket to prevent heat loss across the damaged skin.

THIRD-DEGREE BURNS. The object in treating third-degree burns is to minimize further contamination of the burn and to minimize burn complications, such as vomiting and aspiration, shock, and heat loss. There is no need for cold compresses in third-degree burns, since pain is minimal or absent. The following general guidelines should be observed:

- Place the patient supine or in the stable side position on a STERILE SHEET, and cover the burn with a *dry*, sterile dressing (if the burn is extensive, use another sterile sheet to cover it). Do NOT use goo, and do not use dressings impregnated with goo.
- Do NOT make any attempt to clean the burn wound. That will have to be done surgically in the hospital, and trying to clean the wound simply wastes time in the field.
- Do NOT allow the patient to take anything by mouth. He is very likely to vomit.
- Elevate the patient's legs, unless the injuries preclude it.
- Keep the patient warm; cover the sterile sheet with a clean blanket.
- Treat associated injuries as needed.

It is easier to remember the principles of burn care if you bear in mind the functions of normal skin: protection against bacterial invasion, temperature regulation, and prevention of water loss. When skin is damaged by extensive burns, it cannot carry out those functions properly, and so our treatment is aimed at helping the body to compensate for the functions that have been impaired. We cover burns with sterile dressings to try to keep out as much bacterial contamination as possible. We cover the patient with a blanket to minimize heat loss from the body. And we elevate the patient's legs (and sometimes start intravenous therapy) to make up for some of the fluid that is being lost into and through damaged tissues.

Management of Thermal Burns

1. PUT OUT THE FIRE!
2. Take care of the ABCs—and do not forget OXYGEN.
3. COLD COMPRESSES on first- and second-degree burns, but do *not* put ice directly on a burn.
4. REMOVE RINGS, bracelets, and so forth from a burned extremity.
5. ELEVATE a burned extremity.
6. Do *not* rupture blisters.
7. DO NOT PUT GOO ON A BURN.
8. Cover burns with DRY, STERILE DRESSINGS.
9. Keep the patient WARM.
10. NOTHING BY MOUTH.
11. Treat ASSOCIATED WOUNDS, FRACTURES, and other injuries in the usual fashion.

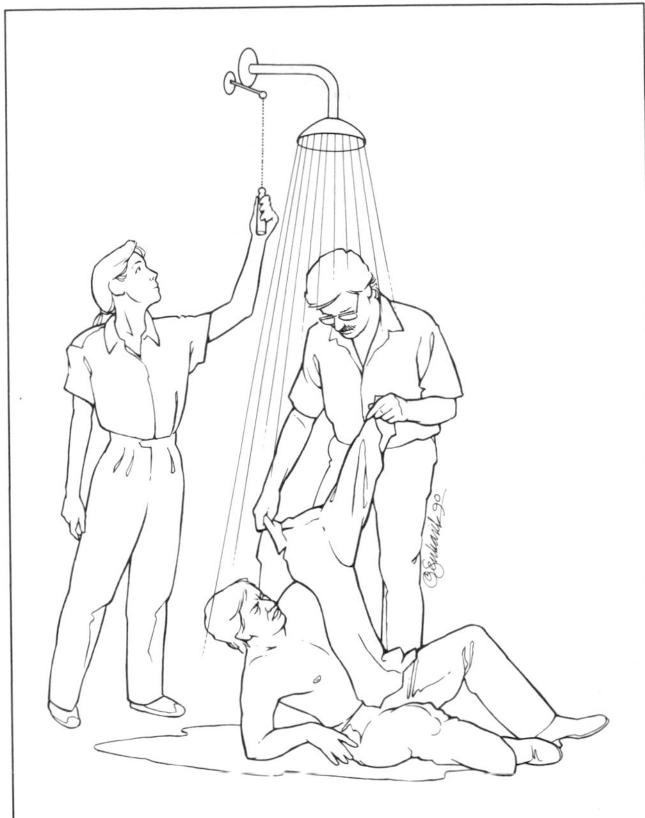

Fig. 13-9. *Treatment of chemical burns. Get the victim immediately into a shower, without initially taking time to remove his clothes.*

CHEMICAL BURNS

Chemical burns occur when the skin comes into contact with strong acids, strong alkalis, or other corrosive materials. These agents eat through the skin and in many cases continue to do damage so long as they remain in contact with the skin. Thus the most important factor in treating a chemical burn is to REMOVE THE CHEMICAL FROM CONTACT WITH THE PATIENT'S BODY AS QUICKLY AS POSSIBLE.

There is no time to waste in dealing with a chemical burn. The patient's history and the rest of the secondary survey will have to be delayed until after treatment has been carried out. If the accidental spill has occurred in a factory or other industrial site, get the patient under a shower immediately (Fig. 13-9). Do not take time initially to remove his clothing, but simply place him fully dressed under a good stream of water. If no shower is available on the premises, use a water hose, but make sure the water is not delivered under high pressure; a blast of water will simply cause further injury to damaged skin. Thus the stream of water should be gentle but full. For accidents in and around the home, put the patient into the shower, or use a garden hose to flush him down. Continue to flush the patient as you remove his clothes, including shoes and socks, which can serve as a reservoir for the spilled chemical. Similarly, watches and jewelry should be removed, for these may hold the chemical in contact with the skin.

Be careful not to get any of the chemical on your own skin while you are flushing the patient. If you do get splashed, immediately rinse off the area where you came in contact with the chemical.

DO NOT WASTE TIME LOOKING FOR SPECIFIC ANTIDOTES to any given chemical. Copious flushing with water is more effective and is usually more available than an antidote. Continue the flushing for 10 to 20 minutes, until you feel that all of the chemical is rinsed off, and then let the patient wash himself down with a mild soap, such as Ivory, before a final rinse.

Once the flushing is complete, allow the patient to dry himself off with clean towels, but instruct him not to rub the towels over any area that hurts. Have him lie down on a clean (preferably sterile) sheet on the stretcher, and do a quick secondary survey, noting the depth and extent of the burns as well as the vital signs. Cover the burned areas with dry, sterile dressings; cover the patient with a clean sheet and blanket; and move on to the hospital. If possible, bring the container of the chemical involved with you to the emergency room.

Management of Chemical Burns

- SPEED IS ESSENTIAL.
- Get the patient under a shower or hose as rapidly as possible.
- Do not take time to remove the patient's clothes until after the flushing is well under way.
- Do not waste time looking for antidotes.
- Flush until you are sure all the chemical is removed.
- Cover all burns with dry, sterile dressings.

Special Cases

There are a few chemicals that require special consideration because they have unusual properties that can affect the way you remove them. One of these is DRY LIME (calcium hydroxide), which forms a highly corrosive substance when combined with water. For this reason, it is preferable to brush as much of the lime off the skin as possible, then remove the patient's clothes and shoes, and *then* flush with copious amounts of water. Use a universal dressing or a gloved hand to brush the patient's skin, to prevent contamination of your own skin with the lime.

PHENOL (carbolic acid) is used widely in industry, and a 10% solution of phenol can produce a deep ulcer of the skin. The problem with phenol is that it is not soluble in water, so it can be more difficult to remove from the skin by flushing than another liquid chemical would be. Phenol is soluble in alcohol or any kind of oil (e.g., vegetable oil, castor oil, cottonseed oil), however, and any of these materials can help dilute the phenol and remove it from the skin surface. Once again, you should not waste time initially searching for one of these solvents. First get the patient under a good stream of water, and get his clothes off. Once he is securely ensconced under the shower, *then* it is worthwhile to try to find some alcohol or oil, which can be spread over the skin in the area of the phenol spill and then flushed off with more water.

SODIUM METAL burns very rapidly and can explode if mixed with water. Its reaction with the skin can be halted, however, by preventing any contact between the sodium metal and the air, which is most easily done by covering the sodium with a thick layer of petrolatum jelly.

Adding water to SULFURIC ACID causes the generation of extreme heat and can even cause an explosion. Thus if at all possible, it is best to start your flushing with a soap solution followed by the usual rinse with *very large amounts* of water so that the acid can be diluted as rapidly as possible.

Special Care of the Eyes

A chemical burn of the eye is an extreme emergency, for permanent damage to the eyes can result from even very short exposure to strong chemicals. The principle of treating a chemical burn to the eye is exactly the same as that for any other chemical burn: FLUSH WITH COPIOUS AMOUNTS OF WATER. The most effective way to do this is to support the patient's head under a swiftly flowing faucet, with the stream of water directed into the affected eye (Fig. 13-10); you may have to hold the eyelid open, for if the patient is in a great deal of pain, he may not be able to keep the eye open voluntarily. If the patient has contact lenses and the initial stream of water does not flush them out, pause for a moment so that the patient can remove the lens from the affected eye—for a contact lens will prevent water from reaching the cornea underneath. Continue to flush the eye for AT LEAST 20 MINUTES, making sure to rinse thoroughly underneath the eyelids, where chemicals may be trapped. Do NOT use any liquid other than water to flush the eyes, and NEVER USE A CHEMICAL ANTIDOTE IN THE EYES. When you finish flushing, gently close the affected eye, and cover it with a soft, bulky patch; soaking the patch with cool sterile water or saline may provide some pain relief to the patient. Transport the patient at once to the emergency department.

DOs and DON'Ts of Surface Burns

Burn Type	Do	Don't
First degree	Apply cold compresses.	Use goo.
Second degree	Immerse in cold water or apply cold compresses. Blot dry. Cover with dry, sterile dressing. Remove rings, bracelets from burned extremities. Elevate burned extremity.	Use goo. Break blisters. Apply ice directly on burn. Cool more than 10% of the body surface.
Third degree	Be alert for other injuries. Cover burns with dry, sterile dressing. Cover patient with a blanket. Elevate patient's legs. Put patient in stable side po-	Use goo. Use wet dressings. Remove charred clothing stuck to the skin. Apply ice. Give anything by mouth.

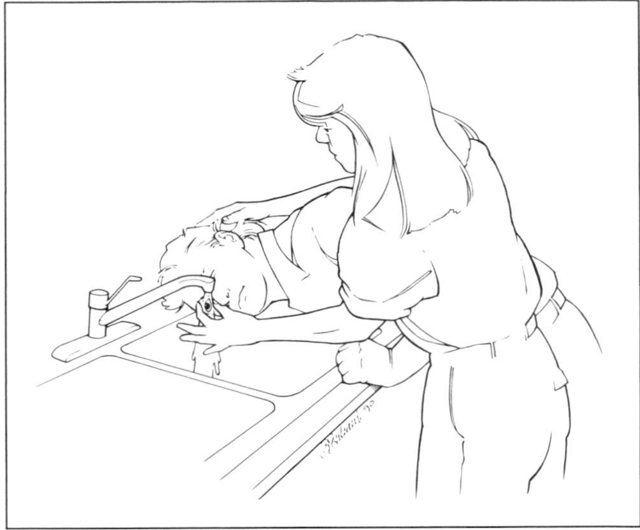

Fig. 13-10. *Chemical burns to the eyes. Flush the affected eye under a gentle stream of water for at least 20 minutes (hold the eyelids open if necessary).*

	sition (other injuries permitting).	
Chemical	Flush with copious amounts of water for 5–15 minutes. Remove contaminated clothing. Cover burns with dry, sterile dressings.	Use acid to neutralize alkali burns or vice versa. Use water on sodium metal. Cover burns with goo. Use "antidotes" in eyes.

ELECTRIC BURNS

Electric burns are very deceptive injuries, for usually the damage visible on the skin from an electric burn is very minimal, while the damage *inside* the body—the damage you cannot see—may be devastating. In order to understand how this damage occurs, we have to learn a little about electricity, which means learning the precise meaning of a few familiar terms.

How Electricity Causes Injury

What kills or damages in electricity is current, which is a flow of electric charge. The *amount* of flow is measured in **amperes** (amps)—the more amperes, the more current that is flowing and the greater the amount of heat that is generated. **Voltage** refers to the *force* that drives the current through the wire. Power stations generate high voltages that are sent out through power lines and then transformed down to about 120 volts for residential circuits. The power lines themselves, however, may carry more than 2,000 volts. Electric *power* is measured in watts, that is, the rate at which a given voltage pushes a given amount of amperes (WATTS = VOLTS × AMPS), and the wattage of most appliances is listed on the appliance label. Suppose, for example, you have an electric hair dryer that uses 1,200 watts, and you operate it out of a regular outlet in your house of 120 volts. Since watts = volts × amps, the current flowing through the hair dryer will be 10 amperes. That may not sound like very much, but if you take into account that a current as small as 0.1 ampere passing through the heart is enough to cause ventricular fibrillation, this means that even a very small current leak from your hair dryer could be fatal.

The amount of current that passes into the body and the path the current takes through the body are also affected by the *resistance* of the skin and internal organs to current flow, which is measured in **ohms**. If you step on an exposed wire, for instance, your calloused foot may offer a very high resistance to current flow—perhaps as much as a million ohms—but the much thinner skin on other parts of the body may be a thousand times less resistant; and if the skin is wet, the resistance to current flow is lowered even further. Once inside the body, current will take the path of least resistance, usually along blood vessels and nerves, and will exit from the body at some point where the body is grounded. If the voltage is high, however (i.e., more than about 1,000 volts), current will take the shortest path through the body, irrespective of the resistance of different tissues.

Electric Dictionary

ampere	*amount* of current flowing along a wire
volt	the *force* driving the current through a wire
watt	the *power* of an electric current (= volts × amps)
ohm	the *resistance* to flow of electric current
AC	alternating current
DC	direct current

Electric current does its damage by generating extremely high temperatures in the tissues through which it passes—sometimes as high as 2000 to 3000°C—and the tissues are quite literally cooked. It is this intense heat following the current flow that causes the enormous damage to deeper tissues, which may lie quite far from a harmless-looking entrance burn. The amount of tissue damage depends on (1) the intensity of the current, (2) the duration of exposure, and (3) the relative resistance of individual types of tissues. A high-voltage current is more destructive than a low-voltage current of the same duration, but even a few seconds of contact with a low-voltage source can cause enormous damage. In this regard, alternating current (AC) is much more dangerous than direct current (DC), for the alternations in current cause spasms of the victim's muscles, which often "freeze" the victim to the electric source until the power is shut off. For this reason, the duration of exposure to alternating current is apt to be prolonged. The resistance of individual tissues and their sensitivity to heat are also factors in determining the type and extent of internal damage. Bone, for instance, is least affected by heat; skin more so; muscle even more so; and nerves are very sensitive to high temperature. Thus one can expect the major direct damage from electric current to occur in muscle and nerve tissues.

The direction of current flow is also important. The most common paths of current flow are from hand to hand (Fig. 13-11), head to hand, hand to foot, head to foot, and thigh to foot. Current flowing from hand to hand is particularly dangerous because it may take a path across the heart, causing not only tissue damage but also ventricular fibrillation.

Four different types of burn are seen as a result of electricity. The most common is the CONTACT BURN, in which the current is most intense at the points where it enters and exits from the body. At *both* these sites—the entrance site and the exit site—you can see a typical burn that looks like a bull's-eye, with a central *black* zone of third-degree burns; a middle zone of cold, *gray*, dry tissue; and an outer *red* zone. A second type of electric burn, the FLASH BURN, occurs when part of the body is close to an electric flash; the flash burn results from the heat of an electric arc explosion and is usually first- or second-degree in depth. The third type of burn, an ARC INJURY, occurs when the patient becomes part of an electric arc, and this type of burn can be very deep. Finally, electricity may cause a garden-variety FLAME BURN, if the patient's clothing is ignited by the electric energy.

Management of Electric Burns

The FIRST step in treating a victim of electric shock is to REMOVE THE VICTIM FROM CONTACT WITH THE CURRENT SOURCE AS QUICKLY AS POSSIBLE. If there is some way to shut off the current quickly, such as closing a main power switch or activating a circuit breaker, do so. Otherwise use a nonconductive item (e.g., wooden broom handle, rope, wooden chair) to try to dislodge the victim from the current source. Be particularly careful around downed electric wires. If a wire is lying on top of an automobile, do NOT encourage anyone inside the automobile to try to jump from the car, since even a slight inadvertent contact with the car's metal frame could be fatal. Also keep bystanders well back from a downed wire, since arcing current can "jump" to objects close to the wire, even if they are not in direct contact with it.

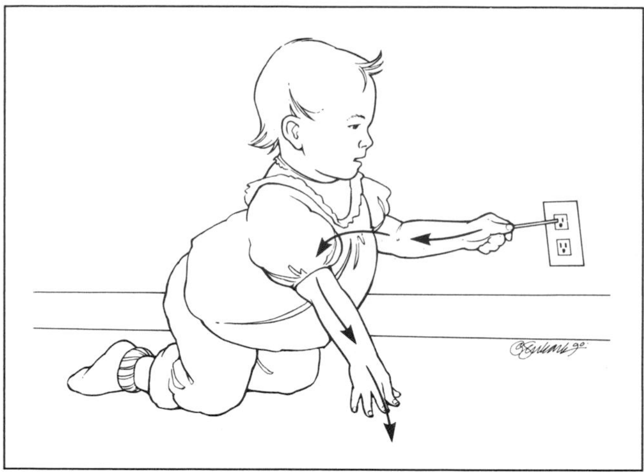

Fig. 13-11. *Electric injuries. One of the most common paths for current is from hand to hand.*

Once you are absolutely certain that the victim is no longer in contact with a live current source, proceed immediately to the PRIMARY SURVEY. Remember, the burn itself is of minor importance initially compared to the possibility of airway obstruction, respiratory arrest, or cardiac arrest. So handle the ABCs first, and give whatever treatment is required.

In the SECONDARY SURVEY, proceed as usual through the general appearance (e.g., state of consciousness, obvious deformities), vital signs, and head-to-toe survey. As you examine the patient from head to toe, LOOK FOR THE BURN ITSELF. Remember, there will usually be at least *two* burns: one where the current entered the body and one where it exited. The hand is the most common place for the entrance wound, and the exit wound is often found on the other hand or on one of the feet—whatever happened to be grounded. Cover both the entrance wound the exit wound with dry, sterile dressings. Check the extremities for PULSES. Remember that beneath normal-looking skin there can be devastating tissue damage and swelling, and the circulation may therefore be compromised. So note whether the distal pulses are full and equal in all four extremities. Check also for FRACTURES, which may occur secondary to a fall (e.g., from a utility pole) or from the violent muscle contractions (tetany) during the shock. Any suspected fracture should be fully immobilized before transport.

Management of Electric Burns

1. REMOVE THE VICTIM FROM CONTACT WITH THE CURRENT SOURCE.
2. Take care of the ABCs.

3. Secondary survey, with special attention to
   a. Entrance and exit WOUNDS.
   b. Distal PULSES.
   c. FRACTURES.
4. COVER BURN SITES with sterile dressings.
5. SPLINT fractures.
6. TREAT FOR SHOCK as necessary.

Remember, never assume that an electric burn is as minor as it looks. The damage is not where you can see it, but it is there. For this reason:

EVERY PATIENT WHO HAS SUSTAINED AN ELECTRIC BURN *MUST* BE EVALUATED IN THE HOSPITAL.

LIGHTNING INJURIES

Lightning injuries are a special kind of electric injury involving special problems. Although lightning injury is usually regarded as rare, in fact lightning causes more deaths than tornados, hurricanes, or any other form of inclement weather. In the United States, there are approximately 1,000 people injured by lightning each year, of whom 250 to 300 die from the injury. These figures indicate an important point: A substantial proportion of people injured by lightning—probably better than 70 percent—do survive. Indeed, there are several cases reported each year of victims who appeared quite dead immediately after being struck by lightning but who recovered completely with minimal resuscitation. Thus every victim of lightning injury deserves energetic rescue efforts, even when the situation at first looks quite hopeless or when CPR has been delayed beyond the "golden period" of 4–5 minutes.

What Is Lightning Made Of?

Lightning strikes when there is a massive discharge of electric energy between two bodies that have different electric charges, as for example between the earth and a storm cloud. Usually during turbulent weather, negative charges build up in the lower layers of the cloud while positive charges accumulate on the surface of the earth. When the attraction between these opposite charges reaches a certain level, lightning occurs to bridge the space between them. Lightning begins with an invisible "leader stroke," in which negative charges from the cloud stream downward, ionizing the air through which they travel and thereby making that air a better conductor of electricity. Sometimes you can "feel" the approach of a leader stroke because the highly charged atmosphere causes your hair to stand on end. As these negative charges near the ground, there is a massive discharge of current and a flash of lightning. While the initial current flow is from the cloud to the earth, the lightning bolt itself actually passes from the earth to the cloud.

The leader stroke will take the path of least resistance and thus will tend to be "attracted" to any object that is a better conductor of electricity than the air, especially if that object is projecting above the earth's surface, such as a flagpole, tree, antenna, or even a person running across an open field.

Lightning carries enormous electric energy—much, much more than even a high-voltage power line. The energy of a lightning bolt can reach 100 *million* volts, and peak currents can be in the range of 200,000 amperes. It is, however, direct, not alternating current, and the duration of exposure is extremely brief—measured in fractions of a second. Thus the severe burns of internal organs are less common in lightning injuries than in injuries produced by household current or high-tension lines. Nonetheless, the powerful shock waves produced by lightning can produce serious *contusion* to internal organs.

A person need not sustain a direct hit from lightning in order to be injured; indeed most victims are not struck directly. Much more commonly, the victim is "splashed" by lightning striking a nearby tree, pole, or other object. Ground current, produced by lightning striking the ground near the victim, can also cause severe injury and accounts for incidents in which there are multiple victims over an extended area, such as on a golf course or baseball field.

An interesting phenomenon that seems to account for the survival of many lightning victims is the so-called flash-over, in which the majority of the lightning energy flows around the outside of the victim's body rather than through it. When this happens, the victim's clothing is quite literally blasted apart and the sweat is instantaneously vaporized from the skin, but internal injury may be minimal.

Prevention of Lightning Injuries

The most effective treatment is prevention, and the EMT—as any other health professional—has a responsibility to educate the public in preventive measures. Obviously, the best prevention of all is to get out of the rain—inside a house or other large building, or in a car (not a convertible), with the windows shut. If, however, you are out of reach of such shelter when a storm threatens, use the following guidelines:

Prevention of Lightning Injuries

- STAY LOW. If you are in an open field and feel the approach of a leader stroke, crouch down and lean forward, with your hands on your knees, so that you are low to the ground but your contact with the ground is minimized. Try to avoid being on a hill or other spot where you will project above the surrounding landscape.

- GET AWAY FROM OPEN WATER.
- STAY AWAY FROM OBJECTS THAT PROJECT ABOVE THE GROUND (e.g., tall trees, poles, high buildings, antennas).
- STAY AWAY FROM ELECTRIC CONDUCTORS. Keep your distance from tractors or other metal farm equipment. Similarly, dismount and get away from a bicycle, motorcycle, golf cart, etc. Do not hold onto a golf club, fishing pole, umbrella, or any other item that could serve as a lightning rod. Also avoid chain link fences, metal pipes, or other conductors from which lightning could "splash" onto you.
- If you are in the woods, head for a LOW-LYING AREA with thick brush and low trees.

Assessment and Management of Lightning Injuries

Lightning injuries differ in several respects from standard high-voltage injuries (Table 13-2). To begin with, as noted earlier, lightning transmits much higher energies, but for much briefer durations and in the form of direct rather than alternating current. And while the exposure to standard AC current is apt to produce major burn of internal organs, lightning more often produces contusion and rupture. Furthermore, when lightning causes cardiac arrest, the type of arrest is likely to be asystole rather than ventricular fibrillation seen after electric shock with household current. The cutaneous burn from lightning does not usually have the black, charred appearance of a standard electric burn, but instead may have a spidery, zigzag, or featherlike appearance. Nonetheless, the *immediate* threats to life are the same in both types of electric injury: airway obstruction, respiratory arrest, and cardiac arrest—and the management of these problems, as always, has priority.

When you are called to the scene of a lightning strike, the FIRST thing to do is MAKE A RAPID EVALUATION OF THE ENTIRE SCENE to determine the number of victims and the condition of each. If there is more than one victim, PRIORITY GOES TO THE VICTIMS WHO ARE NOT BREATHING.

Contrary to what grandmother may have told you, no electricity remains in the body of a lightning victim, and you can touch such a victim without any danger to yourself. If the victim is unconscious, establish an AIRWAY by the jaw thrust method, since you should assume there has been a spine injury until proved otherwise. If BREATHING is absent, start artificial ventilation with oxygen, and proceed to maintain the CIRCULATION with external chest compressions as needed. Often it requires only a few minutes of CPR before the victim regains spontaneous pulse and respirations, even in cases where the victim appeared very dead just moments before.

If the patient is breathing spontaneously, administer oxygen and proceed to the SECONDARY SURVEY, but conduct that survey with the precautions you would use in any potential spine injury. Note and record the patient's STATE OF CONSCIOUSNESS. About 70 percent of lightning victims will lose consciousness for some period, and nearly 90 percent will show some degree of confusion and amnesia (loss of memory). Check the SKIN, and note the location of entrance and exit burns. Record the VITAL SIGNS. A weak, rapid pulse or falling blood pressure suggests that there is internal bleeding from associated injuries. Note whether the PUPILS are equal and react to light. Check the ribs for fractures, and feel the ABDOMEN for rigidity suggestive of internal bleeding or trauma. Note whether the PELVIS is stable. Assess the EXTREMITIES for deformity, swelling, ability to move, sensation, and pulses. Temporary leg paralysis is seen in as many as 70 percent of lightning victims, and arm paralysis occurs in about 30 percent. Marked swelling or deformity suggests the presence of fracture and indicates the need for a splint.

In treating the lightning victim—after managing life-threatening problems—cover any burns with a sterile dressing, splint fractures, and immobilize the patient on a backboard for transport.

Table 13-2. *Lightning Versus High-Voltage Injury*

Factor	Lightning Injury	High-Voltage Injury
Voltage	1 million volts	100 to 10,000 volts
Current	200,000 amps	1 to 100 amps
Type	Direct current	Alternating current
Duration of exposure	Fraction of a second	Often several seconds
Typical skin burn	Spidery, zigzag, or featherlike	Bull's-eye
Typical associated conditions	Contusion to internal organs Asystole Temporary paralysis Confusion, amnesia	Deep muscle burns Ventricular fibrillation

Management of Lightning Injuries

1. EVALUATE THE ENTIRE SCENE to determine the number of victims and the condition of each.
2. TREAT NONBREATHING PATIENTS FIRST.
3. PRIMARY SURVEY, with spine precautions.
4. OXYGEN.
5. SECONDARY SURVEY, with particular attention to
   a. State of consciousness.
   b. Skin: Burn entrance and exit wound.
   c. Vital signs.
   d. Pupils: Equality and reactivity.
   e. Evidence of fractures.
   f. Evidence of paralysis.
   g. Distal pulses.
6. COVER WOUNDS.
7. SPLINT FRACTURES.
8. BACKBOARD.

DRESSINGS AND BANDAGES

Before concluding this chapter, we need to say a few words about the dressings and bandages that we have been applying so liberally to the injuries discussed. To begin with, we need to define what we are talking about, for dressings and bandages are sometimes confused with one another, but they are not the same thing. A **dressing** is a material that is applied directly to a wound, to control bleeding or prevent further contamination, and ideally it should be sterile. A **bandage**, on the other hand, need not be sterile, for its sole function is to hold a dressing in place, and it does not come in contact with the wound.

DRESSING MATERIALS

Most ambulances carry several types of dressings in order to deal with wounds of different shapes and sizes. At a minimum, the ambulance should be supplied with dressings of the following types.

Universal Dressings

The universal dressing is a 9 × 36–inch sheet of thick, absorbent material that is folded into a compact size. It is ideal when bulk is required for a pressure dressing or to stabilize an impaled object. Unfolded, the universal dressing is useful when a relatively large, superficial wound needs to be covered. Sanitary napkins also make very serviceable dressings because of their bulk and absorbency, but they are generally not supplied in sterile form. Thus they need to be distributed into paper bags (2–3 napkins to a bag), with the bags then stapled shut and given to the local hospital to be sterilized and sealed in a plastic wrapper. Army surplus first-aid dressings (Carlisle dressings) are also excellent bulky dressings, for they come with a built-in gauze bandage. They are available in three sizes and can sometimes be purchased very cheaply in large quantities at government surplus auctions.

Gauze Pads

For smaller wounds, separately wrapped, sterile 4 × 4–inch gauze squares are the most convenient type of dressing. An assortment of Band-Aids is also very useful for the minor cuts and scratches that are encountered particularly in very little patients.

Burn Dressing

The ambulance must carry some kind of large dressing for covering extensive burns. Probably the simplest and most economical burn dressing is a standard bed sheet that has been sterilized and sealed in a protective plastic wrapper. Another very effective burn dressing, widely used in Europe and in the military, is the "metalin" dressing, which provides sterile coverage of extensive areas of the body and prevents excessive heat loss. There has been some promising early experience with the Water–Jel burn dressing, which is also worth stocking in the ambulance.

Occlusive Dressings

Occlusive dressings are required for sealing off open wounds of the chest. One of the best materials for an occlusive dressing is aluminum foil, for the entire roll of foil can be sterilized, and the foil itself gives a good seal but does not stick to the wound. Foil has the additional advantage that it is a multipurpose piece of ambulance gear, for it makes a fine "incubator" when wrapped around a premature infant, thereby preventing the baby from losing body heat. Other materials sometimes used as occlusive dressings include household plastic wrap or petrolatum gauze.

Improvised Dressings

In situations where there are multiple casualties, even the most well-stocked ambulance may run short of dressings, and the EMT will have to improvise with whatever can be found at the scene. In most cases, improvised dressings will not be sterile, but at least they should be clean, absorbent, relatively soft, and as free of lint as possible. A handkerchief, towel, diaper, and all sorts of other items can make very serviceable dressings when standard dressing materials are not available. In any case, NEVER NEGLECT A WOUND BECAUSE YOU DO NOT HAVE A COMMERCIAL DRESSING. EMTs are supposed to be resourceful. If you have run out of standard dressings, improvise!

BANDAGING MATERIALS
There are two types of bandaging material that are invaluable on an ambulance. The first is the soft, SELF-ADHERING ROLLER BANDAGE, which is easy to use and eliminates the need for many of the complicated bandaging techniques that are required with standard gauze rolls. The second is the TRIANGULAR BANDAGE, which is a jack-of-all-trades in emergency work—serving as a bandage, a sling, a tourniquet, a means of immobilizing an extremity to a splint, and dozens more handy things as well.

These two types of bandage will handle more than 95 percent of your bandaging needs, but you may also want to carry some standard gauze rolls and adhesive tape. The type of bandage that has *no* place on the ambulance is an elastic bandage, for this type of bandage is frequently applied too tightly and ends up acting as a tourniquet rather than a bandage.

> ELASTIC BANDAGES HAVE NO PLACE IN AN AMBULANCE.

PRINCIPLES OF BANDAGING
Bandages shown in textbooks always look very neat and pretty. That's because the people who draw bandages for textbooks do not have to work under pressure, in the middle of all kinds of blood and gore, with a dozen hysterical bystanders shrieking in the background. The EMT *does* have to work under those conditions, and for that reason, the EMT's bandaging job may not look as pretty as it does in the books. Don't worry about it! SO LONG AS THE BANDAGE DOES ITS JOB PROPERLY, IT DOES NOT HAVE TO BE BEAUTIFUL. Save the pretty knots for your macrame.

Regardless of the technique of bandaging used, certain general guidelines need to be observed:

1. DO NOT MAKE A BANDAGE TOO TIGHT. A bandage applied too tightly can become a tourniquet, cutting off blood flow to the injured extremity. ALWAYS CHECK THE PULSE DISTAL TO THE BANDAGE. If the pulse is not palpable, the bandage is too tight, and you will have to loosen it.
2. As another check on distal circulation, try wherever possible to LEAVE THE FINGERS OR TOES EXPOSED when you are bandaging an extremity. This permits you to keep an eye out for changes in color (pallor or cyanosis in the nail beds) that suggest the blood flow to the extremity is being interrupted.
3. On the other hand, DO NOT APPLY THE BANDAGE TOO LOOSELY. Remember, the purpose of a pressure dressing is to maintain enough pressure to stop bleeding, and you cannot keep pressure on a wound with a loose bandage. Indeed, you cannot even hold the dressing on the wound properly if the bandage is slack. So make sure the bandage is applied snugly and tied or taped securely.

CASE HISTORY

As we promised in Section IV, we shall conclude each chapter with a medical report on a typical patient in order to review both the signs and symptoms of the injuries we have studied and the principles of presenting medical information. Our patient in this chapter is one who has suffered burns in a house fire:

The patient is a 42-year-old man who suffered burns in a house fire. The patient was asleep in his closed bedroom when the fire broke out downstairs and was awakened by a smoke alarm. He found his bedroom full of smoke, and there were flames at the bedroom door, so he jumped from his bedroom window to the ground, about 15 feet below. He complains now of pain in his right leg, face, and right arm. He denies shortness of breath. He has no significant history of medical problems, no previous hospitalizations, and no allergies. He takes no medications regularly.

On physical examination, the patient was found lying on his right side, moaning in pain. He was conscious and alert, and the skin was warm and moist. Vitals are pulse 110, blood pressure 120/88, and respirations 30. The patient's eyebrows and nasal hairs are singed, and he is coughing up sooty sputum. There is no deformity or laceration of the head. There are no burns visible on the neck, and there is no neck tenderness or deformity. No broken ribs are palpated. There are wheezes throughout the chest on auscultation. The abdomen is soft. The pelvis is stable. There is an obvious deformity of the right thigh, at the level of the mid-femur. There are first- and second-degree burns over the face and right arm—we estimate about 9 percent altogether. Distal pulses are full and equal in all extremities.

The patient was given oxygen by nonrebreathing mask at 12 liters per minute. Cold compresses have been applied to the burns, and the right leg has been placed in a traction splint. En route, the patient has developed slight stridor and signs of respiratory distress. Our ETA to your location is 10 minutes.

Questions to think about:

1. Is this patient in danger of developing respiratory complications? If so, what signs would lead you to suspect so?

2. Is this patient in danger of going into shock? If so, what injury would predispose him to shock?
3. Does the patient have a critical burn? Why or why not?
4. Why did the EMTs check the distal pulses?
5. Why did they use a nonrebreathing mask to deliver oxygen (rather than, for example, nasal cannula)?

VOCABULARY

abrasion A wound in which part of the skin surface has been rubbed or scraped away.
AC Abbreviation for *alternating current*.
ampere A unit of electric current.
amputation The severing of a part of the body.
avulsion Injury in which part of the body is partially severed and hangs loose.
bandage Material used to hold a dressing in place.
contusion Closed injury to soft tissues; a bruise.
current Flow of electric charges through a wire or other conductor.
DC Abbreviation for *direct current*.
dermis The inner layer of skin, containing nerves, blood vessels, various glands, and hair follicles.
dressing Material used to cover a wound.
entrance wound Site at which a foreign body or electric current penetrates the skin.
epidermis Outermost skin layer.
exit wound Site at which a bullet, other foreign body, or electric current leaves the body.
first-degree burn The mildest form of burn, affecting only the epidermal layer and producing redness and slight swelling.
hematoma Collection of blood underneath the skin, forming a lump.
impaled object Foreign body that causes a puncture wound and remains embedded in the wound.
incision Wound characterized by a clean cut made with a sharp instrument, such as a knife.
laceration Wound characterized by a ragged cut.
melanin Pigment found in varying amounts in the epidermal layer of the skin.
ohm Unit of electric resistance.
sebaceous glands Glands located in the dermis that produce an oily substance for waterproofing the skin.
sebum Oily substance produced by sebaceous glands that gives the skin its suppleness and waterproof characteristics.
second-degree burn Burn involving the epidermal and dermal layers of the skin, characterized by redness and blistering; partial thickness burn.
subcutaneous Beneath the skin.
third-degree burn Burn involving the full thickness of skin, including the epidermis, dermis, subcutaneous tissue, and sometimes underlying muscle as well.
volt Unit of electric force.
watt Unit of electric power (= volts × amperes).

FURTHER READING

BURNS, GENERAL

Baxter CR, Waeckerle JF. Emergency treatment of burn injury. *Ann Emerg Med* 17:1305, 1988.
Bloch M. Cold water for burns and scalds. *Lancet* 1:695, 1968.
Bourne MK. Fire and Smoke. Managing skin and inhalation burns. *JEMS* 14(9):62, 1989.
Dimick A. The burn at first sight. *Emerg Med* 15(15):129, 1983.
Duda J. Burn wise. *Emergency* 21(6):44, 1989.
Edlich RF et al. Prehospital treatment of the burn patient. *EMT J* 2:42, 1978.
Luterman A, Talley MA. Field management of burn injuries. *Emerg Med Serv* 17(7):30, 1988.
Luterman A, Fields C, Curreri W. Treatment of chemical burns. *Emerg Med Serv* 17(9):36, 1988.
Nordberg M. Questions and controversies in burn care. *Emerg Med Serv* 17(9):24, 1988.
Rodheaver GT et al. Extinguishing the flaming burn victim. *JACEP* 8:307, 1979.
Salisbury R. A burn primer. *Emerg Med* 20(14):155, 1988.
Shulman AG. Ice water as primary treatment of burns. *JAMA* 173:1916, 1960.
Wachtel TL. Major burns: What to do at the scene and en route to the hospital. *Postgrad Med* 85(1):178, 1989.

ELECTRIC AND LIGHTNING INJURY

Amy B. Lightning injury with survival in five patients. *JAMA* 253:243, 1985.
Cooper MA. Lightning injuries: Prognostic signs for death. *Ann Emerg Med* 9:134, 1980.
Cooper MA. Of volts and bolts. *Emerg Med* 15(8):99, 1983.
Dixon G. The evaluation and management of electric burns. *Crit Care Med* 11:384, 1983.
Hammond JS, Ward CG. High-voltage electrical injuries: Management and outcome of 60 cases. *South Med J* 81:1351, 1988.
Hunt JL, Sato RM, Baxter CB. Acute electric burns. *Arch Surg* 115:434, 1980.
Kobernick M. Electrical injuries: Pathophysiology and management. *Ann Emerg Med* 11:633, 1982.
Moran KT et al. Lightning injury: Physics, pathophysiology, and clinical features. *Irish Med J* 79:120, 1986.
Mortenson ML. Electricity sparks multi-system assessment. *Emerg Med Serv* 12(1):15, 1983.
Salisbury R. High-voltage electrical injuries. *Emerg Med* 21(13):86, 1989.
Seward PN. Electrical injuries: Trauma with a difference. *Emerg Med* 19(9):66, 1987.
Solem L, Fischer RP, Strate RG. The natural history of electric injury. *J Trauma* 17:487, 1977.
Wilkinson C, Wood M. High voltage electric injury. *Am J Surg* 136:693, 1978.

14. INJURIES TO THE HEAD, FACE, NECK, AND SPINE

OBJECTIVES

Perhaps nowhere in the spectrum of emergency care can the EMT have so great an impact on a patient's destiny as in the management of patients with injuries to the head and spine. Proper management and handling of such patients in the field can make the difference between a normal existence or a lifetime of total paralysis, and there are more than a few people walking about today who owe their lives and their ability to move to the treatment an EMT gave them in the field. In this chapter, we will examine injuries to the head, face, neck, and spine and learn how to manage such injuries in a way that minimizes the possibility of lifelong disability to the patient. On completion of this chapter, the reader should be able to

1. List the three main subdivisions of the brain and identify the functions of each, given a list of functions
2. Identify the three layers of the meninges, given a diagram or description of the layers
3. Identify two functions of the cerebrospinal fluid, given a list of functions
4. Identify the subdivisions of the spinal column, given a diagram of the spinal column, and indicate which regions of the spine are most vulnerable to injury
5. List at least five questions that should be answered in obtaining the history of a head-injured patient
6. List the signs requiring particular attention when doing the physical assessment of a head-injured patient and indicate how these signs should be checked and recorded
7. Identify the significance of (a) hypertension and bradycardia, (b) hypotension and tachycardia, and (c) hypotension and bradycardia, in the context of head injury
8. Identify the priorities in treating a head-injured patient, given a description of associated injuries and a list of treatment steps
9. Identify the correct treatment of scalp bleeding (a) when there is no skull fracture and (b) when skull fracture is present, given a list of various treatments
10. Identify patients with probable skull fracture, given a description of several patients
11. Identify the correct treatment for bleeding or watery drainage from the ear, given a list of treatments
12. Identify patients with probable increasing intracranial pressure, given a description of several patients
13. Identify the most common cause of death after head injury, given a list of causes
14. Indicate which patients should and should not be covered with a blanket, given a list of patients that includes (a) a head-injured patient and (b) a spine-injured patient in neurogenic shock

15. Identify the optimal position in which to transport (a) an unconscious patient with isolated head injury, (b) a conscious patient with isolated head injury, (c) a conscious patient with epistaxis, (d) a conscious patient with cervical spine injury and neurogenic shock, (e) an unconscious patient with cervical spine injury, and (f) a conscious patient with a severed jugular vein
16. Identify the correct treatment for (a) a penetrating wound of the cheek, (b) an impaled object in the cheek, (c) an avulsed skin flap on the face, and (d) a contusion of the face, given a list of possible treatments
17. Identify the main structures of the eye, given a diagram of the eye or a description of the structures
18. List at least six steps in the examination of an injured eye
19. Identify the correct treatment for (a) a foreign body in the eye, (b) an impaled object in the eye, (c) a laceration of the eyelid, (d) a laceration of the globe, (e) an avulsed eye, and (f) thermal and light burns of the eye, given a list of possible treatments
20. Indicate what preliminary step(s) must be taken before applying pressure to control bleeding from a lacerated eyelid
21. List the measures that should be taken to protect the eyes of any unconscious patient
22. Identify the correct treatment for (a) epistaxis when there is no associated head injury, (b) epistaxis when skull fracture is suspected, and (c) a foreign body in the nose, given a list of possible treatments
23. Identify the correct treatment for (a) laceration of the external ear, (b) bleeding from the ear canal, and (c) a foreign body in the ear, given a list of possible treatments
24. Identify the priorities in treating injuries to the mouth, given a list of treatment steps
25. Identify the correct treatment for (a) an avulsed tooth and (b) a fractured mandible, given a list of possible treatments
26. Identify which patient is likely to have a fractured trachea, given a description of several patients
27. List the steps in treating a patient with an open or closed injury to the larynx or trachea
28. Identify the correct method of treating arterial bleeding from the neck, given a list of methods
29. Identify the principal danger involved in venous bleeding from the neck and list the steps in treating a patient with a severed neck vein
30. List at least eight circumstances or injuries likely to be associated with injury to the spine
31. List at least eight symptoms and signs of spine injury
32. Identify which patients have probable spine injury, given a description of several patients
33. Arrange in the correct sequence the steps in treating a spine-injured patient, given a list of steps in random order
34. Identify errors in handling a spine-injured patient, given a description of several rescue situations.

ANATOMY AND FUNCTION OF THE CENTRAL NERVOUS SYSTEM

The nervous system has three main components: the brain, the spinal cord, and the peripheral nerves. When we talk about injuries to the head and spine, we are concerned chiefly with the first two of these components—the brain and spinal cord—which together make up the **central nervous system (CNS).**

THE BRAIN

The brain is the central computer for the whole body, receiving data from all the sense organs (sight, sound, smell, touch, taste), as well as from internal organs (e.g., position, distention, level of oxygen in the blood); processing the data through hundreds of interconnected programs; and issuing all sorts of orders to various parts of the body ("Move your right leg," or "Breathe faster," or "Run like hell!"). The human brain is by far the most remarkable computer in existence, for it thinks; dreams; provides consciousness and an awareness of the organism's surroundings; invents poems and music and designs for bridges; and all the while manages to keep thousands of processes—such as breathing and temperature regulation—functioning smoothly.

The organ that does all these remarkable things is a soft and very delicate lump of tissue that fits quite snugly inside the cranium, with no room to spare. The brain consists of three components: the cerebrum, the cerebellum, and the brainstem (Fig. 14-1).

The Cerebrum

The **cerebrum** is the largest and smartest part of the brain and is composed of a right and a left hemisphere. Grossly, its surface looks like a big, white peach pit, with deep wrinkles (called convolutions) in its surface. Under a microscope, one can see that brain tissue consists of several different types of cells, each with a highly specialized job. The most significant feature of brain cells differentiates them from most other cells in the body: BRAIN CELLS DO NOT REGENERATE. This means that **once a brain cell is destroyed, it cannot be replaced** by a new brain cell. Scar tissue will take its place, but not its function, which will be lost forever.

The cerebrum is in charge of all higher functions, such as thinking, reasoning, understanding, learning abstract concepts, and feeling nuances of emotion. Specialized areas in the cerebrum process data from the sense organs (e.g., sight, sound) while other specialized areas control the voluntary movements of every skeletal muscle. Because the location of these functions in the brain is known, doctors can often

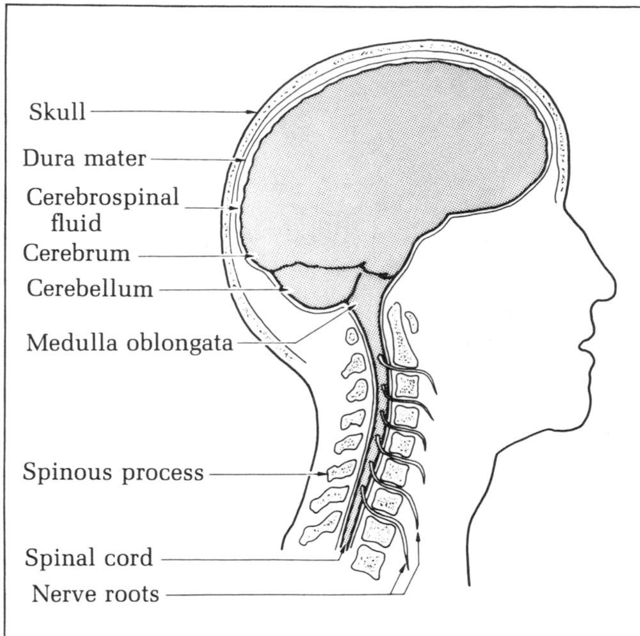

Fig. 14-1. *The brain.*

pinpoint the site of brain injury by determining what function has been impaired or lost. When a person loses the ability to speak, for instance, one knows that damage has probably occurred in the speech center located in the posterior temporoparietal region of the brain.

The motor centers, which control voluntary movement, lie on the side of the brain opposite the side of the body they control; that is, the motor center controlling movement of the left arm and leg is in the right cerebral hemisphere, while that controlling the right arm and leg is in the left cerebral hemisphere. Speech, on the other hand, is regulated by a single center, usually on the same side of the brain as the dominant motor center. Thus the speech center of a right-handed person is usually on the left side of the brain, the side that controls movements of the right hand. For this reason, a person who has a stroke or head injury will be more likely to lose his speech if the injury causes paralysis of the dominant hand; thus in conducting a neurologic examination, it is customary to inquire whether the patient is right-handed or left-handed.

The Cerebellum

The **cerebellum** is located beneath the cerebrum, in the posterior part of the skull. The cerebellum is sometimes called the "athlete's brain," because its job is to ensure balance, muscle tone, and coordination of skilled movements. Riding a bicycle, roller-skating, doing CPR, and even tying a shoelace all require an intact cerebellum.

The Brainstem

At the base of the brain, between the cerebrum and the spinal cord and surrounded by the cerebellum, is the **brainstem**, the old-timer of the brain in terms of evolution. Just about every animal has a structure equivalent to the brainstem, for it is the control center for all vital, automatic functions. The lowermost part of the brainstem, for example, the **medulla**, is the headquarters for control of body temperature, heart rate, breathing, swallowing, and many other critical body functions.

Protective Coverings

The brain is protected from injury by three separate mechanisms: the skull, the meninges, and the cerebrospinal fluid.

The skull, or **cranium,** forms a rigid box that entirely encases the brain; and because of its rigid construction, the skull is somewhat of a mixed blessing for the brain. On the one hand, the solid construction of the skull protects the brain from being contused or squashed by every little bump that a person suffers in the course of normal activity. But on the other hand, precisely because it is a rigid box, the skull cannot expand. Thus if there is any bleeding inside the skull or swelling of brain tissue, the pressure within the skull increases rapidly, often to levels that cause severe brain damage.

Just beneath the skull are three layers of tissue, collectively called **meninges** (Fig. 14-2), that enclose the brain (and the spinal cord) and further protect it from injury. The outermost layer, called the **dura mater** (or just plain dura) is a tough, leathery tissue that helps support and cushion the brain. Just beneath the dura mater is a much thinner, filmy layer called the **arachnoid**, which is rich in blood vessels. Finally, the innermost layer, the **pia mater**, wraps around the surface of the brain like a tight glove. The blood vessels of the arachnoid and the pia mater nourish the outer layers of the brain.

Head injury can result in disruption of blood vessels outside or beneath the meninges. When blood collects between the skull and the dura, it is referred to as an *epi*dural hematoma; if blood collects beneath the dura, the condition is called a *sub*dural hematoma. Either injury produces considerable pressure on the brain tissue, and either can be lethal if not treated promptly.

The spaces between the dura mater and the brain or spinal cord are filled with a clear fluid, called **cerebrospinal fluid (CSF)**, which serves as an additional shock absorber, cushioning any blows that land on the head. The CSF also carries nutrients to the brain and spinal cord. When bacteria or viruses gain access to the CSF, usually through the nose, a severe inflammation of the meninges, called meningitis, can result. In head injuries, when CSF is seen

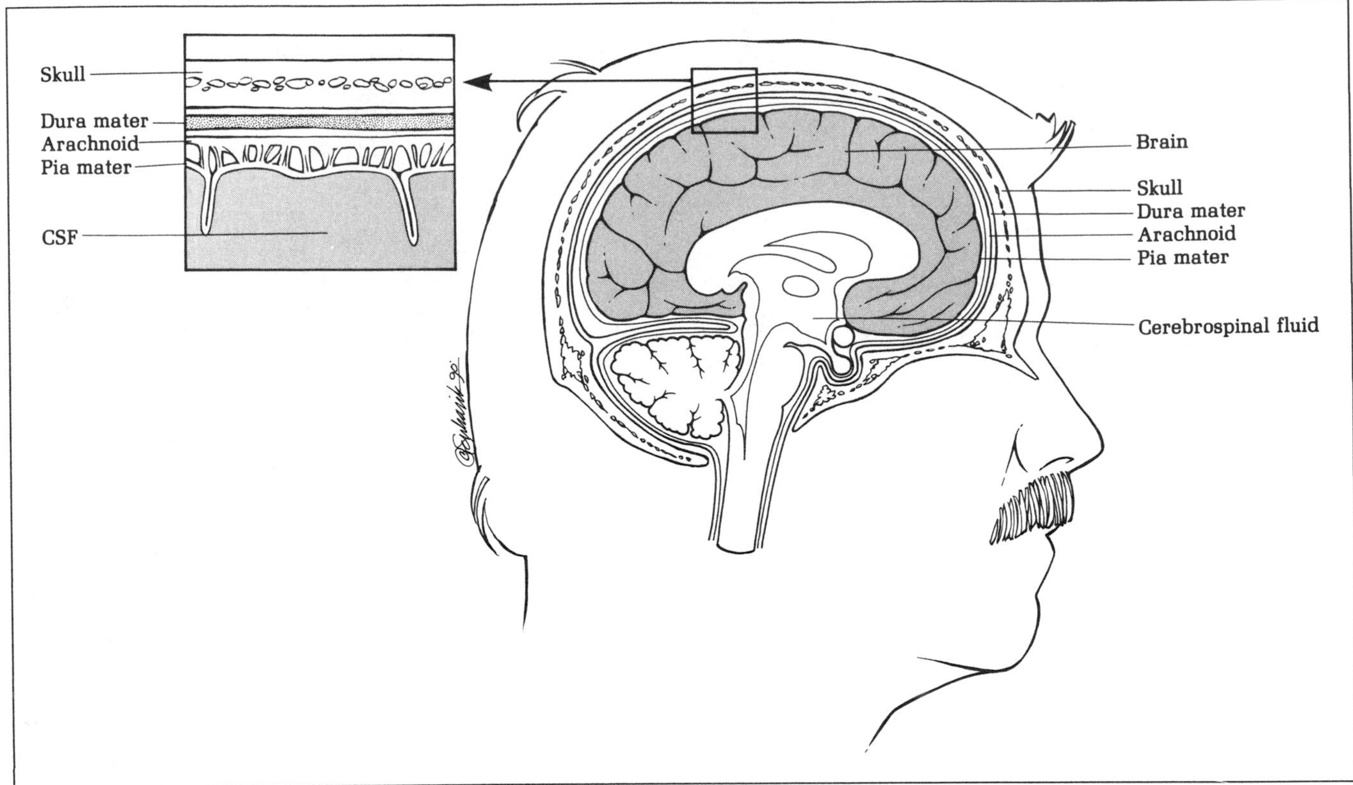

Fig. 14-2. *The fibrous coverings of the brain (meninges).*

leaking from the nose or ears, one can assume that the skull has been fractured and that the underlying dura mater was also lacerated in the process.

THE SPINAL CORD

If the brain is the computer center of the body, the spinal cord is the main cable connecting the computer center to all the remote terminals throughout the organism and carrying data back and forth in both directions. The spinal cord is a continuation of the brain that extends downward from the medulla through the center of the vertebral column, or spine. The bony vertebrae enclose and protect the spinal cord. Between each two vertebrae of the column, a pair of nerve bundles (smaller cables) branch off to the right and left to connect the brain with muscles and other organs at that level. The nerve bundles also contain *sensory* nerves carrying information (e.g., temperature, pressure, position) back from the tissues to the brain. Each vertebra is given a letter and a number according to where it is located (Fig. 14-3). There are seven **cervical vertebrae,** the first of which is called C1, the second C2, and so forth. Beneath the cervical vertebrae are twelve **thoracic vertebrae** (T1–T12), to which the twelve ribs are attached posteriorly. Then come the five **lumbar vertebrae** of the lower back (L1–L5); then the **sacrum**, five fused vertebrae that form part of the posterior pelvis; and finally the **coccyx**, the four fused vertebrae that make up the tail bone. Nerve tracts emerge from the spinal column all the way from the space between C1 and C2 down to the space between L4 and L5, and each nerve bundle carries messages back and forth from a specific part of the body. The most vulnerable areas of the spinal column are the cervical spine and the lumbar spine, for these areas are relatively unsupported by other structures. The thoracic spine is buttressed by the rib cage, but the neck and the lower back have no such lateral struts to keep them stable. Thus they are more vulnerable to bending and twisting forces.

Clearly, the farther up the spinal cord one sustains an injury, the more muscles whose function will be affected. If the spinal cord is damaged in the lumbar region, for example, one would expect to see paralysis and loss of sensation in the legs but not the arms, for the nerves to the arms have already left the main cable at the cervical region. On the other hand, an injury to the neck will damage nerves to *both* the arms and the legs, because both sets of nerves are running in this part of the cable.

The nerve cells in the spinal cord, like those in the brain, are almost entirely incapable of regeneration. A spinal nerve that is destroyed is lost forever, which is the reason that spinal injuries require such extreme precautions in the field.

REMEMBER, QUADRIPLEGIA IS FOREVER.

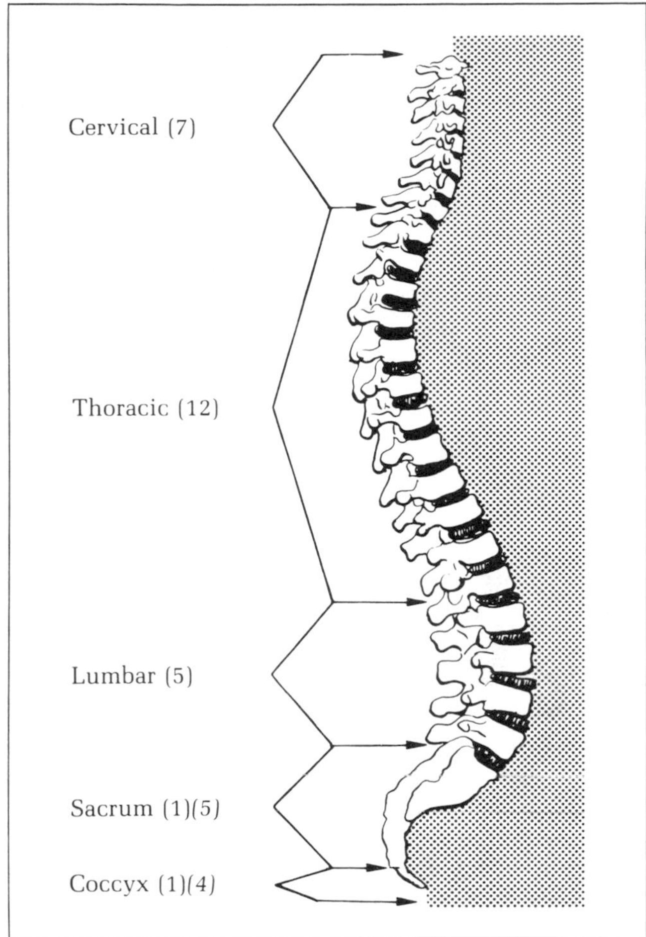

Fig. 14-3. *The spinal column.*

HEAD INJURIES

Injuries to the skull and brain occur quite commonly, especially in vehicular accidents, where head injuries constitute about 70 percent of all injuries sustained and account for about half of all deaths. Head injuries vary in severity from minor scalp lacerations to major brain damage, but for purposes of evaluation and treatment in the field, *every* head injury should be regarded as critical and should be managed accordingly.

ASSESSMENT OF THE PATIENT WITH HEAD INJURY

The assessment of the head-injured patient requires very careful attention to detail and to the recording of repeated observations. The data recorded by the EMT in the field will often play a crucial role in the neurosurgeon's decision whether to operate immediately, and for this reason the EMT should try to be as thorough and accurate as possible in collecting and recording information about the patient.

In reviewing the assessment of the head-injured patient, we will assume for the moment that you have completed the primary survey and have proceeded to the secondary survey of the patient. As always, the secondary survey will consist of the history and physical examination.

The History

The history is a vital part of the assessment of a head-injured patient, and it is usually derived from observations of the scene, from interviews with bystanders, and if the patient is conscious, from the patient himself. At a minimum, one should try to elicit the following information:

- WHEN DID THE ACCIDENT OCCUR? Five minutes ago? Five hours ago? It is very important to be able to relate the patient's present condition to the amount of time elapsed since he sustained the injury. Unconsciousness that develops an hour after a head injury, for instance, is generally more worrisome than a brief period of unconsciousness occurring immediately after a blow to the head.
- HOW DID THE ACCIDENT OCCUR? What were the mechanisms of injury? Was there a direct blow to the head? To which part of the head? Were there strong gravitational forces involved (as in a head-on collision) that would increase the likelihood of associated spine injury? Take a good look at the accident scene, and try to reconstruct what happened and what forces were involved.
- DID THE PATIENT LOSE CONSCIOUSNESS AT ANY TIME? If so, when? Immediately after the accident? After some time had elapsed? How long did he remain unconscious?
- Did the patient VOMIT any time since the accident? Has he had any SEIZURES? Both of these are signs of possible brain injury.
- If the patient is able to communicate, find out his CHIEF COMPLAINT. Is he having PAIN? Where? What about NUMBNESS AND TINGLING? Does he feel WEAKNESS OR HEAVINESS in any of his extremities? Does he feel NAUSEATED? DIZZY? Is he having any PROBLEMS WITH HIS VISION? HAVE HIS SYMPTOMS CHANGED in any way since the injury occurred?
- Are there any possible COMPLICATING FACTORS, such as recent ingestion of ALCOHOL OR DRUGS, or significant UNDERLYING MEDICAL PROBLEMS?

The Physical Assessment

The physical assessment of a head-injured patient must be performed over and over again, for what is important is not the evaluation at any single point in time, but rather CHANGES in the patient's condition as they occur over time. A patient whose state of consciousness is gradually deteriorating, for instance, will probably require surgery very soon after reaching the hospital; whereas a patient who is gradually waking up is much less likely to have a serious head injury and can be kept under observation for a while. The only way to know what changes are occurring is to make frequent checks of the patient and record the time and the findings of each check accurately. In performing the secondary survey, the EMT should give particular attention to the following factors.

GENERAL APPEARANCE. If the patient is conscious, does he appear to be in distress? Is the skin dusky? Is it cold and clammy, suggesting shock from other injuries? What is the patient's STATE OF CONSCIOUSNESS? Be precise. Avoid descriptive terms such as "stupor" or "semicoma," but instead make a careful record of what the patient can and cannot do. Is he oriented, that is, does he know his name, where he lives, where he works, what day it is? If he can speak, make a note of this fact, and record whether SPEECH is clear and logical or whether it is rambling and garbled. If the patient is not fully awake, record WHAT KIND OF STIMULUS IS REQUIRED TO WAKEN HIM. Does he waken in response to a shout? To light pain, such as a pinprick? To stronger pain, such as a pinch? Does he waken at all? If not, does he have ANY REACTION TO PAIN? Is the reaction appropriate, inappropriate, or decerebrate? A reaction is appropriate if the patient tries to move away from the painful stimulus or to push the stimulus away from himself. An inappropriate reaction is one that is ineffective in getting rid of the painful stimulus. In a **decerebrate response**, all of the patient's muscles stiffen spasmodically in reaction to a pinprick or pinch, while in a **decorticate response** the arms flex (Fig. 14-4).

One simple method of describing the patient's level of consciousness is known as the **AVPU Scale.**

AVPU Scale

A The patient is **alert.** He knows his name, where he is, what day it is, and so forth.

V The patient responds to **voice.** He may not be alert or open his eyes spontaneously, but he does respond in an appropriate way when spoken to.

P The patient responds only to a **painful** stimulus, such as a pinch or a pinprick.

U The patient is completely **unresponsive,** even to a painful stimulus.

As noted, you must repeat these observations over and over again during the time the patient is in your care and make a careful record of each observation.

THE MOST IMPORTANT SINGLE SIGN IN THE EVALUATION OF A HEAD-INJURED PATIENT IS A *CHANGING* STATE OF CONSCIOUSNESS.

VITAL SIGNS. Measure and record the vital signs. Note the rate and quality of the PULSE and the magnitude of the BLOOD PRESSURE. A *rising* blood pressure and a *falling* pulse often indicate that the pressure inside the skull (intracranial pressure) is rising, as a result of bleeding within the skull or swelling of the brain. A rapid pulse and a falling blood pressure, on the other hand, are signs of shock and are almost never due to head injury, at least not in adults. Shock means that there is significant injury or hemorrhage *somewhere else* in the body, and it is a signal to the EMT to search for those other injuries.

A FALLING BLOOD PRESSURE IS ALMOST NEVER CAUSED BY HEAD INJURY, AND ONE MUST LOOK FOR SPINAL INJURY OR A SOURCE OF MAJOR BLEEDING ELSEWHERE IN THE BODY.

Note also the quality and rate of RESPIRATIONS, and record any abnormal respiratory patterns. Hyperpnea and tachypnea suggest brain injury, as does Cheyne-Stokes respiration. Measure or estimate the patient's TEMPERATURE as well. Brain injury tends to cause an increase in body temperature, sometimes to very high levels.

Like the assessment of the state of consciousness, the vital signs should be rechecked and recorded frequently. Be especially alert for CHANGES IN PULSE AND BLOOD PRESSURE that may signal shock or increasing intracranial pressure:

Key Changes in Vital Signs

	Increasing Intracranial Pressure	*Shock*
BP	Rising	Falling
PULSE	Slow	Rapid

HEAD-TO-TOE SURVEY. Conduct the head-to-toe survey with extreme care not to move the patient. At least 10 percent of patients with head injury have associated injury to the cervical spine, and thus one should operate in the field under the assumption that spine injury is present:

ANY PATIENT WITH A SIGNIFICANT HEAD INJURY HAS A CERVICAL SPINE INJURY UNTIL PROVED OTHERWISE.

Start the head-to-toe survey by checking the SCALP for bleeding. Palpate the entire scalp gently to check for lumps suggestive of hematoma or depressions suggestive of skull fracture. Look for any clear

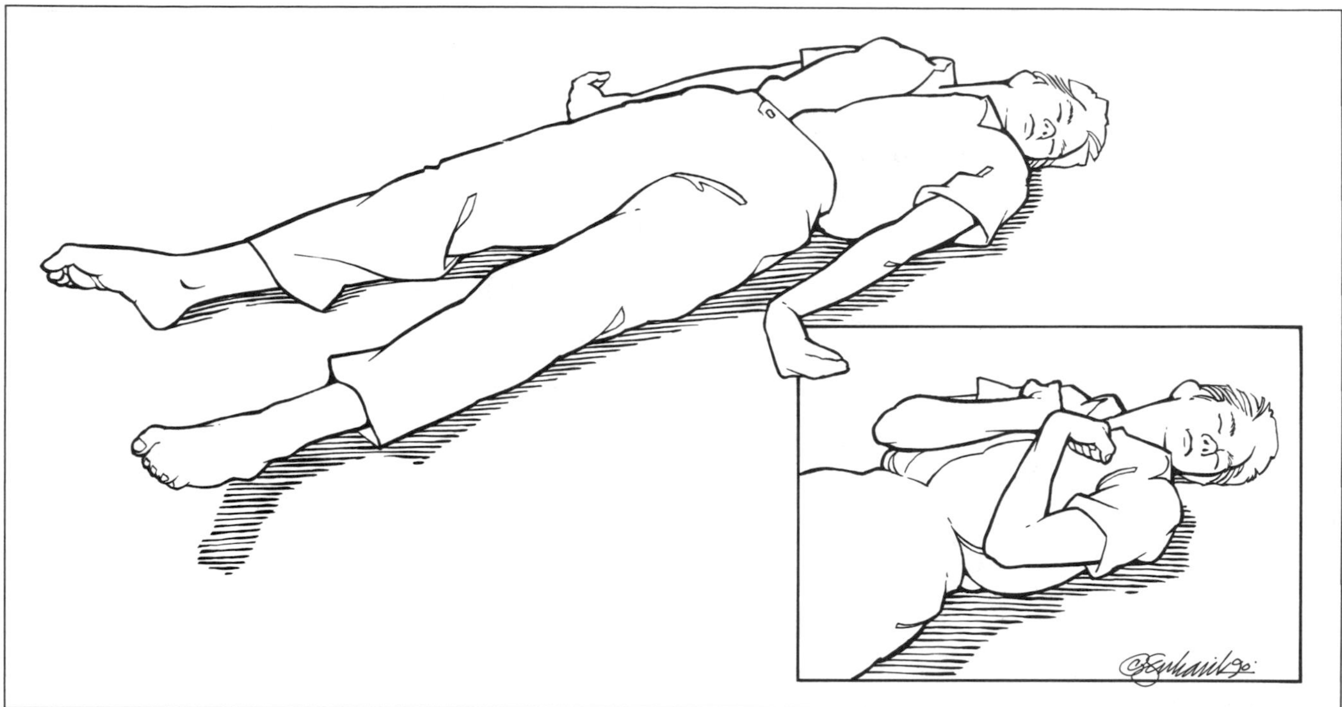

Fig. 14-4. *Responses suggestive of brain injury. A. Decerebrate response (arms and legs extended). B. Decorticate response (legs extended, arms flexed).*

fluid draining from a scalp laceration or from the EARS or NOSE (Fig. 14-5). As we learned earlier, this fluid is cerebrospinal fluid, and its leakage from the ears, nose, or a break in the scalp is a sign that the skull has been fractured and the underlying dura mater has been torn. Other signs of skull fracture include ecchymoses behind the ears over the mastoid (Battle's sign) and around the eyes (raccoon sign), both of which suggest a fracture at the base of the skull.

Examine the FACE for lacerations, bruises, and stability of the facial bones (Fig. 14-6). Make sure to check the MOUTH for blood, broken teeth or dentures, and other foreign materials. Examine the EYES, and make an accurate record of the size and equality of the PUPILS; record as well whether each pupil constricts in response to light. Unequal pupils should be assumed to be a sign of brain injury.

Check the NECK for wounds and any signs of spine injury (we will discuss these signs in greater detail later in this chapter). Survey the CHEST, ABDOMEN, PELVIS, and BACK in the usual fashion. Bear in mind that there may be multiple injuries, and the head injury may be the least serious part of the patient's problem. When you come to the EXTREMITIES, test each extremity for sensation and the ability to move, starting with the toes and working up. Paralysis caused by brain injury is more likely to involve one side of the body (hemiplegia), for instance the right arm and right leg; whereas paralysis from spinal cord injury will usually involve both legs and sometimes both arms as well.

It will be easier to keep an orderly and accurate record of your findings if you carry a special checklist for head-injured patients, such as the NEUROLOGIC EXAMINATION RECORD shown in Figure 14-7. This particular checklist was designed by the Committee on Trauma of the American College of Surgeons, and it provides a relatively simple format for recording very precise observations of a patient's status over time. A record of this type made by the EMT in the field is of inestimable value to the emergency room doctor, for he can see at a glance exactly what changes have occurred in the patient's condition and thus can better appraise the need for urgent surgery. The checklist also helps remind the EMT of what observations need to be made, so the EMT is less likely to forget, in the confusion of the field, to examine the pupils or the movement of each extremity, for example.

GENERAL CONSIDERATIONS IN HEAD-INJURED PATIENTS

No matter what the nature of the head injury, there are certain general considerations that apply to all head-injured patients, and most important among these are our old friends the ABCs, which must be taken care of before any other evaluation or treatment of the patient is undertaken.

The first priority in treating a victim of head injury

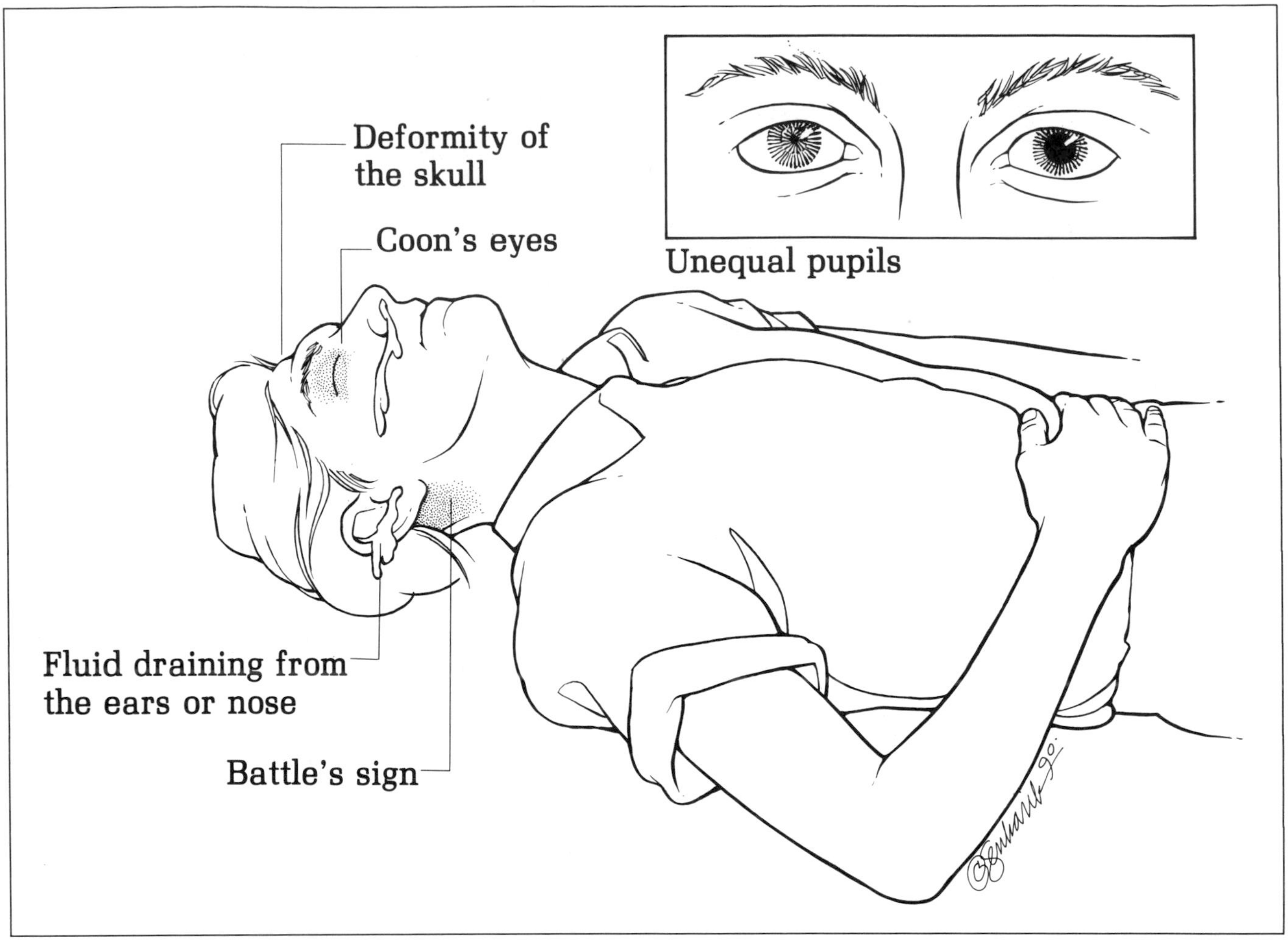

Fig. 14-5. *Looking for signs of injury to the skull or brain: deformity, unequal pupils, raccoon sign, Battle's sign, fluid draining from the ears or nose.*

is to ensure an adequate AIRWAY, which is particularly likely to be in jeopardy if the patient is unconscious. Bear in mind, however, our rule that EVERY HEAD-INJURED PATIENT HAS A CERVICAL SPINE INJURY, and avoid hyperextension of the head and neck; try instead to establish the airway using the *jaw thrust* technique. Make sure that the airway is not blocked by blood clots, vomitus, secretions, or broken teeth, and suction out any accessible foreign material. If the patient is deeply unconscious, use an oropharyngeal airway to keep the airway open. Once the patient has been fully immobilized on a backboard, it is also desirable to tilt the backboard onto its side, leaning slightly forward, so that blood, vomitus, or other secretions can drain out of the patient's mouth rather than down the throat.

Evaluate the patient's BREATHING. In general, isolated head injury does not by itself cause apnea (although apnea may result from airway obstruction or from secondary trauma caused by brain swelling);

Fig. 14-6. *Signs of facial trauma: ecchymoses, deformity, loose or missing teeth, swollen or unstable jaw.*

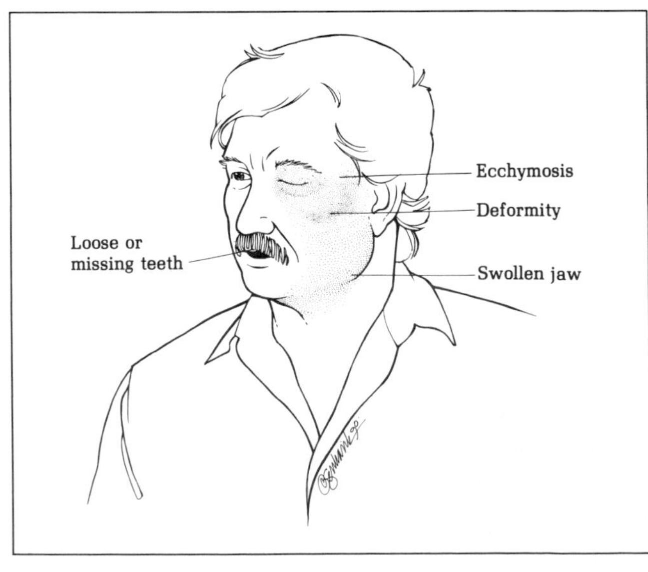

NEUROLOGIC EXAMINATION RECORD

INSTRUCTIONS. Record vital signs in Unit I. If the patient can talk, check (✓) one subdivision in units II, III, and IV. An oriented patient should know his name, age, etc. A moan can be checked as "garbled" speech. If unable to talk, check (✓) "none" in Unit III and one block in Unit V. In an "inappropriate" response, the patient is not effective in removing the painful stimulus; when "decerebrate," the extremities reflexly extend and/or hyperpronate. In Unit VI, draw the size and shape of each pupil and check (✓) for a reaction to light. Under Unit VII, normal strength is scored as "4," slight weakness "3," a 50 percent reduction in strength "2," marked weakness and without spontaneous movement "1," and complete paralysis "0."

UNIT	TIME:					
I Vital Signs	blood pressure					
	pulse					
	respirations					
	temperature					
II Conscious and:	oriented					
	disoriented					
	restless					
	combative					
III Speech	clear					
	rambling					
	garbled					
	none					
IV Will awaken to:	name					
	shaking					
	light pain					
	strong pain					
V Nonverbal reaction to pain	appropriate					
	inappropriate					
	"decerebrate"					
	none					
VI Pupils	size on right					
	size on left					
	reacts on right					
	reacts on left					
VII Ability to move:	right arm					
	left arm					
	right leg					
	left leg					

Fig. 14-7. *Neurologic checklist. (Reproduced courtesy American College of Surgeons.)*

it is more common to see hyperpnea if there is brain damage. Associated spine injury, however, can cause paralysis of the intercostal muscles, in which case the patient will have to rely entirely on his diaphragm to breathe. This kind of breathing is very inefficient and often inadequate to move sufficient quantities of air in and out of the lungs. Thus a patient whose breathing is very shallow may need *gently* assisted ventilations with a bag-valve-mask plus oxygen, but you must take care not to hyperextend the neck and not to force air in under too much pressure. If the patient is breathing adequately on his own, he should be given oxygen by mask or nasal cannula.

Assess the CIRCULATION, and note any signs of shock. Remember that shock is almost never due to head injury, and its presence indicates the need to search for a major source of bleeding elsewhere in the body. Control profuse BLEEDING before moving on to the secondary survey.

Bleeding from the head is usually from disrupted blood vessels in the scalp and can be quite profuse; indeed, it may be sufficient to cause hypovolemic shock, especially in children. The blood vessels in the scalp lie between two tough layers of tissue—a surface skin layer and an inner layer, called the **galea**. When only the surface layer of the scalp is lacerated, bleeding can usually be controlled with a pressure dressing held snugly in place by a circumferential bandage (Fig. 14-8). If, however, the underlying galea has also been lacerated, often the wound will gape open and bleed profusely. The most effective method of controlling this kind of scalp bleeding is to press the bleeding edge of the scalp very firmly against the skull. This method should be used only if the skull beneath the scalp wound is stable, for if there is a skull fracture beneath the laceration, pressure against the skull can push fragments of bone into the brain. If, therefore, there is a depression or instability beneath the scalp wound, simply cover the wound with a bulky dressing and hold it firmly in place with a roller bandage. Pressure point control over the temporal artery can also assist in control of bleeding from scalp wounds.

Having completed the ABCs, it is a good idea to stabilize the cervical spine temporarily, until you can complete the rest of the patient evaluation. Sandbags placed on either side of the patient's head provide a quick and convenient means to limit motion of the head and neck as you proceed through the secondary survey.

Evaluation of the Head-Injured Patient

1. PRIMARY SURVEY
   a. AIRWAY: Use jaw thrust technique, and avoid hyperextension.
   b. BREATHING: Give oxygen; assist shallow respirations gently.
   c. CIRCULATION
      (1) Note signs of SHOCK, which mean injury elsewhere.
      (2) Control BLEEDING.
2. SECONDARY SURVEY
   a. HISTORY
      (1) TIME of injury; MECHANISMS of injury.
      (2) LOSS OF CONSCIOUSNESS?
      (3) NAUSEA or VOMITING?

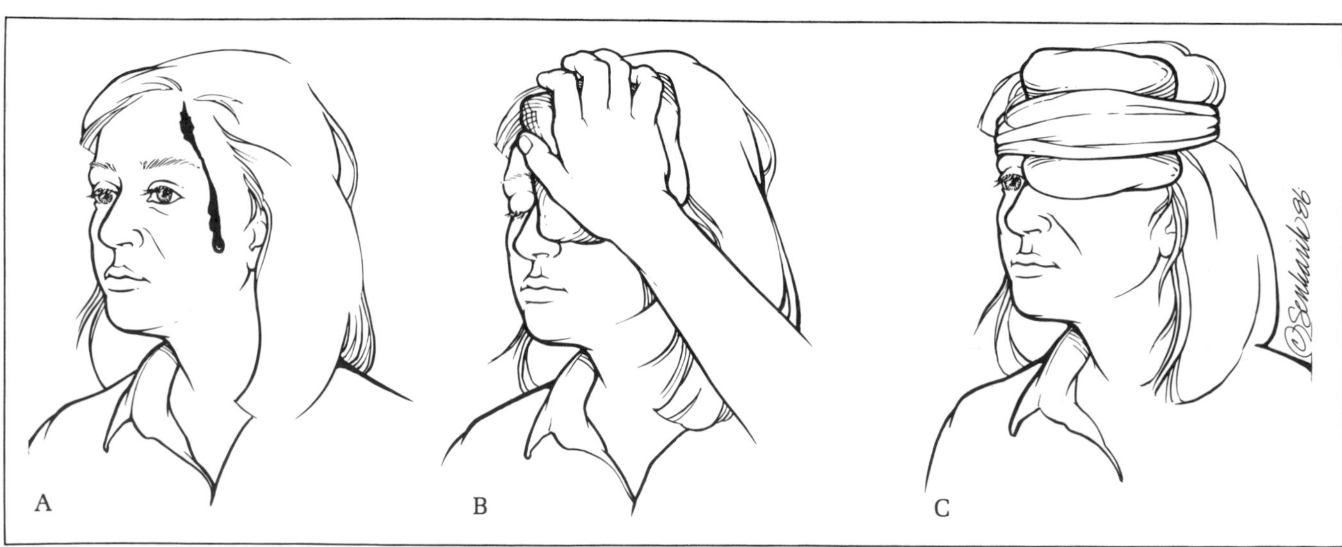

Fig. 14-8. *A. Bleeding from a wound on the forehead. B. Initial control of bleeding by manual pressure. C. Pressure dressing in place.*

(4) SEIZURES?
(5) NUMBNESS, WEAKNESS, PARALYSIS?
(6) Visual disturbances?
(7) Other complaints?
(8) Complicating factors (alcohol, drugs, other illness).

b. PHYSICAL ASSESSMENT (repeat frequently and note changes)
(1) STATE OF CONSCIOUSNESS AND NEUROLOGIC ASSESSMENT
(a) Speech.
(b) Stimulus required to waken.
(c) Response to pain.
(2) VITAL SIGNS
(a) Look for rising BP and falling pulse.
(b) Shock is not due to head injury.
(3) HEAD-TO-TOE SURVEY
(a) *Scalp:* Lacerations.
(b) *Skull:* Deformities.
(c) *Ears, nose:* Leakage of CSF or blood.
(d) Battle's sign; raccoon sign.
(e) *Eyes:* Pupils.
(f) *Mouth:* Blood, vomitus, broken teeth or dentures.
(g) *Mandible:* Stability.
(h) *Neck:* ASSUME A CERVICAL SPINE INJURY.
(i) *Chest:* Breathing movements.
(j) *Extremities:* Sensation and movement.

SKULL FRACTURE

The skull (Fig. 14-9) appears to be a single unit, but actually it consists of 22 bones of the cranium and face, most of which are fused tightly together at joints called sutures. The only moveable bone in the skull is the lower jaw (mandible), which is hinged to the rest of the cranium just below the ears. Fourteen of the bones that make up the skull are facial bones, such as the **zygoma,** or cheek bone. Many of the facial bones contain air spaces, or sinuses, that serve to reduce the overall weight of the skull. Because these sinuses are connected to the nasal cavity, they can become filled with fluid when a person has an upper respiratory infection. The remaining 8 bones of the skull, beside the facial bones, are the cranial bones themselves—frontal, parietal, occipital, and temporal—that form the strong, protective box encasing the brain.

A skull fracture, when present, indicates that a considerable force was applied to the head, but it provides no proof that actual injury to the *brain* has occurred. Paradoxically enough, serious brain injury is more common in trauma in which there is *no* skull fracture. Nonetheless, the possibility of brain injury should be assumed whenever there has been a blow powerful enough to crack the skull.

Recognition of Skull Fracture

Usually the diagnosis of skull fracture requires x-ray examination in the hospital, which can establish whether a fracture is present and, if so, what type of

Fig. 14-9. *The human skull.*

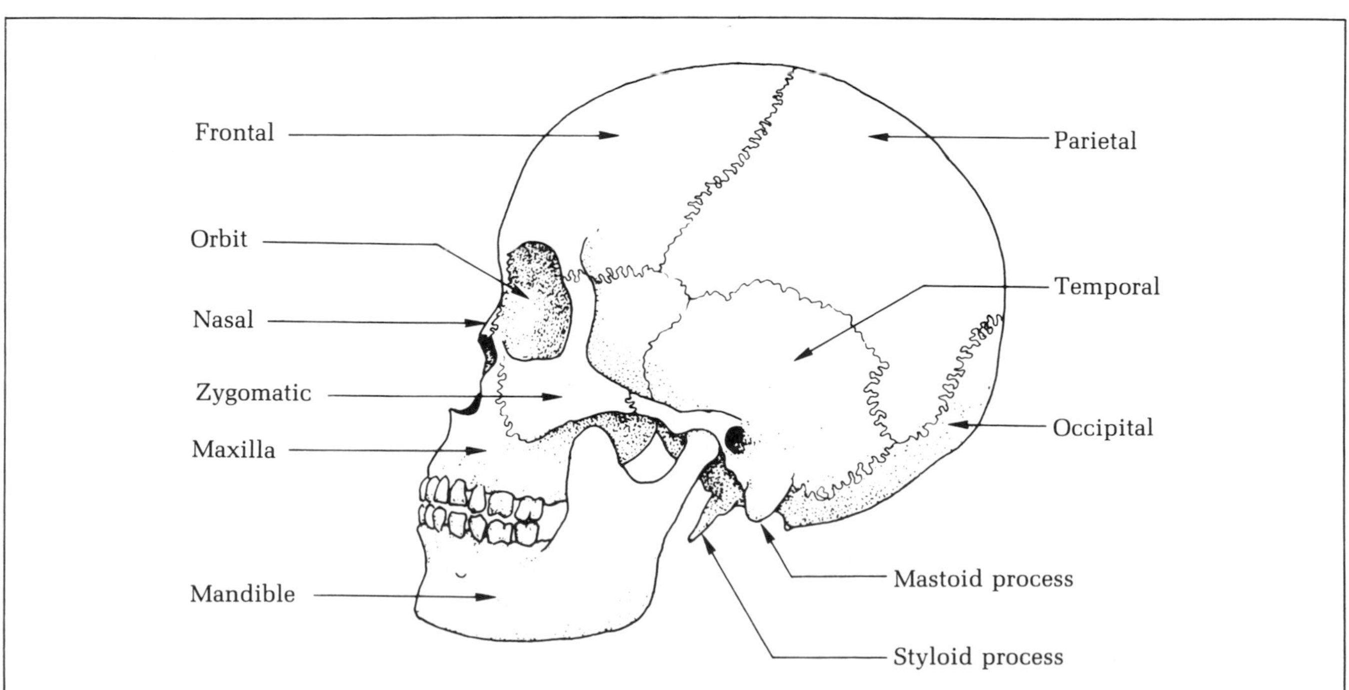

fracture has occurred. Skull fractures are classified as open or closed, depending upon whether underlying tissues are exposed. They are also classified by their appearance on x-ray. Most skull fractures are **linear fractures,** that is, just a thin line or crack in the skull. In a **comminuted fracture,** multiple cracks radiate outward from the point of impact, and the pattern on x-ray may resemble that of a cracked eggshell. A **depressed fracture** is one in which one or more fragments of bone have been pushed inward to press against the brain or sometimes even tear into brain tissue. One type of depressed fracture is a **penetrating injury,** such as that caused by a bullet, in which fragments of the skull may be driven deep into brain tissue, sometimes causing more damage than the bullet itself. Whenever there is a gunshot wound to the head, look for both the *entrance wound* and the *exit wound*. If you do not find an exit wound, the bullet may have ricocheted inside the skull, and you must assume that the bullet is embedded near the spinal cord in the neck until proved otherwise. Finally, a **basal skull fracture** is a crack in the floor of the skull. This type of fracture can be very difficult to detect on x-ray, and often the only indication of its presence is the leakage of spinal fluid from the nose or ear.

Although definitive diagnosis of skull fracture requires x-ray examination, there are several signs that can alert the EMT to the likelihood that a skull fracture is present. To begin with, an obvious depression in the skull is highly suggestive of a skull fracture. Sometimes the fracture may even be visible as a crack seen beneath a lacerated scalp, and in very severe injuries, brain tissue may be seen protruding from an open crack in the skull or from an ear. Penetrating injuries of the head, such as those made by bullets or ice picks, are almost invariably associated with fracture. Clues to the presence of *basal* skull fracture include leakage of watery fluid or blood from the ears or nose and ecchymoses behind the ears or around the eyes.

Signs of Skull Fracture

- DEPRESSION or instability of part of the skull
- Visible CRACK beneath a scalp laceration
- PENETRATING WOUND (e.g., bullet)
- CSF LEAKAGE from the nose, an ear, or a scalp wound
- BLOOD oozing FROM the NOSE or an EAR
- Ecchymosis behind the ear (BATTLE'S SIGN)
- Ecchymosis around the eyes (RACCOON SIGN)

Emergency Care of Skull Fractures

A skull fracture is NOT an immediately life-threatening injury, and if a patient with skull fracture dies, it will be because of associated problems, such as asphyxia or exsanguination. Therefore the care of a patient with skull fracture requires primary attention to the ABCs as well as to the handling of possible associated brain or spinal injury. The principles of treatment in skull fracture are as follows:

Treatment of a Patient with Suspected Skull Fracture

1. Maintain an open AIRWAY (jaw thrust, oropharyngeal airway).
2. Assist BREATHING as required, and give OXYGEN.
3. Maintain the CIRCULATION by CONTROL OF BLEEDING, *but*:
4. DO NOT CONTROL DRAINAGE (do not dam up the flow of blood or CSF from the nose or ear).
5. COVER OPEN WOUNDS with sterile dressings; use pressure bandages only to control profuse scalp bleeding when there is no underlying fracture.
6. DO NOT REMOVE IMPALED OBJECTS FROM THE HEAD. Stabilize the impaled object in place with a bulky dressing.
7. IMMOBILIZE THE CERVICAL SPINE before moving the patient.
8. Maintain a NEUROLOGIC WATCH, using a checklist to record data.

BRAIN INJURY

The brain is a very delicate organ, and injuries to the brain are common. Such injuries may be minor and cause only a temporary loss of function, or they may be severe and even fatal. Brain injuries are frequently classified as concussions, contusions, and hematomas.

The word **concussion** is somewhat vague, and there is a lack of consensus about its precise meaning; but most physicians agree that a concussion involves *temporary* loss of function of some or all parts of the brain. If one could examine the brain of a person who has sustained a concussion, one might not be able to detect any visible damage at all. But nonetheless, the patient shows variable symptoms, ranging from a period of mild confusion to complete loss of consciousness and even apnea of short duration. Usually there is some loss of memory (**amnesia**) for events surrounding the accident, and sometimes the patient cannot remember events that occurred just before the accident either. He may complain of headache, dizziness, nausea, or ringing in the ears. The symptoms of a concussion tend to pass very rapidly and may already have subsided by the time the EMT reaches the scene. Nevertheless, the EMT should maintain the usual neurologic checklist on a patient with an apparent concussion, for changes in the patient's status may indicate that the injury was more severe than originally suspected.

A **contusion** is a bruise of the brain, and like a bruise anywhere else in the body, it involves oozing or bleeding from blood vessels that have been disrupted by the blow and swelling of the underlying brain tissue. The problem is that the brain, unlike a contused muscle, has *no room to swell*, for it is packaged quite snugly inside a closed box. Thus when brain swelling (**cerebral edema**) does occur, the pressure inside the skull builds up, and parts of the brain may be jammed against the bony ridges inside the cranium, causing more brain damage than the original injury. The longer the intracranial pressure is permitted to build up, the greater the likelihood of permanent brain damage or even death.

There are several signs that should alert the EMT to the likelihood of cerebral edema and increasing intracranial pressure (from cerebral contusion or any other cause). To begin with, the patient is likely to have a deteriorating level of consciousness; while on initial examination he may seem merely sleepy, a recheck 10 minutes later may find him completely unconscious and rousable only by painful stimuli. There may be paralysis on one side of the body, and one pupil is apt to become widely dilated and unreactive to light. A conscious patient may complain of headache or nausea, and vomiting may occur. The blood pressure usually starts to climb, while the pulse gets slower, and abnormal respiratory patterns—including apnea—are likely to develop. Any one of these signs is strong evidence of cerebral edema and rising intracranial pressure, and it should be a signal to the EMT to stabilize the patient as quickly as possible and move on to the hospital.

Cerebral hematoma develops when there is significant bleeding within the skull, either between the skull and the dura (**epidural hematoma**) or beneath the dura (**subdural hematoma**). Both of these conditions present the same fundamental problem: bleeding into a closed box that has no room for blood clots. Thus both put pressure on the brain that can be fatal if surgery to evacuate the clots is not performed promptly.

An EPIDURAL HEMATOMA (Fig. 14-10) is usually the result of a blow to the head that produces a linear fracture of the temporal bone. A major artery, the middle meningeal artery, lies in a groove in the temporal bone, and this artery is apt to be disrupted when the temporal bone is fractured. If that happens, there is brisk arterial bleeding into the potential space between the skull and the dura mater, with formation of an epidural hematoma. The patient will often lose consciousness immediately after the blow to the head and then regain consciousness for a variable period, known as a *lucid interval*. However, as the hematoma enlarges and exerts more pressure on the brain, the patient becomes sleepy and then less and less responsive. As the brain is squeezed harder and harder against parts of the skull, the pupil on the affected side dilates and becomes unresponsive to light. Weakness or paralysis becomes evident on the opposite side of the body. If surgery is not performed immediately at this point, pressure on the brainstem will lead to respiratory arrest and death.

In SUBDURAL HEMATOMA (Fig. 14-11), there is venous bleeding beneath the dura. When that happens acutely, as in accidents involving massive deceleration trauma to the head, bleeding is very rapid and the mortality rate approaches 90 percent. More commonly, however, one sees a subacute form of subdural hematoma, in which blood collects more slowly in the subdural space. The signs and symptoms may be very similar to those of an epidural hematoma, for the fundamental problem—increasing intracranial pressure caused by accumulation of blood within the skull—is the same.

In the field, it is often impossible to distinguish between a cerebral contusion with swelling of the brain and a cerebral hematoma. What is important is to recognize the signs of increasing intracranial pressure, common to both, and to understand the urgency that those signs indicate.

Signs of Increasing Intracranial Pressure

- Deteriorating state of consciousness
- Hemiplegia, or sometimes quadriplegia
- Vomiting
- Dilation of one pupil
- Rising blood pressure with slowing pulse
- Abnormal respirations or apnea

Emergency Care of Suspected Brain Injury

In the field, the only thing one can do for an injured brain is to make sure that it gets enough oxygen.

CEREBRAL HYPOXIA IS THE MOST COMMON CAUSE OF DEATH AFTER HEAD INJURY.

Thus we are back once more to basics—and the ABCs.

Ensure an adequate AIRWAY. This means both relieving any obstruction by the base of the tongue and preventing the accumulation of secretions in the back of the throat. To facilitate these objectives, the *unconscious* patient with a head injury should be transported in the STABLE SIDE POSITION, with care taken in turning the patient to ensure that the neck is kept in alignment with the rest of the spine. Remember, vomiting is common in head-injured pa-

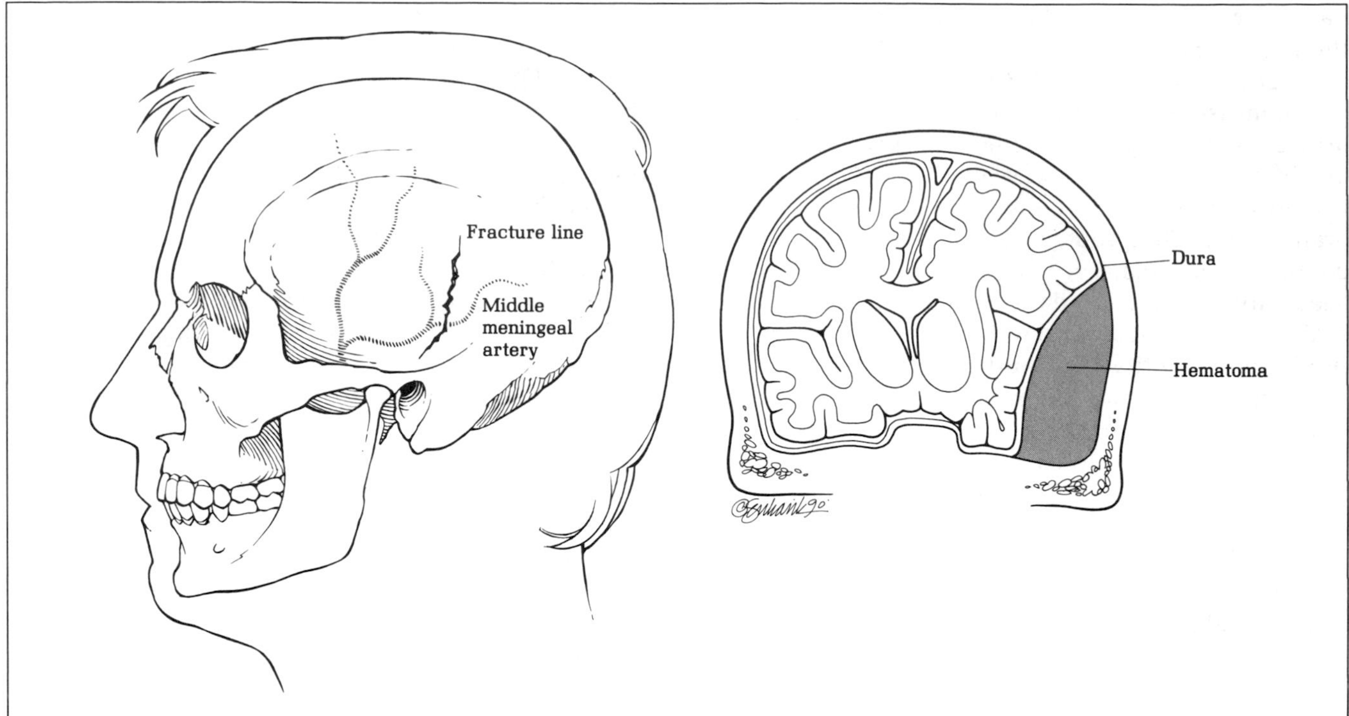

Fig. 14-10. *Epidural hematoma is usually the result of a blow to the head that produces a linear fracture of the temporal bone. Blood collects between the dura and the skull.*

Fig. 14-11. *Subdural hematoma occurs when there is venous bleeding beneath the dura.*

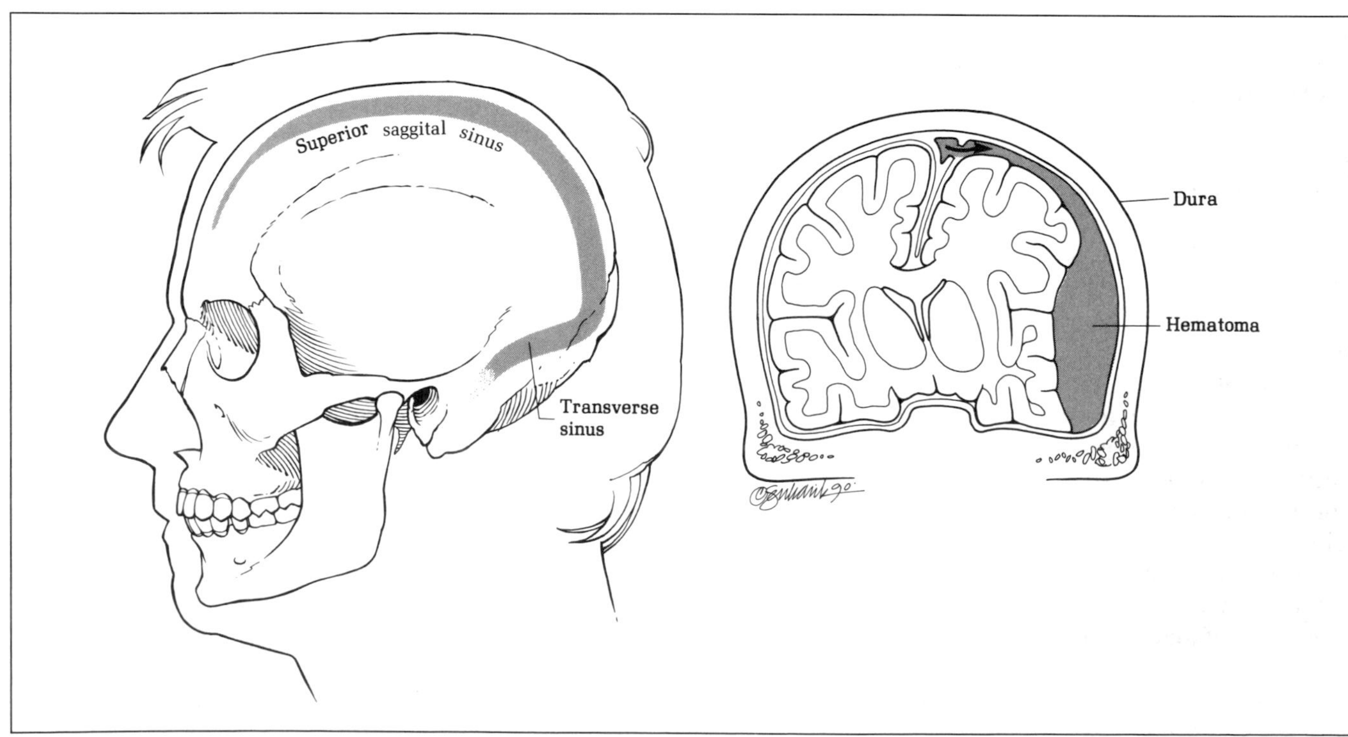

tients (and it may be precipitated by suctioning the back of the throat). An unconscious patient lying supine is a sitting duck (actually, a recumbent duck) for aspiration of vomitus. The stable side position or a semiprone position, on the other hand, permits drainage of secretions and vomitus from the patient's mouth and thereby lessens the chances of aspiration. If the patient is *conscious*, it is preferable that he be transported with his head slightly elevated, which is accomplished by raising the back of the stretcher to about 15 degrees.

Ensure that the patient is BREATHING adequately. Give OXYGEN in high concentration to *every* head-injured patient, and provide assisted ventilation to patients whose respiratory rate is below about 10 per minute. Ideally, head-injured patients should be slightly hyperventilated—about 20 to 25 ventilations per minute—for hyperventilation lowers the level of carbon dioxide in the blood, which in turn constricts cerebral blood vessels and thereby diminishes cerebral edema.

Control BLEEDING as efficiently as possible. Remember, if the patient is in shock, it is NOT from his head injury, and you must look for a cause of shock elsewhere in the body.

COVER ALL OPEN WOUNDS WITH STERILE DRESSINGS. If CSF is oozing from the nose, scalp, or an ear, cover the spot lightly with a dressing, so that it can absorb the flow and prevent contamination without interfering with the flow. Similarly, if there is an open fracture of the skull with brain tissue oozing out, apply a protective sterile dressing *loosely* over the area, and moisten the dressing with sterile saline.

SPLINT ALL FRACTURES before moving the patient.

DO NOT LET THE PATIENT GET TOO HOT! Head-injured patients tend to develop high temperatures, which aggravate the damage to the brain, and their internal temperature will get even higher if they are covered with blankets. Unless the temperature outside (and in the ambulance) is quite chilly, do NOT use a blanket on the patient.

BE ALERT FOR SEIZURES, and be sure to protect the patient's airway if seizures occur.

Head Injury: Points to Remember

- Every patient with a head injury has a CERVICAL SPINE INJURY until proved otherwise. Handle the patient accordingly.
- The most important single sign in the evaluation of a head-injured patient is a CHANGING STATE OF CONSCIOUSNESS.
- HEAD INJURIES DO NOT CAUSE SHOCK. If signs of shock are present, look for injury elsewhere in the body.
- The most common cause of death in head injury is hypoxia. To prevent this, ensure an adequate AIRWAY, and give OXYGEN.
- One of the most valuable contributions an EMT can make to the care of a head-injured patient is to RECORD THE PATIENT'S NEUROLOGIC SIGNS FREQUENTLY AND ACCURATELY.
- BE PREPARED FOR VOMITING AND SEIZURES.

INJURIES TO THE FACE

Injuries to the face occur commonly in the context of road accidents. Seventy-five percent of patients requiring hospital evaluation after a motor vehicle accident have some degree of facial injury. Burns, fistfights, falls, and gunshot wounds are other common sources of facial trauma.

The face is very richly supplied with blood vessels, and injuries to the face are therefore likely to be associated with considerable bruising or bleeding. Facial injuries tend often to be quite disfiguring and grotesque as well, which may lead emergency personnel to rush to apply dressings to facial wounds, forgetting the priorities of treatment in the process. Facial wounds are life-threatening only when they jeopardize the airway or are associated with massive bleeding, and the EMT must therefore control the impulse to cover the facial wounds immediately and should instead follow the usual priorities of ABC.

GENERAL PRINCIPLES IN THE EMERGENCY CARE OF FACIAL INJURIES

The most immediate concern in treating a person with facial injuries is to ensure an adequate AIRWAY. Facial trauma can compromise the airway in a number of ways. First of all, if the patient is unconscious, there is the old troublemaker the base of the *tongue*, which is apt to be resting against the back of the throat and blocking off the pharynx. This type of obstruction is easily relieved by maneuvers learned in earlier chapters, but bear in mind: ANY FORCE STRONG ENOUGH TO HAVE PRODUCED SEVERE FACIAL INJURIES MAY HAVE PRODUCED CERVICAL SPINE INJURY AS WELL. Thus maneuvers to open the airway should avoid hyperextension of the neck. The jaw thrust is the preferred technique when there is any doubt regarding the presence of cervical spine injury. When the lower jaw (mandible) has been fractured, the base of the tongue loses its principal support and is especially prone to fall back against the throat. Pulling the mandible gently forward with a finger hooked inside the mouth or supporting the angles of the mandible with your thumbs will pull the tongue away from the back of the pharynx.

The airway in the victim of facial trauma may also become blocked by *foreign materials*, such as blood clots, avulsed teeth, or broken dentures. Thus it is necessary to open the victim's mouth (gently) and sweep your fingers through the mouth to clear out debris and feel for lacerations or deformities. Intact dentures are best left in place, but broken dentures should be removed and carefully preserved; they may be needed later on to help establish various measurements for reconstructive surgery on the patient's face. Manual clearing of the mouth can be followed by suctioning if there is a lot of blood, vomitus, or other liquid material in the mouth and throat. The patient should also be placed in a semiprone position or in the stable side position, so that blood and vomitus can drain out of the mouth. If there is suspected injury to the cervical spine, the neck should be stabilized before turning the patient, and then the patient should be turned as a unit, with his neck aligned with the rest of the spine. Once he is in the lateral or semiprone position, he should be strapped that way to the stretcher.

Severe injuries to the mouth and nose themselves can also cause airway problems. One should not try to insert an airway into a nose or mouth that has been severely traumatized, for the artificial airway may simply aggravate the damage to soft tissues. Once again, the patient should be turned to a lateral or semiprone position. If the jaw is stable, the mouth can be propped open with a padded tongue depressor inserted between the upper and lower molars to enable mouth breathing and facilitate drainage of blood and secretions from the mouth.

After establishing a good airway, make sure the patient is BREATHING adequately. Respiratory arrest will require artificial ventilation, which can be quite difficult if there is extensive trauma to the face, and rapid transport to the emergency room for insertion of an endotracheal tube may be necessary. If the patient is breathing spontaneously, administer OXYGEN to ensure that the brain (which may have been injured as well) has an adequate supply of that life-giving gas.

Attention to the CIRCULATION means CONTROL OF BLEEDING. Once again, *direct pressure* is the more effective means of hemorrhage control, but use only enough pressure to stop the bleeding, for there may be fractured facial bones beneath the soft tissue injury. If a laceration extends all the way through the CHEEK into the mouth, it will be necessary to apply pressure on *both* sides of the wound, by holding a gauze pad against the inside of the cheek and pressing against it with another gauze pad applied over the outside of the cheek.

Once the ABCs have been taken care of and any associated life-threatening injuries (e.g., a sucking chest wound) have also been attended to, you can turn your attention to DRESSING THE FACIAL WOUNDS. In doing so, there are a few special considerations you need to keep in mind. To begin with, if the wound involves EXPOSED NERVES, TENDONS, OR BLOOD VESSELS, the dressing applied to it should be moistened with sterile saline so that these delicate structures will not dry out and thereby suffer further damage. If there is an AVULSED FLAP OF SKIN on the face or scalp, rinse the wound and the skin flap as free as possible of foreign materials with sterile water or sterile saline, and then gently replace the flap to its normal position, holding it in place with a dressing and bandage. This technique will help control bleeding and will also help keep the flap viable until it can be stitched back into place.

As you examine the face, check to see whether any tissue has been lost altogether. Missing parts—such as pieces of an ear or nose—should be searched for and brought to the emergency room with the patient. Wrap AMPUTATED PARTS in a sterile dressing, and moisten the dressing with cool, sterile saline.

An IMPALED OBJECT IN THE CHEEK represents a special problem, for so long as the object remains impaled in the cheek, it will be impossible to control the profuse bleeding into the mouth and throat, and such bleeding can pose a threat to the airway. For this reason, AN IMPALED OBJECT *SHOULD* BE REMOVED FROM THE CHEEK. This is the *only* situation in the field where it is permissible to remove an impaled object. To do so, probe the inside of the cheek with your fingers to determine whether the object has indeed gone all the way through to the inside of the mouth. If it has, remove it by pulling it out gently in the direction from which it entered the cheek. To stop the bleeding, pack the space between the cheek and the gums with gauze pads, and apply pressure against the packing with a dressing held against the outside of the cheek.

CLOSED SOFT TISSUE INJURIES OF THE FACE are best managed with the application of cold compresses, such as towels or universal dressings that have been soaked in ice water. The local application of cold helps to reduce swelling and control subcutaneous bleeding, and it often provides significant pain relief as well.

General Principles in Caring for Facial Injuries

- Suspect associated HEAD INJURY and CERVICAL SPINE INJURY.
- First priority goes to the AIRWAY:
  1. *Jaw thrust* to pull the tongue forward.
  2. Semiprone or stable side position to facilitate drainage from the mouth (keep the neck stable).
- Administer OXYGEN.
- CONTROL BLEEDING:
  1. *Direct pressure*, but beware of underlying fracture.

2. Remove IMPALED OBJECTS from the cheek.
3. Pressure on the inside *and* outside of penetrating cheek wounds.

- Rinse and replace AVULSED SKIN FLAPS.
- Save AMPUTATED PARTS in moist, sterile dressings.
- Apply COLD COMPRESSES to closed injuries.

INJURIES TO THE EYE

Injuries to the eye are very common and potentially very serious. It is estimated that approximately 1.5 million eye injuries occur in the United States each year (more than half of them in the workplace), 50,000 of which result in some degree of permanent visual loss.

The eye is a delicate and intricate structure that focuses images from the outside world onto specially adapted nerve cells, which then code the images into electric impulses that are transmitted along the optic nerve to a special part of the brain. There the messages are decoded and interpreted, and the net result is what we call "seeing."

The eye is shaped like a large marble, and for this reason the eye as a whole is sometimes called the **globe** (Fig. 14-12). The globe shape is maintained by a jelly-like fluid inside the eye, called the **vitreous humor**, which may be extruded if the globe is lacerated. The anterior part of the globe, the **cornea**, is transparent to enable light to enter the eye. The remainder of the globe is made up of a tough, white tissue called the **sclera**, which forms the "whites of the eyes." A thin layer of smooth mucous membrane, the **conjunctiva**, covers both the anterior sclera and the inner surface of the eyelids. When this membrane becomes irritated or infected, a condition called conjunctivitis, or "pink eye," occurs.

Behind the cornea is a special muscle, called the **iris**, that has an adjustable aperture (the **pupil**). By constricting and dilating, the iris determines the size of the pupil and thus how much light enters the eye, much like the aperture of a camera. Behind the iris is the **lens,** which focuses the image entering the eye onto light-sensitive cells in the back of the eye, in a layer called the **retina**. The cells of the retina translate the visual image into electric signals that are then transmitted to the brain by the **optic nerve**. A salty fluid called the **aqueous humor** fills the space between the cornea and the lens.

The eye is protected in a variety of ways. To begin with, the anterior part of the eye is protected by the eyelids, whose inner surface is lubricated by fluid produced in the lacrimal (tear) glands beneath the lids. Tears keep the globe from drying out and also keep it rinsed free of dust and other irritants. With each blink, the eyelids further sweep the corneal surface free of dust.

The eyeball is also protected by its location within a bony socket, or **orbit**, of the skull. The orbits are lined with a cushion of fatty tissue that acts as a shock absorber to protect the eye from impact. The muscles that enable the eyes to move to the right and left, or up and down, are anchored in the orbits, and these muscles may become nonfunctional if there is a fracture of one of the orbital bones.

Assessment of the Injured Eye

Injury to the eye is always a serious matter, for every eye injury carries the potential for producing blindness. Pay attention to the patient's *complaints*. Any patient who reports pain in the eyes, double vision, blurring, or any other disturbance of vision following injury to the face should be placed immediately at rest on a stretcher and moved without delay to the hospital.

Once you've taken the history of the injury, you need to inspect the eyes for *signs* of trauma. Examination of the eye requires gentle handling (clean hands only!) and careful attention to all the visible structures.

The examination begins with an assessment of the ORBITS, the bony ridges around both eyes. Inspect the orbits for ecchymoses (suggestive of basal skull fracture), swelling, and lacerations. Palpate gently around the orbital rims for tenderness or instability of the bone.

Next inspect the EYELIDS, which may be bruised, swollen, or lacerated, and note any injuries present. If the eyelids appear undamaged, check the CONJUNCTIVAE ON THEIR INNER SURFACES. The conjunctiva of the lower lid can be inspected by pulling the lower lid slightly forward; the conjunctiva of the upper lid is inspected by everting the lid over a cotton-tipped applicator. Note whether the conjunctiva is abnormally red (bloodshot), and check under the lid for foreign bodies, which should

Fig. 14-12. *Structure of the eye.*

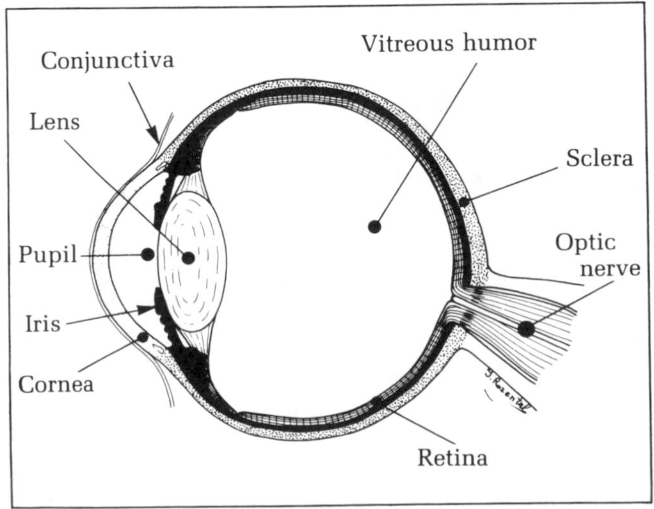

be removed from the underside of the lid with a clean, moist sterile applicator.

Examine the GLOBE, and note the color of the sclera (e.g., white, bloodshot, or yellow). Check for lacerations of the globe or impaled foreign objects. Note whether the globe appears to be "popping out of its socket." If the globe appears uninjured, check the EYE MOTIONS by asking the patient to follow your finger with his gaze as you move your finger 90 degrees right, left, up, and down. The two eyes should move together. Paralysis of upward gaze (i.e., inability to look upward) suggests a fracture of the orbital bone.

Inspect the PUPILS. The entire circle of the iris should be visible, and the pupils should be equal in size and reactive to light. Look carefully for blood overlying the iris and pupil, a sign of hemorrhage within the eye.

Finally, make a rough check of the patient's VISUAL ACUITY by asking the patient to read a few lines of print. It will be very important for the emergency room doctor or eye specialist to know how much vision the patient had immediately after the accident.

Examination of the Injured Eye

- ORBITS: Look for ecchymoses, swelling, lacerations; feel for tenderness, instability.
- LIDS: Ecchymoses, swelling, lacerations.
- CONJUNCTIVAE: Redness, foreign bodies.
- GLOBE: Lacerations, redness, protrusion, impaled objects.
- EYE MOTIONS: Do the eyes move together? Do they move in all directions?
- PUPILS: Size, equality, reaction to light; blood overlying the iris.
- VISUAL ACUITY.

Foreign Bodies in the Eye

Probably the most common eye injury is that due to a foreign body that has been blown onto the outer surface of the cornea. Usually such foreign bodies lodge under the upper lid or on the cornea, and they cause enormous discomfort to the patient. In the majority of cases, the foreign body is washed out of the eye by the patient's own tearing mechanism, but if it remains in the eye, the EMT may have to assist in its removal. The first method to try is gently to rinse the eye by pouring sterile saline over the globe or squirting saline from a squeeze bottle into the eye. If this method does not work, the foreign body is probably stuck under the upper lid, and the lid will have to be everted to get at it. To evert the lid (Fig. 14-13), ask the patient to look down while you grasp the lashes of his upper lid between your thumb and index finger. Place a cotton-tipped applicator horizontally along the outer surface of the eyelid, and then pull the eyelid gently forward and upward so that it folds back upon itself over the applicator. If you can see the foreign body on the undersurface of the lid, remove it with a moistened, sterile applicator. If the foreign body is visible on the sclera, have the patient look down while you flush the sclera with saline. Do NOT, however, use an applicator to remove the foreign body if it is lying on the surface of the cornea; if it cannot be flushed free, it will have to be left as it is until the patient reaches the emergency room.

Impaled Objects in the Eye

An impaled object should NOT be removed from the eye, but like an impaled object anywhere else in the body, it should be stabilized in place. One way to do this is to take a stack of 4 × 4–inch gauze pads and

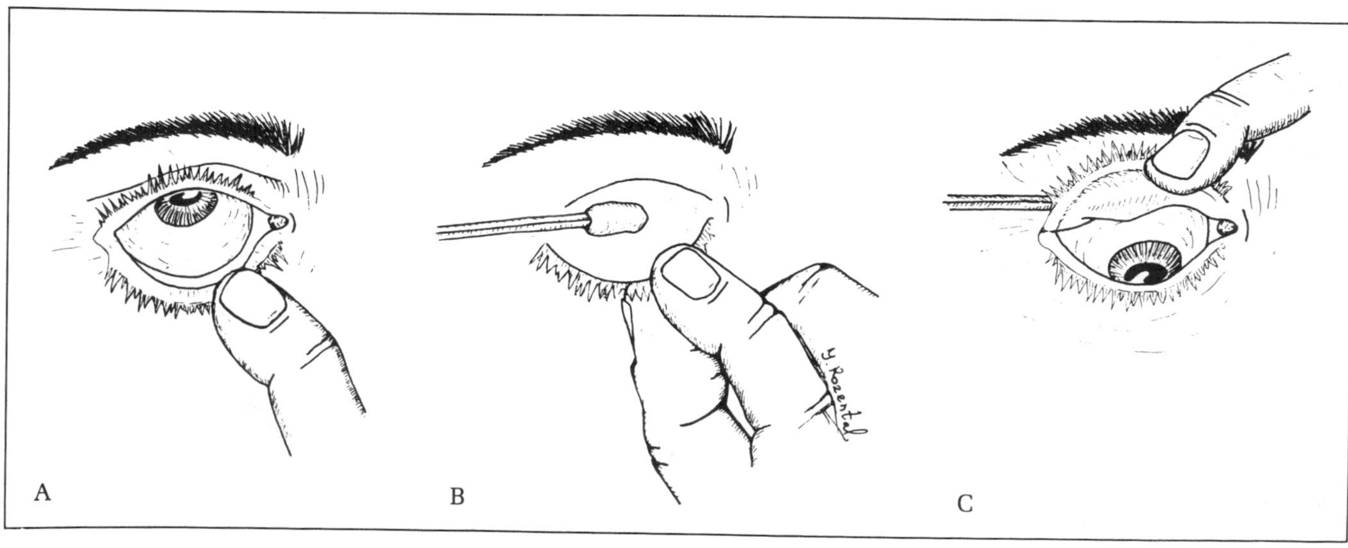

Fig. 14-13. *Examining the eye for a foreign body. A. Pull the lower lid downward to look for a foreign body beneath it. B. Apply a cotton-tipped applicator gently to the upper lid. C. Evert the upper lid over the applicator to examine the eye beneath.*

cut a hole in the center of the stack large enough to fit over the impaled object. Then carefully pass the stack of gauze pads over the impaled object so that the dressing is resting gently against the orbit. To prevent the impaled object from being caught or jarred, next take a paper cup or similar object and position it over the gauze pads so that the impaled object is enclosed within it but not touching it. Fasten the paper cup in place with a circumferential bandage, and PATCH THE OTHER EYE. The reason for patching the uninjured eye is that normally both eyes move together. If the uninjured eye starts looking around to check out the scenery, the eye with the impaled object will move as well, and this can further damage the injured eye. Patching the normal eye thus limits the motion of *both* eyes. Remember, though, a person with both eyes covered cannot see at all, and this can be very frightening, especially to a child. For this reason, it is worthwhile to take a moment before applying the patch to explain to the patient what you are doing and why the patch is necessary. Once the patch is in place, *you* will have to serve as the patient's eyes, explaining to him what is going on, where he is, and so forth. A calm, unhurried, matter-of-fact manner on the part of the EMT can do a great deal to ease the patient's anxiety.

Lacerations and Contusions of the Eye

Lacerations and contusions involving the eye can be minor or severe, depending upon the extent to which the eye itself is involved. Laceration of a lid alone will not impair vision, but lacerations or blunt trauma to the eyeball can result in blindness. The seriousness of an eye injury can be very difficult to gauge in the field, and therefore one must assume that *every* eye injury is serious until proved otherwise.

LACERATIONS OF THE EYELID tend to bleed quite profusely because of the rich vascular supply to the area. Bleeding from a lacerated lid is usually readily controlled by direct pressure, but pressure should not be applied until you have checked the globe to make sure there is no laceration of the eyeball itself. Pressure applied over a lacerated eye can cause the vitreous humor to be squeezed out of the eye, and this will lead to blindness. Thus:

> ALWAYS CHECK THE GLOBE FOR LACERATIONS BEFORE YOU APPLY PRESSURE OVER A BLEEDING EYELID.

If the eyeball is intact, you may apply a pressure dressing over the injured lid. If there is a laceration of the globe—or if there is any doubt—simply apply a sterile dressing *lightly* over the lid to keep the wound protected from further contamination.

An AVULSED EYELID should also be covered lightly with a sterile dressing, which can be moistened with sterile saline. If a piece of the eyelid has been entirely torn off, treat it as any other amputated part; wrap it gently in a sterile dressing, and moisten the dressing with cool, sterile saline.

When the EYEBALL itself has been lacerated or contused, the patient should be kept very still and quiet, lying on his back, and *both* eyes should be covered loosely with protective dressings. If broken fragments of eyeglasses are present, those that are loose around the eye may be removed, but do not attempt to remove any fragments that have penetrated the sclera or cornea. Remember, it will not do much good to tell the patient to keep still if the ambulance is bouncing and careening all over the road, so try to keep the ride as smooth as possible; for jarring motions can cause further damage to the delicate structures of the injured eye.

Avulsion of the Eye

A severe blow to the face can on occasion cause the eyeball to be avulsed from its socket and hang dependent outside the orbit. If you see such an injury, DO NOT ATTEMPT TO PUSH THE EYE BACK INTO ITS SOCKET. Calm the patient (and yourself), and instruct him to remain as still as possible, lying on his back. Cover the extruded eye loosely with a sterile dressing that has been thoroughly moistened with sterile saline, and cover the dressing with a paper cup, just as you would for an impaled object in the eye. Transport the patient supine as gently as possible, for any undue motion or bumps may cause the retina to detach from the injured eye.

Burns of the Eye

The eyes can be burned by exposure to chemicals, heat, or light at certain wavelengths. CHEMICAL BURNS, as noted in the previous chapter, require immediate and copious flushing with water, which should continue for at least 20 minutes. The most effective way to flush the eye under these circumstances is to support the patient's head under a faucet and direct a stream of lukewarm water into the eye.

THERMAL BURNS of the eyes occur when the patient suffers burns about the face from a fire. The eyelids will be burned first, for they will close reflexly in the presence of extremes of heat in an attempt to protect the eyes. Thus what you will see are singed eyelashes and red, swollen eyelids. If there are burns of the eyelids, do not attempt to open the eyes. Simply cover both eyelids lightly with dressings that have been moistened in cool, sterile water. Such dressings will provide some relief of pain and will also help to minimize further swelling of the eyelids.

LIGHT BURNS of the eyes are most commonly caused by exposure to ultraviolet (UV) light, as in the "arc welder's burn," prolonged exposure to a sunlamp, "snow blindness," or even exposure to the UV light used to achieve "psychedelic" effects in certain disco establishments. Generally, pain does not develop until about 3 to 6 hours after exposure to the light, but the pain that does develop can be very severe because of breakdown of the corneal surface. The patient may complain of a gritty feeling in the eyes or of feeling that there is "burning gravel" under the eyelids. Treatment in the field is directed at relieving pain, and this is best accomplished by having the patient lie down and placing moist, cold compresses over the closed eyelids.

General Care of the Eyes in an Unconscious Patient

A patient who is unconscious from any cause may have lost the reflexes that normally protect the eye, such as the blinking reflex that periodically lubricates the eye and sweeps it clean of debris. If the patient cannot protect his own eyes, the EMT must protect the eyes for him. This means keeping the patient's eyes closed, either by taping them closed (with nonallergenic tape) or by covering them with moist dressings.

If an unconscious patient is wearing hard contact lenses, the lenses should be removed; for when hard contact lenses remain in place for prolonged periods with the eyes closed, they can cause irritation and damage to the cornea. (Ask any contact lens wearer who has forgotten to take out his lenses before going to bed!) Every ambulance should be equipped with a specially designed suction cup for removal of contact lenses (these suction cups can be purchased from any optometrist). To use the suction cup, moisten it in sterile saline, squeeze the rubber bulb, and apply it gently to the contact lens while releasing the bulb. When the lens is attached to the suction cup, gently pull it toward you, out of the eye. Take care to put the contact lenses in a safe place, where they will not be lost or damaged, and notify the emergency room staff of where you have put the lenses, so that they can be kept with the patient's other belongings.

INJURIES TO THE NOSE

Injuries to the nose are generally manifested by bleeding, which at times can be very profuse. When EPISTAXIS occurs as an isolated phenomenon and there is no reason to suspect underlying skull fracture, the patient should be placed in a sitting position, leaning slightly forward, and he should be instructed to breathe slowly through the mouth. Meanwhile, control of bleeding may be accomplished either by pinching the nostrils shut or by packing a gauze roll between the upper lip and the teeth. An ice pack applied to the nose may also help control nasal bleeding. Remember, however:

NEVER ATTEMPT TO STOP BLEEDING FROM THE NOSE IF THERE IS ANY REASON TO SUSPECT SKULL FRACTURE.

Closed injuries to the nose can also produce swelling and fracture of the nasal bones. In the field, the only treatment necessary and feasible is to place an ice pack over the injured area and transport the patient in a sitting or semisitting position. When there is an open wound on the nose, control bleeding and dress the wound in the usual fashion. As always, retrieve any amputated parts, and transport them in a cool, moist sterile dressing to the hospital with the patient.

FOREIGN BODIES IN THE NOSE are a problem chiefly among small children, who seem to derive some unique satisfaction from putting peanuts, beans, and similar objects into their nostrils. The field treatment for a foreign body in the nose is to LEAVE IT ALONE! Probing blindly into a nostril without proper lighting or equipment may simply jam the foreign body deeper into the nose or drive it into the nasal tissues, and it is unlikely anyway that the child is going to sit still for these maneuvers. Just try to calm the child and parent, and transport them to the hospital, where the foreign body can be removed by a physician.

INJURIES TO THE EAR

Two parts of the ear are particularly vulnerable to injury: the external ear (**pinna**), which may be contused, lacerated, or avulsed; and the eardrum, which can be ruptured by concussive explosions or by a strong blow to the head.

A simple LACERATION OF THE EXTERNAL EAR should be treated as any other open wound, with application of a sterile dressing, preferably a bulky one, held in place by a circumferential bandage. Any avulsed parts of the ear should be retrieved and brought with the patient to the emergency room.

RUPTURE OF THE EARDRUM can occur when a person is close to an explosion, struck by lightning, or struck forcefully on the side of the head. The ruptured eardrum requires no special treatment in the field except to cover the ear lightly with a sterile dressing to protect it from dirt or further injury.

BLOOD OR CLEAR FLUID DRAINING FROM AN EAR is a sign of basal skull fracture, and the blood or fluid should be allowed to drain freely so that pressure will not build up within the skull.

DO NOT ATTEMPT TO STOP THE FLOW OF BLOOD OR CLEAR FLUID FROM THE EAR CANAL.

Finally, FOREIGN BODIES can get lodged in the ear canal. Once again, this is chiefly a problem in children—usually the same children who put peanuts in their noses. However, adults who use bobby pins, toothpicks, and other questionable devices to clean out their ears are also apt to get a foreign body lodged in the ear canal (and they may succeed in perforating the eardrum as well). As in the case of foreign bodies in the nose, the field treatment for a foreign body in the ear is to LEAVE IT ALONE. Under no circumstances should an EMT insert any instrument into an ear in an attempt to fish out a foreign body. In some ambulance services, the responsible physician may wish to instruct the EMTs in the use of an ear syringe, which is used for flushing out the ear canals, but this device should be used only when there is virtual certainty that the eardrum has not been perforated.

The vast majority of injuries to the ear canal and eardrum can be *prevented* by observing a simple rule:

NEVER PUT ANYTHING SMALLER THAN YOUR ELBOW INTO YOUR EAR.

INJURIES TO THE MOUTH AND JAW

The major consideration in injuries to the mouth is to PROTECT THE AIRWAY. Blood, avulsed teeth, and broken dentures are all potential sources of airway obstruction and should be cleared out of the victim's mouth as quickly as possible. Bleeding from the mouth can sometimes be controlled by packing dressings between the lip and the gum or between the cheek and the gum. If bleeding continues, however, keep the patient in a semiprone or stable side position so that blood can drain out of the mouth and not down the throat. This is important even if the patient is conscious, for swallowing blood often leads to nausea and vomiting, which one would like to avoid if possible.

When TEETH are AVULSED from their sockets, they should be removed from the mouth so that they will not be swallowed or aspirated. The ligament of an avulsed tooth will usually remain alive for about 30 to 60 minutes after the tooth is dislodged from its socket. What this means is that if the tooth can be put back into its socket within about 30 to 60 minutes, the tooth may be saved. Therefore, the decision regarding what to do with an avulsed tooth will depend in part on the distance to the hospital. If you can get to the hospital within about 10 to 15 minutes, then place the tooth in saline or in a carton of milk and bring the patient and the tooth to the emergency room without delay. Handle the tooth gently (pick it up by the crown, not the root). Do not rub, scrape, or try to disinfect it. Put the tooth in a container in which it will not be further damaged by banging against hard surfaces. Notify the emergency room staff by radio, so that they can alert a dentist to be on hand when the patient arrives.

If transport will be delayed by the need to stabilize other injuries (e.g., splinting fractures), or if it is some distance to the hospital, it is worthwhile to try to reinsert the tooth while you are still in the field. To do so, first inspect the tooth to make sure it is intact. Rinse it thoroughly with saline, and rinse out the socket with saline as well. Then line the tooth up in its correct position, and insert it *slowly* and *gently* into the socket, allowing fluid to escape from the socket as you do so. Have the patient bite down firmly with the tooth against a gauze roll for at least 15 minutes. When the patient reaches the hospital, a dentist can construct a special splint to hold the tooth in place until healing is complete.

The lower jaw, or MANDIBLE, may be fractured when there is blunt trauma to the face. Usually when the mandible is fractured, it is fractured in at least two places, and it will be tender and unstable to palpation. In addition, the teeth will appear to be out of line, and the patient's bite will be uneven (maloccluded). If the mandible appears to be fractured and there is no bleeding within the mouth, carefully align the jaw so that the bite is more or less normal, and immobilize the jaw as shown in Figure 14-14. Tie the bandage in such a way that the knots can be released quickly in the event the patient has to vomit.

If a fractured mandible is accompanied by considerable bleeding into the mouth, it is better not to immobilize the mandible in the field, for the risks of jeopardizing the airway with the mouth tied shut outweigh the risks of leaving the fractured mandible unstable.

INJURIES TO THE NECK AND SPINE

The neck is probably the most vital and vulnerable stretch of anatomy in the body, for through it pass the airway, the entire blood supply to the brain, and the nerve supply to the whole body below the head. For this reason, injuries to the neck have enormous potential for damage.

SOFT TISSUE INJURIES TO THE NECK

As elsewhere in the body, soft tissue injuries to the neck can be either closed, resulting from blunt im-

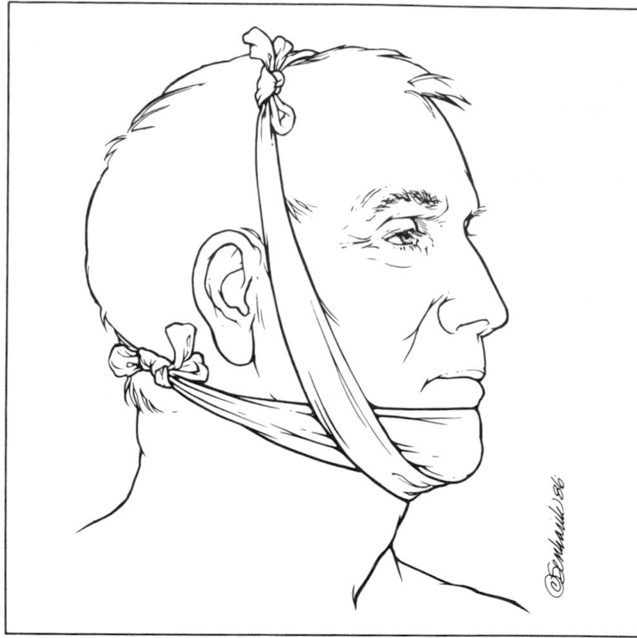

Fig. 14-14. *Immobilization of a fractured mandible.*

pact, or open, from penetration by a sharp object or missile. Each type of injury has its own potential for damage, and each can produce a life-threatening situation.

Blunt Injuries to the Neck

Blunt injury may be sustained in any accident that produces a blow to the neck. A person hurled forward against the steering wheel of a car, for instance, may strike his neck against the wheel with considerable force. A blow to the throat may be sustained in a fight or in a fall against a hard object. In the old cowboy movies, the good guys sometimes used to string a rope between two trees in order to unseat the bad guys from their horses as they galloped by, and this technique must have produced more than a few fatal neck injuries. In any of these cases, the principal danger is FRACTURE AND COLLAPSE OF THE TRACHEA. Once the rigid supporting structure of the trachea has been disrupted, there is nothing to hold the trachea open during inhalation, and the negative pressure of each inhalation tends to collapse and block off the windpipe, making breathing extremely difficult if not impossible.

The *signs* of tracheal fracture are more or less predictable from the nature of the injury. To begin with, there will be marked respiratory distress as the patient struggles to move air through the collapsed windpipe. Usually, the patient will lose his voice because of accompanying injury to the larynx, and the Adam's apple itself may appear to be pushed inward or deformed. A bruise will generally be present on the neck at the point of impact. Furthermore, air leaking out of the disrupted trachea into the surrounding subcutaneous tissues will produce a very characteristic sign called **subcutaneous emphysema**—a swelling of the skin in the neck and sometimes the face and chest that crackles when you touch it because of all the air that has infiltrated into the soft tissue.

Signs of Tracheal Fracture

- Respiratory distress
- Bruise on the neck
- Deformity of the Adam's apple
- Loss of voice
- Swelling and subcutaneous emphysema of the neck and sometimes also the face and chest.

A patient with these signs MUST REACH A MEDICAL FACILITY AS QUICKLY AS POSSIBLE, for urgent surgery will usually be required to open the patient's airway and prevent him from strangling. In the field and en route to the hospital, the important thing is to try to keep the patient calm and instruct him to BREATHE SLOWLY. Slow breaths create less negative pressure on the walls of the trachea and thus decrease the degree of tracheal collapse with each inhalation. OXYGEN should be given in the highest concentration possible, preferably by nonrebreathing mask. And bear in mind, a blow strong enough to fracture the trachea may well have fractured the cervical spine as well; therefore, exercise extreme care not to move the victim's head or neck any more than absolutely necessary, and immobilize the head and neck with sandbags or a backboard and blanket roll.

Treatment of Tracheal Fracture

- Cervical spine precautions: IMMOBILIZE.
- Keep the patient CALM.
- Instruct the patient to BREATHE SLOWLY.
- Administer OXYGEN in high concentration.
- Get the patient to the HOSPITAL as rapidly as possible.

Open Injuries to the Neck

Lacerations of the neck can produce damage to a major artery or vein or to the airway, and any of these injuries is potentially life-threatening.

ARTERIAL BLEEDING from the neck should be controlled by *manual* pressure. Do NOT use a pressure dressing, since a circumferential bandage fastened tightly around the neck can interfere with breathing and with blood flow through the undamaged blood vessels on the opposite side of the neck. Place a bulky, sterile dressing against the wound, and maintain very firm pressure with your hand until you reach the hospital. If the dressing becomes soaked with blood, do not remove it, but simply reinforce it with a fresh dressing on top of it, continuing very firm pressure against the wound. Keep the patient supine, with the legs slightly elevated to compensate for the loss of blood.

VENOUS BLEEDING from the neck is not as brisk as arterial bleeding, but it carries a very special danger all its own—the danger of **air embolism**. When a large vein in the neck is lacerated, there is a tendency for air to be "sucked into" the wound and enter the circulatory system through the injured vein. This tendency is accentuated if the severed vein is higher than the heart, as when the victim is sitting or standing up. If a large enough quantity of air enters the circulation and bubbles through the heart into the lungs, air embolism can be rapidly fatal.

To treat a patient with a severed vein in the neck, immediately get him into a recumbent position, preferably on his left side with the stretcher tilted in a slight head-down angle. This position will help trap any air bubbles that have already entered the circulation in the right side of the heart. Apply pressure on the vein both above and below the bleeding site, and cover the wound with an occlusive dressing, such as household plastic wrap. Tape the wrap down on all sides, so that it forms an airtight seal over the wound, and continue to maintain firm pressure over the severed vein until you reach the hospital. As in all patients with profuse bleeding, a patient with a severed vein in the neck should receive oxygen.

Treatment of a Severed Neck Vein

- LEFT LATERAL RECUMBENT position.
- STRETCHER tilted HEAD-DOWN about 10 to 15 degrees.
- PRESSURE on the vein above and below the bleeding site.
- OCCLUSIVE, AIRTIGHT DRESSING over the wound.
- OXYGEN by nonrebreathing mask at 10 to 12 liters per minute.
- TRANSPORT to the hospital without delay.

LACERATIONS OF THE LARYNX OR TRACHEA present a danger to the airway, for blood clots can form within the airway and cause obstruction. A laceration of the airway may be evident when there is subcutaneous emphysema in the presence of an open wound of the neck; sometimes there will be frothy blood foaming out of the neck wound. First priority should be given to control of bleeding and keeping the airway free of blood, using suction as needed. A semiprone position, with the stretcher tilted slightly head-down, may aid in the drainage of blood out of the pharynx and into the mouth, where it can be spit or suctioned out. Patients with this type of injury should also receive oxygen in high concentration, and transport to the hospital should not be delayed. If there is an IMPALED OBJECT IN THE LARYNX, stabilize it in place with bulky dressings before transport. Remember also to take into consideration the possibility of associated cervical spine injury, and handle the patient accordingly.

INJURIES TO THE SPINE

Each year in the United States, approximately 12,000 people suffer serious spinal cord injury, resulting in permanent paralysis. Eighty percent of those victims are under 40 years of age—most of them young people with their whole lives still ahead of them. Added to the incalculable toll such injuries take on the victims and their families is the enormous economic cost to society: an estimated $1.5 million to support each quadriplegic for the duration of his lifetime.

As we learned earlier, the spine is a column of 33 bones, or vertebrae, that extends from the base of the skull to the tip of the coccyx. By itself, fracture of a vertebra is no more serious than fracture of any other bone, and a vertebral fracture will heal with the same efficiency as any other fracture. The danger in fractures or dislocations of the spine is that they can be associated with damage to nerve roots or to the spinal cord itself. When a fracture or dislocation occurs in the spinal column, the spine often becomes unstable and thus can no longer protect the spinal cord inside. Any movement of the patient may cause the vertebrae to shift position and compress the spinal cord or pinch nerve roots (Fig. 14-15), thereby causing severe damage that can lead to permanent paralysis or even death. For this reason, every potential injury to the spine must be considered serious and must be treated with extreme caution. Every year in the United States, there are at least 5,000 new spinal cord injuries, resulting in immeasurable suffering to the victims and their families and enormous cost to society. Many of these injuries need not have led to paralysis; paralysis occurred because the patient was mishandled at the scene, often by well-meaning people who were simply ignorant of the danger of moving the patient. An EMT should not be ignorant of this danger and should always bear in mind that his or her handling of the potentially spine-injured patient may spell the difference between a normal life or a life spent in total dependency for the patient involved.

Injuries Likely to Cause Spinal Damage

It is critically important for an EMT to maintain a high level of suspicion regarding potential spinal injuries. The EMT should be able to anticipate those injuries that are likely to be associated with spinal

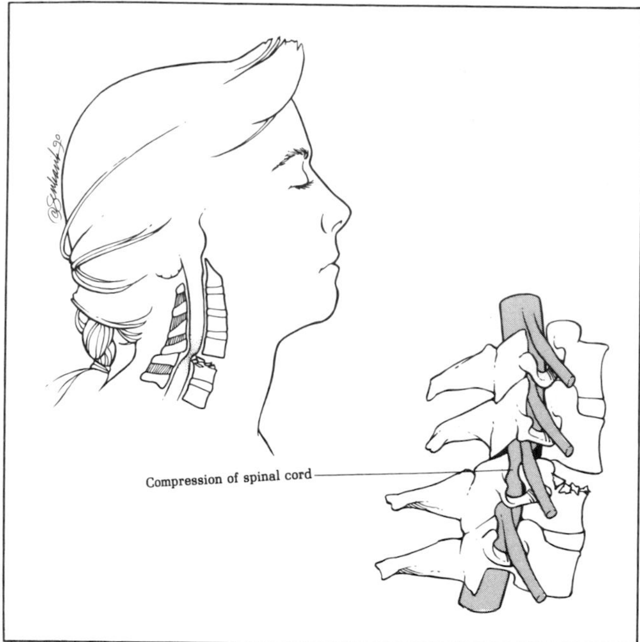

Fig. 14-15. *Compression of the cervical spine. Inset: when the spinal column becomes unstable because of vertebral fracture, very small shifts of one vertebrae with respect to another may crush the spinal cord.*

damage, in order to avoid converting a simple fracture of the vertebra to a case of permanent quadriplegia. For that reason, one needs to be aware of the mechanisms of injury apt to produce spinal damage (Fig. 14-16). In general, those include all injuries involving STRONG ACCELERATION-DECELERATION FORCES; vehicular accidents, falls from a height, and diving accidents are classic examples. ASSOCIATED INJURIES can also give clues to the presence of spinal damage. Any injury that has produced significant trauma to the *head, face, neck,* or *abdomen* should be assumed to have produced spinal injury as well. Similarly, any injury severe enough to produce unconsciousness is likely to have caused damage to the spine. The best general guide is WHEN IN DOUBT, TREAT THE PATIENT AS IF HE HAS A SPINAL INJURY AND IMMOBILIZE HIM ACCORDINGLY. You will not do any harm to a person who has no spinal injury by immobilizing him to a backboard; you can do immeasurable harm to someone who *does* have a spinal injury by *not* immobilizing him. Thus, err on the side of caution.

DO NOT WAIT FOR SIGNS OF QUADRIPLEGIA TO DEVELOP BEFORE YOU SUSPECT SPINAL INJURY. IF THE MECHANISMS OF INJURY SUGGEST POSSIBLE DAMAGE TO THE SPINE, ASSUME THERE *IS* DAMAGE TO THE SPINE AND IMMOBILIZE THE PATIENT ACCORDINGLY.

To summarize, then, the situations in which the EMT should suspect spinal injury are as follows:

Suspect Spinal Injury When:

- There has been a VEHICULAR ACCIDENT.
- There has been a DIVING ACCIDENT.
- There has been a FALL FROM A HEIGHT.
- There has been a CAVE-IN.
- The injury has produced UNCONSCIOUSNESS.
- There is associated INJURY TO THE HEAD OR FACE.
- There is MASSIVE TRAUMA from any source.
- The victim has been struck by LIGHTNING.
- There is any DOUBT whether spinal injury may be present.

Assessment of the Patient with Possible Spinal Injury

The history and physical assessment of the patient can provide valuable clues to the presence of vertebral fracture or injury to the spinal cord. One starts, as usual, with the primary survey, taking precautions not to hyperextend the neck in the process of opening the airway. Once the ABCs have been attended to, it is necessary to obtain more information about the patient and the injury.

First of all, in gathering the HISTORY, examine the scene to try to determine the MECHANISMS OF INJURY. Is the front end of the car accordioned against a tree, suggesting massive deceleration forces that could have snapped the neck violently back and forth ("whiplash" injury)? Does the car seat have a protective headrest to minimize such motion? If the injury was sustained while diving, how shallow is the water? If the patient is simply found unconscious, is there any reason to suspect that the patient might have fallen from a height, such as an overturned ladder? Try to find out from the patient or bystanders how the accident occurred and, equally important, WHEN THE ACCIDENT OCCURRED. Time is an important factor in spinal cord damage, for within a few hours after an accident involving injury to the spinal cord, the chances of restoring lost function are practically nil.

If the patient is conscious, instruct him not to move except when told to do so. Question him about PAIN: Does it hurt anywhere over the spine? Determine if he has any NUMBNESS OR PARESTHESIAS (pins-and-needles feelings). Does he feel WEAKNESS OR HEAVINESS in any of his limbs? Find out whether the patient is experiencing any DIFFICULTY BREATHING. Any of these may be symptoms of damage to the spinal cord.

In doing the PHYSICAL ASSESSMENT, make a

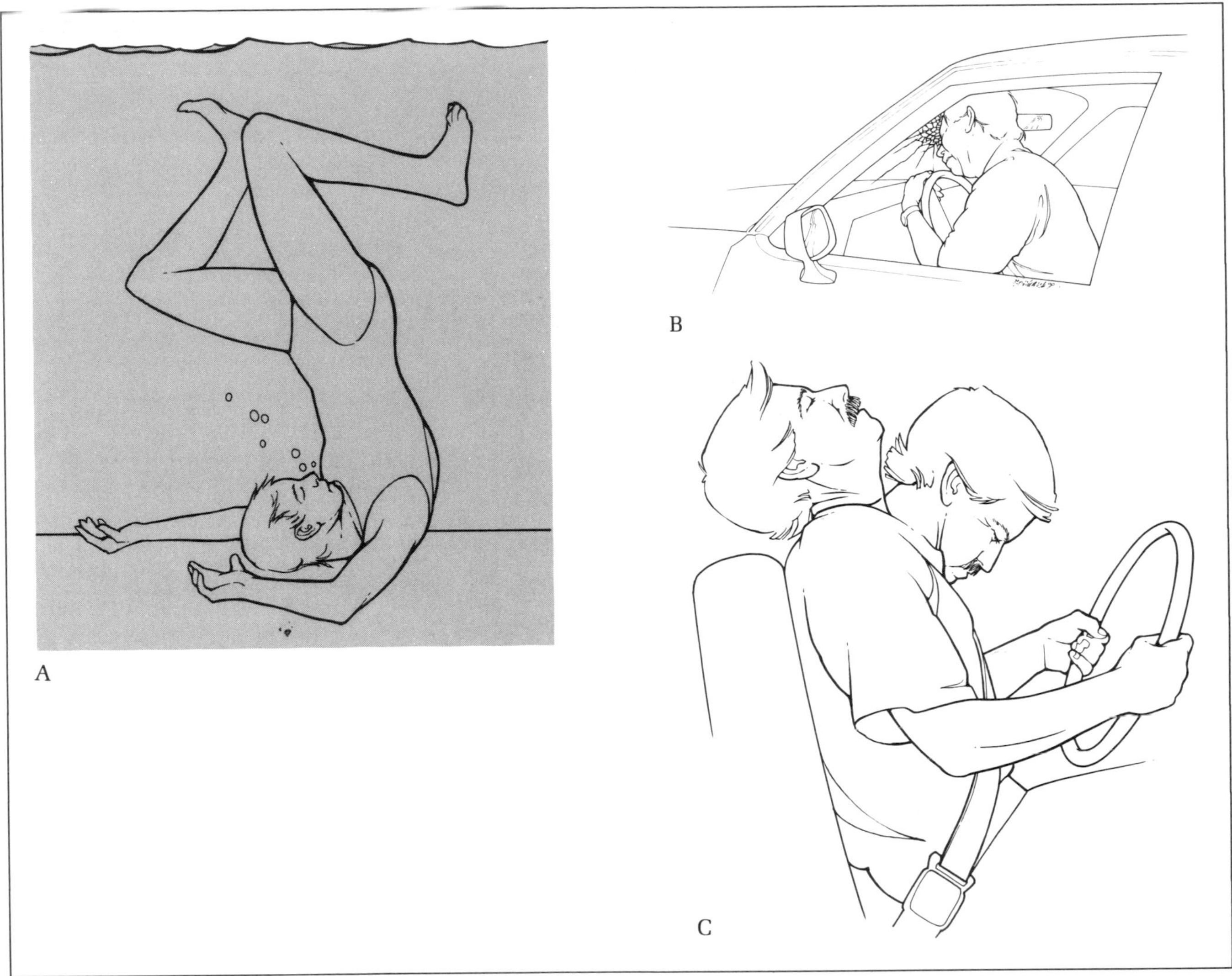

Fig. 14-16. *Typical mechanisms of spinal cord injury. A. Diving injury. B. Forward impact of head. C. Whiplash.*

note of the patient's GENERAL APPEARANCE and the POSITION in which he is found. Do not attempt to change that position unless the airway is in jeopardy. There are some positions that are very characteristic of spinal cord injuries and that should, therefore, immediately arouse suspicion. When there is injury to the spinal cord around C6, for instance, the patient will very often lie with his forearms flexed across his chest, with his hands half closed (Fig. 14-17A). If you straighten out the arm, it will go right back to the flexed position as soon as you let go. Another position characteristic of cervical spine injury is the "stick 'em up" position, where the patient holds his hands half open above his head (Fig. 14-17B).

Measure and record the VITAL SIGNS. Be particularly alert for HYPOTENSION WITHOUT OTHER SIGNS OF SHOCK, for this is highly suggestive of a spinal cord injury producing neurogenic shock (shock from massive dilation of blood vessels). In patients who have sustained injury to the spinal cord, the average *systolic* blood pressure when first examined is around 75 mm Hg. Generally, however, these patients do not show any other evidence of shock (unless there is significant bleeding elsewhere); the pulse is usually slow, and the skin is more apt to be warm and dry than cold and clammy.

Proceed to the HEAD-TO-TOE SURVEY, and check the HEAD AND FACE for cuts and bruises, which are good evidence that strong forces have been exerted upon the patient's head.

> ALMOST ALL PATIENTS WITH A CERVICAL SPINE INJURY WILL HAVE A CUT OR BRUISE ON THE HEAD OR FACE.

The same is true of injuries to other parts of the spine; bruises over the back, abdomen, or shoulders

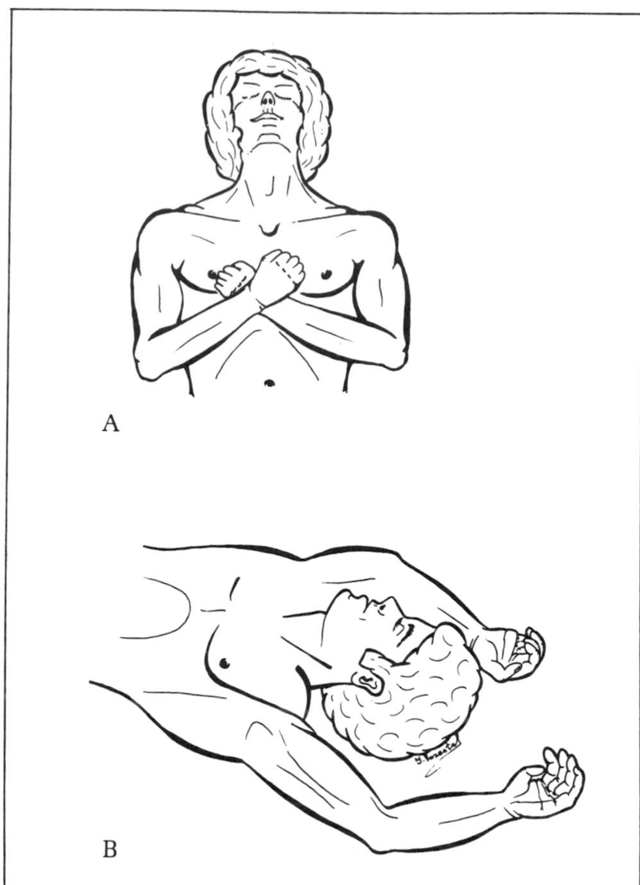

Fig. 14-17. *Positions suggesting spinal cord injury. A. Injury around C6. B. "Stick 'em up" position with cervical spine injury.*

are highly suggestive of strong forces applied to the spinal column. The absence of such visible injuries, however, in no way rules out the possibility that the spine has been injured.

In examining the NECK, palpate gently over the cervical vertebrae, and note any deformity. If the patient is conscious, ask him to report any tenderness he feels as you palpate. Tenderness over the spine should be regarded as strong evidence of spinal injury.

Inspect the CHEST, and observe the PATTERN OF BREATHING. The nerves that control the function of the intercostal muscles exit from the spinal cord around C5 to C6, near the middle of the neck. If the spinal cord is damaged at or above this level, there may be paralysis of the intercostal muscles (together with the arms and legs), and as a result, the patient will be able to breathe only with his diaphragm. Thus the chest of a person with cervical spine injury will move very little with each breath, while the abdomen can be seen to rise and fall slightly with respirations. Diaphragmatic breathing is very inefficient breathing, for only limited amounts of air can be moved in and out of the chest when the diaphragm is working alone. Thus the patient may try to compensate by breathing faster, and the typical patient with cervical spine injury shows *rapid, shallow breathing.*

In examining the ABDOMEN, look for bruises that suggest strong forces applied to that part of the body, and bear in mind the possibility of internal bleeding if the patient is showing signs of hemorrhagic shock. In the male, check for **priapism** (sustained erection of the penis), which is a characteristic sign of spinal cord damage.

Palpate the BACK gently for any irregularity or deformity along the spine. If the patient is conscious, ask him to report any tenderness he feels as you palpate, and note its location.

Test the EXTREMITIES for SENSATION AND MOVEMENT. Start by lightly touching the patient's toes and asking the patient to report when he feels your touch. If sensation is absent at the toes, gradually move up the leg, abdomen, and chest, and make a note of the point at which the patient first begins to feel your touch. As a rough guide, the umbilicus is about at the level of the tenth thoracic nerve (T10); the nipples are roughly at T4, and the clavicles are around C3. Describe the area of **anesthesia** (absence of feeling) as precisely as you can; for instance, "The patient has no sensation to light touch or pinprick from the toes to a point 2 inches above the umbilicus." If sensation is entirely intact, this fact should also be recorded. Once again, as in checking the status of a head-injured patient, it is important to make several observations at regular intervals and to document carefully any *changes* in the patient's function.

If the patient is unconscious, check sensation by applying a painful stimulus (pinprick or pinch) and observing the patient's face for grimaces. Once again, start at the toes and work upward, noting the point at which the patient begins to show some reaction.

After testing sensation, examine the patient's motor function, starting again at the feet. If the patient is conscious, ask him to wiggle his toes. If he can do so, gauge the *strength* in his foot by asking him to push down with the sole of his foot against your hand, and see if he can overcome the resistance of your hand. If there is weakness or paralysis of the foot, ask the patient to try to raise his leg slowly, but instruct him to stop any movement the moment he feels pain and to report the pain to you. Proceed to the examination of the upper extremities, and test motor function by asking the patient to grip your hand as hard as he can with his hand. Note any weakness in either upper extremity.

In an unconscious patient, test for paralysis by applying a painful stimulus first to each foot, then to each hand. If the spinal cord is undamaged, the patient will usually withdraw the extremity to some degree in response to the painful stimulation. If there is no withdrawal, gently try to flex the knee and then the elbow (without moving the patient), and note whether there is resistance to your manipulation. In a normal person, muscles retain a certain amount of tone, even when at rest, and they are slightly resistant to being flexed by the examiner. In a spinal cord injury, the muscles may be **flaccid** (pronounced flasid), that is, soft and completely nonresistant, like a limp rag.

Symptoms and Signs of Spinal Cord Injury

- PAIN and TENDERNESS over the spine
- NUMBNESS or PARESTHESIAS
- WEAKNESS or HEAVINESS in the limbs
- POSITION: arms folded over the chest or "stick 'em up"
- HYPOTENSION WITHOUT OTHER SIGNS OF SHOCK
- CUTS and BRUISES over the HEAD, FACE, NECK, BACK, or ABDOMEN
- DIAPHRAGMATIC BREATHING
- PRIAPISM
- DEFORMITY of the spine
- LOSS OF SENSATION
- WEAKNESS or PARALYSIS; FLACCIDITY

Management of Suspected Spinal Injury

Spinal injury is *not* an immediately life-threatening condition. Airway obstruction, apnea, cardiac arrest, and profuse bleeding are. Thus, as always, the first priorities in treating a patient with suspected spinal injury are the ABCs.

Management of the AIRWAY requires extreme care not to move the patient's neck. If the patient is unconscious, first try to open the airway by inserting a nasopharyngeal airway (or, if that is unavailable, an oropharyngeal airway). If insertion of an artificial airway by itself keeps the patient's airway open, do not move his head or neck in any way. If, however, the patient's airway is still obstructed, the next maneuver to open the airway should be GENTLE JAW THRUST WITHOUT BACKWARD TILT OF THE HEAD. If this is ineffective, the head may be tilted *very slightly* backward, with the neck kept midline with gentle traction. Meanwhile, apply a cervical collar, to minimize subsequent motion of the neck. An oropharyngeal airway should be inserted to keep the patient's airway open.

Injuries to the cervical spine are likely to be associated with inadequate BREATHING, from paralysis of the intercostal muscles. Such breathing will very quickly lead to respiratory insufficiency if steps are not taken to improve the patient's respiratory exchange. If the patient is conscious and has shallow, rapid respirations, his ventilations should be assisted with the demand valve, allowing the patient's inhalations to trigger the valve. Explain to the patient the purpose of the demand valve and how it works—that it will give him a little boost with every breath. Then hold the mask against the patient's face (if his intercostals are paralyzed, chances are his arms will be paralyzed too, so he will not be able to hold the mask by himself), and allow him to trigger the resuscitator with his own inhalations. Be careful not to move the patient's head as you apply the mask. If the patient finds the mask confining, use it only periodically, say, for every third or fourth ventilation.

If the patient with cervical spine injury is unconscious, the demand valve should not be used, for the high pressures it delivers will rapidly inflate the patient's stomach. Assist ventilations instead with gentle squeezes from a bag-valve-mask (with oxygen), timed to coincide with and augment the patient's spontaneous ventilations. Once again, be very careful not to move the patient's head or neck as you assist his ventilations. If the patient has not yet been immobilized on a backboard, kneel at the vertex and stabilize his head and neck between your knees (Fig. 14-18) as you give artificial ventilation.

Attention to the CIRCULATION means CONTROL OF BLEEDING and treatment of NEUROGENIC SHOCK, if present. The latter will require tilting the patient so that his legs are elevated, and this must be deferred until the patient has been properly immobilized. For severe cases of neurogenic shock, where there is evidence of inadequate brain perfusion (e.g., confusion, stupor), the MAST can be used as well.

Immobilization of the Spine

Once the ABCs have been taken care of and any open wounds have been covered, the EMT can turn to immobilization of the spine. EVERY PATIENT SUSPECTED OF HAVING SUSTAINED A SPINAL INJURY *MUST* BE FULLY IMMOBILIZED BEFORE BEING MOVED. The procedures involved in spinal immobilization do *not* require haste. To the contrary, they require slow, careful, and deliberate action by the rescuers. A well-planned and deliberate procedure will also help calm the patient, who is likely to be fearful or panicky on account of his disability.

If the patient is conscious, EXPLAIN THOROUGHLY what you intend to do and why you are doing it. Immobilization means literally being tied down hand and foot, and this can be a frightening experience, especially if a person is simply set upon without warning by a bunch of people with 9-foot straps and a big board. Thus it is necessary to explain to the patient that rigid immobilization is necessary to protect his spine from damage. Also instruct the patient not to move unless you specifically tell him to do so.

For purposes of discussion, we will consider three different patients with definite or suspected spinal injury: (1) a patient found supine on the ground after a fall, (2) a patient found behind the wheel of a car after a head-on collision, and (3) a patient found

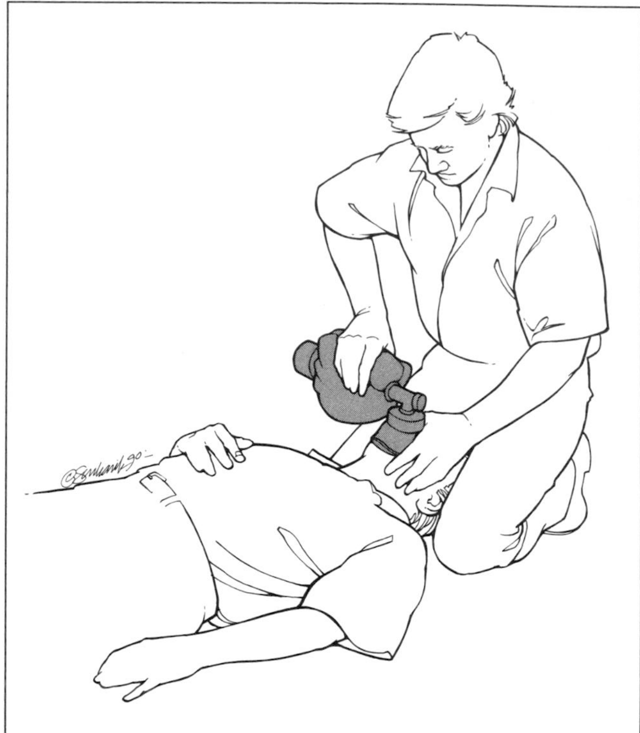

Fig. 14-18. *Stabilize the victim's head and neck between your knees as you give artificial ventilation.*

floating facedown in a swimming pool after a diving accident. Each of these situations requires a slightly different approach, although the underlying principle of immobilization is the same: MAINTAIN GENTLE TRACTION ON THE NECK, AND MINIMIZE MOVEMENT OF THE PATIENT.

PATIENT FOUND SUPINE AFTER A FALL. At least two rescuers should respond to the patient. One of them immediately stabilizes the patient's neck by placing his hands on either side of the patient's head and pulling *gently* backward in a straight line with the spine (Fig. 14-19). The rescuer stabilizing the neck will remain at the patient's head throughout, maintaining gentle traction until the patient has been fully immobilized and directing the activities of the other rescuers. If the patient is conscious, the rescuer at the head should also keep up a running conversation with the patient, to explain what is being done and to calm the patient's anxieties.

While the first rescuer holds the head and neck in a straight line with the spine, the second rescuer conducts the primary and secondary surveys and takes care of whatever problems are detected. The second rescuer or an assistant then gathers the equipment necessary for spinal immobilization.

Equipment for Spinal Immobilization on a Long Backboard

1	long backboard
3	9-foot straps with quick-release buckles
1	blanket that has been folded to about a 12- to 14-inch width, rolled together from both ends, and tied in a roll with two cravats
2 to 3	extra cravats, folded to 3-inch widths
1	cervical collar (preferably Philadelphia or polyethylene collar)

From this point on, more hands will be required—usually more than are present on an ambulance—and the EMT will have to recruit bystanders to help. There should be four or preferably five people to perform backboarding, including at least one EMT to take charge and instruct the assistants on what they are to do.

While the first EMT continues to stabilize the patient's head and neck, the second EMT should gently fasten the cervical collar around the patient's neck (Fig. 14-20). The collar should be snug but not so tight that it strangles the patient. You should just be able to slip two fingers between the collar and the neck. If your whole hand can fit between the collar and the patient's neck, the collar is too loose; if you cannot get two fingers in, it is too tight.

The cervical collar can provide only partial support for the patient's neck. It does *not* replace the support provided by the EMT who is stabilizing the patient's head manually. Thus, the EMT at the vertex should maintain manual support until the patient is fully immobilized to the backboard.

A CERVICAL COLLAR BY ITSELF DOES NOT PROVIDE ADEQUATE IMMOBILIZATION OF THE CERVICAL SPINE. MAINTAIN MANUAL STABILIZATION UNTIL THE HEAD IS SECURED TO A BACKBOARD.

Fig. 14-19. *Holding the neck in line with the spine.*

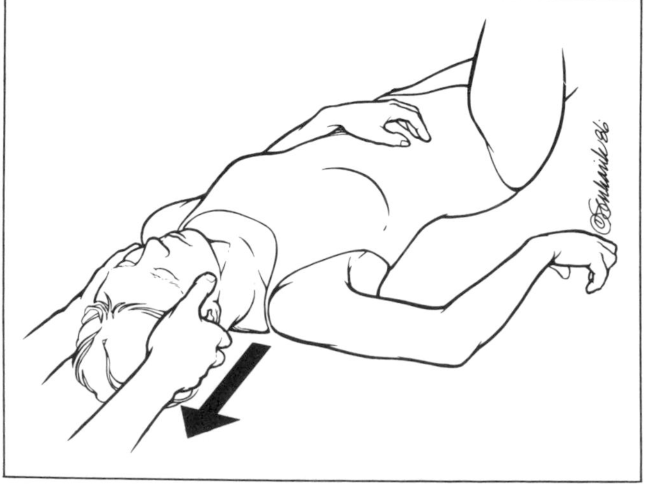

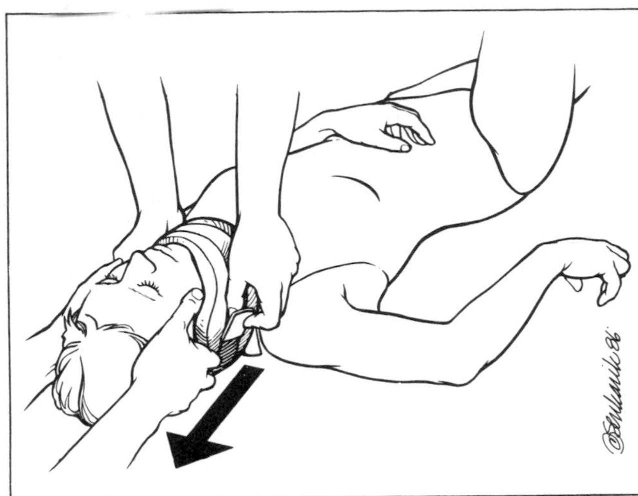

Fig. 14-20. *Application of a cervical collar while one rescuer supports the head and neck.*

Once the collar is in place, the patient must be moved onto the backboard. There are two techniques of accomplishing this: (1) the logroll, in which the backboard is placed alongside the patient; and (2) the straddle-slide, in which the backboard is placed at the patient's vertex. The technique chosen for any given case will depend upon the area in which the patient is found and whether there is more room to work by his side or behind his head. With both techniques, the first EMT remains at the patient's head, supporting the head and neck and directing the activities of the other rescuers.

For the LOGROLL TECHNIQUE, five rescuers are needed, and we shall refer to them as R1, R2, R3, and so forth. The first rescuer (R1), as noted, maintains gentle traction at the patient's head throughout the procedure.

R2 raises the patient's arm above the patient's head on the side to which the patient will be rolled. At the same time, R3 ties the patient's feet together with a cravat. Then R3, R4, and R5 position themselves as follows (Fig. 14-21A):

R3: Kneeling beside the patient's shoulders, with one hand on the patient's opposite shoulder and the other over the patient's opposite arm, just above the beltline.
R4: Kneeling beside the patient's buttocks, with one hand above the patient's opposite buttock and the other hand around the patient's opposite midthigh.
R5: Kneeling beside the patient's knees, with one hand behind the patient's opposite knee and the other hand on the patient's opposite leg, just below the calf. R5's job will be easier if the patient's feet have been tied together with a cravat.

At the command of R1, the other rescuers roll the patient slowly toward them, keeping the patient's body in a straight line. At the same time, R1 supports and turns the patient's head, so that the neck remains in alignment with the rest of the spine. As the patient is being turned, R2 slides the long backboard beside the patient, so that it occupies the place where the patient had been lying (Fig. 14-21B), and holds the backboard in place with his foot to prevent it from slipping. R2 places padding (e.g., folded or rolled towels) on the board where a void will be created by the patient's body (i.e., at the neck, the small of the back, the knees, and the ankles).

At the command of R1, the other rescuers roll the patient back supine onto the board, once again taking care to coordinate their movements so that the patient's spine remains in a straight line. Again, R1 keeps the head and neck in alignment with the body, so that the entire body is turned as a single unit (hence the term "logroll").

Once the patient is lying on the board, three 9-foot straps are slid beneath the board to secure the patient to the board at the chest, thighs, and knees. R2 meanwhile unrolls the blanket to expose about 8 inches of blanket and gently slides the flat part of the roll under the patient's head (while R1 continues to hold the head in traction!), until the two rolled edges of the blanket are pressed firmly on the patient's shoulders (Fig. 14-22). Two cravats are used to fasten the blanket roll in place on the backboard—one cravat over the patient's forehead and the other over his cervical collar—so that the patient's head is sandwiched firmly between the two rolled ends of the blanket. Both cravats should be tied with quick-release knots, and the knots should be placed to a side, over the blanket, not over the patient's face. Once the blanket roll is in place, R1 may release his grip on the patient's head.

Some rescue teams prefer to use sandbags on either side of the patient's head instead of a blanket roll. The sandbags are placed firmly against the sides of the patient's head, and then wide strips of adhesive tape are used to secure the patient's head and the sandbags to the backboard. The disadvantage of sandbags is their weight: If the backboard has to be tilted up onto its side, the sandbags will push the patient's head to a side and thereby drag the neck out of alignment with the rest of the spine. Specially designed, lightweight head supports are now widely available for use with backboards and are to be preferred to sandbags.

The STRADDLE-SLIDE can be performed with four rescuers, positioned as follows:

R1: Crouching at the patient's vertex, maintaining traction on the head.
R2: Behind R1, straddling a backboard that has been placed lengthwise behind the patient's head.
R3: Straddling the patient and facing R1, with his hands beneath the patient's shoulders at the level of the armpits.

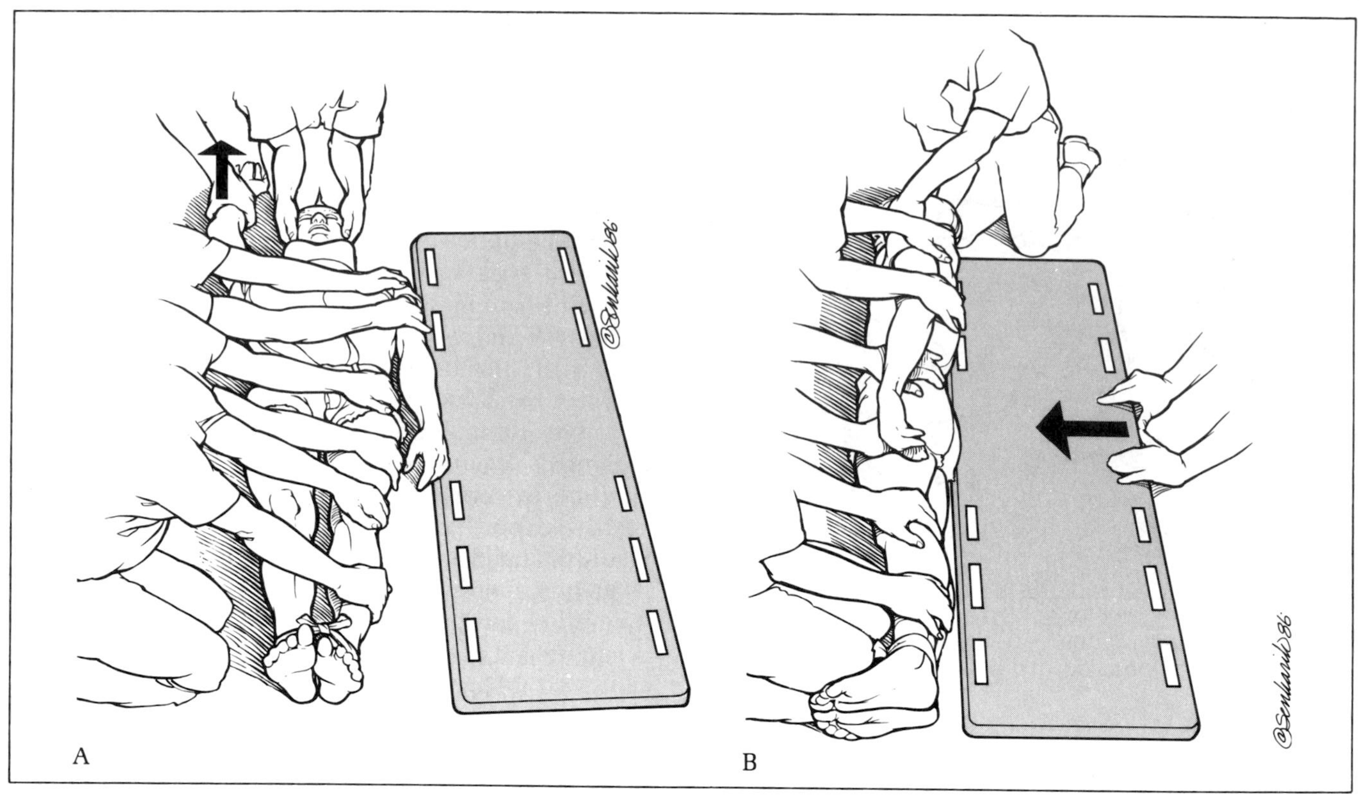

Fig. 14-21. *A. Four rescuers prepare to roll patient. B. Four rescuers roll patient to his side as a unit and backboard is slid beneath him.*

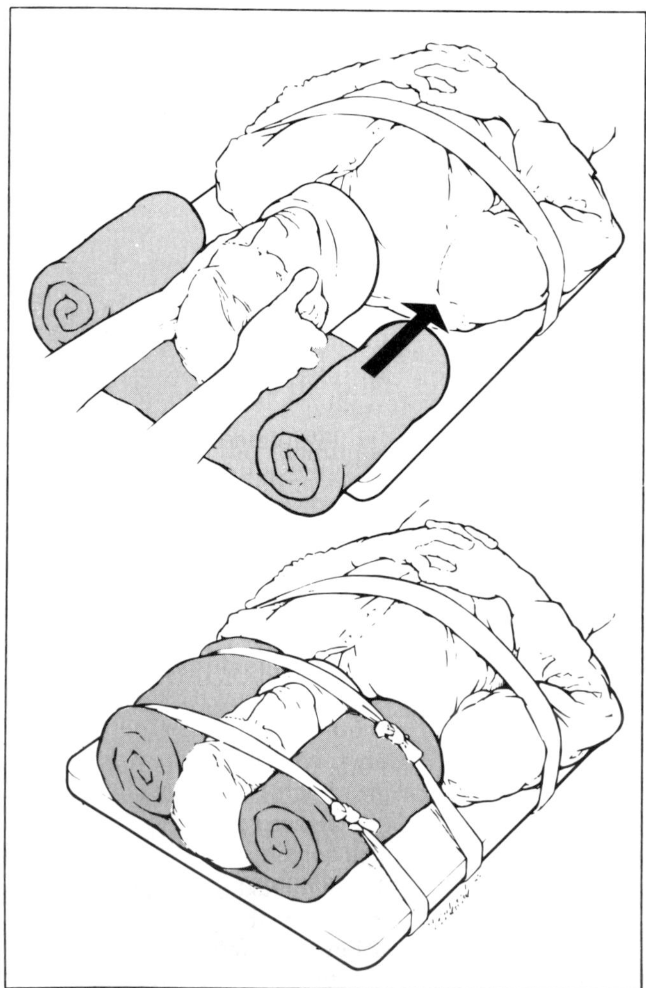

Fig. 14-22. *Blanket roll used to stabilize patient's head.*

R4: Straddling the patient and facing R1, with his hands beneath the patient's waist.

At a command from R1, the patient is lifted *very slightly* off the ground AS A UNIT, just enough to permit R2 to slide the backboard beneath the patient. R1 then gives a command to lower the patient, and once again as a unit, the patient is lowered onto the board. Any voids between the patient and the board (i.e., at the neck, small of the back, knees, and ankles) should be padded with towels. The patient is then secured to the board with straps over the chest, thighs, and knees; and his head is immobilized with a blanket roll as described above.

PATIENT BEHIND THE WHEEL OF A CAR. The patient with suspected spinal injury who is found behind the wheel of a car presents an additional problem: how to get him out of the car without aggravating the damage to his spine, which means getting him out of the car without any motion of his neck or back. One of the most effective ways of accomplishing this is with the use of long and short backboards.

Proper packaging and removal of an injured patient from an automobile requires at least three rescuers for optimal performance. Immediately upon reaching the vehicle, R1 should gain access to the back seat behind the patient and, after explaining who he is, apply gentle manual traction to the patient's head to bring the head into the "eyes-forward" position (Fig. 14-23). R1 will remain in that position throughout the procedure. R2 meanwhile conducts the patient survey and carries out whatever treatment

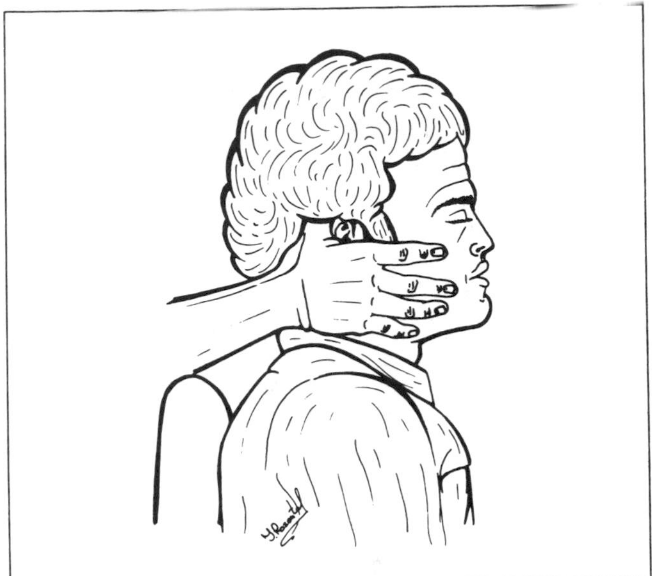

Fig. 14-23. *The patient's neck is maintained in steady axial traction by a rescuer positioned in the back seat.*

is immediately required, such as control of bleeding or administration of oxygen. When finished with those preliminary stabilizing measures, R2 assembles the equipment that will be needed for immobilization and extrication of the patient.

Equipment for Packaging and Removal of a Patient from a Car

1	cervical collar (preferably Philadelphia or polyethylene collar)
1	short backboard
1	long backboard
3 to 5	cravats
5	9-foot straps
1	air splint (forearm size)

R2 gently applies the extrication collar around the victim's neck and checks that the fit is correct. He or she then prepares the short backboard by inserting two straps so that they form an "X" on the back of the board; the buckles are brought out at the top front of the board on either side. R2 positions the board behind the patient (R1 is still maintaining traction on the patient's head and guarding the patient against jarring) so that the "shoulders" of the board are lined up behind the patient's shoulders. The patient is then secured to the board by bringing the lower ends of the straps around the patient's thighs and back up to snap into the respective buckles. R2 tightens the board to the patient by pulling simultaneously on the free ends of both straps.

Once the patient's torso is snugly secured to the short backboard, the head can be secured as well. The air splint is slid behind the patient's neck and inflated slightly. Cravats are then used over the patient's forehead and cervical collar to fasten the patient's head to the board, and the air splint is inflated to the point where it completely fills the void between the patient's neck and the backboard. At this point, R1 may release his traction on the patient's head.

Now that the patient's neck is properly immobilized, there remains the problem of removing the patient from the car. Theoretically, the patient could simply be lifted out, but this is rarely simple, especially if the patient is heavy. Furthermore, lifting the patient upward can cause him to shift position on the board, pushing his trunk upward and squeezing his neck. For these reasons, it is usually preferable to use a long backboard to get the patient out of the car.

R1 and R2 move to opposite sides of the patient, and coordinating their actions, they raise the patient 1 to 2 inches off the car seat by lifting the patient's body (one hand gripping the patient's arm, one under his buttocks), NOT the short backboard. As they do so, a third rescuer slides a long backboard underneath the patient's buttocks and holds the long board in place. R1 then pivots the patient so that the patient's legs are on the passenger seat, while R2 guides and supports the legs (this is easier to do if the feet have been tied together with a cravat). While R3 supports his end of the long backboard, R1 and R2 gently lower the patient—short backboard and all—so that he is lying on the long backboard. At this point, the patient's legs will be flexed in the air, because of the way the straps are fastened around them. R2 will have to loosen the torso straps and—slowly and carefully—lower the patient's legs until they lie flat on the long backboard, at which point the torso straps are retightened. Rolled towels are then placed beneath the small of the patient's back, knees, and ankles; and the patient is secured to the long board with straps over the chest, hip, and lower thigh. The straps are checked for snugness, and the long board is lifted out of the car.

PATIENT FOUND IN THE WATER. Diving accidents are one of the most common causes of cervical spine fracture. In the classic diving injury, a person plunges headfirst into a shallow body of water and strikes his head against the bottom or against some protruding object, such as a rock. Injury to the spinal cord may occur at the moment of impact, but often the spinal cord injury does not occur until later, when the patient's head is allowed to roll about as he is pulled from the water.

Typically, the victim is found floating facedown in the water. Thus the first measure that must be taken is to get the victim safely onto his back and start rescue breathing as needed. The steps in managing this situation are as follows:

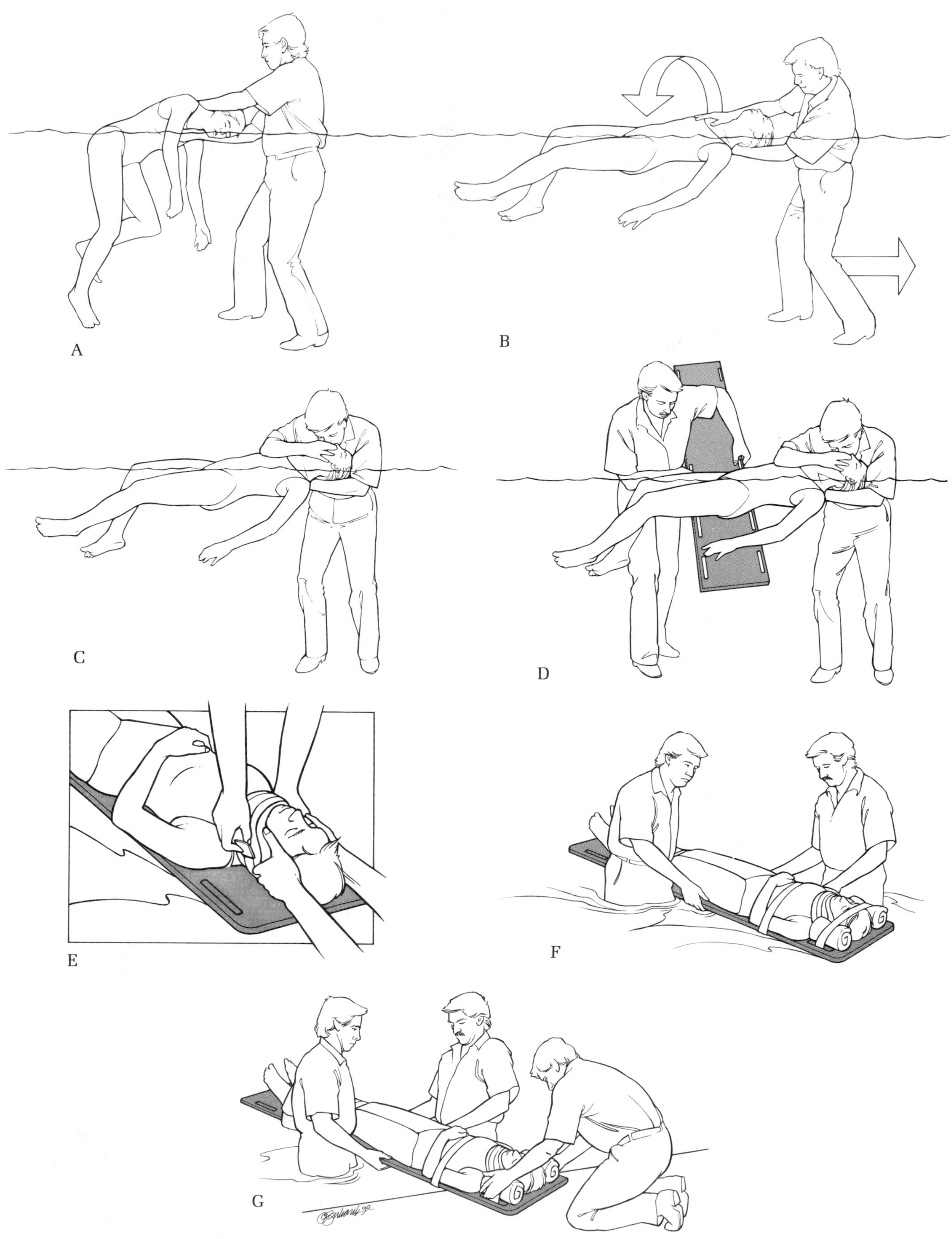

Fig. 14-24. *Extricating a victim found in shallow water (presumed diving accident). A. Splint his head and neck between your arms. B. Pull and rotate. C. Start mouth-to-mouth ventilation. D. Slide backboard beneath victim. E. Apply cervical collar. F. Float board to side of pool. G. Lift victim from water.*

1. R1 enters the water and approaches the victim from the vertex. He places one arm along the victim's spine and the other under the victim's chest, so that the victim's head is firmly sandwiched between the rescuer's arms (Fig. 14-24A). R1 then backs slowly away from the victim while smoothly rotating him into a supine position (Fig. 14-24B). With the victim now on his back in the water, R1 keeps one hand, palm up, under the victim's thoracic spine, so that the victim's head is supported on the rescuer's upper arm. Using the other hand to stabilize the victim's head, R1 begins mouth-to-mouth ventilation as needed (Fig. 14-24C).
2. Meanwhile, R2 has been gathering the necessary equipment from the ambulance, including a long wooden backboard, two to three 9-foot straps, and a blanket roll. R2 enters the water and floats the backboard out to where R1 is working and slides the backboard under the victim (Fig. 14-24D).
3. While R1 maintains traction on the victim's head, R2 applies a cervical collar (Fig. 14-24E), secures the victim's head between the blanket roll and then secures the victim to the board using the 9-foot straps. R1 continues rescue breathing as needed.
4. With artificial ventilation in progress as needed, the backboard is floated to the poolside or to land (Fig. 14-24F) and lifted carefully from the water (Fig. 14-24G). External chest compressions are started if there is no pulse, and CPR is continued as necessary all the way to the hospital.

In any of the above situations, if the patient is unconscious, he should be transported on his side to minimize the risk of aspirating vomitus. To do so, you must first check that the patient is snugly strapped to the long board and then tilt the board up on its left side and slightly forward on the stretcher. Buttress the front of the board with pillows, and strap it in place on the stretcher (Fig. 14-25).

The details of backboarding technique may differ from one region to another, depending on the preferences of local instructors. The fundamental principles remain the same, however, and what is important is to learn a technique and rehearse it until it is second nature.

General Principles of Spinal Immobilization

- EVERY patient suspected of having sustained a spinal injury should be fully immobilized before being moved.
- The object of the exercise is to PREVENT MOVEMENT of the patient's spine.
- DO NOT RUSH! Spinal immobilization should be SLOW, CAREFUL, and DELIBERATE.
- The rescuer at the patient's head is the rescuer in charge.
- Keep the patient's head and neck steady at all times until the patient is fully immobilized.
- If the patient must be moved, he should be moved AS A UNIT.
- Immobilize the patient in the position in which he is found. DO NOT ATTEMPT TO STRAIGHTEN OUT HIS BACK.
- Transport unconscious patients with the backboard on its left side, tilted slightly forward.

Helmets and Their Removal

The victim of an injury found wearing a helmet (e.g., a motorcycle helmet or football helmet) presents a special dilemma: Do you leave the helmet in place and ignore possible injuries beneath it? Or do you remove the helmet and risk moving the victim's neck in the process?

The answer is that the helmet should be removed when its presence interferes with the assessment and management of the victim. In some cases, it may be possible to give adequate care simply by removing *part* of the helmet. For example, access to the airway of an injured football player can usually be obtained by cutting the clips that hold the faceguard to the helmet and lifting the faceguard out of the way. In other cases, however, the helmet may seriously restrict the ability of the rescuers to care for the victim properly. So long as the helmet is in place, it is very difficult to check for and treat any associated head or facial injuries. Vomiting is harder to deal with when the victim is wearing a helmet, especially if

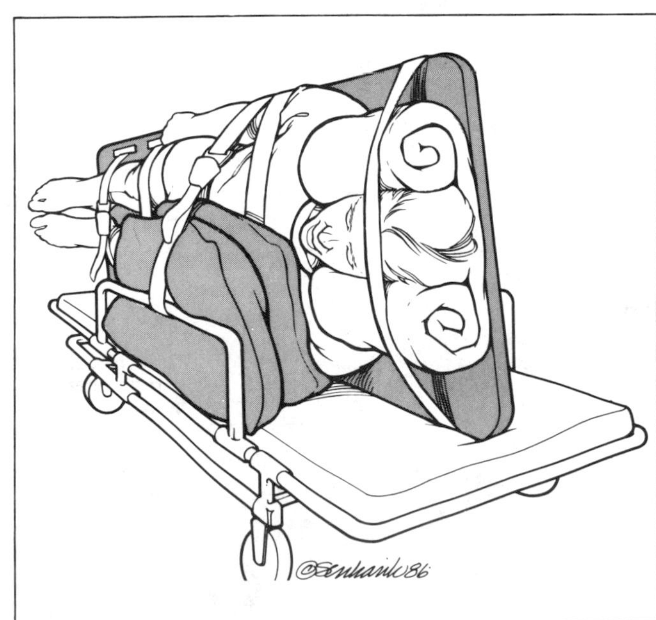

Fig. 14-25. *Backboard propped up and strapped on its side on the stretcher, to permit drainage of secretions from the patient's mouth.*

Types of Helmets

Full face coverage—motorcycle, auto racer

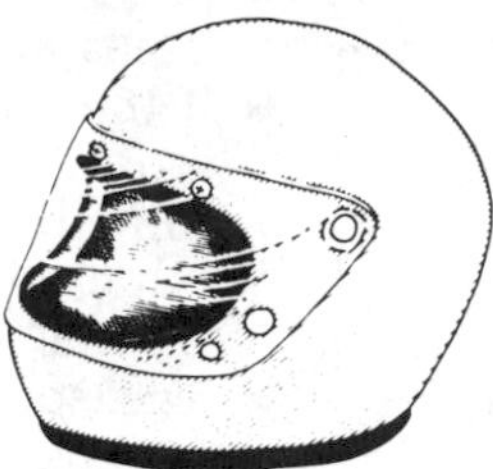

Full face coverage—motocross

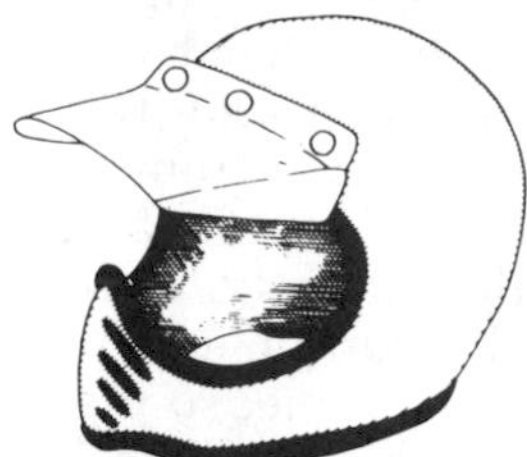

Helmet Removal

1

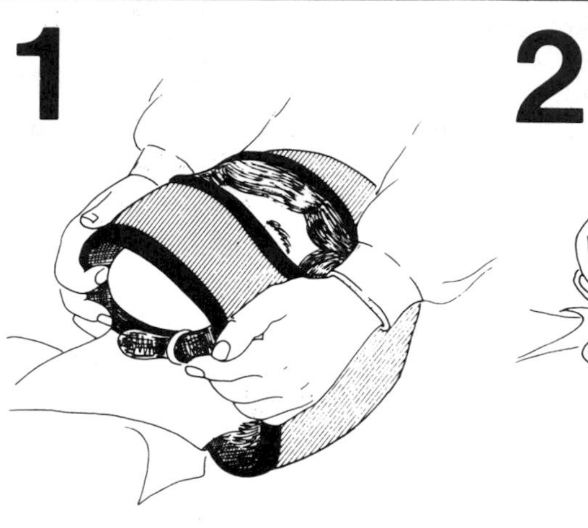

One rescuer applies inline traction by placing his or her hands on each side of the helmet with the fingers on the victim's mandible. This position prevents slippage if the strap is loose.

2

The rescuer cuts or loosens the strap at the D-rings while maintaining inline traction.

The varying sizes, shapes, and configurations of motorcycle helmets necessitate some understanding of their proper removal from victims of motorcycle accidents. The rescuer who removes a helmet improperly might inadvertently aggravate cervical spine injuries.

The Committee on Trauma believes that physicians who treat the injured should be aware of helmet removal techniques. A gradual increase in the use of helmets is anticipated because many organizations are urging voluntary wearing of helmets, and some states are reinstating their laws requiring the wearing of helmets.

American College of Surgeons
Committee on Trauma
July 1980

5

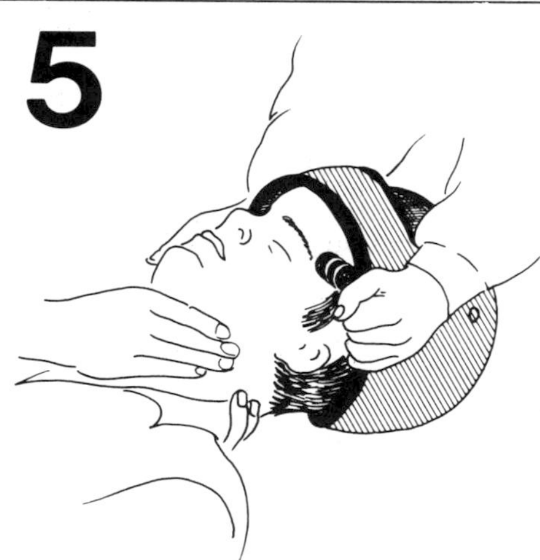

Throughout the removal process, the second rescuer maintains inline traction from below in order to prevent head tilt.

6

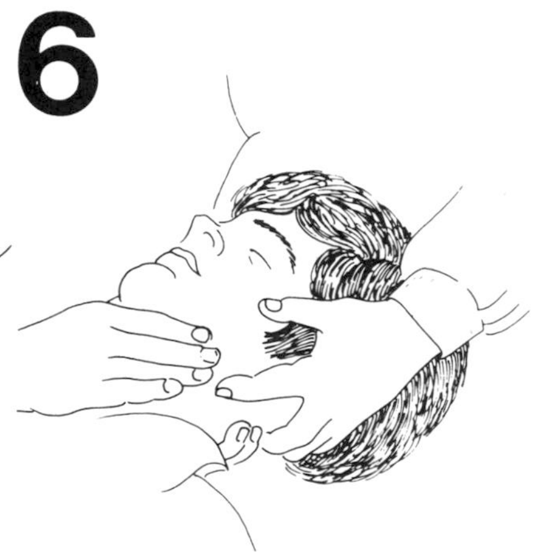

After the helmet has been removed, the rescuer at the top replaces his hands on either side of the victim's head with his palms over the ears.

Fig. 14-26. *Techniques of helmet removal from an injured patient. (Reproduced courtesy American College of Surgeons.)*

Partial face coverage—motorcycle, auto racer

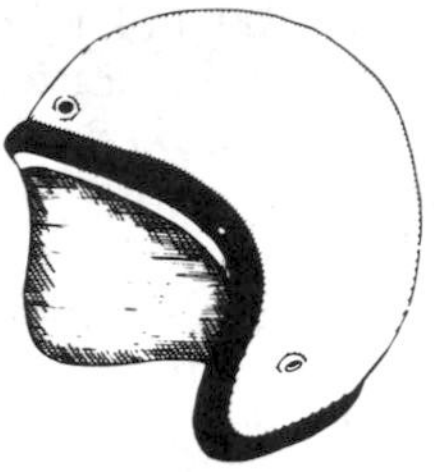

Light head protection—bicycle, kayak

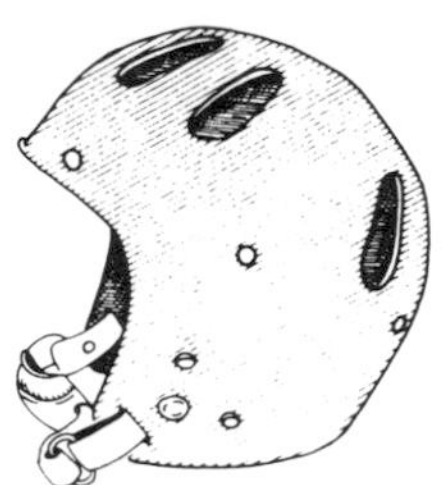

Football

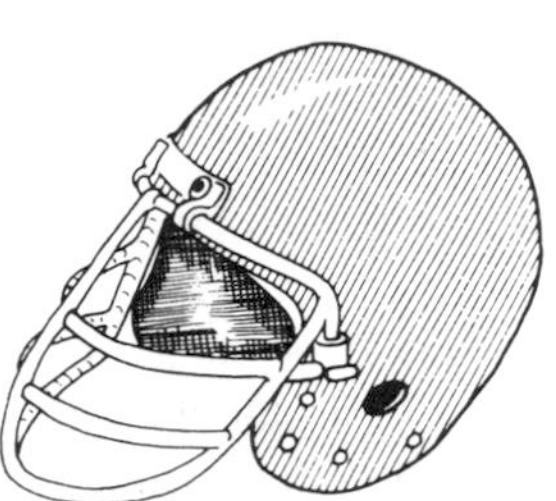

3

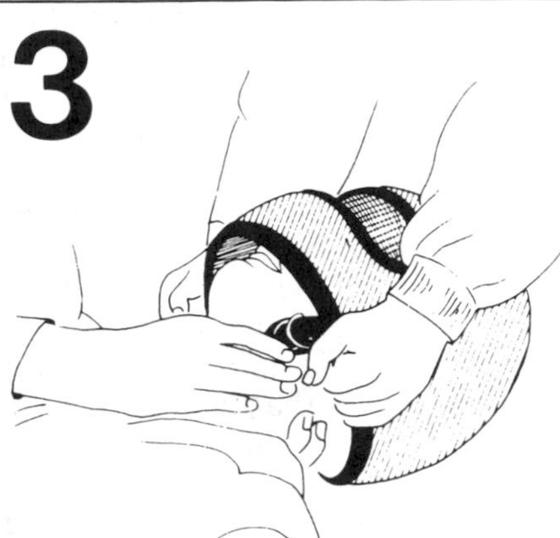

A second rescuer places one hand on the mandible at the angle, the thumb on one side, the long and index fingers on the other. With his other hand, he applies pressure from the occipital region. This maneuver transfers the inline traction responsibility to the second rescuer.

4

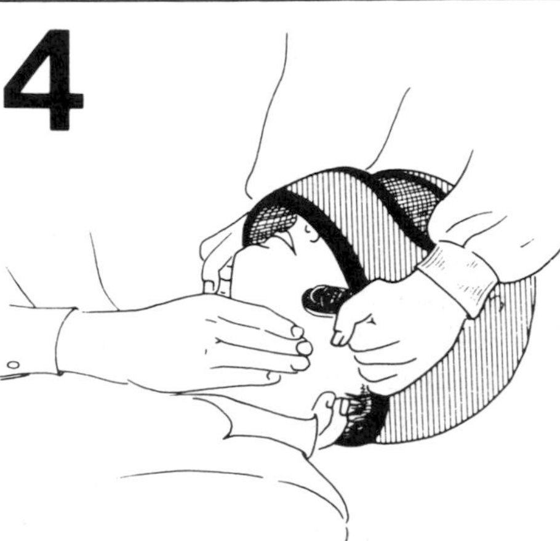

The rescuer at the top removes the helmet. Three factors should be kept in mind:

- **The helmet is egg-shaped, and therefore must be expanded laterally to clear the ears.**
- **If the helmet provides full facial coverage, glasses must be removed first.**
- **If the helmet provides full facial coverage, the nose will impede removal. To clear the nose, the helmet must be tilted backward and raised over it.**

7

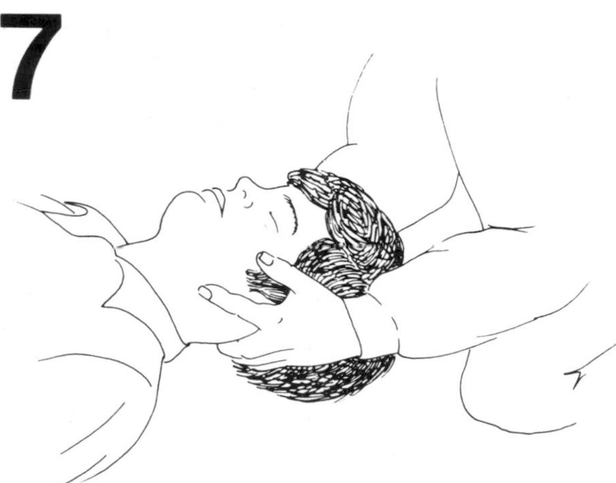

Inline traction is maintained from above until a backboard is in place.

Summary

The helmet must be maneuvered over the nose and ears while the head and neck are held rigid.

- Inline traction is applied from above.
- Inline traction is transferred below with pressure on the jaw and occiput.
- The helmet is removed.
- Inline traction is re-established from above.

the helmet is a full-face model, and the chinpiece can also present problems when it comes to opening the victim's mouth. Needless to say, CPR is virtually impossible on a helmeted victim. Furthermore, the helmet (because of its size and shape) may make it hard to immobilize the victim properly, and the victim's head is more apt to roll about on the stretcher or backboard when it is encased in a bulky sphere of plastic. Finally, it is nearly impossible to apply a cervical collar while the helmet is in place. So for all those reasons, it is often desirable to get the helmet off.

A helmet *can* be removed safely, but only if the rescuer understands how the helmet is constructed and has practiced to perfection the removal techniques. The correct procedures for helmet removal from an unconscious patient, as established by the American College of Surgeons, are shown in Figure 14-26. Note that the victim should be *supine* and that one rescuer constantly supports the head and neck from the vertex. If the victim is wearing glasses, those should be removed before attempting to take off the helmet. The rigid construction of most helmets makes them difficult to spread, but one must spread the helmet base slightly in order to slide it smoothly over the ears. With full-face helmets, take care not to let the chinpiece get hung up on the victim's nose.

As noted, these procedures require practice. The major accident with a badly injured victim is *not* the place to try out helmet removal techniques for the first time. IF YOU ARE NOT SKILLED IN SAFE HELMET REMOVAL TECHNIQUES, LEAVE THE HELMET IN PLACE. Lay the patient in the stable side position on the backboard, with the helmeted head propped up on blankets in order to keep a straight line between the head and the trunk. Then secure the helmet to the backboard. Cravats or roller gauze will be of limited usefulness, since they will slip off the smooth, rounded surface of the helmet. Use adhesive tape instead to fix the helmet to the board. Since it will be virtually impossible to apply a cervical collar, you will have to stabilize the victim's head manually throughout loading and transport; that means that the drive to the hospital must be exceptionally smooth, for a sudden jolt or swerve could cause you to jerk the head at an angle.

If artificial ventilation or full CPR becomes necessary, you will have no choice but to remove the helmet, whether you feel comfortable doing so or not. Thus it is wise to familiarize yourself with the procedures for helmet removal and practice on fellow students until it comes as naturally as any other EMT skill.

CASE HISTORIES

We conclude this chapter with two sample case presentations to review some of the material in the chapter and the method of medical reporting.

CASE ONE

The patient is a 35-year-old man who was injured in an automobile accident. The patient was the driver of a small sedan that struck the back of a truck when his brakes failed. The entire front end of the car was demolished, and the windshield was broken. Bystanders state that the patient was unconscious for 1 to 2 minutes after the impact. The patient himself does not remember the impact, but he does remember that his brakes would not work immediately before the accident. He complains of headache and dizziness. He denies paresthesias or weakness. He denies vomiting or visual problems. He has not taken any alcohol or medications in the past several hours. He has no significant underlying illnesses and has never been hospitalized. He is allergic to penicillin.

On initial examination, the patient was alert and oriented to person and place; he did not know the date. His speech was normal. The skin was warm and dry. Pulse was 100, full and regular; BP 130/80; and respirations 18 and unlabored. There were numerous cuts and bruises of the face, but no discharge from the ears or nose. The pupils were equal, midposition, and reactive to light. The eye motions were full in all directions. There was no neck tenderness. We found no evidence of injury to the chest or abdomen. Sensation and movement were intact in all four extremities.

The patient's wounds were dressed, and he was removed from the car on long and short backboards. He was given oxygen by nasal cannula at 6 liters per minute.

En route to the hospital, the patient began dropping off to sleep, but he could be awakened by shouting his name. His speech became somewhat slurred. Pulse was 60, BP 160/90, and respirations 28. The pupils remained equal.

Questions to think about:

1. Based only on the observations of the scene of the accident, what injuries might you expect the patient to have sustained?
2. What happened to the patient's pulse and blood pressure while he was in the EMTs' care? What is the significance of these changes?
3. Why were backboards used to remove the patient from the car?
4. Why was oxygen given?
5. Did the patient's condition improve or worsen while he was in the EMTs' care? What evidence do you have for your answer?

CASE TWO

The patient is a 28-year-old construction worker who fell from a scaffolding two stories above the ground and landed on his back. He did not lose consciousness. He complains of pain in his neck and a heavy feeling in his arms and legs, and he says the pain gets worse if he tries to move his head. He denies nausea, vomiting, or visual problems. He says he is having trouble breathing. He has no significant past medical history and takes no medications regularly.

On physical examination, the patient was found lying supine and seemed to be in some pain. He was alert and fully oriented. The skin was warm and dry. Pulse was 60, BP 80/40, and respirations 30 and shallow. There was a tender bruise over the back of the head. There was no drainage from the ears or nose, and the pupils were equal and reactive. The midneck was tender to palpation posteriorly. No deformity was felt. The chest did not appear to move with respirations, and there was evidence of diaphragmatic breathing. There was no evidence of injury to the chest, abdomen, or pelvis. Sensation to pinprick was absent from the toes to the clavicles, and the patient could not move his feet or hands.

The patient was given oxygen and immobilized on a long backboard. The foot of the backboard was elevated 10 inches on the stretcher. There were no changes in the patient's condition during transport.

Questions to think about:

1. In view of the mechanisms of injury and the patient's other symptoms, what do you think is the significance of the fact that he complains of difficulty in breathing?
2. What complication should you suspect on the basis of the patient's vital signs and skin condition?
3. At roughly what level of the spine do you think his injury occurred?
4. When a patient is immobilized on a backboard, it is customary to secure the patient's body to the board first, then to secure the head. Why do you think we do things in that sequence? [Hint: Suppose the patient also had a head injury. What complication of head injury might occur while you were in the middle of strapping the patient down?]
5. Why was the foot of the patient's backboard elevated during transport?

VOCABULARY

air embolism A bubble of air in the circulation that can block off a blood vessel and be rapidly fatal.
amnesia Loss of memory.
anesthesia Absence of feeling.
aqueous humor Salty fluid found between the cornea and the lens of the eye.
arachnoid Middle layer of the meninges.
basal skull fracture Fracture of the inferior part of the skull.
brainstem Portion of the brain, located inferior to the cerebrum, that controls automatic functions, such as breathing and body temperature.
central nervous system (CNS) The brain and spinal cord.
cerebellum Portion of the brain, lying inferior to the cerebrum, that controls balance, muscle tone, and coordination of skilled movements.
cerebrospinal fluid (CSF) Watery fluid that bathes the brain and acts as a shock absorber to protect the brain from impact.
cerebrum Largest portion of the brain, responsible for higher functions such as reasoning.
cervical spine First seven vertebrae, located in the neck.
coccyx Lowest portion of the spine; four fused vertebrae that constitute the tail bone.
comminuted fracture Fracture in which several small cracks radiate out from a point of impact.
concussion An injury to the head causing temporary loss of function, usually of very brief duration.
conjunctiva Mucous membrane covering the sclera and inner surface of the eyelids.
cornea Clear, anterior portion of the sclera.
decerebrate response Reaction to a painful stimulus (or sometimes to no stimulus at all) in which the patient's muscles go into spasm, with the legs in extreme extension.
depressed fracture Fracture in which part of the skull is pushed inward toward the brain.
dura mater Tough, outer layer of the meninges.
epidural Lying above the dura (between the dura and the skull).
flaccidity Absence of muscle tone; limpness of an extremity.
galea Tough inner lining of the scalp.
intracranial Within the skull.
iris Circular muscle behind the cornea that regulates the amount of light entering the eye by constricting or enlarging the aperture at its center.
lens Part of the eye, behind the iris, that focuses the image onto the retina.
linear fracture Fracture that appears as a single line or crack.
lumbar spine Part of the vertebral column in the lower back, starting just below the ribs and extending to the pelvis.
medulla Part of the brainstem that regulates breathing, heart rate, and other vital functions.
meninges The three membranes that enclose and protect the brain.
optic nerve Nerve extending from the back of the eye to the brain that carries signals relating to visual images.
orbit Eye socket.
paresthesias Pins-and-needles sensations.
pia mater Innermost layer of the meninges.
pinna The external ear.
priapism Sustained penile erection, seen in patients with spinal cord damage.
retina Layer of light-sensitive cells in the back of the eye.
sacrum Portion of the vertebral column that lies inferior to the lumbar spine and is fused with the pelvis.
sclera Tough, white covering of the eyeball.
subcutaneous emphysema Air in the soft tissues that causes crackling when the skin is palpated.
subdural Beneath the dura.
thoracic spine Part of the spinal column just below

the cervical vertebrae, comprising 12 vertebrae to which the 12 ribs are attached.

vitreous humor Jelly-like substance within the eye that gives the eye its shape.

zygoma Cheek bone.

FURTHER READING

HEAD INJURY

Bachulis BL et al. Patterns of injury in helmeted and non-helmeted motorcyclists. *Am J Surg* 155:708, 1988.

Bouzarth WF. Early management of acute head injury (a surgeon's viewpoint). *EMT J* 2(2):43, 1978.

Cold GE. Does acute hyperventilation provoke cerebral oligaemia in comatose patients after acute head injury? *Acta Neurochir* (Wien) 96:100, 1989.

Jackson FE. The treatment of head injuries. *CIBA Clin Symp* 19:4, 1967.

Javid M. Head injuries. *NEJM* 291:890, 1974.

Jones C, McBride M, Himes L. New protocols for managing the head injured patient. *Emergency* 12(7):53, 1980.

Neifeld GE et al. Cervical injury in head trauma. *J Emerg Med* 6(5):203, 1988.

Saul T, Ducker T. Management of acute head injury. *Emergency* 12(2):59, 1980.

Scali VJ et al. Handling head injuries. *Emergency* 21(11):22, 1989.

Seelig J et al. Traumatic acute subdural hematoma: Major mortality reduction in comatose patients treated within 4 hours. *NEJM* 304:1511, 1981.

Vicario S et al. Emergency presentation of subdural hematoma: A review of 85 cases diagnosed by computerized tomography. *Ann Emerg Med*11:475, 1982.

Weiss MH. Head trauma and spinal cord injuries: Diagnostic and therapeutic criteria. *Crit Care Med* 2:311, 1974.

TRAUMA TO THE FACE, EYES, EARS, NOSE

Chamberlin JG et al. Rationale for treatment and management of avulsed teeth. *J Am Dent Assoc* 10:471, 1980.

Hendler B. The sites and signs of maxillofacial trauma. *Emerg Med* 16(6):23, 1984.

Hoffman J, Neuhaus R, Baylis H. Penetrating orbital trauma. *Am J Emerg Med* 1:22, 1983.

Kalish MA. Airway management in maxillofacial trauma. *Emerg Med Serv* 18(6):42, 1989.

Karesh JW. Ocular and periocular trauma. *Emerg Med Serv* 18(6):46, 1989.

Kirchner JA. Epistaxis. *NEJM* 307:1126, 1982.

Krasner PR. Management of avulsed teeth. *Emerg Med Serv* 18(6):31, 1989.

Kunkel D. Burning issues: Acids and alkalis. Part II. Skin and eye exposures. *Emerg Med* 16(19):165, 1984.

Levitsky L. Ocular examination and contusion injuries. *Emerg Med Serv* 14(1):26, 1985.

Lind G, Spiegel E, Munson E. Treatment of traumatic tooth avulsion. *Anesth Analg* 61:469, 1982.

Manson PN, Kelly KJ. Evaluation and management of the patient with facial trauma. *Emerg Med Serv* 18(6):22, 1989.

Melamed M. A generalist's guide to eye injuries. *Emerg Med* 16(3):99, 1984.

Shingleton BJ. A clearer look at ocular emergencies. *Emerg Med* 21(9):52, 1989.

Shingleton BJ. Opthalmology for the nonophthalmologist. 2. Early management of ocular trauma. *Emerg Med* 19(9):95, 1987.

Thygerson A. Trauma primer: Focus on eye injuries. *Emergency* 13(11):52, 1981.

Wender R et al. Prehospital treatment of dental injuries. *Emerg Med Serv* 8(10):10, 1979.

NECK AND SPINAL INJURY

Anast GT. Fractures and injuries of the cervical spine. *EMT J* 2:36, 1978.

Aprahamian C et al. Experimental cervical spine injury model: Evaluation of airway management and splinting techniques. *Ann Emerg Med* 13:584, 1984.

Aprahamian C et al. Recommended helmet removal techniques in a cervical spine-injured patient. *J Trauma* 24:841, 1984.

Cline JR et al. A comparison of methods of cervical immobilizaiton used in patient extrication and transport. *J Trauma* 25:649, 1985.

Dean D. The child with possible spinal cord injury. *Emerg Med* 14(9):122, 1982.

Graziano AF et al. A radiographic comparison of prehospital cervical immobilization methods. *Ann Emerg Med* 16:1127, 1987.

Herzenberg JE et al. Emergency transport and positioning of young children who have an injury of the cervical spine. *J Bone Joint Surg* 71-A:15, 1989.

Holley J, Jorden R. Airway management in patients with unstable cervical spine fractures. *Ann Emerg Med* 18:1237, 1989.

Howell JM et al. A practical radiographic comparison of short board technique and Kendrick extrication device. *Ann Emerg Med* 18:943, 1989.

Huerta C, Griffith R, Joyce SM. Cervical spine stabilization in pediatric patients: Evaluation of current techniques. *Ann Emerg Med* 16:1121, 1987.

The injured patient's injured neck. *Emerg Med* 16(7):24, 1984.

Little NE. In case of a broken neck. *Emerg Med* 21(9):22, 1989.

McCabe JB, Nolan DJ. Comparison of the effectiveness of different cervical immobilization collars. *Ann Emerg Med* 15:50, 1986.

McGuire RA et al. Spinal instability and the log-rolling maneuver. *J Trauma* 27:525, 1987.

Pal JM et al. Assessing multiple trauma: Is the cervical spine enough? *J Trauma* 28:1282, 1988.

Podolsky S et al. Efficacy of cervical spine immobilization methods. *J Trauma* 23:461, 1983.

Rimel R et al. Prehospital treatment of the patient with spinal cord injury. *EMT J* 3:49, 1979.

Smith M, Bourn S, Larmon B. Ties that bind: Immobilizing the injured spine. *JEMS* 14(4):28, 1989.

Wolf A. Initial management of brain- and spinal-cord injured patients. *Emerg Med Serv* 18(6):35, 1989.

SKILL EVALUATION CHECKLISTS

The following pages contain checklists for some of the skills described in this chapter. The checklists may be used as a guide in practicing the skills involved.

Performance Test
Logroll onto Long Backboard (Conscious Victim)

Students R1: ______________________ Date ______________
R2: ______________________
R3: ______________________
R4: ______________________
R5: ______________________

Instructor: Place an "X" in the Fail column beside any item that is performed incorrectly, out of sequence, or omitted.

Activity	Critical Performance	Fail
Application of cervical traction	R1 approaches victims and instructs him not to move.	
	R1 explains to patient what will be done.	
	R1 grasps either side of the victim's head and holds it steady.	
	R1 keeps head and neck in a straight line with the body.	
Secondary survey	R1 maintains head and neck in a straight line.	
	R2 performs rapid secondary survey, checking: Head: bruises, lacerations, deformity.	
	Ears, nose: drainage.	
	Eyes: pupils.	
	Mandible: stability.	
	Neck: tenderness, deformity.	
	Chest: bruises, fractures, open wounds.	
	Abdomen: bruises, rigidity.	
	Pelvis: tenderness, instability.	
	Extremities: sensation, toe wiggling, hand grip, pulses.	
	R2 applies cervical collar and checks for proper fit.	
Preparation for logroll	R1 maintains head and neck in a straight line.	
	R2 assembles equipment: Long backboard.	
	Blanket roll tied with cravats (or sandbags and tape).	
	Three 9-foot straps.	
	Towels for padding.	
	R3 ties patient's feet together.	
	Rescuers position themselves correctly, on same side of victim: R3 kneeling at victim's shoulders.	
	R4 kneeling at victim's buttocks.	
	R5 kneeling at victim's knees.	

Activity	Critical Performance	Fail
	Rescuers have proper grasp: R2 raises patient's arm above head.	
	R3: one hand on farther shoulder, one hand at beltline.	
	R4: one hand above buttocks, one hand on midthigh.	
	R5: one hand behind knee, one hand behind calf.	
	R2 positions long backboard alongside patient and places towels at neck, small of back, knee, ankle.	
Logroll	R1 gives command (still stabilizing head and neck).	
	Victim is rolled onto his side AS A UNIT, head in alignment.	
	R2 slides board into place.	
	R1 gives command.	
	Victim is lowered onto board as a unit.	
Securing the patient to the backboard	R1 maintains head and neck in a straight line.	
	R5 lifts foot end of board 1 inch off ground.	
	R2 slides three 9-foot straps under board and into position.	
	R5 lowers board back to floor.	
	Straps are secured over chest, thighs, knees.	
	R2 slides flat end of blanket roll beneath victim's head until roll rests firmly against victim's shoulders.	
	R1 adjusts grip so he is holding the victim's head sandwiched within the blanket roll.	
	R2 secures blanket roll to backboard with cravats over patient's forehead and cervical collar.	
	Knots to the side.	
	All straps checked for proper tightness.	

Instructor ______________________________

Performance Test
Straddle-Slide onto Backboard (Conscious Patient)

Students R1: ______________________ Date ______________
R2: ______________________
R3: ______________________
R4: ______________________

Instructor: Place an "X" in the Fail column beside any item that is performed incorrectly, out of sequence, or omitted.

Activity	Critical Performance	Fail
Cervical traction	R1 approaches victim and instructs him not to move.	
	R1 explains procedure to victim.	
	R1 grasps either side of the victim's head and holds it steady.	
	R1 keeps head and neck in a straight line with the body.	
Secondary survey	R1 maintains head and neck in a straight line.	
	R2 performs rapid secondary survey, checking: Head: bruises, lacerations, deformity.	
	Ears, nose: bleeding, drainage.	
	Eyes: pupils.	
	Mandible: stability.	
	Neck: tenderness, deformity.	
	Chest: bruises, fractures, open wounds.	
	Abdomen: bruises, rigidity.	
	Pelvis: tenderness to compression.	
	Extremities: sensation, toe wiggling, hand grip, pulses.	
	R2 applies cervical collar and checks for correct fit.	
Preparation for straddle-slide	R1 maintains head and neck in a straight line.	
	R2 assembles equipment: Long backboard at victim's vertex.	
	Blanket roll tied with cravats (or sandbags and tape).	
	Three 9-foot straps.	
	Towels for padding.	
	R3 ties victim's feet together with a cravat.	
	Rescuers position themselves properly: R2: straddles backboard, behind and facing R1.	
	R3: straddles patient (facing R1), with hands under patient's arms at level of the armpits.	
	R4: Straddles patient (facing R1), with hands under patient's waist.	

Activity	Critical Performance	Fail
Patient is removed from vehicle on long backboard	R1 and R2 on opposite sides of victim; R3 ready with long board.	
	R1 and R2 lift victim (*not* board) 1–2 inches off car seat.	
	R3 slides long backboard beneath victim and supports end of board.	
	R1 and R2 lower victim onto board.	
	R2 ties victim's feet together.	
	R1 pivots victim on board while R2 guides feet.	
	R1 and R2 lower victim so he is supine on long board.	
	R2 loosens torso straps, slowly lowers victim's legs, then retightens straps.	
	Patient is secured to long backboard with straps over chest, thighs, and knees.	
	R1 checks straps for snugness.	
	Backboard is lifted out of vehicle.	

Instructor ____

15. CHEST INJURIES

OBJECTIVES

Within the thoracic cavity, the most important business of the body—the business of breathing and circulating the blood—goes on 24 hours a day. It is in the chest that blood is oxygenated and pumped back out to the waiting tissues. Anything that damages the structures within the chest threatens this operation, and for this reason, injuries to the chest carry a life-threatening potential. Such injuries are relatively common, especially in the eera of the automobile and the handgun, and are responsible for one out of four trauma deaths in the United States. In this chapter, we will look at different types of injuries that can occur when there is trauma to the chest and learn how those injuries should be managed in the field. On completion of the chapter, the reader should be able to

1. Identify the major structures of the chest, given a description of the structures or a diagram of the chest
2. Identify the correct treatment for a sucking chest wound, given a list of treatments
3. Identify the life-threatening complication that can result from treating a sucking chest wound, and indicate how that complication should be managed
4. Identify the correct treatment for an impaled object in the chest, given a list of treatments
5. Identify a patient with (a) simple rib fracture and (b) flail chest, given a description of several patients with various injuries
6. Identify the correct treatment for (a) simple rib fracture and (b) flail chest, given a list of various treatments
7. Indicate the potential danger in using a demand valve to deliver oxygen to a patient who has sustained chest trauma
8. Identify a patient with (a) pulmonary contusion, (b) simple pneumothorax, (c) tension pneumothorax, (d) hemothorax, (e) spontaneous pneumothorax, and (f) traumatic asphyxia, given a description of several patients with various injuries, and list the correct treatment for each of these conditions
9. Identify a patient likely to have suffered a myocardial contusion, given a description of various mechanisms of injury
10. Identify a patient with probable pericardial tamponade, given a description of several patients with various injuries, and indicate the correct treatment for this condition in the field
11. Identify a patient with possible laceration of the great vessels, given a description of several patients, and indicate the correct treatment for this problem in the field
12. Identify those patients who should be transported to the hospital as fast as possible, given a description of various patients with different chest injuries

ANATOMY OF THE CHEST: A REVIEW

Before we look at chest injuries, let us pause a moment to review the structure of the chest wall and the chest contents (Fig. 15-1). Recall that the thorax comprises 12 pairs of ribs that give the chest its structure and protect the vital organs inside. All 12 rib pairs are attached posteriorly to the spine (specifically, to the 12 thoracic vertebrae). In front, the upper 7 rib pairs are attached to the sternum by flexible tissue called cartilage; the next 3 pairs of ribs are attached to cartilage only; while the lowest 2 pairs have no anterior attachment at all and for this reason are called "floating ribs." Note that the first 4 ribs are relatively protected by the shoulder girdle and are thus less likely to be fractured than ribs 5 to 10, which are the most frequently broken as a result of blunt trauma. Another important point regarding the structure of the rib cage itself is that the rib cage tends to become stiffer with age. In a young person, a blunt force applied to the chest is less likely to cause rib fracture than in an older person; but for this very reason, blunt trauma is *more* likely to produce damage to internal organs of the chest, for the pliable rib cage of a young person can more easily be compressed against the lungs or the heart. As a person gets older, calcium collects in the cartilages of the rib cage, stiffening it and making it less and less flexible. In an elderly person, the rib cage is apt to be quite stiff and the ribs themselves very brittle; thus even a small force applied to the thorax of an elderly person (e.g., external cardiac compression) may cause rib fracture or separation of the rib cartilages from the sternum.

Within the rib cage, in the thoracic cavity, we find the heart, the lungs, and the great vessels (aorta and venae cavae). The LUNGS occupy nearly the entire volume of the thoracic cavity. Covering each lung is a smooth, slippery membrane called the **pleura**; a similar membrane lines the inside of the chest cavity. The *potential* space between the two pleural membranes is called the **pleural space**, although normally there is no space there at all and the two pleural surfaces are completely in contact with one another. So long as the lungs and chest wall remain intact, there is negative pressure within the pleural "space." During inhalation, as the diaphragm moves downward and the ribs move upward and outward to expand the volume of the chest, this negative pressure becomes even more negative. The surfaces of the lungs remain in contact with the surface of the inner chest wall, so the net effect is to expand the lungs, thereby creating a negative pressure in the alveoli that "pulls" air into the lungs during inhalation. This system works, however, only so long as both the lungs and chest wall remain intact. If a hole is put in the chest wall or in the lung surface, air is pulled into the pleural space, which then becomes a real space, and effective breathing becomes impossible.

Fig. 15-1. *Anatomy of the rib cage.*

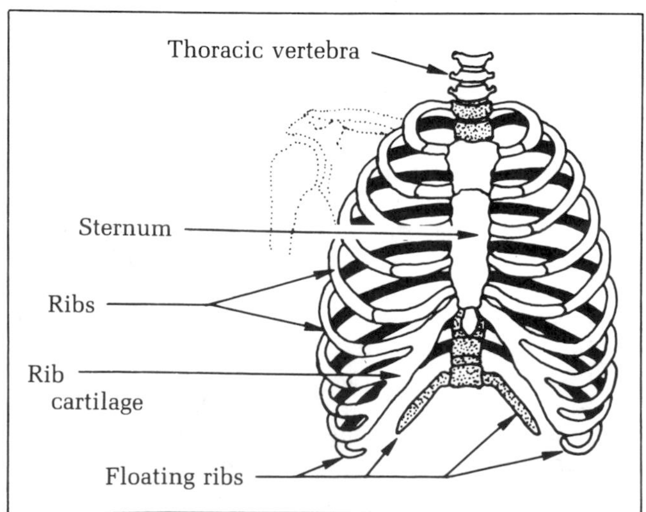

Between the two lungs, in an area called the **mediastinum**, sits the HEART, just behind and partly to the left of the sternum. The heart is enclosed in a tough sac, called the **pericardium** (*peri* = around + *cardium* = heart), that holds the heart in place and gives it some protection. The pericardial sac normally contains between 20 and 60 ml of fluid that lubricates the sac and prevents rubbing as the heart slides against it during each contraction. Because of its position just behind the sternum, the heart is apt to be bruised by blunt impact to the chest, and bleeding from the vessels on the surface of the heart can fill the pericardial sac with blood, thereby preventing the heart from functioning effectively.

The GREAT VESSELS enter and exit the heart within the mediastinum—the venae cavae emptying into the right atrium and the aorta leaving from the left ventricle. These vessels, particularly the aorta, may be subjected to considerable twisting force when there is blunt trauma to the chest, and such force can tear the aorta where it branches into some of its major subdivisions, such as the subclavian or innominate arteries. The venae cavae are subject to another type of problem in chest trauma. Recall that these are relatively thin-walled, low-pressure vessels. If the pressure inside the chest cavity increases—for instance, if the pleural space gets filled with air that cannot get out—the venae cavae can be compressed to the point that they can no longer return blood effectively to the right heart.

One last structure to keep in mind regarding the anatomy of the chest is the ABDOMEN. This may seem paradoxical, but recall that the diaphragm is a dome-shaped muscle that arches up into the chest.

Thus some "abdominal" organs, such as the liver and spleen, are in fact located beneath the ribs and can be injured by trauma to the rib cage. For practical purposes, this means that any injury below the level of the nipples may be an abdominal injury as well as a chest injury.

AN INJURY TO THE CHEST IS AN INJURY TO THE ABDOMEN.

When there is trauma to the chest, the damage may be confined to the chest wall or it may also involve any of the organs within the chest cavity. In the following discussion, we will look first at injuries to the chest wall itself, and then we will consider the types of internal injuries that may accompany chest wall damage.

INJURY TO THE CHEST WALL

As in other parts of the body, injury to the chest wall can be open or closed. Open chest injuries—or penetrating wounds of the chest—are by definition injuries in which the chest wall has been pierced, as for example in injuries caused by a knife, a bullet, or a piece of shrapnel. The chest wall can also be pierced from the *inside,* when the jagged end of a broken rib is driven through the muscle and skin. In closed chest injuries, on the other hand, the skin is not broken, and for this reason the extent of damage within the chest cavity may not be appreciated. Nonetheless, there can be major injury to the lungs, heart, or great vessels in closed chest trauma, and the seriousness of closed injury should not be underestimated. Closed chest injury occurs from blunt impact, such as that suffered when a person is hurled forward against a steering wheel, or from crushing injuries, as might be sustained in a cave-in.

OPEN CHEST INJURIES

Open chest injuries are most commonly caused by knives and bullets, which not only penetrate the chest wall, but also produce varying degrees of damage to the structures within. Indeed, the wound of the chest wall itself may look quite trivial, while within the chest there may be massive damage and profuse bleeding.

When examining the patient who has sustained a penetrating wound of the chest, especially when the injury was caused by a bullet, look carefully for an exit wound (which may or may not be on the chest). If present, the exit wound may give the doctors some information regarding the path taken by the bullet and thus help pinpoint which organs were likely to have suffered damage.

The treatment of open chest injuries follows the usual priorities of ABC. Remember, in any wound of the chest, the main organs of oxygenation and circulation may have been damaged and their effectiveness impaired. Thus in any chest injury, you should ADMINISTER OXYGEN and ANTICIPATE SHOCK.

There are two special circumstances in open injuries of the chest that require particular mention: sucking chest wounds and an impaled object in the chest.

Sucking Chest Wounds

When the chest is penetrated and the hole in the chest wall is larger than the space between the vocal cords, the negative pressure generated during inhalation can cause air to be drawn into the chest through the wound, causing a sucking noise with each inhalation. As the patient exhales, some or all of the air passes back out of the wound. This breach in the chest wall compromises respiration, for so long as the pleural space is open to the air, it cannot develop the negative pressures required to expand the lung. Consequently, the lung on the affected side is not fully inflated during inhalation; to the contrary, the lung on the affected side tends to collapse on inhalation and bulge out on exhalation (Fig. 15-2). Thus there is virtually no air exchange in the affected lung, which soon becomes depleted of oxygen. Furthermore, with each respiration there is progressive collapse of alveoli (**atelectasis**). The net effect is decreased oxygenation of the blood, for red blood cells that are flowing through the affected lung cannot pick up any oxygen during their trip through the pulmonary circuit, and they return to the systemic circulation empty-handed. The result is systemic hypoxia.

The only way to restore the negative pressure within the pleural cavity in this situation is to plug up the hole. In practice, this means sealing the wound with an occlusive dressing. Aluminum foil or household plastic wrap folded several times can be used effectively for this purpose, as can petrolatum gauze. Make sure that the piece of foil, plastic wrap, or gauze is several times larger than the wound, for a small covering is likely to get sucked into the chest with inhalation. Instruct the patient to exhale forcibly, which will cause the lung on the injured side to expand; as the patient reaches the end of that exhalation, cover the sucking chest wound with the occlusive dressing, and tape the dressing to form an airtight seal. The patient should then be positioned on his injured side, to permit the uninjured lung maximal expansion.

There is one significant *danger* in sealing off a

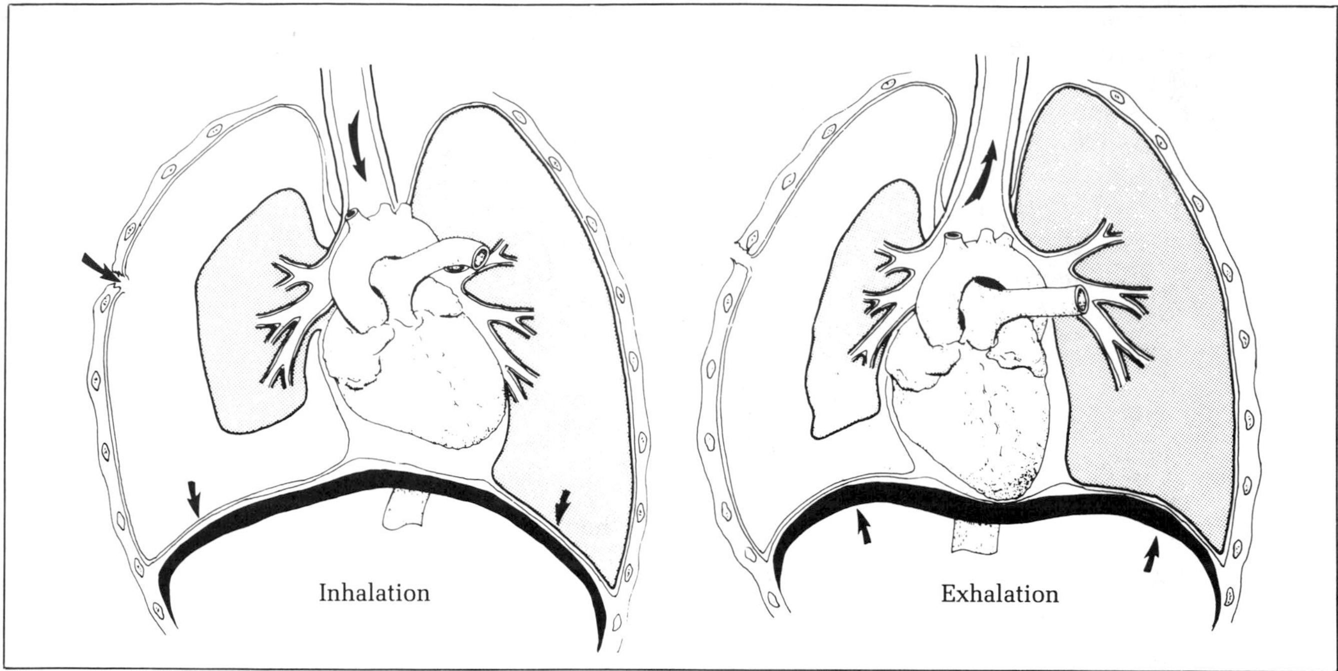

Fig. 15-2. *Sucking chest wound.*

sucking chest wound, and that is the development of what is called a **tension pneumothorax**. If the injury that produced the hole in the chest wall also produced a hole in the lung beneath it, then air entering the lung through the trachea can escape through the hole in the lung into the pleural space. If the wound in the lung is such that it acts as a one-way valve, air will flow into the pleural space during each inhalation, but it will not be able to get back out during exhalation. The result will be a progressive increase in pressure within the pleural space, leading to progressive collapse of the affected lung and compression of the inferior vena cava. If this pressure is not vented quickly, the patient will die.

We will discuss the signs and symptoms of tension pneumothorax in detail later in the chapter. In general, you should suspect a tension pneumothorax if the patient's condition begins to deteriorate any time after you have applied the occlusive dressing. Increasing respiratory distress, falling blood pressure, or distended neck veins (from pressure on the venae cavae) are all clues that tension pneumothorax is occurring. IF THE PATIENT'S CONDITION BEGINS TO DETERIORATE IN ANY WAY, OPEN THE OCCLUSIVE DRESSING. This will enable any air that has built up under pressure in the pleural space to be vented. The wound may then be resealed, but you may have to keep opening the occlusive dressing at intervals until you reach the hospital.

One way to minimize the likelihood of tension pneumothorax developing in such circumstances is to seal the sucking chest wound with a dressing that itself acts as a one-way valve, so that if pressure builds up inside the chest, it can be vented out through the dressing. The simplest way of devising such a vent is to apply the occlusive dressing over the sucking chest wound as described above, but to *tape only three sides closed*, leaving the fourth side untaped. The dressing can then function as a flutter valve: When the patient inhales, the dressing will be pulled tight against the wound, sealing it off so that air cannot enter the thoracic cavity from the outside. But if air enters the pleural space through a tear in the lung, the air can escape through the untaped side of the dressing during exhalation.

Needless to say, any patient who has suffered an injury that compromises the function of an entire lung should be given OXYGEN IN HIGH CONCENTRATIONS, so that red blood cells passing through normally ventilated parts of the lungs can pick up extra oxygen and compensate for their colleagues who return unoxygenated from damaged parts of the lungs. If the patient is breathing spontaneously, do NOT give oxygen under pressure (i.e., do not use the demand valve), for this will only increase the tendency to develop tension pneumothorax. Transport to the hospital should not be delayed.

Sucking Chest Wound: Points to Remember

Definition: A large hole in the chest through which air can be heard being sucked into the chest during inhalation.

Treatment

- Administer OXYGEN (nonrebreathing mask at 10–12 liters/min).
- Seal the wound with an OCCLUSIVE DRESSING applied during forced exhalation.

- If possible, position the patient on his injured side.
- IF THE PATIENT'S CONDITION BEGINS TO DETERIORATE IN ANY WAY, RELEASE THE OCCLUSIVE DRESSING.
- TRANSPORT WITHOUT DELAY to the hospital.

It should be noted that the majority of stab wounds and small caliber gunshot wounds of the chest are NOT sucking chest wounds, for these wounds tend to seal themselves off relatively quickly. In civilian practice, sucking chest wounds are seen chiefly as a result of injury from a high-powered rifle. Blast injuries that propel debris at high velocity can also produce sucking chest wounds.

Impaled Object in the Chest

When there is an impaled object (e.g., a knife or scissors) sticking out of the chest, the usual rule applies: LEAVE IT WHERE IT IS. Removing such an object, particularly if it has a sharp blade, may sever adjacent blood vessels or lung tissue and thereby increase the internal damage. The impaled object should therefore be stabilized in place with bulky dressings built up around it. Secure the dressings with circumferential pressure bandages so that the dressings are pressed down firmly against the chest. In moving the patient, take care that nothing touches or jars the impaled object.

Once again, since there is a likelihood of injury to the underlying lung, the patient with an impaled object in his chest should be given oxygen.

Impaled Object in the Chest

- DO NOT REMOVE THE IMPALED OBJECT!
- Stabilize the object in place with bulky dressings.
- Fasten the dressings with a pressure bandage.
- Administer OXYGEN.
- Transport without delay to the hospital.

CLOSED INJURIES TO THE CHEST WALL

Blunt force applied to the chest wall can cause a variety of chest wall injuries, ranging from mild bruises to multiple fractures with consequent instability of the thoracic cage. The most common source of such injuries is vehicular trauma, but falls from heights, crushing injuries, cave-ins, explosions, and contact sports are all potential causes. The two major categories of chest wall injury likely to result from such accidents are rib fractures and flail chest.

Rib Fractures

Rib fractures are the most common thoracic injury. They are likely to occur when there has been a compression injury or a direct blow to the chest. As noted earlier, the shoulder girdle tends to shield the first four ribs, and for this reason these ribs are rarely fractured, except when the forces involved have been massive. The lowest two ribs are also relatively protected from injury, for as floating ribs they are not anchored in place, and they can "roll with the punch." Thus the most commonly fractured ribs are ribs 5 through 10, anteriorly or laterally.

The most characteristic *symptom* of rib fracture is PAIN localized over the fractured area. Usually the patient will be able to point to the exact site of the fracture, and palpation over this spot will reveal severe tenderness. There may or may not be a bruise over the area. The patient will tend to breathe shallowly and will experience pain on deep breathing, coughing, or any other maneuver that causes motion of the injured rib. For this reason, the patient will usually remain very still and may lean toward the injured side or hold the injured area as a way of splinting it against motion.

Symptoms and Signs of Rib Fracture

- Localized PAIN and TENDERNESS over the fracture.
- Pain aggravated by deep breathing or coughing.
- Patient tries to remain very still.
- Patient leans toward the injured side.
- Patient holds fractured site while breathing.

The principal danger in a simple rib fracture is not from the fracture itself but from the pain it produces. Because of the pain, the patient tends to "splint" the involved side of the chest, and expansion of that side of the chest is limited as a result. This in turn leads to progressive atelectasis (collapse of alveoli), which reduces the efficiency of oxygenation and predisposes the patient to develop pneumonia. Thus the goal of treatment is to encourage the patient to take deep breaths, so that the alveoli can be properly ventilated. However, one must somehow reduce the amount of pain associated with deep inhalation, for the patient is unlikely to comply with a request to breathe deeply if doing so will cause him severe discomfort. In the hospital, pain can be relieved by injecting local anesthesia to block the nerves around the fracture site; in the field, one must rely on somewhat less effective measures.

If the fracture involves only one or two ribs, it should NOT be taped or strapped, for strapping will only cause further limitation of chest expansion. Instead, have the patient hold a pillow against the injured area, and instruct him to take the deepest breaths he can while manually splinting the fracture with firm pressure against the pillow. Explain to the patient the importance of deep breathing in preventing complications such as pneumonia.

If the patient has multiple fractures, manual splinting with a pillow will not be sufficient, and the patient's chest will have to be immobilized. This is best done by using swaths (folded triangular bandages) to strap the patient's arm to his chest, which limits motion on the affected side (Fig. 15-3). The swaths should be secured tightly enough to hold the arm against the unstable part of the chest, but not so tightly that the patient cannot expand his chest on inhalation. If there are fractures on both sides of the chest, both arms may have to be immobilized. Once again, the patient should be encouraged to breathe as deeply as he can manage.

Any patient who has sustained a rib fracture should be assumed to have suffered injury to the underlying lung until proved otherwise. Thus oxygen should be given. In the absence of other injuries, the patient should be transported in a sitting or semisitting position, for breathing is generally easier when sitting up.

Bear in mind that in adults the force required to fracture a rib may be relatively small. In children, however, because of the greater flexibility of their rib cages, a considerably greater force is required to break a rib. Thus a child with a rib fracture is much more likely to have significant damage to underlying structures, and the EMT should be particularly alert for other injuries.

Fig. 15-3. *Sling and swath splint for rib fracture.*

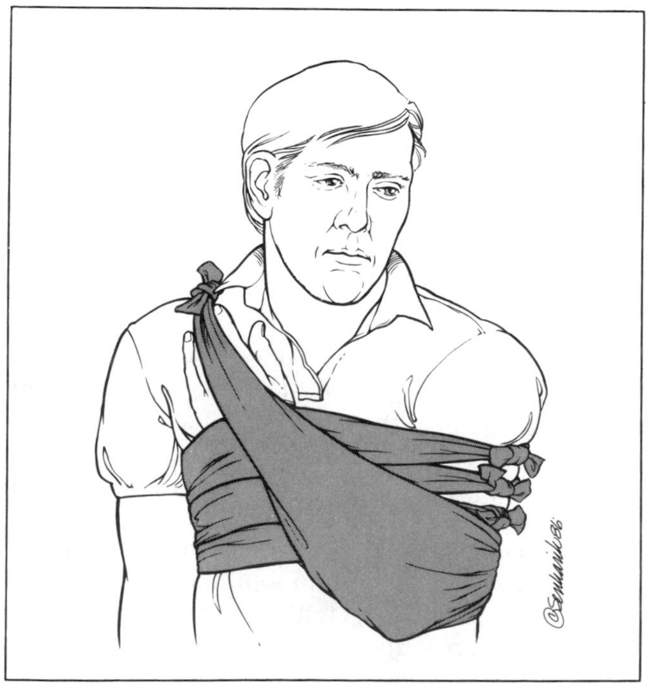

Treatment of Rib Fracture

- For one or two fractures, SPLINT MANUALLY WITH A PILLOW.
- For multiple fractures, SPLINT WITH CROSS-CHEST SWATHS.
- Encourage the patient to take DEEP BREATHS.
- Administer OXYGEN (nasal cannula sufficient).
- Transport the patient in a SITTING POSITION.

Flail Chest

Flail chest occurs when several ribs are broken in several places, so that a portion of the chest wall becomes unstable. When this occurs, the loosened segment of the chest wall no longer moves outward with the rest of the rib cage during inhalation. To the contrary, the "flail segment" is pulled inward by the negative pressure generated during inhalation and protrudes during exhalation—a motion that is called "paradoxical" because it is opposite to the normal motion of the chest wall (Fig. 15-4). Needless to say, as the unstable segment of the chest is flailing in and out, the lung beneath it cannot expand normally and indeed may be further bruised by the motion of the flail segment. Furthermore, the patient will be very reluctant to breathe deeply because of the pain involved, and the shallow breathing will only add to the problem. Thus the flail chest *in itself* will severely compromise respiration. In addition to this, one must keep in mind that any force powerful enough to fracture several ribs in several places has almost certainly produced severe contusion to the lung beneath. Thus oxygenation is further jeopardized by damage to the lung itself. For these reasons, flail chest is a very serious injury and can lead rapidly to life-threatening degrees of hypoxia.

Symptoms and Signs of Flail Chest

- Respiratory distress
- Pain on breathing
- Paradoxical movement of the flail segment
- Possible cyanosis

The treatment of flail chest is aimed at stabilizing the flail segment of the chest wall and providing optimal oxygenation. There are several methods that can be used to stabilize the rib cage, depending on the size and location of the flail segment. When the flail segment is on the anterior chest, a bulky pressure dressing can be taped over it so that the tape is anchored onto the stable parts of the chest. The tape should NOT be circled around the whole chest, however, for this will limit expansion of both lungs.

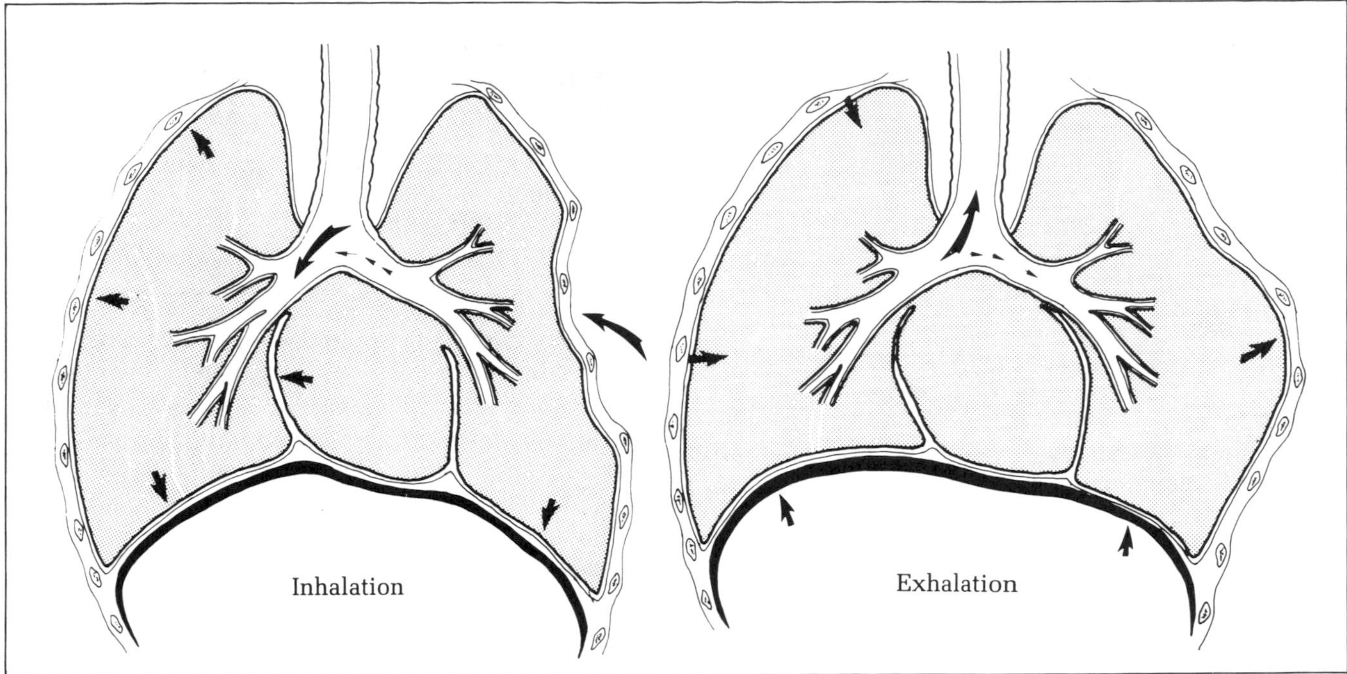

Fig. 15-4. *Flail chest.*

When the flail segment is on the lateral chest, the segment can be stabilized with sandbags piled against it. Alternatively, a pressure dressing can be taped over the flail segment and the patient turned so that he is lying on the affected side. This position splints the flail segment and permits more effective ventilation of the uninjured side of the chest.

Any patient with a flail chest should receive OXYGEN in the highest possible concentration. If the patient appears to be breathing adequately, it is preferable to give oxygen by nonrebreathing mask. If, however, there are signs of inadequate ventilation—such as very shallow respirations, cyanosis, or deterioration of the patient's overall condition—there will be no choice but to assist the patient's ventilations with a demand valve. Use of the demand valve under these circumstances is not without risk, for the oxygen under pressure may rupture damaged lung tissue and thereby cause a pneumothorax. Nonetheless, this risk must be taken if the patient is not capable of ventilating himself adequately, for without oxygen and ventilatory support, such a patient will die.

Transport to the hospital should not be delayed, for definitive treatment of flail chest usually requires endotracheal intubation, placement of chest tubes, and controlled ventilation on a volume respirator—and these measures must be instituted as soon as possible.

Treatment of Flail Chest

- Stabilize the flail segment.
- Administer 100% OXYGEN:
  1. By mask to the patient who is breathing adequately.
  2. By demand valve *only* when breathing is inadequate.
- Transport the patient on the injured side, without delay.

INTERNAL INJURIES TO THE CHEST

Any of the chest wall injuries mentioned above—both open and closed injuries—may be associated with a variety of injuries to the structures within the thoracic cavity. The lungs, the pleural space, the heart, and the great vessels may all be affected in one way or another by trauma that involves strong forces applied to the chest wall.

PULMONARY CONTUSION

Pulmonary contusion is a bruise to the lung tissue that results in edema and hemorrhage within the affected part of the lung. The incidence of pulmonary contusion in patients who have suffered blunt chest trauma has been reported to be as high as 75 percent. The severity of the injury may not be apparent from the outward appearance of the chest, and in a young person with a pliable rib cage, there can be massive contusion to the lungs without even a single broken rib. Pulmonary contusion is a progressive injury; that is, it may produce minimal impairment initially, but as more and more blood and edema fluid collect in the lung, severe respiratory problems gradually develop. This process may take several hours, and thus the patient who says he "feels OK" immediately after sustaining blunt trauma to the chest should nonetheless be evaluated in the hospital—for he may not feel OK at all a few hours later.

Pulmonary contusion should be suspected in every patient who has sustained trauma to the chest. For this reason:

> EVERY PATIENT WHO HAS SUSTAINED AN INJURY TO THE CHEST SHOULD RECEIVE OXYGEN.

SIMPLE PNEUMOTHORAX

Pneumothorax is defined as the presence of air within the pleural space. We have already talked about pneumothorax produced by entry of air through a hole in the chest wall (sucking chest wound). In the *intact* chest (closed injury), pneumothorax can occur when air leaks out of lung tissue that has been lacerated by a fractured rib. A rupture of lung tissue can also occur if the patient's chest was suddenly compressed at a moment when his glottis was closed. Whatever the mechanism that produces the hole in the lung surface, the effect is the same: Air leaks into the pleural space and compresses the lung tissue. In a simple pneumothorax, the hole in the lung then seals itself off, and the degree of respiratory impairment depends upon the amount of air that has meanwhile been trapped in the pleural space. If the volume of air that has gained access to the pleural space is small, there may be few if any symptoms of pneumothorax. If, on the other hand, a large volume of air has entered the pleural space, severe compromise of respiratory function may be evident.

The symptoms and signs of simple pneumothorax can be predicted from the physiology of the injury. To begin with, any time there is some process that interferes with the proper expansion of a lung, the patient is likely to experience DYSPNEA. If there is severe hypoxia from partial or complete collapse of the affected lung, cyanosis may be present, and there is sure to be TACHYCARDIA. Upon head-to-toe examination, you may find that the trachea is slightly deviated *toward* the injured side of the chest, for with each inhalation, the uninjured lung can now expand further in a medial direction, and this will tend to push the trachea into the "empty" side of the thorax. If you tap over the injured side of the chest, it may sound hollow with respect to the normal side, for it is partially filled with air rather than with lung tissue. For the same reason, when you auscultate over the injured side, breath sounds will be much fainter than on the normal side, or they may be absent altogether, because the air exchange in the affected lung is markedly reduced.

> **Symptoms and Signs of Simple Pneumothorax**
> - DYSPNEA
> - TRACHEA may be DEVIATED *toward* the injured side
> - HOLLOW SOUND on percussion over the injured side
> - DIMINISHED BREATH SOUNDS on the injured side

The treatment of simple pneumothorax in the field is to administer OXYGEN in high concentration. Once again, it is preferable to give oxygen by mask to the spontaneously breathing patient, because of the risk of transforming a simple pneumothorax into a tension pneumothorax with use of a demand valve. If, however, the patient's spontaneous respirations are not adequate, a demand valve should be used to assist ventilation, and the patient should be transported without delay to the hospital. Assuming the patient is not in shock, it is preferable that he be transported in a sitting position.

> **Treatment of Simple Pneumothorax**
> - Administer OXYGEN.
> - Assist ventilations if breathing is inadequate.
> - Place patient in sitting position (if not precluded by other injuries).
> - Transport without delay.

TENSION PNEUMOTHORAX

As the name implies, a tension pneumothorax is a pneumothorax in which the air in the pleural space is under pressure, or tension. This situation occurs when the hole in the lung does not seal itself off but rather acts as a *one-way valve* into the pleural space. With each inhalation the patient takes, a little more air is drawn into the pleural space, but the air cannot escape on exhalation (Fig. 15-5). In a very short time, the pressure within the pleural space can build up to the point where the lung on the affected side is entirely collapsed. Furthermore, the heart and the whole mediastinum are pushed over to the uninjured side, thereby restricting the expansion of the normal lung as well. The pressure within the thoracic cavity may indeed be so great as to squeeze the venae cavae shut, preventing them from returning blood to the heart. Because the heart is not filled adequately, the cardiac output drops. The net effect is inadequate ventilation and a kind of cardiogenic shock. If the tension within the pleural cavity is not promptly relieved, the patient will die in a matter of minutes.

The signs of tension pneumothorax follow logi-

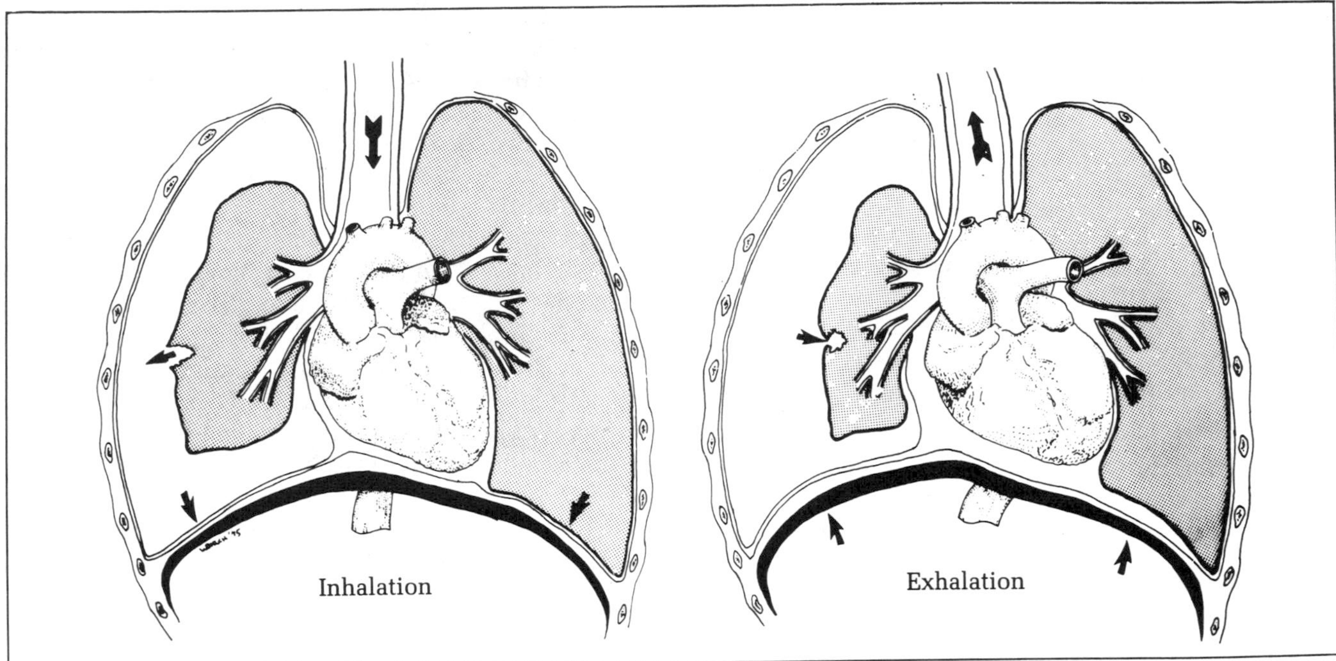

Fig. 15-5. *Tension pneumothorax.*

cally from the mechanisms of the defect. To begin with, the patient can be expected to be in EXTREME RESPIRATORY DISTRESS. As the pressure in the thoracic cavity increases, the patient will find it harder to take a deep breath, and RESPIRATIONS will become SHALLOW AND RAPID. The voice tends to become abnormally high. As hypoxia deepens, CYANOSIS often becomes apparent. The trachea will deviate *away* from the affected side of the chest as the entire mediastinum is shoved toward the uninjured side. Pressure on the venae cavae will result in DISTENTION OF THE JUGULAR VEINS as blood backs up in the venous circuit. Because there is decreased venous return to the heart, the cardiac output falls, reflected in a RAPID, THREADY PULSE and other signs of shock (cold, clammy skin; hypotension). If you tap over the affected side of the chest, it will sound like a hollow drum, for it is filled with air rather than with lung tissue. BREATH SOUNDS will be ABSENT when you listen over the affected side with a stethoscope, for there is no movement of air through the collapsed lung. Often there is also massive SUBCUTANEOUS EMPHYSEMA as air under pressure is forced into the subcutaneous tissues, and this subcutaneous emphysema sometimes extends from the scalp to the toes, giving the patient a grotesque, "bloated-frog" appearance.

Signs of Tension Pneumothorax

- Extreme RESPIRATORY DISTRESS.
- Shallow, rapid respirations.
- High voice.
- Cyanosis.
- Signs of SHOCK: hypotension; tachycardia; cold, clammy skin.
- TRACHEA DEVIATES *away* from the affected side.
- DISTENDED NECK VEINS.
- Chest HOLLOW to percussion on affected side.
- BREATH SOUNDS ABSENT on affected side.
- SUBCUTANEOUS EMPHYSEMA: bloated-frog appearance.

There is only one measure that can save the life of a patient with tension pneumothorax, and that is insertion of a needle or chest tube into the affected side of the chest to vent out the air from the pleural space. TENSION PNEUMOTHORAX IS AN EXTREME EMERGENCY. If the pressure is not vented, the patient will die.

In services where the EMT or EMT-Intermediate is authorized to carry out this procedure, the emergency treatment of tension pneumothorax is to insert a wide-bore (12- or 14-gauge) over-the-needle catheter into the chest cavity between the second and third ribs anteriorly on the affected side. First make a one-way valve by piercing the needle and catheter through a condom. Then insert the catheter through the skin just over the top of the third rib in the midclavicular line. You will know when the needle has entered the pleural space, for air will hiss out through it under pressure. Once the needle has penetrated the pleura, thread the catheter in over the needle, and then withdraw the needle. Tape the catheter securely, and leave it in place until you reach the hospital. Administer oxygen and assist ventilations as needed en route.

If you are not authorized to perform chest decompression, there is no alternative but to get the patient to a medical facility as fast as possible, for death can occur within minutes. Oxygen should be given during transport, but *nothing* should delay moving the patient to the nearest medical facility.

As discussed earlier, when tension pneumothorax occurs in a patient whose sucking chest wound you have sealed with an occlusive dressing, the treatment is simple: Open a corner of the seal immediately, and let the air vent out.

Treatment of Tension Pneumothorax

- If you are authorized to do so, DECOMPRESS THE CHEST with a through-the-needle catheter.
- If you are not, GET THE PATIENT TO A MEDICAL FACILITY AS FAST AS POSSIBLE.
- ADMINISTER 100% OXYGEN by mask en route.

PNEUMOTHORAX WITHOUT TRAUMA

The EMT should be aware of a type of pneumothorax that can occur without injury, called a **spontaneous pneumothorax**. This condition is seen in people who have scattered weak areas in their lung tissue, and occasionally one of these weak areas will rupture by itself, allowing air to leak into the pleural space. The typical patient is a lean, young man, and the pneumothorax typically occurs when the patient is sitting quietly (although it may be precipitated by changes in atmospheric pressure, as in air travel). The patient will usually report that he felt a SUDDEN, SHARP PAIN followed by DIFFICULTY BREATHING. The patient's respiratory distress will be in proportion to the size of the pneumothorax. If the amount of air that has entered the pleural space is small, there may not be any respiratory distress at all; if, on the other hand, a large volume of air leaked into the pleural space before the defect sealed itself off, the patient may be in extreme distress.

The *signs* of spontaneous pneumothorax are the same as for any other simple pneumothorax: respiratory distress, a hollow sound produced by tapping over the affected side of the chest, and decreased or absent breath sounds over the affected lung. The treatment is simply to administer OXYGEN by mask or nasal cannula and transport the patient in a SITTING POSITION to the hospital.

HEMOTHORAX

Hemothorax is the presence of *blood* in the pleural space, and it often accompanies pneumothorax caused by trauma. It may be due to bleeding from vessels in the chest wall, bleeding from vessels in the chest cavity, or less frequently, bleeding from lacerated lung tissue. Bleeding into the pleural space can be massive. Each side of the chest can hold up to 3 liters (about 6 pints) of blood, so a patient can lose half his circulating blood volume into one side of his chest without any bleeding being visible outside the body. The presence of blood in the pleural space has exactly the same effect as the presence of air: It occupies space that should be occupied by the lung and thereby compresses lung tissue—causing atelectasis—and prevents the lung from expanding normally. Like air in the pleural space, blood in the pleural space can also (rarely) push the mediastinum toward the uninjured side and put pressure on the venae cavae thereby decreasing venous return to the heart. Meanwhile, all that blood had to come from somewhere, and the somewhere is the veins or arteries of the vascular system. As far as the cardiovascular system is concerned, massive bleeding into the chest is the same as massive external bleeding: The blood is lost from the circulation, and shock ensues, with all its usual manifestations.

The signs of hemothorax may be very similar to those of tension pneumothorax. There is likely to be RESPIRATORY DISTRESS wtih RAPID, SHALLOW BREATHING. If the amount of blood in the chest is massive enough to push the mediastinum to the opposite side, there will be TRACHEAL DEVIATION *away* from the affected side. The difference between a pneumothorax and a hemothorax may be evident only on tapping over the chest, for a blood-filled chest will sound dull to percussion, while an air-filled chest sounds hollow. That difference may be difficult to appreciate under field conditions, however, and one may only be able to determine that breath sounds are diminished or absent over the affected side. Because of shock, NECK VEINS are likely to be FLAT and the patient may show all the other classic SIGNS OF SHOCK: extreme thirst; restlessness; cold, clammy skin; rapid, thready pulse; and hypotension.

Signs of Hemothorax

- Respiratory distress
- Rapid, shallow breathing
- Possible tracheal deviation *away* from the affected side
- Affected side *dull* to percussion
- Diminished or absent breath sounds on the affected side
- Signs of hemorrhagic shock

The patient with suspected hemothorax should be treated according to his clinical signs. OXYGEN will always be required, in high concentration, and ventilations should be assisted if the patient's breathing is shallow or otherwise inadequate. Associated external bleeding should be promptly controlled. If shock is present, the Military Anti-Shock Trousers may be required. As soon as those basic stabilizing measures have been taken, transport the patient without delay to a medical facility. If authorized to do so, start an IV en route to the hospital and run it wide open.

Treatment of Hemothorax
- Administer OXYGEN.
- Assist ventilations as needed.
- Control external bleeding.
- If shock is present, use the MAST.
- Transport without delay to the hospital.
- Start an IV en route if authorized.

TRAUMATIC ASPHYXIA

Traumatic asphyxia is the name given to a syndrome—that is, a specific collection of symptoms and signs—that is seen in the context of very sudden, severe compression injury to the chest. A classic example is severe steering wheel trauma to the chest. The sudden impact of the wheel against the chest will often cause a CAVED-IN CHEST WALL, with fractures of the ribs and sternum. At the same time, the impact causes an abrupt rise in intrathoracic pressure, which may rupture alveoli in the lung and also force blood out of the right side of the heart up into the veins of the shoulders, neck, and head. The abrupt rise in pressure in the venous system above the chest causes pronounced VENOUS DISTENTION above the shoulders and also causes the EYES to BULGE OUT and look BLOODSHOT. For the same reason, the TONGUE AND LIPS may become SWOLLEN AND CYANOTIC. Stasis of venous blood causes the head, neck, and shoulders to become an alarming shade of blue or purple. RESPIRATORY DISTRESS will be extreme. There may also be hematemesis (vomiting blood) or hemoptysis (coughing up blood), and SIGNS OF SHOCK are almost surely going to be present.

Signs of Traumatic Asphyxia
- CAVED-IN CHEST
- Extreme RESPIRATORY DISTRESS
- VENOUS DISTENTION in the face, neck, and shoulders
- BULGING, BLOODSHOT EYES
- SWOLLEN, CYANOTIC TONGUE and LIPS
- PURPLE FACE, NECK, AND SHOULDERS
- Hematemesis and/or hemoptysis
- Signs of SHOCK

Needless to say, traumatic asphyxia indicates massive injury. The goal of treatment, simply stated, is to try to keep the patient alive long enough to reach the hospital. What this means in practice is moving swiftly to the hospital with strict attention the ABCs en route. Keep the AIRWAY cleared of blood, vomitus, and debris, and administer OXYGEN at high concentration. Controlled or assisted ventilation will probably be required. CONTROL EXTERNAL BLEEDING: Use the MAST garment for shock, if you can apply it en route to the hospital, and start an intravenous infusion with saline if you are authorized to do so. If you have radio contact with the hospital, notify them about the type of case you are bringing in; otherwise have your dispatcher telephone the emergency room, so that the team there can gear up for managing massive trauma.

Treatment of Traumatic Asphyxia
- Ensure an open AIRWAY.
- Assist BREATHING with a demand valve.
- CONTROL external BLEEDING.
- MAST garment for shock, en route.
- Swift transport to the hospital.

INJURIES TO THE HEART

Sitting right behind the sternum, the heart can take a considerable pounding when force is applied to the chest. Penetrating injuries of the chest may also involve the heart, causing lacerations in its surface and sometimes its inner structures as well.

Myocardial Contusion

As the term implies, a myocardial contusion is a bruise of the heart muscle. This kind of injury is usually the result of blunt trauma to the chest, and it does not require much force to bang up the heart. Collisions at speeds as low as 25 miles per hour can produce significant myocardial bruising if the chest is thrown forward against the steering wheel. In such frontal impacts, the diaphragm is forced upward at the same time that the sternum is depressed inward, and the heart gets the squeeze in between. The younger the patient, the more likely that blunt chest trauma has produced myocardial contusion, for as noted earlier, the more flexible rib cage of a young person permits the sternum to be deeply compressed. Myocardial contusion should also be suspected in cases involving blunt trauma to the *abdomen*, for the heart sits on top of the diaphragm only inches away from the abdominal cavity.

A myocardial contusion presents with the SAME SIGNS AND SYMPTOMS AS A MYOCARDIAL INFARCTION ("heart attack")—namely, chest pain, weakness, and diaphoresis (sweating). The chief danger in a myocardial contusion is the development of disturbances in the cardiac rhythm, which are detected by noting an irregular pulse. Rarely, cardiac arrest will occur from ventricular fibrillation, but more commonly the rhythm disturbances are not immediately life-threatening.

The treatment of suspected myocardial contusion requires the administration of OXYGEN, which may in itself prevent the development of serious cardiac rhythm disturbances. The EMT should keep a finger on the patient's pulse throughout transport and make a note of any irregularities in the rhythm. If other injuries do not preclude it, the patient should be transported in a semisitting position, for this position decreases the work the heart has to do in pumping blood.

Treatment of Myocardial Contusion
- Administer OXYGEN (nasal cannula).
- Transport patient in SEMISITTING POSITION.
- Monitor the PULSE throughout transport.

Pericardial Tamponade

Pericardial tamponade is the name given to the condition in which the pericardial sac becomes filled with blood and compresses against the heart. This may occur following severe myocardial contusion, but most commonly pericardial tamponade results from penetrating injuries (e.g., a gunshot or stab wound) that lacerate a coronary artery or one of the cardiac chambers. The result is that blood fills the pericardial sac. The latter is a tough, fibrous bag with very little if any give. As the pericardium fills with blood, it compresses the heart so that the cardiac chambers cannot fill with blood being returned to the heart by the veins. Instead, blood starts to back up in the veins, and they become ENGORGED AND DISTENDED. Meanwhile, with each beat, the heart pumps a smaller and smaller volume of blood, so the pulse grows weaker and weaker. At the same time, the systolic blood pressure begins to fall, and the **pulse pressure** (the difference between the systolic and diastolic pressure) gets narrower and narrower. SHOCK may be present, and it is usually way out of proportion to the amount of blood lost, for it is, in effect, a cardiogenic rather than hemorrhagic shock. If you listen with a stethoscope to the heart of a patient with pericardial tamponade, the HEART SOUNDS will be very soft and DISTANT, for they are muffled by the blood in the pericardial sac.

PERICARDIAL TAMPONADE IS A DIRE EMERGENCY, AND THERE IS NOTHING AN EMT CAN DO FOR THIS CONDITION IN THE FIELD. Emergency treatment requires putting a needle into the pericardium to evacuate the blood, and the patient will die if this treatment is not carried out within several minutes. Therefore, if you suspect pericardial tamponade, GET THE PATIENT TO THE HOSPITAL AS RAPIDLY AS POSSIBLE. Provide 100% oxygen and ventilatory support en route, but DO NOT DELAY AT THE SCENE FOR ANY REASON. Apply the MAST while en route to the hospital and, if authorized to do so, start an IV infusion of normal saline and run it wide open. Radio ahead to the hospital so that the emergency room staff can prepare the necessary equipment.

Signs of Pericardial Tamponade
- Rapid, WEAK PULSE
- DECREASING PULSE PRESSURE
- SHOCK out of proportion to blood loss
- DISTENDED NECK VEINS
- MUFFLED HEART SOUNDS

LACERATION OF THE GREAT VESSELS

The largest blood vessels in the body lie within the thoracic cavity: the aorta, the venae cavae, and the pulmonary veins and arteries. Any of these vessels can be disrupted by trauma, and if one of them is disrupted, exsanguinating hemorrhage into the chest can be rapidly fatal. Usually lacerations of the great vessels occur in association with penetrating injury to the chest, but blunt trauma can also tear a large blood vessel, especially if the injury causes significant torque within the thoracic cavity.

The EMT should suspect laceration of one of the great vessels whenever there is profound shock associated with chest trauma. Once again, the most important aspect of treatment is to MOVE THE PATIENT AS RAPIDLY AS POSSIBLE TO THE HOSPITAL. En route, focus your attention on the ABCs: Keep the AIRWAY open, assist BREATHING with the demand valve, CONTROL external BLEEDING, apply the MAST, and if you are authorized to do so, start at least one intravenous infusion of normal saline, running wide open.

INJURY TO THE BACK OF THE CHEST

Injuries to the back of the chest are of the same general types as those to the anterior chest, although the ribs are more firmly buttressed by powerful muscles in back and thus are less likely to be fractured. The scapula too is buried within a mass of heavy muscle, and if the scapula *is* fractured, this is a signal to the EMT that very strong forces must have been involved in producing the injury.

One of the major concerns in any injury involving the back is the possibility of associated damage to the spine. For this reason, any patient who has sustained significant injury to the back of the chest should be immobilized on a long backboard.

Open injuries or impaled objects involving the back of the chest should be treated just as they are when they occur on the anterior chest.

SUMMARY

In this chapter, we have discussed a variety of injuries to the chest, each of which has its own signs and symptoms. In a multiply injured patient, some of these signs may not be so easy to detect, especially under field conditions. It is MORE IMPORTANT THAT THE EMT RECOGNIZE THAT A SERIOUS CHEST INJURY HAS OCCURRED THAN THAT HE OR SHE MAKE A SPECIFIC DIAGNOSIS. Thus it is a good idea to keep in mind a general list of signs of chest injury and a general plan of action when chest injury is suspected.

Signs of Possible Chest Injury: General

- ANY CHANGE IN THE NORMAL BREATHING PATTERN after injury
- BRUISES over the chest; LACERATION(S) of the chest wall
- TENDERNESS to palpation over the chest
- PAIN on breathing or coughing
- RESPIRATORY DISTRESS
- Diviation of the TRACHEA
- UNEQUAL EXPANSION of the two sides of the chest or PARADOXICAL MOVEMENT of part of the chest wall
- Decreased or ABSENT BREATH SOUNDS on one side of the chest
- MUFFLED HEART SOUNDS
- DISTENDED NECK VEINS
- Hemoptysis
- Cyanosis
- Shock

If any of the above signs is present in a patient who has been subjected to force against the chest, it should be a tip-off to the EMT that significant injury has occurred within the chest and swift treatment must be undertaken.

Treatment of Chest Injuries: General

- Ensure an open AIRWAY.
- Administer 100% OXYGEN.
- Assist breathing *when necessary* with a demand valve.
- CONTROL BLEEDING; treat shock with the MAST applied en route.
- COVER SUCKING CHEST WOUNDS, *but* be alert for developing tension pneumothorax.
- Stabilize flail segments.
- TRANSPORT WITHOUT DELAY to the hospital.

One of the most important lessons of this chapter is one that may sound like heresy:

SOME INJURIES CANNOT BE STABILIZED AT THE SCENE!

Tension pneumothorax, traumatic asphyxia, pericardial tamponade, and laceration of the great vessels are all examples of injuries that require urgent intervention in a medical facility, preferably a trauma center. Trying to "stabilize" a patient with one of those injuries at the scene will only hasten his progress to the most stable condition of all, namely death. Thus the EMT must develop judgment about when it is appropriate to take time at the scene for careful and deliberate treatment, and when to move with all possible speed to the hospital while providing the maximum life support feasible en route. Swift transport to the hospital does not mean panicky transport. It simply means recognizing the urgency of the situation and providing the care you are trained to provide while the driver worries aabout getting you and your patient to the hospital expeditiously.

DON'T DAWDLE WITH SERIOUS TRAUMA!

CASE HISTORY

The patient is a 28-year-old rodeo rider who was kicked in the chest by a steer he was trying to wrestle to the ground. The patient complains of severe pain in the right chest and shortness of breath. He has no significant past medical history.

On physical examination, the patient was restless and in extreme respiratory distress. His skin was cool and dusky. Pulse was 130 and thready, BP 90/60, and respirations 36 and shallow. There was no evidence of injury to the head or neck. The trachea was deviated to the left, and the jugular veins were distended with the patient in a sitting position. There was extreme tenderness over the sixth and seventh ribs on the right side, but no flail chest. Breath sounds were absent on the right. Heart sounds were clear. The abdomen was soft. There was no tenderness over the kidneys. The extremities showed no signs of injury.

The patient was given 100% oxygen by mask. He resisted efforts to place him in a supine position. He was brought rapidly to the hospital for decompression of his right chest.

Questions to think about:

1. What do you think was causing the patient's hypotension?
2. What do the distended jugular veins tell you?
3. What does the absence of breath sounds on the right side of the chest tell you?
4. Why did the EMT making this report mention that the abdomen was soft?

VOCABULARY

atelectasis Collapse of alveoli.
flail chest Condition in which a segment of the chest wall flops inward during inhalation and bulges outward during exhalation, occurring when several ribs are fractured in two or more places.
hematemesis Vomiting blood.
hemoptysis Coughing up blood.
hemothorax The presence of blood in the pleural space.
mediastinum The space within the chest, located between the two lungs, that contains the heart, major blood vessels, trachea, and esophagus.
paradoxical motion Term usually applied to the movement of a flail segment of the chest, which is drawn inward during inhalation and bulges outward during exhalation.
pericardial tamponade Condition in which the pericardial sac becomes filled with blood or fluid to the extent that it compresses the heart and prevents cardiac filling.
pericardium Tough, fibrous sac that surrounds the heart.
pneumothorax The presence of air in the pleural space.
pulse pressure The difference between the systolic and diastolic blood pressures.
simple pneumothorax The presence of a fixed amount of air in the pleural space due to a one-time leak from the lung surface.
spontaneous pneumothorax A pneumothorax occurring without trauma, due to rupture of a congenitally weak area of the lung.
sucking chest wound A large, open wound of the chest wall through which air can be heard to be drawn into the chest during inhalation.
tension pneumothorax A pneumothorax in which air collects in the pleural space under progressively increasing pressure.
traumatic asphyxia Name given to a group of clinical signs associated with severe compression injuries of the chest.

FURTHER READING

Champion HR Trauma score. *Crit Care Med* 9:672, 1981.
Clevenger FW, Yarbrough DR, Reines HD. Resuscitative thoracotomy. The effect of field time on outcome. *J Trauma* 28:441, 1988.
Davis JW et al. Hemodynamic effects of military anti-shock trousers (MAST) in experimental cardiac tamponade. *Ann Emerg Med* 10:185, 1981.
Frame SB, McSwain NE. Chest trauma. *Emergency* 21(7):22, 1989.
Gauthier RK. Thoracic trauma. *Emerg Med Serv* 13(3):28, 1984.
Gervin AS, Fischer RP. The importance of prompt transport in salvage of patients with penetrating heart wounds. *J Trauma* 22:442, 1982.
Ivatury RR et al. Penetrating thoracic injuries: In-field stabilization vs. prompt transport. *J Trauma* 27:1066, 1987.
McGahan JP, Rab GT, Dublin A. Fractures of the scapula. *J Trauma* 20:880, 1980.
Smith MG. Penetrating the complexities of chest trauma. *JEMS* 11(8):50, 1989.
Wilson RF. Averting the worst in chest trauma. *Emerg Med* 14(12):23, 1982.
Woodring JH, Lee C, Jenkins K. Spinal fractures in blunt chest trauma. *J Trauma* 28:789, 1988.

16. INJURIES TO THE ABDOMEN AND GENITOURINARY TRACT

OBJECTIVES

The abdominal cavity contains the major organs of digestion, excretion, and in the female, reproduction. Unlike the chest, it has no bony protection anteriorly, and thus the organs lying within the abdominal cavity are very vulnerable to injury. Either blunt or penetrating trauma can rapidly transform the belly into a reservoir of blood, and fatal shock can occur without a drop of blood ever being spilled outside the abdomen. Because external bleeding may be absent, an examiner who is not alert to the possibility of abdominal injury may miss the signs of intra-abdominal hemorrhage. The purpose of this chapter, then, is to acquaint the EMT with what lies within the abdomen and how the abdominal organs can be damaged by different types of trauma. By the end of this chapter, the reader should be able to

1. Identify the major organs of (a) the abdominal cavity, (b) the pelvic cavity, and (c) the retroperitoneal space, and indicate which are hollow organs and which are solid organs
2. Trace the route food takes through the digestive tract, from the mouth to the anus
3. Identify the functions of the major abdominal organs, given a list of organs and a list of functions
4. Identify the components of the genitourinary system, given a diagram of the system or a description of the components
5. List at least four questions one would like answered in taking the history from a person with possible abdominal injury
6. Indicate the areas of special emphasis in doing the physical examination of a patient with possible abdominal injury
7. Identify the signs and symptoms that should lead one to suspect abdominal injury, given a list of signs and symptoms
8. Identify the correct treatment for (a) closed abdominal injury with shock, (b) an impaled object in the abdomen, and (c) evisceration of abdominal contents, given a list of various treatments
9. Identify injuries likely to be associated with damage to (a) the kidneys and (b) the bladder, given a list of injuries
10. Identify the correct treatment for a patient with (a) suspected kidney injury and (b) suspected bladder injury, given a list of various treatments
11. Identify the correct treatment for (a) blunt trauma to the male genitalia, (b) laceration of the male genitalia, and (c) avulsion or amputation of the male genitalia, given a list of treatments

ANATOMY AND FUNCTION OF THE ABDOMINAL ORGANS

FINDING YOUR WAY AROUND THE ABDOMEN

In this section, we will look first at the location of the major abdominal structures, and then we will review briefly the functions of the digestive and urinary organs in the abdominal cavity.

The abdominal cavity extends from the diaphragm to the groin (on the surface of the body, this means from about the fourth intercostal space, or nipple line, to the groin), and it is lined by a smooth, thin layer of tissue called the **peritoneum.** It is conventional to consider the abdominal cavity in three separate sections: an *abdominal* area, which forms the major part of the cavity; a *pelvic* area, the lowermost portion of the abdomen that is mostly enclosed within the pelvic bones; and a *retroperitoneal* area, the part of the abdomen between the peritoneal lining and the muscles of the back (*retro* = behind + *peritoneum* = the abdominal lining).

In the ABDOMINAL CAVITY proper (Fig. 16-1) are most of the organs of digestion and the spleen. The liver, stomach, and spleen lie tucked up under the ribs and are protected by them. The largest part of the abdominal cavity is occupied by the small intestine and the colon, which comprise about 30 feet of tubing that coils and winds within the space beneath the liver and stomach. Beneath the intestines, in the PELVIC CAVITY, lie the rectum, the urinary bladder, and in the female, the uterus and ovaries. The bladder, in fact, is outside the pelvic cavity, for it lies between the peritoneum and the pubic bone, but it is convenient to regard it as a pelvic organ because it is frequently injured when the pelvis is fractured. The RETROPERITONEAL AREA (Fig. 16-2)—between the peritoneal lining and the back muscles—contains the kidney and their tubes, the ureters; the adrenal glands; the pancreas; and the two major blood vessels of the lower half of the body, the aorta and the inferior vena cava. Nearly all of the organs in the abdomen are loosely suspended from the body walls by a very delicate tissue called **mesentery,** which carries blood vessels and nerves to the internal organs. The mesentery is easily torn, and because it is so richly supplied with blood vessels, it can bleed profusely when lacerated.

Fig. 16-1. *The digestive system—the principal organs of the abdominal cavity.*

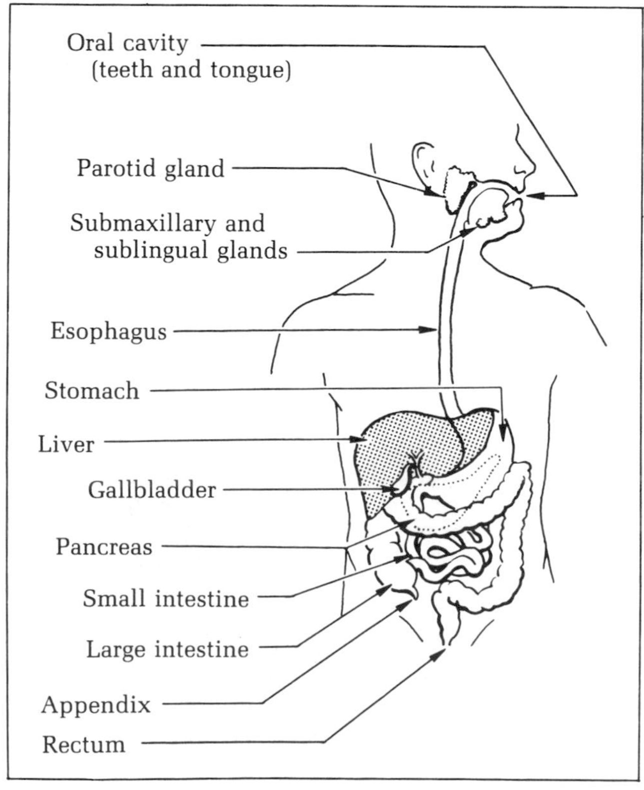

Organs of the Abdominal Cavity

- ABDOMINAL STRUCTURES
  1. Liver and gallbladder (RUQ)
  2. Stomach
  3. Spleen (LUQ)
  4. Small intestine
  5. Large intestine (colon)
- PELVIC STRUCTURES
  1. Rectum
  2. Bladder (in front of the peritoneum)
  3. Uterus and ovaries (in the female)
- RETROPERITONEAL STRUCTURES
  1. Kidney and ureters
  2. Adrenals
  3. Pancreas
  4. Aorta
  5. Inferior vena cava

The abdominal organs are also classified according to whether they are hollow organs or solid organs, for the types of injury are different for each. HOLLOW ORGANS are tubes or sacs through which material is transported. The hollow organs of the digestive tract include the stomach, intestines, and gallbladder, while those in the urinary system are the ureters and bladder. When lacerated, hollow organs spill their contents into the abdominal cavity, which causes an extremely painful inflammation of the peritoneal lining (**peritonitis**). SOLID ORGANS, on the other hand, are firm masses of tissue in which various chemical processes are carried out. The solid organs of the abdomen include the liver, spleen, pancreas, kidneys, and adrenal glands. Solid organs are most susceptible to compression injuries, and they tend to bleed profusely when ruptured or lacerated.

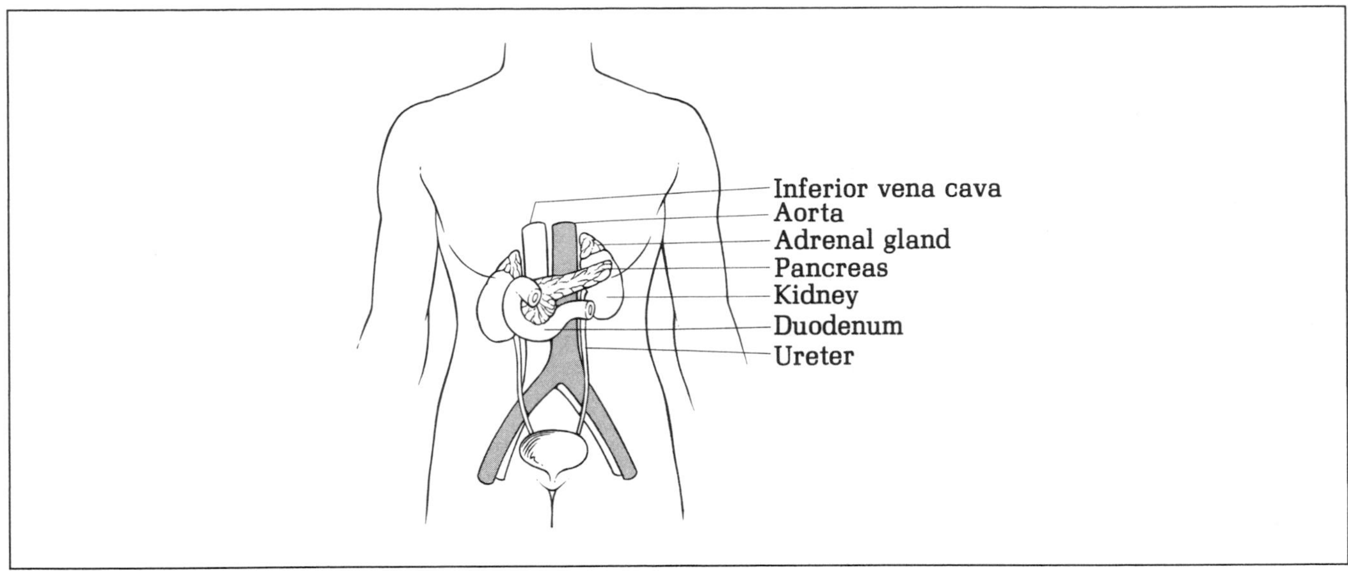

Fig. 16-2. *Contents of the retroperitoneal space.*

Types of Abdominal Organs

Hollow Organs	*Solid Organs*
Stomach	Liver
Small intestine	Spleen
Large intestine	Pancreas
Gallbladder	Kidneys
Ureters	Adrenal glands
Urinary bladder	

THE DIGESTIVE SYSTEM

The job of the digestive system is to take the pizza with double cheese and anchovies that you had for lunch and transform it into basic sugars, fats, and amino acids that the body can use for energy and for various construction projects. This is accomplished by breaking the pizza down into smaller subunits until it is in a form suitable for metabolism. If we follow the pizza on its journey through the body, we can appreciate how this process works.

The MOUTH is the first way station for our pizza. Here the pizza goes through its initial grinding and gets mixed with a fluid produced by the salivary glands. The fluid, saliva, is primarily water, and about 1½ liters of saliva is produced by the salivary glands and emptied into the mouth in a 24-hour period. Saliva serves chiefly to moisten the chewed particles, but it does contain a digestive enzyme, ptyalin, that starts the process of starch breakdown on the pizza dough.

From the mouth, our now chewed-up pizza passes into the PHARYNX, or throat, which, as we learned previously, connects with both the trachea and the esophagus. As swallowing begins, the epiglottis flops over the entrance to the trachea to protect it from aspiration, and the swallowed material is pushed posteriorly into the opening of the ESOPHAGUS. The latter is simply a muscular tube, about 10 inches long, that courses down the back part of the chest, just in front of the spinal column, and connects the pharynx to the stomach. Swallowed materials pass down the esophagus partly by gravity but also by waves of contractions of the esophageal muscles. Thus it is possible to swallow while standing on one's head, although this is not recommended.

Up to this point, the pizza has not yet reached the abdominal cavity. It is only when the bolus of food reaches the STOMACH that it enters the abdomen. The stomach is a J-shaped organ that lies chiefly in the left upper quadrant. In the stomach, our pizza is churned up together with acid and pepsin, a digestive enzyme that begins the breakdown of the cheese and anchovies (proteins). Under normal circumstances, food will be emptied out of the stomach in about 1 to 3 hours, but pain or injury can delay gastric emptying considerably, and for practical purposes it is safest to assume that every injured patient has a full stomach.

When the now emulsified pizza does leave the stomach, it enters the first portion of the SMALL INTESTINE, called the **duodenum.** The duodenum is a tube about a foot long, and it is the most common site for ulcers. As food passes into the duodenum, it is mixed with secretions from the pancreas and liver. The PANCREAS is a flat, solid organ that lies in the retroperitoneal space. It contains two different kinds of glands. One type secretes powerful digestive enzymes that are released into the duodenum to chew up fat, starch, and protein. If the pancreas is torn or otherwise damaged, these enzymes can spill out into the abdominal cavity, where they go to work on the proteins, fats, and starches of body tissues, literally digesting parts of the body itself. The second type of pancreatic gland manufactures the hormone **insulin,** which is released into the bloodstream to regulate the amount of sugar in the blood. When the pancreas fails to produce insulin, a condition called diabetes mellitus occurs (see Chapter 21).

Secretions from the LIVER also enter the duodenum. The liver is a massive solid organ occupying most of the right upper quadrant. It has a number of very important jobs in the body. To begin with, it has a role in digestion, for it produces **bile,** a chemical that is necessary in the absorption of fat. Bile is greenish black in color, and through chemical changes occurring during digestion, it gives the feces their characteristic brown color. The bile produced by the liver is concentrated and stored in a sac called the GALLBLADDER, which discharges the bile into the duodenum when fat is present in the duodenal contents. In some people, stones form in the gallbladder and get stuck in the duct leading to the duodenum, causing a very painful condition called acute cholecystitis. If the duct remains obstructed for any length of time (from a stone or any other cause), the patient becomes jaundiced, that is, his skin takes on a yellow color.

In addition to its digestive functions, the liver is very busy with several other crucial jobs. It produces the proteins necessary for blood clotting, it detoxifies the blood by making chemical changes in poisonous substances that are carried to the liver by the circulation, and it stores sugar so the body can have a source of energy between meals.

The liver is the largest organ in the abdominal cavity, and thus it is the organ most liable to be injured. It is also a very delicate organ, with millions of tiny channels for blood flow, and for this reason, laceration or blunt trauma to the liver can cause massive hemorrhage with rapid death from exsanguination.

We left our pizza in the duodenum, being attacked by digestive enzymes from the pancreas and bile from the liver. The partially digested pizza is now propelled through the second and third segments of the small intestine, the **jejunum** and **ileum** respectively. Together, the jejunum and ileum are about 20 feet long, and within them our pizza goes through the final stages of digestion, being broken down to the most basic chemical building blocks, to be absorbed into the bloodstream. The part that is not absorbed—the waste material—passes on into the LARGE INTESTINE, or **colon,** through a valve between the ileum and proximal colon (the ileocecal valve), which lies in the right lower quadrant. The colon, which is about 5 feet long, sweeps up the right side of the abdomen (ascending colon), crosses the abdomen (transverse colon), and then drops down the left side of the abdomen (descending colon). Stool is formed in the colon and passes out of the body through the rectum and anus. The RECTUM, as noted earlier, is a hollow organ of the pelvic cavity and is designed to store feces until they can be expelled. At its terminal end is the ANAL CANAL.

One pesky little structure in this system of tubing that deserves special mention is the APPENDIX, which is a short, dead-end tube that opens into the cecum in the right lower quadrant. The appendix has no role in digestion. In infancy, it may play a role in the development of normal immunity, but in children and adults it serves no useful function except to provide work for surgeons. When the appendix becomes inflamed (appendicitis), it must be removed surgically or it will rupture and cause the bowel contents to spill into the peritoneum.

The moving force that kept our pizza and later its waste products pushing onward from the throat to the rectum is a process called **peristalsis,** which consists of wavelike contractions of the hollow organs that propel food through the digestive tract. These contractions are reflected in the gurgles and plops, known as "bowel sounds," that one hears when listening over the abdomen with a stethoscope. Bowel sounds are the noises made by gas and liquids being pushed through a hollow tube. When there is injury to the abdomen or severe inflammation of the abdominal cavity, peristalsis often stops altogether, and the belly becomes silent. On the other hand, when there is an obstruction occurring somewhere along the tubing, the body tries to overcome the obstruction by increasing the force of the peristaltic waves in order to ram the obstructed segment open. These forceful contractions produce loud and often high-pitched "tinkling" bowel sounds. In addition, they produce a characteristic, cramping pain called **colic,** which becomes very intense as the bowel contracts and then decreases or disappears as the bowel relaxes. Colicky pain is almost always a sign of obstruction of a hollow tube—be it the intestine or a ureter.

THE SPLEEN

Sitting together with all the digestive organs in the abdomen is the spleen, which is tucked up under the left ribs just below the diaphragm. The spleen is not a digestive organ, and it is not vital for life. Its major function—clearing the circulation of tired, old red blood cells and producing new ones—can be taken over by the liver and bone marrow if the spleen is removed. Like the liver, the spleen is filled with thousands of small channels for blood flow and is very fragile, thus easily injured. Rupture of the spleen is often caused by trauma to the lower left ribs, and when the spleen does rupture, fatal exsanguination into the abdomen can occur very rapidly.

THE GENITOURINARY SYSTEM

Sharing the abdomen with the digestive organs and the spleen are the organs of urine formation and, in the female, the organs of reproduction. The female reproductive system will be described in detail in Chapter 32, and we will deal here only with the urinary system and the male reproductive system.

The urinary system (Fig. 16-3) controls the discharge of waste materials filtered from the blood, and the work of filtration goes on in the KIDNEYS. These are paired organs that sit in the retroperitoneal space, on either side of the spine, just below the diaphragm. The kidneys are vital to survival, for they clear the blood of potentially harmful waste materials and also control the concentrations of various chemical elements (e.g., sodium and potassium) in the body fluids. If something happens to the kidneys so that they can no longer carry out their tasks, waste materials accumulate in the blood, the balance of body chemicals gets out of whack, and death will follow in days to weeks unless an artificial means of filtering the blood is instituted.

When functioning properly, the kidneys must constantly monitor the composition of blood flowing through them. This is an enormous job, for in the course of 24 hours, about 1,500 liters of blood circulates through the kidneys, where water and waste materials are continuously filtered out to form urine. Like other highly vascular organs, the kidneys can bleed heavily when injured, and if disrupted they can also leak urine into the surrounding tissues. Normally, however, urine passes out of each kidney into a small (one-quarter inch wide) tube called a URETER, which connects the kidney to the bladder. Peristalsis of the walls of the ureter propels urine down into the bladder. When a ureter becomes obstructed by a stone, peristalsis can become very intense, producing the excruciating pain of renal colic.

From the ureters, urine passes into the BLADDER, which is tucked just behind the pubic bone of the pelvis. There urine is stored until the bladder becomes relatively full, at which point sensory nerves notify the brain that it is time to empty the bladder. The brain considers this information together with all sorts of other data on the subject (for instance, is there a rest room nearby?), and when the brain decides it is indeed time to urinate, it sends a message back down to the bladder instructing the bladder to relax its sphincter. As the bladder does so, urine is released through a short passage called the URETHRA. In the male, the urethra passes from the base of the bladder through the penis, while in the female it opens at the front of the vagina.

The MALE REPRODUCTIVE SYSTEM (Fig. 16-4) consists of sexual glands, connecting ducts, and the external genitalia. The main sexual glands are called the **testicles,** or **testes,** which lie in a sac, the scrotum, outside the pelvic cavity. The testes produce male hormones, seminal fluid, and sperm. The hormones are absorbed into the bloodstream, while the sperm and seminal fluid (semen) are carried from the testes to a storage area called the **seminal vesicle** through the seminal duct (**vas deferens**). When sex-

Fig. 16-3. *The urinary system.*

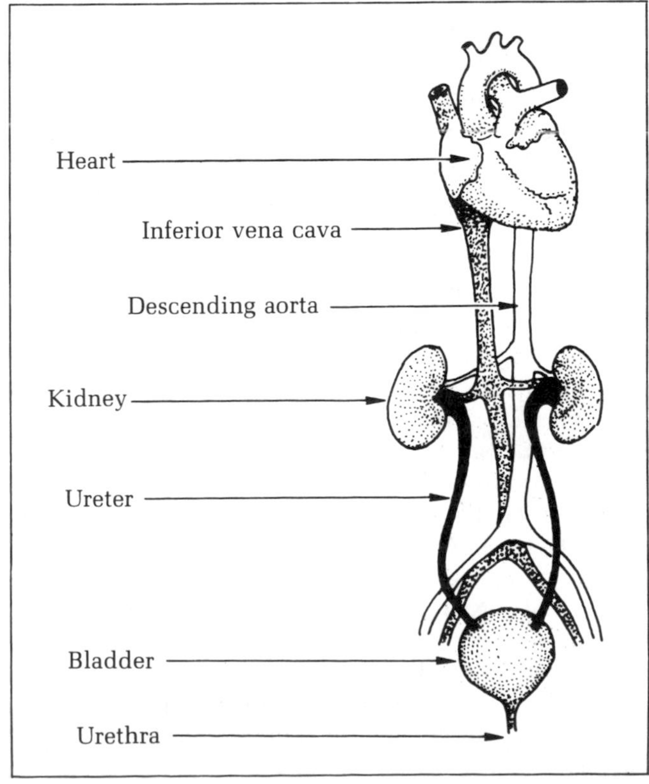

Fig. 16-4. *The male reproductive system.*

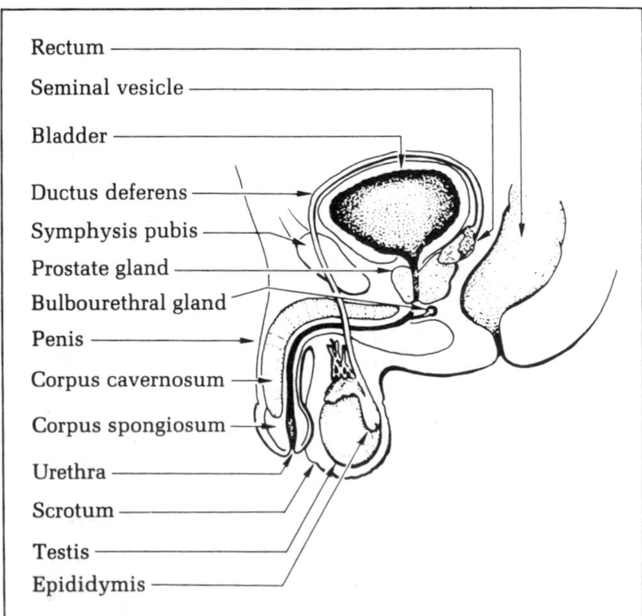

ual arousal occurs, the sperm cells and seminal fluid are released from the seminal vesicle and pass into the urethra, where they are mixed with fluids produced by an accessory gland, the **prostate.** The prostate surrounds the urethra at the point of emergence from the bladder. In later life, the prostate usually enlarges, and as it does so, it may compress and narrow the urethral opening, thereby interfering with urine flow. A man with an enlarged prostate will thus begin to notice difficulty in voiding or a decrease in the force and caliber of his urinary stream, which is gradually reduced to a trickle. Surgery is usually required in such cases to remove the prostate gland.

Having reached the urethra, the semen is then ejaculated out through the penile urethra. The penis serves two functions for the male: during urination it carries urine away from the bladder, and during intercourse it conveys sperm from the seminal vesicle to the vaginal tract of a female. A special mechanism of the nervous system keeps these two functions entirely separate and prevents the passage of urine into the urethra during sexual intercourse, so that only seminal fluid, prostatic fluid, and sperm can pass from the penis into the vagina with ejaculation.

The penis is constructed from a special type of tissue, called erectile tissue, that permits it to become rigid during sexual arousal. Erectile tissue is composed chiefly of channels for blood flow. Normally, these channels remain collapsed, but during sexual stimulation they become engorged with blood, causing the penis to stiffen and enlarge. Recall, however, that the same sequence of events can also occur as the result of spinal injury, which may produce a prolonged and painful erection of the penis called priapism.

ASSESSMENT OF THE PATIENT WITH ABDOMINAL INJURY

As noted earlier, abdominal injuries often are not obvious, and the only way some abdominal injuries can be detected is through a rapid but careful history and physical assessment of the patient. One of the most important elements of the HISTORY is a search for the MECHANISMS OF INJURY, for information of this type is otherwise unavailable to emergency room personnel. The EMT must therefore serve as the eyes and ears of the doctor in the prehospital setting, to collect data that may provide clues regarding what if any organs in the abdominal cavity were injured. If the patient was involved in an automobile accident, find out whether the patient was wearing a SEAT BELT. If so, what kind? Lap seat belts can produce a characteristic injury from abrupt compression of the abdominal cavity during sudden deceleration, and the result is sometimes a laceration of the small intestine or rupture of the diaphragm. When a shoulder harness is worn in conjunction with a lap seat belt, the incidence of this type of injury is reduced, although rib fractures and other injuries to the thorax can occur. Also, check the car for a bent steering column, a smashed front end, or other clues to the type and direction of the forces involved.

When there is an open injury to the abdomen, find out what agent caused the injury. If it was a knife, how long was the blade? What was the angle of thrust? A "pro" will wield a knife underhand and thrust upward into the abdomen, whereas an inexperienced assailant tends to thrust downward with an overhand motion and usually does considerably less damage. If the weapon was a gun, what was the caliber? At what range was the victim shot?

Do not forget to ascertain the patient's CHIEF COMPLAINT, even if it may seem obvious, for the chief complaint may also help reveal unsuspected abdominal injury. If there is PAIN, what is it like? Steady? Colicky? Does it stay in one place, or does it radiate? Blood and especially spilled digestive juices in the abdominal cavity can produce inflammation of the peritoneum, which causes the patient severe, diffuse pain that is made worse by any abrupt movement, even a cough. Pain that radiates into the left shoulder (Kehr's sign) usually indicates blood beneath the left diaphragm, as seen in a patient with a ruptured spleen.

Find out whether the patient has VOMITED. If so, was there blood in the vomitus? When did the patient last eat? When did he last urinate? A full stomach or a full bladder is much more easily ruptured than an empty one.

If the patient sustained blunt trauma, ask whether he had any time to prepare himself for the blow. If a person has time to tense the muscles of his abdomen, he can protect his abdominal organs significantly. Indeed, the famous escape artist Houdini used to challenge the strongest person in the audience to strike him as hard as possible in the abdomen, and for years no one succeeded in causing Houdini any injury, for his tensed muscles repelled the blows. Legend has it, however, that once when Houdini was demonstrating the trick to a medical student, the student struck him before he had completely prepared his abdominal muscles to receive the blow, and Houdini died a few days later, presumably of injuries to his bowel.

In conducting the PHYSICAL ASSESSMENT, note the POSITION in which the patient is found and his degree of distress. A patient with peritoneal irritation, as from spilled digestive juices, will lie very, very still, often with his legs flexed, for the slightest movement will cause him severe pain. If the patient is restless, you must suspect hypoxia or shock or both. Take and record the VITAL SIGNS. A rapid pulse may be one of the earliest signs of shock, and it may be the *only* sign that a patient is bleeding into the abdomen. The pulse, blood pressure, and respirations should be measured early and remeasured periodically thereafter, with an accurate record kept of each reading and the time it was made.

Conduct the HEAD-TO-TOE SURVEY as usual. Pay particular attention to the chest, for any bruise or other injury below the nipples can be considered to involve the abdomen as well (Fig. 16-5). To examine the ABDOMEN itself, you should have the patient lying supine, with the hips and knees flexed to relax the abdominal muscles. The abdomen should be bared, for it is impossible to evaluate any region of the body for injury if the area is clothed. Start with inspection, and LOOK at the abdomen for bruises, distention, or open injuries. Tires, steering wheels, seat belts, armrests, and the like may leave telltale marks on the skin that provide clues to the mechanisms of injury. If there is a penetrating wound from a bullet, look for the exit wound. Other open injuries, such as impaled objects or evisceration of abdominal organs, should be readily evident if present. Next, if conditions permit, LISTEN to the abdomen by letting the diaphragm of your stethoscope rest lightly on the abdominal wall. Listen for a full minute, and make a record of whether bowel sounds are present or absent. When bowel sounds are present immediately after an injury and disappear later, the surgeons have cause for concern, and it is important to document that information when the patient is first examined. Finally, FEEL the abdomen to note tenderness or rigidity. Palpation should be very gentle. If the patient is conscious, ask him to indicate whether it hurts when you push over any given area. Note whether the abdominal wall feels stiff or "boardlike." A rigid abdomen suggests spilled digestive juices or sometimes blood in the peritoneal cavity.

Assessment of the Patient with Possible Abdominal Injury

- HISTORY:
  1. Mechanisms of injury.
  2. Chief complaint.
  3. Associated nausea, vomiting, or hematemesis.
  4. Time to tense the abdominal muscles?
- PHYSICAL ASSESSMENT:
  1. Position of patient.
  2. Signs of shock: Restlessness; cold, clammy skin.
  3. Vital signs, measured and recorded frequently.
  4. Head-to-toe survey, with attention to:
     a. Obvious chest injuries.
     b. Abdomen: bruises or open injuries; bowel sounds; tenderness or rigidity.

It should be emphasized that in severely injured patients, the history and physical assessment must often be carried out simultaneously with initial treatment (e.g., oxygen administration), which in turn may have to be undertaken while en route to the hospital. Like severe chest injuries, severe abdominal injuries sometimes cannot be stabilized in the field, and the patient must be moved with all deliberate speed to the hospital, with life support measures—the ABCs—performed en route.

INJURIES TO THE ABDOMEN

Like injuries elsewhere in the body, abdominal injuries can be open or closed. Open or penetrating injuries are those in which the abdominal wall has been pierced by a foreign object, which may or may not have penetrated all the way into the abdominal cavity. Closed injuries are those in which the abdomen is damaged by a strong blow, such as impact against a steering wheel or a kick in the belly. With either open or closed injuries, both hollow and solid organs may be injured.

In the following discussions, we will look at some specific injuries to the abdomen and the special aspects of their treatment. It is assumed that first priority will be given, as always, to the ABCs.

PENETRATING ABDOMINAL INJURIES

In contemporary American society, the vast majority of penetrating injuries to the abdomen are produced by bullets and knives. In both gunshot wounds and stab wounds, it may be difficult to determine whether the object has penetrated into the abdominal cavity. When a bullet is the agent of injury, the EMT should search for an exit wound, which is usually reliable evidence of abdominal penetration. Stab wounds are usually single and most commonly are inflicted above the umbilicus. About one-third of abdominal stab wounds do not pierce the peritoneal lining, but it is safest to assume that an open injury of the abdominal wall has penetrated into the abdominal cavity.

While penetrating injuries can damage any abdominal organ, it is usually the hollow organs that are lacerated. When this happens, digestive juices spill into the peritoneal cavity, causing inflammation and severe pain. Laceration of solid organs or major blood vessels, on the other hand, will result in massive hemorrhage and signs of shock.

The general treatment of open abdominal injuries requires primary attention to the ABCs. If there are signs of shock, the Military Anti-Shock Trousers should be applied, and when the EMT is authorized to do so, at least one large-bore IV line should be started with saline or Ringer's solution.

Two special cases need particular mention: an impaled object in the abdomen and evisceration of abdominal contents.

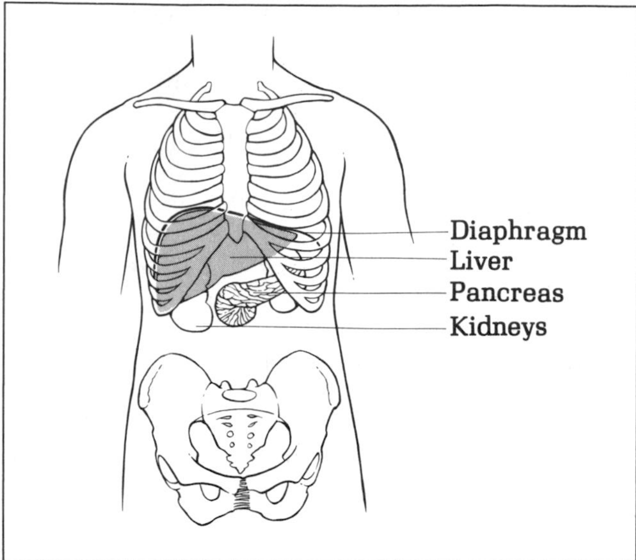

Fig. 16-5. *Intrathoracic abdomen. Some major abdominal organs actually lie beneath the ribs and can be injured if the chest is injured.*

Impaled Object in the Abdomen

If an object such as a knife or ice pick is impaled in the abdominal wall, the usual rule applies: DO NOT TRY TO REMOVE IT. Stabilize the object in place with bulky dressings, and fix the dressings to the abdominal wall with pressure bandages to help control any bleeding around the impaled object. Keep the patient still, and transport him rapidly (but gently!) to the hospital.

Evisceration of Abdominal Contents

A severe laceration of the abdominal wall may produce an evisceration, that is, a protrusion of abdominal organs such as the intestines out of the abdominal cavity. If you see such an injury, the important rule to remember is

DO NOT ATTEMPT TO REPLACE EVISCERATED ABDOMINAL ORGANS BACK INTO THE ABDOMINAL CAVITY.

Cut away any clothing that is in the wound area, and cover the protruding organs either with sterile aluminum foil or with a universal dressing that has been soaked in sterile saline. Do not use dry dressings in direct contact with the protruding viscera, for dry dressings will stick and may be difficult to remove later. Cover the foil or universal dressing with a clean towel or sheet or several additional layers of universal dressings, to help minimize heat loss from the wound.

BLUNT INJURIES TO THE ABDOMEN

Blunt abdominal injuries may have few outward signs, and the EMT must suspect such injuries on the basis of the mechanisms of injury and the patient's overall clinical condition. A person who has been kicked in the abdomen and who is showing signs of shock, for example, should be assumed to have sustained major abdominal damage even if he has no bruises or other outward evidence of abdominal injury. IF YOU DO NOT SUSPECT ABDOMINAL INJURY, YOU WILL NOT FIND IT. BE ALERT.

The treatment for blunt injuries to the abdomen is based on the patient's clinical condition. As always, the AIRWAY must be assured. This means in particular to ANTICIPATE VOMITING and keep the patient's head turned to the side. Give NOTHING BY MOUTH, for eating or drinking will only increase the likelihood of vomiting (and increase the volume of the stomach contents). Administer OXYGEN, and assist breathing as needed. Control any external bleeding. ANTICIPATE SHOCK, and if authorized to do so, get an intravenous infusion started *before* shock occurs. If shock is already present, use the Military Anti-Shock Trousers (leg segments only in the case of an evisceration). Cover open wounds, splint obvious fractures, and move without delay to the hospital.

General Principles of Treating Abdominal Injuries

1. Ensure an open AIRWAY.
   a. Anticipate vomiting.
   b. Give NOTHING BY MOUTH.
2. Administer OXYGEN; assist ventilations as needed.
3. CONTROL EXTERNAL BLEEDING.
4. ANTICIPATE SHOCK: Start at least one intravenous infusion *before* shock develops.
5. If shock is present, use the MAST.
6. Treat the abdominal injury:
   a. Cover open wounds.
   b. DO NOT REMOVE IMPALED OBJECTS.
   c. DO NOT REPLACE EVISCERATED ORGANS.
7. Splint associated fractures.
8. Transport without delay.

INJURIES TO THE GENITOURINARY SYSTEM

INJURIES TO THE KIDNEYS

The kidneys are relatively well protected from injury by the ribs and the heavy muscles of the back, and thus a force powerful enough to damage the kidneys will usually produce other injuries as well, such as fractured ribs or damage to other abdominal organs.

In obtaining the *history* from the patient, once again it will be important to determine the MECHANISMS OF INJURY. A blow to the flank or lower rib cage in the back should lead the EMT to suspect kidney damage. If the patient has urinated since the injury, ask him if he noticed any blood in his urine (**hematuria**). If he has to void while under your care, collect the urine specimen in a container to bring with the patient to the hospital, where the urine can be examined under a microscope for the presence of red blood cells.

In the *physical assessment,* look especially for bruises over the flanks or lower rib cage in back. Penetrating wounds of the lower rib cage, fractures of the lower ribs, or tenderness over the lower thoracic or upper lumbar vertebrae should also arouse suspicion of associated injury to the kidney.

The treatment of suspected kidney injury is based on the patient's clinical signs. Tenderness over the vertebrae requires that the patient be immobilized on a long backboard. Signs of shock demand oxygen, the MAST garment, an IV line, and swift transport to the hospital.

INJURIES TO THE URINARY BLADDER

The urinary bladder, as we learned earlier, sits outside the peritoneum, behind the pubic bone. Because of its location, the bladder is apt to be ruptured or perforated when there is fracture of the pelvis. Blunt injuries to the lower abdomen can also rupture the bladder, especially when it is distended with urine. One of the classic bladder injuries occurs when someone who has been drinking (and thus has a full bladder) is involved in an automobile accident in which sudden deceleration forces literally shear the bladder off at the urethra—another good reason not to drink before you drive. Penetrating injuries to the lower abdomen can also involve the bladder; once again, this is more likely when the bladder is full. In any of these injuries, the net result is that urine is spilled out of the bladder into the surrounding tissues.

The patient with suspected bladder injury should be kept very still. The nature of associated injuries will dictate the treatment given in the field. As always, priority goes to the ABCs. If there is associated pelvic fracture, it should be stabilized with the MAST, which not only provides an excellent pelvic splint, but also helps counter the massive internal hemorrhage that often occurs in the wake of a fractured pelvis.

INJURIES TO THE MALE GENITALIA

Injuries to the male genitalia are rarely life-threatening, but they can be extremely painful, and they are invariably of extreme concern to the patient. These injuries run the entire gamut from abrasions and contusions to lacerations and avulsions, and they may involve the penis or the scrotum or both. Treatment of such injuries requires a calm, professional manner on the part of the EMT, who should also ensure that the patient is properly shielded from the stares of curious onlookers.

Injuries to the Penis and Urethra

BLUNT TRAUMA to an erect penis, as may occur in very active sexual intercourse, can produce a so-called "fracture" of the penis. In fact, this is not a fracture—since there is no bone structure in the penis—but rather an angulation of the penis caused by laceration of the supporting tissue of the organ. It is inevitably associated with severe pain, and the patient will almost certainly be in a state of panic as well. The injured area will show ecchymoses. The field treatment consists of calming the patient and applying cold packs or iced compresses to the injured area to control swelling and alleviate pain. Surgery may be required to repair an injury of this sort, so the patient must be evaluated in the hospital.

LACERATION of the *frenulum* of the penis (the skin below the head of the penis) is another injury that usually occurs when the penis is erect. Bleeding may be very profuse, and it should be controlled quickly by direct pressure on the bleeding area. Lacerations of the *urethra* can occur from pelvic trauma, penetrating wounds of the perineum, or straddle injuries, and they are also often associated with considerable bleeding from the urethral opening. Pressure on the penis to compress the urethra closed will usually control hemorrhage of this type.

A relatively common injury to the penis, particularly in children, is caused when the foreskin becomes caught in the zipper of the victim's trousers. If only one or two teeth of the zipper are involved, you should attempt gently to work the zipper open. If a longer segment of the zipper has entrapped the skin or if the patient is very agitated (as is often the case with children), cut the whole zipper out of the trousers to facilitate transport, and bring the patient and his zipper, suitably draped, to the emergency room. Bleeding from associated tears in the foreskin is usually easily controlled with direct pressure on the wound.

AVULSION of part of the skin of the penis is usually the result of an industrial or farm accident, and is more apt to occur in an uncircumcised individual, when the foreskin becomes entrapped, together with the surrounding clothing, in a piece of machinery. In such cases, the surrounding clothing should be cut away carefully and the denuded area of the penis should be wrapped in a sterile dressing that has been moistened with sterile saline. If at all possible, the avulsed skin should be salvaged and brought to the emergency room in a sterile gauze pad that has also been thoroughly moistened with cold sterile saline.

Probably the most severe injury to the penis is partial or complete AMPUTATION of the penile shaft, which may be the result of an industrial accident or, occasionally, may be self-inflicted by a mentally disturbed person. The most immediate concern in such an injury is to get control of external bleeding, which may be very heavy. Use a moistened dressing to apply firm pressure against the bleeding site as an initial measure. If this is unsuccessful, a tourniquet should be applied around the remaining shaft and tightened just to the point where bleeding can be controlled with direct pressure. If there is a complete amputation, the amputated part should be located and wrapped in a moist, sterile dressing to be brought to the hospital with the patient; the surgeons may be able to make use of the amputated part to reconstruct the penis.

A FOREIGN BODY LODGED IN THE URETHRA should be left in place, just as any other "impaled object."

Injuries to the Scrotum and Testes

Injuries to the scrotum and testes usually produce severe pain and sometimes associated symptoms, such as nausea and vomiting, as well. However, such injuries are almost never life-threatening, and in a multiply injured patient, these injuries should not distract the EMT from the fundamental priorities of care.

BLUNT TRAUMA to the testes can produce considerable internal bleeding within the scrotal sac or even rupture the testes themselves. The injury will be obvious from the patient's extreme pain and the swelling and ecchymosis of the scrotum. Treatment in the field consists of applying a cold pack to the injured area and transporting the patient in a position of comfort to the hospital.

AVULSION of the scrotal skin is most commonly the result of industrial or farm accidents, and the usual principles for care of an avulsion apply. Cover the denuded area with moist, sterile dressings, and preserve the avulsed skin in a sterile pad that has been soaked in cold sterile saline. Bleeding from the injured area should be controlled with direct pressure over the dressing.

If there is an IMPALED OBJECT in the scrotum, leave it alone. Stabilize it in place as best you can, and keep the patient still en route to the hospital.

Injuries to the Male Genitalia: Points to Remember

- These injuries are EXTREMELY PAINFUL, but RARELY LIFE-THREATENING. Remember the priorities of ABC.
- Use MOIST, STERILE DRESSINGS to control bleeding and cover denuded areas.
- PRESERVE AMPUTATED PARTS in sterile dressings soaked with cold sterile saline.
- Use COLD PACKS to relieve pain and minimize swelling.
- DO NOT REMOVE IMPALED OBJECTS.

CASE HISTORY

As usual, we will conclude this chapter with a sample case presentation illustrating some of the significant points in the chapter as well as the method of reporting medical information.

The patient is a 34-year-old man who was injured when the car he was driving left the road and struck a utility pole. The patient climbed from the car after the accident and crawled a few feet. He says he did not lose consciousness. He complains of severe, steady abdominal pain that is made worse every time he coughs or moves. He denies vomiting. He states that he "had a few beers" about 20 minutes before the accident, but he denies the use of any medications. He has no significant past medical history and no known allergies.

On physical examination the patient was conscious and alert, lying very still, supine, with his legs drawn up. He winced every time he moved. His skin was cool and clammy. Pulse was 128 and weak, BP 110/70, and respirations 20 and shallow. There was no evidence of injury to the head or neck. The trachea was midline, and the neck veins were not distended. There were no bruises on the chest, and the chest wall was stable. Breath sounds were equal bilaterally. Heart sounds were clear. The abdomen showed a linear ecchymosis about the width of a seat belt, just above the umbilicus. There were no open wounds. Bowel sounds were not heard. The abdomen was boardlike to palpation and extremely tender in all quadrants. The extremities showed no sign of injury.

The patient was given oxygen at 6 liters per minute by nasal cannula. A 16-gauge Angiocath was inserted in the left arm, and an infusion of saline was begun at a rate of 200 ml per hour. En route to the hospital, the patient vomited bloody material, but his condition was otherwise unchanged. His vital signs remained stable during transport.

Questions to think about:

1. The fact that the patient had a few beers before the accident suggests that he may have been particularly vulnerable to injury of a certain organ. Which organ, and why?
2. This patient is showing symptoms and signs of peritonitis. List at least four of the symptoms and signs of peritonitis mentioned in the case history.
3. What do the skin condition and the pulse suggest to you about the patient's injuries?

VOCABULARY

appendix Wormlike tube projecting from the cecum in the right lower quadrant of the abdomen.

bile Greenish-black fluid secreted by the liver and concentrated in the gallbladder; important in the absorption of fats from the digestive tract.

colic Crampy pain associated with obstruction of a hollow organ.

colon The large intestine.

duodenum The first portion of the small intestine, immediately distal to the stomach.

frenulum Fold on the lower surface of the penis, which bleeds profusely when lacerated.

hematuria Blood in the urine.

ileum Third and final section of the small intestine, which joins with the large intestine at the ileocecal valve.

insulin Hormone produced in the pancreas that regulates the level of sugar in the blood.

jejunum Second portion of the small intestine.

mesentery Delicate tissue that carries blood vessels and nerves to and from the organs of the abdominal cavity.

peristalsis Wavelike contractions of the muscles of hollow organs that propel the contents of the organs forward.

peritoneum Smooth layer of tissue lining the abdominal cavity.

peritonitis Inflammation of the peritoneum.

prostate Accessory sexual gland surrounding the male urethra as it emerges from the bladder.

retroperitoneal Referring to the area behind the peritoneum.

saliva Clear secretion from the glands of the mouth that moistens and softens food and begins the breakdown of starch.

salivary glands Mucus glands of the mouth that produce saliva.

scrotum Sac that contains the testes.

seminal vesicle Structure in which sperm and seminal fluid are stored prior to ejaculation.

testicle Ovoid gland located in the scrotum that produces sperm and male hormones.

testis Another word for testicle (plural, *testes*).

ureter Tube that conducts urine from the kidney to the bladder.

urethra Tube that conducts urine from the bladder to the outside of the body.

vas deferens Seminal duct, which conducts sperm and seminal fluid from the testis to the seminal vesicle.

FURTHER READING

Baxt WG, Moody P. The impact of a physician as part of the aeromedical prehospital team in patients with blunt trauma. *JAMA* 257:3246, 1987.

Cwinn AA et al. Prehospital advanced trauma life support for critical blunt trauma victims. *Ann Emerg Med* 16:399, 1987.

Denis R et al. Changing trends with abdominal injury in seatbelt wearers. *J Trauma* 23:1007, 1983.

Fiedler MD et al. A correlation of response time and results of abdominal gunshot wounds. *Arch Surg* 121:902, 1986.

Majernick TG et al. Intestinal evisceration resulting from a motor vehicle accident. *Ann Emerg Med* 13:633, 1984.

Moore JB, Moore EE, Thompson JS. Abdominal injuries associated with penetrating trauma in the lower chest. *Am J Surg* 140:724, 1980.

Murr PC et al. Abdominal trauma associated with pelvic fracture. *J Trauma* 20:919, 1980.

Pons PT et al. Prehospital advanced trauma life support for critical penetrating wounds to the thorax and abdomen. *J Trauma* 25:828, 1985.

Vayer JS et al. Absence of a tachycardic response to shock in penetrating intraperitoneal injury. *Ann Emerg Med* 17:227, 1988.

17. FRACTURES, DISLOCATIONS, AND SPRAINS

OBJECTIVES

Injuries to the musculoskeletal system—the network of bones, muscles, tendons, and ligaments—are among the most common injuries seen in emergency work. Rarely do such injuries pose a threat to life, but nonetheless the proper handling of musculoskeletal injuries can significantly reduce the amount of pain and subsequent disability the patient suffers. The future function of an injured arm or leg may critically depend upon the way in which the limb is handled immediately after the injury, and the EMT is in a position to make the difference in many cases between restored function and lifelong handicap. In this chapter, we will examine the system of bones and muscles that enables us to move and perform skilled actions. We will see the types of injuries to which the musculoskeletal system is subject, and learn the principles of managing those injuries correctly in the prehospital setting. By the end of this chapter, the reader should be able to

1. Identify the major bones of the human body, given a diagram of the skeleton or a description of the bones
2. Identify the components of major joints, given a list of various bones
3. Identify the function of (a) ligaments, (b) tendons, and (c) cartilage, given a list of functions
4. Identify (a) skeletal muscle, (b) smooth muscle, and (c) cardiac muscle, given a description of types of muscle and their functions
5. Predict the type of musculoskeletal injury likely to be present, given a description of the forces that produced the injury
6. Predict associated injuries likely to be present, given a description of an injury and the way in which it was sustained
7. Indicate the dangers associated with open fractures and describe the special measures that should be taken when there is an open fracture
8. Indicate the areas of special emphasis in examining a patient with suspected musculoskeletal injury
9. Identify a patient with a fracture, a sprain, or dislocation, given a description of several patients with various symptoms and signs
10. Identify the correct sequence of treatment for a multiply injured patient, given a list of treatment steps, and indicate at what point fractures should be treated in this sequence
11. List at least three reasons for splinting injured extremities
12. Identify errors in splinting, given a description of several splinting procedures carried out improperly
13. Identify the correct method of treating various musculoskeletal injuries (including those involving the clavicle, shoulder, humerus, elbow, forearm, wrist, hand, pelvis, hip, femur, knee,

leg, ankle, and foot), given a description of the patient and a choice of alternative treatments

THE MUSCULOSKELETAL SYSTEM

OVERVIEW

The human skeleton is the scaffolding that forms the rigid supporting structure of the body. Without a skeleton, the human organism would be simply a shapeless blob of tissue. The unique human form, however, is largely dictated by the arrangement of its 206 bones.

The skeleton performs several important functions for us. To begin with, it offers considerable *protection* to the delicate internal organs. The brain, for example, is enclosed and protected by the skull; the spinal cord is protected by the bony vertebrae that surround it; the heart and lungs, and much of the liver and spleen, are shielded from injury by the rib cage; and organs of the lower abdomen are partially buttressed by the pelvis. In the second place, the skeleton gives *support* to the body, permitting us to stand erect. And finally, because the skeleton is made up of many separate bones, rather than one fused bone, it permits *motion* of its parts and thereby enables us to do all sorts of extraordinary things such as walking, combing our hair, bending over, and so on.

If we had to design a skeleton from scratch, it would be difficult to improve on the current model. We would want our skeleton to be very strong, so that it could bear a considerable amount of weight, but still we would want it flexible enough that it could absorb impact without shattering. Furthermore, it would have to be relatively lightweight, for one could not get around very well with a skeleton made of structural steel or poured concrete. Fortunately for us, the human skeleton is composed of one of the most remarkable structural materials ever developed—BONE—which meets all the above requirements. Bone is light, strong, and flexible. And even more remarkable, bone has a characteristic that engineers would highly value in structural materials: Bone becomes stronger at points where it is subject to stress. This is because bone is, in fact, more than just a scaffolding. It is a *living* tissue, just like kidney or liver or brain, and it undergoes constant regeneration.

Just like any other living tissue in the body, bone needs oxygen and nutrients, and it has a blood supply to provide these. Bone is a very busy tissue, constantly reshaping and remodelling itself to meet changing stresses—adding a bit of calcium here, subtracting a bit there—and it gets even busier when it is broken, as it undertakes an accelerated rebuilding program. In the process of reconstruction, bone cells divide rapidly to bridge the broken area and surround it with a collar of new tissue called **callus**. As healing progresses, calcium is laid down in the callus, which becomes new bone, and then the callus is gradually whittled down and reshaped to conform to the normal structure of the bone in question.

Wherever two bones come together, or **articulate**, they form what is called a JOINT. Some joints are fused, so that no motion is possible between the component bones. This is the case, for instance, with the joints of the cranial bones (these joints are called **sutures**), which are permanently welded together during childhood into a single unit. Other joints, called SYNOVIAL JOINTS, allow motion, for the component bones are linked together only by bands of tough, fibrous tissue, called LIGAMENTS. The type of motion that occurs between any two bones depends on the type of joint involved. HINGE JOINTS, such as those in the knee, elbow, and fingers, operate like any other hinge and allow motion in only one plane: flexion and extension. A much wider range of motion is permitted by a BALL-AND-SOCKET JOINT, such as in the shoulder or hip. And the SADDLE JOINT of the thumb permits an even larger repertoire of movements. Whatever the type of joint, however, *every* joint has limits to the motion it can allow, and if a joint is forced beyond its limits or in some way made to carry out a motion for which it was not designed, several types of injury can occur. If the joint is relatively mobile, it can become *dislocated*, that is, the ends of its component bones can be displaced so that they are no longer in the proper relationship to one another. This type of injury is especially common in ball-and-socket joints, when a force applied to the bone causes the ball to be popped out of its socket. Alternatively, the ligaments holding the two bones together can be stretched or torn, resulting in an injury called a *sprain*. Or one or both of the bones that make up the joint can break (*fracture*). Any of the above injuries can occur in isolation, or they can occur together. In a fall from a height, for instance, forces applied to the hip can cause both dislocation of the ball-and-socket joint and fracture of the socket, sometimes together with stretching or tearing of the involved ligaments as well.

Synovial joints are cushioned with a material called CARTILAGE, which forms a smooth surface at the bone ends. Cartilage is also present between the vertebrae, where it acts as a shock absorber to buffer the spinal column against jarring, so that the vertebrae do not clatter together every time you take a step.

So far, we have examined the general makeup of the skeleton and how that makeup is designed to permit a wide variety of different movements. But the skeleton would not do very much moving without a system of pulleys that flex a joint here and extend one there. The moving force in this system is supplied by MUSCLE, a very special tissue that has the important property of contracting—and thus becoming shorter—when stimulated. There are three kinds of muscle present in the body: skeletal muscle, smooth muscle, and cardiac muscle. **Skeletal muscle** is the muscle we are concerned with here, for it is the muscle that attaches to and moves bone. It is also called *voluntary* muscle because it is under conscious control; it contracts when you instruct it to contract, for the brain sends orders down through the spinal cord to the muscle, which changes its length in response to those orders. By contrast, **smooth muscle**, which comprises the muscle of most of the internal organs (e.g., stomach, bladder, uterus, gut), is *involuntary* muscle. It goes about its business on its own, under standing orders from the brain, without any conscious instructions from you. And that is just as well, for imagine how complicated life would be if you had to will your stomach to contract or issue orders for each peristaltic wave in your gut or each ripple in the wall of your ureters. **Cardiac muscle** is similar to smooth muscle, but it has one very notable difference: It does not have to take orders from any part of the brain (conscious or unconscious) in order to contract, for it has the property of initiating its own contractions. The heart is, in effect, a self-starter.

As noted, the type of muscle that concerns us here is skeletal, or voluntary, muscle. Most skeletal muscles attach directly to bones by TENDONS, tough cords of fibrous tissue at each end of the muscle. Clearly if the muscle is going to produce movement at a joint, it must attach to *two* bones, so that when the muscle contracts and shortens, a force is created that pulls the two bones into flexion or extension. In order to create an effective fulcrum, most muscles pass across or over a joint, as the biceps muscle crosses the elbow joint, enabling the biceps to flex the elbow on contraction (Fig. 17-1). Once the elbow is flexed, one would like to be able to extend it again, and for this reason, muscle groups tend to come in pairs having roughly equal but opposite functions. The biceps muscle is paired with the triceps muscle, whose job is to extend the elbow. When the biceps contracts, the triceps relaxes, and vice versa.

Muscles are very busy tissues, doing all the lifting, walking, jumping, and other movements of the body; consequently they are hungry tissues. They consume large amounts of oxygen and nutrients, and they produce considerable waste, largely in the form of carbon dioxide and other acids. Thus they need a good blood supply to furnish them with oxygen and food and to cart off the waste products of their metabolism. When the blood supply is not sufficient to carry out these tasks, the muscles become very unhappy, and their unhappiness is manifested in a pain known as "muscle cramps."

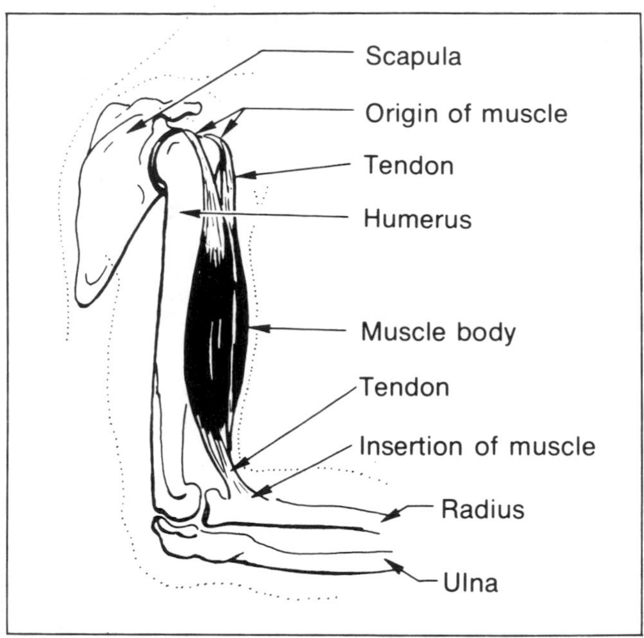

Fig. 17-1. *The biceps muscle.*

THE APPENDICULAR SKELETON

In Chapter 2, we made a brief survey of the human skeleton in order to become familiar with the major bones it comprises. We return now to look at the skeleton in greater detail, with specific attention to the part known as the **appendicular skeleton**, that is, the part of the skeleton that comprises the upper and lower extremities. (The other main division of the skeleton, the **axial skeleton**, comprises the skull, vertebral column, and thorax. Injuries to those regions have been covered in previous chapters.)

The Upper Extremity

The upper extremity is composed of the bones of the shoulder girdle, the arm, the forearm, and the hand. The SHOULDER GIRDLE (Fig. 17-2) is the point of attachment between the upper extremity and the trunk, and it consists of the scapula (shoulder blade) and the clavicle (collar bone). The SCAPULA is a relatively flat bone that is buttressed against the back of the rib cage by powerful muscles, which permit the scapula some freedom of motion to slide across the chest wall and which also buffer the scapula against injury. At the outer, upper end of the scapula is a depression, called the **glenoid**, that forms the socket of the shoulder joint. The second component of the shoulder girdle, the CLAVICLE, is a slender, somewhat S-shaped bone that is attached by liga-

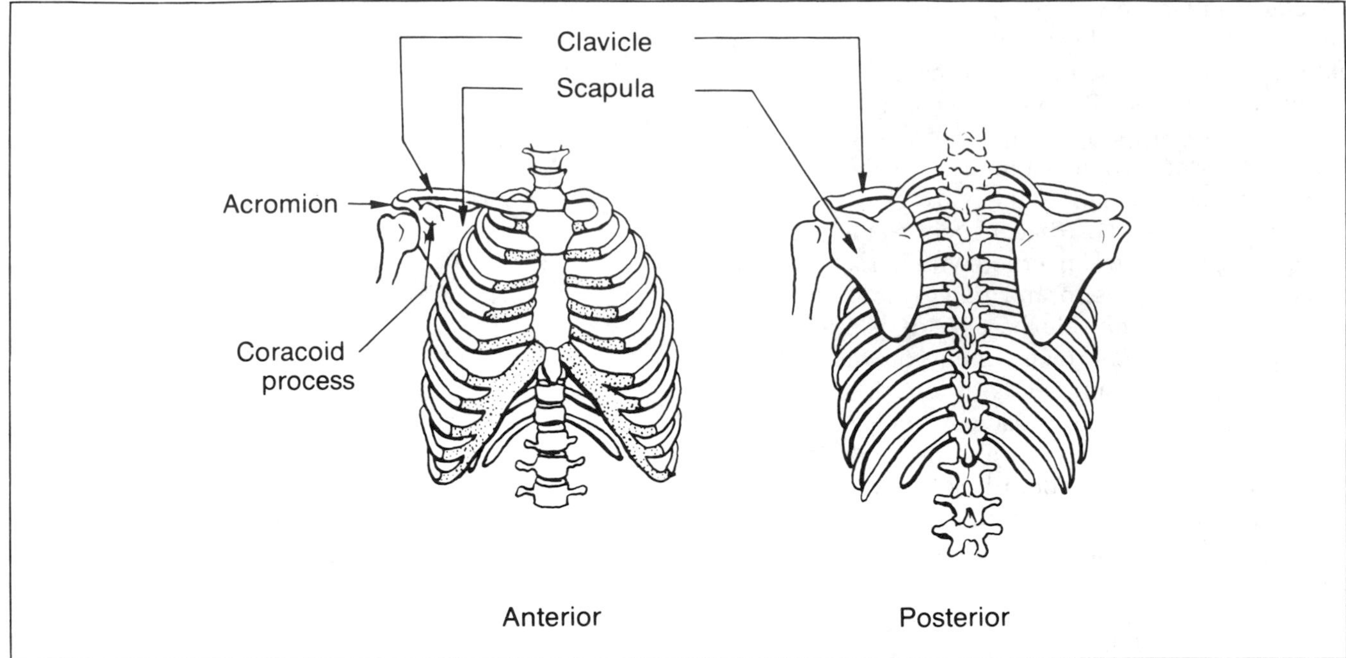

Fig. 17-2. *The shoulder girdle.*

ments to the upper sternum at one end and to the top of the scapula (at a point called the **acromion**) at the other. The clavicle acts as a strut to prop up the shoulder. Being slender and quite exposed, the clavicle is vulnerable to injury from both direct blows and indirect force transmitted through an outstretched arm, and it may be broken or torn away from either of its points of attachment.

Fitting into the socket of the scapula is the rounded proximal end of the HUMERUS, or arm bone (Fig. 17-3), which enjoys a wide range of motion because of the ball-and-socket nature of the shoulder joint. At its distal end, the humerus articulates with the radius and ulna, the two bones of the forearm. The RADIUS is the larger of the two bones, and it lies on the *thumb* side of the forearm (where you find the radial pulse). The proximal end of the ULNA, or **olecranon**, forms part of the elbow joint and can be palpated at the back of the elbow as a bump sometimes called the "funny bone." What makes it "funny" is that the ulnar nerve passes along a groove on the outside of the ulna and is apt to get banged if the elbow is bumped; when this happens, the owner of the elbow experiences tingling sensations (paresthesias). Distally, the ulna is quite narrow and is on the little finger side of the forearm. It serves as a pivot around which the radius turns to rotate the palm up or down. Because the radius and ulna are arranged in parallel, fracture of one of them is often associated with fracture of the other.

At their distal ends, the radius and ulna articulate with the eight CARPAL BONES of the wrist, which resemble eight irregular pebbles. Wrist bones are

Fig. 17-3. *The upper extremity.*

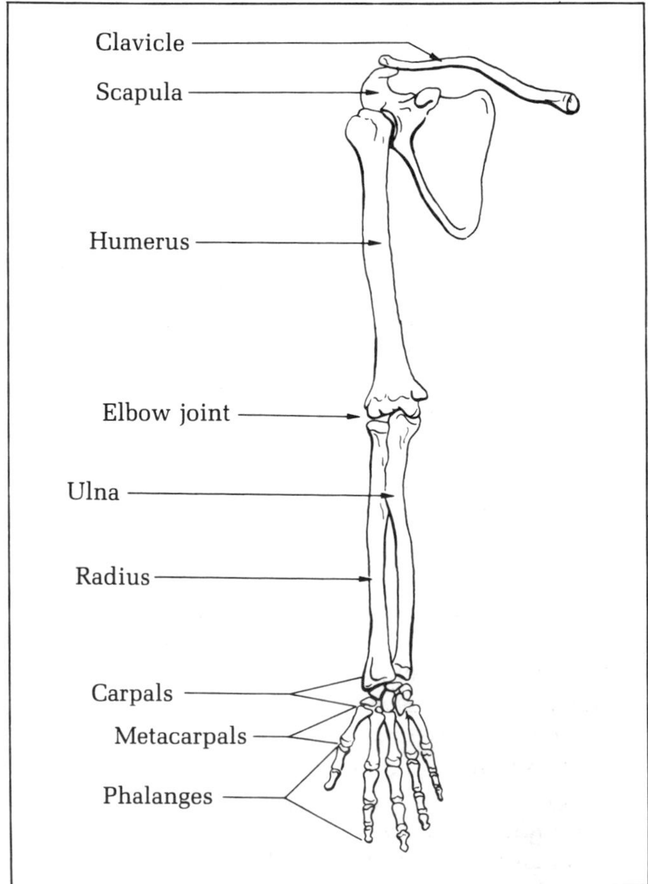

most likely to be broken when a person falls onto an outstetched hand, and one of the more serious fractures of this type involves the **navicular** bone, the carpal bone just distal to the radius.

The carpal bones articulate with the METACARPALS, or hand bones, which in turn articulate with the bones of the fingers, called PHALANGES. The metacarpals, especially that of the little finger, are subject to fracture from blunt impact, while the distal phalanges are more apt to be broken in crush injuries, such as slamming one's finger in a car door.

Before we leave the upper extremity, we need to learn two more terms used to describe the location of injuries. The *back* of the hand and forearm are referred to as the **dorsal** surface, and the *front* as the palmar or **volar** surface. Thus, if there is a bruise on the thumb side of the back of the right wrist, one would say that "the patient has a bruise over the dorsal surface of the right wrist on the radial side."

The Lower Extremity

The lower extremity attaches to the trunk at the PELVIS (Fig. 17-4), a massive ring of bone that forms the lower border of the trunk. The pelvis is in fact made up of several bones fused solidly together. The back of the pelvis is formed by the SACRUM, the lower five vertebrae of the spinal column. The sacrum is attached on both sides by strong ligaments to the two winglike pelvic bones, and the point where the sacrum and pelvic bones come together is called the SACROILIAC JOINT. Each of the two pelvic wings is itself made up of three fused bones: the broad, heavy ILIUM superiorly; the ringlike ISCHIUM inferiorly; and the PUBIS in front. The point where the two pubic bones come together can be felt in the midline of the lower abdomen and is called the PUBIC SYMPHYSIS, which is directly in front of the bladder. The posterior portion of the ischium, known as the ISCHIAL TUBEROSITY, forms a hard bump that can be palpated in each buttock and is an important landmark in applying a traction splint to the lower extemity, for it is used to buttress the top of the splint.

The three pelvic bones—ischium, ilium, and pubis—come together laterally to form a hollow depression, called the **acetabulum**, which serves as the socket for the hip joint. The fusion between these bones must be very strong, for when a person is standing, the entire weight of the body is transmitted across the hip joints into the legs.

The acetabulum receives the rounded head of the FEMUR, or thigh bone (Fig. 17-5). The femur is the longest bone in the body and one of the strongest bones as well. It is usually referred to in three parts: At its proximal end are the head and neck of the femur, the *head* being the ball-shaped part that fits into the acetabulum, and the *neck* a short stretch of bone, about 3 inches long, that comes off at an angle from the long part of the femur, the femoral *shaft*. The neck of the femur is set off from the shaft by two bumps, called **trochanters**. The femoral neck is a common site for fractures, especially in the elderly.

Fig. 17-4. *The pelvis.*

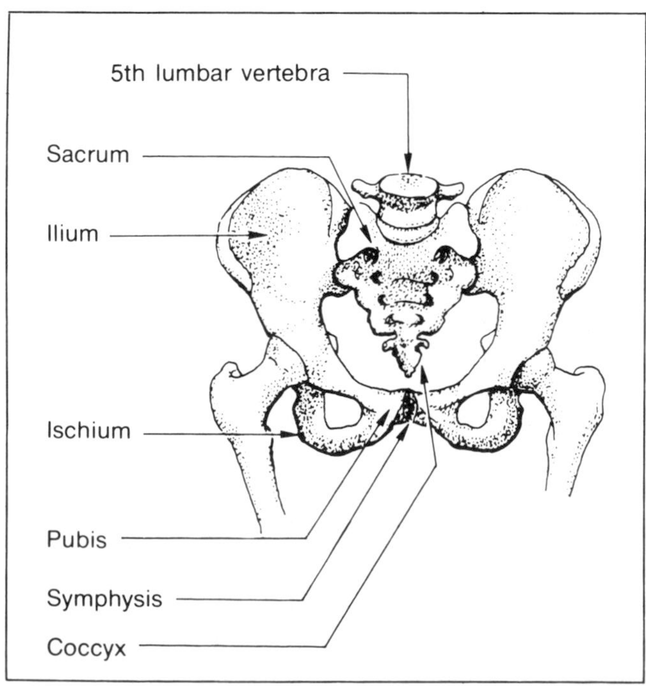

Fig. 17-5. *The lower extremity.*

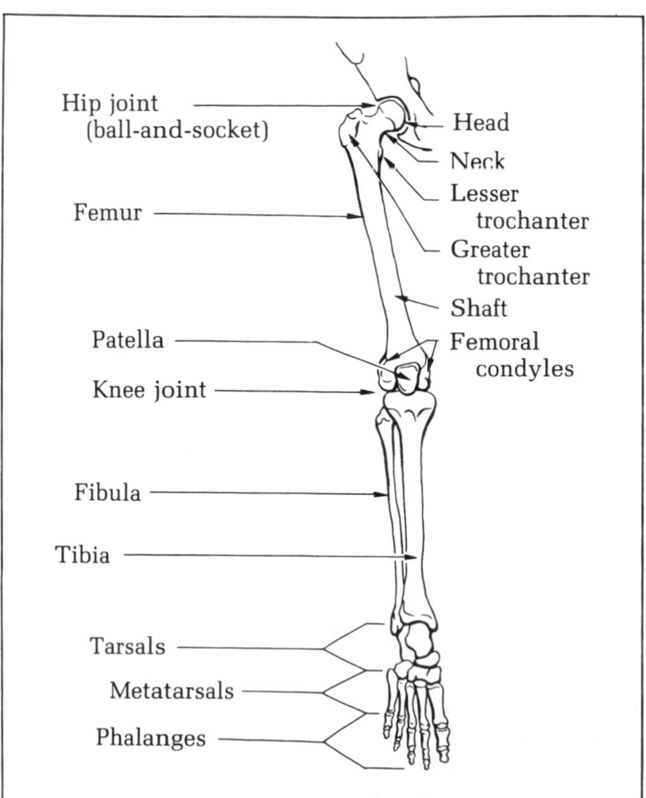

At the distal end of the femoral shaft are two rounded structures called **condyles**, which articulate with the upper end of the tibia to form the knee joint.

The *knee joint* is the largest joint in the body, and it is supported by a complex network of ligaments that are subject to all sorts of injury, especially when twisting forces are applied to the knee. On the front of the knee joint sits a small, moveable bone, the PATELLA (knee cap), which is anchored down by the tendon of the quadriceps muscle. The knee cap can be fractured, especially when the knee is flexed and force is applied horizontally to the knee.

The lower leg is made up of two bones, the tibia and the fibula. The TIBIA, or shin bone, is the larger of the two, and its broad, proximal end forms part of the knee joint. The tibia runs down the front of the leg, very close to the skin, and because of its superficial location, it is very susceptible to open fracture (fracture in which the skin is broken). At its distal end, the tibia articulates with the bones of the foot to form the ankle joint, and the distal part of the tibia can be palpated as a bony knob at the inner surface of the ankle, called the **medial malleolus**.

The FIBULA is considerably more slender than the tibia, and it runs down the back of the leg, where its shaft is relatively protected from direct impact. The fibula is not part of the knee joint, but at its distal end it does make up the lateral knob of the ankle joint, the **lateral malleolus**.

Heavy ligaments strap the lower ends of the tibia and fibula to the TARSAL BONES. These are seven very strong, irregularly shaped bones that support the weight of the body. The tibia articulates with one of the tarsal bones, called the talus, which in turn rests on the largest of the tarsal bones, the **calcaneus**, or heel bone. The calcaneus may be fractured when a person falls from a height and lands squarely on his feet, and a fracture of this sort is a tip-off that powerful shock waves must also have been transmitted up through the spine.

The tarsals arch upward to join with the five METATARSAL BONES of the foot, which in turn articulate with five of the PHALANGES of the toes. The metatarsals are a common site for stress fractures, or "march fractures," which occur in people who undertake a long hike or long-distance run when they are unaccustomed to that kind of exercise.

MUSCULOSKELETAL INJURIES: GENERAL CONCEPTS

Musculoskeletal injuries fall into three general categories—fractures, dislocations, and sprains—and any of these can occur alone or in association with another type of injury. A **fracture** is a break anywhere in a bone; it may be just a small crack, or it may involve complete separation of the bone into two or more pieces, but in each case there is some degree of disruption in the continuity of the bone. A **dislocation** is an injury that occurs at a joint when one of the bone ends that make up the joint is pushed out of its proper position so that the two joint surfaces are no longer in normal contact with one another. A **sprain** also occurs at a joint and involves stretching or partial tearing of one or more of the ligaments that strap the bones of the joint together.

MECHANISMS OF INJURY

A variety of different types of forces can cause musculoskeletal injury, and often if the type of force involved is known, it is possible to predict the injury that was sustained. To begin with, injury to the musculoskeletal system can be caused by a DIRECT BLOW, in which the injury occurs at the point of impact. A direct blow is most likely to result in a fracture, as when a person is thrown forward against the dashboard and breaks the collar bone at the point where it makes contact with the dash. By contrast, an injury caused by an INDIRECT BLOW does not occur at the point of impact but rather at a point some distance away, due to forces transmitted along the bone. Indirect blows can cause either fractures or dislocations or both. For instance, the proximal end of the humerus (at the shoulder) can be *fractured* when a person falls onto his outstretched hand; in this case, the impact is applied at the hand, but the force is transmitted along the line of the arm bones and does its damage as the head of the humerus is rammed into the shoulder socket. Similarly, the hip can be *dislocated* when the patella strikes the dashboard of a car and the forces are transmitted backward along the line of the femur (Fig. 17-6).

TWISTING FORCES, such as commonly occur in football or skiing, can cause fractures, dislocations, or sprains. Typically, the distal part of the lower extremity remains fixed—as when football cleats anchor the foot to the turf—while torsion develops in the more proximal part of the limb, causing a spiral-type fracture in the bone or a shearing of the ligaments in the involved joint. Many knee and ankle injuries occur by this mechanism.

Less commonly, fractures or dislocations can be caused by VIOLENT MUSCLE CONTRACTIONS, as occur in some lightning injuries or seizures. The sudden shortening of a powerful muscle can tear the tendon away from the bone or actually yank off the part of the bone to which the tendon is attached.

FATIGUE FRACTURES, or stress fractures, are caused by repeated stress to an area of bone, usually when the bone is not accustomed to the stress in question. When fatigue fractures occur in the bones of the feet, they are often called march fractures, because they commonly occur in new recruits forced to undertake long marches.

Finally, fractures can occur after very minimal force in certain PATHOLOGIC CONDITIONS that weaken areas of bone. When cancer spreads to bone, for instance, it can produce localized areas of thinning of the bone structure so that a very trivial blow may be sufficient to break the bone in those areas. AGE by itself causes changes in bone that make it more susceptible to fracture; thus, for example, an elderly person is much more likely than a young person to suffer hip fracture from a fall, because the elderly person's bones are much more brittle.

Mechanisms of Musculoskeletal Injury

- DIRECT FORCE (injury at the point of impact)
- INDIRECT FORCE (injury distant from the point of impact)
- TWISTING FORCE
- Violent MUSCLE CONTRACTIONS (e.g., seizures)
- Repeated STRESS (fatigue fractures)
- PATHOLOGIC CONDITIONS and AGE

When examining a patient who has sustained a musculoskeletal injury, it is important to try to determine the nature of the forces that produced the injury, for this information often provides clues to other unsuspected injuries. In evaluating musculoskeletal trauma, the EMT needs to think like a physicist or engineer and try to picture the direction in which forces were transmitted. Some injuries commonly come in pairs, based on the way forces were applied. For instance, a fractured patella in a patient who was seated in a car is often paired with a fractured or dislocated hip, for the impact of the dashboard against the knee is trasmitted back along the femur (see Fig. 17-6). Similarly, a fractured calcaneous (heel bone) should alert the EMT to the possibility of a spine injury, for anyone who has come down hard enough to fracture his heel has inevitably given his spine a tremendous jolt. Pain in the navicular bone of the wrist means that the patient fell hard against his outstretched hand and suggests the possibility of associated fractures anywhere along the axis of the forearm and arm, especially near the elbow and shoulder. Thus when you find evidence of an injury that is commonly paired with another injury, look for its mate!

Look for Paired Injuries

- Fractured PATELLA: dislocated HIP
- Fractured CALCANEUS: fractured LUMBAR SPINE
- Fractured carpal NAVICULAR: fractures of the forearm, ELBOW, arm, or SHOULDER

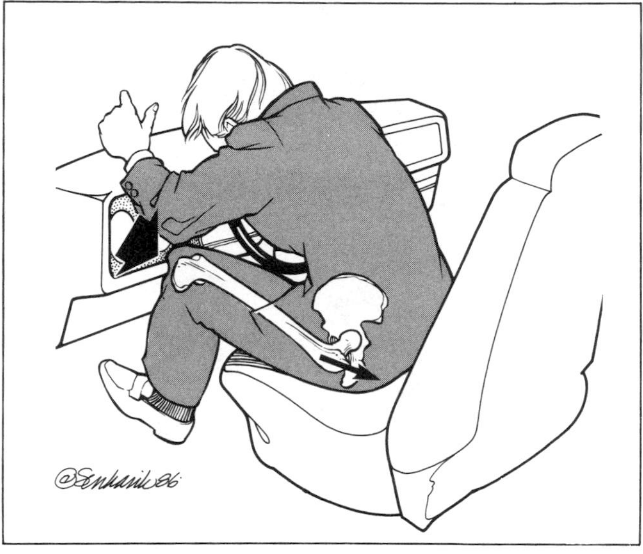

Fig. 17-6. *Mechanism by which a force applied to the patella can result in fracture/dislocation of the hip.*

FRACTURES

A fracture is an interruption in the continuity of a bone. Any bone in the body can be fractured if sufficient stress is applied to it, although some bones are more prone to fracture than others because of the nature of their location. The shaft of the tibia, for example, coursing down the front of the leg, is much more apt to be broken by a direct blow than is the shaft of the fibula, which is buried deep within the leg muscles.

Classification of Fractures

Fractures are commonly divided into two major categories: closed and open (Fig. 17-7). A CLOSED FRACTURE, or *simple fracture*, is one in which there is no break in the overlying skin. In an OPEN FRACTURE, or *compound fracture*, a bone end has pierced through the skin or some other open wound penetrates down to the area of the injured bone. An open fracture has a much greater potential for complications than a closed fracture, for contamination of the wound can lead to severe infection in the underlying bone, preventing proper bone healing. Furthermore, bleeding may be much more profuse from an open fracture because the tissues that would ordinarily exert pressure over the fracture site and tend to limit bleeding have been disrupted.

Fractures are also classified according to their appearance on x-ray (Fig. 17-8), and although the EMT will not have an x-ray machine available in the field, it is sometimes possible to make an educated guess at the x-ray appearance of the fracture based on the mechanisms of injury. A TRANSVERSE FRACTURE divides the bone in two in a line that cuts straight across the bone at right angles to its long axis. A GREENSTICK FRACTURE is also a break straight across the bone, but it goes only partway through the

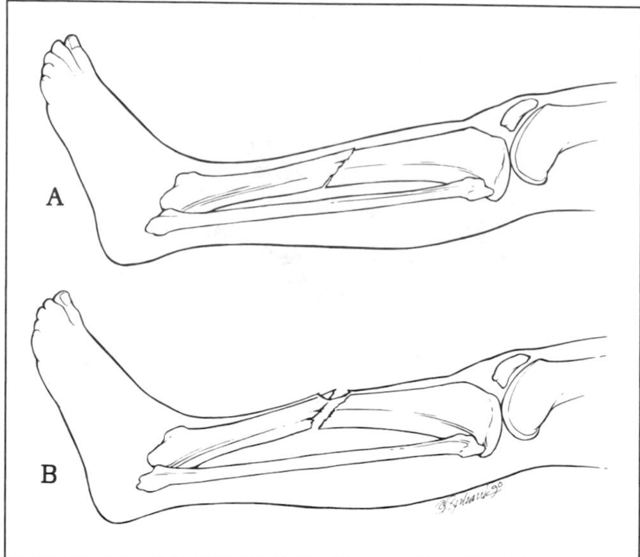

Fig. 17-7. *Categories of fractures. A. Closed fracture: there is no break in the skin above the fracture. B. Open (compound) fracture: the skin overlying the fracture is broken and sometimes bone is seen protruding through the wound.*

bone and is thus an incomplete fracture. Greenstick fractures occur mainly in small children, whose bones are pliable (like green sticks) and can bend considerably without breaking all the way through. In an OBLIQUE FRACTURE, the fracture line crosses the bone at an angle to the shaft, suggesting that the force that produced the fracture was also applied at an angle. SPIRAL FRACTURES usually result from twisting injuries, and the fracture line has the appearance of a coil or spring. In an IMPACTED FRACTURE, the broken bone ends are jammed into one another; this type of injury tends to occur from indirect forces, when a bone is trapped along its long axis between the proverbial "rock and a hard place." Very powerful *direct* forces, on the other hand, are likely to produce a COMMINUTED FRACTURE, in which the bone is fragmented into more than two pieces.

For practical purposes in the field, the most important classification to make is whether the fracture is open or closed, for this determination will influence the way in which the fracture is handled in the prehospital setting.

Symptoms and Signs of Fractures

The chief complaint of a person who has sustained a fracture is almost invariably PAIN, usually quite localized to the area of the injury. Sometimes the patient will be able to report that he actually felt the bone break or that he heard a sudden crack or snap at the moment of injury.

On physical examination, there are several signs that should alert the EMT to the likelihood of fracture. One of the most reliable of these is DEFORMITY; that is, the extremity may lie in an unnatural position or be bent or have motion at a place where there is no joint. Deformity is best appreciated by **comparing the injured extremity to the uninjured extremity** on the other side. Comparison of one side to the other will also permit one to notice any SHORTENING of the injured limb, which can occur with either fracture or dislocation.

TENDERNESS is almost invariably present when there is a fracture, and it is usually localized to the site where the bone is broken. SWELLING is also a nearly constant feature of fractures, and it is due to

Fig. 17-8. *Types of fracture.*

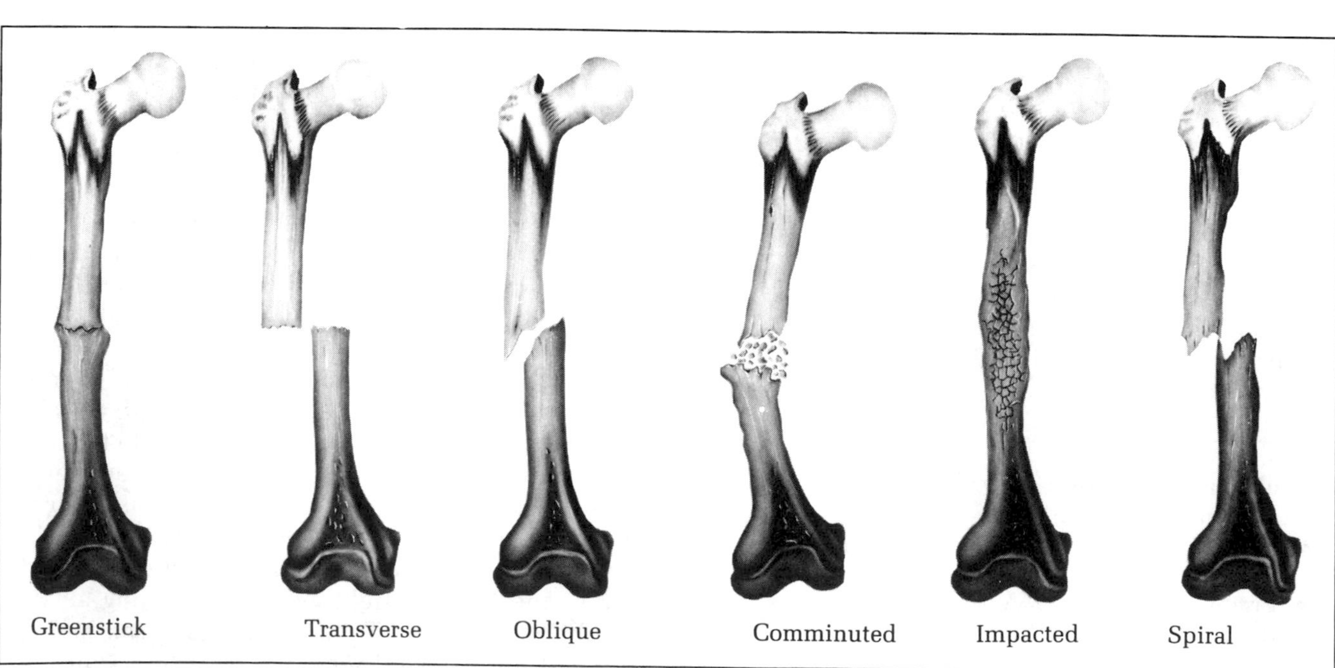

Fig. 17-7. *Types of fracture.*

bleeding into the surrounding tissues and, over a period of several hours, the accumulation of edema fluid in the injured area. When bleeding is considerable and blood infiltrates into the tissues just beneath the skin, ECCHYMOSIS is also seen.

GUARDING and LOSS OF USE are characteristic of most fractures. The patient with a fractured extremity will attempt to keep the fractured part very still and will avoid any stress on the area. Thus if the fracture involves a leg, the patient will avoid bearing weight on the leg; when an arm is involved, the patient will often support the injured part with his other hand. Sometimes the position the patient assumes to keep from moving the injured part is itself a clue to the type of injury he has sustained. For instance, the patient who walks toward you holding the dorsum of one wrist in his other hand can be predicted with about 80-percent accuracy to have sustained a type of fracture to the distal radius and ulna called a Colles' fracture. A patient who stands with one shoulder slumped and his head cocked to that side probably has a fracture of the clavicle.

If the patient does attempt to move the injured extremity, you may be able to feel GRATING or CREPITUS, which is caused by broken fragments of bone ends grinding together. NEVER ATTEMPT TO ELICIT THIS SIGN BY INTENTIONALLY MOVING THE INJURED AREA, for you will only cause the patient severe pain in doing so, and you may increase the damage to surrounding soft tissue as well.

Finally, an *open* fracture may be evident from the presence of EXPOSED BONE FRAGMENTS protruding from the skin or visible within an open wound.

Symptoms and Signs of Fracture

- PAIN at the fracture site.
- Patient may have HEARD THE BONE SNAP.
- DEFORMITY or UNNATURAL MOTION.
- SHORTENING of the extremity.
- TENDERNESS over the site of fracture
- SWELLING.
- ECCHYMOSIS.
- GUARDING and LOSS OF USE of the injured part.
- GRATING or CREPITUS.
- EXPOSED BONE ENDS (open fracture).

Not all of the above signs will be present in every fracture, but in nearly all cases there will at least be some degree of pain, tenderness, and swelling.

Potential Complications of Fractures

In previous chapters, we learned that fractures can be associated with damage to internal organs, damage to the spinal cord, and severe hemorrhage. In dealing with fractures of the extremities, there are two additional complications of which the EMT should be aware: damage to blood vessels and damage to nerves.

The major blood vessels of an extremity tend to run close to bone, which means that any time a bone is broken, the adjacent blood vessel is at risk of being torn by bone fragments or pinched off between the broken bone ends. Needless to say, if a major artery is completely severed or pinched off for any length of time, the whole limb distal to the injury is in danger. For like tissues elsewhere, the tissues of the arms and legs cannot survive without a continuing supply of oxygen and nutrients. The only way to determine whether the blood supply to an extremitiy is intact is to **palpate for a pulse distal to the injury.** In injuries to the upper extremity, one should always determine whether the radial pulse is present in the injured arm (Fig. 17-9A), while the survey of an injured lower extremity should always include a check for one of the pedal pulses (dorsalis pedis or anterior tibial, Fig. 17-9B). Use a ballpoint pen to mark the spot where you found each pulse so that you can locate it again quickly for frequent rechecking.

ALWAYS CHECK THE PULSE DISTAL TO AN INJURY.

When distal pulses are absent—and remain absent after a fracture has been straightened—urgent treatment in the hospital is required, and the patient's transport should not be delayed.

A second potential complication of fracture is injury to nerves, which may come about in a manner similar to that in which blood vessels are injured. Major nerve pathways also travel close to bone and are thus also susceptible to being torn or pinched when adjacent bone is broken. Nerve injury should be suspected whenever the patient complains of NUMBNESS or TINGLING distal to the fracture site. In addition, the survey of every fracture should include a check for SENSATION and MOVEMENT in the extremities, comparing the injured side to the uninjured side.

ALWAYS CHECK SENSATION AND MOVEMENT DISTAL TO AN INJURY.

The absence of sensation or movement in the distal extremity is also a very serious sign and should be a signal to the EMT to move expeditiously to the hospital.

While considering the potential complications of fractures, it is worth reemphasizing that fractures can produce major blood loss—enough to cause hy-

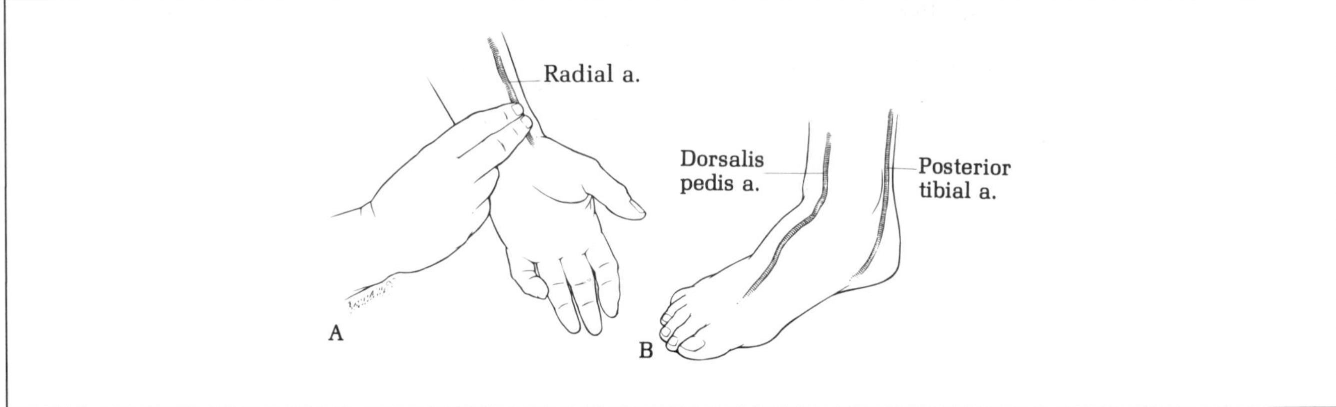

Fig. 17-9. *Checking the pulses distal to an injury. A. In an injured arm, check for a radial pulse. B. In an injured leg, check for a posterial tibial or dorsalis pedal pulse.*

povolemic shock. This is particularly true of fractures of the pelvis and femur, but significant blood loss can occur from other fractures as well; for when a bone breaks, bleeding occurs from both the bone itself and from vessels in the surrounding tissues. So remember:

FRACTURES BLEED—SOMETIMES MASSIVELY.

DISLOCATIONS

A dislocation occurs when one of the bone ends making up a joint is displaced from its normal position (Fig. 17-10). When that happens, there is usually associated stretching or tearing of the ligaments that ordinarily hold the bone end in place. There may also be damage to the joint capsule, a layer of fibrous tissue that encloses the two bone ends composing the joint and helps stabilize them in place. The most commonly dislocated joints are the ball-and-socket joints of the shoulder and hip. Dislocations at the elbow, fingers, and ankle also occur frequently. Less commonly, a wrist or knee may be dislocated.

The symptoms and signs of dislocation are similar to those of a fracture. To begin with, there is usually PAIN in the affected area, and the patient will generally report that the pain is AGGRAVATED BY ATTEMPTED MOVEMENT of the joint in question. On physical examination, marked DEFORMITY is evident at the site of the dislocated joint, which appears obviously out of its proper alignment. TENDERNESS and SWELLING may be present as well, but it is unusual to see ecchymosis unless there is an associated fracture. One highly characteristic sign of dislocation is LOSS OF MOVEMENT at the joint, which tends to become "locked" in a deformed position.

Symptoms and Signs of Dislocation

- PAIN, aggravated by attempts to move the injured joint
- DEFORMITY
- TENDERNESS; sometimes SWELLING
- LOSS OF MOTION

When evaluating and describing dislocations, one needs some special terminology relating to position and motion of a limb. **A*b*duction** is movement of a limb *away* from the body, whereas **a*d*duction** is movement of the limb *toward* the body. When a limb is turned outward (laterally), it is said to be **externally rotated**; when it is turned inward, it is **internally rotated**. These terms are helpful in describing dislocations, for they encompass the types of positions one is likely to see in dislocated extremities.

Fig. 17-10. *Dislocation of the elbow joint.*

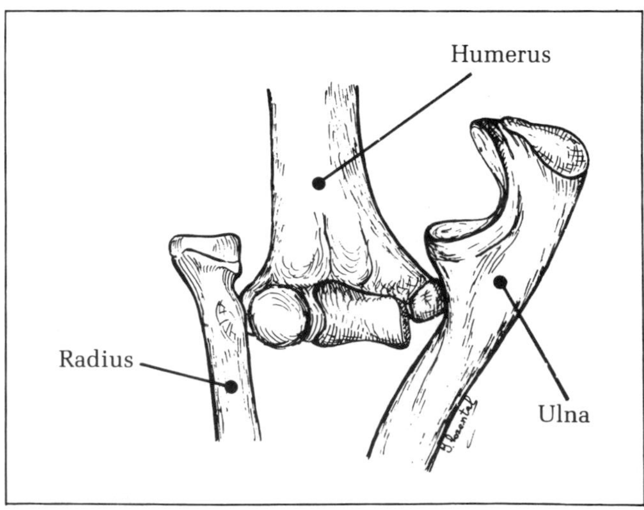

For example, when the head of the femur is popped backward out of its socket in the hip joint (posterior dislocation of the hip), the patient typically lies with his leg bent at the hip and knee, his thigh turned inward and pushed toward the midline of the body. Thus one would say that the thigh was "in internal rotation and adducted."

Dislocations can produce the same complications as fractures, namely damage to adjacent blood vessels or nerves that are pinched or stretched as the dislocated bone end impinges against them. Thus the survey of every suspected dislocation must also include an inquiry about numbness and tingling and a check of distal pulses, sensation, and movement.

SPRAINS

A sprain is the stretching or tearing of a ligament (Fig. 17-11), and it occurs when a joint is forced beyond its normal range of motion, usually as the result of twisting forces. Sprains most commonly involve the ankle or the knee. In ankle sprains, the mechanism is usually a sudden inward twisting (**inversion**) or outward twisting (**eversion**) of the foot, which places the person's body weight squarely on the stretched ligament. Knee injuries are more apt to occur when the foot remains fixed and the leg is subjected to a sudden twist.

Sprains vary in severity from very mild stretching of a ligament to complete separation of the ligament from one of the bones to which it attaches. When such separation occurs, the sprain may be accompanied by dislocation. A severe sprain may present signs and symptoms very similar to those of fractures or dislocations, that is, PAIN, TENDERNESS, SWELLING, REDNESS or sometimes ecchymosis, and GUARDING OR PAINFUL MOVEMENT. In general, however, deformity is *not* a feature of sprains unless there is associated dislocation, and the absence of deformity can sometimes assist in making a distinction between sprains and other musculoskeletal injuries.

Symptoms and Signs of Sprains
- PAIN, aggravated by motion
- TENDERNESS
- SWELLING AND REDNESS

Sometimes it will be impossible in the field to distinguish between a fracture, a dislocation, and a sprain. For this reason, a good rule of thumb is

WHEN IN DOUBT, TREAT THE INJURY AS A FRACTURE.

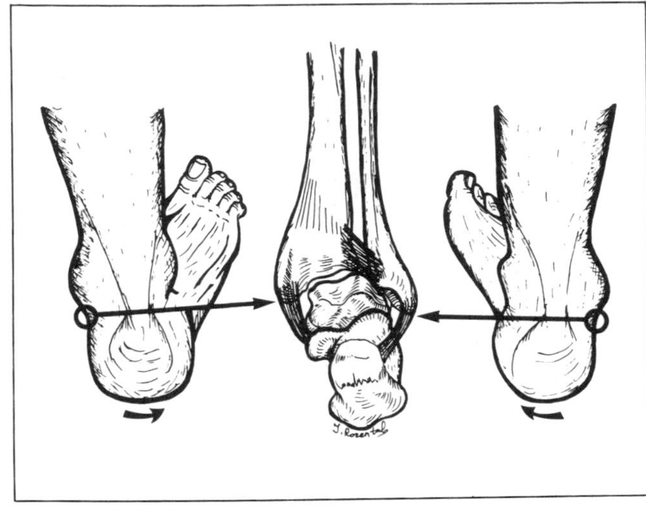

Fig. 17-11. *Mechanism of inversion* (left) and eversion (right) *injury to the ankle.*

Let us summarize, then, the principal points of emphasis in evaluating a patient for musculoskeletal injury:

Evaluation of Musculoskeletal Injury: Points to Remember
- History:
  1. MECHANISMS OF INJURY: What FORCES were applied and in what direction?
  2. Is there PAIN? If so, where?
  3. Did the patient feel a SNAP, CRACKLE, OR POP?
  4. Does the patient feel NUMBNESS OR TINGLING in the injured limb?
- Signs of Musculoskeletal Injury:
  1. TENDERNESS.
  2. DEFORMITY or UNNATURAL MOTION.
  3. SHORTENING of the extremity.
  4. SWELLING and REDNESS or ECCHYMOSIS.
  5. PAINFUL or ABSENT MOTION.
  6. GRATING of bone ends.
  7. BONE ENDS VISIBLE protruding from a wound.
- Signs of Complications:
  1. ABSENT DISTAL PULSE.
  2. ABSENT SENSATION OR MOTION distal to the injury.
  3. Signs of SHOCK.
- LOOK FOR INJURIES THAT COME IN PAIRS.

GENERAL PRINCIPLES IN TREATING MUSCULOSKELETAL INJURIES

The title of this discussion is somewhat misleading, for in medicine we do not treat injuries; we treat people. This is more than a matter of playing with words, for it brings us to a very important principle regarding fractures, dislocations, and sprains:

MUSCULOSKELETAL INJURIES ARE RARELY, IF EVER, AN IMMEDIATE THREAT TO LIFE.

One must look at the *whole* patient, not just the twisted arm or leg. Granted, a grotesquely deformed limb may be the most obvious and dramatic injury in a victim of multiple trauma, but it is unlikely to be the most serious injury, and it should not distract the EMT from fundamental priorities.

A FRACTURE CAN WAIT. THE AIRWAY CANNOT.

Thus the first principle in treating fractures, dislocations, and sprains is that they are relatively *low priority injuries*—way down the list after airway, breathing, circulation, bleeding, and wounds. Indeed, in the severely injured patient, stabilizing fractures is usually the last thing you do before moving the patient to the hospital.

This is not to imply that the treatment of musculoskeletal injuries is unimportant. As noted in the introduction to this chapter, the EMT can significantly shorten a patient's hospital stay and minimize subsequent disability by proper handling of fractures and related injuries in the field. Musculoskeletal injuries *are* important, but in general you have plenty of time to treat them.

THE REASONS FOR SPLINTING

The basic principle in treating musculoskeletal injuries is to splint them; that is, to secure the injured part to a supporting object in order to prevent movement of the part. Immobilization accomplishes several useful objectives. First of all, it tends to alleviate pain, which is always a primary goal in treatment. Pain is not only undesirable in itself, but it can also aggravate shock, and thus it must be minimized. In the second place, immobilization limits further damage to muscles, nerves, and blood vessels surrounding broken bone ends. A fractured extremity allowed to flop about freely is susceptible to significant secondary damage, as the jagged edges of broken bones continue to shred nearby tissues. Immobilization prevents this from happening. By the same token, a splint will prevent a closed fracture from becoming an open fracture, which can otherwise easily occur if the limb is further jarred and a bone end is jammed through the skin. Finally, splinting reduces local hemorrhage and swelling, and indeed in some cases it may not be possible to control bleeding from a fractured extremity until a splint has been applied.

Reasons for Splinting

- To minimize pain
- To prevent further damage to muscle, nerves, and blood vessels
- To prevent a closed fracture from becoming an open fracture
- To reduce bleeding and swelling

PRINCIPLES OF SPLINTING

Regardless of the location of the injury or the type of splint used to immobilize it, there are certain rules that apply to splinting in general. To begin with, the EMT has to be able to *see* precisely what kind of injury is involved—how extensive it is, whether it encompasses a joint, whether it is open or closed. This means that clothing must be cut away from any suspected fracture or dislocation, for you cannot properly visualize an injured area when it is covered with clothes. So the first step in evaluating and treating a musculoskeletal injury is to VISUALIZE THE INJURED AREA.

Once the area is visible, take time to make a careful check of the injured extremity. Note and record (1) the position in which the extremity is found; (2) the presence of swelling, ecchymosis, or open injury; (3) the presence or absence of pulses distal to the injury; and (4) the presence or absence of sensation and movement distal to the injury. Feel the injured limb, and note whether it seems colder than the opposite limb.

Having finished your examination of the injured extremity, COVER ALL OPEN WOUNDS WITH STERILE DRESSINGS before proceeding with immobilization. Then choose a suitable splint (see following discussion). If it is a rigid splint, it should be fully padded so that it will not apply undue pressure to any given area of the limb.

FRACTURES THAT ARE SEVERELY ANGULATED SHOULD BE STRAIGHTENED WITH GENTLE TRACTION. When a bone is broken, there is a tendency for muscle attached to the broken bone to contract, which may in turn cause the two broken bone ends to override (that is one reason that a fractured limb may appear shorter than the opposite limb). Overriding of bone ends generally produces angulation of the fracture. An angulated fracture is by nature unstable. The purpose of traction, then, is to counter the tendency for the limb to be angulated and thereby minimize the damage from overriding bone ends. Traction *does not* attempt to pull the limb back in perfect alignment. That process—called *reduction* of a fracture—is carried out in the hospital, with x-rays to assist in visualizing the exact position of the broken bone ends.

In order to apply traction, first explain to the patient that straightening the fracture may cause a momentary increase in pain, but that pain relief will be significant once the fracture is straightened and splinted. Then grasp the injured extremity firmly with both hands—one hand proximal and the other distal to the injury—and exert steady, *gentle* traction in a line with the bone (Fig. 17-12). DO NOT USE EXCESSIVE FORCE!

Dislocations or fractures involving joints require particular caution. An attempt may be made—very gently!—to straighten the deformity, but if the maneuver meets resistance or causes the patient an increase in pain, leave the injury as it is, and "splint it as it lies," that is, splint it in the position in which it was found. Attempts to force an injured joint back into position can cause severe damage to the nervous and vascular structures around the joint.

When dealing with open fractures, DO NOT ATTEMPT TO PUSH EXPOSED BONE ENDS BACK BENEATH THE SKIN, for this will simply guarantee that all the dirt and bacteria on the skin surface are dragged deep into the wound. Cover the bone ends with a sterile dressing that has been slightly moistened with sterile saline. Sometimes the process of straightening an angulated fracture will itself tend to pull bone ends back into the wound. In general, try to avoid letting this happen and apply traction only to the point that the bone ends are not drawn beneath the skin. If despite these precautions bone fragments should return to the soft tissue during splinting, notify the emergency room staff of this fact when you arrive with the patient.

In any fracture, always IMMOBILIZE THE JOINT ABOVE AND BELOW THE SITE OF INJURY. For example, if you are dealing with a fracture of the shaft of the radius, your splint should be long enough and shaped properly to immobilize the wrist and the elbow. If you immobilize the wrist only, the radius still has a great deal of play every time the elbow is turned. When a *joint* is injured, immobilize the bone above and below the joint; for instance, in an elbow injury, the splint should be secured at both the forearm and upper arm.

SPLINT FIRMLY, BUT NOT SO TIGHTLY AS TO OCCLUDE THE CIRCULATION. Always try to leave the distal part of the extremity out of the bandage so that you can check the circulation after the splint has been applied. If the distal pulses are inaccessible (e.g., in our radial fracture, whose splint encompassed both the elbow and wrist joints), at least leave the tips of the fingers or toes accessible to check for

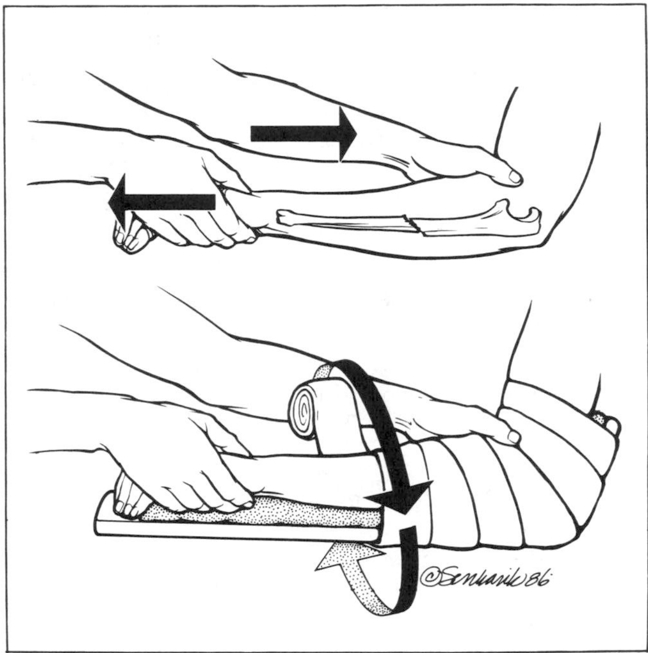

Fig. 17-12. *A fractured arm is held in traction and splinted while traction is maintained.*

CAPILLARY REFILL. To do so, press down on the fingernail or toenail until it blanches, and then release it. If circulation is intact, the nail bed should immediately "pink up" as it quickly refills with blood. If pulses were present before you applied your splint and the pulse or capillary refill is absent afterward, the splint is too tight.

ALWAYS CHECK AND RECHECK DISTAL CIRCULATION AFTER YOU HAVE APPLIED A SPLINT. THEN CHECK AGAIN.

If the patient's condition is stable, IMMOBILIZE ALL FRACTURED OR DISLOCATED EXTREMITIES BEFORE ATTEMPTING TO MOVE THE PATIENT. When there are multiple fractures, this may take some time, but it is time well spent—even though your diplomatic resources may be taxed by impatient bystanders or police who demand to know why you are "hanging around" at the scene. Simply explain that you are "hanging around" because your job is to make sure the patient's injuries are not aggravated and that moving the patient without proper splinting could cause serious additional damage.

For the patient who has multiple, serious injuries, emphasis must be on expeditious transport to the hospital. Such a patient will fare better with minimal splinting at the scene (MAST plus spinal immobilization) and rapid evacuation than with painstaking, time-consuming immobilization of every potential fracture. As we will learn in Chapter 18, salvage of life always takes precedence over salvage of limb.

What about the injury you are not sure about? It could be a fracture, but then again it could be a sprain. You will not do any harm to a sprained limb by immobilizing it in a splint, but you could do considerable harm to a fractured limb by failing to immobilize it. Thus, WHEN IN DOUBT, TREAT THE INJURY AS A FRACTURE AND SPLINT IT.

Wherever possible, ELEVATE AN INJURED EXTREMITY. A patient with an injured ankle, for example, is best transported supine or semisitting, with his splinted ankle elevated on pillows. This promotes drainage from the limb by gravity and thereby minimizes swelling.

General Principles of Splinting

- VISUALIZE THE INJURED AREA: Cut away clothing as needed.
- RECORD STATUS OF PULSES, SENSATION, and MOTION distal to the injury.
- DRESS WOUNDS BEFORE SPLINTING FRACTURES.
- STRAIGHTEN SEVERELY ANGULATED FRACTURES.
    1. Use extreme caution for injuries involving joints.
    2. NEVER USE FORCE.
- DO NOT PUSH BONE ENDS BACK BENEATH THE SKIN.
- PAD RIGID SPLINTS GENEROUSLY.
- IMMOBILIZE THE JOINTS ABOVE AND BELOW THE INJURY.
- CHECK AND RECKECK THE DISTAL PULSE AFTER APPLYING A SPLINT.
- IMMOBILIZE ALL FRACTURES BEFORE MOVING THE PATIENT.
- Where possible, ELEVATE THE INJURED EXTREMITY.
- In major trauma, THE AXIAL SKELETON IS ALWAYS SPLINTED ON A LONG BACKBOARD.
- WHEN IN DOUBT, SPLINT.

TYPES OF SPLINTS

Splints are of two general types: those that come supplied with the patient and those that do not. By a splint that comes with the patient, we mean any part of the patient's body that is used to support and immobilize an injured part. An injured arm, for example, can be secured to the chest, or an injured leg can be secured to the uninjured leg. The use of the patient's own body as a splint can be a very handy and effective method for immobilizing certain types of fractures, especially in mass casualty situations, for this kind of splinting requires a minimum of equipment.

Besides the patient's own body, there exist a large variety of devices that can be used to immobilize a fracture, sprain, or dislocation. We will confine our discussion here to commercially available, professional splints, for this is the equipment the EMT will be using in the bulk of his or her work. It is, however, a worthwhile exercise now and then to stage a multicasualty drill and see how well you can improvise without the commercial splints. Any device that can hold an injured extremity still in the proper position can be used as a splint: a rolled newspaper, a cane, an umbrella, a broom handle, and so forth. The possibilities are limited only by the limits of the EMT's imagination, and lack of a commercially made splint should NEVER prevent a well-trained EMT from properly immobilizing an injured patient. Not long ago, a young farmer who suffered a cervical spine injury when his tractor overturned arrived in the emergency room of an Israeli hospital immobilized to a barn door—attesting to the fact that a good EMT will find a way to get the job done even if the standard equipment is not available.

Rigid Splints

A rigid splint is a device that is applied along the side, front, or back of an injured extremity to give the extremity stability. It can be a board, a piece of heavy cardboard, a molded sheet of aluminum, or a wire "ladder" splint. Whatever its construction, it must (1) be SUFFICIENTLY LONG to be secured beyond the joints above and below the fracture site and (2) be GENEROUSLY PADDED to make sure that there is uniform pressure between the limb and the splint along their entire line of contact.

To use a rigid splint for immobilizing a *fracture*, first grasp the injured extremity above and below the fracture site as shown in Figure 17-12, and apply gentle, steady traction in line with the limb. While you continue to hold the limb in traction, have an assistant place the well-padded splint alongside the limb and wrap the limb and splint securely with self-adhering bandage. The fingers or toes should be left out of the bandage so that the nailbeds can be checked periodically for capillary refill. Remember:

A RIGID SPLINT IS EFFECTIVE ONLY IF IT IS LONG ENOUGH TO IMMOBILIZE THE JOINTS ON EITHER SIDE OF THE FRACTURE.

When a rigid splint is used to immobilize a *dislocation* that must be left in the position in which it was found, the splint should be secured to the bones on either side of the dislocated joint. If, for instance, the elbow is dislocated in a flexed position, the splint will have to cross the elbow at an angle and be secured at the mid-arm above and the mid-forearm below (Fig. 17-13). In some types of dislocations, as we shall see, it is more convenient to use the patient's body as a splint.

Soft Splints

A soft splint, as the name implies, is made of relatively soft material and is usually applied *around* the injured extremity. Soft splints include air splints, pillow splints, and slings.

The AIR SPLINT is an inflatable plastic cylinder that comes in a variety of sizes and is useful primarily for fractures of the *forearm* and *lower leg*. It is an excellent splint for injuries of these areas, for it provides good stabilization, is easy to apply, is comfortable for the patient, and has the added advantage of exerting uniform, circumferential pressure on the injured limb, which helps control bleeding.

To describe application of an air splint, let us consider as an example a forearm fracture. If the air splint is the type without a zipper, slide the deflated air splint backward up your own forearm (i.e., so that the wider part is closest to your wrist). With the same hand, grasp the patient's hand (injured arm side), and pull gently toward you while an assistant holds countertraction at the patient's shoulder or upper arm (Fig. 17-14). If there is an open wound on the extremity, the assistant should cover the wound with a sterile dressing before you proceed further. Then slide the air splint over your hand and up along the patient's arm until the proximal end of the splint is well above the patient's elbow and the distal end is just above his knuckles. The splint should be wrinkle-free. While you continue to maintain traction, your assistant should inflate the splint *by mouth*. NEVER USE ANY TYPE OF PUMP TO INFLATE AN AIR SPLINT—LUNG POWER ONLY! A mechanical pump can overinflate the splint and cause damaging levels of pressure to be exerted on the limb. Inflate the splint just to the point at which finger pressure will make a slight dent in it. Do not forget to check the nail beds for capillary refill once the splint has been inflated.

Fig. 17-13. *A rigid splint used to stabilize an injured (e.g., dislocated) elbow.*

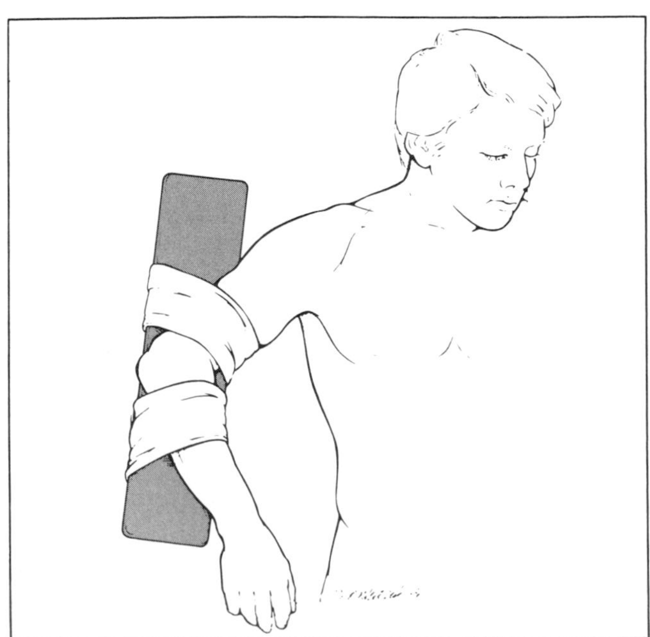

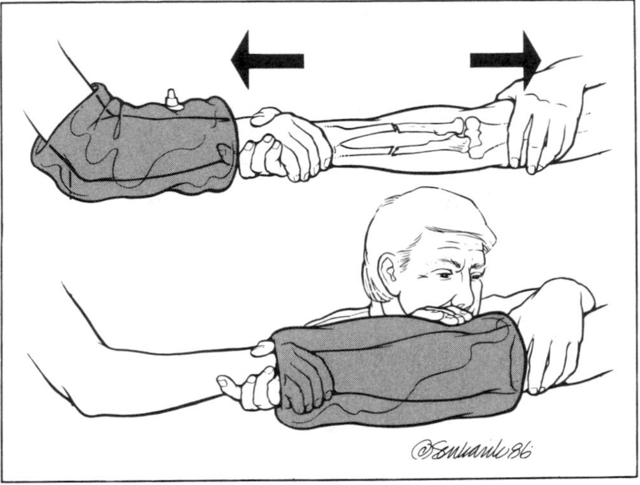

Fig. 17-14. *Application of an air splint. A. The rescuer pushes the splint up his own arm and then holds the patient's arm in traction; a second rescuer maintains countertraction. B. The air splint is slid across to the patient's arm and is inflated by the second rescuer, while the first rescuer maintains traction.*

If the air splint is of the type equipped with a zipper, simply apply it to the fractured limb while an assistant holds the limb in traction proximally and distally; then zip it up, and inflate it as described.

When it is anticipated that the air splint will have to remain in place for more than about an hour, and especially in hot weather, it is desirable to place some material between the plastic splint and the patient's skin, for sweating within the splint can cause maceration of the skin. Ideally, the ambulance should be stocked with a roll of orthopedic stockinette, a length of which can simply be rolled onto the patient's arm or leg in a manner similar to that in which the air splint itself is slid into place. The air splint is then slid onto the limb on top of the stockinette, which will absorb some of the perspiration and keep the skin from direct contact with the plastic.

Air splints must be watched closely to make sure they do not lose pressure or become overinflated. Overinflation is particularly apt to occur when the patient is moved from a cold environment to a warm environment (e.g., from a ski slope to the heated ambulance), for as the air inside the splint warms, it will expand. Theoretically, this effect can also be seen if the patient is moved to an area of lower atmospheric pressure, as in aircraft transport. Recheck capillary refill frequently, and if the patient tells you that the splint feels tighter, listen to him! If capillary refill disappears, or if you can no longer indent the splint with pressure from your finger, the splint has become too tight, and you need to release some of the air.

Among other soft splints, a PILLOW makes an excellent support to immobilize an injured foot or ankle (Fig. 17-15). When a pillow is used for this purpose, it is molded around the injured foot and secured in place with cravats. A pillow is also useful as a means of providing padding and stability when placed between two legs that are being secured together or beneath a dislocated arm that is being secured to the chest. A small pillow secured to the chest with cravats is sometimes useful in stabilizing a flail segment.

Soft splinting materials also include SLINGS, which are used, sometimes in conjunction with a rigid splint, to immobilize injuries of the upper extremity. The sling supports the injured extremity and elevates it so that it does not hang dependent. For greater stability, a sling is usually used with one or two swaths to bind the sling to the patient's trunk (Fig. 17-16).

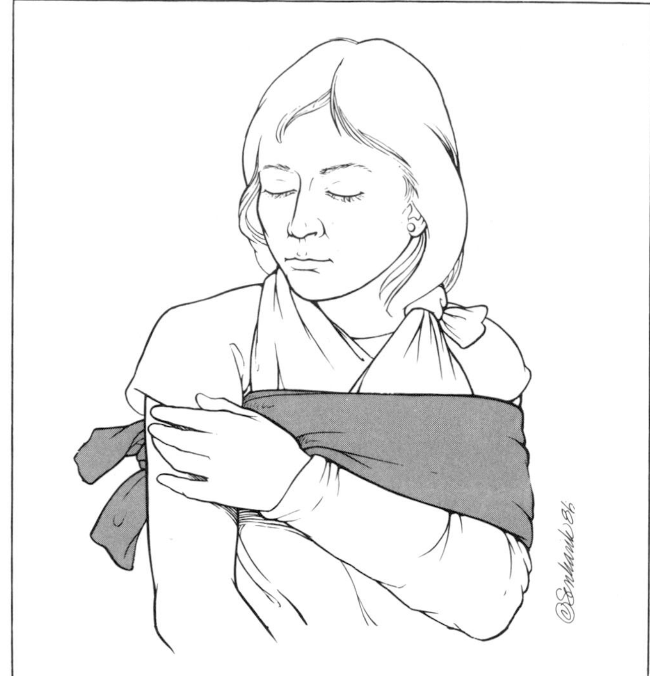

Fig. 17-16. *Sling and swath.*

Traction Splints

A traction splint is a device used to provide constant, steady traction on an injured extremity and thereby prevent broken bone ends from overriding as a result of muscle contractions. It is simply a mechanical means to accomplish the traction that is always a part of immobilization of a fracture. In practice, traction splints are used only for *lower* extremity fractures (chiefly fractures of the hip and femur), where countertraction is applied by seating the proximal part of the splint against the ischial bone of the pelvis. In the upper extremity, this is not feasible, for in order to develop countertraction, one would have to jam the proximal end of the splint into the armpit, where it could damage the complex of nerves and blood vessels passing through the axilla.

Fig. 17-15. *Pillow splint.*

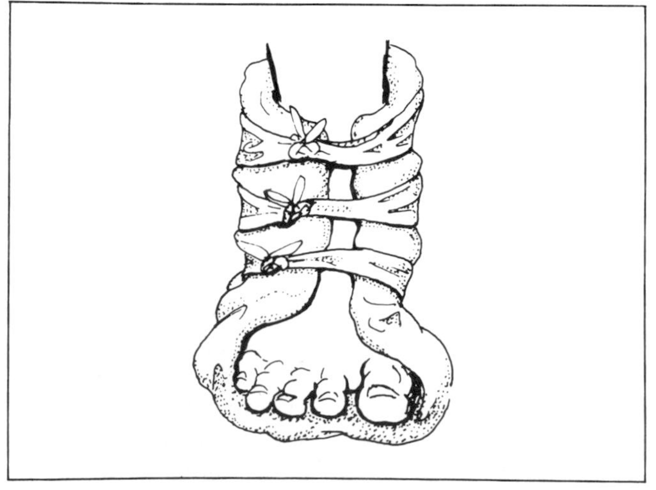

The traction splint was developed around the turn of the century by Sir Hugh Owen Thomas, an orthopedic surgeon, and nearly all traction splints in use today are based on Dr. Thomas's concept. The two basic types of traction splint found in ambulances are the Thomas half-ring splint, which is simply a metal frame with a padded half-ring at the top, and a mechanical version of the Thomas splint, which uses a ratchet mechanism instead of a Spanish windlass to tighten traction. The basic principles of application are the same for all traction splints, and for our discussion here we will use the simple Thomas half-ring splint as our model, since it is the least expensive and requires the fewest accessories.

Proper application of a traction splint is *not* easy and requires a great deal of practice (Fig. 17–17). The patient's injured leg should be exposed, by cutting open the trouser leg if necessary. Most authorities recommend that the patient's shoe be left on, to reduce the amount of pressure applied directly to the patient's foot. In general, this is a good idea, although the disadvantage in leaving the shoe in place is that the distal pulse and capillary refill cannot be checked. Bulky padding around the patient's instep can give some protection to the foot and at the same time permit visualization of the toes for checking distal circulation.

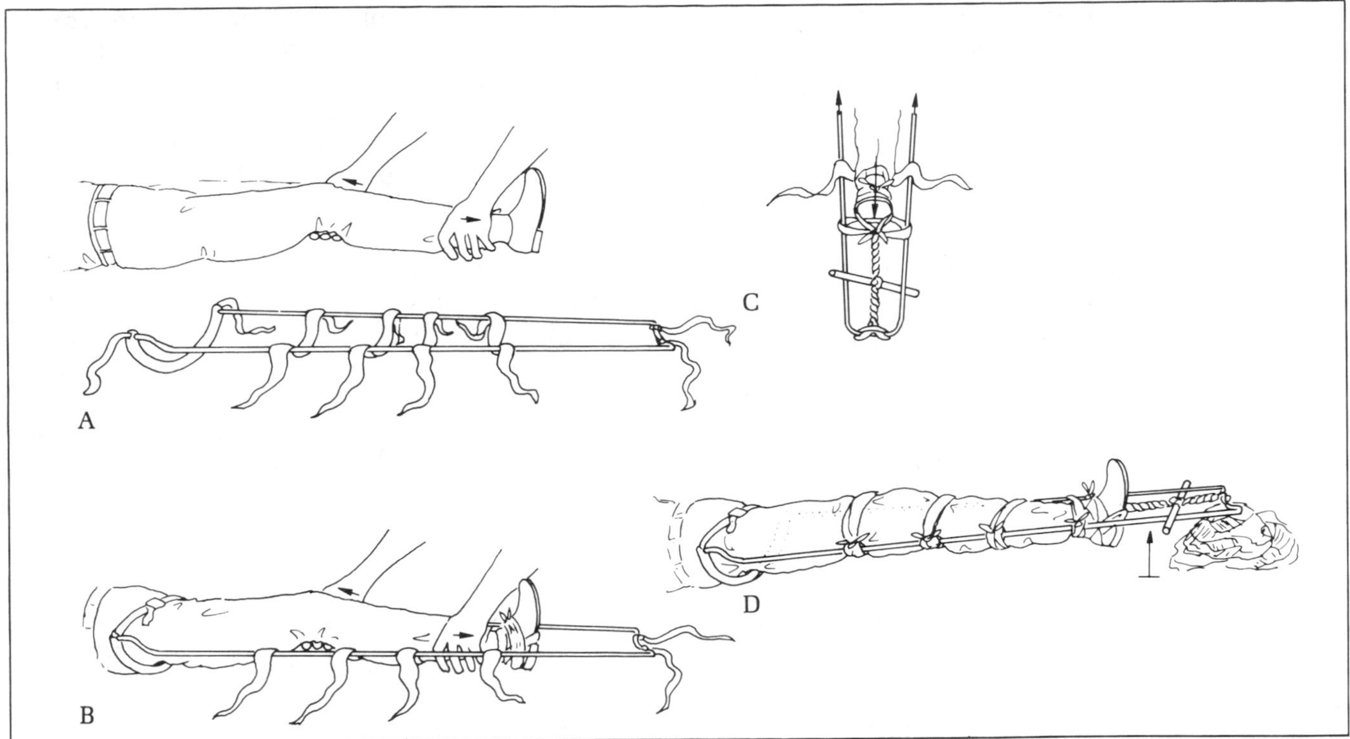

Fig. 17-17. *Application of a Thomas splint. A. Apply traction; prepare splint. B. Secure splint. C. Secure ankle hitch; develop traction. D. Secure support cravats; elevate splint.*

One rescuer (R1) applies traction to the injured leg by grasping the ankle and calf and exerting a gentle but steady *longitudinal* pull. As the first rescuer maintains traction, the second rescuer (R2) attaches an ankle hitch over the patient's ankle and foot. Commercial, padded ankle hitches are preferable, but if these are not available, a Collins hitch can be devised using a cravat. Rope, wire, tape, or other narrow materials should *not* be used to improvise an ankle hitch, for they can act as a tourniquet to cut off the circulation at the ankle. Once the ankle is secured, R2 exerts longitudinal traction with the hitch, while R1 releases his grip on the patient's leg and proceeds to prepare the splint.

R1 measures the splint alongside the patient and adjusts it to the correct length, which is about 12 to 18 inches longer than the distances from the patient's groin to the heel. A cravat is secured as a lock hitch to the distal end of the splint, as shown in Figure 17-18. Then while R2 elevates the injured leg slightly (still maintaining traction through the ankle hitch), R1 slides the splint beneath the leg so that the padded half-ring is snugly seated against the patient's ischial tuberosity. The patient's groin should be well padded, and care must be taken that the splint is not jammed up against the genitals (a conscious patient will usually let you know quite promptly if this happens!). With the splint properly seated, R1 secures the splint in position by fastening the ischial strap. R1 then moves to the foot end of the splint and fastens the loops of the ankle hitch to the lock hitch at the bottom of the splint. All this while, R2 continues to maintain longitudinal traction from the foot.

Fig. 17-18. *Lock hitch for half-ring splint.*

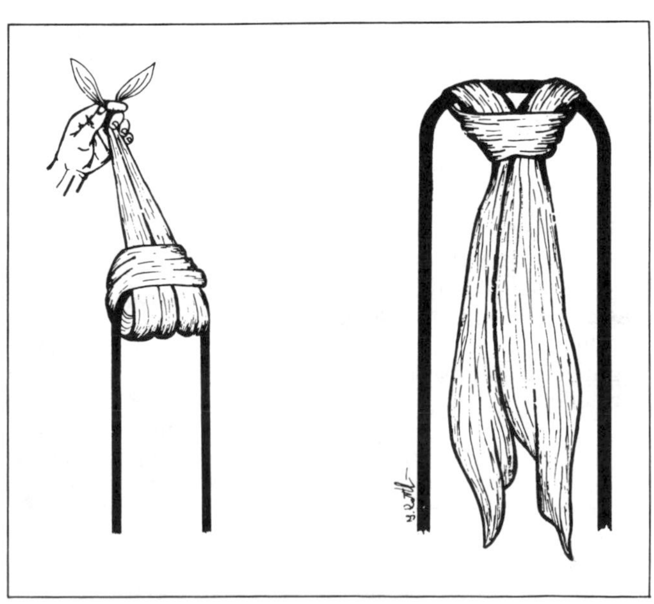

At this point, traction is developed by placing a stick between the loops of the lock hitch and twisting the stick (Spanish windlass technique), which in turn shortens the lock hitch and pulls the foot toward the distal end of the splint. If a mechanical traction splint is used, the ratchet knob is turned by hand to develop traction. The amount of traction that should be applied is that necessary to hold the limb in a secure, correct position and alleviate the patient's pain. At that point, the stick should be secured. The support slings (which may be either cravats or Velcro fasteners) are then secured in place above and below the knee and at the midcalf, in order to fasten the limb closely to the length of the splint. Finally, the splint is elevated so that the patient's foot is kept clear of the ground. The application of a traction splint is summarized in Table 17-1.

Vacuum Splints

The vacuum splint was developed in Europe and only recently has come into use in the United States. It consists of a sealed mattress that is filled with air and thousands of small plastic beads. The mattress is laid out on the stretcher, and the patient is placed on top of it and allowed to settle into a comfortable position. Then a suction pump attached to the mattress is used to evacuate all the air from inside the mattress. This creates a vacuum inside the mattress, which compresses the beads in such a way that the whole splint becomes rigid—like a plaster cast that has been molded to conform to the contour of the patient's entire posterior surface. Thus the vacuum splint in effect provides a tailor-made posterior body cast for each patient.

The vacuum mattress is an excellent splint, but it has several significant drawbacks that limit its usefulness. To begin with, the mattress-type vacuum splint is quite bulky and thus not only takes up a lot of storage room in the vehicle but also can be difficult to work with in cramped quarters. Furthermore, it requires that one carry along a mechanical suction pump, yet another piece of equipment. Finally, the vacuum mattress is relatively expensive and may not be within the means of every ambulance company. Smaller vacuum splints, for upper and lower extremities, are available however; and these can be a valuable addition to the EMT's gear.

Table 17-1. *Application of a Traction Splint: Summary*

First Rescuer	Second Rescuer
Cuts trouser leg as needed.	
Applies traction, grasping ankle and calf.	
	Attaches ankle hitch, and takes over traction at the foot.
Releases grip on leg.	Maintains longitudinal traction.
Measures and adjusts splint.	
Attaches lock hitch.	
Seats half-ring properly, and fastens ischial strap.	
Fastens ankle hitch to lock hitch.	
Tightens windlass or ratchet.	
	Gradually releases manual traction as splint develops traction.
Secures windlass or ratchet.	Fastens support slings.
Elevates end of splint.	

TREATMENT OF UPPER EXTREMITY INJURIES

The upper extremity extends from the shoulder girdle to the fingertips and can be injured just about anywhere in between.

SHOULDER INJURIES

Shoulder injuries involve the clavicle, scapula, or the head of the humerus, and the sling and swath will be your handiest splint in stabilizing the majority of these injuries.

Injuries to the Clavicle

The clavicle has a quite superficial location and is relatively vulnerable to trauma. Injury to the clavicle is usually caused by indirect force, such as a fall onto the shoulder or onto an outstetched hand, although the clavicle can also be broken by a direct blow, as in contact sports.

FRACTURES OF THE CLAVICLE (Fig. 17-19A) are seen in all age groups, but most commonly in children. The patient will complain of pain in the area of the injury and will not raise his arm on the injured side. Indeed, often the patient will hold the arm of the injured side against his chest with the other hand in order to prevent motion in the shoulder and the pain it causes. Typically, the patient cocks his head toward the injured side to loosen the pull of his neck muscles on the fractured area. Swelling, tenderness, deformity, and sometimes crepitus will be evident over the fracture. As with any extremity fracture, the distal pulses should be checked when the patient is first examined and again later, after the injury has been splinted.

A *sling and swath* provides adequate temporary splinting for a fractured clavicle. It should be applied so that the forearm is well supported and does not droop downward. In the hospital, the fracture

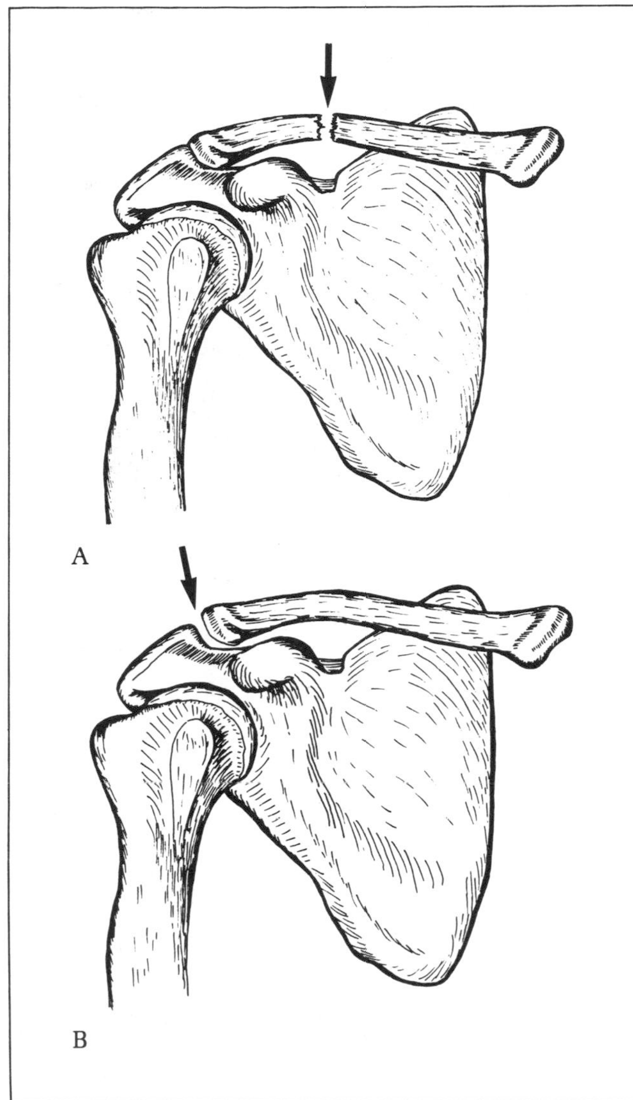

Fig. 17-19. *A. Fracture of the clavicle. B. Dislocation of the clavicle.*

may be reduced with a figure-of-eight bandage, but there is no need to attempt reduction in the field. Cold compresses applied to the injured area may provide significant relief of pain.

DISLOCATIONS OF THE CLAVICLE (Fig. 17-19B) most commonly involve the acromioclavicular joint, that is, the joint where the lateral end of the clavicle attaches to the acromial projection on the scapula. Separation of the acromioclavicular joint—sometimes called a "knocked down shoulder"—occurs commonly in athletes from a fall or a jar at the point of the shoulder. Usually the patient will be in considerable pain and will not be able to lift his arm or to bring his arm across his chest. The deformity tends to be quite obvious, and the skin may be stretched outward by the lateral end of the clavicle poking into it. Tenderness, swelling, and local ecchymosis may also be present.

Shoulder separations should be treated in the field with a *sling and swath*. Once again, a cold pack over the injured area may give substantial pain relief.

Injuries to the Scapula

FRACURE OF THE SCAPULA usually results from a direct blow to the shoulder blade. Because the scapula is buttressed by heavy muscles, it takes a very powerful blow to break it; thus the presence of a scapular fracture should be a tip-off to the EMT that strong forces were involved in the accident, and associated injuries (e.g., rib fracture, lung contusion) are likely. The injured area will be swollen, tender, and often ecchymotic. There may be noticeable deformity if the bone has been displaced. The patient's chest should be examined carefully, with special attention to the stability of the ribs and the presence of breath sounds on both sides. In the absence of other injuries, the fractured scapula can be adequately splinted with a *sling and swath*.

Dislocations of the Shoulder Joint

Dislocations of the shoulder account for about half of all major joint dislocations. The vast majority of shoulder dislocations are anterior; that is, the head of the humerus pops *forward* out of the socket. ANTERIOR DISLOCATIONS are most common in the under-30 generation and are often associated with athletic injuries. The mechanism of injury is one in which force is applied along the arm when it is abducted (held away from the body) and externally rotated, as for instance when someone falls backward onto an outstretched arm. The resulting force drives the head of the humerus forward and pops it out in front of the shoulder joint.

The patient with an anterior dislocation of the shoulder will usually resist any attempt to move his arm on the injured side and often grasps the arm of the injured side to protect it from motion. The shoulder itself looks obviously deformed, with a very prominent acromion, and the head of the humerus can usually be palpated anteriorly. The arm tends to be abducted and externally rotated. Recall that the major nerves and blood vessels to the upper extremity travel just beneath the shoulder joint, in the axilla; thus it is crucial to check the distal pulse, sensation, and movement in patients with shoulder dislocation. Some degree of nerve injury occurs in about 10 percent of patients with anterior shoulder dislocation.

The anterior shoulder dislocation presents an awkward target for splinting because the patient's arm is fixed in abduction. Probably the most comfortable splinting method is to place a *pillow* between the involved arm and the chest, to fill the space created by abduction of the arm, and then use *cravats* or roller bandage to secure the arm against the chest. The patient may be more comfortable if the arm is support in a sling before being strapped (Fig. 17-20).

POSTERIOR DISLOCATION OF THE SHOULDER is a relatively rare occurrence, accounting for only about 5 percent of all shoulder dislocations. Often the history seems unrelated to the shoulder. The majority of cases, for example, occur during seizures; after the patient regains consciousness, he complains of stiffness in his shoulder or inability to raise his arm—complaints that rescuers may tend to brush aside in their concern over the seizures themselves. The shoulder deformity in a posterior dislocation is not as obvious as that in an anterior dislocation—another reason why this injury is frequently missed. Careful examination will usually reveal that the arm is *internally* rotated, and if you palpate the head of the humerus, it is clear that it is not where it should be.

A posterior dislocation should be splinted in a position of comfort, which is usually best accomplished with a *sling and swath.*

FRACTURES OF THE HUMERUS

Fractures of the humerus can occur in any part of the bone, from its proximal articulation in the shoulder to its distal end at the elbow.

The same type of forces that produce a dislocated shoulder in a young person are apt to produce a FRACTURE OF THE PROXIMAL HUMERUS in an elderly person. The injury tends to be very painful and usually produces marked swelling, deformity, and discoloration in the area of the shoulder. The patient will not be able to move his upper arm. Once again, the trusty friend of the upper extremity, the *sling and swath,* makes a good splint for this type of injury.

FRACTURES OF THE SHAFT OF THE HUMERUS can be caused by either a direct blow or an indirect force, such as falling on an outstretched hand. The humeral shaft may also be fractured in association with a shoulder dislocation. When a direct blow is involved, the chest wall is frequently injured as well, and the EMT should be alert to this possibility when examining the patient. The fracture itself is usually obvious from swelling, deformity, and discoloration. It is very important to check the pulses and neurologic status distal to this fracture, for *injury to the radial nerve* is very common in association with fractures of the humeral shaft. The radial nerve supplies the muscles that extend the hand and fingers; when the radial nerve is damaged, these extensor muscles no longer receive signals to contract, so the hand cannot be extended. What one sees is a condition called "wrist drop"; that is, the patient's hand hangs like a limp rag from the wrist. Wrist drop is an important sign that radial nerve damage has occurred, and it should be carefully recorded on the

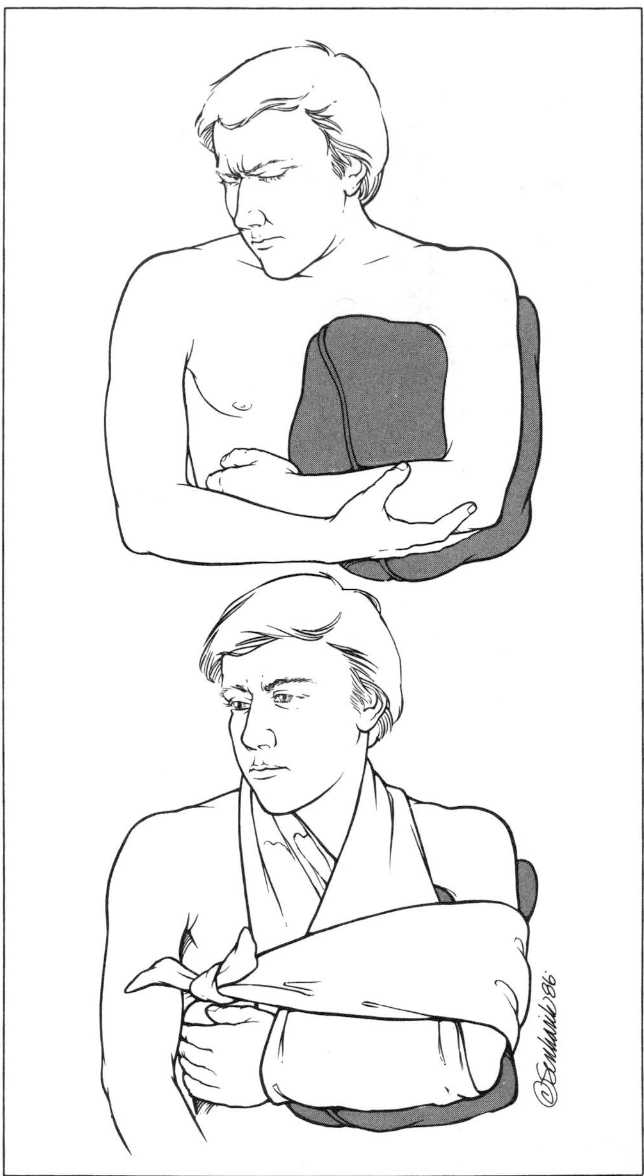

Fig. 17-20. *Pillow, sling, and swath for a shoulder dislocation.*

patient's trip sheet, along with the status of distal pulses and sensation.

Fracture of the humeral shaft is best managed with a *sling and swath.* First support the forearm in a sling, with the hand elevated above the elbow; then use roller gauze to bandage the entire arm, sling and all, to the chest. Keep the fingers out of the sling and bandage, so that you can check the nail beds periodically for capillary refill. If the fracture is severely angulated, it should be gently straightened and held in position with a *padded board splint* rather than sling and swath. Do not forget, the board splint must be long enough to be fastened well below the elbow and at the shoulder. If there is any question of associated chest injury, be sure to administer oxygen.

FRACTURES OF THE DISTAL HUMERUS, just above the elbow, are extremely serious injuries because they are often accompanied by severe damage to the nerves and blood vessels that supply the forearm and hand (Fig. 17-21). If not handled properly, this injury can result in a dreaded complication called **Volkmann's ischemic contracture**, in which the fingers become contracted and powerless from hypoxic damage to tissue. The mechanism of distal humeral fracture is a fall on an extended or flexed elbow, and the advent of the skateboard has made this a fairly frequent injury. Fractures of the distal humerus produce marked to extreme deformity of the elbow, with massive swelling; it is not uncommon for these fractures to be open, with bone fragments protruding through the skin. A careful assessment should be made of the radial and ulnar pulses and of sensation and movement in the fingers; the findings should be recorded accurately. Absent pulses or absence of capillary refill indicates an urgent situation.

The method chosen to splint a fracture of the distal humerus will depend somewhat on the position in which the extremity is found. If the arm is in extension, it should be immobilized on a long *padded board splint* that extends from the axilla to at least the fingertips. Keep the fingertips out of the bandage, however, so that the nail beds can be checked. If the arm is found flexed at the elbow, it can be immobilized to the chest with a *sling and swath* or held in position with a padded board splint that is fixed at the mid-arm and mid-forearm (see Fig. 17-3). Before you immobilize the arm in a flexed position, however, make sure the radial pulse is present; if it is not, slightly extend the elbow, and recheck for a radial pulse. When the pulse reappears or the color improves in the distal extremity, you need not extend the arm further and can immobilize it in position.

Patients with injuries to the upper arm or shoulder girdle will in general be more comfortable sitting up and should be transported in a sitting position unless shock or other injuries preclude this.

Fig. 17-21. *Fracture of the distal humerus with impingement of the brachial artery and radial nerve.*

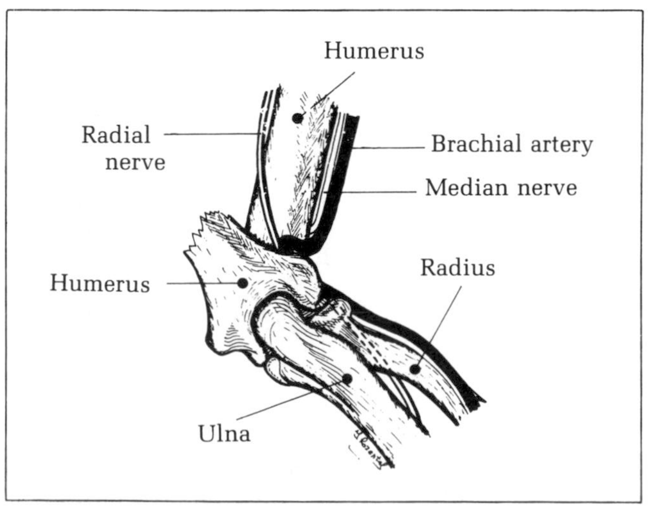

INJURIES TO THE ELBOW, FOREARM, AND WRIST

Dislocations of the Elbow

Dislocation of the elbow (see Fig. 17-10) usually occurs from a fall on a hyperextended arm. It may also be seen in a small child who has been lifted roughly by the elbows. The patient with a dislocated elbow complains of pain that is aggravated by any attempt to move the joint. He may also say that his elbow feels "locked" in position. The elbow itself is likely to be extremely deformed and may look very alarming. The wrist pulses should be checked, as well as sensation and movement of the fingers. Bear in mind that if the patient fell on an outstretched hand, the force transmitted to the elbow was also transmitted to the wrist; thus you should check for associated wrist fractures.

A dislocated elbow is best splinted in the position in which it is found, using either *sling and swath* or *padded board splint* secured above and below the joint, as for a fracture of the distal humerus.

Fractures of the Proximal Ulna and Radius

The proximal ulna—the part that hooks around the humerus and forms the "funny bone"—is called the olecranon, and it is usually fractured from a direct blow. Radial head fractures, on the other hand, are more likely to be due to indirect forces, such as the famous fall on the outstretched hand. In practice, these fractures can be difficult to distinguish in the field from other injuries to the elbow, and they should be treated the same way as elbow dislocations: SPLINT IT WHERE IT LIES, using *sling and swath, padded board splint*, or a *pillow splint*, whichever works best given the position in which the limb is found.

Fractures of the Forearm

Fractures of the forearm usually involve both the radius and the ulna and can be the result of either an indirect force or a direct blow. Once again, severe pain, swelling, and often marked deformity at the injured site are the hallmarks of forearm fracture. A fractured forearm is best immobilized with an *air splint*, applied with the arm held in traction as described earlier. To be effective, the splint must extend well above the elbow and below the wrist (IMMOBILIZE THE JOINTS ABOVE AND BELOW A FRACTURE—remember?). If the patient is transported supine, the splinted arm should be propped up on pillows to keep it elevated.

Fractures of the Wrist

The wrist can be fractured at one of the carpal bones, the distal radius, distal ulna, or any combination of these. The most common mechanism of injury is a fall onto an outstretched hand, especially in the elderly. One classic type of wrist fracture is called a Colles' fracture (after Abraham Colles, who first described the injury in 1814). In a Colles' fracture, the distal tips of the radius and ulna are broken (Fig. 17-22), and the hand and wrist are displaced. The Colles' fracture is also sometimes called a "silver fork" deformity, because when viewed from the side, the curve of the fractured wrist resembles that of a dinner fork.

Regardless of whether they involve the radius, ulna, or a carpal bone, wrist fractures should be immobilized in the same fashion. Either an *air splint* or *padded board splint* can be used, but in either case the elbow must be included in the splint to eliminate pronation and supination of the forearm, for these motions cause movement of the injured bones. The wrist should be gently straightened and secured with the splint. An air splint has the advantage that it may help minimize swelling in the wrist, which is apt to be considerable. For this reason, it is also a good idea to transport the patient supine, with the splinted wrist propped up on pillows.

Dislocations of the Wrist

Wrist dislocations are most commonly encountered in athletes, and a dislocated wrist is usually fractured as well. As in many of the other injuries we have considered, the mechanism is most often a fall onto an outstretched hand. In the field, a dislocated wrist can be difficult to distinguish from a fractured wrist, and as mentioned, fracture is likely to be a component of the injury anyway. Therefore a dislocated wrist should be treated as a fractured one, with gentle straightening and splinting with an *air splint* or *padded board splint*.

Fig. 17-22. *Colles' fracture with "silver fork" deformity.*

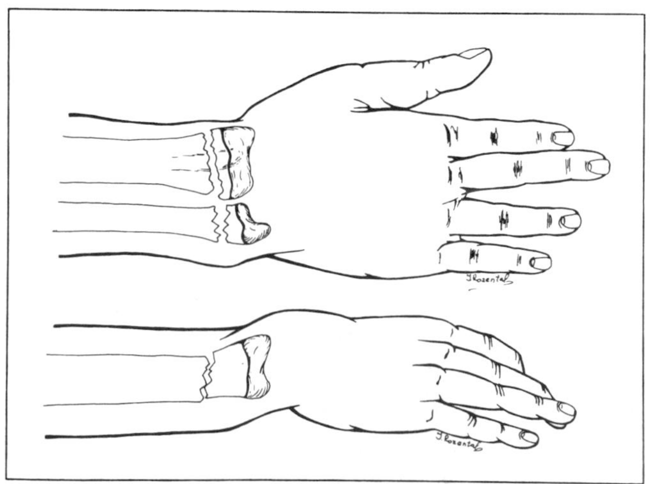

INJURIES TO THE HAND AND FINGERS

FRACTURE OF THE CARPALS OR METACARPALS can result from direct trauma or from force transmitted through the phalanges. Fracture of the fifth metacarpal head, for instance, is often called a "boxer's fracture," because it is commonly sustained when the closed fist is jammed into a hard object, such as someone's chin. Carpal and metacarpal fractures tend to be associated with a great deal of swelling in the hand, in addition to the pain and limitation of motion that characterize most fractures. The most important rule in managing fractures involving the hand is to SPLINT THE HAND IN A POSITION OF FUNCTION, which means with the fingers relaxed and slightly flexed. One way to do this is to fluff up some gauze pads into a large, soft ball and place these in the palm of the injured hand, with the fingers flexed around them. Then use self-adhering roller gauze to secure the hand around the ball of gauze. Once this is done, a padded board splint can be applied to immobilize the hand, wrist, and forearm. If the patient is sitting, the splinted hand should be placed in a sling tied so that the hand is held elevated above the heart. The pressure bandage around the hand, the splint, and elevation will all help to reduce the swelling of the injured hand, which may be massive.

FRACTURES OF THE PHALANGES are quite common, and about half of them occur as a result of industrial or athletic accidents. The car door is also a frequent offender, and as many as 10 percent of phalangeal fractures are sustained when a finger is slammed in a car door. When there is a fracture of the phalanx, the finger should be immobilized in a position of comfort. If the finger is relatively straight, it may be secured to a padded tongue depressor. If it is flexed, one of the more useful devices available commercially for splinting this type of finger injury is a strip of aluminum and foam rubber that can be cut to the desired length and bent to the desired curvature. Two words of caution are necessary regarding the splinting of finger fractures:

- DO NOT TAPE THE FINGER CIRCUMFERENTIALLY TO SECURE THE SPLINT. Fractured fingers swell, and tape applied around a finger can act as a tourniquet once swelling sets in. So do not bring the tape all the way around the finger; just have enough skin contact so that the tape holds the splint in position (Fig. 17-23).
- DO NOT USE ALUMINUM SPLINTS THAT REQUIRE "FEET" TO BE BENT AROUND THE FINGER ("frog splints"), for these splints can damage the skin and create a tourniquet effect if the finger swells.

As in hand injuries, a fractured finger should be kept elevated above the level of the heart to minimize

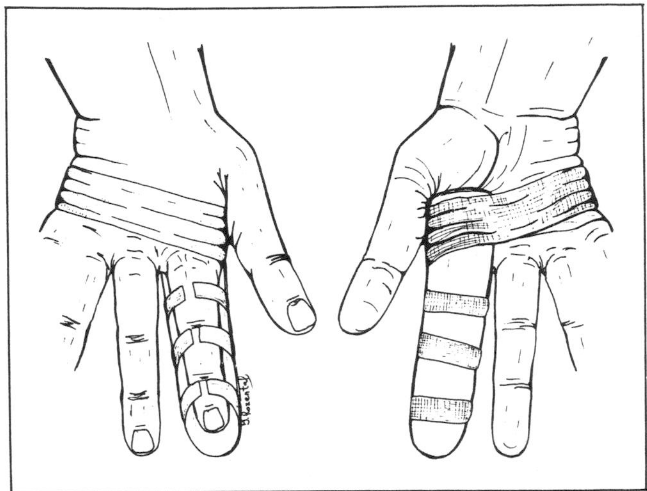

Fig. 17-23. *Finger splint. Note that tape is not circumferential, thus leaving room for the finger to swell.*

swelling. This is easily accomplished with a properly applied sling.

TREATMENT OF LOWER EXTREMITY INJURIES

FRACTURES OF THE PELVIS

Pelvic fracture is one of the most common causes of traumatic death—not because the fracture itself poses a threat to life, but because of the other serious problems likely to be associated with a fractured pelvis. About two-thirds of pelvic fractures are complicated by other fractures and/or soft tissue injury; nearly half of patients with pelvic fracture are in hemorrhagic shock by the time they reach the emergency room. Since these are usually closed fractures, the extent of bleeding may not be readily apparent, and early signs of shock may be missed if the EMT is not alert for them.

Conditions Commonly Associated with Pelvic Fracture

- HEMORRHAGIC SHOCK, due to bleeding into the pelvic cavity
- LUMBOSACRAL SPINE injury
- BLADDER laceration or rupture
- Damage to OTHER ABDOMINAL ORGANS
- Fractures of the LOWER EXTREMITIES

Pelvic fracture is usually the result of compression injury, in which the pelvic bone is crushed between two hard objects, and by far the most common scenario for this type of injury is the vehicular accident. Falls from heights also cause a significant number of pelvic injuries. The amount of force necessary to produce a pelvic fracture is considerably less in old people than in young people, and in an elderly person, even a fairly trivial fall can cause pelvis injury.

Pelvic fracture can involve any of the pelvic bones. Common sites for pelvic fracture are shown in Figure 17-24. The patient with a pelvic fracture will usually complain of pain in the injured area. The hallmark of a fractured pelvis is PAIN FELT WHEN THE PELVIS IS COMPRESSED (Fig. 17-25), and often this pain is experienced in the pubic area. The pelvis may feel unstable as well, and sometimes deformity will be evident.

In treating a patient with pelvic fracture, priority must be given to associated life-threatening injuries. Ten to thirty percent of patients with pelvic fracture die from hypoxia or hemorrhage. Thus securing the AIRWAY, administration of OXYGEN, and CONTROL OF BLEEDING must be the first steps of treatment. Bear in mind too that forces powerful enough to disrupt the massive pelvic ring are likely to have produced spinal injury as well, and the patient must be immobilized accordingly.

The most effective means of immobilizing a pelvic fracture is with the *Military Anti-Shock Trousers*, and if the patient is showing signs of shock, the MAST should be applied and inflated without delay. If the patient is stable and not showing signs of shock, it is a good idea to apply the MAST anyway, so that it can be rapidly inflated should shock develop. Meanwhile, the patient should be secured to a *long backboard*, with his knees slightly flexed and supported on a pillow.

INJURIES TO THE HIP

Dislocations of the Hip

Dislocation of the hip is a major injury, for the forces necessary to displace the head of the femur from its socket can be expected to produce considerable soft

Fig. 17-24. *Possible sites of pelvic fracture.*

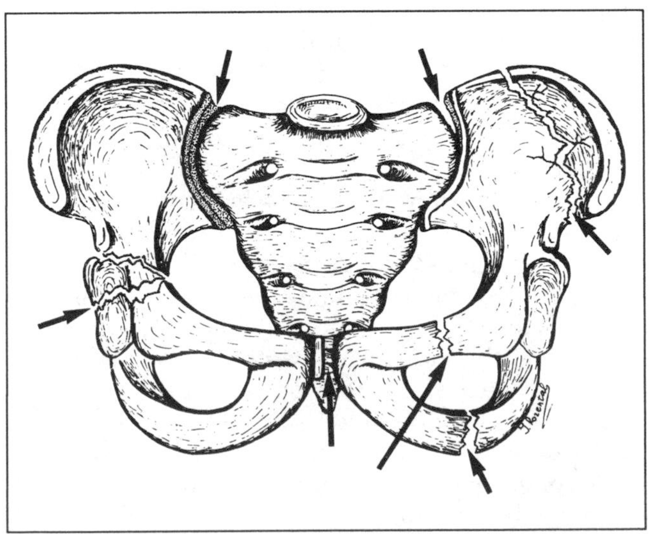

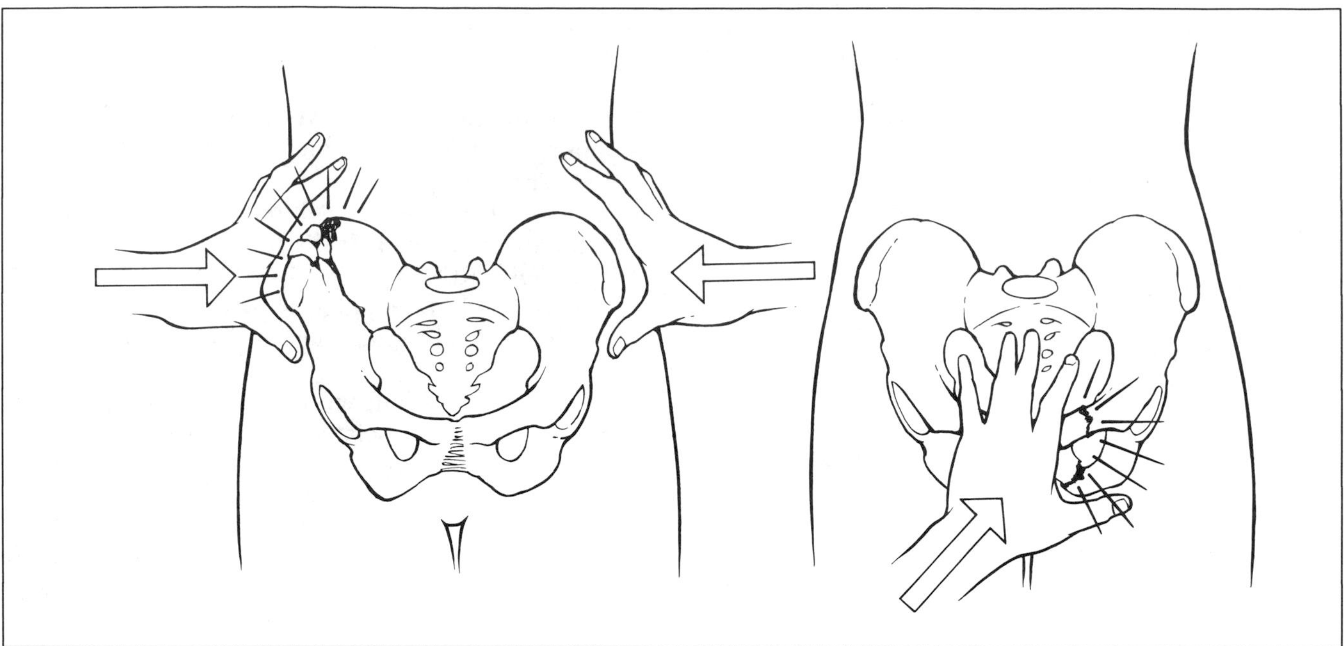

Fig. 17-25. *Pelvic fracture. When the pelvis is fractured, compression of the iliac crests or the pubic symphysis elicits pain.*

tissue damage as well. There is frequently associated fracture of one of the components of the joint. Furthermore, hip dislocation is most commonly caused by vehicular trauma, and thus there is usually a likelihood of additional injury elsewhere.

Dislocations of the hip are classified as anterior or posterior, depending upon whether the head of the femur pops out in front of the acetabulum or behind it. POSTERIOR DISLOCATIONS occur when a force is applied to the flexed knee while the hip is also in flexion, as when the knee strikes the dashboard during a head-on collision (see Fig. 17-6). The impact on the patella is transmitted backward and rams the head of the femur out of the acetabulum. On examination, a patient with posterior hip dislocation will be found lying with the hip flexed, *adducted*, and *internally rotated*, so that the knee crosses over the midline (Fig. 17-26A). The affected limb will also usually appear shorter than the normal limb. It is not uncommon for posterior hip dislocation to be complicated by *injury to the sciatic nerve*, which lies behind the hip joint and can be bruised or stretched when the head of the femur is forced out of its socket posteriorly. The sciatic nerve controls movement of muscles below the knee, and when it is damaged, the patient may develop "foot drop"; that is, the foot just hangs, and the patient is unable to raise his toes or flex his ankle. Posterior dislocation of the hip is also liable to disrupt the blood supply to the femur and lead to necrosis of the femoral head. This underscores once more the importance of checking the distal extremity for pulse, sensation, and movement. IF YOU DON'T CHECK FOR NEUROLOGIC OR PULSE DEFICIT YOU WON'T FIND IT.

ANTERIOR HIP DISLOCATIONS are relatively rare and tend to occur in automobile accidents, falls, or other situations in which the leg is forcefully abducted into a kind of involuntary "split." On examination, the hip is slightly *flexed*, *abducted*, and *externally rotated* (Fig. 17-26B). Thus the knee on the injured side points *away* from the midline of the body.

Effective splinting of hip dislocations is difficult because of the awkward position in which the affected extremity is fixed. The patient should be transported strapped on a *long backboard*, with pillows used to support the dislocated limb in the position in which it is found.

Fractures of the Hip

A hip fracture is a fracture of the proximal end of the *femur*—either in the head of the femur, in the neck of the femur, or in the region of the trochanters. Hip fractures are most common in the elderly, in whom they can occur as a result of relatively mild trauma, such as a fall from a chair. In younger individuals, much more force is required to fracture the hip, and thus hip fractures in the young tend to be seen in the context of severe multiple injury, as in vehicular trauma.

A patient with an *impacted* fracture of the femoral neck may complain of only slight pain in the groin and may actually be up walking around on the injured hip. In such cases, there is no obvious defor-

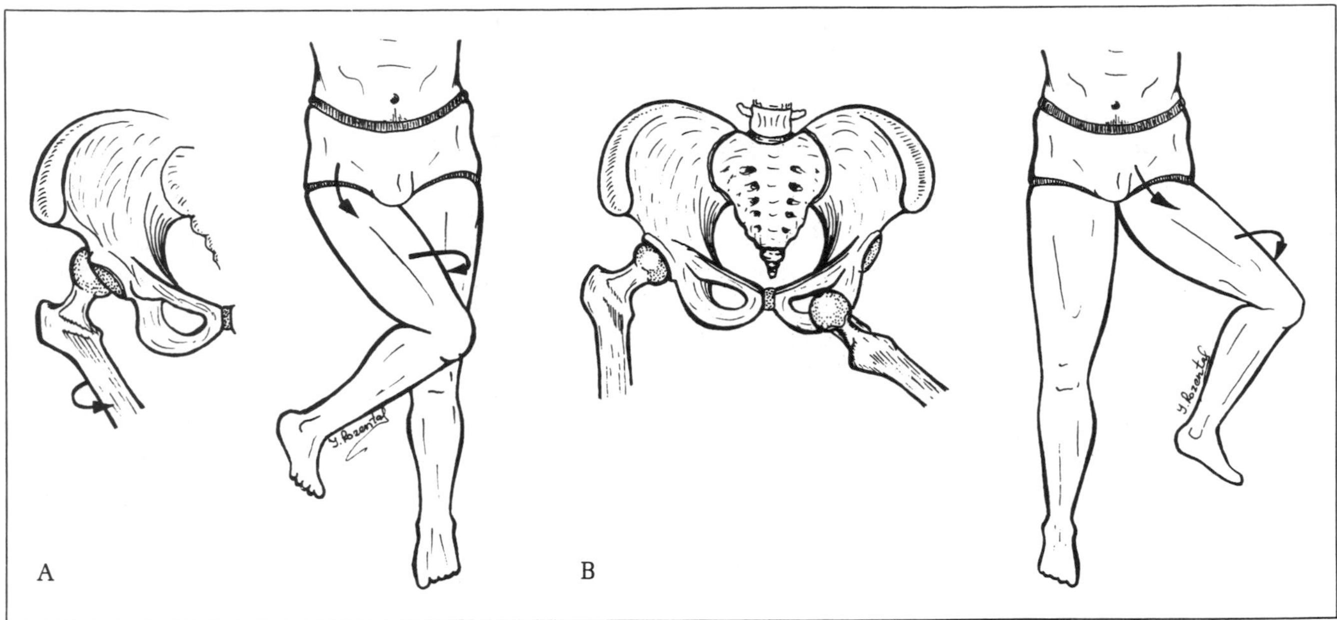

Fig. 17-26. *A. Posterior dislocation of the hip. B. Anterior dislocation of the hip.*

mity, and one can only suspect the diagnosis based on the history and mechanisms of injury. The classic hip fracture in the elderly is the intertrochanteric fracture, and it typically occurs from a fall in which the patient lands directly on the hip joint. A patient with this type of hip fracture will be in considerable pain and will lie with the leg *externally rotated*. Usually the injured leg will appear shortened, and there is apt to be swelling in the hip region.

The best method of immobilizing a hip fracture is with a *traction splint*. If a traction splint is not available, two alternative methods are use of the patient's own body or use of a rigid splint. In the former, pillows or folded blankets can be placed between the patient's legs for padding, and then the injured leg is strapped securely to the uninjured leg. The patient should then be immobilized on a long backboard for posterior support. Alternatively, *padded boards* can be used to stabilize a hip fracture. Two boards are necessary—one of which, placed between the victim's legs, should extend from the groin to the foot; and the other, placed along the victim's side, should extend from the armpit to the foot. The boards must be well padded along their entire length and over the ends and should be secured with cravats so that the injured extremity is sandwiched between them (Fig. 17-27). Once again, the patient and the splint should be immobilized on a *long backboard* for transport.

Bear in mind that hip fracture can be associated with a great deal of internal bleeding—enough to cause shock. If the patient is showing signs of shock, the method of choice for managing the hip fracture is to immobilize the patient first in the *Military Anti-Shock Trousers*, and apply a *traction splint* to the injured extremity over the inflated MAST leg.

FRACTURES OF THE SHAFT OF THE FEMUR

Fracture of the femoral shaft usually presents no difficulty in diagnosis, for the patient's pain is se-

Fig. 17-27. *Board splint for femoral fracture.*

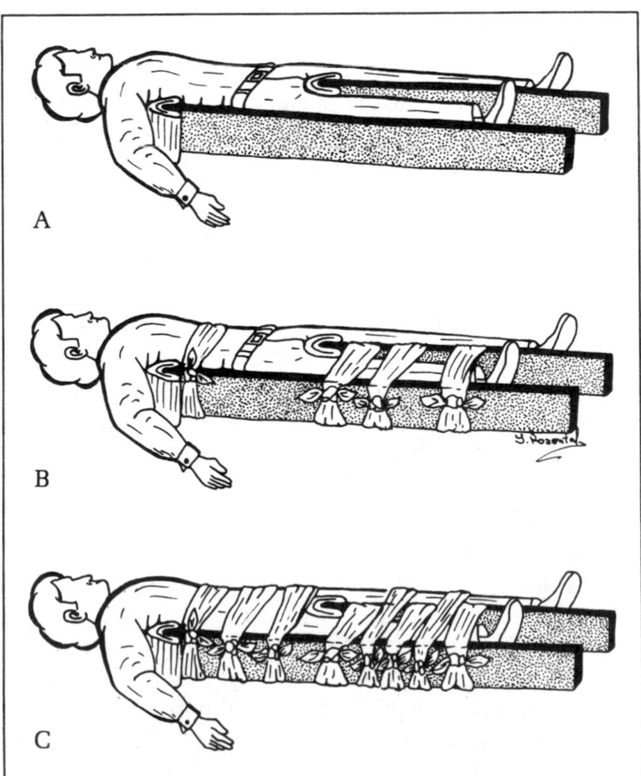

vere, and the deformity tends to be marked; open fractures are common as well. Often the fractured extremity will appear shorter than the uninjured limb, due to overriding of bone. Femoral fractures are the result of major trauma, and for this reason, associated injuries are common. Even when a fractured femur occurs in isolation, however, *shock* should be anticipated, for blood loss of 3 to 4 units is the rule with femoral fracture, whether closed or open.

The treatment of choice for a femoral fracture is the *traction splint*. If the fracture is open, care should be taken to avoid pulling exposed bone fragments back into the wound as traction is developed, and the wound should be covered with a sterile dressing that has been slightly moistened in sterile saline.

When shock is present in association with a femoral fracture, the limb should first be held in traction manually while the *Military Anti-Shock Trousers* are applied and inflated. Then, while the leg is still held in traction, a traction splint should be applied over the inflated MAST leg.

Damage to blood vessels is not uncommon in association with fractures of the femoral shaft. Such damage is suggested by the absence of a distal pulse or by a pale, cold foot that has poor capillary refill. Often, straightening the fracture and splinting it under traction will restore distal circulation, and the foot will "pink up" again. A careful record must be made of the circulatory status both before and after the splint was applied. A pedal pulse that does not return after the fracture has been straightened means a leg in severe jeopardy, and the patient must reach a medical facility as rapidly as possible.

Note that in those cases cited where both the MAST and a traction splint are required, we have specified that the MAST be applied *first* and then the traction splint applied *over* the MAST. This sequence follows logically from the priorities we learned earlier: Control of bleeding and treatment of shock take precedence over splinting of fractures. So if a patient is bleeding—internally or externally—from a femoral fracture or is in imminent danger of shock, we have to deal with those problems first, by applying the MAST. The fracture can wait; shock cannot.

KNEE INJURIES

Sprains of the Knee

The ligaments of the knee are among the most commonly injured ligaments in the body. Knee sprains occur frequently in athletes and usually involve ligaments on the medial side of the knee. A sprained knee is painful and may be swollen and deformed as well. It should be immobilized on a *long padded board splint* or wrapped in a *pillow splint*. Cold packs applied to the knee may give substantial relief of pain.

Dislocations of the Knee

Dislocation of the knee joint is a relatively rare but very serious injury. It presents with severe pain and swelling, considerable deformity, and inability to move the joint. The danger in knee dislocation is in associated *injury to the popliteal artery*, which lies behind the knee joint and supplies the entire lower leg. Nearly half of patients with knee dislocations have some impairment of the blood supply to the foot, and if such impairment is not corrected rapidly, the tissues of the lower leg will become ischemic and suffer irreversible damage. A cold, pale foot is a sign that the popliteal artery has been damaged or pinched off.

In examining the patient with a dislocated knee, first determine whether the pedal pulses are present. If so, splint the knee in the position in which it is found. If the pulses are absent, or if the foot is pale and cold, try *gently* to straighten the knee—but only to the point where you do not cause the patient an increase in pain. Occasionally the knee will pop back into place during this straightening maneuver. Should the pulse fail to return after the attempt to straighten the knee, the leg should be splinted as is with a *long padded board* or *long-leg air splint* and the patient transported without delay to the hospital. If at all possible, the hospital should be notified of the type of case being transported and the estimated time of arrival, so that an orthopedic surgeon can be on hand in the emergency room to give immediate treatment to the patient.

Dislocations of the Patella

Dislocation of the patella, or knee cap, is a common injury among athletes, and it usually occurs when the knee is forcibly twisted while the foot remains planted on the ground. It can also occur from a direct blow to the lateral aspect of the knee. In either case, the dislocation is almost always to the lateral side. A patient with this injury usually complains of pain and holds his knee in a flexed position. There may be an abnormal bulge on the medial side of the knee, which is the femoral condyle suddenly made prominent because the knee cap is displaced from above it. There is apt to be considerable swelling as well.

The EMT can try *gently* to straighten the leg—but only to the extent that doing so does not cause the patient increased pain. The leg should be splinted with a long padded board for transport to the hospital.

Fractures of the Knee

Fractures of the knee can involve the distal femur, proximal tibia, or the patella, and they are usually the result of a direct blow. Such fractures can be difficult to distinguish in the field from dislocation injuries, and they carry the same potential hazard: compression or damage to the popliteal artery. For this reason, they should be treated in the same fashion as suspected knee dislocations; that is, *gentle* straightening and splinting with a *long padded board splint* or long-leg air splint. The status of distal pulses must be monitored and recorded frequently, both before and after splinting.

Do not forget that a PATELLAR FRACTURE sustained when the knee and hip are in flexion (e.g., dashboard injury) is often a signpost pointing toward associated hip injury. Check the hip on the involved side carefully, and if there is any doubt, splint the hip as well.

FRACTURES OF THE SHAFT OF THE TIBIA AND FIBULA

Fractures of the tibial and/or fibular shaft are relatively common. The tibia can be injured either by a direct blow or by twisting forces, and because the tibia lies so close to the skin, tibial fractures are often open fractures. The fibula is less vulnerable to direct violence because it is buried within heavy muscles, and thus fibular fractures more commonly result from twisting forces, as in ski injuries.

Fractures of the lower leg are often severely deformed and angulated, and they may be associated with loss of distal pulses. These fractures should be gently straightened, and the leg splinted in an *air splint* that extends from the foot to the upper thigh. If the fracture is open, the wound must be covered with a moist, sterile dressing before the air splint is applied, and the fracture should be straightened just to the point where pulses return to the foot.

INJURIES TO THE ANKLE

Ankle injuries are among the most common musculoskeletal problems, and usually they result from twisting forces. Such forces can produce the entire spectrum of musculoskeletal damage—from tears in the ligaments to fractures of the bones that constitute the joint; often more than one type of injury is present (e.g., sprain plus dislocation, or fracture plus dislocation). In most cases, it is nearly impossible in the field to differentiate between a severe ankle sprain, a dislocation, and a fracture, for there is likely to be marked swelling, deformity, and limitation of motion in all three. For this reason, ALL ANKLE INJURIES ARE TREATED AS IF THEY WERE FRACTURES.

A *pillow splint* or an *air splint* provides good immobilization for an injured ankle. If for some reason these materials are not available, a cravat tied in a figure-of-eight can be used to support the ankle (Fig. 17-28). No matter what form of splint is used, the ankle should not be permitted to hang dependent, for this position will only promote further swelling. The patient should be transported supine or semisitting, with the injured ankle and leg propped up on pillows. Cold packs applied to the ankle may provide pain relief.

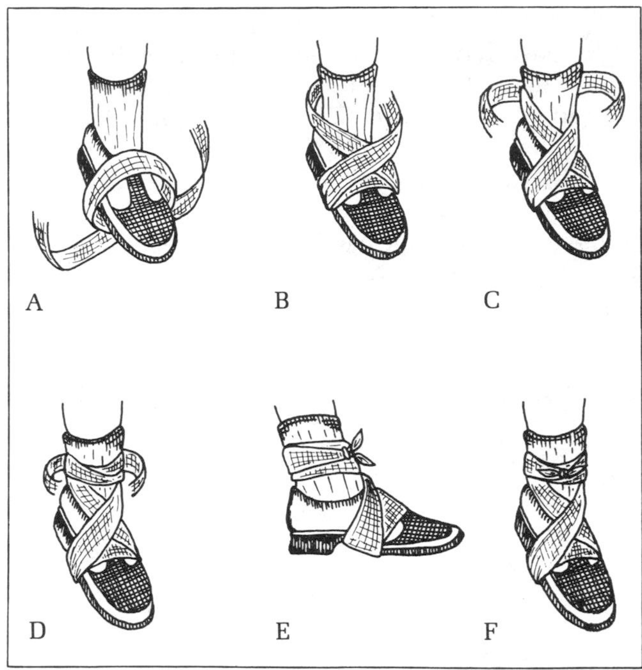

Fig. 17-28. *Figure-of-eight tie to support sprained ankle.*

FRACTURES OF THE FOOT

The HEEL (calcaneus) is the most frequently fractured tarsal bone. Calcaneus fractures usually occur when a person jumps or falls from a height and lands on his heels, and very often *both* heels are broken. The patient will complain of pain and tenderness in the heel(s), and often ecchymoses are visible on the sole of the foot beneath the heel bone. Because of the mechanism of injury, FRACTURES OF THE CALCANEUS TEND TO BE ASSOCIATED WITH COMPRESSION FRACTURES OF THE LUMBAR SPINE, and thus immobilization of the patient on a *long backboard* is the most important aspect of splinting. The calcaneus fracture itself can be adequately immobilized in a *pillow splint.*

FRACTURES OF THE METATARSALS occur from crushing injuries or sometimes from repeated stress (march fractures). The patient will complain of pain in his foot and will avoid bearing weight on the injured part. If there has been a crush injury, severe swelling will be present as well. The foot is best immobilized in a *pillow splint* or air splint and should be kept elevated to minimize further swelling.

FRACTURES OF THE TOE are most often seen after the toe has been jammed into a hard object or a heavy object has been dropped on it. A broken toe is tender, swollen, and discolored. In the field, elevation of the foot and cold packs over the toe are usually sufficient treatment. Taping the injured toe to an adjacent toe can wait until the patient has been evaluated in the hospital; if taping is undertaken immediately after the injury, before swelling reaches its maximum, the tape can become too tight and constrict the injured toe.

SUMMARY

The treatment of specific musculoskeletal injuries is summarized in Table 17-2. While this chapter seems to have covered a great many injuries, in fact the principles of treating those injuries are very few and relatively simple, and the reader is urged to recite the principles of splinting on p. 305 each night at bedtime until they are indelibly burned into memory.

Table 17-2. *Treatment of Musculoskeletal Injuries*

Region	Injury	Commonly Associated Injuries	Treatment
Spine	Fracture		Long backboard
Clavicle	Fracture or dislocation		Sling and swath
Scapula	Fracture	Rib fracture; lung contusion	Sling and swath
Shoulder	Anterior dislocation	Nerve injury (brachial plexus)	Sling; pillow and cravats
	Posterior dislocation		Sling and swath
Humerus	Proximal or shaft fracture	Radial nerve injury (wrist drop); chest injury	Sling and swath with or without rigid splint
	Distal fracture	Volkmann's ischemic contracture	Sling and swath with rigid splint
Elbow	Dislocation	Wrist fracture	Rigid splint
Ulna/radius	Proximal fracture	Wrist fracture	Rigid splint
	Midshaft fracture		Air splint
Wrist	Fracture	Elbow or shoulder injury	Air splint or rigid splint
	Dislocation		Air splint or rigid splint
Carpals or metacarpals	Fracture or dislocation		Rolled gauze in palm plus rigid splint; hand in position of function
Phalanges	Fracture or dislocation		Tongue depressor or padded aluminum
Pelvis	Fracture	Injury to bladder, lumbosacral spine, abdominal organs, lower extremities; shock	MAST; long backboard
Hip	Posterior dislocation	Sciatic nerve injury (foot drop)	Long backboard and pillows
	Anterior dislocation		Long backboard and pillows
	Fracture	Shock	Traction splint or rigid splint, with MAST if shock is present; long backboard
Femoral shaft	Fracture	Shock; damage to blood vessels	Traction splint, with MAST if shock is present
Knee	Sprain		Rigid splint or pillow splint
	Dislocation	Injury to popliteal artery, nerves to leg; tibial fracture	Rigid splint or long-leg air splint
	Fracture	Popliteal artery injury; hip dislocation	Rigid splint or air splint
Tibia/fibula	Mid-shaft fracture	Damage to blood vessels	Long-leg air splint; elevation
Ankle	Fracture, dislocation, or sprain		Pillow splint or air splint; cold packs; elevation
Heel	Fracture	Lumbar spine fracture; knee or hip injury	Long backboard; pillow splint
Metatarsal	Fracture		Pillow splint; elevation
Toe	Fracture		Cold pack; elevation

It should be stressed that EVERY INJURY IS DIFFERENT, and each case will present a different challenge to the EMT, for splinting is not carried out in isolation but rather must reflect the overall situation of the patient. Open wounds, burns, shock, and a host of other factors will influence the decision regarding how any given musculoskeletal injury should be immobilized, and ingenuity is a great asset for anyone performing emergency care in the field.

CASE HISTORY

The patient is a 38-year-old woman who was the front seat passenger in a car that struck a utility pole at 40 miles per hour. The patient was loosely restrained by a lap seat belt and was hurled forward, striking her knee against the dashboard before the seat belt halted her forward momentum. She complains of pain in her knee. She is under a doctor's care for diabetes and takes insulin regularly. She has no known allergies.

On physical examination, the patient was sitting up in the seat of the car, still strapped in by the seat belt, and she was in obvious distress. She was oriented to person, place, and time. The skin was somewhat pale and cool. Vitals were pulse 124, BP 110/60, and respirations 28 and shallow. There was no evidence of head injury. Pupils were equal and reactive. There was no neck tenderness. The trachea was midline, and the jugular veins were not distended. No bruises were seen over the chest. The chest wall was stable. Breath sounds were equal bilaterally, and heart sounds were normal. On examination of the abdomen, there was a horizontal seat belt mark crossing the umbilicus. The abdomen was rigid and tender to palpation. Bowel sounds were absent. The pelvis was stable, and there was no pain on compression of the iliac wings. The right leg was held flexed, adducted, and internally rotated. There was pain, ecchymosis, and swelling over the right patella. The right foot hung limply, and the patient was unable to flex the foot. Sensation to touch was diminished on the sole of the right foot. The peripheral pulses were full and equal, and the extremities were warm.

The patient was given oxygen by nasal cannula at 6 liters per minute and was removed from the car on short and long backboards. The right knee was wrapped in a pillow splint, and the hip was buttressed with pillows. There were no changes in the patient's vital signs during transport, and the right dorsalis pedis pulse remained palpable.

Questions to think about:

1. What clues do you have that this patient has suffered an abdominal injury?
2. What injuries to the lower extremity are present? What is the evidence?
3. What is the significance of the fact that the right foot hung limply and the patient was unable to flex it?
4. What do the pulse and the condition of the skin suggest to you?

VOCABULARY

abduction A movement of a limb *away* from the midline of the body.

acetabulum Depression in the pelvic bone that serves as the socket for the hip joint; formed from the junction of the ilium, ischium, and pubis.

acromion An extension of the scapula that forms the highest point of the shoulder and articulates with the clavicle.

adduction A movement of a limb *toward* the midline of the body.

appendicular skeleton The part of the skeleton comprising the shoulder girdle, upper extremity, pelvis, and lower extremity.

articulation Point where two or more bones come together to form a joint.

axial skeleton The part of the skeleton comprising the skull, vertebrae, and thorax.

calcaneus Heel bone.

callus Tissue that forms a collar joining two ends of a broken bone, which is gradually replaced by new bone as fracture healing progresses.

cardiac muscle Involuntary muscle found only in the heart that has the property of initiating its own contractions.

cartilage Connective tissue that lines synovial joints and provides structure and cushioning elsewhere in the body.

Colles fracture Fracture of the distal radius and ulna.

comminuted fracture Fracture in which a bone is broken into three or more pieces.

compound fracture An open fracture; a fracture in which the bone ends are visible in or protruding from a wound.

condyle A rounded projection at the end of a bone.

dislocation The displacement of a bone end from a joint.

dorsal Referring to the back surface.

eversion Twisting of the foot *outward*.

external rotation Turning of an extremity laterally.

fracture A break in the continuity of a bone.

glenoid The depression in the scapula that serves as the socket of the shoulder joint.

greenstick fracture An incomplete fracture, extending only partway through a bone.

ilium One of two large bones that form the wings of the pelvis.

impacted fracture Fracture in which the bone ends are jammed into one another.

internal rotation The turning of an extremity medially.

inversion Twisting of the foot *inward*.

ischial tuberosity The most inferior and posterior portion of the ischium, which can be palpated as a bump in the buttocks.

ischium One of the two bones that form the inferior portion of the pelvic ring.
joint Place where two or more bones come together.
ligament Band of fibrous tissue that connects *bone* to *bone*.
malleolus The rounded knob on either side of the ankle; the medial malleolus is formed by the distal tibia, and the lateral malleolus by the distal fibula.
march fracture Type of stress fracture involving the metatarsal bones, caused by prolonged walking.
navicular One of the carpal bones, located just distal to the radius.
oblique fracture Fracture in which the fracture line is at an angle to the shaft of the bone.
olecranon Proximal end of the ulna that hooks around the distal humerus to form the elbow.
pubis One of two bones that form the anterior portion of the pelvic ring.
radial nerve A nerve of the arm that controls the muscles of extension in the hand.
reduction The restoration of a broken bone to its proper alignment.
sacroiliac joint Joint between the sacrum and the ilium.
sciatic nerve Major nerve of the lower extremity that runs behind the hip and down the length of the leg.
simple fracture A closed fracture; a fracture in which the skin is not broken.
skeletal muscle Voluntary muscle that is attached to bone and permits locomotion.
smooth muscle Involuntary muscle that makes up the walls of hollow organs.
spiral fracture Fracture caused by twisting forces that looks like a coil or spring on x-ray.
splint Any device used to immobilize an injured part.
sprain Injury involving the stretching or tearing of a ligament.
suture Fused joint at which two or more bones of the skull come together.
symphysis pubis Point at which the two pubic bones come together.
synovial joint Joint that permits movements of its parts.
tendon Fibrous tissue that connects *muscle* to *bone*.
Thomas splint Splint developed by Sir Hugh Owen Thomas for applying traction to the lower extremity.
traction Pulling or drawing, with the aim of bringing an injured part into a straighter condition.
transverse fracture Fracture perpendicular to the long axis of a bone.
trochanter Either of two processes below the neck of the femur.
volar Pertaining to the palm side of the arm.
Volkmann's ischemic contracture Contracture and loss of function in the fingers and wrist due to tissue hypoxia; may be a complication of fractures of the humerus or elbow.

FURTHER READING

Anast GT. Fractures and splinting. *Emergency* 10(11):42, 1978.

Bostian LC et al. Survey of common athletic injuries. *EMT J* 5(4):265, 1981.

Burtzloff HE. Splinting closed fractures of the extremities. *Emerg Med Serv* 10(3):70, 1981.

Connolly JF. Fracture pitfalls: General principles. *Emerg Med* 14(17):161, 1982. [Note: This article is the first of an excellent series on fractures that appeared in *Emergency Medicine* during 1982 through 1984.]

File D, Barancik C. Northeastern Ohio trauma study III: Incidence of fractures. *Ann Emerg Med* 14:244, 1985.

Gustafson JE. Contraindications to the repositioning of fractured or dislocated limbs in the field. *JACEP* 5:184, 1976.

Martina K. Management of joint fractures. *EMT J* 3(4):46, 1979.

Rayburn BK. Prehospital care of fractures and dislocations of the extremities. *EMT J* 4(2):61, 1980.

Sherman M. Hot or cold: Which treatment to recommend. *Am Pharm* 20(8):46, 1980.

Sloan JP et al. Inflatable splints—what are they doing? *Arch Emerg Med* 1:151, 1984.

Stanley D, Norris SH. Recovery following fractures of the clavicle treated conservatively. *Injury* 19:162, 1988.

Tomford W. Basics of broken bones for the nonorthopedist. 1. The fundamental principles. *Emerg Med* 19(15):25, 1987.

Wald DA, Ziemba TJ, Ferko JG. Upper extremitiy injuries. *Emergency* 21(3):25, 1989.

SKILL EVALUATION CHECKLISTS

The following pages contain skill checklists for application of an air splint, padded board splint, and traction splint. The checklists may be used as aids in practicing the skills involved.

Performance Test
Air Splint (Forearm Fracture)

Students R1: ______________________ Date ______________
R2: ______________________

Instructor: Place an "X" in the Fail column beside any item that is performed incorrectly, out of sequence, or omitted.

Activity	Critical Performance	Fail
Primary survey	(Instructor states that patient is conscious.) Checks for profuse bleeding.	
Secondary survey	Vital signs.	
	Head-to-toe survey. (Instructor states patient has a closed fracture of the forearm.)	
	Exposes victim's forearm without moving it.	
	Checks radial pulse.	
	Checks sensation and movement in the fingers.	
	Palpates elbow and shoulder for associated injury.	
Splinting (splint without zipper)	R1 explains procedure to patient.	
	R1 draws air splint backward onto his own arm.	
	R1 grasps victim's hand and exerts gentle traction.	
	R1 slides air splint onto victim's arm: Proximal end at least 5 in. above elbow.	
	Distal end over knuckles.	
	Splint wrinkle-free.	
	R2 inflates splint by mouth.	
	Splint inflated to correct pressure (will indent with finger).	
	R1 releases grip.	
Checking the splint	Asks patient if he feels numbness or tingling in splinted hand.	
	Checks nail beds for capillary refill.	
Transport	Patient placed supine or at 30-degree head elevation on stretcher.	
	Splinted arm elevated on pillows.	

Instructor ______________________

Performance Test
Padded Board Splint (Leg Fracture)

Students R1: ______________________ Date ______________
R2: ______________________

Instructor: Place an "X" in the Fail column beside any item that is performed incorrectly, out of sequence, or omitted.

Activity	Critical Performance	Fail
Primary survey	(Instructor states that patient is conscious.) Checks for profuse bleeding.	
Secondary survey	Vital signs.	
	Head-to-toe survey. (Instructor states patient has deformity and wound at mid-calf).	
	Exposes victim's leg without moving leg.	
	Checks pedal pulses (removes shoe and sock without moving leg).	
	Checks sensation and movement in the toes.	
	Compares temperature of foot to foot on uninjured side.	
Splinting	R1 dresses and bandages wound.	
	R1 explains splinting procedure to patient.	
	R1 grasps ankle and exerts gentle, steady, longitudinal traction.	
	R2 lines up padded board along side of leg.	
	Board long enough to extend from foot to mid-thigh.	
	R2 adds padding as needed to fill in spaces between board and leg.	
	R2 secures board to leg with cravats above and below the fracture and at the ends of the board.	
	No motion of leg during procedure.	
Checking the splint	Checks for presence of pedal pulse.	
	Asks patient if he feels numbness or tingling in foot.	
Transport	Patient moved to stretcher (preferably on backboard).	
	Injured leg elevated on pillows.	

Instructor ______________________

Performance Test
Traction Splint (Thomas Half-Ring)

Students R1: ______________________ Date ______________
R2: ______________________

Instructor: Place an "X" in the Fail column beside any item that is performed incorrectly, out of sequence, or omitted.

Activity	Critical Performance	Fail
Primary survey	(Instructor states that patient is conscious.) Checks for profuse bleeding.	
Secondary survey	Vital signs.	
	Head-to-toe survey. (Instructor states there is a closed fracture of the mid-femur.)	
	Checks pedal pulses (removes shoe).	
	Checks sensation and movement in foot.	
	Compares temperature of foot to foot on uninjured side.	
Splinting	R1 explains procedure to the patient.	
	R1 grasps victim's ankle and exerts gentle longitudinal traction.	
	R2 attaches ankle hitch to victim's ankle.	
	R2 takes over traction, using ankle hitch.	
	R1 measures splint alongside victim and adjusts length.	
	R1 attaches locking hitch to bottom of splint and cross hitches for support slings.	
	R2 lifts victim's leg slightly, maintaining traction.	
	R1 slides splint into position: Seated properly against ischial tuberosity.	
	Groin adequately padded.	
	Not pressing against genitals.	
	R1 secures ischial strap.	
	R1 fastens ankle hitch to locking hitch.	
	R1 develops traction using stick to twist locking hitch.	
	R2 releases grip slowly as splint takes over traction.	
	R2 fastens support slings.	
	R2 secures stick and elevates end of splint.	
Checking the splint	R2 checks pedal pulse or capillary refill.	
	R2 asks patient if he feels numbness or tingling in foot.	

Instructor ______________________

18. TRIAGE

OBJECTIVES

Triage (pronounced *tree-ahzh*) is the French word for "sorting." In medicine, it is used to refer to the sorting of casualties to establish priorities of treatment and evacuation. Although in general triage is applied to situations in which there are several casualties, the word can also refer to the assessment of a single patient with multiple injuries for the purpose of deciding which injury should be treated first. In this chapter, we will examine both aspects of triage: triage of a single, multiply injured patient and triage when there are many casualties. We will also look at strategies for dealing with mass casualty situations and the special problems such situations pose. By the end of this chapter, the reader should be able to

1. State the fundamental principles that guide all triage activities
2. Arrange in the correct sequence the steps in managing a multiply injured patient, given a list of the patient's injuries and steps of treatment in random order
3. Identify those conditions that necessitate immediate transport to the hospital ("load-and-go" situations) given a list of various injuries and their consequences.
4. Identify situations in which compromises must be made in the usual priorities in order to save the patient's life
5. List the information the dispatcher should obtain upon receiving a call regarding a multicasualty incident
6. Identify the correct position in which to station the first ambulance to arrive at a disaster scene, given a description of several possible locations
7. Identify an appropriate triage area, given a description of the disaster scene and several alternative triage areas
8. State the reasons for centralizing the ambulances in a staging area away from the triage area
9. Identify (a) first-priority patients, (b) second-priority patients, and (c) third-priority patients, given a description of several patients with different injuries
10. Estimate how many ambulances will be needed at a multicasualty incident, given a description of the patients at the scene
11. Indicate the proper order of evacuation, given a list of patients with different conditions
12. Identify common emotional reactions to mass casualty situations, and indicate how to deal with people manifesting these reactions
13. List at least three ways in which bystanders can be put to use in mass casualty situations

PRINCIPLES OF TRIAGE

Whether one is dealing with a single patient who has multiple injuries or a score of injured people, the fundamental principles of triage are the same:

Principles of Triage

- SALVAGE OF LIFE TAKES PRECEDENCE OVER SALVAGE OF LIMB.
- THE TWO *IMMEDIATE* THREATS TO LIFE ARE ASPHYXIA AND HEMORRHAGE.

These two principles guide all of our work with critically injured patients and dictate the priorities of treatment; for each time we ask the question "Can this injury wait?" or "Can this patient wait?" the answer will be based upon the principles stated above.

TRIAGE OF THE MULTIPLY INJURED PATIENT

By now, the process of triage of the multiply injured patient should be entirely familiar to us. We have not used the *word* "triage" before, but every time we dealt with the ABCs and the proper sequence of treatment, we were in essence talking about triage—sorting out the patient's problems according to priorities. In the foregoing chapters, we have considered a great many injuries to various organ systems. In this discussion, we will draw together some of the concepts of trauma learned in previous chapters and consider **basic trauma life support** (BTLS), the overall approach to the patient with multiple injuries.

THE GOLDEN HOUR

Trauma experts often talk about the "golden hour" for critically injured casualties. Studies have shown that seriously injured patients who manage to reach the operating room within one hour of the time of injury have the highest rate of survival. So we call that hour—the hour after the victim is injured—the golden hour, and we try not to waste even one minute of that golden hour. Response times must therefore be prompt. Equipment must be assembled and ready before you even reach the patient. And every action in the field must have a lifesaving purpose—for everything you do before transport eats up minutes of the golden hour.

The very first action to take upon reaching the scene of any sort of accident is to MAKE A QUICK SURVEY OF THE SCENE. Look for HAZARDS to yourself or to the victim(s). Are there downed electric wires? Is a vehicle lying on its side in an unstable position? Is there a risk of fire or explosion? Try also to get an idea of the MECHANISMS OF INJURY: Is a car accordioned against a tree? Is there damage to the passenger compartment? What sort of damage?

Make it a habit to CARRY ALL ESSENTIAL EQUIPMENT TO THE PATIENT as you first approach him, so you won't have to waste time afterward running back and forth to the ambulance for things you left behind. While you are still en route to the call, assemble everything you might need for a major trauma case:

Equipment to Carry to a Trauma Victim

- Long backboard with straps, cervical collar, and device for immobilizing the head
- Airway equipment
- Oxygen
- MAST (unfolded and laid out on the backboard)
- Trauma kit (see Table 38-4)

When you reach the victim, there are four steps that must be carried out as expeditiously as possible:

1. **Primary Survey:** to identify and treat injuries that could kill the patient if not managed imediately.
2. **Transport decision** and **critical interventions:** to decide if there is a "load-and-go" situation and if any lifesaving actions must be taken before transport
3. **Secondary survey:** to find the patient's injuries and establish baseline observations
4. **Communications with medical control:** to prepare the receiving hospital for the patient's arrival

THE PRIMARY SURVEY

Triage of the multiply injured patient begins, as always, with the primary survey: the ABCs and, in basic trauma life support, there is a D and an E as well.

AIRWAY (AND CERVICAL SPINE CONTROL)

The airway remains the first consideration, and in the victim of trauma, the airway can be jeopardized in several ways. If the patient is unconscious, there is, to begin with, the usual problem of obstruction by the base of the tongue. But the usual solution—backward tilt of the head—will not do; for as we learned earlier, EVERY SEVERELY INJURED ACCIDENT VICTIM HAS A CERVICAL SPINE INJURY UNTIL PROVED OTHERWISE. So we have to modify our approach and try to get the airway open with JAW THRUST or with an artificial airway, avoiding any motion of the head or neck.

Besides the tongue, blood, vomitus, avulsed teeth, or broken dentures may be obstructing the airway of the trauma victim. All such foreign materials need to be swept out manually or suctioned out. Once the spine is properly stabilized, the patient should be kept turned to a side so that foreign material drains out of the mouth rather than down the throat.

Facial trauma that produces fractures to the maxilla or mandible can also produce problems in getting the airway open. If the mouth cannot be opened for suctioning and there is foreign material in the airway, the patient must reach a medical facility as quickly as possible, for a tracheostomy may be required. Similarly, direct trauma to the neck that causes fracture of the trachea presents an extreme airway emergency—and one that cannot be adequately managed in the field. In such cases, the patient must be moved with all possible speed to the hospital so that endotracheal intubation or a surgical procedure can be performed to establish an airway and prevent asphyxia.

Ensuring the Airway in the Trauma Victim

- Open the airway by JAW THRUST; avoid moving the head or neck.
- Clear out FOREIGN MATERIALS manually or with suction; anticipate VOMITING.
- Keep the unconscious patient TURNED TO A SIDE, so that foreign materials can drain from the mouth.
- Facial fractures about the mouth and tracheal fractures are EXTREME EMERGENCIES: Get to the hospital without delay!

BREATHING

Once we have the airway under control, our next concern is to ensure that the patient is breathing adequately. Needless to say, if the patient is not breathing at all, artificial ventilation must be started promptly and supplemented as soon as possible with high concentrations of oxygen. (Keep the victim's back immobilized between your knees as you ventilate with a bag-valve-mask.) Even if the patient is making respiratory efforts, however, there are a number of injuries that can sabotage the effectiveness of the respirations. We have seen, for instance, how SUCKING CHEST WOUNDS prevent adequate expansion of the lung. Thus, open chest wounds must be closed without delay. If there are signs of TENSION PNEUMOTHORAX and the EMT is not authorized to decompress the chest, the only thing that will save the patient is to get him to a medical facility with all possible speed, so that decompression can be performed there. FLAIL CHEST should also be noted during the primary survey, although its stabilization can wait until other more urgent tasks have been accomplished. Finally, *every* severely injured patient should be assumed to have some degree of respiratory insufficiency and should therefore be given OXYGEN—whether the injuries are primarily to the head, chest, abdomen, extremities, or any combination thereof.

Ensuring Respiration in the Trauma Victim

- For APNEA, start artificial ventilation promptly.
- Close SUCKING CHEST WOUNDS.
- For TENSION PNEUMOTHORAX, decompress the chest at once, or move the patient to the hospital without further delay.
- Note the presence of FLAIL CHEST (stabilize it later).
- EVERY SEVERELY INJURED PATIENT NEEDS OXYGEN.

CIRCULATION

To assess the circulation in the primary survey of a trauma victim, we need to check the pulse and the degree of peripheral perfusion. If the carotid PULSE is present, check for a pulse at the wrist. A palpable radial pulse means that the patient's systolic blood pressure is at least 80 mm Hg. If you can feel a pulse at the neck but *not* at the wrist, the systolic pressure is somewhere between 60 and 80 mm Hg—usually an indication of advanced shock. A quick and easy way to check PERIPHERAL PERFUSION is by the **capillary blanch test:** Press on the palm of the victim's hand until it blanches (turns white), then release the pressure. In a normally perfused person, the color will return within 2 seconds. If the area you pressed stays blanched for more than 2 seconds, it is a sign of shock.

When we discuss circulation in the context of trauma, we are talking principally about CONTROL OF BLEEDING and TREATMENT OF SHOCK, both of which must be accomplished as rapidly as possible once the airway and breathing have been ensured. Recall that an adequate circulation requires three intact components: a functioning PUMP (the heart), intact PIPES (veins and arteries) capable of constricting in response to changes in volume, and an adequate VOLUME (blood) to fill the pipes. Clearly any or all of these components can be damaged in trauma. The pump can be bruised or be prevented from functioning properly by blood in the pericardial sac. PERICARDIAL TAMPONADE is, in effect, a form of *cardiogenic shock* and is a dire emergency, requiring immediate transport to the hospital. Another factor that can prevent the heart from pumping effectively is AIR EMBOLISM, which may result from an open wound in the neck. Such wounds must be sealed off with an occlusive dressing as part of step C of the ABCs.

The *pipes* too can be affected, directly or indirectly, by trauma. The arteries, for example, can be rendered incapable of constriction by injury to the spine—that is, in *neurogenic shock*—and restoration of effective circulation in such cases will require intravenous fluids and often the MAST garment.

Finally *volume* can be lost—in the form of blood, in either an open or a closed injury, or as plasma, from burns—and in either case the resulting *hypovolemic shock* must be treated with the MAST and intravenous fluids. As a general rule, whenever there is serious injury involving the chest, abdomen, pelvis, or thigh, shock is very likely, and the EMT should not wait for signs of shock to develop in order to begin treatment. Intravenous fluids should be started at the earliest possible moment. Recall also that HEAD INJURIES *DO NOT* CAUSE SHOCK. If shock is present in a head-injured patient, look for serious injury elsewhere.

If the patient does have signs of shock, do a MAST SURVEY; that is, do a quick check of the abdomen, pelvis, and legs (the areas of the body that will be covered as soon as the MAST is applied and therefore no longer accessible for examination during the secondary survey). Remember: In order to examine a part of the body, you must be able to *see* it; so cut away any clothing from the legs and pelvis. Check the abdomen, pelvis, and lower extremities. Make a note of any injuries detected, then apply the MAST.

Ensuring Circulation in the Trauma Victim

- If there is no pulse, start EXTERNAL CARDIAC COMPRESSIONS.
- CONTROL BLEEDING with direct pressure.
- ANTICIPATE SHOCK in every severely injured patient, and START AN INTRAVENOUS INFUSION of saline or Ringer's.
- For hypovolemic or neurogenic shock, use the MAST garment after doing a MAST survey.
- For PERICARDIAL TAMPONADE, get the patient to a hospital fast!
- Seal off OPEN NECK WOUNDS as quickly as possible.
- Shock in a head-injured patient means injury elsewhere.

DISABILITY (NEUROLOGIC)

In basic trauma life support, we add two more letters to the primary survey alphabet: D and E. D stands for *disability assessment*, specifically neurologic disability. And in the primary survey, checking for neurologic disability means looking at just two things: the patient's pupils and level of consciousness. Check the PUPILS for size, equality, and reactivity to light. For assessing the LEVEL OF CONSCIOUSNESS in the primary survey, use the AVPU Scale (further described in Chap. 14):

AVPU Scale

A **A**lert
V Responds to **v**oice
P Responds only to **p**ain
U **U**nresponsive to any stimulus

EXPOSURE

The E of the BTLS primary survey is to *expose* the whole patient, in preparation for further assessment. Just opening the patient's shirt or cutting a trouser leg is not sufficient to make a thorough examination. Cut through the front of the victim's garments so that the sleeves, trouser legs, and torso sections fall away. (If the patient is out in the open, delay this step until you've moved him into the ambulance.)

TRANSPORT DECISION AND CRITICAL INTERVENTIONS

Properly conducted, the primary survey will give you all the information you need to decide whether a critical situation is present. If so, the patient must be transported *at once* ("load-and-go"), according to our first principle of triage: SALVAGE OF LIFE TAKES PRECEDENCE OVER SALVAGE OF LIMB. What that means in practice is that sometimes you will not be able to stabilize the patient to the degree you might wish before moving him. A spine-injured casualty in a burning car, for example, must be pulled from the car as fast as possible, even at the risk of aggravating his spinal injury. A patient with pericardial tamponade must be moved with all possible speed to the hospital, even if his fractures have not been fully splinted. THE HIGHEST PRIORITY IS TO KEEP THE PATIENT ALIVE. Everything else is secondary.

Load-and-Go Situations

- AIRWAY OBSTRUCTION that cannot be relieved (e.g., tracheal fracture, laryngeal edema)
- RESPIRATORY IMPAIRMENT
  1. tension pneumothorax
  2. sucking chest wound
  3. traumatic asphyxia
  4. flail chest
- SHOCK
  1. hemorrhagic
  2. neurogenic
  3. pericardial tamponade
  4. cardiac arrest
- DECREASED LEVEL OF CONSCIOUSNESS

In all "load-and-go" situations, only a bare minimum of CRITICAL INTERVENTIONS are carried out at the scene—those that are immediately required to save the patient's life:

Critical Interversions
- Manual opening of the airway
- Control of bleeding
- Sealing off sucking chest wounds
- Starting artificial ventilation or CPR as needed
- Decompressing a tension pneumothorax if trained and authorized to do so

All other procedures, such as bandaging wounds or splinting fractures, must be carried out en route. Remember: Every procedure you carry out in the field is taking up precious minutes of the patient's golden hour. Make sure the procedure is worth it!

NONLIFESAVING PROCEDURES SHOULD NEVER DELAY THE TRANSPORT OF A CRITICALLY INJURED PATIENT.

If the patient falls into the "load-and-go" category, then carry out the critical interventions: log-roll the patient onto a long backboard/MAST; start oxygen; load; and GO! Continue your assessment and care en route.

THE SECONDARY SURVEY

If the primary survey does not identify a "load-and-go" situation, you can proceed at the scene to the secondary survey and assess the patient for other injuries. Whether done at the scene or en route to the hospital, the secondary survey should be accomplished in less than five minutes.

An important element of the secondary survey is the patient's HISTORY. One useful way to remember what information you need about a trauma patient is to think of taking an AMPLE history:

A allergies
M medications
P past medical history (or other illnesses)
L last meal (how long ago?)
E events preceding the injury (what happened?)

Now is the time to get a full set of VITAL SIGNS, and record your findings accurately. Then proceed to the HEAD-TO-TOE SURVEY:

Head-to-Toe Survey in BTLS: Points of Emphasis
- HEAD: Raccoon sign, Battle's sign, drainage of blood or fluid from the nose or ears, lacerations. *Reassess* the airway and the pupils.
- NECK: Lacerations, contusions, tenderness, distended neck veins, deviation of the trachea. *Recheck* the carotid pulse. Then apply a cervical collar.
- CHEST: *Recheck* for open wounds or flail. Check for bruises, tenderness, equality of breath sounds. Stabilize any flail segments manually or with a pillow.
- ABDOMEN: Look for contusions or open wounds. Feel for tenderness or rigidity (a distended, tender abdomen means internal bleeding. Treat for shock and **transfer immediately**).
- PELVIS AND EXTREMITIES: Stablity of the pelvis (if the pelvis is unstable, apply the MAST and **transfer immediately**); swelling or deformity of any extremity; sensation and pulses distal to any injury.

If the patient is stable, finish bandaging wounds and splinting fractures before moving him. Continue to monitor his condition constantly. If at any time his condition starts to deteriorate, START ALL OVER AGAIN FROM THE PRIMARY SURVEY. Repeat every step. Record all of your observations, along with the times.

The priorities of treatment in trauma patients are summarized in Figure 18-1.

COMMUNICATIONS WITH MEDICAL CONTROL

The more severely injured the patient, the earlier you need to contact medical control so that the receiving hospital can prepare for your arrival. Remember the patient's golden hour. It takes time to summon the appropriate surgeon and to mobilize an operating room team. If the patient reaches the hospital promptly but then has to wait for the surgical team to get ready, crucial minutes of the golden hour may slip away. Therefore, when you are coming in with a critically injured patient, give the receiving hospital as much advance notice as possible.

If the patient is not in critical condition, radio communication can wait until you are ready to transport.

Use the standard format for reporting your findings about the patient (see Chap. 12). Keep your transmissions brief and to the point.

MULTIPLE CASUALTY INCIDENTS

The accident or disaster involving several casualties presents the EMT with the most difficult and challenging situation he or she is likely to face. Not only does the multiple casualty incident (MCI) require the EMT to deploy many different skills of judgment and emergency care, it also demands that these skills be exercised under extremely difficult conditions, which may involve hazards to safety, mass panic, and general confusion. Simply knowing how to maintain an airway or apply a traction splint is not

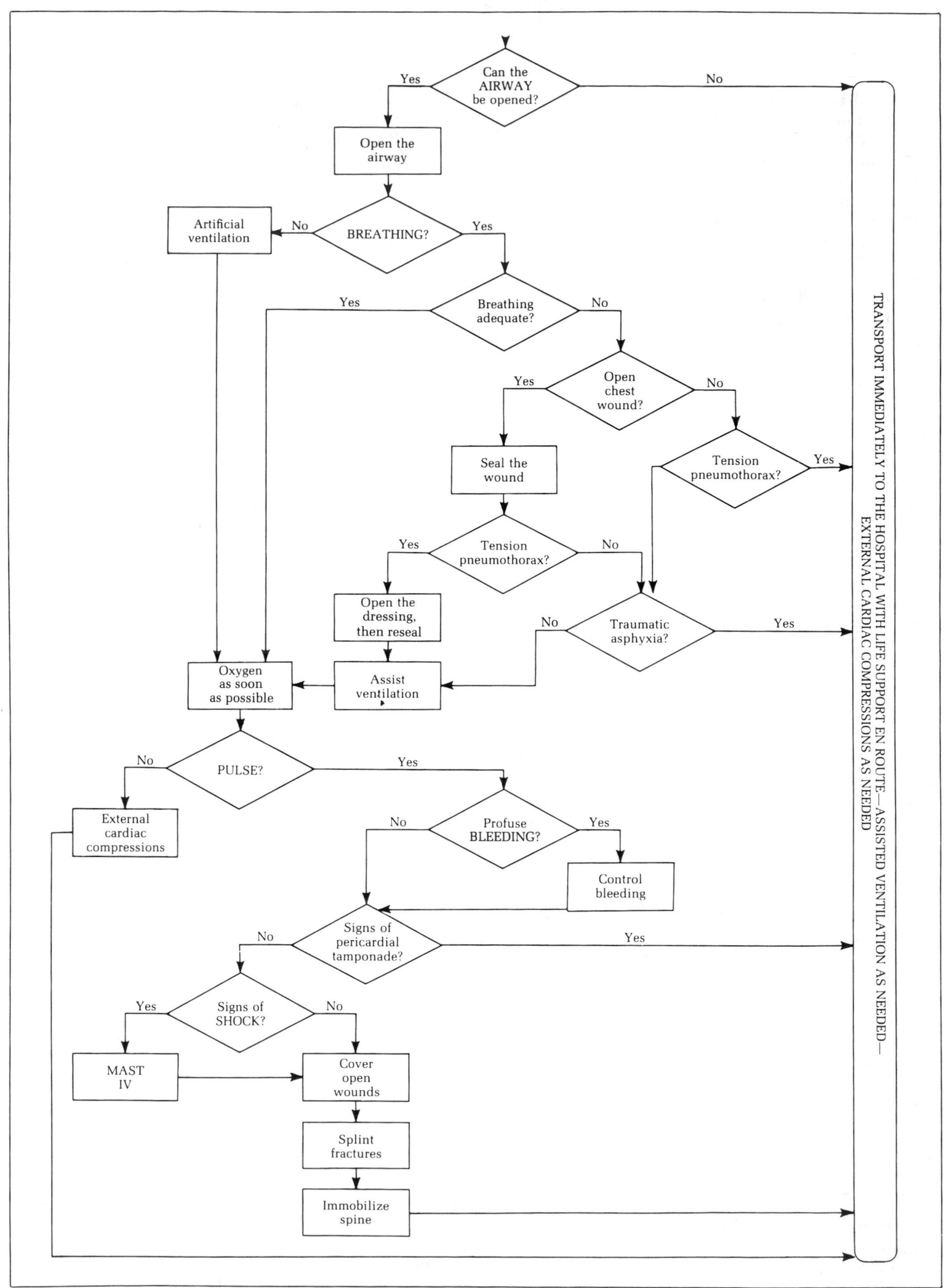

Fig. 18-1. *Priorities in the multiply injured patient.*

enough when dealing with multiple casualties. One must also know whom to treat first, whom to pass by, how to deal with hysterical bystanders, how to coordinate one's efforts with those of other rescue workers, and most important, how to stay cool. The slickest EMT in the squad may go to pieces when faced with a dozen or more severely injured or mutilated victims of a major accident—unless that EMT has rehearsed over and over again the actions that must be taken in such a situation.

The response to a multiple casualty incident involves several distinct phases: (1) receiving the call for help, (2) arriving at the scene, (3) establishing a triage area, (4) sorting and initial treatment of casualties, (5) secondary treatment of casualties, and (6) evacuation of casualties. If these steps are to go smoothly in the chaotic circumstances of an MCI, each step needs to be carefully planned and practiced ahead of time, and mass casualty drills should be carried out regularly by every ambulance service.

RECEIVING THE CALL FOR HELP

The first phase of triage begins the moment the dispatcher receives the call for emergency assistance. While the first ambulance heads out toward the scene, the dispatcher should try to obtain at least the following information from the caller:

Information Required from the Caller

- The exact LOCATION of the accident or disaster:
  1. Specific directions; landmarks.
  2. Telephone number of caller (which may help pinpoint location).
- If it is a vehicular accident, the number and types of VEHICLES involved:
  1. If there are trucks, what are they carrying? Are there hazardous cargoes?
  2. Are there any buses involved?
  3. In what condition are the vehicles? Is any vehicle on fire?
- NUMBER OF VICTIMS and estimated extent of injuries.
- HAZARDS at the scene:
  1. FIRE.
  2. Downed ELECTRIC WIRES.
  3. HAZARDOUS MATERIALS carried by involved vehicles.
  4. TRAFFIC hazards.
  5. Vehicles in unstable or precarious positions.
  6. Debris.
  7. Armed or dangerous persons.

A printed dispatch form that covers the above questions can facilitate gathering this information (Fig. 18-2), which should be relayed by radio to the ambulance en route to the scene. Based on this information, the dispatcher must also make some preliminary estimates regarding the need for more ambulances and for ancillary services (e.g., police, fire companies, utility workers).

ARRIVING AT THE SCENE

Upon reaching the scene, the EMT must make several quick decisions even before the ambulance pulls to a stop. The first of these decisions is made instantly and almost unconsciously, and that is the decision WHERE TO POSITION THE AMBULANCE. The position may have to be altered later, when a staging area has been organized, but in selecting the initial position for the vehicle, the driver should take into account the following principles:

Positioning the Ambulance

- The ambulance should be positioned OFF THE ROAD, out of the flow of traffic.
- If the ambulance is facing oncoming traffic, the HEADLIGHTS SHOULD BE TURNED OFF. Revolving or flashing warning lights should remain on to alert oncoming traffic of the hazard ahead.
- The ambulance should be parked BEYOND THE REACH OF ANY DOWNED WIRES and AT LEAST 30 TO 40 METERS FROM ANY BURNING VEHICLE. If there is spilled gasoline flowing along the road, the ambulance should be placed *upstream* from the flow.
- The ambulance should be parked UPWIND FROM ACCIDENTS INVOLVING SPILLAGE OF DANGEROUS CHEMICALS.
- The ambulance should not be closer than 700 to 1,000 METERS FROM an accident involving EXPLOSIVE CARGOES.

The second decision that is made upon arrival at the scene requires the EMT to determine IF THERE IS A HAZARD AT THE SCENE TO THE SAFETY OF THE RESCUERS. A situation in which there are multiple casualties is often a situation in which there is danger to those at the scene. Fire, downed wires, toxic chemicals—all of these must be managed before proper sorting and care of patients can begin. The EMT who rushes blindly into a mass casualty scene without first checking for hazards simply creates more problems for his colleagues, for that EMT is likely to become yet another victim who must be sorted and treated.

The initial, rapid assessment of the scene should also permit a preliminary estimate of HOW MUCH MORE HELP WILL BE NEEDED. In general, one can figure that one vehicle and at least two EMTs will be required for every seriously injured patient. Ongoing

Date ____________ Log # ____________

Times
Call received ____________ A.M./P.M.
Car out ____________
Arrived at scene ____________
Left scene ____________
Arrived at hospital ____________
Back in service ____________

Patient's name ____________
Address ____________
City/town ____________

Patient status
Conscious ____________
Breathing ____________
Bleeding ____________
Other ____________

If vehicular accident
Number and kinds of vehicles involved
____cars ____trucks ____buses ____________other
Number of persons injured ____________
Extent of injuries ____________
Are persons trapped? ____________
Hazards
____traffic ____wires down ____fire ____hazardous cargo
____unstable vehicle ____debris ____submerged vehicle

Caller: Name ____________ Phone no. ____________

Vehicle dispatched ____________
Crew ____________ Other units called ____________

Fig. 18-2. *Dispatch record.*

triage will permit a more accurate estimate of the need for help, but a quick look around should enable the EMT to radio in regarding *immediate* needs for help. It is clear, for instance, that a single ambulance with a crew of three will not be sufficient to handle forty casualties from an overturned bus, and in such a situation, several more vehicles should be summoned at once. Wherever possible, a physician should also be summoned to the scene to act as senior triage officer and provide medical command.

From this point on, several activities must proceed simultaneously: (1) establishing a triage area, (2) initial sorting of casualties, and (3) initial treatment of immediately life-threatening conditions. The ambulance crew will have to split up and pursue these tasks separately until help arrives (Fig. 18-3). Let us assume the first ambulance on the scene has a crew of three. One member of the crew will start at once to establish a triage area.

ESTABLISHING A TRIAGE AREA

The triage area will be the place to which all casualties are brought as they are removed from the accident scene. It should be a large, well-lighted area at a safe distance from any known hazards, and it must be arranged in such a way that the triage officer will be able to check the entire area at a glance. Furthermore, the triage area should be located *between* the place from which the casualties are being removed and the place where the evacuation vehicles are parked (staging area), so that the triage officer can ensure an orderly sequence of triage, treatment, and evacuation (Fig. 18-4). If ambulances are scattered all over the scene, there is a tendency to grab patients willy-nilly and rush them off to the hospital, without proper regard to which patients should be evacuated first and without adequate means of documenting who has left the scene.

In the triage area, all necessary equipment should be arranged so that it is immediately visible and ac-

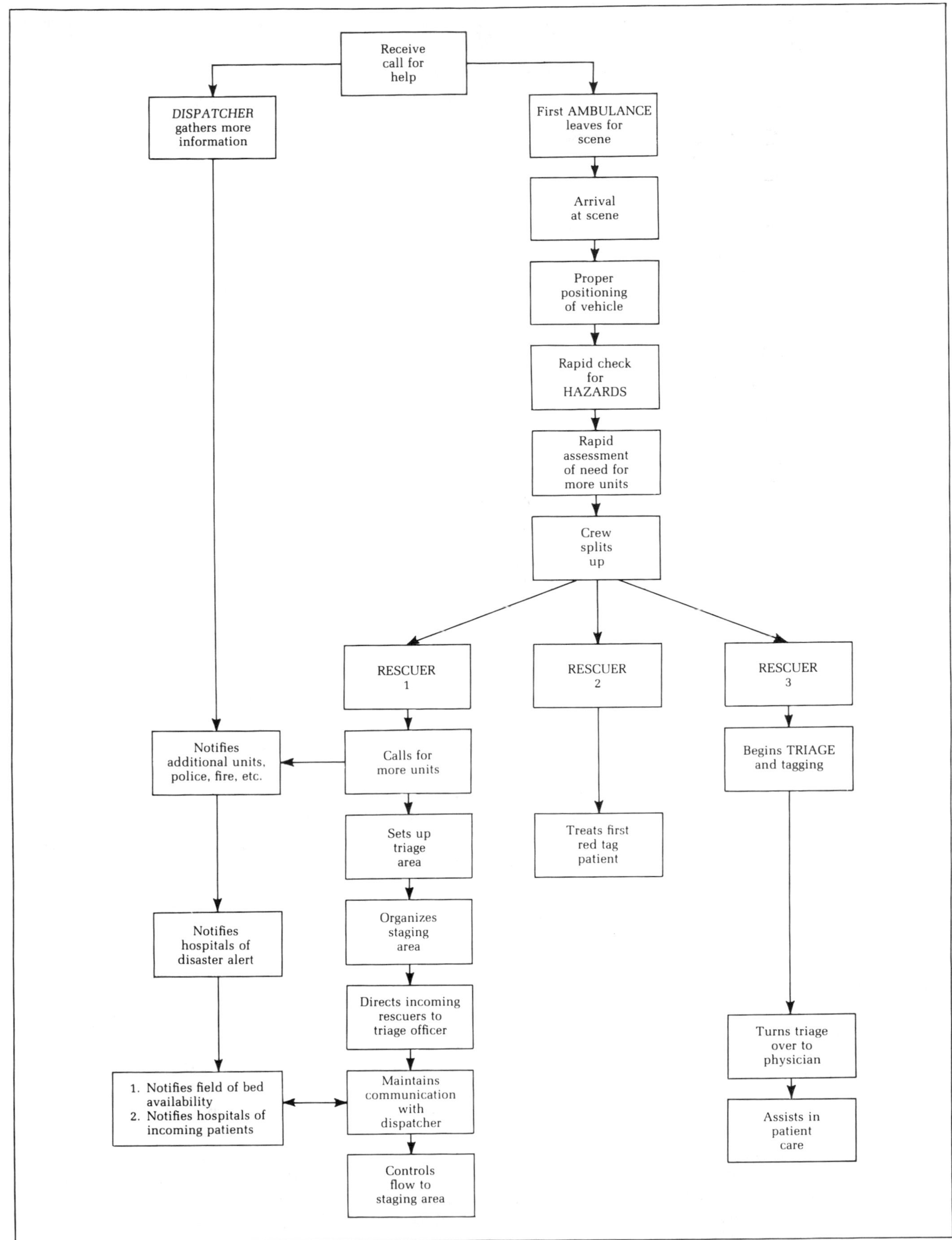

Fig. 18-3. *Steps in responding to a multiple casualty incident.*

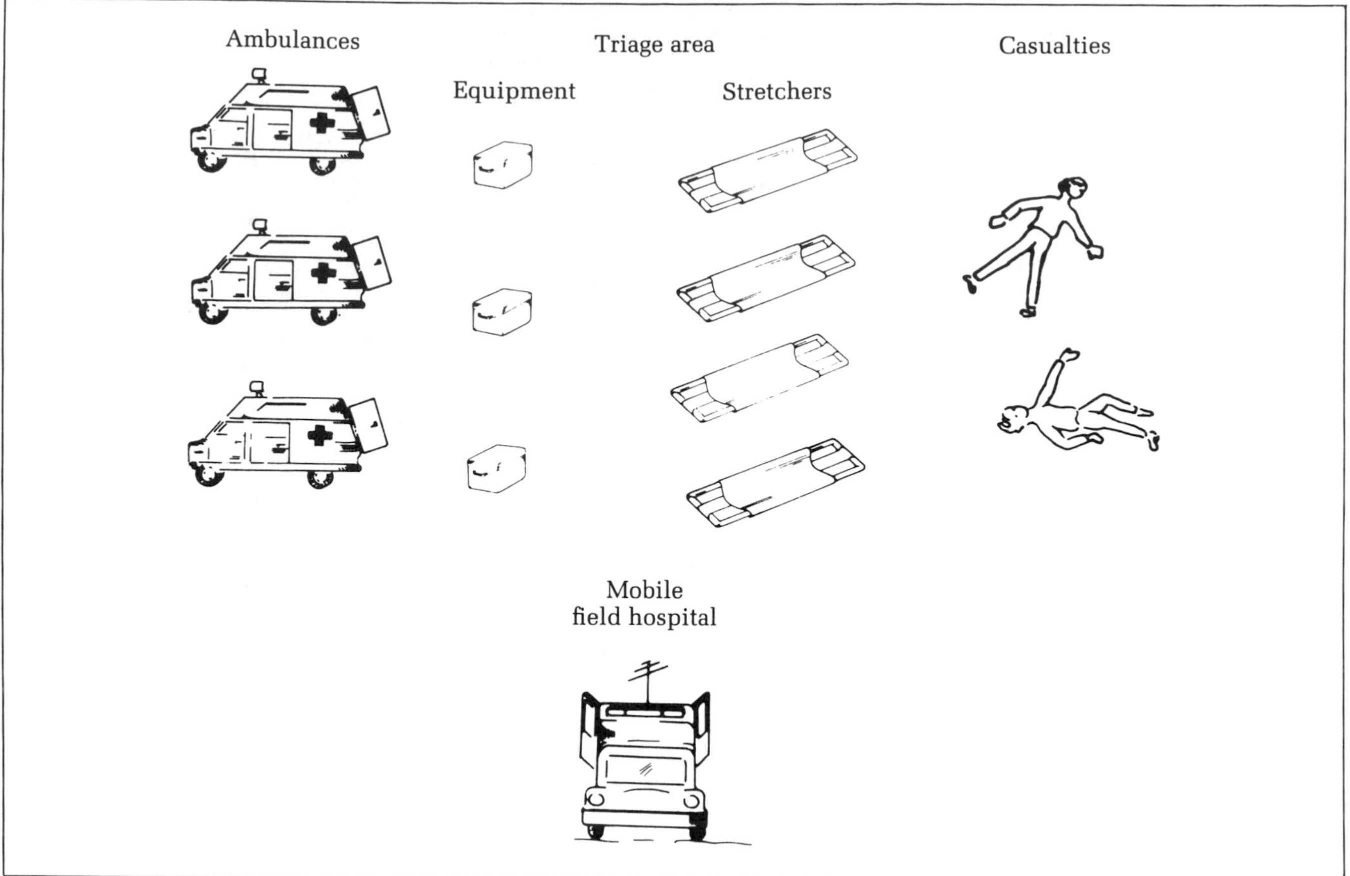

Fig. 18-4. *Triage area.*

cessible. As more ambulances arrive, their crews should be directed to unload their gear in the triage area, where it can be pooled and arranged in an orderly manner. Between each set of two stretchers there should be a small equipment center with at least the following:

Equipment at Each Stretcher Position
- OXYGEN
- Portable SUCTION
- Bag-valve-mask or pocket mask
- Oropharyngeal airways
- Bandages and dressings
- Intravenous infusion kit
- Stethoscope and sphygmomanometer

In addition, cervical collars, backboards, splints, and Military Anti-Shock Trousers should be conveniently placed and readily visible. As soon as there are sufficient rescuers present, one rescuer should be put in charge of controlling the equipment in the triage area and ensuring that each stretcher position is kept properly supplied.

Although we have been referring here to *stretchers*, in fact, it is preferable that long backboards be used from the outset at every stretcher position. The process of triage requires frequent movement of the casualty: from the disaster site to the triage area; from row to row within the triage area during re-evaluations; and from the triage area to the ambulance. Since many of the casualties will have mutiple trauma, *how* you move them is critically important: Canvas stretchers are *not* adequate.

Since thee probably won't be enough buckled straps to go around, you can use cravats (fashioned from triangular bandages) to secure patients to backboards. Five cravats—one tied across the chest just under the armpits; one tied below the waist holding down the wrists as well; one tied just above the knees; one tied just above the ankles; and one joining the feet together to prevent outward rotation of the legs—will give adequate stabilization for most fractures of the appendicular skeleton. (If spinal injury is suspected, the usual procedures for spinal immobilization should be carried out, as described in Chap. 14).

The process of setting up the triage area is greatly facilitated if the ambulance carries special MCI boxes, each of which contains a specified complement of equipment for two stretcher positions. These boxes can be loaded aboard the ambulance as it leaves for the scene or can be permanently stored in a special vehicle that is dispatched only to mass casualty situations. When such boxes have been prepared in advance, they simply need to be distributed among the stretcher positions, together with oxygen and suction, and they can be opened as patients are brought to the triage area. In this way, the triage area can be completely laid out in a matter of 1 or 2 minutes. Sturdy cardboard cartons are adequate as MCI boxes, and each should contain at least the following equipment:

Contents of MCI Carton

- 10 universal dressings
- 20 4 × 4–inch sterile gauze pads
- 15 triangular bandages
- 1 roll sterilized aluminum foil
- 2 sterile sheets
- 2 envelopes petrolatum gauze
- 20 safety pins
- 4 oropharyngeal airways (2 adult, 2 child)
- 1 heavy-duty scissors
- 2 intravenous infusion kits, including:
  - 2 administration sets
  - 4 intravenous catheters (over-the-needle)
  - 10 povidone-iodine swabs
  - 10 alcohol swabs
  - 2 tourniquets
  - 1 roll adhesive tape
  - 4 liter bags of normal saline or Ringer's
- 1 ball-point pen and small pad of paper
- 6 armbands for rescue workers

SORTING OF CASUALTIES

While one EMT is setting up the triage area, the other two EMTs begin the process of sorting casualties. The goal of this process is to accomplish THE GREATEST GOOD FOR THE GREATEST NUMBER, and for this reason, the decisions involved may be very difficult ones. The hopelessly injured must be passed by, and this goes against the grain for most health professionals, who are accustomed to giving their best efforts to saving each patient. But when there are many casualties, one must operate according to a different philosophy. For if the EMTs get tied up trying to save one hopelessly injured patient, several other patients who could have been saved with simple interventions—such as opening the airway or controlling hemorrhage—may die needlessly.

Triage decisions require very sophisticated judgment. Ideally these decisions should be made by a senior surgeon; but until more highly trained personnel reach the scene, the first EMT to arrive must assume the role of triage officer and begin sorting the patients. Whoever is triage officer should be clearly identified by a color-coded helmet or similar means, so that there can be no doubt as to who is in charge.

Triage is conducted in several rounds. On the first round, the triage officer simply identifies those patients who require immediate attention, according to the familiar priorities of airway, breathing, and circulation. First-priority patients are those in danger of asphyxia or shock.

First-Priority Patients (Red Tag)

- Patients in DANGER OF ASPHYXIA:
  1. Obstructed AIRWAY
  2. APNEA
  3. SUCKING CHEST WOUNDS
  4. TENSION PNEUMOTHORAX
  5. TRAUMATIC ASPHYXIA
- Patients in SHOCK or IMPENDING SHOCK:
  1. Major external or internal HEMORRHAGE
  2. BURNS over more than 20 percent of body surface
  3. PERICARDIAL TAMPONADE

The triage officer should not stop to treat any one patient but should keep moving from one patient to the next, assigning other EMTs to manage those with first-priority injuries. This process is greatly facilitated if the triage officer is equipped with a supply of color-coded TRIAGE TAGS, such as that shown in Figure 18-5. A red triage tag affixed to the victim indicates a need for immediate treatment; yellow means urgent; green nonurgent; and black indicates dead or hopelessly injured. The tag should be brightly colored and large enough to be visible from a distance, so that rescuers arriving at the scene can proceed directly to patients with high-priority tags. The tags should also be durable enough to withstand wet weather and dirt, and they should have a string or wire for attaching to the patient's wrist or clothing.

On successive rounds, the triage officer identifies patients with second- and third-priority injuries and tags them accordingly.

Second- and Third-Priority Patients

- SECOND-PRIORITY PATIENTS (Yellow Tag):
  1. Visceral injuries (e.g., evisceration) without shock
  2. Vascular injuries (all injuries that require a tourniquet)
  3. Head injuries with decreasing level of consciousness
  4. Burns less than 20 percent but involving the face, hands, feet, or genitalia
  5. Brain and spinal cord injuries
  6. Compound (open) fractures
- THIRD-PRIORITY INJURIES (Green Tag)
  1. Soft tissue injuries without shock
  2. Musculoskeletal injuries without shock or loss of pulses

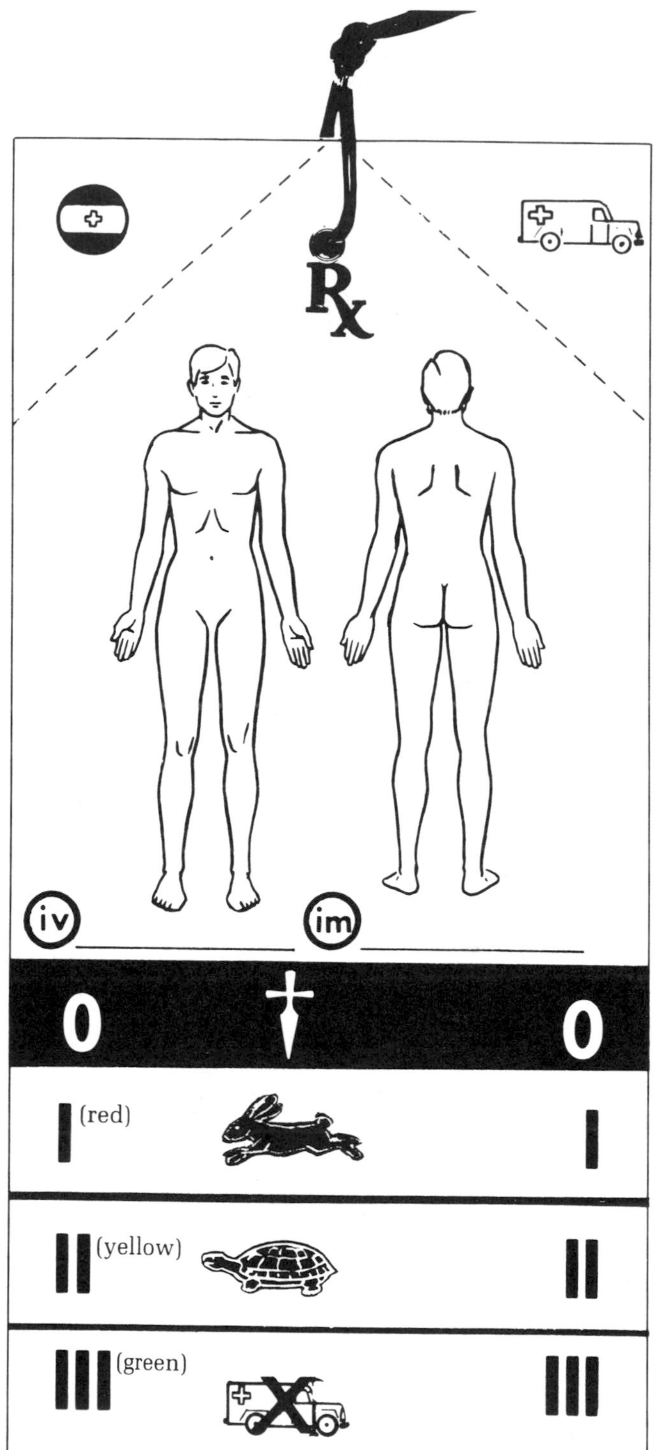

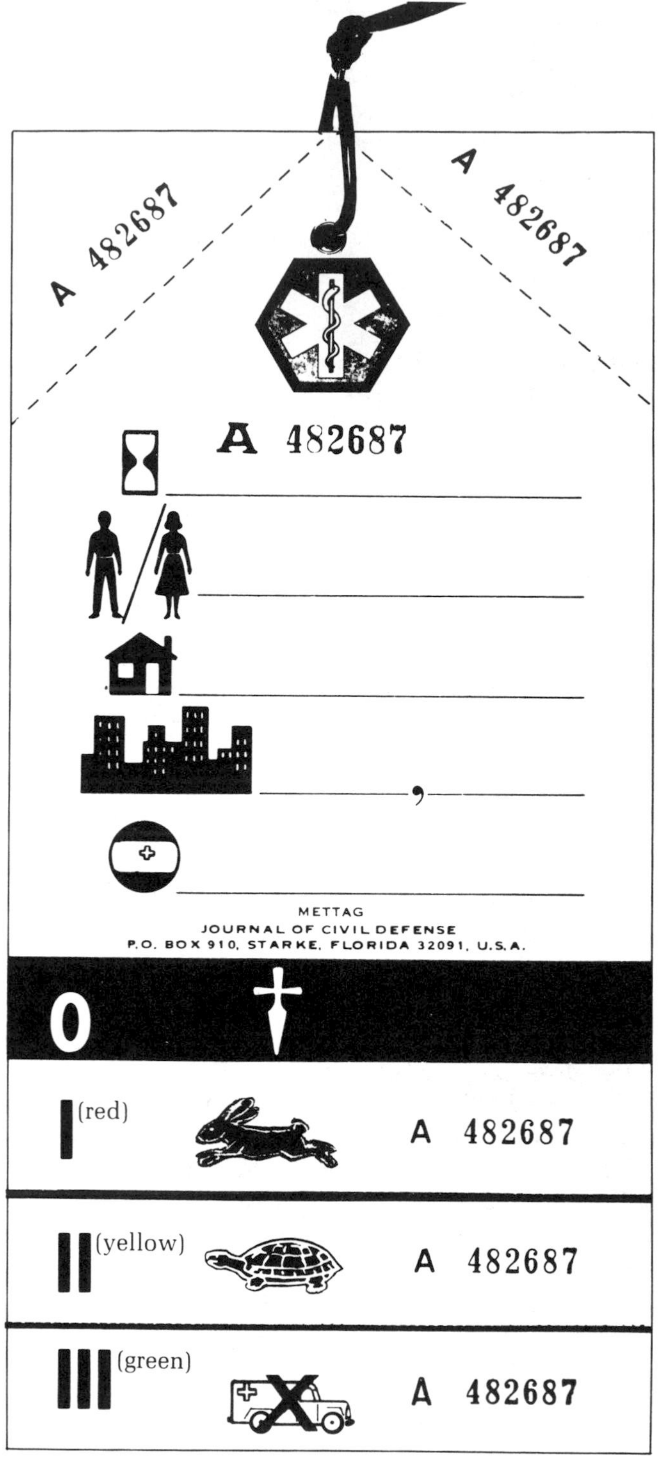

Fig. 18-5. *Triage tag, front and back. (Reproduced courtesy* Journal of Civil Defense, *Starke, Florida.)*

3. Injuries of the eye
4. Burns of other locations, under 20 percent

As the triage officer proceeds on the rounds of triage, he or she should make sure that all patients with red tags are being attended to before rescuers start working on patients with yellow tags and that all those with yellow tags are being cared for before those with green tags are seen. By the end of the first or second triage round, the triage officer should be able to make a better estimate of how much additional help is needed, and this information should be radioed back to the dispatcher.

As mentioned, patients who are obviously dead or hopelessly injured should be tagged as such and at the earliest convenience covered with a sheet and removed from the triage area. Hopelessly injured patients are those whose injuries are such that survival is considered impossible—for instance, a patient whose head has been amputated or whose brains are spilled out all over the ground.

As rapidly as possible, all of the injured should be centralized in the triage area, where they should be arranged in rows according to the severity of their injuries. Thus, red-tag patients will be in row 1, yellow-tag patients in row 2, and so forth. The initial triage is rapid and inevitably imprecise. The main purpose is to break down a large group of casualties into smaller, more manageable groups, but the initial classification of a casualty is not the final verdict. Frequent reassessment will enable the triage officer to reclassify casualties whose condition has improved or deteriorated or who were intitially misclassified, and to move them to a different row, as indicated. When victims must be removed from wreckage, one would ideally like to have the victims removed according to the severity of their injuries—the most severely injured brought out first. That is rarely feasible, however, and in practice those victims who can be freed readily must be removed as quickly as possible to clear the wreckage for more difficult extrication procedures. Triage thus usually begins as victims are brought from the wreckage to the triage area.

CONTINUING TREATMENT

Only when the immediately life-threatening conditions are under control can personnel be assigned to the patients with second-priority injuries, who will meanwhile have been tagged by the triage officer to indicate their status. While efforts continue to stablize the critically injured (e.g., initiation of IV lines, MAST garment), those with urgent but not life-threatening injuries are assessed, and their treatment is begun. At this stage, plans for evacuation need to be made.

EVACUATION OF THE INJURED

The priorities for evacuation will depend upon the number of ambulances available at the scene. If the number of ambulances equals or exceeds the number of victims, there is no problem, and the principle of evacuation is simple: THOSE WHO ARE STABILIZED FIRST ARE EVACUATED FIRST. If, however, there are more casualties than there are ambulances, priority for evacuation must be given to those patients who are most critically injured. There are various systems for assigning such priorities. The following system is adapted from that used by the military in NATO countries:

Priorities for Evacuation

- Priority I: Patients in persisting danger of asphyxia or exsanguination, including patients with
  1. THORACIC INJURIES, such as
     a. Persistent intrapleural hemorrhage
     b. Pericardial tamponade
     c. Thoracoabdominal injuries
  2. Unstable maxillofacial injuries that threaten the airway
  3. Shock
- Priority II:
  1. Stabilized patients in danger of shock, such as
     a. Blunt abdominal trauma
     b. Burns
  2. Patients with closed head injuries and decreasing level of consciousness
- Priority III: Patients with
  1. Spinal cord injuries
  2. Eye injuries
  3. Hand injuries
  4. Major compound fractures and injuries involving large areas of muscle
- Priority IV: Patients with lesser fractures and soft tissue injuries
- Priority V: "Walking wounded" (i.e., no systemic injury)

Whatever priority system is chosen for evacuation, it is critical that there be a *single* person in charge of assigning those priorities and controlling the flow of patients from the triage area to the staging area. Usually the triage officer assumes this responsibility, and he should be assisted by a transport/communications officer who (1) maintains contact with the receiving hospitals to determine which hospital is prepared to receive another casualty at any given time, (2) summons the ambulances from the staging area as they are needed, and (3) logs out *every* patient leaving the scene, with a record of the patient's name, the ambulance unit, and the hospital destination. The last is determined by the triage officer and not by the ambulance driver. Wherever possible, patients should be sent directly to special care centers that exist in a given region (e.g., burned patients to a burn center if close by; spinal injuries to a spinal cord center when available). In all instances, contact must be maintained with the receiving hospitals to notify them of incoming patients and to update information regarding which hospitals are already filled to capacity. Too often in mass casualty incidents, one hospital gets swamped with victims while a nearby hospital is completely overlooked. There is no reason for that to happen in a properly planned and organized mass casualty response.

Ambulances leaving the scene should be used to full capacity. High-priority injuries will usually require one ambulance per patient to permit adequate care of the patient en route to the hospital. But patients with less severe injuries can often be accommodated two or three to a vehicle, especially if the patients are in a condition to sit on the squad bench. Patients with minor injuries in stable condition can also be evacuated in vehicles other than ambulances. It may be possible, for instance, to commandeer a bus to transport the "walking wounded"; but at least one EMT should accompany the group, for responsibility for the patients continues until their care has been formally transferred to another medical professional.

The phases of triage are summarized in Figure 18-6.

DEALING WITH VICTIMS AND BYSTANDERS

In situations of mass casualties, both victims and bystanders may react by becoming dazed, confused, panicky, or otherwise overwhelmed. In general, there are five types of reaction that the EMT is likely to encounter in such situations. The NORMAL REACTION to a disaster is extreme anxiety, often with physical symptoms such as sweating, weakness, nausea, vomiting, and trembling. A person having such a reaction may recover control of himself relatively quickly and be able to provide assistance to the EMTs if properly directed.

A second type of reaction seen during mass casualties is BLIND PANIC. A person in this condition seems to lose all judgment and may behave entirely irrationally. What makes blind panic particularly dangerous is that it tends to be contagious, and the panic may spread quickly from one person to another. The person showing signs of blind panic must therefore be isolated from the rest of the bystanders and, if necessary, restrained. Preferably this job should be assigned to a responsible, calm bystander so that the EMTs can remain free to deal with the seriously injured.

DEPRESSION is seen in the person who sits or stands as if numbed, looking dazed or overwhelmed. It is important to try to get a person who is in such a state to "snap out of it," which can sometimes be accomplished by issuing a firm order to carry out some task (e.g., "Hold this IV bag for me."). In contrast to the bystander with depression, the person who manifests OVERREACTION tends to talk compulsively, joke inappropriately, and race back and forth from one task to another without accomplishing anything useful. The person who is overreacting will not be of any help to the rescue team, but will simply get in the way. He should be diverted to some activity that places him well out of the triage area or should be placed under the supervision of a more responsible, calmer bystander. Finally, a person may react to mass disaster with a condition known as CONVERSION HYSTERIA, in which the person converts his anxieties into bodily symptoms. He may become unable to see or hear or incapable of moving an arm or a leg. Such a patient can be difficult to distinguish from one who has actually been injured and should simply be categorized as nonurgent and managed accordingly.

Needless to say, rescue personnel are not immune to the reactions listed above. Even an experienced EMT can become momentarily dazed, panicky, or overreactive at the sight of several dozen bodies strewn all over the road. If this happens to one of your crew, give him or her a sharp command to carry out a specific task; for instance, "Go take care of that fracture—get moving!" Both EMTs and bystanders tend to function more effectively when they have a specific, well-defined job to carry out, and the skilled triage officer will assign tasks to all able-bodied personnel at the scene. The goal in doing so is to free up the EMTs from nonmedical assignments (e.g., directing traffic, crowd control) so they can use their skills to care for the injured.

The following guidelines, then, should be observed in dealing with mass casualty incidents:

Guidelines for Behavior in Mass Casualty Situations

- THE TREATMENT OF SERIOUS INJURIES HAS PRIORITY, but psychologic treatment should not be neglected altogether.
- When a member of the rescue team appears dazed or stunned, GIVE HIM OR HER A SPECIFIC JOB TO DO.
- MAKE MAXIMAL USE OF RESPONSIBLE BYSTANDERS to carry out nonmedical tasks.
  1. Calming and comforting other bystanders and the lightly injured.
  2. Crowd control; keeping spectators away from patients.
  3. Directing traffic.
- MAKE MAXIMAL USE OF EMTS FOR MEDICAL TASKS. Leave hazard control, rescue, crowd control, traffic control to other authorities wherever possible.
- Do not permit bystanders or officials from other agencies to interfere with medical care.
- ACCEPT THE CASUALTY'S LIMITATIONS AS REAL, including emotional limitations.
- ACCEPT YOUR OWN LIMITATIONS!

DISASTER PLANNING

As noted earlier, the response to a multicasualty incident is unlikely to go smoothly unless it has been planned and rehearsed well in advance. Planning for such incidents must involve *all* applicable agencies (rescue services, public safety organizations, hospitals, and so forth), for the success of the venture depends critically upon how well individuals from different organizations can work together and coordinate their efforts. Lines of authority and lines of communications must be clearly established and

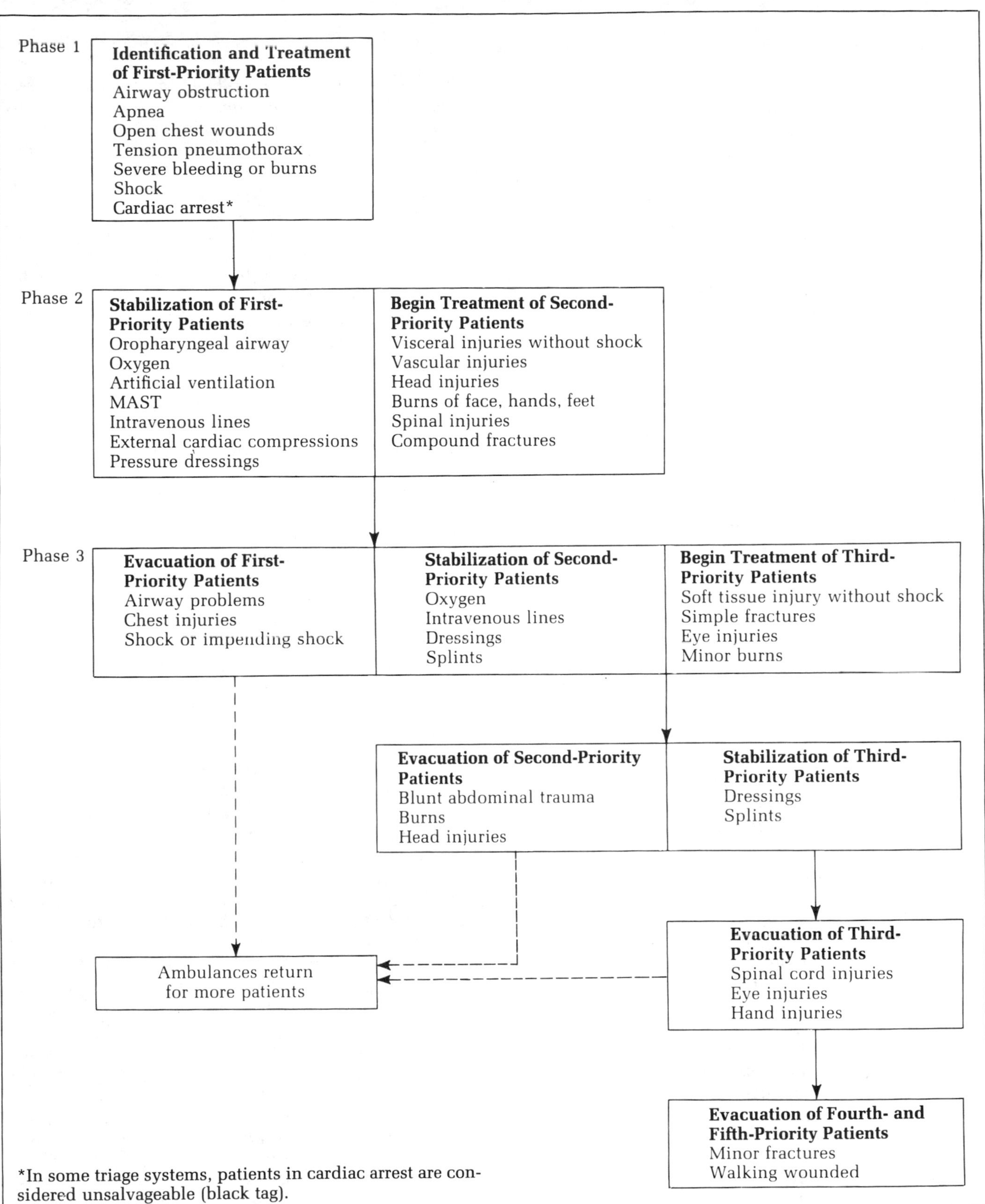

Fig. 18-6. *Phases of triage and evacuation.*

agreed upon *before* the disaster occurs. There is no time at the scene of a mass casualty incident to argue over who is in charge.

In addition, certain types of disasters require special considerations, and these must be identified in advance. In radiation incidents, for example, decontamination will assume first priority (see Chapter 31). In aircraft crashes, special care must be taken to mark the location of each victim before the victim is removed to the triage area. All of these actions require planning and drill. A multicasualty incident may occur only once in a few years, but when it does occur, the EMS system must be ready.

It should be stressed that the plan for managing victims of a disaster must be built around the existing EMS system in a given community. Insofar as possible, individuals should function in their usual roles in order to minimize confusion. Hospital personnel, for example, should remain at the hospital, with the possible exception of a mobile triage team dispatched from the hospital to the scene. Communications should go through the usual channels, and the dispatcher should "clear the air" of all unnecessary transmissions. Radio discipline must also be rehearsed during disaster drills.

CASE HISTORY

To summarize the concepts in this chapter, let us look at a hypothetical mass casualty incident in which a commuter train has been derailed near a large field and two passenger cars are overturned. The screams of the passengers can be heard from the forward, overturned cars as the first ambulance arrives at the scene. Passengers from the cars farther to the rear are meanwhile straggling out to see what is going on.

The driver of the ambulance parks the vehicle about 50 meters upwind from the engine car, lest it catch fire—near one of the more rearward passenger cars. Meanwhile, one EMT is radioing back to headquarters requesting assistance from the fire department, the police, and at least another five ambulances, to start. Then, switching the microphone over to the public address system, the EMT instructs passengers in the rear cars to remain seated and stay calm. He requests one volunteer in each upright car to survey the passengers in the car and make a list of those who will need treatment.

While one EMT remains near the ambulance to begin setting up a triage area, the other two EMTs head for the overturned cars. Two more ambulances arrive in the meanwhile and are directed to drop off their equipment at the triage area and park 100 meters away, in the staging area. Doing so, five of the incoming EMTs join the triage team, while a sixth remains behind to help establish the triage area.

The first EMT begins sorting through those patients who have crawled out or have been thrown clear of the cars and tags those with immediately life-threatening problems. The EMTs behind him begin splitting off to attend to the tagged patients. Meanwhile several engine companies arrive and begin bringing victims out of the wreck to the triage area. These victims are assessed and tagged as they reach the triage point. A surgeon arriving at the scene takes over as triage officer. By now, there are enough rescuers that one or two can go back with MCI boxes to check the rearward cars for injured. Mostly they find only minor injuries, but one elderly man showing signs of a heart attack is tagged for early evacuation and carried to the triage area. He is given oxygen and placed in a semisitting position on a stretcher. Several passengers are recruited to help tend to the patients with minor injuries and to calm the other passengers. A few young, sturdy types among the uninjured passengers are asked to come help carry stretchers and are given armbands to identify them as delegates of the rescue team.

Meanwhile, some of the first victims seen are in need of evacuation, so the triage officer begins summoning ambulances one by one from the staging area. After checking with the receiving hospitals—all of which were already notified to put their own disaster plans into effect—the triage officer instructs the driver of each ambulance regarding the hospital destination, and each patient is logged out by a bystander who has been recruited to act as scribe. The scribe records the name of each patient leaving the scene, the number of the ambulance in which the patient is being transported, and the hospital to which the patient is being sent. He also keeps a running update of information regarding hospital capabilities, as it is relayed from the dispatcher. For instance, "Montefiore: can take 3 more. Mercy: full. University Hospital: can take 5 more."

One of the EMTs who has been going through the rear cars reports that he has 26 "walking wounded" ready to be evacuated. The dispatcher is notified and asked to arrange for a bus to be sent to the scene and also to check which hospital can receive this volume of minor casualties. Meanwhile, treatment and evacuation continue. A separate area is set aside, out of view, for the dead. Police have now roped off the whole scene and are assisting in keeping spectators back from the triage area. Ambulances returning from the hospital report back to the staging area to await another assignment.

One hour after the first ambulance has arrived at the scene, all of the injured have been evacuated to the hospital. Six critically injured, 11 seriously injured, and 32 with mild to moderate injuries were distributed among 9 hospitals, all of which were on alert and prepared for the arrival of each patient. All casualties are accounted for, and relatives can be informed of which hospitals family members were evacuated to. Care given immediately to the most seriously injured saved half a dozen lives, and rapid evacuation of those most critically in need of immediate surgical treatment ensured that the lives saved in the field were not lost en route to the hospital.

The above is an idealized account of a multiple casualty incident response. There is no reason, however, why actual incidents should not be handled just as smoothly if adequate planning and drill has been carried out periodically in the community.

Questions to think about:

1. What tasks were given to bystanders in this incident? Can you think of any other jobs that bystanders could have performed?
2. Why were armbands issued to bystanders who were helping to carry stretchers?
3. Why was every patient "logged out" before being evacuated from the scene?
4. Why is it important for the triage officer or the dispatcher to maintain contact with the area hospitals?

VOCABULARY

MCI Abbreviation for *multiple casualty incident.*

staging area Area in which ambulances are stationed until they are needed for evacuation; it should be located beyond the triage area so that patients must pass through triage before being evacuated.

triage The sorting of patients according to the seriousness of their injuries.

FURTHER READING

MULTIPLY INJURED PATIENTS

Baxt WG et al. The failure of prehospital trauma prediction rules to classify trauma patients accurately. *Ann Emerg Med* 18:1, 1989.

Champion HR et al. The effect of medical direction on trauma triage. *J Trauma* 28:235, 1988.

Elling R. Expanding your trauma patient's primary assessment: Are you prepared? *Emerg Med Serv* 18(1):33, 1989.

Ferko JG. The triage factor. *Emergency* 20(8):44, 1988.

Gervin AS et al. The importance of prompt transport in salvage of patients with penetrating heart wounds. *J Trauma* 22:443, 1982.

Ivatury RR et al. Penetrating thoracic injuries: In-field stabilization vs. prompt transport. *J Trauma* 27:1066, 1987.

Jurkovitch GJ et al. Paramedic perception of elapsed field time. *J Trauma* 27:892, 1987.

Knoff R et al. Mechanism of injury and anatomic injury as criteria for prehospital trauma triage. *Ann Emerg Med* 17:895, 1988.

Knudson P, Frecceri CA, DeLateur SA. Improving the field triage of major trauma victims. *J Trauma* 28:602, 1988.

Koehler JJ et al. Prehospital index: A scoring system for field triage of trauma victims. *Ann Emerg Med* 15:178, 1986.

Moreau M et al. Application of the trauma score in the prehospital setting. *Ann Emerg Med* 14:1049, 1985.

Morris JA et al. The trauma score as a triage tool in the prehospital setting. *JAMA 256:1319, 1986.*

NATO. Emergency War Surgery. United States Issue. Washington, D.C.: U.S. Government Printing Office, 1975.

Rogers LF. Common oversights in the evaluation of the patient with multiple injuries. *Skel Radiol* 12:103, 1984.

Smith JP et al. Prehospital stabilization of critically injured patients: A failed concept. *J Trauma* 25:65, 1985.

Stewart C. Mechanisms of injury. *Emerg Med Serv* 18(1):21, 1989.

Timberlake GA. Trauma in the golden hour. *Emerg Med* 19(20):79, 1986.

Trunkey DD. Is ALS necessary for pre-hospital trauma care. *J Trauma* 24:86, 1984.

Werman H et al. Basic trauma life support. *Ann Emerg Med* 16:1240, 1987.

Wilder RJ. How much time should a paramedic spend examining the patient? *Emerg Med Serv* 7(2):74, 1978.

MULTIPLE CASUALTY INCIDENTS

Borden F. Earthquake planning and preparedness. *Emerg Med Serv* 14(3):12, 1985.

Boyd-Dernocoeur K, Wells-Mackie J. Disaster equipment: A weak link in the rescue chain. *Emergency* 12(12):56, 1980.

Butman AM. The challenge of casualties en masse. *Emerg Med* 15(7):111, 1983.

Caroline NL. EMS response to a terrorist attack. *Emerg Med Serv* 7(5):21, 1978.

Fisher CJ. Mobile triage team in a community disaster plan. *JACEP* 6:10, 1977.

Garcia B. Picking and choosing. *Rescue* 2(4):15, 1989.

Haynes BE et al. A prehospital approach to multiple-victim incidents. *Ann Emerg Med* 15:458, 1986.

Jacobs L. When disaster strikes in Boston. *Emerg Med* 15(10):28, 1983.

Kelly R. Mass casualty incident preparedness: Can you plan for disasters? *Emerg Med Serv* 14(3):16, 1985.

McKenna R. Hazardous materials incidents and the EMT. *EMT J* 5(6):400, 1981.

Orr S, Robinson W. The Hyatt-Regency skywalk collapse: An EMT based disaster response. *Ann Emerg Med* 12:601, 1983.

Saner P, Wolcott B. Stress reactions among participatns in mass casualty situations. *Ann Emerg Med* 12:426, 1983.

Stutz DR, Janusz SG. *Hazardous Materials Injuries: A Handbook for Pre-Hospital Care* (2nd ed.). Beltsville, MD: Bradford Communications, 1988.

U.S. Department of Transportation. *Hazardous Materials Emergency Response Handbook.* Washington, D.C.: U.S. Government Printing Office, 1980.

VI. MEDICAL EMERGENCIES

Medical emergencies are those caused by sudden acute illness or sudden deterioration in a chronic illness. They make themselves known to the patient in the form of symptoms*—pain, dyspnea, nausea, dizziness, and so forth—uncomfortable feelings that tell the patient something is not as it should be. Medical emergencies also produce clinical* signs*—objective changes in the patient's appearance or bodily functions that can be observed by an examiner.*

What the EMT finds on reaching a patient with a medical emergency is a person with a certain combination of symptoms and signs. What the EMT does not *find is a handy label attached to the patient with a diagnosis inscribed on it. This is not as serious a drawback as it might seem, for in practice, it is seldom necessary or even useful to come to a precise diagnosis in the field for purposes of giving basic life support. Every patient with chest pain will be treated as if he or she is suffering a heart attack, for in the early hours of chest pain this is the safest assumption to make. Every patient with difficulty breathing will receive oxygen, whether the respiratory distress is due to asthma, pneumonia, or another cause.*

For this reason, we have divided up the unit on medical emergencies according to the chief complaint—dyspnea, chest pain, belly pain, and so forth—for in large measure, it is the patient's chief complaint and overall condition that will determine the prehospital management. Within each category of chief complaint, however, there is a discussion of the different illnesses that may give rise to the complaint in question. For as part of the health care team, the EMT should have a basic understanding of the illnesses he or she is treating, in order to communicate effectively about the patient with other members of the medical team.

We begin this unit with a consideration of one of the most common chief complaints: shortness of breath.

19. DYSPNEA

OBJECTIVES

Dyspnea is the **sensation** of being short of breath. It may be experienced in a variety of conditions, all of which share one common feature: that the respiratory mechanism has become insufficient to supply the body's need for oxygen delivery and carbon dioxide removal at a given moment. All of us have experienced dyspnea under circumstances of exertion—that feeling of being unable to catch your breath after running to catch a bus or bolting up a few flights of stairs. But the dyspnea we are talking about here is not that caused by strenuous exercise. In this chapter, we are concerned with dyspnea that results from some disturbance or failure of the circulatory or respiratory system, and we shall examine several illnesses that commonly make their presence known by shortness of breath. By the conclusion of this chapter, the reader should be able to

1. Describe the principal drive that stimulates breathing in healthy individuals
2. Identify patients likely to be suffering from (a) hypoxia and (b) hypercarbia, and indicate how each of these patients should be managed, given a description of several patients
3. List at least five causes of dyspnea
4. Identify patients suffering from (a) left heart failure, (b) acute asthmatic attack, (c) decompensated chronic obstructive pulmonary disease, (d) pneumonia, and (e) pulmonary embolism, given a description of several patients with different signs and symptoms, and indicate the appropriate treatment for each
5. Identify symptoms and signs indicative of life-threatening danger in an asthmatic attack
6. Describe the special precautions that are necessary when administering oxygen to patients with chronic obstructive pulmonary disease and explain the reason for these precautions
7. Identify persons at risk of having suffered inhalation injury in a fire, given a description of several fire victims
8. Identify patients at risk of rapidly life-threatening complications after smoke inhalation, given a description of several smoke inhalation victims
9. Identify (a) first-priority victims, (b) second-priority victims, and (c) third-priority victims of chlorine gas exposure, and indicate the correct treatment for each
10. List the steps in treating a victim of hydrogen sulfide gas exposure
11. Identify correct and incorrect steps of managing tear gas exposure, given a list of various steps
12. Identify a patient suffering from hyperventilation syndrome, given a description of several patients with various respiratory disorders, and describe the management of this condition

THE PURPOSE OF BREATHING

Before we consider the various conditions that may interfere with normal respiration, let us review for a moment why we breathe in the first place and how breathing is adapted to changing needs. As we learned in an earlier chapter, breathing has two objectives: (1) to supply the body with oxygen, and (2) to blow off the carbon dioxide produced during metabolism. In a healthy person, the levels of both oxygen and carbon dioxide in the blood are constantly monitored by special receptors. The primary mechanism to control breathing is based on the level of CARBON DIOXIDE in the blood. If this level begins to *rise*, signals are sent to the lungs to increase the rate and depth of breathing, which enables the body to blow off more carbon dioxide and thereby drop the CO_2 level back toward normal. As a backup mechanism, the body also keeps tabs on the OXYGEN levels in the blood, and if these levels *fall* below a certain critical minimum, once again the lungs are instructed to speed up their operation.

When illness or injury interferes with the normal process of gas exchange, two possible disturbances may develop, either or both of which may cause serious problems for the patient. To begin with, any time that the *volume* of respiration—that is, the amount of air moved in and out of the lungs each minute—is insufficient, carbon dioxide will begin to build up in the blood, a situation called **hypercarbia.** High concentrations of carbon dioxide act in a manner very similar to narcotic drugs and can produce drowsiness or even unconsciousness. The only way to correct the problem of hypercarbia is to increase the volume of respiration, that is, to assist the patient's ventilations so that his breathing is deeper and more rapid. On the other hand, if for any reason an insufficient amount of oxygen is supplied to the blood and thence to the tissues—because of fluid in the alveoli, anemia, or various other reasons—the levels of oxygen in the blood begin to fall, and hypoxia results. The only way to correct hypoxia is to administer oxygen (Table 19-1).

Dyspnea occurs when either or both of these two disturbances are present: an acute rise in the level of carbon dioxide in the blood or a fall in the level of oxygen in the blood.

Table 19-1. *Disturbances in Gas Exchange*

Blood Chemistry	Term	Treatment
Rise in carbon dioxide	Hypercarbia	Assisted ventilation, to increase the rate and volume of breathing
Fall in oxygen	Hypoxemia	Oxygen administration

CAUSES OF DYSPNEA: OVERVIEW

As noted, the symptom of dyspnea may come about either because there is too much carbon dioxide in the blood or too little oxygen reaching the tissues, and those disturbances in turn may be caused by many types of problems, not just by problems with the lungs. In general, the causes of dyspnea can be put into three main categories: (1) respiratory, (2) cardiac, and (3) all the rest.

RESPIRATORY CAUSES OF DYSPNEA

Problems in the upper airway, the lower airways, and the lungs themselves are probably the most common causes of respiratory distress. As we recall the structure of the respiratory system, it is clear that there are several points at which disruption of normal breathing may occur. First, if the UPPER AIRWAY becomes blocked by a foreign body or by swelling, the flow of air to the lungs may be severely restricted or cut off altogether, and the patient will experience extreme, terrifying shortness of breath. Similar obstruction may occur in the LOWER AIRWAYS (the bronchi or bronchioles) because of spasm, swelling, or plugs of mucus, as seen in asthma. Here again, the flow of air into and out of the lungs is diminished, hypoxia and hypercarbia occur, and the patient experiences this reduction of air flow as dyspnea. In the lungs themselves, the ALVEOLI may become nonfunctional in a variety of ways: They may *collapse* (atelectasis) because of failure to take sufficiently deep breaths, as often occurs after rib fracture; they may become filled with *fluid* (pulmonary edema), *pus* (pneumonia), or even *blood* (after pulmonary contusion); or they may become filled with *gases* other than air during exposure to smoke or toxic fumes. In any of these situations, hypoxia is bound to follow, for red blood cells passing by an alveolus that is collapsed or filled with fluid will not be able to pick up oxygen and will thus return to the systemic circulation empty-handed. And as hypoxia occurs, the patient will become aware that something is wrong by a sensation of dyspnea, or air hunger, that hypoxia produces. Finally, respiratory distress may be the result of disruption of the PULMONARY CIRCULATION. If, for instance, a large blood clot lodges in one of the main pulmonary arteries (pulmonary embolism), blood flow through the lungs will be partially blocked. Even if the alveoli are functioning normally, they will not be able to deliver oxygen to the circulation, for there will be no red blood cells traveling past the alveoli to pick up oxygen.

CARDIAC CAUSES OF DYSPNEA

The most common cardiac cause of dyspnea is CONGESTIVE HEART FAILURE. As we shall discuss in more detail later, when the left side of the heart does not pump effectively, blood backs up in the lungs and seeps out of the lung capillaries into the alveoli, producing pulmonary edema. As in pulmonary edema from any other cause, when there is fluid in the alveoli due to left heart failure, oxygen cannot reach the blood, and hypoxia results.

OTHER CAUSES OF DYSPNEA

Even when there is normal respiratory and cardiac function, dyspnea may occur if the delivery of oxygen to the tissues is insufficient to meet their needs or if the rate and depth of breathing cannot keep up with an increased production of carbon dioxide. When there is acute ANEMIA, for instance, the loss of red blood cells from the circulatory bucket brigade may result in inadequate oxygen delivery to the tissues; and sometimes the first clue that a patient is suffering internal bleeding is the development of shortness of breath. The tissues do not know that the lungs are functioning properly; all they know is that they are not getting enough oxygen, so that the message they broadcast is "More air!" And the only way the body knows to get more air is to breathe deeper and faster. Increases in the production of carbon dioxide or other acids have a similar effect. There are several conditions, such as diabetes, which may cause METABOLIC ACIDOSIS, that is, a rise in the level of acid in the body. The only way the body can quickly rid itself of acid is to blow it off in the form of carbon dioxide. Thus patients with metabolic acidosis have deep, rapid respirations in an attempt to excrete more CO_2 through the lungs.

The various causes of dyspnea are summarized in Table 19-2. In this chapter, we shall examine in detail some of the more common cardiac and respiratory causes. Noncardiopulmonary disorders associated with dyspnea are covered elsewhere in this book.

LEFT HEART FAILURE

The job of the left side of the heart—the left atrium and left ventricle—is to pump oxygenated blood forward into the systemic circulation. If for any reason the left heart cannot pump out blood rapidly enough to keep up with the inflow of blood from the lungs, blood begins to back up in the pulmonary circuit. The pulmonary capillaries start to bulge; and plasma, mixed with a few red blood cells here and there, starts to leak out of the capillaries into the adjacent alveoli. The result is pulmonary edema, filling of the alveoli with fluid.

What causes the left heart to fail in the first place? One of the most common predisposing factors is chronic high blood pressure, or HYPERTENSION. When the arteries are constantly in a state of constriction, the left side of the heart has to work much harder to pump blood against the resistance these constricted arteries impose. After months and years of having to work so hard, the left heart simply gives out from the strain. A heart attack, or MYOCARDIAL INFARCTION, may also cause left heart failure, especially if there is extensive damage to the heart muscle, for a damaged heart cannot pump effectively.

The CHIEF COMPLAINT of a patient with left heart failure is almost always dyspnea. The patient will often give a HISTORY of having awakened from sleep because of difficulty breathing, and he may report that this has been going on for several nights—that each night he had to get up and walk around

Table 19-2. *Causes of Dyspnea*

Cause	Examples	Principal Disturbance	Treatment
RESPIRATORY CAUSES			
Upper airway obstruction	Laryngeal edema Foreign body (choking)	Hypoxia	Eliminate obstruction Oxygen
Lower airway obstruction	Asthma Emphysema Chronic bronchitis	Hypercarbia Hypoxia	Assisted ventilation Oxygen
Alveolar malfunction			
Atelectasis	Rib fracture	Hypoxia	Oxygen
Fluid in alveoli	Drowning, aspiration, toxic inhalations	Hypoxia	Oxygen
Pus in alveoli	Pneumonia	Hypoxia	Oxygen
Blockage of pulmonary circulation	Pulmonary embolism	Hypoxia	Oxygen
CARDIAC CAUSES			
Left heart failure	Pulmonary edema	Hypoxia	Oxygen
Total pump failure	Cardiogenic shock	Hypoxia	Oxygen
OTHER CAUSES			
Acute anemia	Internal or external bleeding	Hypoxia	Oxygen
Metabolic acidosis	Diabetic ketoacidosis Some poisonings	Accumulation of organic acids	Intravenous fluids

because of difficulty breathing, or that he had to sleep sitting up, propped up with pillows. This type of dyspnea that is worse when lying down is called **orthopnea,** and it is very characteristic of left heart failure. When the patient is recumbent, fluid tends to pool in the lungs, thereby adding to the excess fluid already there. When the patient gets up and walks around, some of that fluid drains by gravity out of the lungs and thereby helps relieve the patient's symptoms.

On PHYSICAL EXAMINATION, the patient in left heart failure shows signs of hypoxia and the presence of fluid in the lungs. To begin with, there is likely to be marked RESPIRATORY DISTRESS, as the patient struggles to get more oxygen. Terror and hypoxia may make the patient extremely AGITATED, CONFUSED, and even COMBATIVE. If hypoxia is marked, CYANOSIS may be evident. BREATHING is DEEP and LABORED, and in severe cases, the patient may cough up PINK, FROTHY SPUTUM—the edema fluid from the alveoli. Auscultation of the lungs will reveal loud, bubbling RALES and sometimes whistling WHEEZES as well—the sounds of air passing through edema fluid and narrowed airways. As the body tries to compensate for hypoxia, the pulse speeds up (TACHYCARDIA) and the blood pressure rises (HYPERTENSION). If there is failure of the right side of the heart as well, distention of the jugular veins and edema in the feet will indicate that blood is also backing up in the systemic side of the circulation.

Pulmonary edema due to left heart failure is a CRITICAL MEDICAL EMERGENCY and requires immediate treatment and prompt transport. The patient should be placed in a SITTING POSITION WITH LEGS DANGLING, in order to promote the drainage of fluids by gravity out of the lung. For this reason, it is preferable that the patient be transported in a chair stretcher, and the ambulance should be arranged in such a way that a chair stretcher can be secured to the front wall of the patient area for transport.

OXYGEN IN THE HIGHEST POSSIBLE CONCENTRATION is a must. If the patient will tolerate it, the demand valve is the best means of delivering 100% oxygen in this situation, for the positive pressure delivered by the demand valve may help drive fluid out of the alveoli. Often, however, patients in left heart failure are so frantic from hypoxia that they will not tolerate any kind of mask at all, because they feel as if they are suffocating when a mask is placed over their faces. In such cases, one may have to compromise and give oxygen by two-pronged nasal cannula. That is not ideal, for even at 6 liters per minute, a nasal cannula will deliver only about 40% oxygen. It is better, however, than not giving any supplemental oxygen at all, and if the patient keeps flinging away the demand valve or tearing off a nonrebreathing mask, there may be no choice.

Definitive treatment of left heart failure requires the administration of drugs that will help the patient excrete some of his excess fluid as urine. These drugs cannot be given by EMT-As, and thus it is imperative to TRANSPORT THE PATIENT PROMPTLY TO THE HOSPITAL, where further treatment may be initiated.

Left Heart Failure: Summary

- HISTORY
  1. Chronic hypertension or chest pain
  2. Severe DYSPNEA; often ORTHOPNEA
- PHYSICAL FINDINGS
  1. Patient in MARKED DISTRESS; may be AGITATED, CONFUSED, and COMBATIVE
  2. TACHYCARDIA and ELEVATED BLOOD PRESSURE
  3. Pink, FROTHY SPUTUM
  4. CYANOSIS
  5. RALES and WHEEZES
  6. Sometimes signs of right heart failure (pedal edema, jugular distention)
- TREATMENT
  1. SIT THE PATIENT UP with legs dangling
  2. 100% OXYGEN, preferably by demand valve
  3. Prompt transport

OBSTRUCTIVE AIRWAYS DISEASE

Among the *pulmonary* disorders that can lead to respiratory distress, probably the most common are a group of diseases that cause narrowing and obstruction of the *lower* airways. These diseases include asthma and chronic obstructive pulmonary diseases (emphysema and chronic bronchitis).

ASTHMA

Asthma is an episodic disease that afflicts about six million Americans. It is characterized by acute attacks of **bronchospasm,** in which the airways become swollen, constricted, and filled with mucous plugs. Between attacks, the patient is usually free of symptoms. In taking the HISTORY from the patient with asthma, one will often find that the patient has had SIMILAR ATTACKS IN THE PAST, some of which may have required treatment in the emergency room. Try to determine whether there was some particular PREDISPOSING FACTOR for this attack: Acute asthmatic attacks are frequently precipitated by respiratory infection, inhaled pollutants or allergens (such as dust, smoke, pollen), or even emotional stress. Be sure to inquire as well what MEDICA-

TIONS the patient takes and how much medication he or she has already taken for this attack. Most asthmatics use inhalers or bronchodilator pills when they feel an attack coming on, and patients with severe asthma are sometimes prescribed steroid medications as well.

On PHYSICAL EXAMINATION, the patient with an acute asthmatic attack will be in obvious RESPIRATORY DISTRESS. The patient is usually found sitting up, leaning forward, and fighting for air. Often he is very FRIGHTENED. He may have spasms of COUGHING without bringing up any sputum. USE OF ACCESSORY MUSCLES to assist respiration is prominent, and thus one will see retractions of the muscles above the clavicles during respiration. The nature of bronchial obstruction in asthma is such that the patient finds exhalation more difficult than inhalation. For this reason, the asthmatic having an acute attack tends to exhale a slightly smaller volume than he inhaled, so with each breath there is progressive air trapping in the lung. This leads to HYPERINFLATION OF THE CHEST, which will sound unusually hollow if you tap over it. Upon auscultation of the chest, one usually hears WHEEZING, the sound of air whistling through narrowed airways. But wheezes may be absent if the attack is very severe and very little air is moving in and out of the lungs. Anxiety and the struggle to breathe will almost invariably produce TACHYCARDIA, and the blood pressure may be slightly elevated for the same reason.

One very severe form of acute asthmatic attack is called **status asthmaticus,** which is a prolonged asthmatic attack that does not "break" with the use of the usual medications. The history will reveal that the attack has been going on for hours, perhaps days. The patient is usually exhausted and severely dehydrated; he may be very sleepy as well, for as air exchange decreases, carbon dioxide builds up in the blood and acts as a narcotic to sedate the patient. The chest is likely to be very distended from air trapping, and breath sounds, even wheezes, may be completely inaudible because there is virtually no air moving through the swollen, constricted bronchi.

A SLEEPY ASTHMATIC WITH A SILENT CHEST IS A DIRE MEDICAL EMERGENCY.

There are 4,000 to 5,000 deaths from asthma each year in the United States, and many of these deaths result from hypoxia and hypercarbia—strangulation at the bronchial level.

TREATMENT of the patient with an acute asthmatic attack requires that the rescuer maintain a CALM, REASSURING MANNER. Remember, the patient is likely to be terrified because of his inability to get enough air, and his agitation only makes the situation worse. He needs to feel that you have everything under control. Allow the patient to remain SITTING UP, for this is the position in which it is easiest to breathe, and administer humidified OXYGEN, preferably by mask. If the patient is not moving very much air in and out of his chest, you may have to give him an occasional assisted breath with the demand valve. Do not use the demand valve constantly, for the very dry gases it delivers will cause further hardening of mucous plugs obstructing the airways. If the patient is a young person, without any history of heart disease, and if you are authorized to do so, start an INTRAVENOUS INFUSION to combat the patient's dehydration. Determine whether the patient has taken his prescribed medications and, if not, assist him in doing so. TRANSPORT WITHOUT DELAY to the hospital.

Acute Asthmatic Attack: Summary

- HISTORY
  1. Previous attacks
  2. Precipitating factors (flu, allergy, emotional stress)
  3. Medications (inhalers, bronchodilator pills, steroids)
  4. Severe DYSPNEA
- PHYSICAL FINDINGS
  1. Severe RESPIRATORY DISTRESS; patient sitting up, leaning forward, fighting for air
  2. ANXIETY
  3. Unproductive COUGH
  4. Use of ACCESSORY MUSCLES to assist breathing
  5. HYPERINFLATED CHEST
  6. WHEEZES (Note: A SILENT CHEST MEANS DANGER!)
  7. DROWSINESS (Note: A SLEEPY ASTHMATIC IS AN ASTHMATIC IN TROUBLE!)
- TREATMENT
  1. Calm, reassuring manner
  2. Humidified OXYGEN
  3. Keep the patient SITTING UP
  4. Intravenous fluids (for patient under 35 years old)
  5. Assist patient in taking his medications
  6. PROMPT TRANSPORT

CHRONIC OBSTRUCTIVE PULMONARY DISEASE (COPD)

The two most common chronic obstructive pulmonary diseases—emphysema and chronic bronchitis—are characterized by destructive changes in the lungs and progressive dyspnea. These are very common diseases, affecting between 10 and 20 percent of the adult American population. The most important factor known to play a role in causing COPD is CIGARETTE SMOKING. In 1986, there were 71,099 deaths from COPD in the United States, 82 percent of those deaths attributable to smoking.

In EMPHYSEMA, there is distention and destruction of the air spaces in the lungs. The patient with emphysema gives a history of increasing dyspnea on exertion that has caused more and more limitation of his activities. On physical examination, he tends to be THIN and may appear somewhat wasted (Fig. 19-1). Cyanosis is unusual in emphysema, except during severe decompensation, and for that reason these patients are sometimes called "pink puffers," which describes both the color of their mucous membranes and the fact that they often PURSE THEIR LIPS on exhalation. The CHEST in emphysema tends to be BARREL-SHAPED and sounds hollow when you tap on it, owing to air trapping in the lungs. BREATH SOUNDS are usually distant.

CHRONIC BRONCHITIS is characterized by excessive mucus production in the bronchial tree, with a CHRONIC PRODUCTIVE COUGH. The patient with chronic bronchitis is almost invariably a HEAVY CIGARETTE SMOKER. He tends to be obese and often has a rather BLUISH COMPLEXION—features that have led to the term "blue bloater" to describe this type of patient. Upon auscultation of the patient's chest, one is likely to hear a symphony of rales, rhonchi, wheezes, and squeaks, due to bronchospasm and mucus rattling about in the airways. Right heart failure is not uncommon in these patients and, when present, is manifested by distended jugular veins and pedal edema.

In actual practice, the pink puffer and the blue bloater are usually not so sharply differentiated, and most patients with COPD have elements of both emphysema and chronic bronchitis. All of these patients live in a state of very marginal compensation, the damaged respiratory mechanism being just barely adequate to take care of their resting needs for oxygen. They have very little respiratory reserve, and for that reason even a small stress such as a bout of the flu or other illness may plunge the patient into sudden respiratory failure. And it is when this kind of acute decompensation occurs that the patient is likely to call for medical help.

The HISTORY of a patient in acute decompensation of COPD will usually reveal that there has been INCREASING DYSPNEA over the past several days, often in the wake of some illness. Frequently the patient will report that the dyspnea has begun to interfere with his sleep, and that he has to get up

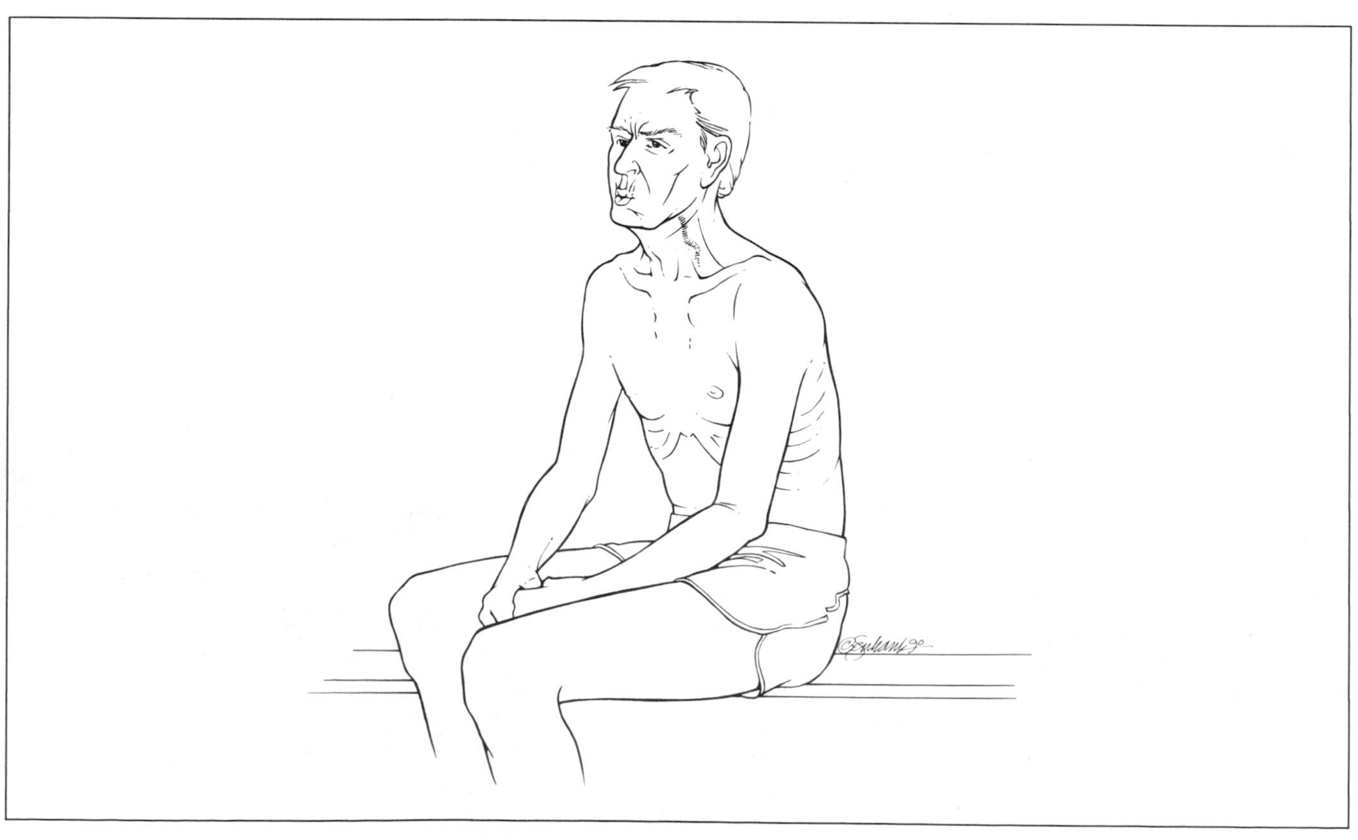

Fig. 19-1. *Typical patient with emphysema. Note the posture (leaning forward), wasted muscles, retractions of the intercostal and supraclavicular muscles, distended neck veins, and pursed lips.*

several times during the night on account of it. He may note INCREASING COUGH or a CHANGE IN HIS SPUTUM, which becomes more voluminous and yellow-green instead of white.

On PHYSICAL EXAMINATION, the patient is likely to be in MARKED RESPIRATORY DISTRESS. Hypoxia and hypercarbia may produce CONFUSION, AGITATION, and MUSCULAR TWITCHING. CYANOSIS is often present. The chest is likely to be full of noisy RALES, RHONCHI, and WHEEZES. If right heart failure is present, the jugular veins will be distended and the feet swollen.

The most critical aspect of the TREATMENT of a patient in respiratory failure from COPD is to ADMINISTER OXYGEN, for the major threat to the patient's life is hypoxemia. In giving oxygen, it is important to be aware that oxygen can depress the respirations of such patients. This is because many patients with COPD are chronically underventilated and walk around with very high levels of carbon dioxide in their blood. After a while, the body gets used to these high CO_2 levels, and hypercarbia no longer serves as a stimulus to breathe as it would in a healthy person. Instead, such patients breathe on what is called a hypoxic drive; that is, their stimulus to breathe is a fall in the *oxygen* content in the blood rather than a rise in the carbon dioxide content. Now, if you give such a patient oxygen, and the level of oxygen in his blood rises back toward normal, his stimulus to breathe is abolished, and he may actually stop breathing altogether! THIS IS *NOT* A JUSTIFICATION TO DEPRIVE THE PATIENT OF OXYGEN THERAPY, FOR HE MAY DIE WITHOUT IT. It simply means that when you administer oxygen to a patient with known COPD, you must watch him like a hawk! If his respiratory rate starts to slow, coach him to breathe deeply, and if he continues despite your coaching to show signs of respiratory depression, whip out the bag-valve-mask (with oxygen) or demand valve, and start assisting ventilations.

This point is often misunderstood and bears reemphasis. It is true that oxygen may depress the respirations of a patient with COPD and even cause apnea. This does *not* mean that such patients should not receive oxygen. It does mean that when you do administer oxygen to a patient with COPD, you must **monitor the patient closely** and be prepared to **assist ventilations as needed.**

> NEVER, NEVER, NEVER WITHHOLD OXYGEN THERAPY FROM A PATIENT IN RESPIRATORY DISTRESS, EVEN A PATIENT WITH COPD.

Allow the patient to remain SITTING UP, and ENCOURAGE HIM TO COUGH in order to bring up some of the sputum obstructing his airways.

Acute Decompensation of COPD: Summary

- HISTORY
  1. CHRONIC DYSPNEA, recently worse
  2. Heavy CIGARETTE SMOKING
  3. Recent respiratory infection
  4. CHANGE IN the amount and color of SPUTUM
- PHYSICAL FINDINGS
  1. RESPIRATORY DISTRESS
  2. CONFUSED and AGITATED; *or* SLEEPY and STUPOROUS
  3. Muscular TWITCHING
  4. CYANOSIS
  5. PURSED-LIP breathing
  6. Use of ACCESSORY MUSCLES to breathe
  7. Noisy chest: RALES, RHONCHI, and WHEEZES
  8. Sometimes signs of right heart failure
- TREATMENT
  1. Keep the patient SITTING UP
  2. Give OXYGEN (nasal cannula, 4–6 liters/min)
  3. MONITOR respirations closely, and ASSIST VENTILATIONS as needed
  4. Encourage the patient to cough
  5. Prompt transport

PNEUMONIA

Pneumonia is a general term applied to a group of illnesses characterized by inflammation and often consolidation of the lungs. Fluid or pus accumulates in the alveoli and interferes with the oxygenation of the blood. Pneumonia may be caused by bacteria, viruses, aspirated vomitus, or inhaled chemical agents. The typical patient with a *bacterial* pneumonia, one of the more common types, is elderly or debilitated. The HISTORY will usually reveal the SUDDEN ONSET OF SHAKING CHILLS AND FEVER. In addition, CHEST PAIN, DYSPNEA, and PRODUCTIVE COUGH are usually part of the clinical picture. On PHYSICAL EXAMINATION, the patient will appear very ill with hot dry skin. The TEMPERATURE is likely to be quite elevated, and there may be evidence of RESPIRATORY DISTRESS, especially tachypnea. RHONCHI may be audible upon auscultation of the chest.

In the field, the only TREATMENT feasible for a patient with suspected pneumonia is to allow him to assume a POSITION OF COMFORT, and administer OXYGEN.

Pneumonia: Summary

- HISTORY
  1. Elderly or debilitated patient
  2. SUDDEN ONSET of shaking CHILLS
  3. Productive COUGH; sometimes chest pain, belly pain

- PHYSICAL FINDINGS
  1. Hot, dry skin; FEVER
  2. TACHYPNEA
  3. Rhonchi may be audible
- TREATMENT
  1. POSITION OF COMFORT
  2. OXYGEN (nasal cannula or mask)
  3. Transport to hospital

PULMONARY EMBOLISM

Gas exchange in the lungs requires functional alveoli to provide oxygen to and take up carbon dioxide from the blood. But this is only half of the picture. The other half comprises the pulmonary vessels that carry venous blood to the lungs to be "aired out." In the preceding sections, we have looked at some conditions that interfere with alveolar function. But even normal alveoli will be of little use if blood cannot reach them. This is the situation in pulmonary embolism.

A pulmonary embolism is the sudden blocking of a pulmonary artery or one of its branches by some obstructing plug that is swept into the pulmonary circulation by blood currents. Probably the most common form of pulmonary embolism is a BLOOD CLOT, arising in the veins of the legs or the pelvis and then breaking loose to flow downstream, through the right heart, into the lungs. This is particularly likely to occur in patients who have been confined to bed for long periods or who have inflammation of the veins in their legs (thrombophlebitis). Young women taking birth control pills are also at greater risk to develop wandering blood clots. Pulmonary emboli may, however, arise from other sources besides blood clots. FAT PARTICLES released from broken bone ends may cause pulmonary embolism in a patient who has suffered massive skeletal trauma. In a difficult childbirth, AMNIOTIC FLUID may find its way from the amniotic sac into the mother's circulation and be swept into the lungs, causing obstruction of the pulmonary arteries. Even AIR entering the circulation, as from an open wound of the neck, can lodge in a pulmonary vessel and effectively block blood flow through it.

The typical patient with a pulmonary embolism presents with the SUDDEN ONSET OF SEVERE DYSPNEA. In many cases, this will be the only symptom, but sometimes that patient will also report SHARP CHEST PAIN, and very occasionally he will cough up blood. On PHYSICAL EXAMINATION, there is likely to be evidence of RESPIRATORY DISTRESS. TACHYCARDIA is almost always present, and in severe cases a falling blood pressure may suggest the presence of shock. Usually the rest of the physical examination is unremarkable when the patient is first seen.

TREATMENT in the field for suspected pulmonary embolism consists of giving OXYGEN in high concentrations and transporting the patient without delay to the hospital.

Pulmonary Embolism: Summary

- HISTORY
  1. Prolonged bedrest; thrombophlebitis; birth control pills
  2. SUDDEN ONSET of severe dyspnea
- PHYSICAL FINDINGS
  1. RESPIRATORY DISTRESS
  2. TACHYCARDIA
  3. Hypotension in severe cases
- TREATMENT
  1. POSITION OF COMFORT
  2. OXYGEN (nonrebreathing mask)
  3. Prompt transport

TOXIC INHALATIONS

The inhalation of smoke, toxic fumes, or various gases may produce a variety of untoward effects on both the respiratory tract and the body as a whole. Sometimes these effects may not become evident until several hours after the exposure, so in general the EMT must assume that victims of toxic inhalation have suffered respiratory damage until proved otherwise.

It is beyond the scope of this book to elaborate the specific effects produced by every toxic gas, and we will confine ourselves here to consideration of some of the more common or more dangerous exposures. The general principles of management do not differ significantly for other toxic inhalations, and the rule of thumb is always:

GET THE PATIENT AWAY FROM THE BAD GAS, AND GIVE HIM THE GOOD GAS (OXYGEN).

SMOKE INHALATION

Smoke inhalation injury occurs in 15 to 25 percent of burn victims and accounts for approximately half of the mortality from fires. Smoke inhalation is a sneaky saboteur of the respiratory tract, for it may produce fatal pulmonary damage with minimal external evidence. For this reason, the EMT must have a clear idea of WHO IS AT RISK of having suffered significant inhalation injury, so that such patients may be identified and treated early, before the respiratory problems become life-threatening. In the section on burns, we have already mentioned some of the factors that should alert the EMT to the possibility of respiratory damage after exposure to smoke.

Who Is at Risk for Inhalation Injury After Fire

- Persons whose exposure was of LONG DURATION
- Persons trapped in a CLOSED SPACE during the fire
- Persons who LOST CONSCIOUSNESS in a smoky environment
- Victims of fire with any of the following
  1. DYSPNEA
  2. HOARSENESS
  3. WHEEZING
  4. BRASSY COUGH
  5. SOOTY SPUTUM
  6. FACIAL BURNS
  7. SINGED NASAL HAIRS, beard, moustache, or eyebrows

Remember: At the scene of a fire, inhalation injuries may occur in both victims who have suffered burns and victims who have not suffered burns.

Every victim of fire having any of the above risk factors *must* be treated as a victim of smoke inhalation and evaluated in the hospital, even if the victim has no present difficulty breathing. Respiratory symptoms may take hours to develop, and the victim of smoke inhalation may leave the scene feeling fine only to go into fulminant pulmonary edema upon reaching home.

In evaluating the persons at risk, it is also important for the EMT to try to determine WHAT THE PATIENT INHALED, which means finding out WHAT WAS BURNING. Most serious respiratory injury after smoke inhalation is caused by toxic products of combustion present in the smoke (Table 19-3). The burning of many commonly used structural materials or home furnishings produces a variety of harmful chemicals and gases, which can wreak havoc throughout the respiratory tract causing upper airway obstruction (by edema), bronchospasm, and chemical pulmonary edema. In addition, the combustion of many materials produces a dangerous respiratory poison, carbon monoxide, which prevents adequate oxygenation of the blood (see Chapter 26).

The TREATMENT of victims of smoke inhalation requires first of all REMOVAL OF THE VICTIM FROM THE TOXIC ENVIRONMENT. Victims of fire should be brought to a triage area *upwind* from the fire, where there is good ventilation. Humidified OXYGEN should be administered as soon as possible to *every* person (including fire personnel) suspected of significant smoke exposure. Those victims already showing signs of pulmonary edema (e.g., rales) should receive 100% oxygen by demand valve. Victims with potential for upper respiratory tract burns—that is, patients with burns about the face and neck; patients with hoarseness or stridor—should be TRANSPORTED AT ONCE to the hospital, for laryngeal edema may develop extremely rapidly in such patients, closing off the whole airway in a matter of minutes.

Smoke Inhalation: Summary

- Identify PATIENTS AT RISK.
- Determine WHAT WAS INHALED.
- TREAT AND TRANSPORT *ALL* PATIENTS AT RISK, even if they do not have respiratory distress at present.
  1. Remove victims from exposure to smoke.
  2. Give humidified OXYGEN.
  3. First priority for transport: patients with facial burns, hoarseness, or stridor.

CHLORINE GAS EXPOSURE

Accidents involving chlorine gas are relatively common because of the widespread use of chlorine compounds both in the home and in industry. Household exposures usually occur when someone mixes a cleaning agent containing sodium hypochlorite (such as bleach) with some strong acid in an overzealous attempt to "really clean" a toilet bowl. The resulting chemical reaction releases chlorine gas, often in high concentrations. Most cases of chlorine gas exposure occur outside the home, however, in situations of mass exposure. The chlorination of large swimming pools (where the gas rather than the liquid or solid forms of chlorine tends to be used) has led to numerous cases of mass exposure at hotels and community recreation centers. Leakage from industrial storage tanks or from trucks or trains carrying chlorine has also resulted in virtual epidemics of chlorine gas exposure. Thus, in the majority of instances in which the EMT has to deal with chlorine gas inhalation, there will be a LARGE NUMBER OF VICTIMS, and the usual principles of triage must be applied.

The SYMPTOMS AND SIGNS of chlorine gas inhalation depend on the concentration of the inhaled gas and the duration of exposure. Chlorine gas is extremely irritating to all mucous membranes, and when it comes in contact with the moisture on these surfaces, it can form hydrochloric and other acids that are very damaging to body tissues. With *minor exposures*, the patient will experience BURNING SENSATIONS in the eyes, nose, and throat and

Table 19-3. *Toxic Products of Combustion*

Substance	Found in	Products of Combustion	Effects of Exposure
Polyvinyl chloride	Plastic bottles, electric insulation, car and aircraft upholstery, wall coverings, phonograph records	Hydrogen chloride, phosgene, chlorine, carbon monoxide	Pulmonary edema, mucosal irritation, chest tightness
Polyurethane	Thermal insulation, mattresses, carpets, seat cushions	Hydrogen cyanide, isocyanate, CO	Asphyxia
Acrylics	Textiles, paints, aircraft windows	Acrolein, acetic acid, formic acid	Mucosal irritation, asphyxia
Nylon	Clothes, carpeting, upholstery	Ammonia, hydrogen cyanide	Pulmonary edema, asphyxia
Wood, cotton, paper	Furniture, structural materials, paper products, clothing	Acrolein, acetaldehyde, formaldehyde, acetic acid, formic acid	Mucosal irritation

perhaps a slight cough. *More intense exposure* to chlorine gas causes CHEST TIGHTNESS, CHOKING, PAROXYSMAL COUGH, HEADACHE, NAUSEA, and sometimes WHEEZING. Patients with the *most severe exposure* are apt to manifest, in addition, CYANOSIS, RALES, SHOCK, CONVULSIONS, and COMA.

In treating the victims of chlorine gas inhalation, once again the first priority is to REMOVE THE VICTIMS FROM EXPOSURE TO THE GAS. In order to do so, the EMT must take proper precautions to prevent his or her own exposure, which means the use of an appropriate gas mask. A makeshift gas mask, for both rescuers and victims, may be fashioned from a piece of cloth soaked in water and held over the face.

As soon as the victims have been removed to a safe environment, upwind from the gas spill, they must be rapidly TRIAGED (Table 19-4). Oxygen cylinders and demand valves will usually be in short supply, so the most seriously affected must have priority for oxygen therapy. Those with dyspnea, wheezing, severe cough, or other signs of respiratory distress should receive humidified oxygen by mask; the demand valve should be reserved for victims with rales or other indications of pulmonary edema. Once these patients have been treated and their evacuation to the hospital is under way, less serious problems may be addressed. Burning or itching eyes should be irrigated with tap water, as should any areas of the skin that may have come in contact with the chlorine.

Chlorine Gas Exposure: Summary

- PROTECT YOURSELF! Wear appropriate gas mask or breathing apparatus.
- REMOVE VICTIMS FROM EXPOSURE.
- TRIAGE.
- OXYGEN to those with respiratory distress.
- Transport to hospital.

HYDROGEN SULFIDE GAS EXPOSURE

With its highly pungent and characteristic odor of rotten eggs, hydrogen sulfide gas is hard to miss. It is found in sewer gas, cesspools, and other areas of putrefaction. Industrial exposure may occur in the shale oil industry and in the manufacture of some fertilizers. Hydrogen sulfide is a very toxic gas, and it may be lethal in a matter of minutes if inhaled in high concentrations. With *mild exposure*, the patient experiences burning sensations in the eyes, a tight feeling in the chest, cough, and skin irritation. More *intense exposure* causes TACHYPNEA FOLLOWED BY RESPIRATORY ARREST, weakness, headache, and SUDDEN UNCONSCIOUSNESS. The main principles of TREATMENT involve protection of the rescuers, removal of the patient from exposure, and basic life support as needed.

Treatment of the Victim of Hydrogen Sulfide Inhalation

- PROTECT YOURSELF! Don your breathing apparatus before entering the rescue environment.
- REMOVE THE VICTIM IMMEDIATELY TO FRESH AIR, UPWIND.
- Keep the victim still.
- Administer OXYGEN in high concentration.
- If apnea occurs, perform artificial ventilation.
- If the eyes are affected, irrigate them thoroughly with tap water.
- Transport to hospital.

Table 19-4. *Triage of Chlorine Gas Victims*

Category	Signs and Symptoms	Treatment
First priority	Severe respiratory distress Cyanosis Rales Shock Convulsions Coma Respiratory arrest	OXYGEN via demand valve Prompt transport to hospital Sitting position if not in shock or coma
Second priority	Chest tightness, air hunger Paroxysmal cough, wheezing Nausea, headache, or both	Humidified oxygen by mask Transport to hospital in sitting position
Third priority	Burning or itching eyes Burning sensations in nose, throat	Irrigate eyes with tap water Throat lozenges Transport to hospital when ambulance or other means is available

TEAR GAS EXPOSURE

With increasing levels of urban unrest over the past few decades, both law enforcement agencies and private citizens are resorting to the use of tear gas or Mace to disperse unruly crowds or to ward off would-be attackers. The EMT may be called on to treat and transport persons contaminated with these agents, and thus it is important for EMS personnel to understand the characteristics of the tear gases and the precautions they require.

The properties of the principal tear gases are summarized in Table 19-5. Probably the most widely used of these is chloroacetophenone (CN), a white solid substance that produces a blue-white powder with an apple blossom odor on release. CN is also the active ingredient in Mace, which uses kerosene as a propellant to permit the CN to be sprayed rather than burned or detonated.

Whatever the type of tear gas used, its effects will be influenced by a variety of factors, including wind direction, temperature, and humidity. The PHYSICAL ACTIVITY OF THE CONTAMINATED PERSON is also an important factor in determining the effect of tear gas exposure: Exertion, hyperpnea, excitement, or sweating will all markedly increase the toxic effects of a given "dose" of tear gas. In general, intense exposures to tear gas are likely to produce TEARING, SALIVATION, DYSPNEA, and COUGH. Very high concentrations of these gases may cause pulmonary edema.

In responding to a tear gas incident, EMS personnel should maintain CLOSE COMMUNICATIONS WITH THE POLICE to determine (1) the boundaries of the hostile environment; (2) the optimal approach routes, triage area, and staging area for ambulances; and (3) the police plan of action. Rescuers will be of little help if they find themselves directly in the path of an onrushing wave of riot police, and EMTs may become victims if close communications with the police are not maintained.

In order to minimize contamination of rescue personnel, the fewest number of EMTs possible should enter the contaminated environment to remove patients. Those who do enter should wear breathing apparatus, helmet with face shield, turnout coat, and gloves to reduce skin and respiratory exposure.

As victims are removed from the contaminated area, they should be taken to a place upwind where there is maximal EXPOSURE TO FRESH AIR. Victims in obvious respiratory distress should be treated first, with OXYGEN. Those with burning and tearing of their eyes may get considerable relief from looking into the wind; these victims must be cautioned against rubbing their eyes. Contaminated clothing should be removed, especially if it is wet, and contaminated skin should be flushed thoroughly with cool water or 5% sodium carbonate solution. No salves or oils should be applied to the skin, for they may simply prolong contact between the toxic agent and the skin surface.

It is very important to NOTIFY THE EMERGENCY ROOM well in advance of taking in victims contaminated with tear gas, so that the hospital can make adequate preparations to manage the situation. Such preparations will include closing off common ventilation systems that could circulate air from the emergency room throughout the hospital and setting up fans to vent the ER air directly out the windows. Whenever possible, the patient should be washed down in a shower facility outside the emergency room proper before being taken into the ER. Under no circumstances should an ambulance crew take a contaminated victim to an emergency room without giving advance notice.

Ambulances used for the transport of contaminated victims should be thoroughly decontaminated

Table 19-5. *Characteristics of Tear Gases*

Type of Gas	Characteristics	Effects	Comments
CN (chloroacetophenone)	Blue-white powder Apple blossom odor	Tearing, red eyes Burning sensation of nose, skin Increased salivation Headache	Most widely used by law enforcement agencies Active ingredient in Mace
CS (chlorobenzalmalononitrile)	White cloud Pungent, pepper odor	As above, but faster, more intense Spasmodic coughing Chest tightness Feeling of suffocation Rhinorrhea Panic	Standard riot control agent of U.S. armed forces
DM (diphenylaminechlorarsine; Adamsite)	Yellow cloud Licorice odor	Severe dyspnea Severe nausea, vomiting Sneezing, coughing, gasping, choking Diarrhea	Used chiefly by the military
CR (dibenzoaxepine)		Severe tearing Spasm of the eyelids Rhinorrhea Elevated blood pressure	Being tested in U.S.

after the run. All blankets, sheets, towels, and similar items should be removed in sealed plastic bags. The temperature inside the vehicle should be raised to about 95°F for a few minutes, and then the air should be circulated out with fans. After that procedure has been repeated 3 or 4 times, the vehicle interior should be thoroughly vacuum-cleaned and washed down with a dilute bleach solution.

Management of Tear Gas Exposure: Summary

- Maintain a close LIAISON WITH POLICE.
- PROTECT YOURSELF! (Breathing apparatus, protective clothing).
- REMOVE VICTIMS FROM CONTAMINATED AREA and TRIAGE.
- Turn victims' FACES TO THE WIND.
- KEEP VICTIMS STILL.
- OXYGEN for those in respiratory distress.
- Caution victims against rubbing their eyes.
- Remove CONTAMINATED CLOTHING.
- FLUSH SKIN with cool water; do *not* apply salves, ointments, or similar agents.
- NOTIFY EMERGENCY ROOM as early as possible.
- Decontaminate ambulance after the run.

HYPERVENTILATION SYNDROME

The EMT should be aware of a syndrome that occurs chiefly in anxious young patients as a result of "overbreathing." The chief complaint may or may not be dyspnea, and usually the patient is entirely unaware that he or she is breathing abnormally, deeply, or rapidly. The SYMPTOMS of this syndrome include MARKED ANXIETY, sometimes to the point of panic. The patient may say that he feels as if he is suffocating or dying. In addition, such patients usually experience NUMBNESS OR TINGLING around the mouth and in the hands and feet. They often complain of DIZZINESS and may also report STABBING CHEST PAINS, which elicit further anxiety and sometimes lead the patient to conclude that he or she is suffering a heart attack. When DYSPNEA is a major complaint, it is unlikely to be related to exertion.

On PHYSICAL EXAMINATION, the patient will usually demonstrate HYPERPNEA and TACHYPNEA, with deep, sighing respirations. Anxiety produces TACHYCARDIA, and one may also observe CARPOPEDAL SPASM, a contorted position of the hands, in which the fingers are flexed like claws and the thumb curls in toward the palm. If hyperventilation has continued for any length of time, FAINTING may occur.

All of these signs and symptoms are brought about by the lowering of carbon dioxide levels in the blood. When CO_2 levels fall significantly below normal, various derangements occur in the body's chemical systems, and these derangements lead to the characteristic signs of hyperventilation. It should be emphasized that not every patient who is breathing deeply and rapidly is hyperventilating. By definition, hyperventilation means breathing at a rate or depth *in excess of the need to blow off carbon dioxide*, so that the CO_2 level in the arterial blood falls below normal. A diabetic in metabolic acidosis will breathe very deeply and rapidly, but this is *not* hyperventilation. The hyperpnea and tachypnea of the diabetic are an attempt to blow off *surplus* CO_2; the blood levels of carbon dioxide are elevated, not reduced. The same picture may be seen in certain poisonings, such as poisoning with methyl alcohol. So keep in mind:

> NOT EVERY PATIENT WHO IS BREATHING VERY DEEPLY OR RAPIDLY IS ACTUALLY HYPERVENTILATING.

In evaluating the patient with suspected hyperventilation, one must be careful to rule out organic causes of the patient's symptoms. The patient's age and lack of cardiac history will usually make a diagnosis of heart attack unlikely. But in a young patient, one must still consider asthma, spontaneous pneumothorax, pulmonary embolism, and diabetic acidosis. The history and physical examination should aim specifically to rule these possibilities out (Table 19-6).

TREATMENT of hyperventilation is aimed at restoring the patient's CO_2 levels to normal. Since most ambulances do not carry cylinders of compressed Co_2, we used to believe that the next best source of CO_2 for administration to a hyperventilating patient was the patient's own exhaled air. Thus, medical workers were taught to have the patient breathe in and out of a paper bag—the idea being that the patient would thereby rebreathe his own exhaled carbon dioxide, which in turn would help to raise the CO_2 levels in his blood back toward normal.

Recently, however, "paper bag therapy" has been called into question. When a person rebreathes his own exhaled air from a paper bag, the oxygen content of his inspired air progressively falls. After the patient has taken several breaths, the air in the paper bag will contain only a very low concentration of oxygen. Continuing to breathe that oxygen-poor air could be dangerous, especially if the patient is already suffering from some degree of hypoxemia (e.g., a patient with an unsuspected pulmonary embolism). The only way to be really sure that the patient is not hypoxemic is to measure the amount of oxygen in his blood—a procedure that is neither practical nor worthwhile in the field. For that reason, it is probably safest *not* to use "paper bag therapy" outside the hospital. Instead, try to calm the patient verbally ("Okay, I want you to breath s-l-o-w and e-a-s-y, s-l-o-w and e-a-s-y . . . ") and help him to take conscious control of his breathing.

It is important to bear in mind that patients who are hyperventilating become extremely panicky, and by the time you arrive, the patient's panic is likely to have infected several bystanders, so that the whole scene is one of near hysteria. In such circumstances, a calm, reassuring manner on the part of the EMT is one of the most crucial elements of the treatment.

Once the patient's symptoms have subsided and the patient has calmed down, it is worthwhile to explain and demonstrate how the symptoms came about. Hyperventilation tends to be a chronic problem, and unless the patient learns to recognize the early signs and take measures to abort the attack, you are likely to be getting frequent calls to the same address. Take a few minutes to explain how the distressing feelings are produced. Reassure the patient that many people suffer from this problem and learn to control it, and that the symptoms, while real, are not indications of serious illness. Then have the patient intentionally hyperventilate under your supervision, so that he or she can see that this maneuver reproduces the symptoms. Some people never entirely overcome the tendency to hyperventilate, but they do learn to take conscious control of their breathing when they feel the symptoms of hyperventilation coming on.

Hyperventilation Syndrome: Summary

- HISTORY
  1. Young, anxious patient; may be panicky
  2. No history of cardiac or respiratory disorders
  3. NUMBNESS or TINGLING around the mouth, in the hands and feet
  4. DIZZINESS
  5. STABBING CHEST PAINS
- PHYSICAL FINDINGS
  1. HYPERPNEA and TACHYPNEA
  2. FAINTING
  3. CARPOPEDAL SPASM
  4. Normal breath sounds
  5. No fruity odor to the breath
- TREATMENT
  1. Reassurance
  2. Rebreathing into a paper bag
  3. After the acute attack subsides, explain and demonstrate the cause

CASE HISTORY

The patient is a 52-year-old man who called for an ambulance because of severe dyspnea. The patient states that he felt relatively well when he went to bed, but that he woke about 4 hours later with a feeling that he could not get enough air. He got some relief from getting up and walking around the room. He says he has had similar episodes during the past two or three nights, but they were not as severe as this one. He denies chest pain and has no known history of heart problems. He is, however, under treatment at Elmview Hospital clinic for hypertension, and he takes Diuril pills. He has never been hospitalized and has no known allergies.

Table 19-6. *Dyspnea in a Young Person*

Causative Condition	History	Physical Findings	Treatment
Asthma	Dyspnea Previous attacks Allergic history Attack brought on by flu, stress	Respiratory distress Wheezing Hyperinflated chest Use of accessory muscles to breathe	Oxygen Intravenous fluids
Spontaneous pneumothorax	Tall, thin patient Sudden, sharp chest pain Sudden dyspnea	Respiratory distress Decreased breath sounds on affected side	Oxygen
Pulmonary embolism	Sudden, sharp chest pain Sudden dyspnea History of birth control pills, sickle cell disease	Respiratory distress Tachypnea Tachycardia Hypotension	Oxygen
Diabetic ketoacidosis	Known diabetic Takes insulin Nausea, vomiting Increased urination Extreme thirst Abdominal pain	Sweet, fruity odor on breath Deep, rapid breathing Sometimes shock	Intravenous fluids
Hyperventilation syndrome	No history of significant cardiac or respiratory disease ± Dyspnea Numbness, tingling in hands, feet, around lips Dizziness Stabbing chest pains	Tachypnea Hyperpnea Carpopedal spasm Fainting Breath sounds normal No abnormal breath odors	Reassurance Rebreathing into paper bag

On physical examination, the patient was very anxious, restless, and in marked respiratory distress. He appeared intermittently confused and agitated. His skin was clammy and cyanotic. Pulse was 130 and regular, BP 200/130, and respirations 40 and labored. The patient was coughing up pink, foamy sputum. Neck veins were not distended. There were noisy, bubbling rales on both sides of the chest, from the diaphragms to the clavicles. Heart sounds were difficult to hear. The abdomen was soft. There was no pedal edema.

The patient was placed in a sitting position with his legs dangling and given 100% oxygen by demand valve. His color improved with oxygen treatment, but his condition remained otherwise unchanged en route to the hospital.

Questions to think about:

1. Why do you suppose the patient was confused?
2. Why was the pulse rapid?
3. What was the source of the pink, foamy sputum? How did this fluid get into the lungs?
4. Why was the patient placed sitting up with his legs dangling?

VOCABULARY

bronchospasm Violent contraction of the muscles in the bronchial walls, causing marked constriction of the bronchi.

carpopedal spasm Contorted position of the hand in which the fingers flex in a clawlike attitude and the thumb curls toward the palm; may be caused by hyperventilation.

congestive heart failure Inadequate pumping by the heart, leading to back up of blood behind the affected atrium.

COPD Abbreviation for chronic obstructive pulmonary disease.

chronic bronchitis Form of chronic obstructive pulmonary disease characterized by excessive production of mucus, chronic cough, and often cyanosis.

emphysema Form of chronic obstructive pulmonary disease characterized by destructive changes in the terminal air spaces of the lung.

hypercarbia Abnormally high level of carbon dioxide in the blood.

hyperventilation Abnormally deep or rapid breathing that causes the level of carbon dioxide in the blood to fall below normal.

hypoxic drive The primary stimulus to breathe in some patients with COPD, in which a fall in the levels of oxygen in the blood is the sole spur to increase respirations.

metabolic acidosis An abnormal increase in the amount of acid in the body.

orthopnea Dyspnea made worse by the recumbent position.

status asthmaticus A very severe asthmatic attack that does not respond to the usual medications; may be fatal.

FURTHER READING

GENERAL

Hunt D. Common respiratory emergencies. *Emerg Med Serv* 19(1):19, 1990.

Nixon RG. The respiratory system: An overview. *Emerg Med Serv* 19(1):18, 1990.

LEFT HEART FAILURE

Levy DB, Pollard T. Failure of the heart. *Emergency* 20(12):22, 1988.

Tresch D et al. Out-of-hospital pulmonary edema: Diagnosis and treatment. *Ann Emerg Med* 12:533, 1983.

OBSTRUCTIVE AIRWAYS DISEASE

Balskus MT, Niersbach C. Matters of life and breath. *Emergency* 21(4):12, 1989.

British Thoracic Association. Death from asthma in two regions of England. *Br Med J* 285:1251, 1982.

Johnson AJ et al. Circumstances of death from asthma. *Br Med J* 288:1870, 1984.

Sly RM. Mortality from asthma in children 1979–1984. *Ann Allergy* 60:443, 1988.

PULMONARY EMBOLISM

Bell WR, Simon TL, DeMets DL. The clinical features of submassive and massive pulmonary embolism. *Am J Med* 62:355, 1977.

Turner R, Gusack M. Massive amniotic fluid embolism. *Ann Emerg Med* 13:359, 1984.

Valenzuela T. Pulmonary embolism. *Ann Emerg Med* 17:209, 1988.

TOXIC INHALATIONS

Barber J. EMT checkpoint: Burns and related inhalation injuries. *EMT J* 3(3):68, 1979.

Bascom R, Kennedy K. Toxic gas inhalation. *Emerg Med Serv* 13(7):17, 1984.

Cohen M, Guzzardi L. Inhalation of products of combustion. *Ann Emerg Med* 12:628, 1983.

DiVencenti F et al. Inhalation injuries. *J Trauma* 11:109, 1971.

Done A. The toxic emergency: It's a gas. *Emerg Med* 8:305, 1976.

Fein AM. Toxic gas inhalation. *Emerg Med* 21(7):53, 1989.

Fine K, Bassin R, Steward M. Emergency care for tear gas victims. *JACEP* 6:144, 1977.

Hedges J, Morrissey W. Acute chlorine gas exposure. *JACEP* 8:59, 1972.

Heimbach DM, Waeckerle JF. Inhalation injuries. *Ann Emerg Med* 17:1316, 1988.

Hu H et al. Tear gas—harassing agent or toxic chemical weapon. *JAMA* 262:660, 1989.

Jelenko C, McKinly J. Postburn respiratory injury. *JACEP* 5:455, 1976.

Landa J, Avery W, Sackner M. Some physiologic observations in smoke inhalation. *Chest* 61:62, 1972.

Leonard RB. Chemicals in transit: Be prepared. *Emerg Med* 16(18):17, 1984.

Trunkey DD. Inhalation injury. *Surg Clin North Am* 8:1133, 1978.

HYPERVENTILATION SYNDROME

Callaham M. Hypoxic hazards of traditional paper bag rebreathing in hyperventilating patients. *Ann Emerg Med* 18:622, 1989.

Chelmowski MK, Keelan MH. Hyperventilation and myocardial infarction. *Chest* 93:1095, 1988.

Demeter SL, Cordasco EM. Hyperventilation syndrome and asthma. *Am J Med* 81:989, 1986.

Grossman JE. Paper bag treatment of acute hyperventilation syndrome (letter). *JAMA* 251:2014, 1984.

Pfefer JM. Hyperventilation and the hyperventilation syndrome. *Postgrad Med* 60 (Suppl. 2):47, 1984.

Stoop A et al. Hyperventilation syndrome: Measurement of objective symptoms and subjective complaints. *Respiration* 49:37, 1986.

Wheatley CE. Hyperventilation syndrome: A frequent cause of chest pain. *Chest* 68:195, 1975.

20. CHEST PAIN

OBJECTIVES

Chest pain is a chief complaint that must always be taken seriously, for in many cases it is a distress signal from a severely hypoxic or damaged heart. In this chapter, we will examine the circumstances that lead to chest pain and the characteristics of heart attack victims. We shall also learn what the EMT can do to help the patient with chest pain and improve his or her chances of reaching the hospital alive. By the conclusion of this chapter, the reader should be able to

1. Identify the vessels that provide the blood supply to the heart muscle
2. Identify the disease process that may interfere with the blood supply to the heart muscle, and indicate the consequences of a reduced or absent myocardial blood supply
3. List at least five risk factors for heart attack, and indicate which of these risk factors an individual can control by changes in habits or lifestyle
4. Identify a patient with angina pectoris, given a description of several patients with various symptoms
5. Identify a patient with a probable heart attack, given a description of several patients with various symptoms and signs
6. Identify the correct steps in managing a patient with chest pain, and indicate the proper sequence in which those steps should be performed
7. Identify common complications of a heart attack, given descriptions of patients with signs of various complications, and indicate the correct management of each in the prehospital setting

THE BLOOD SUPPLY TO THE HEART

Recall that the heart is a muscle, and like any other muscle, it requires a blood supply to furnish it with oxygen and nutrients. In the case of the heart, this blood supply must be constant and must not be interrupted, even for a few moments, for the heart muscle, or **myocardium,** is working all the time—contracting 60 or more times a minute, 60 minutes an hour, 24 hours a day. That is about 86,000 beats a day, and each beat requires oxygen and glucose to fuel the pump. Furthermore, the blood supply to the heart must be adaptable to changing needs. During exercise, for instance, when the heart pumps fast, the myocardium needs more oxygen to fuel the increased effort (just as a car engine needs more gas when it runs faster), so the blood flow to the heart muscle must increase as the heart increases its level of work.

The heart gets its oxygen from a special set of arteries, the **coronary arteries,** that originate from the aorta and spread out over the entire heart muscle (Fig. 20-1). When the heart increases its level of work, as during exertion, these arteries dilate, per-

COMPLICATIONS OF ACUTE MYOCARDIAL INFARCTION

A heart attack may lead to several serious and even life-threatening complications, and the EMT should be alert for signs that such complications are developing.

The most serious potential complication of AMI is CARDIAC ARREST. Sometimes cardiac arrest will occur suddenly, without any warning, especially during the first few minutes of the infarction. Often, however, the patient will develop disturbances in cardiac rhythm first—a few extra beats here and there—and if these disturbances are detected and treated in time, cardiac arrest may be prevented. For this reason, it is essential to keep a finger on the patient's pulse at all times. Any irregularities in the pulse should be regarded as a danger signal and should indicate the need for prompt transport to a medical facility, where drugs may be administered to correct the rhythm disturbance before it deteriorates to cardiac arrest.

Another possible complication of acute myocardial infarction is CONGESTIVE HEART FAILURE (see Chapter 19). If a large portion of the left ventricle is damaged in an infarction, the left ventricle may not be able to contract forcefully enough to pump blood out effectively. When this occurs, blood backs up behind the left side of the heart into the lungs, and one sees all the usual signs of left heart failure: tachypnea; pink, frothy sputum; rales. A patient with these signs must be treated as any other patient in congestive heart failure; that is, he should be placed in a sitting position with legs dangling and given high concentrations of oxygen (nonrebreathing mask or demand valve).

A heart attack may also be complicated by CARDIOGENIC SHOCK. When cardiogenic shock occurs, it is a sign of massive damage to the myocardium, which can no longer pump forcefully enough to maintain adequate perfusion of the body tissues. The signs of cardiogenic shock are similar to those of other types of shock: tachycardia; cold, clammy skin; confusion; and low blood pressure. A patient in shock should be kept supine and given high concentrations of oxygen. The base station physician should be consulted for possible orders to use the Military Anti-Shock Trousers, which have been reported to be effective in some cases of cardiogenic shock.

The potential complications of AMI* are summarized in Table 20-2.

Table 20-2. *Potential Complications of Acute Myocardial Infarction*

Complication	Warning Signs	Field Management
Cardiac arrest	May be preceded by irregular pulse, or may occur without warning	Cardiopulmonary resuscitation
Congestive heart failure	Dyspnea, tachypnea Pink, frothy sputum Wheezes or rales	Patient in sitting position with legs dangling 100% oxygen
Cardiogenic shock	Tachycardia Confusion Cold, clammy skin Hypotension	Patient in supine position 100% oxygen Consult physician regarding possible use of MAST

OTHER CAUSES OF CHEST PAIN

Needless to say, not every case of chest pain is a heart attack. Chest pain may be due to many other factors, including inflammation of the lungs, pleura, or rib cartilages; gastrointestinal disturbances; and even hyperventilation. For purposes of prehospital emergency care, however, it is safest to assume that every patient over 30 years old with chest pain has a serious cardiac problem until proved otherwise.

> TREAT EVERY ADULT WITH CHEST PAIN AS A HEART ATTACK VICTIM.

CASE HISTORY

The patient is a 44-year old business executive who called for an ambulance because of chest pain. The patient states that the pain started about an hour ago, while he was watching television. He describes it as a "heavy pressure in my chest" that radiates down the left arm. Nothing he has done to relieve the pain—including lying down and taking a Tums—has helped. He has also noted nausea and a cold sweat. He denies dyspnea, dizziness, or palpitations. He has never had any pain like this before and states that up to now he has been in perfect health. He has no history of diabetes or hypertension. He is a nonsmoker. He jogs five miles every day. His father died at the age of 48 of a heart attack.

On physical examination, the patient was pale and apprehensive. He was fully oriented and appeared in moderate distress. The skin was cold and clammy. Pulse was 110 and regular, although an occasional extra beat was noted when the patient was first examined. BP was 120/70, and respirations were 18 and unlabored. There was no distention of the neck veins. The chest was clear. There was no pedal edema.

The patient was placed in a semireclining position and given 6 liters of oxygen per minute by nasal

* It is recommended that students in the EMT-Intermediate course go back and review defibrillation (Chap. 9) at this point.

cannula. His color improved considerably with oxygen therapy, and no further extra beats were noted in the pulse after oxygen administration was begun. Vital signs remained unchanged en route to the hospital.

Questions to think about:

1. Did this patient have any risk factors for heart attack? If so, which risk factors?
2. Why did the EMT making this report bother to mention that the chest was clear?
3. Suppose the chest had not been clear but had been full of rales. What would that suggest?
4. Why was the patient placed in a semisitting position rather than supine?

VOCABULARY

angina pectoris Characteristic pain due to myocardial hypoxia; usually substernal, squeezing, brought on by exertion, relieved by rest.

anorexia Loss of appetite.

atherosclerosis Disease that causes narrowing and hardening of the coronary and cerebral arteries.

coronary arteries Vessels that carry oxygenated blood to the heart muscle.

denial Psychologic mechanism by which a person attempts to minimize or ignore serious illness.

diaphoresis Profuse sweating.

myocardial infarction Death of a segment of heart muscle, due to interruption of the blood supply to the area.

myocardium Heart muscle.

nitroglycerin Medication used by patients with angina pectoris for relief of chest pain, usually taken as a small white tablet that is placed under the tongue.

palpitations Sensation of very forceful heartbeats or of the heart skipping a beat.

risk factor Factor that increases a person's susceptibility to a given disease.

FURTHER READING

Assey ME. Ischemia without symptoms. *Emerg Med* 20(7):26, 1988.

Bayer AJ et al. Changing presentation of myocardial infarction with increasing old age. *J Am Ger Soc* 34:263, 1986.

Chatterjee K. Unstable angina. *Emerg Med* 15(14):271, 1983.

Click RL. What causes chest pain in young adults? *Emerg Med* 21(2):60, 1989.

Conti R, Christie L Jr. Sorting out chest pain. *Emerg Med* 14(15):113, 1982.

Cooke DH. When angina destabilizes. *Emerg Med* 20(9): 143, 1988.

Cousins N. *The Healing Heart*. New York: WW Norton, 1983.

Goldberg RJ et al. Recent changes in attack and survival rates of acute myocardial infarction (1975 through 1981). *JAMA* 20:2774, 1986.

Gore JM et al. Feasibility and safety of emergency interhospital transport of patients during early hours of acute myocardial infarction. *Arch Int Med* 149:353, 1989.

Hargarten KM et al. Limitations of prehospital predictors of acute myocardial infarction and unstable angina. *Ann Emerg Med* 16:1325, 1987.

Ho MT et al. Delay between onset of chest pain and seeking medical care: The effect of public education. *Ann Emerg Med* 18:727, 1989.

Kannel WB, Abbot RD. Incidence and prognosis of unrecognized myocardial infarction: An update on the Framingham study. *N Engl J Med* 311:1144, 1987.

Kaplan L, Walsh D, Burney RE, Emergency aeromedical transport of patients with acute myocardial infarction. *Ann Emerg Med* 16:55, 1987.

Maydayag T. Emergency cardiac assessment. *Emerg Med Serv* 7(6):42, 1978.

O'Doherty M et al. Five hundred patients with myocardial infarction monitored within one hour of symptoms. *Br Med J* 286, 1405, 1983.

Smith HWB et al. Acute myocardial infarction temporally related to cocaine use. *Ann Intern Med* 107:13, 1987.

Solomon CG et al. Comparison of clinical presentation of acute myocardial infarction in patients older than 65 years of age to younger patients: The multicenter chest pain study experience. *Am J Cardiol* 63:772, 1989.

Turzi ZG et al. Implications for acute intervention related to time of hospital arrival in acute myocardial infarction. *Am J Cardiol* 58:203, 1986.

Wiederhold R. Cardiovascular anatomy review. *Emerg Med Serv* 18(9):58, 1989.

Wroblewski M et al. Symptoms of myocardial infarction in old age: Clinical case, retrospective and prospective studies. *Age & Aging* 15(2):99, 1986.

Note: The American Heart Association (AHA) produces a wide selection of excellent educational materials on heart attack, coronary risk factors, healthy cardiac living, and related subjects. These materials are available, usually free of charge or for a very nominal price, from most AHA chapters. Your local Red Cross chapter is also a good source of printed materials on cardiac emergencies.

21. UNCONSCIOUS STATES

OBJECTIVES

An unconscious patient is a patient in danger. No matter what the cause, by its very nature being unconscious places a person in jeopardy. The unconscious person is mute and defenseless. He cannot explain what has happened to him. He cannot indicate if anything hurts. And, more important, he cannot rely upon protective reflexes that ordinarily defend him while awake—such as the gag reflex that guards the airway from aspiration, or the blinking reflex that shields the cornea of the eye from foreign bodies. In caring for an unconscious patient, the EMT must substitute for these lost protective reflexes and defend the patient's vital functions until definitive treatment can be provided.

In this chapter, we will look first at some general principles that apply to the care of *any* unconscious patient, regardless of the cause of unconsciousness. Then we shall consider a few of the more common illnesses or circumstances that can lead to loss of consciousness, and we will examine the special considerations relevant to the treatment of each. By the conclusion of this chapter, the reader should be able to

1. Identify the dangers that threaten every unconscious patient
2. Indicate the priorities of management of the unconscious patient, given a list of treatment steps in random order
3. Identify the most likely cause of unconsciousness (coma), given a list of clues found at the scene or during examination of the patient
4. Indicate the correct management of an unconscious patient who smells of alcohol, given several alternative courses of action
5. Identify the hormone that normally facilitates the uptake of sugar from the bloodstream, given a list of hormones
6. Identify a patient with (a) diabetic ketoacidosis and (b) insulin shock, given a description of several patients with various signs and symptoms, and indicate the correct field treatment for each
7. Indicate the correct management of a diabetic in coma when the cause of coma is not known
8. Identify the correct steps in managing a person who has fainted
9. Identify the correct steps in managing a person who is having a seizure
10. Indicate under what circumstances seizures are a life-threatening emergency, and what measures are necessary in this situation

GENERAL PRINCIPLES OF CARE FOR THE UNCONSCIOUS PATIENT

An unconscious, or **comatose,** person is defenseless—defenseless against extremes of temperature, against painful positions, against aspiration. This is true whether the unconscious state was brought on

Table 21-1. *Major Causes of Coma and Clues to Their Detection*

Cause	Clues	Detailed discussion in
Head trauma	Mechanism of injury Bruises, lacerations, blood in ear canals	Chapter 14
Drug overdose	Empty medication bottles, syringes Vomitus containing undigested pills Needle tracks, pinpoint pupils (heroin user)	Chapter 25
Diabetes	Insulin in refrigerator, syringes at home Hyperpnea, fruity odor to breath Needle marks on thighs, abdomen Medical identification tag	Chapter 21
Seizures	Evidence of tongue biting, incontinence Seizure medications (Dilantin, Mysoline, Tegretol, phenobarbital)	Chapter 21
Stroke	Asymmetry of the face One side of body weak or flaccid Medications for high blood pressure (e.g., Diuril, Lasix, Catapres, Apresoline, Aldomet)	Chapter 22
Meningitis	High fever Rigid neck	Chapter 27

detail later in this chapter; others are covered in other sections of this book. For our purposes here, we shall simply review briefly some of the conditions that may lead to an unconscious state.

TRAUMA may or may not be evident from examination of the patient. Absence of visible bruises does not rule out the possibility of head injury, and if any doubt exists, the patient should be treated with the precautions appropriate to any potential victim of head trauma, which means, among other things, spinal immobilization.

DRUG OVERDOSE is a frequent cause of coma. The presence at the scene of empty medication bottles or syringes, vomitus containing undigested pills, or needle tracks on the patient's arm is suggestive that drugs may be at least a factor in the patient's condition. POISONING should be suspected when noxious substances are found near the patient, especially if the patient is a small child.

UNDERLYING MEDICAL CONDITIONS, such as DIABETES, thyroid problems, and others, may be signalled by a medical identification tag. EPILEPSY is suggested when the patient was seen having a seizure prior to becoming unconscious or if he is carrying medications used to control chronic seizures.

Coma may occur as a result of a STROKE, which may be suspected in an elderly patient, especially if there is a known history of high blood pressure. MENINGITIS, an acute infection of the membranes covering the brain, is a possibility if the comatose patient has a high fever and rigid neck.

Finally, unconsciousness may occur as a result of ALCOHOL INTOXICATION. A word of caution, however: Just because an unconscious person has alcohol on his or her breath does not necessarily mean that the person is unconscious *because* of alcohol. A person who smells of alcohol may be in coma from any of the causes listed above, and tragic errors have been made by assuming that an unconscious person was "just drunk." Remember

EVERY UNCONSCIOUS PERSON IS IN DANGER—EVEN A PERSON WHO SMELLS OF ALCOHOL.

The "drunk" you save may turn out to be a diabetic, an epileptic, or a victim of stroke. The "drunk" you neglect may wind up in the morgue.

Some of the major causes of coma and the clues to their detection are summarized in Table 21-1. One way to remember the most common causes of coma is to think of the vowels A-E-I-O-U and the word "TIPS":

Common Cause of Coma

A Alcohol
E Epilepsy, endocrine system
I Insulin (too much or too little, in diabetics)
O Opiates (or other drugs)
U Uremia (or other kidney problems)

T Trauma, temperature extremes (hypo-, hyperthermia)
I Infection (e.g. meningitis)
P Poison
S Shock, stroke, subdural or subarachnoid hemorrhage

In the following sections, we will consider three causes of coma in detail: diabetic states, fainting, and seizures.

DIABETES MELLITUS

Diabetes mellitus, sometimes called sugar diabetes, is a chronic, systemic disease affecting many organ systems in the body. Among the organs severely impaired is the pancreas, which becomes incapable of producing **insulin,** the hormone that normally promotes the efficient utilization of sugar by body cells. Without insulin, sugar, in the form of glucose, cannot enter body cells. Instead, it accumulates in the blood, leading to excessively high concentrations of blood sugar (**hyperglycemia**). Hyperglycemia in turn leads to a variety of serious derangements in the body's fluid and chemical balance, and if uncorrected, these derangements can proceed to dehydration, cardiac rhythm disturbances, and death.

Diabetes ranges in severity from mild cases, in which there is still some pancreatic function and low level insulin production, to very severe cases, in which the pancreas has ceased to produce insulin altogether. Patients with mild diabetes may be able to control their disease by limiting their dietary intake of sugar and by taking pills (e.g., Orinase, Tolinase, Diabinase, and Dymelor) that stimulate the pancreas to put out more insulin. Those with severe diabetes, however, are entirely dependent upon insulin injections, which the patient usually administers to himself once or twice a day. The insulin given by injection has the same action as insulin produced by a normal pancreas, so it helps to compensate for the absence of pancreatic function.

In the normal person, the amount of insulin released by the pancreas at any given time is finely regulated in such a way as to maintain the level of blood sugar relatively constant. A diabetic who must take insulin by injection has to try to achieve this same regulation by gauging the insulin dose according to food intake. If the diabetic takes too little insulin with respect to sugar intake, his blood sugar will be too high; if he takes too much, his blood sugar will fall to dangerously low levels.

Diabetics get into trouble when their blood sugars become too high (hyperglycemia) or too low (hypoglycemia). Either of those abnormalities can lead to coma.

DIABETIC KETOACIDOSIS (HYPERGLYCEMIC COMA)

When a diabetic's blood sugar becomes too high, a condition called **diabetic ketoacidosis,** or diabetic coma, is likely to follow. In general, ketoacidosis occurs when a diabetic has not taken a sufficient dose of insulin to cover increased food intake. Infection or other stress may also precipitate diabetic ketoacidosis.

As the concentration of sugar in the blood rises, there is an excessive loss of both sugar and water in the urine, leading to dehydration and severe thirst. Two of the most classic signs of early diabetic ketoacidosis are POLYURIA (frequent urination) and POLYDIPSIA (frequent intake of liquids). Meanwhile, the body cells are literally starving in the midst of plenty, for the high levels of sugar in the blood are of no use to the cells without insulin to move the sugar from the blood into the cells. So the cells have to switch to some other fuel, and they begin to burn fat instead of sugar. The metabolism of fat produces acid waste products, which in turn greatly increase the acidity of the blood (hence "acidosis"). The only means the body has of getting rid of acid quickly is to blow it off in the form of carbon dioxide. Thus as the blood becomes more and more acid, the patient begins breathing very deeply and rapidly (KUSSMAUL BREATHING) in an attempt to eliminate the excess acid in the blood. Another group of waste products of fat metabolism, ketones, are excreted both in the breath and in the urine (hence *keto*acidosis). In the breath, ketones produce a characteristic FRUITY ODOR. The chemical imbalance in the patient's body often leads to ABDOMINAL PAIN, NAUSEA, and VOMITING, the last of which only serves to worsen the already severe dehydration. This dehydration is reflected in WARM, DRY SKIN, TACHYCARDIA, and SUNKEN EYES. Dehydration sometimes results in fever and hypotension as well. If the condition is allowed to progress, the patient sinks into coma, due to a combination of dehydration and high acid levels in the blood.

The sequence of events described above usually develops *gradually*, over a period of 12 to 48 hours, with the patient growing sicker and weaker until he or she slowly slips into unconsciousness.

INSULIN SHOCK (HYPOGLYCEMIC COMA)

At the other end of the spectrum is the diabetic whose blood sugar is too low. This usually occurs because the patient has taken too much insulin with respect to food intake. He or she may, for instance, have taken the usual insulin dose but then skipped a meal or exercised more strenuously than usual. As the blood sugar falls, the first organ to notice that something is wrong is the brain, for the brain relies exclusively on sugar for its fuel supply. Sugar is as critical to the brain as oxygen is, and the moment the amount of sugar available in the blood decreases, the brain cannot function properly. Thus the patient with hypoglycemia begins to notice a HEADACHE and DIZZINESS. Sometimes he may develop weakness or paralysis on one side of the body, as if he were having a stroke. He may become CONFUSED and DISORIENTED, and sometimes the hypoglycemic patient will show marked DISTURBANCES IN BEHAVIOR. He may become hostile, belligerent or even appear drunk. Indeed, more than one diabetic has died of insulin shock in a police lockup after being detained overnight because of "drunken and disorderly behavior." WEAKNESS and INCOORDINATION also tend to make the hypoglycemic patient resemble an intoxicated person, and profuse DROOLING contributes to this impression as well. If the patient does not receive sugar promptly, CONVULSIONS and COMA will swiftly occur. The patient's skin usually becomes COLD AND CLAMMY, as in shock, and often the body temperature is abnormally low.

The sequence of events in insulin shock, as distinct from those in diabetic ketoacidosis, occurs very rapidly—sometimes within minutes. The patient becomes suddenly irritable and belligerent, begins to stagger and drool, and then collapses.

It should be pointed out that hypoglycemia may also occur in nondiabetics. Chronic alcoholics, for example, are prone to episodes of hypoglycemia, as are some patients suffering from cancer, liver disease, or chronic kidney disease. Hypoglycemia may also occur as a result of some poisonings—for example, aspirin overdose in children.

How Do You Tell the Difference?

Often by the time the EMT reaches the scene, the patient is already in coma or near coma, and the EMT does not have the opportunity to observe the events that led up to that state. Under such circumstances, it may be very difficult to distinguish the coma produced by hyperglycemia and diabetic ketoacidosis from that produced by hypoglycemia and insulin shock. Nonetheless, the patient's history and physical signs may provide clues to help differentiate between the two conditions.

If the patient is still conscious, the EMT should ask (1) Have you eaten today? and (2) Did you take your insulin today? The answers to these two questions may provide the first clue to the patient's problem.

	Diabetic ketoacidosis	*Insulin shock*
Has the patient eaten?	Yes	No
Has the patient taken his insulin?	No	Yes

The diabetic will usually have a pretty good idea of what the problem is, so it pays to listen to what the patient has to say on the subject.

If the patient is unconscious, the EMT must rely on the report of relatives or bystanders and on the physical assessment of the patient to determine what has caused the coma. The key differences between diabetic ketoacidosis and insulin shock are summarized in Table 21-2.

Table 21-2. *Differentiating Diabetic Emergencies*

Characteristic	Diabetic Ketoacidosis	Insulin Shock
Blood sugar	Hyperglycemia	Hypoglycemia
History		
Onset of symptoms	Gradual (12–48 hr)	Rapid (minutes to an hour)
Food intake	Excessive	Inadequate; may have skipped a meal
Insulin intake	Inadequate	Excessive
Other precipitating factors	Infection, illness, stress	Strenuous exercise
Symptoms	Polyuria, polydipsia, nausea, vomiting, abdominal pain	Headache, dizziness, irritability, hostile or bizarre behavior, confusion, tremors, drooling, weakness, staggering
Physical findings		
Skin	Warm, dry	Cold, clammy
Pulse	Rapid, thready	Rapid, may be weak
Blood pressure	Hypotension	Usually normal
Respirations	Kussmaul (hyperpnea, tachypnea)	Normal or shallow
Temperature	May have fever	Normal or depressed
Neurologic	Restless	Weak, uncoordinated, tremulous, sometimes seizures
Urine test		
Sugar	Present	Absent
Acetone	Present	Absent
Treatment	Intravenous infusion of large amounts of normal saline; insulin at the hospital	Sugar—by mouth if conscious, 50 ml of 50% dextrose IV if unconscious

Why bother to make the distinction? The answer is that the treatment of the two conditions is very different. The patient in DIABETIC KETOACIDOSIS needs a lot of FLUIDS, best given in the form of an intravenous infusion of normal saline solution. The patient in INSULIN SHOCK, on the other hand, needs SUGAR and needs it fast! A brain deprived of sugar is in as much jeopardy as a brain deprived of oxygen; with every minute that passes in severe hypoglycemia, brain cells die. If the patient is still conscious and able to swallow, sugar should be given in the form of candy, sugar cubes, or fruit juice to which sugar has been generously added. If the patient is unconscious, however, liquids or solids should not be placed in his mouth because they may be aspirated into the lungs. The most effective means of administering sugar to an unconscious patient is to inject 50 ml of 50% dextrose solution intravenously (along with 100 mg of thiamine), through an established, free-flowing intravenous line. EMT-Intermediates should be trained and authorized to administer 50% dextrose in this manner, since it is a simple procedure that can prevent permanent neurologic damage in the hypoglycemic patient and even save his life. There are few cures in medicine more dramatic than that seen when a hypoglycemic patient is given sugar: The comatose patient wakes up in seconds; the hostile, confused, drooling patient is suddenly transformed into a pleasant and alert human being.

If intravenous dextrose is not available, some benefit may be achieved by smearing a thick, sweet substance, such as honey, on the membranes inside the patient's cheeks. Some sugar may be able to pass through these membranes into the bloodstream. Definitive treatment, however, will require intravenous dextrose, and thus transport to the hospital should not be delayed. Remember

> HYPOGLYCEMIC COMA IS A DIRE MEDICAL EMERGENCY. DO NOT DELAY THE ADMINISTRATION OF DEXTROSE OR TRANSPORT OF THE PATIENT TO A FACILITY WHERE DEXTROSE CAN BE GIVEN.

What if you are not sure? That is, what if you find the diabetic in coma and you cannot be certain whether the coma is from hyperglycemia or hypoglycemia? The answer is a simple rule of thumb.

> WHEN IN DOUBT, GIVE SUGAR.

The administration of sugar to a patient with hyperglycemia is unlikely to do any harm, for the patient already has so much sugar in his blood that a little more will not appreciably change his blood sugar concentration. The patient in hypoglycemic coma, on the other hand, is in grave danger of sustaining brain damage; failure to give this patient sugar may result in permanent injury to the brain or even death. Thus, if you are not sure whether the patient is hyperglycemic or hypoglycemic, assume that it is the more critical of the two—*hypoglycemia*—and give sugar.

What about the patient who is simply found unconscious, without medical identification tags, without relatives or friends nearby to give you a history—a patient who is unconscious from unknown cause and you do not even know whether he is a diabetic at all? Once again, one should treat the patient for the most critical possibility, and that means, GIVE SUGAR. If the patient is not a diabetic, a little sugar will not do him any harm. If he is a diabetic (or, for that matter, even a nondiabetic) in hypoglycemic coma, the sugar will save his life. Our general rule is, then

> *EVERY* UNCONSCIOUS PATIENT SHOULD RECEIVE 50% DEXTROSE INTRAVENOUSLY AT THE EARLIEST POSSIBLE MOMENT—EVEN IF THE PATIENT IS NOT KNOWN TO BE A DIABETIC.

The principles of treating the diabetic in coma are summarized in Figure 21-2.

FAINTING

The medical term for fainting is **syncope**, and it is characterized by a sudden, temporary loss of consciousness. There are a variety of conditions that may bring about syncope—pain, fright, disturbances in cardiac rhythm, hypoglycemia, certain drugs—but all of them have one thing in common: They produce a temporary decrease in blood flow to the brain. It is this reduction in cerebral blood flow that causes the person to lose consciousness. Nature's wisdom dictates that when a person faints, he falls down, for by assuming the recumbent position, the victim of syncope improves the blood flow to his brain (the heart does not have to pump uphill if the patient is lying flat). If something should prevent the fainting person from falling—for instance, fainting in a confined space, such as a phone booth—this improvement in cerebral blood flow will not take place, and the patient may suffer permanent brain damage.

Sometimes a person can feel a fainting spell coming on, especially when syncope is caused by some stress, such as the sight of blood. The patient may experience warning symptoms, including dizziness, weakness, blurred vision, a pounding sensation in the head, nausea, and abdominal discomfort. The pulse may become very slow and the skin cold and clammy. If a person tells you that he or she feels faint, the syncopal episode may be prevented by quickly having the person lie down and elevating his or her legs. Elevation of the legs increases blood return to the heart, while the recumbent position facilitates blood flow to the brain.

If the patient has already fainted and is unconscious or semiconscious when you arrive, KEEP HIM FLAT and elevate his legs. Under no circumstances

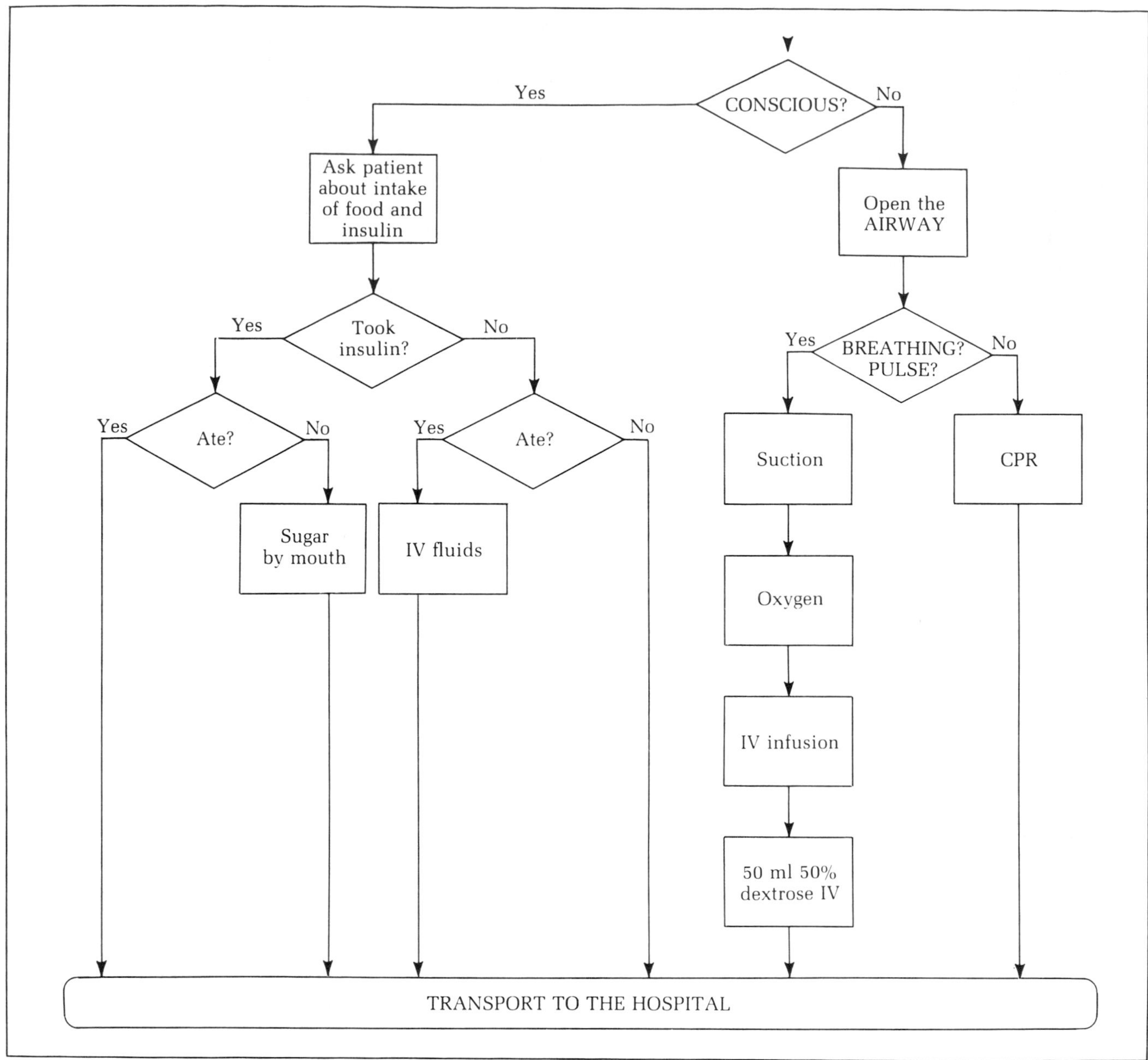

Fig. 21-2. *Treatment of diabetic emergencies.*

should a patient who has fainted be lifted into a sitting position, for this will simply further reduce blood flow to the brain and could lead to a stroke.

Make sure the patient has an open AIRWAY, and administer OXYGEN by nasal cannula. Most syncopal episodes are not dangerous and are not caused by serious illness, but until the cause of the faint has been established, one must assume that cerebral hypoxia may have been a factor—and therefore one must give oxygen.

LOOSEN ANY TIGHT CLOTHING on the patient, and check the VITAL SIGNS. A very slow pulse or any irregularities in the pulse should be noted. Also CHECK FOR INJURIES that may have been sustained when the patient fell.

When the patient regains consciousness, keep him flat, and move him to the stretcher in a horizontal position. Do not allow the patient to get up and walk around. Try to find out from the patient what caused the fainting episode. Did he or she feel it coming on? Was there some stressful event that preceded the faint? What position was the patient in when fainting occurred? Is the patient on any medications?

Once the secondary survey is complete and any injuries have been stabilized, transport the patient supine to the hospital.

Management of Fainting

1. KEEP THE PATIENT FLAT, WITH LEGS ELEVATED. Never lift a person who has fainted into a sitting position.
2. Open the AIRWAY.
3. Administer OXYGEN by nasal cannula.
4. LOOSEN ANY TIGHT CLOTHING on the patient.
5. Measure and record VITAL SIGNS. Recheck frequently.
6. CHECK FOR INJURIES sustained in the fall.
7. Obtain a HISTORY.
8. TRANSPORT to hospital in SUPINE position.

SEIZURES

Seizures, or convulsions, are the most common serious neurologic disorder. Approximately 4 million Americans have suffered at least one seizure during their lives. Seizures occur when there is a massive discharge of a group of nerve cells in the brain from any of a wide variety of causes, including stroke, old or recent head injury, withdrawal from drugs or alcohol, hypoxia, hypoglycemia, and meningitis. Most commonly, though, seizures occur in persons with a condition called **epilepsy.** The causes of epilepsy are not well understood. Often it begins in childhood or young adulthood, and it is manifested by episodic convulsive attacks. Most known epileptics take medications that keep their seizures under good control, but seizures may still occur if the patient neglects to take a prescribed medication or if the dose of medication is inadequate.

The typical generalized motor seizure—also called a **grand mal seizure**—is a very dramatic and sometimes frightening spectacle. The patient may feel the convulsion coming on, or it may occur without warning. Sometimes the patient will let out a short, high-pitched cry as he or she collapses and loses consciousness. The patient's muscles become extremely rigid for about 15 to 30 seconds, and then there is a period of violent muscle contractions all over the body, during which the patient may lose bowel and bladder control. Spasmodic contractions of the jaw muscles may cause the patient to bite his tongue or lips, while the violent movements of the arms and legs may lead to injury of the back and extremities. Sometimes spasms of the chest muscles result in temporary apnea, during which the patient turns an alarming shade of blue.

As these violent muscle contractions subside, usually within a minute or two, the patient begins to drool and hyperventilate. The pulse is very rapid at this point. Following the seizure, the patient is apt to remain unconscious or stuporous for some time, and when he does awaken, he is likely to be confused and to complain of headache.

The treatment of a simple seizure is aimed at protecting the patient from injury during the phase of violent muscle contractions. As the patient loses consciousness, he or she should be placed on a wide bed or on the floor, away from any furniture or other objects. Try to protect the patient's head and extremities from banging into hard surfaces, but DO NOT FORCIBLY RESTRAIN THE PATIENT, for this may simply result in injury to both of you. If his jaws are not already clenched shut, insert a padded tongue blade or other soft "bite stick" between the patient's back teeth to prevent tongue biting. Do not place your fingers in the patient's mouth, unless you want to lose them. If the patient's mouth is already clamped shut, DO NOT TRY TO JAM A BITE STICK BETWEEN CLENCHED TEETH, for this is liable to damage or dislodge teeth. Try as best as possible to maintain the patient's AIRWAY, but do not force the head backward while the patient is seizing. A nasopharyngeal airway may be useful in such circumstances. Bearing in mind that some seizures are caused by hypoxia, administer OXYGEN by nasal cannula as soon as possible.

Once the seizure activity has subsided, obtain VITAL SIGNS, and CHECK THE PATIENT FOR INJURIES that might have been sustained during the convulsive phase of the attack. Be particularly alert for posterior dislocation of the shoulder, which is easily missed if one is not specifically looking for it. Turn the patient to the side to minimize the danger of aspiration.

Try to obtain whatever information you can at the scene. Ask bystanders to describe the seizure. Did it start in one particular part of the body? Did the patient's eyes deviate in one direction or the other? Search the patient for medical identification tags and for medications that might indicate a chronic history of seizures. Such medications include Dilantin, Tegretol, Mysoline, and phenobarbital. Take any medications you find to the hospital with the patient.

When you have completed the survey, transport the patient to the hospital, even if he or she has recovered consciousness and feels fine. A seizure in a nonepileptic needs thorough investigation in the hospital to determine the cause, and a seizure in a known epileptic indicates a need to re-examine the patient's medication dosage. In either case, the seizure patient must be evaluated in a medical facility.

Management of an Isolated Seizure

1. PROTECT THE PATIENT FROM INJURY by keeping him clear of furniture or other objects. DO NOT FORCIBLY RESTRAIN HIM.
2. If the mouth is still slack, insert a bite stick

22. STROKE

OBJECTIVES

The term *stroke* is a very vivid description of the process it depicts: a sudden striking down of the patient. One moment the person is relatively well and able to function, the next moment he or she is struck dumb or unable to move one or more extremities. There are few illnesses that cause more anxiety and despair in the victim and that therefore require so much tact and consideration on the part of those caring for the victim. In this chapter, we will examine some of the causes of stroke and the ways in which stroke manifests itself. We will also learn how to manage a patient with suspected stroke in the prehospital phase. By the conclusion of this chapter, the reader should be able to

1. Identify the correct definition of stroke, given a list of definitions
2. Distinguish between the three major causes of stroke, given a description of each
3. Identify the factors that predispose to different types of stroke, given a list of factors
4. Identify a patient with a stroke, given a description of several patients with different symptoms
5. List the points to be emphasized in the evaluation of a patient with suspected stroke
6. List the steps in caring for a stroke victim in the prehospital phase

DEFINITION AND CAUSES OF STROKE

The term stroke refers to the sudden loss of some neurologic function such as speech, movement, or sensation for an extended period (i.e., more than 24 hours). A stroke is also sometimes called a **cerebrovascular accident**, or **CVA**, although that term is inaccurate and misleading, for there is nothing accidental about it. Stroke occurs when, for whatever reason, there is an interruption in the blood flow to a region of the brain. Any part of the brain that is deprived of its blood supply for more than a few minutes will suffer irreversible damage, and the function carried out by that part of the brain will be lost. As we learned earlier, different regions of the brain are specialized to carry out different specific tasks. A portion of the temporal lobe, for instance, is in charge of speech; visual images are processed in the occipital lobe; voluntary movement is controlled by centers in the frontal lobe. The effects of a stroke will depend, therefore, on the region of the brain whose blood supply was interrupted. If the speech center is damaged, the patient may be unable to speak or write; damage to the motor center in one of the cerebral hemispheres may result in weakness or paralysis on one side of the body.

In general, interruption of the blood supply to a part of the brain may come about in one of several ways (Fig. 22-1). To begin with, a clot, called a

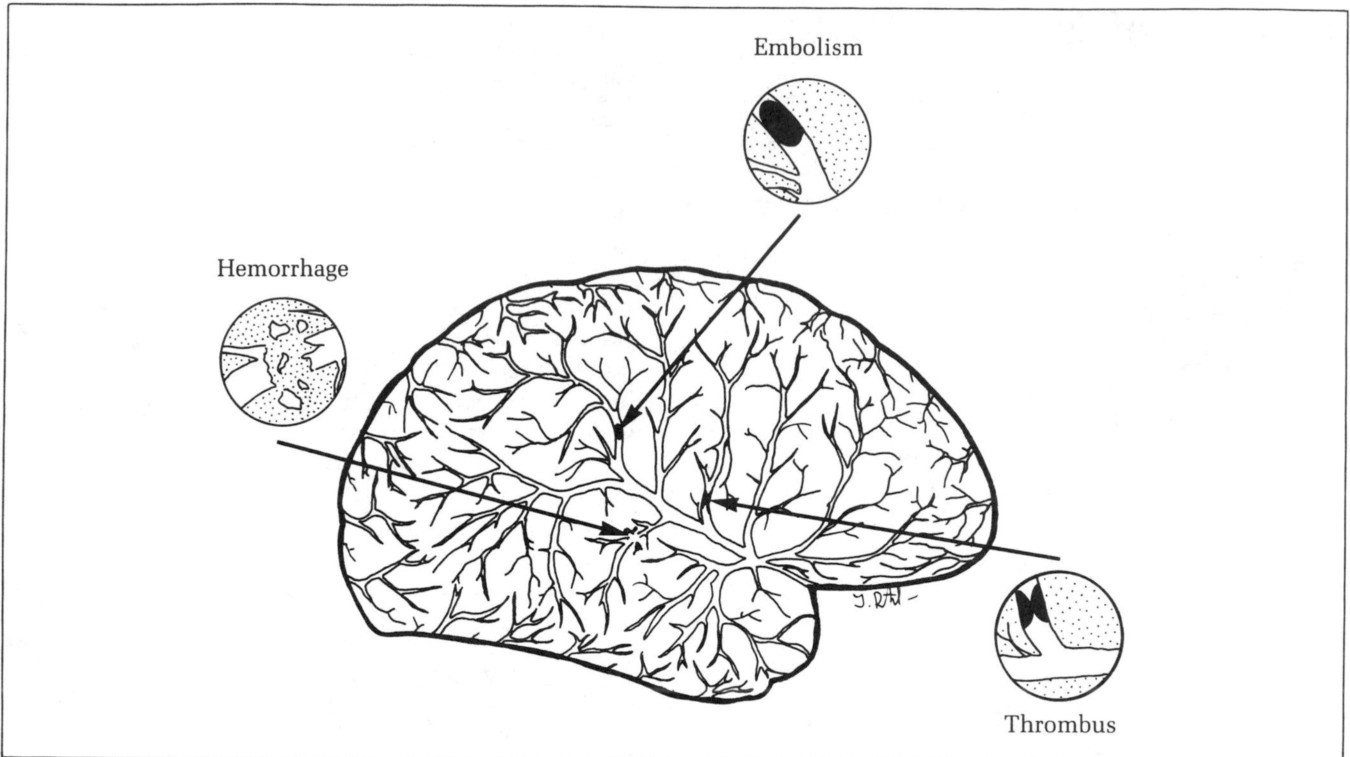

Fig. 22-1. *Mechanisms of stroke.*

thrombus, may form within one of the cerebral arteries, thereby clogging up the artery and preventing blood flow through it. This process is called **cerebral thrombosis**, and it generally occurs in people over 50 years of age who have widespread atherosclerosis. We have already learned how the atherosclerotic process causes narrowing and hardening of the coronary arteries. The same process can and does occur in the cerebral arteries, and a scarred, narrowed cerebral artery is very prone to develop a thrombus. When a thrombus becomes large enough to completely occlude an artery, blood flow through the artery is shut off and the brain tissue beyond the thrombus is deprived of its blood supply. Cerebral thrombosis is the most common cause of stroke, accounting for about 70 to 80 percent of stroke cases.

A similar problem develops when a clot that has formed elsewhere in the body breaks loose and gets swept into the cerebral circulation. When such a wandering clot—called an **embolus**—finally lodges in one of the cerebral arteries (an event called a **cerebral embolism**), there is a sudden cut-off of the blood flow through the artery involved, and once again the part of the brain supplied by that artery is left without its vital blood supply. Wandering emboli of this sort are particularly apt to develop in people who have rheumatic heart disease or other conditions that affect the valves of the heart. When the valves of the left side of the heart are scarred, blood clots tend to form on them. Eventually these blood clots break loose, as emboli, and go whizzing out into the arterial circulation. Such blood clots also tend to form in the heart after myocardial infarction or during a kind of chronic cardiac rhythm disturbance called atrial fibrillation. Finally, the formation of emboli is enhanced in black patients with sickle cell disease and in women taking birth control pills. Whatever their cause, emboli that form in the left side of the heart or elsewhere in the arterial circulation have a good chance of ending up in one of the cerebral arteries.

A third type of stroke is that which occurs when one of the cerebral arteries ruptures—a **cerebral hemorrhage**. Cerebral hemorrhage may occur in young people if there is an aneurysm—a weakened, bulging area—in one of the cerebral arteries. In older people, cerebral hemorrhage is usually associated with high blood pressure.

Major Causes of Stroke

- CEREBRAL THROMBOSIS: the formation of an obstructing clot (thrombus) within one of the cerebral arteries
- CEREBRAL EMBOLISM: the obstruction of a cerebral artery by a clot formed elsewhere in the body that breaks loose and floats free
- CEREBRAL HEMORRHAGE: bleeding into brain tissue caused by rupture of a cerebral artery

Table 22-1. *Major Causes of Stroke*

Characteristic	Cerebral Thrombosis	Cerebral Embolism	Cerebral Hemorrhage
Age group	Usually over 50, incidence increases with age	Young or middle-aged adults	Incidence increases with age, over 50
Underlying factors	Atherosclerosis	Rheumatic heart disease, cardiac arrhythmias, AMI, oral contraceptives, sickle cell disease	Hypertension
History of TIAs	80% of cases	Occasional	Rare
Onset	Acute or gradual	Acute	Acute, precipitous
Headache	Occasional, mild	Sometimes, moderate	Frequent, severe
Stiff neck	Rare	Rare	Frequent
Typical early signs	Difficulty in speech, weakness of an arm or leg	Very abrupt onset	Severe headache, rapid loss of consciousness, abnormal breathing

CLINICAL PICTURE OF STROKE

The initial signs and symptoms of stroke vary somewhat depending on the mechanism by which blood flow to part of the brain was interrupted (Table 22-1). In CEREBRAL THROMBOSIS, the onset of symptoms may be gradual. Often the patient will give a history of having experienced a series of "little strokes"—called **transient ischemic attacks,** or **TIAs**—in the months preceding the present attack. TIAs are temporary losses of neurologic function such as paralysis or loss of speech lasting anywhere from a few moments to several hours. Between attacks, the patient may feel perfectly normal. The present symptoms are likely to be similar to those experienced in the past, but this time those symptoms do not go away. Cerebral thrombosis most commonly presents at night or first thing in the morning with difficulty in speech or weakness of an arm or leg.

CEREBRAL EMBOLISM is most apt to occur very suddenly, "out of the blue," often during exertion, and it may start with a seizure or abrupt paralysis. The victim of cerebral embolism is apt to be younger than the typical victim of cerebral thrombosis, and there may be a known history of valvular heart disease or other risk factors.

CEREBRAL HEMORRHAGE often makes its presence known by an excruciating headache followed rapidly by loss of consciousness. A typical scenario for intracerebral hemorrhage is that of a patient sitting on the toilet, straining, who suddenly gets a severe headache and collapses. The patient's blood pressure is apt to be extremely elevated—sometimes with systolic pressures above 200 mm Hg—and the neck may be rigid due to irritation of the meninges by blood seeping into the CSF.

Whatever the mode of onset of the stroke, the eventual clinical picture is made up of a variable combination of signs and symptoms that depend chiefly on the area of the brain that has been damaged. Often the signs are quite obvious; sometimes they are very subtle. In general, one must maintain a high index of suspicion in any patient, especially an elderly patient, who presents with a sudden change in behavior, speech, or motor function.

Among the most classic signs of stroke is HEMIPARESIS, weakness on one side of the body, or HEMIPLEGIA, paralysis of one side of the body. Sometimes the motor disorder will be evident at a glance, for there may be paralysis of the facial muscles on one side that causes the whole face to look lopsided. Other times, hemiparesis may not become evident until you test the patient for strength in the arms and legs and notice that one side is markedly weaker than the other. In some patients, both sides of the body may be affected, and on examination you will find generalized weakness.

SPEECH DISTURBANCES are also very common in stroke. They may take the form of slurred speech, inability to name objects, inability to speak at all, or inability to understand what other people are saying. A word of caution

> DO NOT ASSUME THAT BECAUSE A PATIENT CANNOT SPEAK, HE OR SHE CANNOT UNDERSTAND.

The areas for speech production and speech comprehension are located in different parts of the brain, and there is every possibility that the mute patient understands perfectly. If the patient is unable to speak, try to assess comprehension by giving a simple command, such as, "Squeeze my hand," in order to see if the patient can comply. In general, it is safest to assume that the patient *does* understand what you are saying and to talk to the patient accordingly.

LACK OF COORDINATION may be a prominent feature in some strokes. The patient may stagger and lose his balance easily or may be unable to perform a simple maneuver such as buttoning a shirt. Some stroke patients will complain of HEADACHE and BLURRING OF VISION. In others, there may be CHANGES IN THE STATE OF CONSCIOUSNESS, ranging from CONFUSION to outright COMA. SEIZURES may occur, especially with cerebral embolism, and abnormal respiratory patterns are seen in severe cases.

Signs and Symptoms That May Be Seen in Stroke

- HEMIPARESIS or HEMIPLEGIA
- SPEECH DISTURBANCES
- INCOORDINATION
- HEADACHE
- VISUAL DISTURBANCES
- CONFUSION
- SEIZURES
- COMA

It is important to bear in mind that every stroke is different, and not all of the above signs will be present in any given patient. Any one of the signs listed, however, should alert the EMT to the possibility that the patient is suffering a CVA.

MANAGEMENT OF THE PATIENT WITH SUSPECTED STROKE

In caring for the patient with a stroke, one of the most important things to keep in mind is that the patient is likely to be very frightened and very depressed—and with good reason. Imagine what it feels like to find yourself suddenly paralyzed and, even worse, to be unable to communicate your distress because even though you know what you want to say, the words just won't come out. Clearly such a patient requires kind, considerate care. Even if the patient cannot talk, assume that he or she is an intelligent person who *can* understand. Explain to the patient that you realize how frustrating it must be to be unable to communicate, but that there is every chance that this problem is only temporary. A large number of stroke victims regain some or all of their ability to function, and it is important to maintain a hopeful attitude in talking to these patients. This does not mean engaging in cheerful platitudes such as, "Everything is going to be all right," for such statements will simply convince the patient that you do not understand the seriousness of the situation. But it is possible to offer honest reassurance and to tell the patient that there is usually a very good prospect for regaining lost functions.

As you examine the patient, make a careful note of what the patient can and cannot do. Use the neurologic checklist (see Fig. 14-7) to document your findings. Check the PULSE in both wrists and both carotids, and note whether the pulses are of equal strength on both sides. Also be alert for irregularities in the pulse that may give a clue to underlying heart disease and a possible source of cerebral emboli. Record the BLOOD PRESSURE. Recall that an elevated blood pressure with a slow pulse is often a sign of brain swelling with increasing intracranial pressure, an occasional and dangerous complication of stroke. Note any abnormalities in RESPIRATIONS, and be prepared to assist breathing if respirations are very shallow or if there are periods of apnea. Continue the secondary survey, paying special attention to the PUPILS, MUSCLE STRENGTH, and SENSATION.

Administer OXYGEN by nasal cannula, and place the patient in a comfortable position, preferably semi-recumbent, on the stretcher, taking care to PROTECT PARALYZED EXTREMITIES from injury. Give NOTHING BY MOUTH, since the throat may be paralyzed, and the patient may thus be unable to swallow properly. Transport the patient smoothly to the hospital, avoiding the use of sirens, which are likely to increase the patient's anxiety.

Needless to say, if the patient is unconscious, first priority must be given to supporting vital functions, and all of the principles of managing an unconscious patient apply: Maintain the AIRWAY, and guard against aspiration; support respiration as needed; keep a finger on the patient's pulse; and move swiftly to the hospital.

Management of the Patient with a Stroke

- TENDER LOVING CARE: Calm, considerate, hopeful attitude.
- Administer OXYGEN by nasal cannula.
- Measure and record VITAL SIGNS.
- NEUROLOGIC CHECKLIST.
- NOTHING BY MOUTH.
- PROTECT PARALYZED EXTREMITIES.
- Transport without undue haste to the hospital. Avoid sirens.

CASE HISTORY

The patient is a 76-year-old woman who was found unable to move at home. The patient could not speak, so part of the history was obtained from her son, who called for the ambulance. Apparently the patient was well last night when she was at a family dinner, but this morning, when the family could not reach her by phone, her son became worried and came to her apartment to find her lying paralyzed in bed. According to the son, the patient has had a few episodes of slurred speech during the past month, but these lasted only a few minutes. She has a history of myocardial infarction two years ago, and she is also under treatment for hypertension.

On physical examination, the patient appeared alert and upset; she cried periodically when she was questioned. She was unable to speak or write, but she could follow simple commands. The skin was warm and moist. Pulse was 100 and regular, equal at both wrists, BP was 180/110, and respirations were 16 and unlabored. The pupils were equal and reactive to light. The right side of the face was drooping. There was no distention of the neck veins, and the neck was not rigid. The chest was clear. The patient could not move her right arm or right leg at all, and she did not wince in response to pinprick on the right side.

She was given 4 liters of oxygen per minute by nasal cannula and transported in a semisitting position to the hospital. Vital signs and state of consciousness were unchanged en route.

Questions to think about:

1. What is the significance of the fact that the patient had a few episodes of slurred speech during the past month?
2. Is there any evidence in the patient's history that she has atherosclerosis and might therefore be predisposed to cerebral thrombosis? If so, what is the evidence?
3. On which side of the brain did the ischemic damage occur?
4. Do you think the patient was right-handed or left-handed? Why? (If you are unsure about the answers to questions 3 and 4, go back and review p. 247.)
5. Why was the patient given oxygen?

VOCABULARY

cerebral embolism Free-floating blood clot that lodges in one of the cerebral arteries.

cerebral hemorrhage Bleeding into brain tissue caused by rupture of a cerebral artery.

cerebral thrombosis Obstruction of a cerebral artery by a blood clot that arises within the artery, usually in an area scarred by atherosclerosis.

cerebrovascular accident (CVA) Another term for stroke.

embolus Free-floating blood clot.

stroke Sudden loss of some neurologic function, due to the interruption of the blood supply to a part of the brain.

thrombus Blood clot that forms within a blood vessel.

transient ischemic attack (TIA) Temporary loss of some neurologic function, often a warning sign of impending stroke.

FURTHER READING

Barber JM. EMT checkpoint: Management of the patient with suspected stroke. *EMT J* 4(3):69, 1980.

Edmeads J. Strategies in stroke. *Emerg Med* 15(4):163, 1983.

Jacobs FL. Stroke: Emergency management and assessment. *Emerg Med Serv* 14(2):41, 1985.

Klag MJ et al. Decline in U.S. stroke mortality: Demographic trends and antihypertensive treatment. *Stroke* 20:14, 1989.

Mikolich JR et al. Cardiac arrhythmias in patients with acute cerebrovascular accidents. *JAMA* 246:1314, 1981.

Myers MG et al. Cardiac sequellae of acute stroke. *Stroke* 13:838, 1982.

Samuels MA. All about stroke. *Emerg Med* 18(6):94, 1986.

Walshaw MJ, Pearson MG. Hypoxia in patients with acute hemiplegia. *Br Med J* 288:15, 1984.

23. ANAPHYLAXIS

OBJECTIVES

An acute anaphylactic reaction is an overwhelming allergic response, and it is one of the most dramatic and dangerous medical emergencies. Within moments of being stung by a bee or receiving an injection of medication, a susceptible person may become massively swollen, develop severe respiratory distress, and suffer an abrupt drop in blood pressure. If treatment is not given immediately, asphyxiation and cardiovascular collapse will lead rapidly to death. In this chapter, we will look at the mechanisms by which anaphylaxis occurs and the signs and symptoms by which it is manifested. We will also learn what measures should be taken to treat the patient who is suffering an anaphylactic reaction. By the conclusion of this chapter, the student will be able to

1. Define anaphylaxis, given a list of alternative definitions
2. Identify substances commonly responsible for anaphylactic reactions, given a list of substances
3. Identify a patient experiencing an anaphylactic reaction, given a description of several patients with different symptoms and signs
4. Indicate the principal life-threatening complications of an anaphylactic reaction, and identify the signs of these complications
5. List the correct measures in the prehospital treatment of an anaphylactic reaction

CAUSES OF ANAPHYLAXIS

Anaphylaxis is the most severe form of allergic reaction, and it is responsible for some 2,000 deaths per year in the United States. Anaphylaxis occurs when a physiologic system designed to protect the body goes haywire. The physiologic system in question is the immune system, whose job it is to spot foreign substances (**antigens**), such as those present on viruses or bacteria, and produce specific proteins, called **antibodies,** to inactivate the intruders. The normal immune response has three phases. In the first phase, the foreign substance—the antigen—is introduced into the body; it may be injected, inhaled, or eaten. During the next phase, lasting several days to weeks, the immune system processes the antigen and produces specific antibodies against it. Should the antigen ever be reintroduced into the body—and this is the third phase—it will be rapidly inactivated by the antibodies previously programmed to deal with that specific foreign substance. The immune response is the reason that most people do not get measles, for example, more than once: During the first exposure to the measles virus, the body develops antibodies against the virus. And should the measles virus ever be reintroduced into the body—say after exposure to a person in the contagious stage of measles—the antibodies formed during the first exposure will rapidly wipe out the invading measles viruses. This is also the principle behind vaccination. When you vaccinate, or immunize, a person against a particular disease—polio, for instance—what you are doing is introducing a harmless form of the polio virus into the body, so that the immune system can become acquainted with the virus and develop antibodies against it. Subsequently, if the immunized person should ever be exposed to the dangerous form of the polio virus, he will not become infected, because the polio virus will be spotted and wiped out by antibodies specifically assigned to tackle that particular antigen. In this way, the immune system protects us against a whole host of microorganisms, and without such a system, life would be simply a series of infections. (This, in fact, is precisely what happens in acquired immunodeficiency syndrome [AIDS], a disease in which the immune system no longer functions properly: The patient with AIDS is susceptible to a whole range of bacteria and other microorganisms that healthy people easily resist. A more detailed discussion of AIDS can be found in Chap. 28.)

In the allergic reaction, however, this protective system gets out of control. The word *anaphylaxis* literally means "without protection," and it refers to the fact that in an affected individual, exposure to certain antigens does *not* produce immunity, or protection, from the antigen but instead produces a markedly increased sensitivity to it. Upon reexposure to the antigen to which one is allergic—say, penicillin—the individual experiences a violent reaction. As the antigen is captured by the antibody, the two of them together prompt the release within the body of several chemical substances that cause capillaries to leak, respiratory smooth muscle to constrict, and arteries to dilate. The results of these reactions are the typical signs and symptoms of anaphylaxis, which we will discuss in the next section.

Who is susceptible to an anaphylactic reaction? The answer is that just about anyone may suffer this massive allergic response, although the incidence seems to be higher in individuals who have a history of multiple allergies. An immediate family history of similar reactions also suggests increased susceptibility, and certainly any person who has already experienced one severe allergic reaction is at risk of similar, if not more severe reactions in the future.

What sorts of materials can act as antigens to stimulate an anaphylactic reaction? Probably the most common offender is PENICILLIN. About 4 out of every 10,000 people receiving penicillin can be expected to have some sort of anaphylactic reaction, and about 2 of every 100,000 people given penicillin will die from anaphylactic shock. This does not sound like a very large figure until one considers that literally millions of doses of penicillin are dispensed in the United States each year. Thus the chances of an ambulance team seeing an anaphylactic reaction from this source are relatively high. OTHER DRUGS, such as other antibiotics, aspirin, or local anesthetics, are also frequently implicated in severe allergic responses.

Another common source of anaphylactic reactions is INSECT STINGS, particularly the stings of insects in the Hymenoptera family, which includes hornets, wasps, honeybees, and yellow jackets. Anaphylactic reactions to insect stings occur in susceptible persons within 5 to 30 minutes after the sting and are often very severe—sometimes fatal. Usually the intensity of the reaction is related to the number of stings, but even a single sting may cause a severe reaction in a very sensitive person.

FOODS may also give rise to severe allergic responses in sensitized individuals, with shellfish and nuts being common antigens in this category.

Although the above materials are the most common sources of anaphylaxis, it is important to realize that nearly any substance taken into the body by injection, inhalation, or ingestion can cause an anaphylactic reaction in a sensitized person. Drugs, foods, pollen, venoms—any of these may be responsible for anaphylaxis in a given case.

Materials Commonly Causing Anaphylaxis

- DRUGS
  - Penicillin and other antibiotics
  - Aspirin
  - Local anesthetics
- INSECT STINGS
  - Hornets
  - Wasps
  - Yellow jackets
  - Honeybees
- FOODS
  - Shellfish and other seafoods
  - Nuts
  - Berries

SIGNS AND SYMPTOMS OF ANAPHYLAXIS

The characteristic signs and symptoms of anaphylaxis are a direct result of the action of chemical mediators released during the antigen-antibody response. These signs and symptoms fall into three general categories: (1) cutaneous, (2) respiratory, and (3) cardiovascular.

The SKIN, first of all, becomes red and FLUSHED, and the patient experiences diffuse ITCHING (**pruritus**). As fluid oozes out of leaky capillaries into the subcutaneous tissues, there is widespread SWELLING and HIVES (**urticaria**), especially around the eyes, lips, ears, and in the hands and feet.

Meanwhile, in the RESPIRATORY SYSTEM there

Table 23-1. *Symptoms and Signs of Anaphylaxis*

Pathologic Process	Resulting Symptoms and Signs
Constriction of bronchial smooth muscle (bronchospasm)	Dyspnea Chest tightness Wheezes (silent chest in severe cases)
Laryngeal and glottic edema	Feeling of a lump in the throat Hoarseness or stridor
Arterial dilation	Hypotension (neurogenic-type shock) and reflex tachycardia
Leakage of plasma into subcutaneous tissues	Swelling of eyelids, tongue, lips Relative hypovolemia, contributing to hypotension
Edema of GI tract	Nausea, vomiting, cramps, diarrhea
Chemical mediators	Pruritus Urticaria

is violent spasm of the bronchial tubes, causing the patient to feel a TIGHTNESS IN THE CHEST and DYSPNEA. Auscultation of the chest will reveal WHEEZES, reflecting the passage of air through severely narrowed airways. If, however, bronchospasm is very intense, the chest may be silent altogether, indicating that air is unable to traverse the bronchi at all. Farther up the airway, massive SWELLING OF THE LARYNX (laryngeal edema) and glottis is signalled by HOARSENESS or STRIDOR. The patient may complain of a lump in his throat or of feeling as if his throat is closing. When laryngeal edema is extreme, the upper airway may be shut off entirely, and the only way to save the patient's life if that happens is via tracheostomy.

The CARDIOVASCULAR RESPONSE is one of shock. HYPOTENSION results from both leakage of fluid out of the vascular system and widespread dilation of small arteries—thus there are components of both hypovolemic and neurogenic shock. The fall in blood pressure elicits a reflex TACHYCARDIA, as the heart seeks desperately to compensate for hypotension by beating faster.

Swelling of the hollow organs within the gastrointestinal tract may lead as well to BLOATING, NAUSEA, VOMITING, CRAMPS, and DIARRHEA.

The symptoms and signs of anaphylaxis, and the mechanisms that produce them, are summarized in Table 23-1.

In the usual sequence of events, the patient first begins to feel a vague uneasiness or apprehension, a sensation of warmth, and itching of the palms of the hands and soles of the feet. Soon thereafter, he may notice a scratchy sensation in his throat and tightness in his chest, followed rapidly by the eruption of hives and facial swelling. There may be spasms of coughing or sneezing, with increasing respiratory distress, along with abdominal cramps and nausea. Flushing and tachycardia signal the approach of cardiovascular collapse. This sequence of events—from the first vague feeling of apprehension to full-blown shock—may occur within minutes.

TREATMENT OF ANAPHYLACTIC REACTIONS

Anaphylaxis is a dire medical emergency. While anaphylaxis may range in severity from a mild reaction to a life-threatening crisis, it is difficult to predict, even in apparently mild attacks, which reactions will progress to very severe ones. Thus every anaphylactic reaction must be regarded as potentially life-threatening. Airway obstruction from laryngeal edema or cardiovascular collapse from massive vasodilation may lead to death at any moment if swift action is not taken.

The single most important step in the treatment of anaphylaxis is the administration of a drug called EPINEPHRINE, or Adrenalin. Epinephrine works by opening up the lower airways **(bronchodilation)** and causing the peripheral arteries to constrict **(vasoconstriction)**; it also stimulates the heart to beat more forcefully. Epinephrine is the only thing that can save the life of a patient in anaphylactic shock, and even basic life support ambulances should carry epinephrine in the form of an inhaler (like that used by asthmatics) for use in this situation. EMT-As should be trained and authorized to administer epinephrine by aerosol inhaler for cases of anaphylactic shock, for if administration of this drug must be delayed until the patient reaches the hospital, the chances of the patient surviving are markedly reduced.

THERE IS NO TIME TO WASTE IN ANAPHYLACTIC SHOCK.

Epinephrine administered by inhaler is absorbed rapidly across mucous membranes and works nearly as fast as when it is injected directly into the bloodstream. To give epinephrine in this fashion, have the patient open his mouth wide, and instruct him to inhale as deeply as he can while you spray the epinephrine into the back of his throat. This procedure should be repeated once or twice to ensure that an adequate dose reaches the lower respiratory tract, where it can be absorbed into the blood.

KEEP THE PATIENT FLAT, WITH LEGS ELEVATED. If hypotension is severe, apply the MILITARY ANTI-SHOCK TROUSERS and, if authorized to do so, start an INTRAVENOUS INFUSION with normal saline. (When anaphylaxis is the result of an injection or sting on one arm, use the other arm for the IV.)

Administer OXYGEN by nasal cannula. Be alert for hoarseness or stridor, for these are signs of laryngeal edema and indicate the possibility of impending airway obstruction. If these signs are present, move the patient to a medical facility as fast as possible, as tracheostomy may be required to prevent death from asphyxia.

If anaphylaxis is due to an injection or insect sting on an extremity, apply a TOURNIQUET around the extremity proximal to the injection site or sting, in order to slow absorption of the antigen from the injection site into the systemic circulation. The tourniquet should be tight enough to obstruct venous return from the extremity, but not so tight that it cuts off the arterial circulation into the extremity. Check the pulse distal to the tourniquet, and if the pulse is absent, loosen the tourniquet until the pulse becomes palpable.

Once the anaphylactic reaction has subsided, some PATIENT EDUCATION is in order. First of all, the patient should be strongly urged to wear a medical identification tag that specifies the substance to which he is allergic and indicates that he is prone to anaphylaxis. He should also be advised to carry an emergency kit consisting of an automatic epinephrine syringe or epinephrine inhaler with him at all times, for use at the first sign of an anaphylactic attack. Remind him that when the next anaphylactic attack occurs, the ambulance might not get there in time to save him, and a personal emergency kit may be his only chance to survive.

Treatment of Anaphylactic Reactions

1. KEEP THE PATIENT FLAT, with legs elevated.
2. Administer EPINEPHRINE by inhaler.
3. Administer OXYGEN by nasal cannula.
4. *If* the patient is in *shock*
   a. MILITARY ANTI-SHOCK TROUSERS.
   b. INTRAVENOUS INFUSION of normal saline.
5. *If* anaphylaxis is due to injection or sting on an extremity, place a venous TOURNIQUET proximal to the injection site.
6. *If* the patient has *hoarseness* or *stridor*, MOVE WITH ALL POSSIBLE SPEED TO THE EMERGENCY ROOM.
7. After the emergency, PATIENT EDUCATION
   a. Medical identification tag.
   b. Personal emergency kit.

CASE HISTORY

The patient is a 32-year-old woman who was stung by a bee while working in her garden. She states that about 10 minutes after being stung, she began to feel warm all over and noticed an itchy sensation in the back of her throat. Minutes afterwards, she broke out in hives all over her body, but it was not until she started feeling a tightness in her chest that she became sufficiently alarmed to call for an ambulance. She states that once before, about a year ago, a bee sting led to her breaking out in hives, but the reaction was not nearly this severe. She denies any other allergies, but she says that her father and brothers are very allergic, and that one brother once collapsed after getting a shot of penicillin.

On physical examination, the patient appeared flushed and apprehensive. The skin was warm and dry. There was severe swelling around her eyes and lips, and hives were present all over her body. The pulse was 120 and regular, BP 110/60, and respirations 28 and somewhat labored. There was some hoarseness, but no stridor. Wheezes were heard throughout the chest, and bowel sounds were hyperactive. The site of the bee sting was visible on the left forearm.

The patient was placed supine with her legs elevated and given 6 liters per minute of oxygen by nasal cannula. Epinephrine was administered by inhaler. An intravenous infusion was started in the right arm with normal saline, at 180 ml per hour, and a venous tourniquet was placed on the left arm proximal to the site of the sting. The patient's wheezes and respiratory distress diminished during transport, and the blood pressure rose to 120/80. Her condition was generally improved upon arrival at the hospital.

Questions to think about:

1. Did this patient have any risk factors for anaphylaxis? If so, what were they?
2. Is she showing any signs that her airway is in jeopardy?
3. What caused the patient's wheezes (i.e., what was happening in the lungs)? What helped alleviate them?
4. Why was the intravenous infusion started in the right arm rather than in the left arm?
5. Why was oxygen given?
6. Could this woman ever suffer another attack of anaphylaxis? If so, is it likely to be more or less severe the next time?

VOCABULARY

Adrenalin Trade name for epinephrine.

anaphylaxis An exaggerated allergic reaction characterized by bronchospasm, laryngeal edema, urticaria, and sometimes cardiovascular collapse.

antibody A protein produced in the body in response to a specific antigen (foreign protein) that destroys or inactivates the antigen.

antigen An agent that, when taken into the body, stimulates the formation of specific protective proteins called antibodies.

bronchodilation Widening of the bronchial air passages brought about by relaxation of the muscles in the bronchial walls.

bronchospasm Violent contraction of the muscles of the bronchial walls, causing marked narrowing of the bronchi.

epinephrine A drug or hormone that promotes bronchodilation and vasoconstriction.

pruritus Itching.

tracheostomy A surgical opening into the trachea, through the anterior neck, to provide an airway.

urticaria Hives.

vasoconstriction Narrowing of the caliber of the arteries, brought about by contraction of muscles in the arterial walls.

vasodilation Widening of the caliber of the arteries, brought about by relaxation of muscles in the arterial walls.

FURTHER READING

Austen KF. Systemic anaphylaxis in the human being. *NEJM* 291:661, 1974.

Barach EM et al. Epinephrine for treatment of anaphylactic shock. *JAMA* 251:2118, 1984.

Barr SE. Allergy to hymenoptera stings. *JAMA* 288:718, 1974.

Bickel W, Dice W. Military antishock trousers in a patient with adrenergic-resistant anaphylaxis. *Ann Emerg Med* 13:189, 1984.

Frazier C. Food allergy emergencies. *Emerg Med Serv* 12(2):71, 1983.

Kaliner MA. Calling a halt to anaphylaxis. *Emerg Med* 21(16):51, 1989.

Levy DB. Anaphylaxis. *Emergency* 21(4):42, 1989.

Lucke WC, Thomas H. Anaphylaxis: Pathophysiology, clinical presentations, and treatment. *J Emerg Med* 1:83, 1983.

Oertel T, Loehr M. Bee sting anaphylaxis: The use of medical antishock trousers. *Ann Emerg Med* 13:459, 1984.

Schwartz H, Sher T. Anaphylaxis to penicillin in a frozen dinner. *Ann Allergy* 52:342, 1984.

Vanselow NA. Minutes to counter anaphylaxis. *Emerg Med* 20(15):121, 1988.

Yunginger JW et al. Fatal food-induced anaphylaxis. *JAMA* 260:1450, 1988.

24. ABDOMINAL PAIN

OBJECTIVES

Abdominal pain varies from the simple bellyache due to dietary indiscretion to the severe distress due to rupture of an internal organ. In this chapter, we shall be chiefly concerned with what is called the *acute abdomen*. This term is somewhat vague, but in general it is used to refer to conditions in which there is inflammation of the abdominal lining and resulting intense abdominal pain. We will look at some of the causes of the acute abdomen, the typical signs and symptoms, and the measures that can be taken in the field to ensure that the patient with an acute abdomen reaches the hospital in optimal condition. By the conclusion of this chapter, the reader should be able to

1. Identify conditions that may lead to an acute abdomen, given a description of several medical conditions
2. Identify the type of illness or possible organ involved in an acute abdomen, given a description of the nature and location of the abdominal pain
3. Indicate what aspects of the history and physical examination should be emphasized in evaluating a patient with abdominal pain
4. Identify the specific significance of various symptoms and signs of possible life-threatening problems in a patient with abdominal pain
5. Indicate the correct prehospital management of a patient with abdominal pain

CAUSES OF THE ACUTE ABDOMEN

Most textbooks of surgery list anywhere from 80 to over 100 causes of severe abdominal pain. Obviously it is not feasible for the EMT to study all of these different illnesses that produce abdominal pain, nor would it be particularly useful to do so. The EMT should, however, have a general idea of the types of illnesses that can manifest themselves as an acute abdomen and the possible dangers associated with these illnesses.

Recall that there are several organ systems, or portions of organ systems, located in the abdominal cavity, and disease in any one of these systems may lead to an acute abdomen. Most prominently represented in the belly is the GASTROINTESTINAL SYSTEM, and among the gastrointestinal organs, those most likely to give rise to an acute abdomen are the stomach, small or large bowel, pancreas, and gallbladder. Problems arising in the STOMACH include inflammations of the stomach (gastritis) and gastric **ulcer**, an erosion of the stomach lining that may lead to internal bleeding as well as pain. Ulcers also commonly occur in the DUODENUM, the first portion of the small intestine. If an ulcer erodes all the way through the stomach or duodenal wall, that is, it if perforates, gastrointestinal contents, such as enzymes and acids, spill out into the peritoneal cavity, causing inflammation of the peritoneum itself (**peritonitis**) and often excruciating pain. Peritonitis of this sort may also occur when there is inflammation of the PANCREAS (**pancreatitis**), for when the pancreas becomes inflamed, the very powerful digestive enzymes it produces often leak out into the abdominal cavity, resulting in severe peritoneal irritation. Obstruction of a hollow organ may also give rise to intense belly pain. When the GALLBLADDER becomes obstructed by a gall stone, for instance, there may be severe pain in the right upper quadrant of the abdomen. Obstruction of the BOWEL from any cause may also cause marked abdominal distress. Even the tiny, worm-like appendage to the cecum, the APPENDIX, can be the culprit, bringing about intense right lower quadrant pain.

The CARDIOVASCULAR SYSTEM is another organ system well-represented in the abdomen, in the form of a rich blood supply to abdominal organs. The AORTA, the largest artery in the body, courses through the abdomen, and disease in the aorta may thus give rise to abdominal pain. If, for instance, there is a weakened, bulging area of the aortic wall (called an **aneurysm**), such an area may develop a leak or may rupture altogether, causing blood to escape into the abdominal cavity. Like digestive enzymes, blood is very irritating to the peritoneum, and its presence in the peritoneal cavity thus produces intense pain. The many ARTERIES supplying gastrointestinal organs are also not immune from disease. A narrowed, atherosclerotic artery in the mesentery, for example, may cause angina and infarction of the bowel in exactly the same way that atherosclerosis of a coronary artery can lead to infarction of the heart.

Organs of the GENITOURINARY SYSTEM, even though they are located outside the peritoneal cavity, may also give rise to abdominal pain. Stones originating in the KIDNEY may lead to excruciating pain when they get hung up in the corresponding ureter. Infections of the BLADDER and of the FEMALE REPRODUCTIVE ORGANS can also cause intense abdominal pain.

To make matters even more complicated, abdominal pain can result from disease in ORGANS OUTSIDE THE ABDOMEN. Some cases of pneumonia, for example, present as belly pain, and even an occasional myocardial infarction may be experienced as pain in the upper abdomen rather than the chest. So too, the clinical picture in metabolic disorders, such as diabetic ketoacidosis, may be dominated by severe abdominal distress.

SYMPTOMS AND SIGNS OF THE ACUTE ABDOMEN

With such a large range of possible causes, how does one sort it all out? To begin with, one can get some clues from the LOCATION OF THE PAIN (Fig. 24-1). Pain in the right upper quadrant of the abdomen, for instance, suggests that the problem may be in the gallbladder or duodenum, while pain in the right lower quadrant is more likely to be due to appendicitis or sometimes a kidney stone on the right. RADIATION OF THE PAIN may provide further clues. Pain radiating into the right shoulder again suggests a problem in the gallbladder. Pain boring through into the back may be due to pancreatitis, while that radiating into the groin can be caused by a kidney stone. Also check WHETHER THE PAIN HAS SHIFTED IN LOCATION since it began. Pain from appendicitis typically starts in the midabdomen and gradually moves to the right lower quadrant.

The patient's description of the NATURE OF THE PAIN can also be enormously helpful. COLICKY PAIN is crampy and comes in waves, rising to a peak of intensity, then subsiding, then growing more intense again. Such pain is characteristic of obstruction—for instance, obstruction of the bowel or obstruction of a ureter by kidney stone. Patients with colicky pain are apt to thrash about in bed, trying to find a position of comfort. PERITONEAL PAIN, by contrast, tends to be steady. It may be very severe, and it is usually aggravated by even the slightest movement. For this reason, a patient with peritoneal pain will lie very still and will cry out if jolted, as when the ambulance goes over a bump. This kind of pain can come about from any condition that permits gastric juice, intestinal contents, urine, blood, pus, or dead tissue to enter the peritoneal cavity.

Finally, it is important to know about the ONSET AND DURATION of the pain. Did it come on abruptly, from one minute to the next, or did it creep up on the patient gradually? A sudden, severe pain suggests perforation of a hollow organ, while inflammatory processes, like appendicitis, usually take some time to develop. As regards duration, abdominal pain that has been present more than about six hours must be considered serious, and any extremely severe abdominal pain—no matter how long it has been present—should also be considered a potentially grave emergency.

Besides obtaining an accurate description of the pain, what else do we want to know when questioning the patient whose chief complaint is abdominal pain? Perhaps most important is to try to determine whether there have been any SIGNS OF INTERNAL BLEEDING. Blood present in the stomach or duodenum, as from a severe ulcer, acts as an irritant;

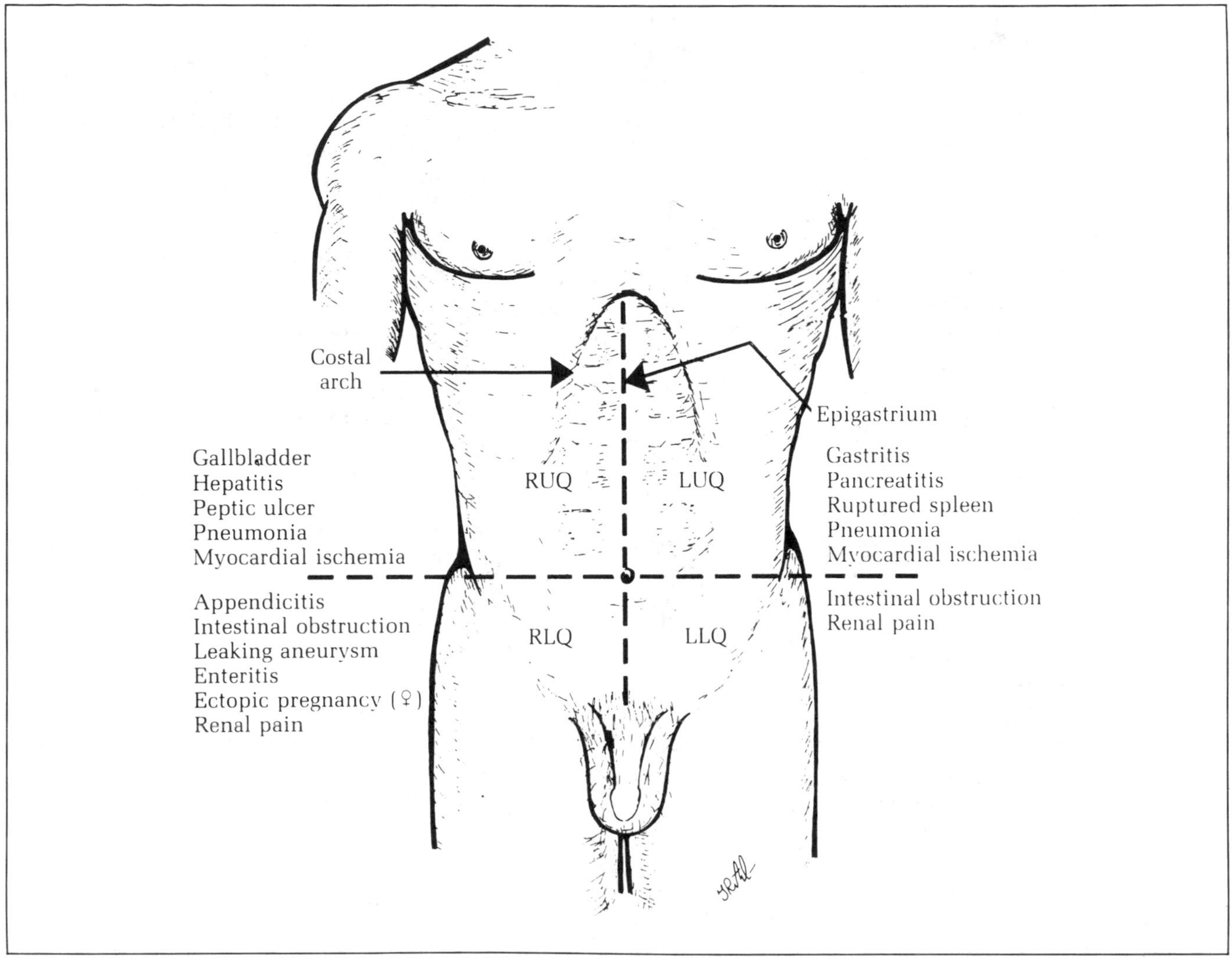

Fig. 24-1. *Some typical sources of abdominal pain.*

there may be resulting VOMITING OF BLOOD (**hematemesis**), and the patient with abdominal pain should be asked specifically whether this occurred. If blood sits around for a while in gastric juices before being vomited, it may not be red—indeed, it may not look like blood at all, but rather like coffee grounds. Thus, if the patient reports that he has vomited, ask what the vomitus looked like. If he vomits in your presence, try to save a sample of the vomitus in a container to take with the patient to the emergency room. Blood may also pass out of the gastrointestinal tract via the rectum, and blood leaving the gastrointestinal tract through this orifice may be red or may turn the stool a tarry, black color. Thus one needs to ask the patient about the COLOR OF HIS STOOL. Any signs that the patient has vomited blood or passed blood through the rectum should alert the EMT to the danger of impending hemorrhagic shock. Even if there has not been any evidence of bleeding, severe vomiting or diarrhea may in themselves have led to significant dehydration, and for this reason, one must always inquire about these symptoms.

On PHYSICAL EXAMINATION, the most important things to look for are SIGNS OF IMPENDING SHOCK. Shock may occur in the acute abdomen from several mechanisms. We have already mentioned vomiting and internal bleeding as possible sources of shock. In addition, severe hypovolemia may result from peritonitis itself. When the peritoneum is inflamed, large amounts of body fluids leak out of the blood vessels into the abdominal cavity. This fluid is lost from the circulation just as irrevocably at if it were lost by vomiting or diarrhea. Whatever the source of hypovolemia—internal bleeding, vomiting, peritonitis, or any combination of these—the signs are the same: RESTLESSNESS; TACHYCARDIA; COLD, CLAMMY SKIN; and eventually FALLING BLOOD PRESSURE. Remember

SIGNS OF HYPOVOLEMIA ARE SIGNS OF DANGER.

Such signs indicate that the patient is at the brink of shock, and he or she must be stabilized swiftly and moved as expeditiously as possible to a medical facility.

As you examine the patient, also make a note of his GENERAL APPEARANCE and POSITION. A patient with an acute abdomen *looks* very ill. Furthermore, his position in bed may provide additional clues to the cause of his problem. As noted earlier, patients with diffuse peritonitis will usually lie very still. The patient with pancreatitis tends to curl up on his right side, while the patient with appendicitis may lie with his right leg flexed. In each case, the position is one that relaxes the muscles in the inflamed area and thereby reduces pain.

Up to this point, we have mentioned nothing about EXAMINATION OF THE ABDOMEN itself. This was not an oversight. In the hospital, examination of the abdomen is one of the most important aspects of evaluating a patient with severe abdominal pain. In the field, the overall condition of the patient and his vital signs are most important considerations. This is because field management and hospital management have different goals. In the field, we ask, "How *severe* is the patient's problem?" in order to determine what measures must be taken to stabilize the patient and enable him to reach the hospital in optimal condition. In the hospital, the doctors need to ask, in addition, "What is *causing* the patient's abdominal pain?" That is, they have to make a diagnosis.

THERE IS NO NECESSITY OR USEFULNESS IN DIAGNOSING THE CAUSE OF ABDOMINAL PAIN IN THE FIELD.

Thus there is no need to make a painstaking examination of the abdomen in the field. Furthermore, in the patient with peritonitis, an additional session of prodding and poking at his belly just means additional pain. For these reasons, the EMT should confine his or her examination of the patient's abdomen to the following:

1. LOOK at the abdomen, and note whether there appears to be any DISTENTION.
2. LISTEN with the diaphragm of the stethoscope resting lightly on the abdominal wall for the PRESENCE OF BOWEL SOUNDS. Listen for at least 1 to 2 minutes, and record whether or not you heard bowel sounds during this period.
3. FEEL VERY GENTLY to determine (a) whether the abdomen is SOFT OR RIGID and (b) whether palpation elicits any TENDERNESS. If tenderness is present, note whether it is diffuse or localized to a particular spot. (Note: If the patient complains of localized pain, always examine the painful part of the abdomen *last*.)

Assessment of the Patient with Abdominal Pain

- HISTORY
  1. Description of the PAIN
     a. Onset and duration
     b. Location: shifts in location; radiation
     c. Type of pain; steady? colicky? sharp? dull?
  2. Has the patient been VOMITING? If so, was there blood or "coffee-ground" material in the vomitus? (Save sample.)
  3. Changes in BOWEL HABITS? (Constipation or diarrhea?) Were stools bloody or tarry black?
- PHYSICAL ASSESSMENT
  1. GENERAL APPEARANCE: Does the patient look ill?
  2. POSITION and MOVEMENT: Is the patient thrashing about or lying still? How is he lying?
  3. SIGNS OF IMPENDING SHOCK
     a. Restlessness
     b. Cold, clammy skin
     c. Tachycardia
     d. Tachypnea
     e. Hypotension
  4. ABDOMINAL SIGNS
     a. Distention
     b. Bowel sounds
     c. Tenderness or rigidity

TREATMENT OF THE ACUTE ABDOMEN

The goals of the prehospital management of the patient with an acute abdomen are (1) to prevent life-threatening complications, such as shock or aspiration, (2) to make the patient as comfortable as possible, and (3) to move the patient expeditiously to the hospital.

To begin with, place the patient in a recumbent POSITION OF COMFORT. If the patient feels nauseated, it is preferable that he or she lie on the left side (i.e., facing the squad bench in the ambulance) to minimize the risk of aspiration should vomiting occur. Have an emesis basin ready, and keep suction handy.

Administer OXYGEN by nasal cannula at 4 to 6 liters per minute. Avoid the use of oxygen masks, for a mask becomes a problem if there is vomiting.

If you are authorized to do so, start an INTRAVE-

NOUS INFUSION with normal saline or Ringer's solution. Use a good sized intravenous catheter—16- or 18-gauge—for if signs of shock develop, the patient will need a lot of fluid fast.

DO NOT PERMIT THE PATIENT TO TAKE ANYTHING BY MOUTH, and do not allow the patient to be given any medications by any route. The addition of food or liquids to the patient's stomach simply increases the likelihood of vomiting and aspiration and may aggravate the patient's underlying condition as well. Medications can mask the patient's symptoms and make it more difficult for the doctor to evaluate those symptoms in the hospital.

In moving the patient, AVOID ROUGH HANDLING. Every jolt of the stretcher and every bump along the road can be a torment to a patient with peritonitis. Handle the patient with this in mind, and try as well to keep the ride to the hospital as smooth as possible.

DO NOT DELAY TRANSPORT. The secondary survey and stabilization should be accomplished rapidly and efficiently.

Make a DETAILED RECORD of the patient's history and physical findings. The patient may not be in any shape to tell his story all over again by the time you reach the hospital, or his physical findings may have changed markedly by then. Thus your report may provide the doctors with crucial information about the onset and course of the patient's illness.

Treatment of the Acute Abdomen

- Place the patient in a POSITION OF COMFORT.
- BE ALERT FOR VOMITING. Have an emesis basin and suction ready.
- Administer OXYGEN by nasal cannula.
- Start an INTRAVENOUS INFUSION with normal saline, if so authorized.
- NOTHING BY MOUTH.
- GENTLE HANDLING.
- TRANSPORT to the hospital WITHOUT DELAY.
- Keep an accurate, DETAILED RECORD of the secondary survey.

CASE HISTORY

The patient is a 43-year-old man who called for an ambulance because of severe abdominal pain. He states that he has been having such pain on and off for about a year, and usually he can get some relief from drinking a glass of milk or taking an antacid. But for the past day or so, the pain has gotten much worse, and nothing seems to relieve it. He describes the pain as steady and dull. It is located in the epigastrium and does not radiate. This afternoon, he vomited some coffee-ground material, and he has also noticed that his stools have become black. He has no known history of significant illnesses and takes no medications except antacids.

On physical examination, the patient appeared pale and apprehensive. His skin was cold and moist. The pulse was 132 and thready, BP was 100/60, and respirations were 28 and shallow. The neck veins were collapsed. The chest was clear. The abdomen appeared slightly distended. Bowel sounds were not heard during two minutes of auscultation. There was diffuse tenderness to light palpation, and the abdomen wall felt rigid.

The patient was placed on his left side and given 6 liters per minute of oxygen by nasal cannula. As per orders of Dr. Tums, an intravenous infusion was started with normal saline with a 16-gauge angiocath placed in the right forearm, and fluids were infused at 200 ml per hour. Vital signs were unchanged during transport.

Questions to think about:

1. What is the significance of the fact that the patient has vomited "coffee-ground material" and that his stools have become black?
2. What potentially life-threatening complication is the patient already manifesting? What is the evidence that he has developed this complication?
3. Does this patient have any signs of peritonitis? If so, what signs?
4. Why was the patient transported on his left side (as opposed to his right side)? (Hint: Think about the layout of an ambulance.)
5. Why was oxygen given?
6. Why was an infusion started?

VOCABULARY

aneurysm Sac or bulge resulting from the weakening of the wall of a blood vessel.

hematemesis Vomiting of blood.

pancreatitis Inflammation of the pancreas.

peritonitis Inflammation of the membrane lining the abdomen.

ulcer An open lesion or erosion in the skin or in a mucous membrane.

FURTHER READING

Fontanarosa PB. Acute abdominal pain: Exploring the gut-level causes. *JEMS* 14(11):28, 1989.

25. ALCOHOL AND DRUG ABUSE

OBJECTIVES

Abuse of alcohol and abuse of drugs together comprise one of the most widespread medical and social problems in the United States. It is a problem that has few boundaries in terms of age, sex, or social and economic status. It is a safe generalization that virtually every ambulance team will sooner or later have to deal with a patient who is suffering the ill effects of alcohol or other drugs; indeed, in large urban areas, such cases may constitute a significant proportion of ambulance runs. In this chapter, we will examine the medical problems caused by alcohol and various other types of drugs. We shall look at some of the potentially life-threatening conditions such substances may induce, and we will discuss the means of evaluating and treating patients who have been poisoned by excessive intake of these substances. By the conclusion of this chapter, the reader should be able to

1. Identify the correct definitions of (a) drug dependence, (b) compulsive drug use, (c) tolerance, and (d) addiction
2. Identify the untoward effects of alcohol on various organ systems and the illnesses to which alcoholics are therefore more susceptible
3. Indicate the areas of special emphasis in the secondary survey of a patient with alcohol on his breath
4. List at least three potentially life-threatening emergencies that may be directly due to excessive alcohol consumption, and indicate the treatment in the field for each
5. Identify patients suffering from (a) delirium tremens, (b) narcotic overdose, (c) amphetamine overdose, and (d) hallucinogen reaction, given a description of several patients with various signs and symptoms
6. Correctly classify various commonly abused substances as "uppers," "downers," or hallucinogens, given a list of such substances
7. List the major threat(s) to life in a person rendered unconscious by alcohol or drugs
8. Indicate the areas of special emphasis in evaluating a patient who has taken an overdose of drugs
9. Identify those patients in whom vomiting should NOT be induced, given a description of several patients who have ingested an overdose of a drug
10. Identify the correct method for inducing vomiting, including the medication used and the correct dosage
11. Indicate in the correct sequence the steps in treating a person found unconscious from an overdose of an unknown drug
12. Identify any special measures that should be taken in the treatment of patients who have overdosed with (a) depressant drugs, (b) stimulant drugs, (c) hallucinogens

THE TERMINOLOGY OF SUBSTANCE ABUSE

Before we can begin our discussion of the effects of alcohol and other drugs, we need to acquire some vocabulary. The substances we shall be talking about all produce certain effects upon the user, which cause varying degrees of chronic preoccupation with the substance in question. These effects may be classified as follows:

1. **Dependence** occurs when the user needs the drug in order to "keep going," and dependence may be psychological or physical or both. In *psychological dependence,* the user needs the drug in order to maintain his or her feeling of well-being. *Physical dependence* occurs when the altered physiologic state produced by the drug requires repeated administration of the drug in order to prevent withdrawal symptoms.
2. Dependence leads to a situation called **compulsive drug use**, in which the user becomes extremely preoccupied with the procurement and use of the drug in question. The heroin user, for example may spend the bulk of his waking hours planning how and where he will get his next "fix."
3. In the chronic drug user, **tolerance** to the drug may develop; that is, it may take larger and larger doses of the drug to achieve the desired effect. A barbiturate user who could once obtain soothing effects from a single Seconal, for instance, may find that he is requiring five, ten, or twenty Seconals to reach the same state, and thus his intake of Seconal increases proportionally.
4. Dependence, compulsive drug use, and tolerance are part of the syndrome of **addiction**, which is characterized by an overwhelming involvement in the use of a drug. For the addicted person, nearly everything in life revolves around the drug. All his or her energies are invested in procuring and taking the drug, often in increasing doses, and should the addict be prevented from taking the drug, severe and sometimes fatal withdrawal reactions may occur.

ALCOHOL ABUSE

"If you arrive at a bad auto collision at 2 A.M. and neither driver appears drunk, then someone is missing!"

—*Mike Taigman, EMT-P*

Alcohol is the most frequently abused drug in most industrialized nations today. In the United States alone, there are an estimated 9 million alcoholics, and for each alcoholic, there are at least another 3 or 4 people who are in some way adversely affected by alcohol consumption. In addition to the more than 30,000 deaths in the United States each year due directly to alcohol, there are many times that number of deaths due to the harmful effects of alcohol on various organs, such as the stomach, liver, pancreas, and central nervous system. That makes alcohol one of the leading causes of death in America. Furthermore, alcohol is estimated to be a factor in about half a million injuries from road accidents annually and to be responsible for nearly half of all road traffic fatalities.

The price tag to the nation of alcohol abuse is enormous. It is now costing the United States approximately $15 billion a year to treat alcoholism and alcohol-related illness. And this figure does not take into account indirect costs of alcoholism: the costs of lost life and productivity, property loss, alcohol-related crime, and so forth—costs estimated to be as high as $100 billion a year.

ALCOHOLISM is a form of addiction and has all of the attributes of addiction discussed above. Usually true alcoholism is preceded by a phase of PROBLEM DRINKING, during which alcohol is used with increasing frequency to relieve tensions or deal with other emotional difficulties. The stage of true addiction is reached when the user can no longer abstain from alcohol without suffering symptoms of withdrawal.

Alcoholism is a problem at all levels of society, and only a very small minority of alcoholics—probably less than 5 percent—are "skid row" types. The roster of alcoholics includes housewives, professionals, manual laborers, and even refined little old ladies. Most alcoholics are working men (alcoholism occurs three times more frequently in men than in women) who do not regard themselves as alcoholics at all, but rather as social drinkers. As they become more and more dependent on alcohol, however, their performance at work begins to suffer, as do their personal relationships. Alcohol-related illness and injury begin to occur with increasing frequency, and alcoholic binges—so-called lost weekends—bring on further deterioration in the drinker's physical and social condition. This alcoholic syndrome produces the same overall effects regardless of the form in which alcohol is taken—whether it is beer, wine, or hard liquor. It is important to bear in mind also that many alcoholics are dependent on other drugs in addition to alcohol, especially sedative drugs such as tranquilizers and barbiturates.

Alcoholism is an illness and should be treated as such. It is very important that the EMT and other health professionals refrain from passing moral judgment on patients with alcohol-related problems. It is no more justified to look down on an alcoholic than to condemn a diabetic or an epileptic. Alcohol-related problems are true medical emergencies that may, in some cases, be fatal if not handled appropriately. Thus the alcoholic should be approached with the same professional attitude accorded any other seriously ill or injured person.

HARMFUL EFFECTS OF EXCESS ALCOHOL

Chronic overindulgence in alcohol produces a variety of untoward effects on the body, which in turn render the alcoholic more susceptible to a wide range of illnesses and injuries. To begin with, alcohol is a strong CENTRAL NERVOUS SYSTEM DEPRESSANT. That is, it slows down many functions of the brain and thereby leads to *sleepiness, mental confusion,* and related symptoms. Problems with balance and coordination result in *frequent falls* and other trauma, rendering the alcoholic much more prone to serious injury. *Subdural hematoma,* for instance, is common in alcoholics, due to repeated head trauma sustained while intoxicated. Furthermore, as we shall see later, severe intoxication may in itself produce *coma, respiratory depression,* and *loss of protective reflexes.*

In addition to its effects on the CNS, alcohol also attacks the GASTROINTESTINAL TRACT. Its irritant effects on the lining of the STOMACH, for example, may lead to massive *gastrointestinal bleeding.* Damage to the LIVER due to chronic alcohol abuse results in impairment of many vital functions normally carried out by the liver, such as the production of clotting factors and the mobilization of sugar from storage areas into the blood. Thus the alcoholic is more apt to *bleed profusely,* even from minor trauma, and is also prone to *hypoglycemia.* Untoward effects of alcohol on the PANCREAS lead to a high incidence of *pancreatitis* in the alcoholic population. The types of medical problems seen frequently in alcoholics are summarized in Table 25-1.

Table 25-1. *Medical Problems Frequently Seen in Alcoholics*

Condition	Contributing Factors
Subdural hematoma	Frequent falls, impaired clotting mechanisms
Gastrointestinal bleeding	Irritant effect of alcohol on the stomach lining, impaired clotting mechanisms, cirrhosis of the liver leading to engorgement of esophageal veins (esophageal varices)
Pancreatitis	Indirect effect of alcohol on the pancreas
Hypoglycemia	Damage to the liver, which normally mobilizes sugar into the blood
Pneumonia	Aspiration of vomitus occurring during intoxication and coma, made worse by suppression of immune mechanism by alcohol
Burns	Relative insensitivity to pain occurring during intoxication, falling asleep with lit cigarette while intoxicated
Hypothermia	Insensitivity to extremes of temperature while intoxicated, falling asleep outside in the cold
Seizures	Effect of withdrawal from alcohol

ALCOHOLIC EMERGENCIES

Any of the conditions mentioned above—gastrointestinal hemorrhage, pancreatitis, subdural hematoma—may lead to a medical emergency in the alcoholic patient. In addition, however, there are a number of alcoholic emergencies that are directly related to the consumption of or abstinence from alcohol itself. These include severe alcoholic intoxication, withdrawal seizures, and delirium tremens.

Severe Alcoholic Intoxication

Severe alcoholic intoxication is, in essence, a form of poisoning, and as such it carries all of the lethal potential of poisoning with any other CNS depressant. The seriousness of intoxication depends on a number of factors, including the amount of alcohol consumed, the speed with which it was consumed, the presence of other drugs in the patient's system, and underlying illnesses. Death from alcohol intoxication has been reported at blood alcohol levels of 4000 mg per liter, which can be attained by the relatively rapid consumption of half a pint of whiskey. The most immediate danger to an acutely intoxicated person is DEATH FROM RESPIRATORY DEPRESSION. Because reflexes are suppressed, ASPIRATION OF VOMITUS and resulting pneumonia are also significant dangers. Furthermore, alcoholic intoxication may be, and often is, complicated by a variety of coexisting conditions—subdural hematoma, drug overdose, hypoglycemia—and the EMT must be alert for signs of these problems. As we learned in a previous chapter, the presence of alcohol on a patient's breath does *not* prove that his condition is solely or even partially the result of alcohol intoxication, and other possible causes of coma should be carefully considered. Remember

THE PATIENT WHO ACTS DRUNK MAY BE ILL FROM OTHER CAUSES.

The treatment of the acutely intoxicated patient is aimed at protecting the patient from injury and safeguarding his vital functions. If the patient is conscious and agitated, he must be prevented from injuring himself and others. If possible, this should be accomplished without the use of physical restraints, which are apt to aggravate rather than diminish the patient's agitation. A kind but firm approach, with attempts to orient the patient and help him understand what is happening, can sometimes do much to calm agitated behavior.

If the patient is unconscious, he must be treated with the same measures that apply to any other unconscious patient. Protection of the AIRWAY has first priority, and the patient should be positioned on his side to minimize the danger of aspiration. Suction should be close at hand. As any other comatose patient, the victim of severe alcohol intoxication should receive OXYGEN, preferably by nasal cannula. If there is marked respiratory depression, as manifested by slow, shallow breathing, ASSISTED VENTILATION with a bag-valve-mask unit and oxygen will be required.

CHECK the patient carefully FOR SIGNS OF INJURY. In evaluating the VITAL SIGNS, recall that a rising blood pressure and slow pulse are indicative of increased intracranial pressure and may therefore give a clue to coexisting subdural hematoma. As for any other unconscious patient, fill out a NEUROLOGIC CHECKLIST (see Fig. 14-7), and recheck the vital and neurologic signs frequently.

EVERY INTOXICATED PATIENT MUST BE TRANSPORTED TO THE HOSPITAL. It is outright negligence to leave a patient at the scene on the assumption that he is just drunk, even if the patient is one of your "regulars."

Treatment of Acute Alcohol Intoxication

- *If the patient is conscious*, PROTECT THE PATIENT FROM INJURY. Avoid restraints wherever possible.
- *If the patient is unconscious*
  1. Open and maintain the AIRWAY.
  2. PREVENT ASPIRATION: Stable side position and suction.
  3. Administer OXYGEN by nasal cannula.
  4. CHECK FOR INJURY.
  5. Monitor VITAL SIGNS, and maintain a NEUROLOGIC CHECKLIST.
- TRANSPORT EVERY SEVERELY INTOXICATED PATIENT TO THE HOSPITAL.

Withdrawal Seizures

When a person who has been drinking heavily over an extended period suddenly stops drinking—because he ran out of alcohol, decided to turn over a new leaf, or for any other reason—a variety of signs and symptoms of withdrawal may occur. One of the more common manifestations of withdrawal from alcohol is seizures, sometimes referred to as alcoholic epilepsy, or rum fits. Alcoholic seizures generally occur, if they are going to occur at all, from about 12 to 48 hours after the patient had his last drink. They are typically grand mal seizures, and are usually only one or two in number, although status epilepticus may occur.

Withdrawal seizures should be treated as seizures from any other source (see Chapter 21). PROTECT THE PATIENT FROM INJURY. Guard the AIRWAY from aspiration. Administer OXYGEN. Check the patient carefully for injuries, and transport to the hospital.

Delirium Tremens

One of the most serious syndromes resulting from alcohol withdrawal is delirium tremens (DTs). Not every alcoholic who stops drinking will experience DTs, but in those in whom DTs do occur—perhaps 5 to 10 percent of alcoholics in withdrawal—the symptoms usually start somewhere between 48 and 72 hours after the patient's last drink. In occasional cases, however, the onset of DTs may be delayed as long as 7 to 10 days from the time the patient stopped drinking.

Delirium tremens is a serious and potentially fatal syndrome, carrying a mortality rate as high as 15 percent. It is characterized by CONFUSION, TREMORS, RESTLESSNESS, and HALLUCINATIONS, the latter often very frightening (snakes, spiders, rats). FEVER, SWEATING, and a greatly INCREASED METABOLIC RATE lead to significant dehydration, and cardiovascular collapse due to HYPOVOLEMIC SHOCK is an ever-present danger in these patients.

On physical examination, check carefully for SIGNS OF INJURY, especially injury to the head. Record VITAL SIGNS and general neurologic signs (e.g., state of consciousness, response to stimuli) on a NEUROLOGIC CHECKLIST. Recheck these signs frequently.

In managing the patient with DTs, it is essential to PROTECT THE PATIENT FROM INJURY. Terrifying hallucinations may render the patient severely agitated and combative, and every effort should be made to reassure the patient and calm him down by verbal means. AVOID THE USE OF RESTRAINTS if at all possible, for these are likely to worsen the patient's agitation, especially if he feels himself menaced by snakes and spiders. If authorized to do so, start an INTRAVENOUS INFUSION with normal saline, to combat dehydration and lesson the risk of hypovolemic shock. Explain the intravenous procedure before you jab the patient with a needle, and secure the IV well (wrap it with layers of roller bandage) to guard it from being accidently yanked out.

Keep talking to the patient throughout transport, to help orient and reassure him. Snakes and spiders are not quite so frightening when there is a calm person at one's side, so let the patient know that he or she is not alone.

Treatment of the Patient with Delirium Tremens

- PROTECT THE PATIENT FROM INJURY.
- AVOID RESTRAINTS. Use verbal reassurance.
- Start an INTRAVENOUS INFUSION with normal saline, if authorized to do so.
- Monitor VITAL SIGNS, and maintain a NEUROLOGIC CHECKLIST.
- TRANSPORT the patient to the hospital.

DRUG ABUSE

Drug abuse refers to the self-administration of a drug or drugs for other than approved medical purposes—usually for stimulatory, sedative, or hallucinatory effects. The problem of drug abuse is extremely widespread, varying only in degree from the businessman or housewife who drinks a dozen cups of coffee a day for the stimulant effects of caffeine to the junkie who spends all of his or her waking hours preoccupied with procuring and taking heroin.

The prevalence of drug abuse at all levels of society means that drugs may be a factor in many illnesses and injuries. For this reason, certain general guidelines are warranted in the evaluation of *every* patient.

- ALWAYS inquire about the USE OF MEDICATIONS, whether prescribed or self-administered. If the emergency occurs in the patient's home, check out the medicine cabinet, and note what drugs are present.
- When dealing with any unconscious patient, look for medication containers on his person or in his surroundings, and take all such containers with the patient to the hospital.
- Be particularly alert for the possibility of drug use in any patient presenting with unexplained CHANGE IN BEHAVIOR, STUPOR, COMA, or SEIZURES.

EVALUATION OF THE DRUG USER

In general, the drug-related complaint most likely to elicit a call for an ambulance is OVERDOSE, and the EMT should have a clear idea of the kinds of information that should be obtained in any overdose case.

In obtaining the HISTORY from the patient or bystanders, it is most important, first of all, to try to determine WHAT WAS TAKEN? That may not be as simple as it sounds, for drugs obtained from illicit sources may be improperly labelled or have been sold to the user under false claims. Various filler substances may have been used to "cut" (dilute) the drug, and often such fillers are more toxic than the drug itself. There is not, after all, any consumer protection agency to set standards for purity of street drugs. Furthermore, drug users tend to employ a bewildering street slang to refer to various drugs, and the EMT may be mystified when the patient reports having ingested "two peaches, a red devil, and some angel dust." Some of the street slang for drugs is listed in Table 25-2, but such terms vary with time and place, and the EMT should keep a notebook of street terminology current in his or her own community. In any case, if there are any medication bottles at the scene, be sure to take them along with the patient to the hospital. Also save a sample of any vomitus containing pills.

In addition to finding out what drug was taken, it is very important to know WHEN the drug was taken since this information will influence the decision whether to induce vomiting. Vomiting is much more likely to be effective in removing the drug if it was ingested within the previous half hour. In addition, try to determine HOW MUCH drug was taken, for this will give some indication of the potential danger of the overdose; the patient who has swallowed 100 barbiturate pills could be in life-threatening jeopardy, while the patient who took only 5 such pills is much less likely to develop serious problems.

Inquire whether ANY OTHER DRUGS (INCLUDING ALCOHOL) WERE TAKEN BY ANY ROUTE. Patients who have taken more than one drug are likely to be in grave danger. Each drug may heighten the effects of the others, and the resulting combined effect is often much greater than that of any one of the drugs when taken alone. The combination of drugs and alcohol is particularly common—and particularly dangerous.

Find out WHETHER ANYTHING HAS ALREADY BEEN DONE FOR THE PATIENT. Street resuscitation techniques are sometimes as dangerous as the overdoses they seek to treat. A patient who has taken an overdose of narcotics, for example, may have received an injection of uppers from well-meaning friends who were trying to reverse the depressant effects of the overdose.

In carrying out the PHYSICAL EXAMINATION, make a careful note of the patient's GENERAL APPEARANCE and STATE OF CONSCIOUSNESS. Does he seem very sleepy, suggesting overdose of depressant drugs, or is he restless and wild-eyed, as in amphetamine overdose? Record the VITAL SIGNS, and be particularly alert for SIGNS OF RESPIRATORY DEPRESSION and SIGNS OF SHOCK, both of which may complicate drug overdose. Examine the PUPILS and note whether they are constricted or dilated. Constricted, "pinpoint" pupils suggest narcotics overdose, while widely dilated, unreactive pupils may occur in barbiturate poisoning.

Listen to the CHEST, and note any abnormal breath sounds. Some cases of heroin overdose are complicated by pulmonary edema, which can be detected by the characteristic rales heard on auscultation. Finally, examine the EXTREMITIES for needle tracks along the veins that suggest chronic heroin use.

Evaluation of the Overdose Victim

- HISTORY
  1. WHAT WAS TAKEN? (Take medication containers to the hospital with the patient.)
  2. WHEN was it taken?
  3. HOW MUCH was taken?
  4. Were ANY OTHER DRUGS taken by any route?

5. What has already been done for (or to) the patient?

- PHYSICAL EXAMINATION
  1. STATE OF CONSCIOUSNESS
  2. VITAL SIGNS: Be alert for respiratory depression, shock
  3. PUPILS
  4. Signs of pulmonary edema
  5. NEEDLE TRACKS on the extremities

MANAGEMENT OF OVERDOSE: GENERAL PRINCIPLES

If the overdose victim is still conscious, the first consideration is WHETHER TO INDUCE VOMITING. The purpose of making the patient vomit is to empty his or her stomach of any pills that have not yet been absorbed and thereby reduce the dose of drug that reaches the bloodstream. But ingested drugs do not remain in the stomach forever; sooner or later they are absorbed or move on into the intestine. So the more time that has elapsed since the patient took the drug, the less the chance of retrieving a significant amount of the drug by induction of vomiting. As a general rule, it is worthwhile to induce vomiting if the patient ingested the drug(s) sometime within the past 30 minutes. There are, however, several important exceptions. Vomiting should *not* be induced in patients who are already very sleepy or stuporous, for such patients may not be able to protect their airways against aspiration. For the same reason, vomiting should not be induced in a patient having seizures. Nor should vomiting be stimulated when the patient has overdosed on **anti-emetic** drugs (drugs that prevent vomiting), for the patient will simply end up with a stomach dangerously full of water and medications given to induce vomiting, and he may go on to regurgitate and aspirate the contents of his stomach as he gets sleepier. The most common anti-emetic drugs are tranquilizers, such as Thorazine, Phenergan, or Tigan. Finally, vomiting should not be induced in a pregnant woman, for the straining associated with forceful vomiting may threaten the pregnancy.

Do Not Induce Vomiting In
- a STUPOROUS or COMATOSE patient
- a patient having SEIZURES
- a patient who has taken ANTI-EMETIC DRUGS
- a PREGNANT woman

When, in the absence of the above contraindications, the decision is made to induce vomiting, the patient should initially be in a sitting position, to facilitate swallowing the medication and fluid required. The medication used to induce vomiting is a substance called SYRUP OF IPECAC, which works by irritating the lining of the stomach. The dosage for an adult is 30 ml (2 tablespoons) by mouth. After the syrup of ipecac has been given, wait a couple of minutes, then give the patient a glass or two of lukewarm water to drink, for patients do not readily vomit when the stomach is empty. Allow the patient to move about as he or she wishes, for movement enhances the action of ipecac. Vomiting should occur within 20 minutes of syrup of ipecac administration. When the patient reports an urge to vomit, position him with his head lower than his trunk, to minimize the danger of aspiration, and be prepared to suction vomitus from his mouth and throat.

Even with effective vomiting, 60 to 70 percent of the ingested drug may be left in the patient's stomach, and for that reason it is necessary to take additional measures to prevent further absorption of the remaining drug. Once the patient has finished vomiting he or she should therefore be given ACTIVATED CHARCOAL, a compound that absorbs many drugs to its surface and thereby inactivates them. There is, in fact, recent evidence that activated charcoal in the stomach helps to clear the body of ingested drugs even after the drugs have been absorbed into the bloodstream. So it is worth giving activated charcoal even several hours after a drug ingestion. To administer activated charcoal, mix at least 2 tablespoons of the charcoal with tap water to make a slurry, and then have the patient drink it (That may take a bit of persuading, since the mixture does not look very appetizing!).

Induction of Vomiting
1. Have the patient SIT UP.
2. Administer 15 ml (3 teaspoons) of SYRUP OF IPECAC by mouth.
3. Wait a few minutes, then give LARGE AMOUNTS OF FLUIDS by mouth.
4. Allow 15 to 20 minutes for the syrup of ipecac to work.
5. When the patient needs to vomit, assist him to a HEAD-DOWN POSITION. Have SUCTION ready.
6. After the patient has ceased vomiting, give 2 to 3 tablespoons of ACTIVATED CHARCOAL in water.

Some authorities now recommend giving activated charcoal *together with* syrup of ipecac, rather than waiting until the patient has vomited—the rationale being to enable the charcoal to start detoxifying the patient immediately. Indeed, authors of some recent studies have proposed skipping the syrup of ipecac altogether, especially if the ingestion occurred more than 30 minutes earlier. Until there is concensus on these matters, EMTs should follow the guidelines issued by their local poison control centers.

If the overdose victim is unconscious, treat him or her as any other unconscious patient, with special attention to the AIRWAY and the PREVENTION OF ASPIRATION. Administer OXYGEN by nasal cannula. Since respiratory depression is common in overdoses, be prepared to ASSIST VENTILATIONS if breathing is abnormally slow or shallow. If authorized to do so, start an INTRAVENOUS INFUSION with normal saline, so that a line will be available for rapid fluid administration in the event of cardiovascular collapse.

TYPES OF DRUGS COMMONLY ABUSED

Drugs commonly abused fall into three general categories, according to the effects they produce: (1) stimulant drugs ("uppers"), (2) depressant drugs ("downers"), and (3) hallucinogens (Table 25-2).

Stimulant Drugs

Uppers are central nervous system stimulants and include drugs such as amphetamines, cocaine, caffeine, decongestants, and certain antiasthma preparations. The use of such drugs induces a typical set of symptoms, all of which are related to CNS stimulation. Excitement, jitters, restlessness, talkativeness, irritability, and sleeplessness are all characteristic. A case in point is the amphetamine user, or "speed freak," who can usually be recognized by his wild-eyed appearance and hyperactive behavior. The speed freak gives a history of SLEEPNESSNESS and LOSS OF APPETITE. On physical examination, he usually shows TACHYCARDIA, HYPERTENSION, DILATED PUPILS, and TREMORS. Occasionally SEIZURES occur. The patient may be hostile or combative and often has delusions of being persecuted. He may thus regard the EMT, and anyone else, with great suspicion. Withdrawal from amphetamines may lead to severe emotional depression and consequent suicidal behavior.

Nowadays, by far the most commonly abused stimulant drug is cocaine, thirty to sixty tons of which (with a street value of $55 billion) are imported into the United States every year. An estimated 25 million Americans have tried cocaine at least once; 5,000 try it for the first time each day; and four million Americans use it regularly. What that means is that there is scarcely an ambulance service in America that will not have to deal with patients who are cocaine users.

Until recently, cocaine was most commonly sold as a fine, white crystalline powder, which was taken either intranasally by inhalation ("snorting") or by injection into the skin, muscle, or a vein. Within the past few years, however, a much cheaper but more powerful form of cocaine, called **crack**, has become available that can be taken via the intrapulmonary route (smoked, or "freebased"). When cocaine powder is "snorted," the user feels a "high" within one or two minutes, which peaks around 15–60 minutes after use. When crack is smoked, by contrast, the user experiences a very intense "high" in 8–10 *seconds*. It is probably because of the speed and intensity of the "high" it produces that crack is so highly addictive.

When the effect of a dose of cocaine, in whatever form, wears off, the user experiences a "crash," a period of depression, irritability, sleeplessness, and exhaustion. In order to try to avoid the crash, the user will often seek more cocaine until he no longer has funds to buy more of the drug. At that point he may try to escape the unpleasant effects of crashing by taking some kind of sedative drug (e.g., alcohol, heroin, Valium). Thus, the chronic cocaine user is likely to be dependent on more than one drug—cocaine and a combination of sedatives—and he may present to emergency services overdose from "uppers" *or* "downers."

If the user has overdosed on cocaine, he may show any of the signs and symptoms described previously for stimulant drugs in general. Cocaine, furthermore, has been increasingly reported to cause a variety of very serious, sometimes fatal, complications, including acute myocardial infarction, lethal cardiac dysrhythmias, seizures, stroke, apnea, hyperthermia, and a variety of psychiatric symptoms. What all that means in practice is that the EMT must maintain a high index of suspicion regardless of the patient's chief complaint. Nowadays, a young person complaining of chest pain may indeed be suffering a myocardial infarction if that person has been freebasing crack during the past hour. Make it a habit, therefore, to check out the patient's surroundings for drug paraphernalia and report any evidence of drug use to the doctor at the receiving hospital.

The field management of adverse reactions to stimulant drugs is aimed primarily at ensuring the safety of the rescuers and calming the patient. If the patient is obviously violent and unresponsive to attempts to talk with him, the EMTs probably should not try to handle the situation without police assistance. If the patient *is* controllable, and if his vital signs are normal, what he needs most is a reassuring friend and a quiet, supervised environment in which to "crash." Usually the hospital is *not* a very good place for this; a hospital emergency room tends to be noisy and intimidating. A quiet room in a detoxification center or in the home of a reliable friend may be preferable. The physician at the base hospital should be consulted for advice regarding where to transport the patient. Bear in mind that if there are any significant abnormalities in vital signs, or if the patient is completely out of control, hospitalization will be necessary. Complications, such as seizures or shock, should be treated as described in previous chapters.

Table 25-2. *Classification of Commonly Abused Drugs*

Type of Drug	Examples	Street Names	Signs of Overdose
Uppers			
Amphetamines	Benzedrine	A's, Bennies, Benzies, cartwheels, hearts, peaches, roses, speed	Restlessness, agitation, jitters; incessant talking; insomnia; anorexia Tachycardia, tachypnea, hypertension Extreme depression on withdrawal
	Dexedrine	Dexies, footballs, oranges	
	Methadrine	Bonita, bambita	
	MDMA	Ecstasy, Adam, MDM	
	MDEA	Eve	
Cocaine		Bernice, big C, blow, burese, C, carrie, cecil, charlie, cholly, coke, corine, crack (freebase cocaine), dama blanca, dynamite, flake, gin, girl, gold dust, green gold, happy dust, happy trails, heaven dust, jet, joy powder, lady, liquid lady (cocaine and alcohol), nose candy, paradise, rock (freebase cocaine), snort, snow, speedball (cocaine and heroin), stardust, star-spangled powder, sugar, toot, white dust, white girl	
Antiasthmatics	Aminophylline		
	Isoproterenol		
	Adrenalin		
Caffeine	Coffee, cola		
Downers			
Alcohol	Wine, beer, whiskey	Rosy (wine), sneaky Pete (wine)	Slurred speech, incoordination
Narcotics	Heroin	Horse, Harry, smack, stuff, big H, blanco, China white	Constricted, "pinpoint" pupils, marked respiratory depression, needle tracks (heroin user), decreased response to pain
	Morphine	Unkie, Miss Emma, hard stuff, big M	
	Codeine	Fours	
	Dilaudid	Dillies	
	Methadone	Amidone, dollies	
	Opium	Auntie, black stuff, Greece	
Barbiturate	Phenobarbital (Nembutal)	Yellow jackets, hellows, nimbies, nebbies	Respiratory depression, hypotension, dilated pupils
	Amobarbital (Amytal)	Blue devils, blue birds, blue heaven, blue bullets, jack-up	
	Seconal	Red birds, red devils, pinks, bala, M&Ms	
Chloral hydrate		Mickey Finn, Mickey, Peter, chlorals, hog	Coma
Tranquilizers	Thorazine		Incoordination, slurred speech; coma
	Valium		
	Librium	Roche-tens	
Marijuana type	Marijuana	Grass, pot, Acapulco gold, ace, Aunt Mary, bo-bo, broccoli, duby, gage, Mary Jane, tea, reefer, weed, joint, roach, spliff, nickel	Sedative effects; may cause hallucinations
	Hashish	Black Russian, blue cheese, gram, hash, heesh	
	THC		
Hallucinogens			
Lysergic acid diethylamide (LSD)		Acid, blue cheers, California sunshine, crackers, cubes, ghost, heavenly blue	Hallucinations Panic reactions Agitation Sometimes hostile, aggressive, or destructive behavior
Phencyclidine (PCP)		Elephant, PeaCee Pill	
Mescaline		Cactus buttons	
Peyote		Bad acid, bad seed, big chief, button, half-moon	

Management of the Patient Overdosed on Uppers

- SYMPTOMS
  1. Jitters, excitement, hyperactivity
  2. Loss of appetite
  3. Sleeplessness
- SIGNS
  1. Restlessness, irritability, talkativeness
  2. Tachycardia, tachypnea, hypertension
  3. Dilated pupils
  4. Tremor
- TREATMENT
  1. "Talking down"
  2. If the patient is overtly violent, summon police assistance

Depressant Drugs

Downers include narcotics, sedatives, tranquilizers, hypnotics, and alcohol. All share the characteristic of producing depressant effects on the central nervous system. The most dangerous of these effects is RESPIRATORY DEPRESSION, and patients who have taken an overdose of depressant drugs often have very slow, shallow respirations and sometimes even apnea. HYPOTENSION is also common in this type of overdose, especially in cases of barbiturate poisoning (Nembutal, Seconal, Amytal). Loss of protective reflexes renders the patient susceptible to ASPIRATION, while decreased sensitivity to pain may permit the patient to lie for long periods in an unnatural position, leading to ischemia and damage to the muscles of an extremity.

The patient who has taken an overdose of depressant drugs is likely to be found stuporous or unconscious. *If he or she is still fully conscious,* and if the drug was taken by mouth, vomiting should be induced as described earlier. Every attempt should be made to maintain the patient's level of consciousness by stimulating him to stay awake. Keep the patient sitting up or moving about, and shake him or shout at him if he begins to nod off. Once the patient loses consciousness, the likelihood of respiratory depression and apnea increases markedly.

If the patient is groggy or unconscious, do not attempt to induce vomiting. First priority, as always, goes to MAINTAINING THE AIRWAY and PREVENTING ASPIRATION. Anticipate regurgitation, and keep suction handy. OXYGEN should be given by nasal cannula, and VENTILATIONS should be ASSISTED as necessary if the patient's spontaneous breathing is abnormally slow or shallow. When severe hypotension is present, it is a good idea to start an INTRAVENOUS INFUSION with normal saline, if authorized to do so. CHECK THE PATIENT CAREFULLY FOR INJURIES. Be particularly alert for a COLD, SWOLLEN, CYANOTIC EXTREMITY—a sign of ischemic damage to muscle and nerves caused by lying for an extended period in a contorted position. The presence of a damaged limb is an acute emergency, for the limb may require immediate surgery. The EMT should reposition and splint the limb, elevate it, and keep it cool (but not cold). Transport to the hospital should be as prompt as possible.

Keep a close check on VITAL SIGNS, and maintain a NEUROLOGIC CHECKLIST.

Treatment of the Patient Overdosed on Downers

- *If the patient is fully conscious:*
  1. Induce vomiting
  2. Stimulate the patient to keep him awake.
- *If the patient is stuporous or unconscious:*
  1. Maintain an OPEN AIRWAY.
  2. PREVENT ASPIRATION: Stable side position (if no injuries); have suction handy.
  3. Administer OXYGEN by nasal cannula.
  4. INTRAVENOUS INFUSION with normal saline, if authorized.
  5. *If there is an ischemic extremity:*
     a. Reposition the limb in normal alignment and splint.
     b. Elevate the ischemic extremity.
     c. Keep the ischemic extremity cool.
  6. Monitor VITAL SIGNS; maintain a NEUROLOGIC CHECKLIST.
  7. TRANSPORT WITHOUT DELAY to the hospital.

Hallucinogens

Hallucinogens are drugs that cause hallucinations, and the most commonly abused drugs in this category are lysergic acid diethylamide (LSD) and phencyclidine (PCP). The use of hallucinogens rarely results in coma. It is more likely that the EMTs will be summoned because the user is experiencing a "bad trip" or other adverse reaction.

The patient having a bad trip with LSD may exhibit panic and agitation. Frequently he or she will report having very vivid hallucinations and unusual bodily sensations. There may be rapid swings of mood and loss of motor coordination. On physical exam, the patient often has tachycardia and elevated blood pressure. The pupils are frequently dilated. Chills and shivering may be prominent.

PCP intoxication sometimes presents with the sudden onset of bizarre, "crazy" behavior. A diminished sensitivity to pain may permit the patient to carry out various self-destructive acts, such as gouging out his own eyes, and violent behavior is not uncommon. On examination, the PCP patient characteristically has a blank stare, with small pupils. His muscles may be very rigid, and he may show markedly decreased sensation to pinprick. Fever, sweating, and hypersalivation are also common.

The treatment of a patient having a bad trip requires first and foremost EMOTIONAL SUPPORT. Particularly in the case of an LSD user, the technique of talking the patient down may be very effective in alleviating some of the patient's panic. Keep talking to the patient, reassuring and orienting him to where he is, who you are, and so on. Encourage him to express his feelings and to talk about what he is experiencing. Talking down is less likely to be effective in the victim of PCP intoxication, but it should be attempted. The EMT should maintain a calm, sympathetic attitude and reassure the patient that his condition is the result of the drug and that he will feel greatly improved once the drug has been eliminated from the body. Wherever possible, AVOID THE USE OF RESTRAINTS, for these will only increase the patient's panic. Keep stimulation to a minimum, which means NO SIRENS and NO WILD RIDES TO THE HOSPITAL. Finally, once you have responded to the call, DO NOT LEAVE THE PATIENT ALONE for any reason until he has been transferred to the care of another medical professional.

Management of the Patient on a Bad Trip

- Provide EMOTIONAL SUPPORT; use talking down technique.
- AVOID RESTRAINTS whenever possible.
- Keep stimulation to a minimum: NO SIRENS.
- DO NOT LEAVE THE PATIENT ALONE.
- Prevent the patient from harming himself or others.

CASE HISTORY

The patient is a 22-year-old woman who was found unconscious in her apartment. Friends stated that the patient has been very depressed lately and that she took an overdose of "nebbies." An empty phenobarbital bottle was found on the bathroom sink, and there was a suicide note on the bedside table.

On physical examination, the patient was deeply unconscious and unreactive even to painful stimuli. Pulse was 132 and thready, BP 80/50, and respirations 10 and shallow. There was no evidence of head injury. The pupils were widely dilated and unreactive to light. There was no smell of alcohol on the patient's breath. The neck was not rigid. The chest was clear, and the abdomen soft. There were no needle tracks on the patient's arms.

The patient's mouth and throat were suctioned, and she was given assisted ventilation with bag-valve-mask and oxygen. An intravenous infusion was initiated with normal saline and was run at 200 ml per hour, as per orders of Dr. Sleeper. The patient was transported in the left lateral position. Vital signs remained unchanged during transport, and the patient remained entirely unresponsive throughout.

Questions to think about:

1. Why did the EMTs check to see if the patient's neck was rigid? What condition(s) were they trying to rule out?
2. Why were the patient's ventilations assisted?
3. Why was the intravenous infusion started?
4. Why was the patient transported in the left lateral position (as opposed to supine)?

VOCABULARY

activated charcoal Substance used to adsorb ingested drugs or poisons.
addiction An overwhelming involvement in the use of a drug, characterized by physical and psychologic dependence, compulsive drug use, and tolerance.
alcoholism An addiction to alcohol.
anti-emetic Agent used to control or stop vomiting.
compulsive drug use Situation in which a drug user becomes extremely preoccupied with the procurement and use of a given substance.
delirium tremens (DTs) Potential complication of alcohol withdrawal, characterized by frightening hallucinations, agitation, and sometimes cardiovascular collapse.
downer Depressant drug.
drug dependence State in which repeated administration of a given drug is necessary to maintain a person's feeling of well-being and to prevent withdrawal symptoms.
hallucinogen Drug that has the capacity to stimulate hallucinations, that is, perceptions not founded on objective reality.
ischemia Tissue anoxia from diminished blood flow, caused by a narrowing or occlusion of the artery supplying the tissue.
syrup of ipecac Agent used to induce vomiting.
tolerance Progressive decrease in susceptibility to the effects of a drug after repeated doses.
upper A stimulant drug.
withdrawal Symptoms produced by abstinence from a drug to which one is addicted.

FURTHER READING

ALCOHOL AND ALCOHOLISM

Barber JM. Recognition of alcohol-related problems—alcohol withdrawal. *EMT J* 5(1):48, 1980.

Best J, Lawrence KE. Alcoholism in EMS: A management challenge. *Emerg Med Serv* 17(8):17, 1988.

Blume SB. Women and alcohol: A review. *JAMA* 256:1467, 1986.

Brown CG. The alcohol withdrawal syndrome. *Ann Emerg Med* 11:276, 1982.

Clark D, McCarthy E, Robinson E. Trauma as a symptom of alcoholism (editorial). *Ann Emerg Med* 14:274, 1985.

Criteria Committee, National Council of Alcoholism. Criteria for the diagnosis of alcoholism. *Ann Int Med* 77:249, 1972.

Johnson MW. Alcohol-related emergencies. *Emerg Med Serv* 12(3):51, 1983.

Kassirer JP et al. A comatose alcoholic. *Hosp Pract* 20:26, 1985.

Knott D, Fink R, Morgan J. Beware the patient with alcohol on breath. *Emerg Med Serv* 6(3):40, 1977.

Lerner WD, Fallon HJ. The alcohol withdrawal syndrome. *N Engl J Med* 313:905, 1985.

Lowenfels AB et al. Alcohol and trauma. *Ann Emerg Med* 13:1056, 1984.

Maull KI. Alcohol abuse: Its implications in trauma care. *South Med J* 75:794, 1982.

Niven RG. Alcoholism—a problem in perspective. *JAMA* 252:912, 1984.

Scarano SJ. Emergency response—alcohol-intoxicated patient. *Emerg Med Serv* 8(5):78, 1979.

Sellers E, Dalant H. Alcohol intoxication and withdrawal. *NEJM* 294:757, 1976.

Taigman M. The battle scars of booze: Treating the chronic alcoholic. *JEMS* 14(10):45, 1989.

Taigman M. Just another drunk. . . . *Emerg Med Serv* 17(8):8, 1988.

Thrasher M, Thrasher C. Prehospital treatment of acute adolescent alcoholism. *Emerg Med Serv* 14(1):32, 1985.

Waller PF et al. The potentiating effects of alcohol on driver injury. *JAMA* 256:1461, 1986.

DRUG ABUSE AND OVERDOSE

Aronson JK. The treatment of self-poisoning. *Emerg Med Serv* 18(5):51, 1989.

Cregler LL et al. Medical complications of cocaine abuse. *N Engl J Med* 315:1495, 1986.

Dowling GP, McDonough ET, Bost RO. "Eve" and "ecstasy": A report of five deaths associated with the use of MDEA and MDMA. *JAMA* 257:1615, 1987.

Fauman G et al. Psychosis induced by phencyclidine. *JACEP* 4:233, 1975.

Fontanarosa PB, DiBartolomeo A. Cracking the case of the cocaine user. *JEMS* 14(5):42, 1989.

Fortenberry JD. Gasoline sniffing. *Am J Med* 79:740, 1985.

Gay GR. Clinical management of acute and chronic cocaine poisoning. *Ann Emerg Med* 11:562, 1982.

Haddad L. Management of hallucinogen abuse. *Am Fam Phys* 14:82, 1976.

Kunkel DB. Marijuana: A few new thoughts on an old subject. *Emerg Med* 17(9):134, 1985.

Leisner K. The EMS addict: Chemically dependent providers. *Emerg Med Serv* 17(8):12, 1988.

Lowenstein DH et al. Acute neurologic and psychiatric complications associated with cocaine abuse. *Am J Med* 85:841, 1987.

McCarron MM et al. Acute phencyclidine intoxication: Incidence of clinical findings in 1,000 cases. *Ann Emerg Med* 10:237, 1981.

Mittleman R, Wetli C. Death caused by recreational cocaine use. *JAMA* 252:1889, 1984.

Roehrich H, Gold MS. Emergency presentations of crack abuse. *Emerg Med Serv* 17(8):41, 1988.

Rothenberg R. Cocaine. *Emerg Med Serv* 13(2):29, 1984.

Sternback G, Moran J, Eliastam M. Heroin addiction: Acute presentation of medical complications. *Ann Emerg Med* 9:161, 1980.

Turner BM. Drug use: Myths, reality, and problems for EMS. *Emerg Med Serv* 12(4):49, 1983.

NOTE: References regarding the use of activated charcoal and syrup of ipecac can be found at the end of Chapter 26.

26. POISONING

OBJECTIVES

One million poisonings occur in the United States each year, and a substantial number of these incidents elicit a frantic call for an ambulance. Arriving at the scene, the EMT may confront a very cheerful, robust 3-year-old who has just wolfed down his mother's cold cream or a comatose toddler having seizures after ingesting a bottle of silver polish. In each case, the EMT will have to make rapid decisions regarding the appropriate management of a specific ingestion or exposure. In this chapter, we shall look at some general principles in the prevention, detection, and management of poisoning. Clearly the number of toxic materials to be found even in the home is nearly limitless, and it would be impossible to deal in detail here with each potential poison. Instead, we shall look at a few illustrative examples of different types of poisoning and learn how these relatively common poisonings are managed. By the conclusion of this chapter, the reader should be able to

1. Identify safe and unsafe practices in storing household chemicals and medications, from the point of view of prevention of poisoning
2. Identify the organ systems most commonly affected by poisoning and the symptoms and signs commonly produced
3. Indicate what materials should be brought to the hospital with the patient in a case of poisoning
4. Identify poisoning victims (a) for whom induction of vomiting is recommended and (b) for whom induction of vomiting is forbidden
5. Identify a patient poisoned by (a) aspirin, (b) a petroleum product, (c) carbon monoxide, and (d) an organophosphate insecticide, given a description of several poisoning victims
6. Indicate the special considerations in the evaluation and treatment of a person who has swallowed a potentially toxic plant

OVERVIEW

A poison is a substance that produces harmful effects upon the body. While the word *poison* usually conjures up an image of an agent like arsenic or cyanide used for diabolical purposes, in fact the vast majority of poisonings are caused by common household substances ingested accidentally. Cleaning agents, pesticides, waxes and polishes, petroleum products, and nonprescription medications account for a large proportion of poisoning cases seen in emergency medical facilities.

PREVENTION OF POISONING

The victim of poisoning is usually a child, 2 to 3 years of age, whose spirit of adventure and curiosity have sent him poking about in the cleaning closet or medicine cabinet in search of something new and interesting to put into his mouth (Fig. 26-1). A toddler will injest just about anything he or she can lay hands on, even substances whose taste or smell would strongly discourage the average adult. Nor is the toddler likely to be the least bit inhibited by a previous episode of poisoning; as a matter of fact, a significant number of poisoned children are repeated offenders.

All of this underscores the importance of taking appropriate measures to remove potential sources of poisoning from the child's environment. Since 80 percent of childhood poisonings occur in the home, what we are talking about is poison-proofing the home. This is as much the concern of the EMT as it is of public health officials. Even if the EMT is not himself or herself a parent, as a health care professional, the EMT has an obligation to try to prevent needless injury and death.

The key word, then, is *prevention*, and prevention can be greatly facilitated by following a few simple guidelines.

- Keep all drugs, pesticides, household cleaners, and other potentially dangerous substances out of the reach of children. Since small children are ingenius in climbing, crawling, and getting into places where they do not belong, this means keeping drugs in a *locked* medicine cabinet and household chemicals in a *locked* cupboard.

Fig. 26-1. *A curious toddler will try to taste any substance he or she can lay hands on. Cabinets containing toxic substances should be childproofed.*

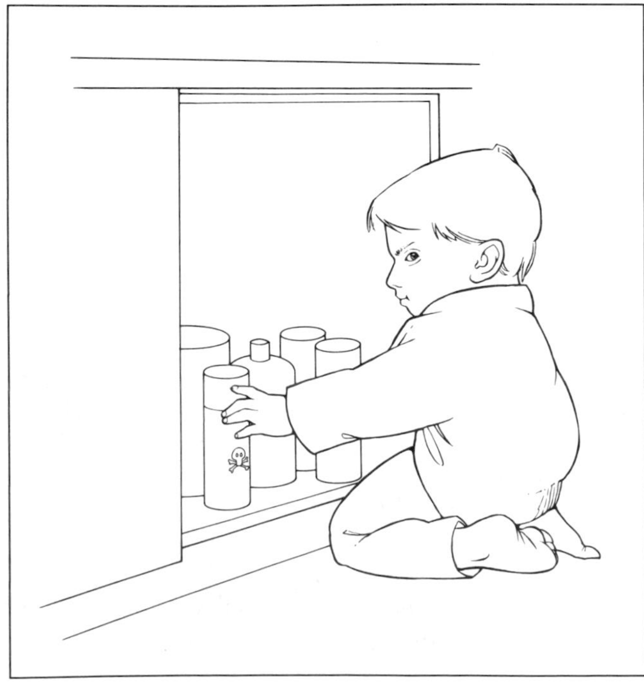

- Do not transfer drugs or chemicals to containers other than those in which they were purchased, especially not to food containers. One of the most common scenarios for kerosene ingestion occurs when kerosene has been poured into a soft drink bottle, and the familiar bottle encourages the child to drink the contents.
- Insist upon safety packaging (that is, child-proof bottles) for any medications that are to be kept in a home frequented by small children.
- Never tell a child that medicine is candy, for the child is quite likely to believe you! The administration of medicine to a child should be treated in a serious, matter-of-fact way and not made a game.
- Parents who take medications of one sort or another should do so in private and not in the presence of small children, who are notorious imitators.
- Each poisoning incident should prompt a thorough study of the situation in which it occurred, so that measures may be taken to prevent a similar incident from occurring again in the same home. Just as many fire departments offer fire safety inspections as a service to homeowners, EMTs trained in poison control can utilize slack hours to conduct "poison safety inspections" in their community.

POISON CONTROL CENTERS

Many large communities have poison control centers whose function is to maintain a detailed file on toxic materials and on the ingredients in literally hundreds of thousands of household, industrial, and medical products. These centers offer first aid advice to callers and detailed information to medical personnel managing a poisoning case. Wherever possible, direct radio contact or telephone patch between the ambulance service and the local poison control facility is desirable, to enable the EMT to get prompt advice regarding the emergency treatment of any given poisoning. The telephone number of the poison control center should also be widely advertised in the community, as a resource for lay persons to consult regarding what to do until help arrives.

GENERAL EFFECTS OF POISONS

Poisons may enter the body in several ways. Probably the most common way in which poisons gain access to the body is INGESTION; that is, the poison is taken by mouth and swallowed. Poisoning by ingestion is particularly common among small children, who put just about anything they can get their hands on into their mouths. Adults too, however, may swallow very toxic materials, especially when there is suicidal intent. Poisons may also enter the body by INHALATION of toxic fumes. Vapors from insecticides, leaky gas appliances, automobile exhaust, and the like are all potential sources of poisoning by inhalation.

Besides reaching the bloodstream by ingestion and inhalation, a poison may find its way into the body through ABSORPTION across the surface of the skin. That is particularly apt to occur with certain kinds of insecticides, which may penetrate the skin very rapidly when an exposed individual is not wearing protective clothing. Finally, poisons may enter the body through INJECTION, via the bite or sting of a poisonous spider, snake, or marine animal.

Once within the body, poisons exert their effects in a variety of ways. Some poisons, such as cyanide or carbon monoxide, interfere with the oxygen transport system of the blood and produce a kind of suffocation at the cellular level. Some, like certain insecticides or strychnine, cause intense stimulation of the nervous system, while others, like sleeping pills taken in excess, produce profound CNS depression. Finally, certain poisons produce direct tissue damage; strong acids or alkalis, for instance, eat away at tissues with which they come in contact, causing severe chemical burns.

The signs and symptoms of poisoning are as variable as the agents responsible for poisoning. Common among these signs and symptoms are GASTROINTESTINAL DISTURBANCES (abdominal pain, nausea, vomiting, diarrhea) and CENTRAL NERVOUS SYSTEM DISTURBANCES (pupillary changes, hypersalivation, sweating, seizures, coma, respiratory depression). Some of these signs are outlined in Table 26-1. In general, one should suspect poisoning whenever there is an unexplained onset of gastrointestinal and neurologic symptoms, and one should make a careful search of the patient's environment for a possible source. An improperly vented wood stove, a can of insecticide, an empty medicine bottle—any of these may provide a valuable clue to the cause of the problem. If you have even the slightest suspicion of poisoning, *always* take the container of the suspected toxic substance with the patient to the emergency room. Do not simply write down the name of the product, for you may not get it right and, besides, the label may contain a great deal of additional information useful to the emergency room staff—such as the components of the product, the name of the manufacturer, and sometimes even a telephone number to call for further information. So remember

> ALWAYS TAKE THE CONTAINER OF A SUSPECTED POISON TO THE EMERGENCY ROOM WITH THE POISONED PATIENT.

In the remainder of this chapter, we will look at a few illustrative types of ingested, inhaled, and absorbed poisons. Poisoning by injection will be taken up in Chapter 27, Bites and Stings.

INGESTED POISONS

The most common portal through which poisons enter the body is the mouth, and thus the vast majority of poisonings the EMT will encounter will involve ingested poisons.

GENERAL PRINCIPLES OF EVALUATION AND MANAGEMENT

In evaluating the patient who has swallowed a potentially toxic substance, one needs first to find out, just as in the case of drug overdose

- WHAT was ingested
- HOW MUCH was ingested
- WHEN was it ingested

Those questions are crucial, for the answers will help determine whether vomiting should be induced, and that is a decision that must be made rapidly. Other factors that will influence the decision on vomiting are the patient's state of consciousness and the presence or absence of seizures. Thus in the first few minutes at the scene, the EMT should quickly ascertain the nature of the poisoning and the patient's overall neurologic status. The remainder of the assessment may be deferred until treatment has been started.

The two basic rules for dealing with an ingested poison may be summarized as follows.

> DILUTE THE POISON, AND GET IT OUT.

The conscious patient should immediately be given 1 or 2 glasses of water or milk to drink, as a means of diluting any poison that is still in the stomach. If there are no contraindications to doing so, the patient should then be induced to vomit. As a general rule, any patient who has swallowed a potentially toxic substance within the past 30 minutes should be made to vomit, but there are some important exceptions. To begin with, the CONDITION OF THE PATIENT is a primary consideration. Just as in the case of drug overdose, vomiting should *not* be induced in a poisoned patient if the patient is less than fully alert or is having seizures; for under such circumstances there is considerable danger of aspiration. The TYPE OF SUBSTANCE INGESTED must also be taken into account. Vomiting should *not* be induced if the patient has swallowed a caustic or corrosive compound, such as acid, lye, ammonia, drain cleaner, or any other substance that has caused burns of the lips, mouth, or throat. The damage done

Table 26-1. *Common Signs and Symptoms of Poisoning*

Sign or Symptom	Possible Causative Agents
Odor	
Bitter almonds	Cyanide
Garlic	Arsenic, organophosphates, phosphorous
Acetone	Methyl alcohol, isopropyl alcohol, aspirin, acetone
Wintergreen	Methyl salicylate
Pears	Chloral hydrate
Violets	Turpentine
Camphor	Camphor
Alcohol	Alcohol
Pupils	
Constricted	Narcotics, organophosphates, jimson weed, nutmeg, Darvon
Dilated	Barbiturates, atropine, amphetamines, Doriden, LSD, cyanide, carbon monoxide
Mouth	
Salivation	Organophosphates, arsenic, strychnine, mercury, salicylates
Dry mouth	Atropine (belladonna), amphetamines, Benadryl, narcotics
Burns in mouth	Formaldehyde, iodine, lye, toxic plants, phenols, phosphorous, pine oil, silver nitrate, acids
Skin	
Pruritus	Jimson weed, belladonna, boric acid
Dry, hot skin	Atropine (belladonna), botulism, nutmeg
Sweating	Organophosphates, arsenic, aspirin, amphetamines, barbiturates, mushrooms, naphthalene
Respiratory	
Depressed respirations	Narcotics, alcohol, Darvon, carbon monoxide, barbiturates
Increased respirations	Aspirin, amphetamines, boric acid, cyanide, kerosene, methyl alcohol, nicotine
Pulmonary edema	Organophosphates, petroleum products, narcotics, carbon monoxide
Cardiovascular	
Tachycardia	Alcohol, amphetamines, arsenic, atropine, aspirin, cocaine, some antiasthma drugs
Bradycardia	Digitalis, gasoline, nicotine, mushrooms, narcotics, cyanide, mistletoe, rhododendron
Hypertension	Amphetamines, lead, nicotine, antiasthma drugs
Hypotension	Barbiturates, narcotics, tranquilizers, house plants, mistletoe, nitroglycerin, antifreeze
Central nervous system	
Seizures	Amphetamines, camphor, cocaine, strychnine, arsenic, carbon monoxide, petroleum products, scorpion sting
Coma	All depressant drugs (e.g., narcotics, barbiturates, tranquilizers, alcohol), carbon monoxide, cyanide
Hallucinations	Atropine, LSD, mushrooms, organic solvents, PCP, nutmeg
Headache	Carbon monoxide, alcohol, Antabuse
Tremors	Organophosphates, carbon monoxide, amphetamines, tranquilizers, poisonous marine animals
Weakness or paralysis	Organophosphates, botulism, eel, hemlock, puffer fish, pine oil, rhododendron
Gastrointestinal	
Cramps, nausea, vomiting, and/or diarrhea	Many if not most ingested poisons

by such an agent en route to the stomach will only be compounded if the substance is vomited back up again. Vomiting should also *not* be induced if the patient has ingested any kind of petroleum product such as gasoline, kerosene, lighter fluid, or liquid furniture polish since such substances are readily aspirated into the lungs, where they may cause severe chemical pneumonia. (A possible exception is the case in which someone has swallowed a very large quantity of a petroleum product. In such a case, the risk of toxic systemic effects from the product may outweigh the risk of aspiration, and vomiting should be induced. Consult the base station physician for advice in such a situation.) Finally, vomiting should *not* be induced in patients who have swallowed products containing strychnine (e.g., some rat poisons), for such patients are very prone to seizures.

Do Not Induce Vomiting If

- The patient is STUPOROUS or UNCONSCIOUS.
- The patient is having SEIZURES.
- The patient ingested:
  1. A CORROSIVE or CAUSTIC SUBSTANCE, such as a strong acid, alkali, or drain cleaner.
  2. A PETROLEUM PRODUCT (gasoline, kerosene, lighter fluid).
  3. A substance containing STRYCHNINE (some rat poisons).

If you are not sure whether it is safe to induce vomiting in a given case, check with the local poison control center or with the physician at the base hospital. If the patient is not fully conscious or has swallowed a substance that precludes the induction of vomiting, he must be transported without further delay to the hospital.

If the decision is made to induce vomiting, administer 2 tablespoons (30 ml) of SYRUP OF IPECAC followed by one or two glasses of water, just as for the drug overdose. While waiting for the ipecac to work, complete the secondary survey, and record the patient's vital signs and any other findings. Vomiting should occur within 15 to 20 minutes. If it does not, the same dose of syrup of ipecac may be repeated *once only*.

When the ipecac takes effect and the patient feels the urge to vomit, position him on his side, with his head lower than his trunk, to facilitate emptying the stomach and to minimize the risk of aspiration. Save a sample of the vomitus in a closed container, to take with the patient to the hospital.

Once the patient has finished vomiting, administer ACTIVATED CHARCOAL—1 to 2 tablespoons mixed thoroughly in a glass of water.

The steps in treating the pateint who has ingested a poison are summarized in Figure 26-2.

SPECIFIC INGESTIONS

We will look now at a few common ingestions to see how the principles discussed above are applied in specific cases.

Aspirin Ingestion

One of the most commonly ingested poisons is not usually regarded as a poison at all, and that is standard aspirin. Aspirin and other salicylates were involved in nearly 19,000 poisonings reported in the United States in 1986. The passage of federal regulations limiting to 36 the number of tablets contained in a single bottle of baby aspirin has somewhat reduced the incidence of severe aspirin poisoning; but aspirin remains a great favorite among the 3-year-old set, and many of the poisonings occur when the child gets hold of a bottle of adult aspirin preparation. In addition, a large number of aspirin poisonings in small children—perhaps as many as 50 percent—occur when an overzealous parent gives the child too many aspirins in the course of an illness.

Aspirin is an acid (acetosalicylic acid), and consumption of large amounts of aspirin therefore leads to an increased level of acid in the body (**acidosis**). As we learned earlier, when studying diabetic ketoacidosis, the only way the body can get rid of excess acid quickly is to blow it off in the form of carbon dioxide. Thus the most characteristic early sign of aspirin poisoning is DEEP BREATHING. Indeed, this sign is so typical that it should suggest the possibility of aspirin overdose in any child who presents with unexplained hyperpnea (with or without tachypnea).

SUSPECT ASPIRIN POISONING IN ANY CHILD WITH UNEXPLAINED HYPERPNEA.

Besides changes in respirations, most victims of aspirin overdose will have significant FEVER and SWEATING, both of which contribute to the development of DEHYDRATION. As more aspirin is absorbed into the system, SEIZURES may occur, and in severe cases, the victim lapses into COMA.

Management of aspirin overdose is aimed at emptying the stomach and providing general supportive measures. If the victim is alert and has had no seizure activity, INDUCE VOMITING with syrup of ipecac (2 tablespoons for patients over 1 year of age) as described earlier. When vomiting has ceased, administer ACTIVATED CHARCOAL (1–2 tablespoons mixed thoroughly in a glass of water). If the patient's temperature is above 104°F (40°C), sponge his body with cool but not cold tap water. Particularly in children, high fever is apt to provoke seizures, and for this reason the temperature should be brought down. Do not, however, allow the child to become chilled or to start shivering.

Recognition and Management of Aspirin Overdose

- SIGNS
  1. TACHYPNEA and HYPERPNEA.
  2. FEVER and SWEATING.
  3. COMA in severe cases.
- TREATMENT
  1. *If the patient is alert and without seizures:*
     a. INDUCE VOMITING with SYRUP OF IPECAC.
     b. When vomiting has ceased, give ACTIVATED CHARCOAL.
  2. *If the patient has high fever,* SPONGE WITH TAP WATER.

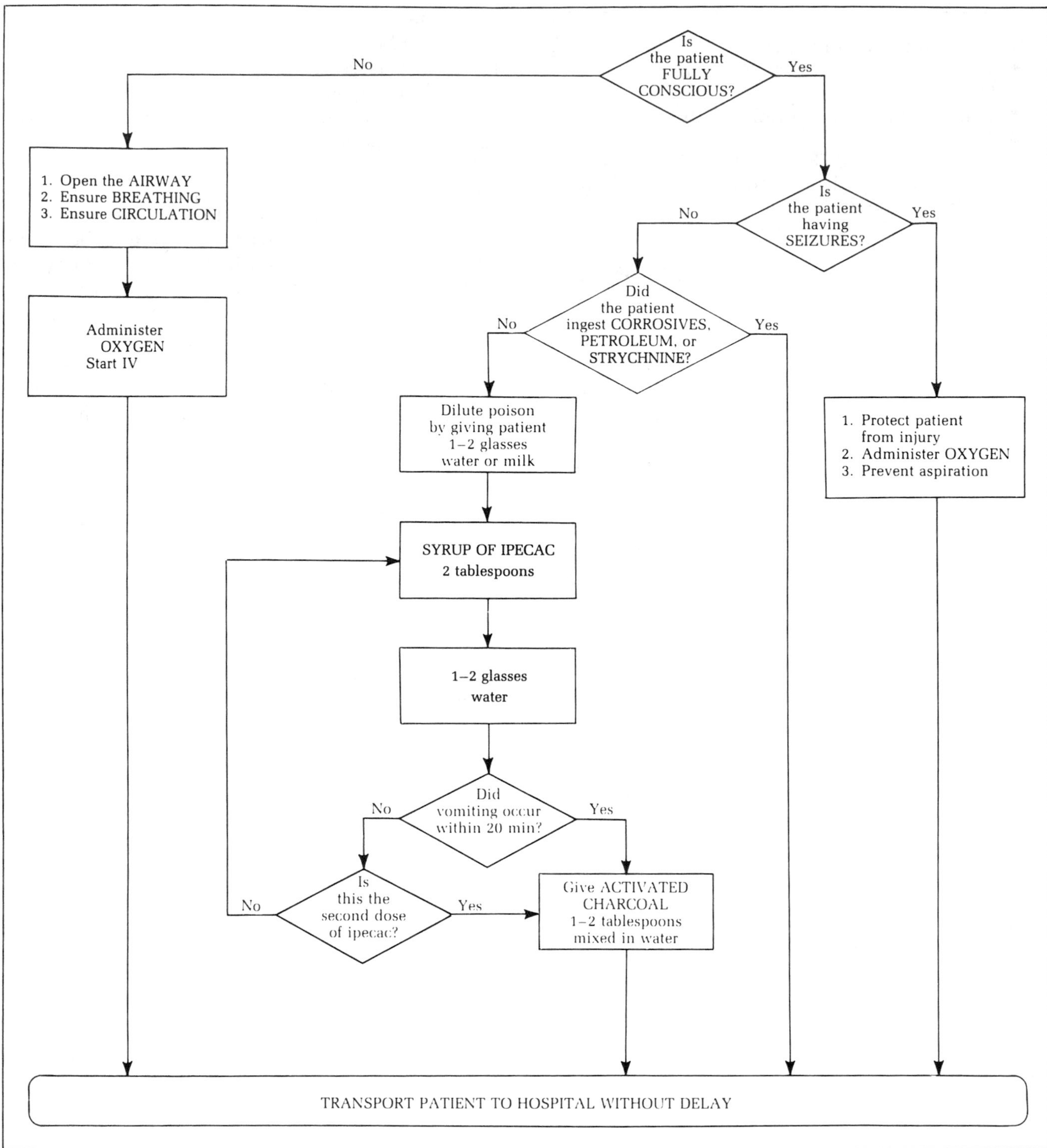

Fig. 26-2. *Management of poisoning by ingestion.*

3. *If the patient is stuporous or in coma:*
   a. Do NOT induce vomiting.
   b. Maintain the AIRWAY.
   c. Stable side position.
   d. Administer OXYGEN.
4. TRANSPORT without delay to the hospital. Bring the medication container with the patient to the hospital.

Ingestion of Petroleum Products

About 10 percent of hospitalizations for poisoning in childhood are the result of ingestion of petroleum products. Commonly, kerosene or gasoline that has been stored in a soft drink bottle is mistaken by the child for something good to drink, and it is quite extraordinary how a small child can down a whole bottle of kerosene without noticing that it tastes a bit different from the standard carbonated beverage. Other commonly involved substances include lighter fluid, turpentine, and gasoline. One particularly dangerous substance is red seal-oil furniture polish, the pretty color of which is very enticing to children and whose low viscosity makes it easily aspirated.

Patients who have ingested petroleum products typically present with PULMONARY SIGNS AND SYMPTOMS, including COUGH, CHOKING, RALES, and RHONCHI, and in severe cases CYANOSIS. ABDOMINAL PAIN is not uncommon. In addition, these patients often show signs of central nervous system involvement, ranging from IRRITABILITY and SEIZURES to COMA. Occasionally, HYPOGLYCEMIA is present, and DISTURBANCES OF CARDIAC RHYTHM may occur.

In managing a patient who has ingested a petroleum product, the first rule is DO NOT INDUCE VOMITING, since these highly volatile substances are very apt to be aspirated as they travel back up into the throat. As noted earlier, the only possible exception to this rule is the case in which a large quantity (more than a few ounces) of kerosene or a similar product has been ingested. In this situation, the danger of toxicity to the central nervous system is probably greater than the danger of aspiration. In such circumstances, the physician at the base hospital should be consulted for advice.

Because there is likely to be respiratory distress and sometimes even pulmonary edema, patients who have ingested petroleum products should receive OXYGEN in high concentration. Suction should be readily available to take care of the greatly increased secretions produced by these patients.

En route to the hospital, keep a finger on the patient's pulse, and note any irregularities. Be alert for seizures, and be prepared to protect the patient and his airway if seizures occur.

Recognition and Management of Poisoning with Petroleum Products

- SIGNS AND SYMPTOMS
  1. RESPIRATORY DISTRESS: cough, choking, air hunger
  2. RALES and RHONCHI on auscultation
  3. CYANOSIS
  4. ABDOMINAL PAIN
  5. IRRITABILITY and SEIZURES
  6. LETHARGY or COMA
  7. IRREGULAR PULSE
- TREATMENT
  1. DO NOT INDUCE VOMITING (If a large volume has been ingested, consult physician for orders)
  2. Administer OXYGEN, preferably by nonrebreathing mask
  3. Have SUCTION handy
  4. BE PREPARED FOR SEIZURES
  5. TRANSPORT without delay

Ingestion of Poisonous Plants

You have just finished poison-proofing your home. The medicine cabinet in the bathroom is securely locked; all the household cleaners, pesticides, and similar products are carefully stashed away in a locked cabinet. So now Junior is safe, right? Wrong. Not so long as the philodendron is trailing along the living room window, the dieffenbachia is thriving in the den, the English ivy is creeping up the front of the house, and the narcissus bulbs are out in the garage, waiting to be planted. The average home and garden are apt to be full of unsuspected poisons lurking in some of the most common cultivated plants (Table 26-2). While these plants may not seem particularly tempting to the average adult, at least 12,000 children every year find toxic plants sufficiently appetizing to ingest them and be poisoned by them.

What do you do, then, when you respond to a call from a frantic parent who reports that a 2-year-old ate one of the house plants or something growing in the garden? First, find out WHEN the plant was eaten. If more than 12 hours has passed since the ingestion and the child is without symptoms, it is unlikely that the plant ingested was a toxic one. If untoward effects are going to occur, they usually make themselves evident within about four hours. Next, find out WHAT PLANT was eaten, and WHAT *PART* OF THE PLANT. The latter information is crucial, for some plants contain both edible parts and toxic parts. The rhubarb stalk, for instance, is quite edible, while the leaf is highly toxic. The American diet would be almost unthinkable without the potato, but new potato sprouts may cause severe gastrointestinal symptoms, respiratory depression, and circulatory collapse. If you are not a botanist, TAKE WHAT IS LEFT OF THE PLANT TO THE EMERGENCY ROOM WITH THE PATIENT, so that a definitive identification of the plant can be made.

What should you do for the patient until he or she reaches the hospital? If the child—it *is* usually a child—is without symptoms and ingested the plant within the previous four hours, induce vomiting. Even if you are not sure the plant is toxic, or you do not know precisely what plant the victim swallowed, be on the safe side and get it out of his or her stomach. If the child is already showing signs of poisoning, however, it is best *not* to induce vomiting at the scene. In some plant poisonings, seizures may occur suddenly, and one does not want the patient to have a stomach full of ipecac and water when a seizure comes on. Thus if the patient is already symp-

Table 26-2. *Poisons in Some Common Plants*

Plant	Poisonous Part	Poison	Signs and Symptoms of Poisoning
Apricot	Seeds	Cyanide	Headache, dizziness, weakness, nausea, vomiting, coma, seizures
Autumn crocus	Entire plant	Colchicine	Cramps, nausea, hematuria, diarrhea, coma, shock
Bird of paradise	Pod	Multiple	Vomiting, diarrhea
Bloodroot	Root	Sanguinarine	Cramps, diarrhea, dizziness, paralysis, coma
Buttercup	Entire plant	Protanemonin	Gastroenteritis, seizures
Caladium	Leaves and roots	Calcium oxalate	Burning of mucous membranes, swelling of tongue and throat, salivation, gastroenteritis
Cherry	Bark, leaves, seed	Amygdalin	Stupor, vocal cord paralysis, seizures, coma
Dieffenbachia	Leaves and roots	Calcium oxalate	Same as for caladium
Daffodil	Bulb	Multiple	Gastroenteritis
Deadly nightshade	Berry, leaf, root	Atropine	Fever, tachycardia, dilated pupils, hot, red, dry skin
Elderberry	Leaf, shoot, bark	Sambunigran	Gastroenteritis
Holly	Berries	Ilicin	Gastroenteritis, coma
Hyacinth	Bulb	Multiple	Severe gastroenteritis
Jack-in-the-pulpit	All parts	Calcium oxalate	Severe gastroenteritis, burning of oral mucosa
Jimson weed	All parts	Atropine	Dry mouth, hot, red skin, headache, hallucinations, tachycardia, hypertension, delirium, seizures
Laurel	All parts	Andromedotoxin	Salivation, lacrimation, rhinorrhea, vomiting, seizures, bradycardia, hypotension, paralysis
Lily of the valley	Leaf, flowers	Glycosides	Cardiac dysrhythmias, nausea
Mistletoe	All parts	Tyramine	Bradycardia, gastroenteritis, hypertension, dyspnea, delirium, sweating, shock
Morning glory	Seeds	LSD	Hallucinations
Narcissus	Bulb	Multiple	Gastroenteritis
Oleander	Entire plant	Oleanin	Cramps, bradycardia, dilated pupils, bloody diarrhea, coma, apnea (One leaf is lethal.)
Philodendron	Entire plant	Calcium oxalate	Edema of tongue, throat
Poinsettia	Leaves, stem, sap	Multiple	Contact dermatitis, gastroenteritis
Potato	Green tubers, new sprouts	Solanine	Severe gastroenteritis, headache, apnea, shock
Rhododendron	Entire plant	Andomedotoxin	Salivation
Rhubarb	Leaves only	Oxalic acid	Cramps, nausea, vomiting, anuria
Wisteria	Pods	Glycoside	Severe gastroenteritis, shock

tomatic, simply take him and the reamins of the plant promptly to the emergency room (Fig. 26-3).

INHALED POISONS

The most frequently encountered poisoning by inhalation is that due to **carbon monoxide (CO)** gas. CO is the commonest cause of poisoning *death* in the United States, and at least half of all adult suicide fatalities are from this souce. Furthermore, CO poisoning is the most common killer in fires, accounting for half of all burn deaths.

Carbon monoxide is a *colorless, odorless, tasteless* gas that is produced by the incomplete burning of organic materials such as gasoline, wood, paper, charcoal, coal, and even natural gas. Thus substantial concentrations of carbon monoxide may be present when there are poorly maintained heating systems, inadequately vented sterno or wood stoves, or even an hibachi used in a closed trailer or tent. An automobile sitting with the engine running can generate a lethal concentration of carbon monoxide inside a closed garage in about 15 to 30 minutes. Virtually any large fire also generates significant amounts of carbon monoxide, and thus CO poses a particular danger to fire fighters and fire victims. Because it is entirely odorless, CO is a silent killer. The victim of accidental exposure usually has no idea that he or she is being poisoned by a toxic gas, and even the development of severe symptoms does not give the victim any clue as to the source of the problem. Thus the exposure victim is apt to remain in the exposure environment, suffering even further and perhaps fatal inhalation of the gas.

Carbon monoxide produces its toxic effects by combining with hemoglobin, the pigment in red

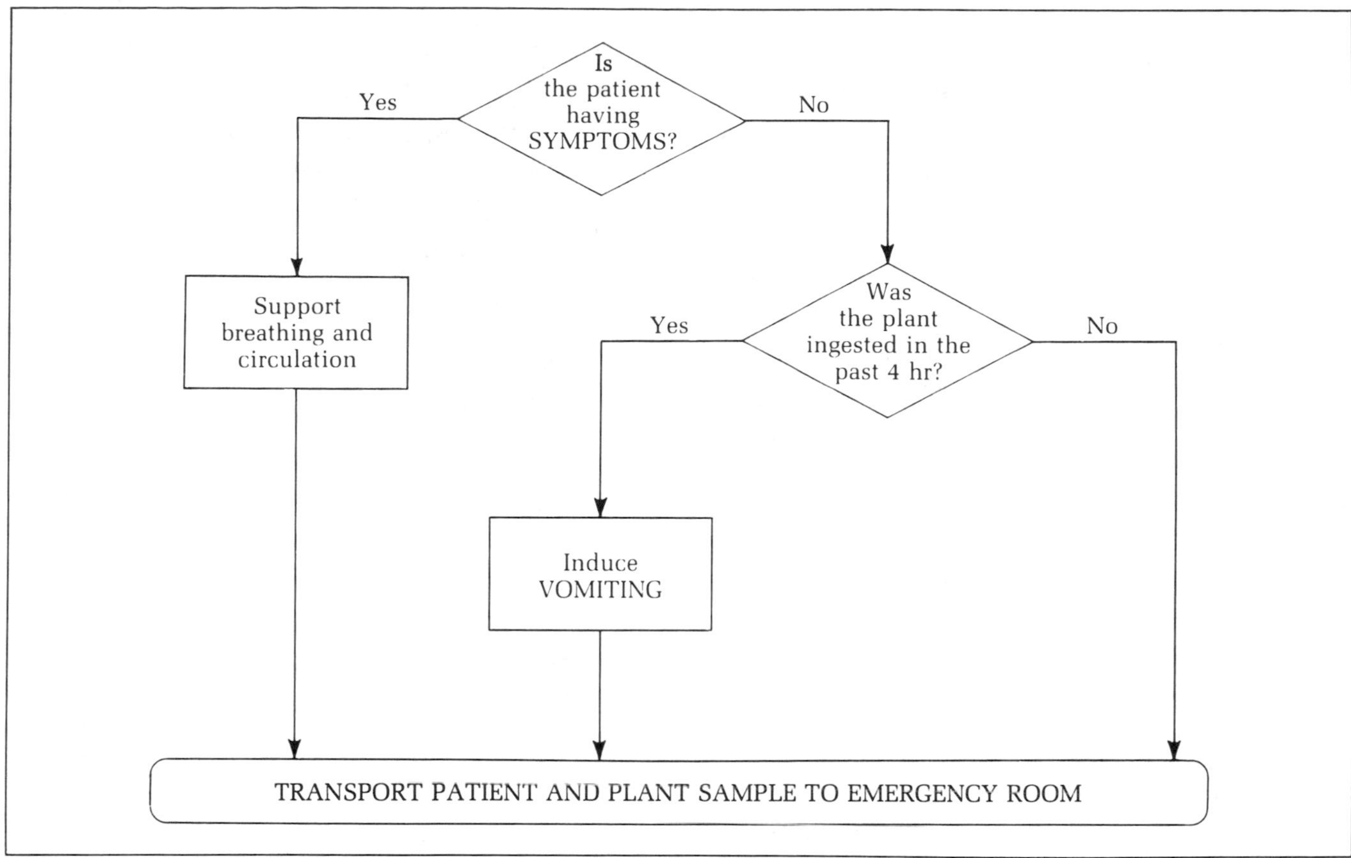

Fig. 26-3. *Management of plant ingestion.*

blood cells that normally carries oxygen to the tissues. When combined with CO, hemoglobin (now in a form called **carboxyhemoglobin**) cannot carry oxygen. If a significant percentage of the blood hemoglobin is in the form of carboxyhemoglobin, the overall ability of the blood to bring oxygen to the tissues is reduced, and the tissues begin to feel the effects of hypoxia.

The signs and symptoms of carbon monoxide poisoning are extremely variable and depend on a whole host of factors, such as the intensity of the exposure, the duration of the exposure, and so forth. Even if you take half a dozen people who all had the same exposure—say they were all together in a closed room in which there was a badly vented stove—you are likely to hear half a dozen different stories. Who will suffer the worst effects? Anyone whose perfusion is marginal will be among the first to experience symptoms. For example, a patient with chronic angina, whose heart is getting barely enough oxygen under the best of circumstances, will be very sensitive to the decrease in his blood oxygen, and this person may experience angina as his first symptom. Anything that increases the need of the body for oxygen will also increase one's susceptibility to carbon monoxide. Thus if one of the people in our closed room is doing pushups or has a fever, he will experience symptoms sooner than someone sitting quietly. Similarly, small children and household pets, whose metabolic rate and oxygen requirements are higher than those of an adult, are apt to get much sicker from a given dose of CO. In general, it is a good rule of thumb that

WHEN YOU SEE A BUNCH OF PEOPLE WITH A BUNCH OF SYMPTOMS AND THEY HAVE ALL BEEN IN THE SAME PLACE, SUSPECT CARBON MONOXIDE POISONING.

The symptoms a given person experiences are usually directly related to the amount of carbon monoxide that has found its way into the blood. The level of CO in the blood is usually expressed as percent carboxyhemoglobin, that is, the percent of the hemoglobin in the body that is carrying carbon monoxide instead of oxygen. Table 26-3 shows the relationship between the level of CO in the blood and the patient's signs and symptoms.

Most victims of carbon monoxide poisoning present with a confusing combination of symptoms that will not make much sense unless the EMT is alert enough to connect the patient's symptoms with the circumstances in which the patient is found.

Table 26-3. *Symptoms and Signs of Carbon Monoxide Poisoning*

Percent Carboxyhemoglobin	Symptoms and Signs
10	Dyspnea on exertion, tight feeling in the head
20	As above, plus throbbing headache at the temples, nausea, vomiting
30	As above, plus irritability, dizziness, impaired judgment, dimness of vision, drunk behavior
40–50	As above, plus tachycardia, tachypnea, confusion, cardiovascular collapse, incontinence
60–70	Coma, seizures, respiratory failure
80 or more	Rapid death

Suspect carbon monoxide poisoning in:

- Patients rescued from structural fires
- Firefighters overcome by smoke
- Patients found in warm, poorly ventilated places in winter
- Patients found in a closed car or garage
- Patients with winter headaches

The aims of treating carbon monoxide poisoning are to get the victim out of the exposure environment and get the carbon monoxide out of his blood. The FIRST step of management is to REMOVE THE VICTIM FROM EXPOSURE TO CARBON MONOXIDE. If he is in a closed room or an automobile, get him out immediately. Should there be extrication problems involved, don an air tank for yourself and clamp an oxygen mask on the victim's face until he can be removed from the toxic environment. The next and most crucial step in management is to administer 100% OXYGEN by tight-fitting nonrebreathing mask. When a person is breathing room air, the half life of CO in the blood is about 5 to 6 hours. Breathing 100% oxygen reduces this half life to about 1¼ hours. The only way to get rid of the carbon monoxide in the blood even faster is to deliver oxygen at greater than atmospheric pressure in a hyperbaric chamber, such as those used to treat divers with decompression sickness. In a hyperbaric chamber at 3 atmospheres pressure, the elimination of CO can be speeded up to about 30 minutes. If such a facility exists in your community, that is the place to which the CO victim should be transported.

Recognition and Management of Carbon Monoxide Poisoning

- SIGNS AND SYMPTOMS
  1. THROBBING HEADACHE, DIZZINESS, BLURRED VISION, IRRITABILITY, CONFUSION.
  2. NAUSEA, VOMITING.
  3. SEIZURES, COMA, RESPIRATORY DEPRESSION.
- TREATMENT
  1. REMOVE THE VICTIM FROM EXPOSURE.
  2. Administer 100% OXYGEN by tight-fitting, nonrebreathing mask.
  3. Be prepared to support respirations.
  4. Transport to a hospital with a HYPERBARIC CHAMBER, if one exists in the community.

ABSORBED POISONS

As noted earlier, some poisons may find their way into the body by absorption across the skin or mucous membranes. We will take as our example of this type of poisoning the case of organophosphates, which are a major component of many insecticides (e.g., Buthion, trithion, malathion, parathion). Poisoning with organophosphates is most likely to occur in people who are involved in the manufacture or use of these products, but occasionally children have been poisoned by organophosphates merely from handling gloves or work clothes contaminated with the insecticide. In general, the incidence of this kind of poisoning is higher in farm areas, but urban dwellers are also at risk, in view of the large number of pesticides available in the average home. Pilots who do crop-dusting have a particularly high incidence of organophosphate poisoning.

The SYMPTOMS AND SIGNS of organophosphate poisoning depend on how large a dose of the insecticide the victim received. In *mild poisoning,* the patient complains of HEADACHE, FATIGUE, DIZZINESS, NUMBNESS, TIGHTNESS IN THE CHEST, NAUSEA, and ABDOMINAL PAIN. He is usually DIAPHORETIC and SALIVATING excessively. The patient is apt to smell like GARLIC. With *moderate poisoning,* the patient is so WEAK he cannot even walk. There may be FASCICULATIONS (a kind of rippling twitching of the muscles), and the PUPILS tend to be CONSTRICTED. With *severe poisoning,* the patient goes into COMA. There is MUSCLE PARALYSIS, with resulting FLACCIDITY. RALES are heard in the lungs, and there may be marked CYANOSIS.

In treating the victim of organophosphate poisoning, the goals are to terminate the exposure and support vital functions. Start by giving 100% OXYGEN. Use the demand valve if you hear rales in the victim's lungs. Then DECONTAMINATE THE PATIENT. Make sure you are wearing protective clothing and rubber gloves when you do so, for otherwise you may be the next victim. Get the patient out of the exposure environment, and remove his shoes and clothing, which should be placed in a plastic bag. Then wash him down from head to toe with plenty of soap and water. That is best accomplished in a shower in the home, but, weather conditions and screening permitting, even a garden hose will do. The best agent for decontamination is tincture of green soap, which contains alcohol. If you do not have green soap, use any soap and rinse with dilute alcohol. Then repeat the whole procedure.

If the patient is already experiencing severe weakness and/or respiratory distress, you will have to accomplish the decontamination very quickly. The cause of death in organophosphate poisoning is respiratory arrest, so BE PREPARED TO ASSIST VENTILATIONS, and HAVE SUCTION HANDY to take care of the massive secretions seen in these patients.

Recognition and Management of Organophosphate Poisoning

- SYMPTOMS AND SIGNS
  1. Mild: HEADACHE, FATIGUE, DIZZINESS, NUMBNESS, TIGHTNESS IN THE CHEST, NAUSEA, ABDOMINAL PAIN, DIAPHORESIS, HYPERSALIVATION, GARLIC ODOR.
  2. Moderate: Above signs plus CANNOT WALK, CONSTRICTED PUPILS, FASCICULATIONS.
  3. Severe: COMA, PULMONARY EDEMA, CYANOSIS, FLACCIDITY, APNEA.
- TREATMENT
  1. PROTECT YOURSELF FROM EXPOSURE: mask, surgical gown, gloves.
  2. Administer 100% OXYGEN; use demand valve for pulmonary edema.
  3. SUCTION as needed. Be prepared to ASSIST VENTILATIONS.
  4. DECONTAMINATE THE PATIENT
     a. Remove all the patient's clothing.
     b. Wash patient with soap and water, alcohol rinse. Repeat.
  5. Expeditious transport to the hospital.

CASE HISTORY

The patient is a 2½-year-old boy whose mother called for an ambulance because the child was panting. The mother stated that the child has been in good health and she could not imagine what was wrong; she just found him breathing very deeply after his nap. A search of the house produced an empty aspirin bottle on the bathroom floor. The mother stated the bottle had been purchased last week and was nearly full when last seen.

On physical examination, the child appeared ill but alert. His skin was hot and wet. Pulse was 160 per minute, and respirations were 40 and deep. Oral temperature was 104°F (40°C). The pupils were slightly dilated but reactive. The chest was clear. The abdomen was slightly tender.

The child was sponged down with tepid water to lower his temperature. One tablespoon of syrup of ipecac was administered, followed by a glass of lukewarm water, and vomiting occurred in 12 minutes. The vomitus contained fragments of pills, and a sample of the vomitus was saved in a closed container to take to the hospital. When he stopped vomiting, the child was given 2 tablespoons of activated charcoal mixed in a glass of water. Vital signs were unchanged en route to the hospital.

Questions to think about:

1. What was causing the child's hyperpnea?
2. Why was it important to try to lower the child's fever?
3. Why was a sample of vomitus saved to take to the hospital?
4. What was the purpose of giving activated charcoal?
5. Could this poisoning have been prevented? Is there any advice you could give the child's mother to try to ensure that something like this does not happen again?

VOCABULARY

acidosis Condition in which the level of acid in the body is increased above normal.

carbon monoxide Colorless, odorless, tasteless gas produced by incomplete combustion of organic materials; a highly toxic gas.

carboxyhemoglobin Hemoglobin that is combined with carbon monoxide instead of oxygen.

fasciculations Rippling, twitching movements in the muscles.

organophosphate Class of chemicals used in insecticides and nerve gases.

FURTHER READING

GENERAL POISONING

Arena JM. Poisoning. *Emerg Med* 8:171, 1976.

Caroline NL. Poison patrol. *Emerg Med Serv* 11(2):80, 1982.

Centers for Disease Control. Poisoning among young children—United States. *MMWR* 33:129, 1984.

Done AK. The basic approach. *Emerg Med* 6:205, 1974.

Done AK. The toxic emergency: How are we faring? *Emerg Med* 14(9):39, 1982.
Flomenbaum N. Toxicology by system: The GI front. *Emerg Med* 15(17):152, 1983.
Goldfrank L, Weisman R, Flomenbaum N. Teaching the recognition of odors. *Ann Emerg Med* 11:684, 1982.
Henry J et al. ABC of poisoning: Immediate measures outside the hospital. *Br Med J* 289:39, 1984.
Nelson R, Wilson P, Kelley M. Caustic ingestion. *Ann Emerg Med* 12:559, 1983.
Penner GE. Acid ingestion: Toxicology and treatment. *Ann Emerg Med* 9:374, 1980.
Throckmorton K, Throckmorton D. Pills, plants, and poisonings. *Emergency* 20(9):53, 1988.
The toxic effects of agriculture. *Emerg Med* 21(3):151, 1989.
United States Department of Health, Education, and Welfare. *Handbook of Common Poisonings in Children.* HEW Pub (FDA) 76-7004, 1976.
Veltri JC, Litovitz TL. Annual report of the American Association of Poison Control Centers national data collection system. *Am J Emerg Med* 2:420, 1984.
Walton WW. An evaluation of the poison prevention packaging act. *Pediatrics* 69:363, 1982.

SYRUP OF IPECAC AND ACTIVATED CHARCOAL

Albertson TE et al. Superiority of activated charcoal alone compared with ipecac and activated charcoal in the treatment of acute toxic ingestions. *Ann Emerg Med* 18:56, 1989.
Auerbach PS et al. Efficacy of gastric emptying: Gastric lavage versus emesis induced with ipecac. *Ann Emerg Med* 15:692, 1986.
Dean BS, Krenselok EP. Syrup of ipecac . . . 15 ml versus 30 ml in pediatric poisonings. *Clin Toxicol* 23:165, 1985.
Flomenbaum NE, Hoffman R. GI evacuation: Is it still worthwhile? *Emerg Med* 22(2):80, 1990.
Freedman G, Pasternak S, Krenselok EP. A clinical trial using syrup of ipecac and activated charcoal concurrently. *Ann Emerg Med* 16:164, 1987.
Grande GA et al. The effect of fluid volume on syrup of ipecac emesis time. *Clin Toxicol* 25:473, 1987.
Greensher J et al. Ascendency of the black bottle (activated charcoal). *Pediatrics* 80:989, 1987.
Ipecac syrup and activated charcoal for treatment of poisoning in children. *Med Letter* 21:70, 1979.
Katona BG et al. The new black magic: Activated charcoal and new therapeutic uses. *J Emerg Med* 5:99, 1987.
King WD. Syrup of ipecac: A drug review. *Clin Toxicol* 17:353, 1980.
Kulig K et al. Management of acutely poisoned patients without gastric emptying. *Ann Emerg Med* 14:562, 1985.
Levy D. Activated charcoal update. *Emergency* 20(6):16, 1988.
Levy G. Gastrointestinal clearance of drugs with activated charcoal. *NEJM* 307:676, 1982.
McNamara RM et al. Efficacy of charcoal cathartic versus ipecac in reducing serum acetaminophen in a simulated overdose. *Ann Emerg Med* 18:934, 1989.
Mofenson HC. Benefits/risks of syrup of ipecac. *Pediatrics* 77:551, 1986.
Park GD et al. Expanded role of charcoal therapy in the poisoned and overdosed patient. *Arch Intern Med* 146:969, 1986.
Tenenbein M. Inefficacy of gastric emptying procedures. *J Emerg Med* 3:133, 1985.
Tenenbein M, Cohen S, Sitar DS. Efficacy of ipecac-induced emesis, orogastric lavage, and activated charcoal for acute drug overdose. *Ann Emerg Med* 16:838, 1987.

ASPIRIN POISONING

Bailey RB, Jones SR. Chronic salicylate intoxication: A common cause of morbidity in the elderly. *J Am Geriat Soc* 37:556, 1989.
Burton B et al. Comparison of activated charcoal and gastric lavage in the prevention of aspirin absorption. *J Emerg Med* 1:411, 1984.
Kearney TE. Salicylate poisoning: Recognition and management. *Emerg Med Serv* 18(5):39, 1989.

POISONING BY PETROLEUM PRODUCTS

Dice WH et al. Pulmonary toxicity following gastrointestinal ingestion of kerosene. *Ann Emerg Med* 11:138, 1982.
Machado B, Cross K, Snodgrass WR. Accidental hydrocarbon ingestion cases telephoned to a regional poison center. *Ann Emerg Med* 17:804, 1988.

PLANT POISONS

Arena JM. The peril in plants. *Emerg Med* 6:221, 1974.
Arena JM. Plants that poison. *Emerg Med* 21(11):20, 1989.

CARBON MONOXIDE POISONING

Burney R, Wu S, Nemiroff M. Mass carbon monoxide poisoning: Clinical effects and results of treatment in 184 victims. *Ann Emerg Med* 11:394, 1982.
Dan BB. The twilight zone: Death on a Sunday morning (editorial). *JAMA* 261:1188, 1989.
Heckerling PS. Occult carbon monoxide poisoning. A cause of winter headache. *Am J Emerg Med* 5:201, 1987.
Jackson DL et al. Accidental carbon monoxide poisoning. *JAMA* 243:722, 1980.
Kirkpatric JN. Occult carbon monoxide poisoning. *West J Med* 146:52, 1987.
Levy DB. A breath of dead air. *Emergency* 20(11):18, 1988.
Mofenson HC et al. Carbon monoxide poisoning. *Am J Emerg Med* 2:254, 1984.
Myers RA et al. Carbon monoxide poisoning: The injury and its treatment. *JACEP* 8:479, 1979.
Olson KR. Carbon monoxide poisoning: Mechanisms, presentation, and controversies in management. *J Emerg Med* 1:233, 1984.
Wharton M et al. Fatal carbon monoxide poisoning at a motel. *JAMA* 261:1177, 1989.
Zeller WP et al. Accidental carbon monoxide poisoning. *Clin Ped* 23:694, 1984.

27. BITES AND STINGS

OBJECTIVES

In the year 3000 B.C. Memes, the Pharaoh of Egypt, succumbed to the sting of a wasp. Doubtless he was not the first person to be dispatched from this world by the bite or sting of one of nature's little creatures, and certainly he was not the last. Every year in the United States, man's unhappy encounters with things that fly, swim, crawl, bark, and even things that walk upright lead to more than a million emergency room visits. In this chapter, we will look at some of the more commonly encountered bites and stings and how these injuries should be managed in the field. By the conclusion of the chapter, the reader should be able to

1. Identify a poisonous snake, given a picture or description of several snakes
2. Identify the signs and symptoms of an envenomed snake bite, given a description of various snakebite victims
3. Identify correct and incorrect methods of treating a victim of an envenomed snake bite
4. Indicate what information in the history of a patient who suffered an animal bite points to the probability that the animal was rabid
5. Identify the correct treatment of an animal bite, given a list of possible treatments
6. Identify the correct treatment of a human bite, given a list of possible treatments
7. Identify the symptoms and signs of (a) a local reaction and (b) an anaphylactic reaction to hymenoptera stings, and indicate the correct treatment for each
8. Identify the signs and symptoms of a bite by a poisonous spider, and indicate the correct treatment for this problem
9. Identify a patient who has suffered (a) the sting of a poisonous scorpion, (b) tick paralysis, given a description of several patients, and indicate the correct treatment for each
10. Identify the signs, symptoms, and correct treatment of common injuries inflicted by marine animals

ANIMAL BITES

Just about any creature with a good set of teeth, including man, can inflict a bite, but some bites are more serious than others owing to the injection of venom into the wound or the possibility of serious infection. In this section, we will examine the bites inflicted by three types of creatures: snakes, furry animals, and man—each of which has its own unique potential to cause significant bodily harm.

SNAKE BITES

Approximately 50,000 snake bites occur in the United States each year, of which about 8,000, or 16 percent, are caused by poisonous snakes. Among those 8,000, only half to two-thirds of the victims actually receive any snake venom when bitten, and among those who do suffer envenomed bites, about 12 to 14 die each year. We can see, then, that only a small proportion of snakebites are inflicted by poisonous snakes, and even those bites that *are* inflicted by poisonous snakes may not contain poison. What this means for the EMT is that it is important (a) to be able to distinguish poisonous from nonpoisonous snakes and (b) to be able to recognize the signs of **envenomation** (injection with poison).

Among the 120 or so species of snakes in the United States, only about 20 are poisonous. The poisonous species fall into two general categories, pit vipers and coral snakes, about who we shall have more to say in a moment. Venomous snakes are widespread throughout the United States, particularly in the South and Southwest and also in major mountain range areas on both coasts. Only Alaska, Hawaii, and Maine are entirely free of poisonous snakes.

Poisonous and nonpoisonous snakes often look very similar. If the snake has a rattle on its tail, you can be certain it is poisonous no matter what it looks like. Otherwise, definitive identification often requires a careful examination of the snake for distinguishing features, and cross-checking in a good reference book. A casual glance at the creature in the field is usually not sufficient. For practical purposes, this means that wherever possible, you should try to take the snake to the ER with the patient. Needless to say, it is highly desirable that the snake be dead—preferably dead for some time—before you undertake to transport the creature. Quite aside from the hazard to your own safety, there are few emergency room staffs that will appreciate the arrival on the premises of an active eight-foot diamondback rattler or one of its cousins.

WHEREVER POSSIBLE, KILL THE SNAKE AND TAKE IT WITH THE PATIENT TO THE HOSPITAL FOR DEFINITIVE IDENTIFICATION.

The local zoo or science museum is a good place to become familiar with some of the snakes that reside in your area. Zoos are also a good resource to know about when a snake bite case occurs, for many larger zoos stock snake **antivenin** (a serum used to counteract the toxic effects of a given snake venom) and will provide this material to an emergency room if there is a case requiring it.

Sometimes the specific type of antivenin needed to treat a particular snake bite is not available locally and has to be flown in from another part of the country. For this reason, the ambulance team dealing with a snakebite victim should always radio ahead to the receiving hospital with details of the type of snake thought to be involved. This advance notice gives the hospital personnel a chance to get started right away in checking for a source of antivenin.

The Poisonous Snakes and the Effects of Their Poisons

As noted, all poisonous snakes in the United States fall into two general categories: the pit vipers and the coral snakes.

PIT VIPERS. Pit vipers are so named because they have a deep depression, or pit, between the eye and the nostril on either side of the head. The pit is a special sense organ that detects heat, thereby enabling the snake to track and strike accurately at a warm-blooded target, even in the dark. Pit vipers also have characteristic folding fangs in the upper jaw, and when the snake bites, those fangs pop forward to inject venom through their hollow centers. Thus the bite of a pit viper leaves a distinctive mark (Fig. 27-1) that can be used to differentiate this kind of bite from that of nonpoisonous snakes: two puncture wounds in front, with one row of teeth marks extending behind each. Other characteristics of pit vipers include a thick body, a broad, flat, almost triangular head, and vertical, slit-like pupils.

The pit viper family includes RATTLESNAKES, COPPERHEADS, and WATER MOCCASINS. Rattlers are by far the most common, present throughout the United States except in Delaware, District of Columbia, and the three snake-free states mentioned earlier. Rattlers are larger and more venomous than

Fig. 27-1. *A. Pit viper. B. Nonpoisonous snake.*

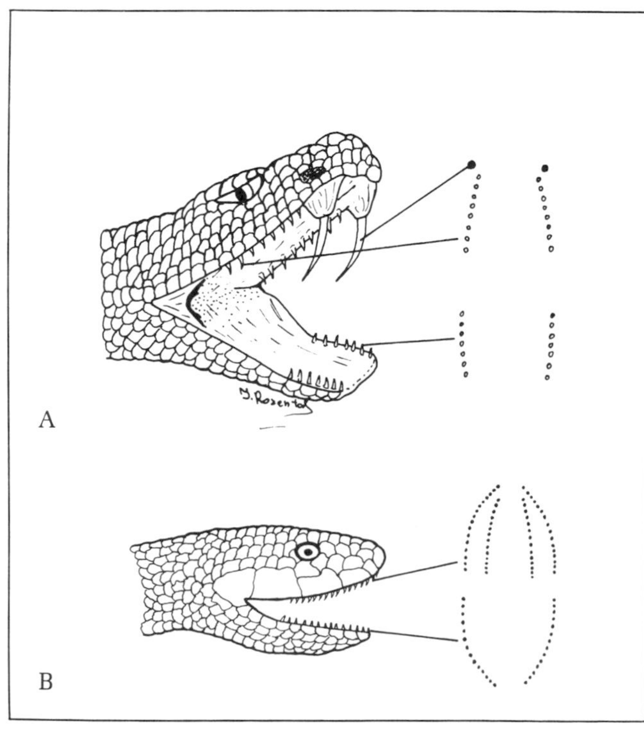

other types of pit vipers. The most impressive is the diamondback rattlesnake, which can reach a length of 8 feet and a weight of 30 pounds. The water moccasin (also called the cottonmouth, because of its white mouth) and the copperhead are southern snakes, found primarily in the sunbelt from Texas to the Old South.

Few snakes are naturally aggressive, although some, such as the diamondbacks, are more irritable than others. Pit vipers will, however, strike in self-defense, and when a pit viper does bite, it does so with lightning speed. As its fangs spring forward and penetrate the victim's skin, the pit viper injects a variable amount of venom—ranging from no venom at all to a lethal dose—through its fangs into the wound. The venom produced by these snakes contains very powerful enzymes that can digest all sorts of tissues; thus, pit viper venom wreaks widespread destruction of skin and muscle in the bitten area.

The classic SYMPTOMS AND SIGNS of pit viper envenomation are instantaneous, severe, BURNING PAIN in the area of the bite. SWELLING around the fang marks follows within a few minutes, and untreated, the swelling may spread to involve the whole extremity within one to several hours. Remember, a SNAKE BITE DOES NOT AUTOMATICALLY MEAN ENVENOMATION. If you want to be sure, look for fang marks and swelling. If there are no fang marks, there is no envenomation. Pain is *not* a reliable indicator, because *every* snake bite hurts, whether it was inflicted by a poisonous or a nonpoisonous snake. If you see swelling around the fang marks, you can be fairly confident the patient got a dose of venom, especially if the fang marks themselves continue to ooze nonclotting blood.

ECCHYMOSIS is also characteristic within the first few hours after the bite, and the skin becomes shiny, taut, and black and blue. A few hours later, HEMORRHAGIC BLISTERS appear, and the patient may notice NUMBNESS at the site.

Meanwhile, as the venom is absorbed into the bloodstream, SYSTEMIC SYMPTOMS begin to appear. NAUSEA and VOMITING along with WEAKNESS, FAINTNESS, and SWEATING may occur within the first 15 minutes after the bite. As more of the venom is absorbed, DIZZINESS, TACHYCARDIA, and HYPOTENSION occur, and in severe cases, these signs may be followed by DELIRIUM, SEIZURES, COMA, and DEATH.

The speed with which these signs and symptoms develop, and their intensity, are directly related to the amount of venom that was injected. The bigger the dose, the faster and more intense the development of symptoms. Injections deep into the muscle (as opposed to a bite that just penetrates the skin) will also speed the arrival of symptoms.

CORAL SNAKES. Coral snakes belong to the Elapid family, which also includes cobras, mambas, and all the Australian poisonous snakes (e.g., taipans, tiger snakes). The eastern coral snake is found throughout the southern states, from North Carolina to Florida, and westward to the Mississippi. The habitat of the Texas coral snake is chiefly Texas, Arizona, and New Mexico. Coral snakes are considerably smaller than the average pit viper—usually only about 10 to 18 inches long—and much more shy. Thus although its venom is extremely toxic, the coral snake is responsible for few serious snakebites. Its tendency is to slither away rather than hang around and fight. Besides matters of size and temperament, the coral snake also differs from pit vipers in the arrangement of its fangs, which are short and fixed in position. For this reason, the coral snake cannot launch the kind of lightning-swift strike that a pit viper performs, but rather must hang onto the victim and chew its venom into the wound.

Coral snakes are brightly colored, with circumferential bands of yellow, red, yellow, and black (in that order), although the yellow is sometimes nearly white. There are many harmless snakes with similar coloration, so one has to take a close look at the arrangement of the bands to be sure the snake is really a coral snake. In a true coral sake, the red band is *always* next to the yellow band; if the red band borders a black band, the snake is harmless. A jingle well-known in first aid courses helps in remembering this color arrangement.

RED ON YELLOW, KILL A FELLOW.
RED ON BLACK, VENOM LACK.

The venom of coral snakes is quite different from that of pit vipers, for it produces a minimum of local tissue destruction. Coral snake venom acts instead on the central nervous system, and thus the classic SYMPTOMS AND SIGNS of envenomation by a coral snake are related primarily to CNS depression. Usually, there is LITTLE OR NO PAIN at the site of the bite, and swelling is also minimal. There may, however, be some local bruising, due to mechanical damage sustained when the snake was chewing its venom into the wound. Other symptoms are usually delayed anywhere from one to twelve hours after the bite. Often MOOD is affected first, and the mood may change to EUPHORIA, ANXIETY, or DEPRESSION. The patient may note marked DROWSINESS and increased SALIVATION. As the venom begins to get a strong grip on the nervous system, paralysis of various muscle groups occurs. This PARALYSIS commonly involves the EYELIDS, the MUSCLES OF SWALLOWING, and RESPIRATORY MUSCLES—the latter involvement leading to respiratory insuffi-

Table 27-1. *Poisonous Snakes in the United States*

Category	Examples	Distinctive Features	Signs and Symptoms of Envenomation
Pit viper	Rattlesnakes diamondback, prairie, red timber, Mojave, sidewinder Copperhead Water moccasin	Pits between eyes and nostrils Erectile fangs Flat, triangular head Slit-like, vertical pupils Thick body, may be very large	Local: Burning pain, fang marks, edema, ecchymoses, blisters, numbness. Systemic: Nausea, vomiting, weakness, sweating, tachycardia, hypotension, dizziness. In severe case, delirium, seizures, coma, and death.
Coral snakes	40 to 50 species	Tricolor: Black, red, and yellow (or white) Small (10–18 in.) Fixed fangs Less aggressive than pit vipers	Local: Minimal pain or swelling at site. Systemic: Symptoms come on 1–12 hours after bite. Euphoria, depression, or anxiety; drowsiness; paralysis of eyelids, throat muscles, respiratory muscles; respiratory failure; seizures, coma.

ciency. SEIZURES and COMA may follow, and death may occur, usually within 24 hours of the bite.

As in the case of pit viper envenomation, in coral snake bites, the speed with which symptoms develop and the severity of the symptoms reflect the amount of venom the victim received. As a general rule, you should suspect that the victim got a big dose of venom if he complains of numbness at the site of the injury or around the lips, tongue, or scalp. Yellow vision is also an ominous sign. These symptoms often herald the onset of generalized paralysis and respiratory failure, so the EMT should be alerted that assisted ventilation may be required at any moment.

The characteristics of pit vipers and coral snakes are summarized in Table 27-1.

Treatment of Envenomed Snake Bites

The goals of field treatment of envenomed snake bites are to retard the absorption of the venom and to support the patient's vital functions until he or she reaches the hospital. Since about 98 percent of snake bites involve the extremities, we will direct our discussion here to management of a patient bitten on an arm or leg, but the general principles are similar for bites elsewhere on the body.

The *first* step in managing the snakebite victim is to GET THE PATIENT AWAY FROM THE SNAKE! There is no code of ethics among snakes that says a snake may bite only once, and you or the victim may be the recipient of bite number two if you do not get out of the way. When you reach the patient who has been bitten by a poisonous snake, you are likely to find him or her in a highly excited, panicky state. Thus the next measure to take is to CALM AND REASSURE THE VICTIM. Panic and moving about will increase the rate at which venom is absorbed from the wound, so the patient should be persuaded to SIT OR LIE QUIETLY. Calming the patient should be accomplished through verbal means. DO NOT PERMIT THE PATIENT TO TAKE ANY ALCOHOL as a means of calming down, for this may simply aggravate CNS depression.

Flush the area of the bite with plenty of water, and WASH THE WOUND THOROUGHLY with soap and water or antiseptic solution to remove any venom still on the skin surface. Since considerable swelling can be anticipated, REMOVE ALL RINGS, BRACELETS, and any other potentially constricting items from the bitten extremity. Once swelling does occur, jewelry of this sort will be very difficult to remove and may serve as a tourniquet, cutting off arterial circulation to the distal part of the limb. It was previously recommended that constricting bands be placed above and below the fang marks to retard absorption of snake venom. However, experts now question the usefulness of *any* sort of tourniquet or constricting band in snake bites. There is no evidence that venous tourniquets do indeed retard the absorption of venom, and a constricting band applied too tightly may actually increase the damage to the bitten extremity. Constricting bands, therefore, are generally out of favor, although the matter is still somewhat controversial.

As noted, movement increases the rate of absorption of the venom by increasing circulation, so SPLINT THE BITTEN EXTREMITY, just as if it were broken. Keep the extremity below heart level, to discourage drainage of the venom by gravity into the trunk, but do not let the arm or leg hang completely dependent. DO NOT PERMIT THE PATIENT TO WALK ON A BITTEN LEG.

For many years, rescuers were taught to apply ice to a snake bite (so-called *cryotherapy*), on the theory that cold decreases swelling and slows the action of harmful enzymes contained in the venom. Experience showed, however, that application of cold packs or immersion of the bitten extremity in ice water usually did more harm than good—often causing frostbite injuries that required amputation of the limb. For that reason, cryotherapy is now considered to be contraindicated in snake bites.

Another controversial measure is the incision and suction technique for removal of snake venom, and the EMT should follow local protocols regarding its use. The incision and suction technique is effective only if applied very soon after the bite was inflicted—within about the first 10 minutes. *If* the patient was bitten by a pit viper, within that time period, and *if* there are signs of envenomation, and *if* you receive a physician's orders to do so, apply the incision and suction technique as follows: Use a sterile surgical scalpel to make a lengthwise incise—about 1/2 inch long and 1/4 inch deep—directly through each fang mark. Then apply a suction cup (available in any snakebite kit) over the incisions and leave it there, up to an hour if necessary. Do NOT use your mouth to apply suction unless no other means is available, for the human mouth is teeming with nasty bacteria that could enter the wound and cause infection.

Keep the patient warm, and monitor VITAL SIGNS. Treat for shock, seizures, or coma if they occur, as outlined elsewhere in this book. BE ALERT FOR SIGNS OF RESPIRATORY INSUFFICIENCY, and be prepared to assist ventilations if breathing becomes slow or shallow.

GET THE VICTIM TO THE HOSPITAL AS RAPIDLY AS POSSIBLE. Field treatment must be accomplished deliberately but swiftly, and it should not delay transport by more than a few minutes. Use judgment about which measures are necessary in the field. If you are three minutes from a hospital, do not spend 10 minutes on incision and suction!

TAKE THE DEAD SNAKE WITH YOU TO THE HOSPITAL for identification. The emphasis is on the word *dead*. If you are not versed in killing snakes, however, do not take on a diamondback rattler, for it may have plenty of venom left for you. Indeed, if you are not versed in snakes, do not handle even a dead snake, for the snake's striking reflex persists for several hours after its death; for all practical purposes, a dead snake *can* still inflict a venomous bite. So if you are not an expert on snakes, just get a good look at the snake and let it be.

Management of Envenomed Snake Bites

1. GET THE PATIENT AWAY FROM THE SNAKE!
2. *If possible,* KILL THE SNAKE AND TAKE IT WITH YOU, BUT do not waste time chasing the snake, and do not put yourself in danger.
3. CALM AND REASSURE THE PATIENT.
4. DO NOT PERMIT THE PATIENT TO MOVE AROUND.
5. CLEAN THE AREA AROUND THE BITE THOROUGHLY.
6. REMOVE ALL JEWELRY from the bitten extremity.
7. SPLINT THE BITTEN EXTREMITY, and keep it below heart level. Do not permit the patient to walk on a bitten leg.
8. Consult base hospital physician for orders regarding incision and suction.
9. ANTICIPATE RESPIRATORY PROBLEMS: Be prepared to assist ventilations.
10. MONITOR VITAL SIGNS. Treat for shock as needed.
11. MOVE RAPIDLY TO THE HOSPITAL.

Please note that none of the treatment measures described above require any special equipment other than that which would be routinely stocked on any ambulance. Therefore, you can save your service some money by *not* purchasing a special "snakebite kit." Most of the commercially available snake bite kits simply contain a collection of hazardous or useless items (suction devices, ammonia perles, cloth straps) together with instructions that are seldom correct.

ANIMAL BITES

Man's best friend, Fido, is responsible for at least one million bites in the United States each year. Another million or so bites are inflicted by other domestic and wild animals. Rarely are these bites life-threatening, nor is the treatment any more complicated than that of any other soft tissue injury. Where the EMT can make a vital contribution to the patient's management, however, is in obtaining a careful history at the scene. In many cases, the circumstances of the bite will determine whether the patient must be subjected to the expensive and repeated treatment with rabies vaccine. There is only about one case of rabies in humans in the United States annually, but about 30,000 people each year undergo treatment with rabies vaccine. Often this treatment is undertaken simply because the circumstances of the bite are not clear enough to rule out the possibility that the animal was rabid. Thus, the more accurately those circumstances can be documented, the better the chances of avoiding an unnecessary course of rabies treatment.

In taking the HISTORY from the victim, first determine WHAT KIND OF ANIMAL INFLICTED THE BITE. Rabies in dogs is relatively rare nowadays—fewer than 400 cases per year in the United States—but the incidence of rabies in certain species of wildlife is still significant. Skunks, raccoons, foxes, and especially bats are much more frequently infected than dogs, and it is a good idea to keep tabs, through state public health officials, on what species of animals, if any, have been found to be rabid in your region.

Next, find out the CIRCUMSTANCES OF THE BITE. What precisely happened? Was the biting animal a dog that suddenly and without any apparent reason turned upon the victim? If a wild animal was involved, WAS THE BITE PROVOKED? If a wild—or for that matter, a domesticated—animal has attacked without provocation, there is a much greater likelihood that the animal was rabid, for most wild animals avoid humans or use other means of protection than biting. The skunk, for instance, has a very effective method for discouraging unwanted attentions; only a rabid skunk would forego his usual means of defense and attack a human with his teeth. If the wild animal that did the biting is still in the vicinity, it should be killed and sent to local health authorities for examination.

When considering the bite of a *domesticated animal*, such as a dog, find out whether the IDENTITY OF THE ANIMAL'S OWNER is known, and if so, make a record of the address and phone number. It will be very important to contact the owner and find out whether the animal has been vaccinated against rabies, for an effectively immunized animal is unlikely to transmit rabies virus. If the animal was not vaccinated, it must be confined and kept under observation for ten days.

In examining the patient, look carefully to see whether the bite has PENETRATED THE SKIN. The patient is at risk of getting rabies only if saliva from a rabid animal has entered his body, and this can occur only if the bite breaks the skin surface or the animal's saliva somehow enters another open wound.

In treating the victim of an animal bite, meticulous care of the wound is essential. In an uncomplicated dog bite, thorough washing of the dog bite wound reduces the incidence of infection. Where the biting animal is suspected to be rabid, attention to the wound is crucial. The incidence of rabies can be markedly reduced by meticulous cleansing of the bite wound. WASH THE WOUND THOROUGHLY with lots of soap and water, then rinse it with strong alcohol. If you do not carry alcohol stronger than 40% in the vehicle, whiskey or a similar product that may be available in the patient's home will do. If the bite is on an extremity, splint the injured limb, and take the patient to the hospital.

Management of Animal Bites

1. TAKE A VERY CAREFUL HISTORY to determine
   a. the TYPE OF ANIMAL RESPONSIBLE (if wild, call police to search for the animal and kill it).
   b. WHETHER THE BITE WAS PROVOKED.
   c. whether the biting animal was BEHAVING STRANGELY.
2. EXAMINE THE WOUND to see whether the skin was broken.
3. WASH THE WOUND THOROUGHLY with soap and water; rinse with alcohol.
4. SPLINT a bitten extremity.
5. TRANSPORT the patient to the hospital.

HUMAN BITES

Among the nastiest bites a person can suffer are those inflicted by another human. In actuality, most human bites are not really bites at all, but occur when a person's knuckles come in contact with another person's teeth during an altercation. The reason that human bites are so serious is that the human mouth is a septic tank of noxious bacteria. Thus any wound caused by a human bite is, by its very nature, heavily contaminated, and the risk of infection is high.

Given the above considerations, the most important principle in treating a human bite wound is to GET THE WOUND AS CLEAN AS POSSIBLE AS QUICKLY AS POSSIBLE. Use lots of soap and water or antiseptic solution and *scrub!* Then cover the injury lightly with a sterile dressing, and move the patient on into the hospital. Even if the wound appears to be a minor one, the patient *must* be evaluated in the hospital, since severe infectious complications may occur if the wound is not properly taken care of, particularly if the wound is on the hand.

EVERY VICTIM OF A HUMAN BITE MUST BE EVALUATED IN THE HOSPITAL.

BITES AND STINGS OF ARTHROPODS

The phylum Arthropoda includes at least a million and a half known species of "joint-footed" animals, ranging from the lobster to the mite. The arthropod classes of medical importance, because of the possibility of envenomation, are principally the Arachnida (including spiders, scorpions, ticks), Chilopoda (centipedes), and Insecta (including the hymenoptera: bees, hornets, wasps, ants). In this section, we will consider the injuries caused by hymenoptera, spiders, scorpions, and ticks.

HYMENOPTERA STINGS

The hymenoptera family of insects includes bees, wasps, hornets, yellow jackets, and ants. Members of this family kill more people each year than all other venomous animals, including snakes. When death occurs, it is usually due to a severe anaphylactic reaction, the signs and treatment of which have been discussed in Chapter 23. We will confine our remarks here to the recognition and management of the sting itself.

When a person is stung by one of the hymenoptera clan, there is almost always an immediate local reaction of burning PAIN, REDNESS, SWELLING, and sometimes ITCHING. In examining the site, one will usually see a raised, white area in the middle of a larger, red, swollen area. If the culprit was a honeybee, chances are that the stinger and its venom sac are still attached to the victim's skin because the honeybee is a kamikaze: Its attack is a suicidal one. A wasp or ant, on the other hand, can remove its stinger from the victim after the evil deed is done and thus can make a clean getaway or even sting again if so inclined.

The treatment of an uncomplicated bee sting is aimed at relieving the victim's pain and preventing infection. First, DETERMINE WHETHER THE STINGER IS STILL ATTACHED TO THE SKIN. If so, use a knife blade to scrape the stinger and its sac sideways out of the wound. Do *not* try to pluck the stinger out with a tweezers or similar instrument. Squeezing will only pump more venom into the wound.

Once the stinger is out, CLEAN THE WOUND THOROUGHLY with soap and water or antiseptic solution. COLD PACKS applied to the sting will help relieve pain. Not every victim of a bee sting needs to be treated in the hospital, and the majority of bee stings cause no serious complications. If, however, there is even the slightest suspicion of a systemic reaction—symptoms such as headache, weakness, generalized itching—the patient must be brought to the hospital with all possible speed, and treatment for anaphylaxis (see Chapter 23) should be initiated en route.

Be on the lookout for the patient who has suffered MULTIPLE STINGS, as may occur when someone disturbs a hornets' nest and the angry inhabitants come swarming out en masse. Even in a nonallergic individual, a large dose of hymenoptera venom can cause severe systemic poisoning, with violent vomiting and diarrhea and sometimes coma. It is estimated that about 500 stings are enough to kill the average adult, but life-threatening poisoning may occur with considerably fewer stings. Thus the patient with more than a few stings should be checked in the hospital. The same goes for the patient who has been stung about the eyes, for severe swelling may occur in such cases.

If the patient is without systemic symptoms and is left at home, instruct him or her in the warning signs of anaphylaxis and the urgency of getting to a hospital if any of those symptoms occur. Also tell the patient to have the wound rechecked it if is not markedly improved in 24 hours. Secondary infections are common after bee stings, and usually such infections require antibiotic therapy.

Treatment of Hymenoptera Stings

1. REMOVE THE STINGER, if present.
2. CLEAN THE WOUND THOROUGHLY.
3. Apply a COLD PACK to the wound.
4. TRANSPORT to the hospital if
   a. There is ANY SUSPICION OF A SYSTEMIC REACTION.
   b. There are MULTIPLE STINGS.
   c. There are STINGS AROUND THE EYES.

SPIDER BITES

In the United States, three types of spiders prompt visits to the emergency room: the black widow spider, the brown recluse spider, and the tarantula. In fact, only the first two of these harbor poisonous venom, but the imposing appearance of the tarantula and the popular mythology associated with it often impel the victim of a tarantula bite to call for emergency assistance. Let us take these creatures one by one.

Black Widow Spider

It is the female black widow spider that causes all the problems, for she is the one that does the biting. Her body is button-shaped and glossy black; on average, it is about 1/2 inch long, and the leg span adds another inch or so to the overall length. Her abdomen is marked by a characteristic red or orange "hourglass" (Fig. 27-2).

The black widow is found almost everywhere throughout the United States but particularly in the Ohio valley, the South, and the West Coast. She likes to hang around rocks, debris, basements, garages, and outhouses—and her presence in the last-mentioned habitat makes for some painful bites in sensitive places.

The bite of the black widow spider may not be very painful initially. Most victims recall only a small pinprick of pain, if they recall anything at all. Very soon after the bite occurs, however, a DULL, NUMBING PAIN develops in the bitten area and rapidly spreads, within 15 to 20 minutes, to neighboring muscle groups. If the bite is on a lower extremity, muscle spasm of the abdomen will usually occur, causing a RIGID, BOARDLIKE BELLY that may be mistaken for an acute abdomen. If an upper extremity is bitten, the spread of pain and muscle spasm is more apt to be into the shoulder, back, and chest. NAUSEA, VOMITING, HEADACHE, and SWEAT-

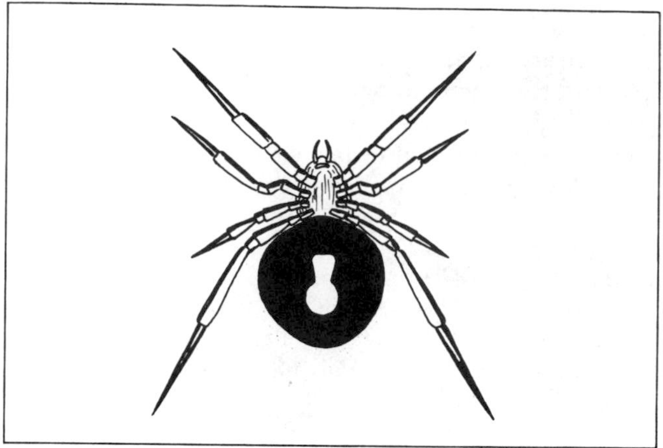

Fig. 27-2. *Black widow spider.*

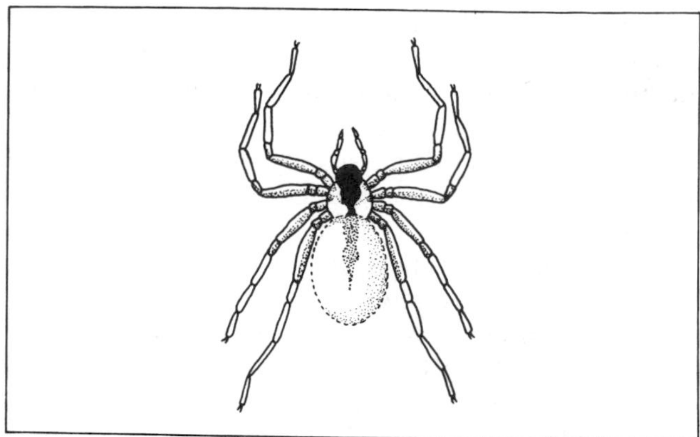

Fig. 27-3. *Brown recluse spider.*

ING are common systemic symptoms. In severe cases, these symptoms may progress to PARALYSIS, SEIZURES, SHOCK, and RESPIRATORY ARREST.

In evaluating the victim of a suspected black widow spider bite, first of all, try to LOCATE THE BITE, which may or may not be obvious. Look for an area of swelling, and scrutinize such an area closely for tiny red fang marks. Note the patient's overall condition, and record the VITAL SIGNS.

In managing the patient, first of all, CLEAN THE BITE AREA THOROUGHLY. If the bite is on an extremity, SPLINT THE EXTREMITY, for movement of an envenomed limb hastens the absorption of the poison. APPLY A COLD PACK to the wound, to provide pain relief and to slow absorption of the venom. Needless to say, if there are seizures, shock, coma, or respiratory arrest, these must be given priority and treated as outlined in previous chapters.

The cornerstone of treatment is the administration of a specific antivenin that neutralizes the effect of the black widow's venom, and to receive this therapy, the patient must reach the hospital. Radio ahead, so that the hospital staff can begin to hunt around for the closest source of antivenin.

If at all possible, TAKE THE SPIDER TO THE ER for definitive identification. Usually the spider gets away, but occasionally it is killed while in the act of biting, and its earthly remains should be preserved and taken to the hospital.

Brown Recluse Spider (Brown Fiddleback)

The brown recluse spider is smaller than the black widow, and it can be identified by a fiddle-shaped marking on its back (Fig. 27-3). It is found throughout the southern and upper midwestern United States, but its common presence in warehouses makes it a frequent interstate traveller; the brown recluse may arrive in virtually any part of the country after hitch-hiking in a freight shipment from one region to another. The brown recluse likes to hang out in closets, attics, trunks, stored shoes and clothing; outdoors, it prefers to be in woodpiles or beneath rocks.

The bite of the brown recluse is usually painless, and often the victim does not notice the spider or realize that a bite occurred. Pain begins several hours later, when the bitten area becomes red and tender, and one or more small blisters start to form. Over several days, as the venom continues its local tissue destruction, the bitten area becomes dark and ulcerated. A black scab forms, which is later sloughed off leaving a depressed, ugly scar.

Systemic reactions are uncommon, but when they occur, they usually come on about 24 hours after the bite and consist of headache, weakness, drowsiness, joint pains, fever, and measles-like rash. Such symptoms tend to be more severe in children.

Emergency treatment at the scene consists of CLEANING THE WOUND THOROUGHLY and applying COLD PACKS to relieve pain. It is enormously helpful if the spider can be retrieved and taken to the hospital for identification, but this is seldom feasible for, by the time symptoms develop, the culprit is generally long gone.

Tarantula

The tarantula is a large, hairy spider—its body alone is about 2 inches long!—with a very sinister reputation, owing in part to its imposing size and appearance. North American tarantulas, found principally in the Southwest, are relatively harmless to man, although some of their Central American cousins may be poisonous.

The bite of a tarantula produces a local reaction of PAIN and EDEMA. If the victim saw what bit him, there is also likely to be considerable panic. Field treatment, then, consists first of REASSURANCE. Calm the victim down, and explain that the bite, while painful, is not dangerous. CLEAN THE WOUND, and apply a COLD PACK to it for relief of pain.

Management of Spider Bites: General Principles

1. CALM AND REASSURE THE VICTIM.
2. CLEAN THE WOUND THOROUGHLY.
3. If the bite is on an extremity, SPLINT the bitten extremity.
4. Monitor VITAL SIGNS.
5. Wherever possible, TAKE THE SPIDER in with the patient.

SCORPION STINGS

Among the 30 or so species of scorpion that live in the United States, only two possess a dangerous venom, and these two make their homes chiefly in very dry areas of the Southwest, especially Arizona and vicinity. The other scorpions produce a painful but harmless sting that can be managed with simple measures, such as cleansing and application of cold packs.

The venom of the Arizona-type scorpion has a very strong affinity for nervous system tissues. The sting is quite painful and produces a PINS-AND-NEEDLES SENSATION that spreads to involve the entire limb. Systemic reactions begin in about an hour and may be heralded by itching in the nose, mouth, and throat together with difficulty in speech. The victim first becomes exicted, then DROWSY AND NUMB. There is markedly increased SALIVATION. The muscles begin to twitch, and severe MUSCLE SPASMS follow. NAUSEA, VOMITING, and SEIZURES are common. In severe cases, RESPIRATORY ARREST may occur. In untreated patients, if the victim survives more than three hours, he or she will usually recover spontaneously.

There is a specific antivenin available for treatment of an envenomed scorpion bite, and field management is aimed at supporting vital functions until the patient can reach a facility where such antivenin can be administered. APPLY COLD PACKS to the bitten area, and apply a CONSTRICTING BAND about 2 inches proximal to the bite, to retard absorption of the venom. RADIO AHEAD to the receiving hospital so that arrangements can be made to obtain the appropriate antivenin. En route to hospital, be alert for seizures and respiratory problems, and treat accordingly.

TICKS

Ordinarily, the bite of a tick is not a medical emergency. Occasionally., however, the bite of a tick—especially on the back of the head, neck, or spine—may produce a potentially life-threatening paralysis, which cannot be reversed unless the tick is removed. Any case of unexplained weakness in a child or in someone who has been out in the woods should prompt a close inspection of the patient's body for the presence of one of these pesky creatures. Even when ticks are not a medical emergency, they should be removed promptly, for ticks can transmit a variety of serious illnesses, including Lyme disease, Rocky Mountain spotted fever, and tularemia.

Ticks attach themselves very doggedly to their victims by their mouth parts, and attempts to remove them forcibly may leave the mouth parts embedded in the skin. If a tick is found, it should not be twisted or squeezed. Instead, use a curved forceps (or *gloved* fingers) to grasp the tick by the head as close to the skin as possible and pull straight upwards. Use even pressure as you pull: avoid twisting or jerking the tick. Do not squeeze or crush the tick's body. Do not handle the tick with bare hands (handling ticks or crushing them can result in disease transmission even without a tick bite). Use gloves or, better still, a forceps. Dispose of the tick in a container of alcohol, or flush it down the toilet. Once the tick has been removed, wash the wound thoroughly with soap and water. In the case of tick paralysis, provide supportive treatment as needed en route to hospital.

The recognition and management of various arthropod bits and stings are summaried in Table 27-2.

STINGS OF MARINE ANIMALS

The beach is a nice place to spend a weekend. It is also a good place to run afoul of mother nature in the form of creatures that inhabit the local waters. There are a large variety of marine animals that produce harmful reactions in man when they bite, sting, puncture the skin, or are eaten. We will deal here with a few representative examples of different types of injuries produced by these creatures. The EMT is advised to become familiar with the potentially harmful marine animals in his or her region. Also, please note that the treatment of some of these injuries requires materials not ordinarily stocked on an ambulance (e.g., meat tenderizer), and the ambulance service operating in an area where marine animal hazards are present should modify its equipment lists accordingly.

COELENTERATES (STINGING MARINE ANIMALS)

The coelenterates are characterized by tentacles equipped with **nematocysts**, or stinging cells. The group includes the JELLYFISH, PORTUGUESE MAN-OF-WAR, ANEMONES, and STINGING CORALS. Stings from these creatures usually occur on the legs. There is intense, sometimes excruciating pain, which may be so severe that it disables a swimmer and causes him to drown. Systemic symptoms may also occur, including faintness, weakness, chills, fever, and even shock and death.

Table 27-2. *Common Arthropod Bites and Stings*

Arthropod	Identification	Signs and Symptoms of Sting	Emergency Treatment
Hymenoptera	Biwinged, three body segments	Painful sting Multiple stings produce gastrointestinal symptoms, coma Anaphylactic reactions	Local reaction: Remove stinger, clean wound, apply cold. Anaphylactic reactions: basic life support, oxygen, epinephrine, intravenous fluids.
Spiders			
Black widow	Shiny, black body, red hourglass on belly	Violent pain and muscle spasms, headache, nausea, sweating, paralysis, seizures, shock	Clean wound, apply cold, treat for seizures, shock, respiratory depression as needed.
Brown recluse	Small, brown, fiddle-shaped mark on back	Very painful, ulcerated wound; sometimes headache, weakness, drowsiness, fever, rash	Clean the wound, transport.
Tarantula	Large, black, long hairy legs	Pain and edema at site of bite	Reassurance, clean the wound, apply cold pack.
Scorpion	Crablike, with long segmented tail	Painful sting Arizona type may cause drowsiness, numbness, salivation, muscle spasms, nausea, vomiting, seizures	Nontoxic: Wound care, cold pack. Toxic: Immobilize extremity, constricting band, cold pack, basic life support as needed.
Tick	Ovoid, fused body, six legs	Rare cases of paralysis	Remove tick with gasoline, clean wound, basic life support as needed.
Puss caterpillar	Teardrop shape, furry pointed tail	Severe burning pain radiating into armpit or groin; redness, swelling, blisters	Apply cold pack to point of "hair" contact.
Fire ant	Large, bright red	Multiple bites in clusters with intense burning; systemic effects in allergic persons, or as in black widow spider bites	Clean wound, cold packs. Anaphylactic reaction: basic life support, oxygen, epinephrine, intravenous fluids.

In treating the victim of a coelenterate sting, first RINSE THE INJURED PART IN SEA WATER. Do not use fresh water. Do not scrub the injured area. Inspect the wound and TRY TO REMOVE ANY TENTACLES adhering to it (wear gloves!). Then POUR VINEGAR OVER THE WOUND to fix the nematocysts onto the skin and prevent further stinging. If vinegar is not available, use 40 to 70 percent alcohol. For sea nettles, use a slurry made from baking powder and water instead of vinegar or alcohol. After several rinses with vinegar, apply a DRY POWDER to the area, which will make the nematocysts stick together. A MEAT TENDERIZER is ideal because it also neutralizes the acid venom. Then use a knife or spatula to SCRAPE THE NEMATOCYSTS OFF THE SKIN. The best way to remove the nematocysts, in fact, is to *shave* them off, using a razor and shaving cream. Once the nematocysts have been removed, rinse the injured part again with ocean water.

Treat any systemic reactions as needed. Any patient who does have a systemic reaction to a coelenterate sting (e.g., hypotension, wheezing, vomiting) should be taken to the hospital for observation. Be alert for anaphylactic reactions in individuals who are frequent beach-goers and have suffered similar stings in the past.

ECHINODERMS AND OTHER PUNCTURING ANIMALS

Echinoderms are spiny sea creatures—such as sea urchins and spiny starfish—that produce their harmful effects by puncturing the victim's skin with a toxic material. Stingrays and salt water catfish operate according to a similar mechanism. Generally injury occurs when one of these creatures is accidentally stepped on or unwisely handled, and the resulting puncture may be extremely painful. Numbness and muscle weakness also occur. Because of the usual mechanism of injury, most of these wounds occur on the feet.

In managing a puncture wound from an animal of this type, first check to see whether any of the creature's little spines have broken off in the wound; if so, TRY TO REMOVE THE SPINE from the wound. The next step is to inactivate the venom, and this is done by taking advantage of the fact that most of these venoms are destroyed by high temperatures. A bucket of quite hot water (up to 45°C, or 113°F) should be prepared, and the patient should immerse *both* the injured and the uninjured foot in HOT WATER for 30 to 90 minutes. The reason for immersing the uninjured foot is to protect the injured foot from burns; the injured extremity may be relatively numb and insensitive to excessively high temperature, so the uninjured foot serves as a safety device to warn the patient if the water is too hot.

POISONOUS FISH

There are a variety of different marine animals that may produce poisoning if ingested, including puffer fish, ciguatera, contaminated shellfish, and many otherwise harmless fish (such as mackerel and tuna) that have been improperly preserved. Symptoms of these poisonings usually involve headache, muscle pains, nausea, vomiting, and sometimes respiratory distress. In the case of poisoning due to paralytic shellfish (i.e., shellfish—usually bay clams, muscles, or certain oysters—that have been feeding on poisonous plankton), there is burning and tingling about the face, lips, and tongue; intense thirst; weakness; salivation; and paralysis.

The treatment of such poisonings in the field is supportive. Provide basic life support as needed, and transport to the hospital. Be alert for signs of laryngeal edema (hoarseness, stridor), and move with all possible speed to a medical facility if these signs are present.

CASE HISTORY

The patient is a 31-year-old man who was bitten on the right calf by a rattlesnake while hiking. His companion killed the snake and went for help. The ambulance arrived at the scene about 45 minutes after the bite was sustained. The patient at that time complained of burning pain in his right leg, weakness, and nausea. He had no significant past medical history and no known allergies.

On physical examination, the patient appeared pale and apprehensive. He was sweating profusely. Pulse was 124 and regular, BP was 100/70, and respirations were 28 and somewhat shallow. Positive findings were limited to the right calf, where there was considerable swelling. Fang marks were visible.

The wound was washed with green soap solution. The right leg was splinted. On orders from Dr. Jones, an intravenous infusion was started with normal saline at a rate of 200 ml per hour. The patient was carried to the ambulance and transported supine to the hospital with his injured leg slightly dependent. En route, the patient became somewhat delirious, but vital signs remained unchanged.

Questions to think about:

1. Is the patient showing any signs of envenomation? If so, what signs?
2. Why was the right leg splinted?
3. Why was an intravenous infusion started and run at such a rapid rate?
4. Why was the right leg kept slightly dependent (i.e., below the level of the rest of the body) during transport?
5. Did the EMTs forget anything?

VOCABULARY

antivenin Serum containing antibodies to a specific animal venom, administered to counteract the effects of a venom.

envenomation Process by which a venom or toxin is deposited in a wound.

hymenoptera Class of insects that includes honey bees, hornets, wasps, yellow jackets, and ants.

nematocyst Stinging cell at the end of a tentacle in jelly fish, stinging corals, and similar animals.

toxin Poison produced by a living creature, such as bacteria, poisonous snakes.

venom Poisonous substance produced by a snake, spider, bee.

FURTHER READING

BITES OF REPTILES

Anker R et al. Retarding the uptake of "mock venom" in humans: Comparison of three first aid techniques. *Med J Australia* 6(5): 212, 1982.

Arnold R. Controversies and hazards in the treatment of pit viper bites. *South Med J* 72:909, 1979.

Of bites and stings. *Emerg Med* 15(11):121, 1983.

Boyden TW. Snake venom poisoning: Diagnosis and treatment. *Ariz Med* 37:639, 1980.

Gill KA. The evaluation of cryotherapy in the treatment of snake envenomization. *South Med J* 65:552, 1970.

Kitchens CS et al. Envenomation by the eastern coral snake (*Micrurus fulvius fulvius*): A study of 39 victims. *JAMA* 258:1615, 1987.

Kunkel DB et al. Reptile envenomations. *J Toxicol Clin Toxicol* 21:503, 1984.

Kunkel DB. Treating snake bites sensibly. *Emerg Med* 20(12):51, 1988.

Pearn J et al. Efficacy of a constrictive bandage with limb immobilization in the management of human envenomation. *Med J Australia* 6(6):293, 1981.

Podgorny G. Snakebite in the United States. *Ann Emerg Med* 12:651, 1983.

Russell FE. *Snake Venom Poisoning*. Philadelphia: Lippincott, 1980.

Stewart ME et al. First-aid treatment of poisonous snakebite: Are currently recommended procedures justified? *Ann Emerg Med* 10:331, 1980.

Streiffer RH. Bite of the venomous lizard, the Gila monster. *Postgrad Med* 79:279, 1986.

Wasserman GS. Wound care of spider and snake envenomations. *Ann Emerg Med* 17:1331, 1988.

Watt CW. Snakebite: Don't cool it. *Emerg Med Serv* 8(3):10, 1979.

Wingert WA. Rattlesnake bites in southern California and rationale for recommended treatment. *West J Med* 148:37, 1988.

MAMMALIAN BITES

Aghababian V et al. Mammalian bite wounds. *Ann Emerg Med* 9:79, 1980.

Anderson LJ et al. Human rabies in the United States, 1960 to 1970: Epidemiology, diagnosis, and prevention. *Ann Intern Med* 100:728, 1984.

Baker MD, Moore SE. Human bites in children: A six-year experience. *Am J Dis Child* 141:1285, 1987.

Burdge D., Scheifele D, Speert D. Serious Pasteurella multocida infections from lion and tiger bites. *JAMA* 253:3296, 1985.

Callaham ML. Dog bite wounds. *JAMA* 244:2327, 1980.

Callaham ML. When an animal bites. *Emerg Med* 20(11):119, 1988.

Centers for Disease Control. Compendium of animal rabies vaccines 1985. *MMWR* 33(51–52). 1984.

Faralli VJ. Human bite wounds of the hand. *J Okla State Med Assoc* 79:87, 1986.

Libby J., Meislin H. Human rabies. *Ann Emerg Med* 12:217, 1983.

Lindsey D et al. Natural course of the human bite wound: Incidence of infection and complications in 434 bites and 803 lacerations in the same group of patients. *J Trauma* 27:45, 1987.

Ordog GJ et al. Rat bites: Fifty cases. *Ann Emerg Med* 14:131, 1985.

Paisley JW, Lauer BA. Severe facial injuries to infants due to unprovoked attacks by pet ferrets. *JAMA* 259:2005, 1988.

Sacks JJ, Sattin RW, Bonzo SE. Dog bite-related fatalities from 1979 through 1988. *JAMA* 262:1489, 1989.

Tahzib A. Camel injuries. *Trop Doc* 14:187, 1984.

The who and how of rabies prophylaxis. *Emerg Med* 16(14):159, 1984.

ARTHROPOD BITES AND STINGS

Curry SC et al. Envenomation by the scorpion centruroides sculpturatus. *J Toxicol Clin Toxicol* 21:417, 1984.

Fire ants—too hot to handle. *Emerg Med* 17(12):75, 1985.

Frazier CA. Emergency treatment of insect stings and bites. *Emerg Med Serv* 6(4):8, 1977.

Ginsburg CM. Fire ant envenomation in children. *Pediatrics* 73:689, 1984.

Green VA et al. Bites and stings of hymenoptera, caterpillar, and beetle. *J Toxicol Clin Toxicol* 21:491, 1984.

Jonas M., Cunha B. The ticks of summer. *Emerg Med* 14(12):146, 1982.

Kobernick M. Black widow spider bite. *Am Fam Phys* 29:241, 1984.

Kunkel DB. The myth of the brown recluse spider. *Emerg Med* 17(5):124, 1985.

Kunkel DB. The sting of the arthropod. *Emerg Med* 20(12):41, 1988.

Needham GR. Evaluation of five popular methods for tick removal. *Pediatrics* 75:997, 1985.

Rauber A. Black widow spider bites. *J Toxicol Clin Toxicol* 21:473, 1984.

Thygerson A. Tick bites. *Emergency* 13(6):26, 1981.

BITES AND STINGS OF MARINE ANIMALS

Auerbach PS. Stings of the deep. *Emerg Med* 21(12):26, 1989.

Burnett JW, Calton GJ. Jellyfish envenomation syndromes updated. *Ann Emerg Med* 16:1000, 1987.

Kizer KW. Marine envenomations. *J Toxicol Clin Toxicol* 21:527, 1984.

Kizer KW et al. Scorpaenidae envenomation: A five-year poison center experience. *JAMA* 253:807, 1985.

Raynor AC et al. Alligator bites and related infections. *J Flor Med Assoc* 70:107, 1983.

Rosson CL et al. Management of marine stings and scrapes. *West J Med* 150:97, 1989.

Schultz K. Hazardous marine life. *Emerg Med Serv* 14(3):62, 1985.

Stein MR et al. Fatal Portuguese man-o'-war (Physalia physalis) envenomation. *Ann Emerg Med* 18:312, 1989.

Stings of the sea. *Emerg Med* 14(13):183, 1982.

28. COMMUNICABLE DISEASES

OBJECTIVES

Because of the nature of the job, an EMT routinely comes in contact with a great many sick people, some of whom have illnesses that are communicable, that is, illnesses that can be transmitted to another person. The EMT must have a general familiarity with such illnesses, so that he or she can take appropriate measures to avoid personal illness and to prevent the vehicle and its equipment from becoming sources of infection to other patients. In this chapter, we shall look at the general nature of communicable diseases and the precautionary measures that these diseases require. By the conclusion of this chapter, the reader should be able to

1. List the ways in which communicable diseases can be transmitted, and indicate how the risks of each type of transmission can be minimized
2. Identify the correct definition of (a) contamination, (b) carrier, (c) reservoir, (d) communicable period, (e) incubation period, given a list of definitions
3. Identify a patient with probable (a) meningitis, (b) active tuberculosis, (c) viral hepatitis, given a description of several patients with various signs and symptoms, and indicate how each of these illnesses is transmitted
4. List the ways in which AIDS is known to be transmitted, and list the precautions necessary when transporting a patient known to have AIDS
5. List the routine immunizations every EMT should have and explain the importance of immunization against German measles for women and immunization against mumps for men
6. List the routine measures that should be taken to minimize the spread of communicable diseases by ambulance personnel
7. List the steps in decontaminating the vehicle, its equipment, and exposed personnel after transporting a patient known to have a communicable disease

TRANSMISSION OF COMMUNICABLE DISEASES

A communicable disease is a disease that is "catching," or contagious, by virtue of being caused by a microorganism (such as a virus or bacteria) that can be transmitted from one person to another. Such transmission can take place in a variety of ways. The most obvious is by DIRECT CONTACT with the infected person—for instance, a handshake during which bacteria pass from one person's hand to that of another. In some instances, this direct contact may be of a very intimate nature, as in diseases transmitted by SEXUAL CONTACT. Alternatively, the viruses or bacteria may be transmitted by CONTACT WITH CONTAMINATED MATERIALS, such as a handkerchief, clothing, or bedding. Germs can also be acquired by INHALATION OF INFECTED DROPLETS that are propelled through the air by the sneeze of an infected person (that is why you should cover your mouth and nose when you sneeze or cough!). BITES FROM INFECTED ANIMALS (including man) OR INSECTS can effectively deposit microorganisms in the victim's body, as can dirt falling into an open wound or contaminated food taken into the stomach.

A distinction must be made here between contamination and infection. Any person, animal, or thing that has harmful microorganisms on it or in it is **contaminated**. This applies to water, food, dressings, bedding, other equipment, and even the ambulance itself. A person is not **infected**, however, unless the microorganisms cause an illness or other abnormal state. Some people walk around all the time with harmful microorganisms residing happily in their bodies and are not sick from those microorganisms. Such individuals are called **carriers**; that is, they carry an infectious agent and, although they are not themselves ill, they can transmit the illness to others.

Another concept that is important is that of a reservoir. In the context of communicable diseases, a **reservoir** is a place where germs live and multiply. In the ambulance, for instance, the oxygen humidifier is a common reservoir of infection.

Once a person is exposed to a harmful microorganism, it takes a variable amount of time for that microorganism to multiply in the person's body and produce symptoms. That time period—between exposure to the germ and the first appearance of symptoms—is called the **incubation period.** In chicken pox, for instance, it takes 2 to 3 weeks from the time a susceptible person is exposed to the chicken pox virus until the beginnings of fever and headache are felt. It should be pointed out that a given infectious disease is generally contagious only during a portion of the illness. A person may, for instance, be sick with measles for a couple of weeks, but he is capable of transmitting measles to someone else only for a part of that time. The portion of an illness during which an infected person is capable of transmitting the illness is called the **communicable period.**

The risks of handling people who have communicable diseases should not be exaggerated. The risks are there, granted, and the EMT needs to be aware of them. But these risks can be kept to a minimum by taking appropriate precautions, and the fact that a patient has a communicable disease should not cause undue worry or reluctance to transport the patient.

In the following section, we will look briefly at a few common or worrisome communicable diseases to illustrate some of the concepts discussed here.

EXAMPLES OF COMMUNICABLE DISEASES

There are many communicable diseases to which the EMT may be exposed in the course of work. We will look here at a few of those illnesses that often cause particular concern among exposed personnel. A more extensive summary of commonly encountered communicable diseases may be found in Table 28-1.

MENINGITIS

Meningitis is an inflammation of the membranes that cover the brain and spinal cord. Few other illnesses, except perhaps AIDS, elicit so much panic among ambulance personnel, although in the majority of cases, there is little need for exposed personnel to exercise anything more than routine precautions.

Meningitis may be caused by a variety of different bacteria, viruses, and other microorganisms, and the contagiousness of the disease depends to some extent on the type of microorganism involved. Meningitis caused by the bacteria *meningococcus* is probably the most worrisome from the point of view of contagion, and this type of meningitis is especially likely to spread rapidly in places where many people are confined, such as military barracks.

In general, TRANSMISSION of bacterial meningitis occurs through droplet spread (i.e., bacteria expelled in a sneeze or cough) or *direct* contact with an infected person or carrier. Indirect transmission—through contact with objects recently soiled with the patient's secretions—is insignificant since the meningococcus is not a very hardy bacteria and is easily killed by chilling or drying. Meningococcal meningitis occurs most frequently in children and adolescents, but it is also seen occasionally in adults. The greatest incidence is in winter and spring.

The classic SIGNS AND SYMPTOMS of meningitis include FEVER, HEADACHE, and STIFF NECK AND BACK. Often there are CHANGES IN THE STATE OF CONSCIOUSNESS, ranging from apathy to delirium. VOMITING is common. In meningococcal meningitis, as opposed to that caused by other bacteria, the onset of symptoms is often quite sudden, and, in addition, there is frequently a characteristic RASH, which may be blotchy red or bluish. Other types of meningitis tend to come on more slowly, preceded by a few days of sore throat, runny nose, and other upper respiratory symptoms.

The INCUBATION PERIOD for meningococcal meningitis ranges from 2 to 10 days (the average is 3 to 4 days). The COMMUNICABLE PERIOD is variable and lasts as long as the bacteria are present in the patient's nasal and oral secretions. Usually the meningococcus disappears from the patient's upper respiratory tract within 24 hours after antibiotic treatment has been started.

If you are transporting a patient with suspected meningitis, you can minimize your risk of infection by wearing a disposable surgical mask while in contact with the patient and by washing your hands thoroughly once that contact is terminated. The vehicle should then be thoroughly aired and cleaned, and all linen or bedding that the patient came in contact with should be laundered. Stay in touch with the hospital to find out what type, if any, meningitis was diagnosed; if it was meningococcal, consult your physician about any other measures you should take. Sometimes a course of antibiotics is given as a preventive measure.

TUBERCULOSIS

Tuberculosis, or TB, was once a widespread and dreaded disease that took an enormous toll among young people. Today, its incidence in the United States is very low, and effective treatment is available for those who do contract the illness.

TRANSMISSION of the bacteria that cause tuberculosis usually occurs by droplet spread, that is, by inhaling droplets expelled in a sneeze or a cough by a person with active TB. In general, this type of spread occurs chiefly among people who have continued and intimate exposure to the infected individual, such as those living in the same household. For the EMT, such exposure is likely to occur only in the case where mouth-to-mouth ventilation has been given to a patient with active tuberculosis. TB is *not* spread on hands, dishes, utensils, or other such objects.

The SIGNS AND SYMPTOMS of a person's initial infection with TB may be minimal. In fact, there may be no symptoms at all, and usually the disease lies dormant for many years before the signs that are commonly associated with TB—night sweats, headache, cough, weight loss—occur. Early infection with TB can, however, be detected with a special skin test, called a **tuberculin test**, and also with chest x-rays. Every health care worker should have a tuberculin test at the beginning of employment and annually thereafter and should be x-rayed if the tuberculin test becomes positive.

Since the INCUBATION PERIOD for tuberculosis is 4 to 8 weeks, the EMT who suspects he or she has been exposed to TB should wait about two months from the time of exposure before getting a tuberculin test. If it is found that the tuberculin test has become positive, the individual will usually be given a year's course of antibiotic therapy. The vehicle and fixed equipment used in the transport of a patient with suspected active TB should be thoroughly aired and cleaned. Linens should be laundered, and disposable equipment that was in contact with the patient, such as an oxygen mask, should be incinerated.

VIRAL HEPATITIS

There are several forms of viral hepatitis. *Type A* (formerly called *infectious hepatitis*) accounts for about 30 percent of hepatitis cases in the United States. Type A hepatitis generally occurs in young people and may break out in epidemics. TRANSMISSION is most commonly through fecal-oral contamination, that is, by touching something that has been in contact with the patient's excretions (such as the patient's hands or bathroom utensils). The ingestion of contaminated water, milk, or other foods such as uncooked shellfish, is also responsible for some outbreaks. Finally, accidental puncture with a needle that has been used in a patient with hepatitis can also transmit the disease. Infectious hepatitis has an INCUBATION PERIOD of 15 to 50 days (usually around 30 days). The COMMUNICABLE PERIOD is variable, for some patients may remain carriers for many months after their symptoms have disappeared.

A second major type of viral hepatitis, called *Type B* (formerly called *serum hepatitis*) accounts for 50 percent of cases in the United States and has a much longer INCUBATION PERIOD—anywhere from 14 to 180 days. In the vast majority of cases, TRANSMISSION is by sexual contact or by needle: accidental puncture with a contaminated syringe, sharing of needles among drug addicts, or use of contaminated tattooing instruments. Thus the EMT is unlikely to contract serum hepatitis unless he or she is inadvertently stuck by a needle that was used on an infected person.

A third type of viral hepatitis is called *non-A, non-B hepatitis*—a name that reflects our relative ignorance about the virus that causes it. Non-A, non-B hepatitis is most commonly transmitted by transfusion or accidental puncture with a contaminated needle.

All types of viral hepatitis have similar SIGNS AND SYMPTOMS. There is usually a period of vague systemic symptoms: loss of appetite, generalized fatigue and the "blahs," fever, abdominal discomfort, and sometimes flu-like symptoms, lasting anywhere from 2 to 14 days. Smokers often report a sudden distaste for cigarettes during this period. After about a week of vague symptoms, the patient usually notices that his or her URINE BECOMES DARK. A few days later, JAUNDICE—a yellowing of the skin and the sclerae of the eyes—becomes evident. It should be noted that NOT EVERY CASE OF JAUNDICE IS DUE TO HEPATITIS. Many other, noncontagious illnesses may produce jaundice, but the presence of jaundice should nonetheless alert the EMT to take special precautions.

What kind of PRECAUTIONS are necessary? To begin with, all emergency medical personnel should be immunized with the hepatitis B vaccine. This is a

Table 28-1. *Profiles of Communicable Diseases*

Disease	Characteristics	Transmission	Incubation Period	Communicable Period	Necessary precautions	
					For personnel	For vehicle
AIDS	Decreased resistance to many infections	Sexual contact; contaminated needles or blood products	May be months to years	Not known	Mask, gloves, gown, wash hands	Air, scrub, launder linen
Chicken pox	Usually in children, fever	Oral and nasal secretions; direct and droplet contact	2–3 wk	1 day before rash to 6 days after	Shower, change clothes	Air, scrub, boil linen
Diphtheria	Severe sore throat, fever	Oral and nasal secretions; direct or indirect contact	2–5 days	2–4 wk	Mask if not immune	Air, scrub, disinfect, launder linen
German measles	Fever, rash, sore throat	Oral and nasal secretions; direct, indirect, or droplet contact	14–21 days	7 days before rash to 4 days after	Mask if not immune	Air, scrub, launder linen
Gonorrhea	Yellow urethral discharge	Sexual intercourse	3–4 days	Until treated	Routine	Air, launder linen
Hepatitis Infectious	Loss of appetite, lethargy, jaundice, dark urine, fever	Oral and fecal secretions, contaminated food, water, contaminated needles	15–50 days	Variable	Care in handling IV equipment	Air, scrub, launder linen
Serum		Contaminated needles	50–180 days	Variable		
Influenza	Fever, myalgias, sore throat, upper respiratory symptoms	Droplet spread	1–3 days	7 days	Wear mask	Air, scrub, launder linen
Measles	Fever, rash, cough	Droplet spread	10 days	4 days before rash to 5 days after	Mask if not immune	Air, scrub, launder linen
Meningitis	Fever, headache, stiff neck, vomiting, coma	Droplet spread	2–10 days	Variable	Wear mask, antibiotic treatment if close contact	Air, scrub, disinfect linen
Mononucleosis	Fever, swollen glands, sore throat, fatigue	Mouth-to-mouth	2–6 wk	Unknown	Routine	Disinfect equipment soiled with oral secretions
Mumps	Fever, swollen parotid glands, orchitis in adult men, sometimes pancreatitis	Saliva, droplet spread	12–26 days	9 days after swelling	Mask if not immune	Air, scrub, launder linen

Table 28-1. Continued

Disease	Characteristics	Transmission	Incubation Period	Communicable Period	Necessary precautions	
					For personnel	For vehicle
Pneumonia	Fever, chills, cough, chest pain	Respiratory secretions, direct or indirect contact, carriers	Variable	Variable	Routine	Air, scrub, launder linen
Scarlet fever	Fever, sore throat, rash, headache, vomiting	Respiratory secretions	2–5 days	Unknown	Mask, shower, change clothes, boil dirty clothes	Air, scrub with germicide, boil linen
Spotted fevers	Fever, headache, rash on palms and soles	Infected tick	3–10 days	Tick's life span	Gloves, remove ticks	Destroy all ticks
Syphilis	First lesion a sore, later rash, final stage cardiac and cerebral symptoms	Saliva, semen, vaginal discharge, sexual intercourse	10 days–10 wk	Variable	If scratched or bitten, consult doctor	Air, launder linen
Tuberculosis	Weight loss, night sweats, cough, hemoptysis, fatigue	Droplet spread	4–8 wk	Until treated	Mask, annual tuberculin test	Air, scrub, launder linen
Typhoid fever	Anorexia, diarrhea, fever	Feces and urine, direct and indirect	2 wk	Until treated	Wash hands	Air, scrub, incinerate soiled linen
Whooping cough	Violent, stridorous cough, fever	Droplet spread	1–3 wk	1–3 wk	Shower, boil clothes	Air, scrub, boil linen

very effective vaccine, but it gives protection only against serum hepatitis. Thus care is still required in handling patients with undiagnosed jaundice. It is vital, then, that all needles and intravenous equipment used for a patient with jaundice be handled and disposed of carefully. The EMT should also wash his or her hands thoroughly after contact with a jaundiced patient. The vehicle and equipment used in the transport should be aired and cleaned. Stay in touch with the receiving hospital to find out whether a diagnosis of infectious (Type A) hepatitis was made. If so, consult your physician about getting a shot of immune globulin.

COMMON CHILDHOOD DISEASES

We need to say one or two words about some of the common childhood illnesses—measles, mumps, chicken pox—for while these illnesses generally are not dangerous, there are some special circumstances of which the EMT should be aware. First, let us consider GERMAN MEASLES, or rubella. In children, this is a relatively mild illness, with an incubation period of 2 to 3 weeks, characterized by fever, sore throat, runny nose, and a red rash. It is highly contagious and is spread by droplets sneezed or coughed into the air by an infected person. Where German measles becomes dangerous is in women during the first three months of pregnancy, for the rubella virus may cause very serious birth defects in the developing fetus. For this reason, every woman who has not had German measles should be vaccinated against rubella before puberty. Women working as EMTs should make certain they are properly immunized against rubella before beginning employment as an EMT.

The other viral illness we need to mention is a problem for men, and that is MUMPS. In children, mumps is usually a mild and self-limited illness, characterized by fever, swelling of the parotid glands, sore throat, and similar symptoms. In adult men, however, mumps can be an extremely painful illness, with severe swelling of the testicles (**orchitis**) that can lead to sterility. For this reason, male EMTs who have not had mumps as children should be immunized against mumps before beginning employment.

AIDS

Few illnesses since the Black Plague of the Middle Ages have caused as much hysteria as the acquired immunodeficiency syndrome, or AIDS—a hysteria all out of proportion to the present incidence and communicability of the disease. As of July 31, 1989, there had been approximately 100,000 reported cases of AIDS in the United States, and among those known to have AIDS, there had been a mortality rate of about 59 percent since reporting of the disease first began, in 1981. Compare these figures to the 165,000 deaths per year from trauma, or the 500,000 deaths per year from cardiovascular disease, and one begins to wonder what all the hysteria is about. Nonetheless, there is an enormous fear of AIDS among the public; 70 perent of Americans surveyed in a 1987 Gallup poll believed AIDS to be *the* most urgent health problem in the United States. Every day newspapers report incidents in which patients suffering from AIDS were refused ambulance services or hospital admission or even the services of funeral homes because of other people's fear.

Why has AIDS caused so much panic? First of all, it is a relatively new disease. And even though medical science has made extraordinary progress in discovering its cause, there are still many things about AIDS that remain unknown. It is that element of the unknown that inspires a great deal of the fear. In addition, AIDS seems to strike mostly at young people in the prime of life, people with whom it is easy to identify. Finally, a very high percentage of those who develop clinically evident AIDS die, and we do not at present have any effective cure for the condition.

The intense fear of AIDS, then, comes about mostly from ignorance about the illness. There is no excuse, however, for medical personnel to remain ignorant about the disease or to act out of ignorance toward patients who are suffering from AIDS. So what, then, *do* we know about AIDS?

- AIDS is caused by a virus—human immunodeficiency virus (HIV)—either alone or in combination with other microorganisms.
- In the Western world, AIDS is primarily a disease of male homosexuals and intravenous drug users.
- In the majority (about 55–60 percent) of cases, AIDS is transmitted by sexual contact. Another 20–25 percent of AIDS patients acquire the disease through sharing contaminated needles during intravenous drug use.
- Approximately 12,000 people in the United States contracted AIDS from transfusion of HIV-contaminated blood or blood products before routine HIV screening of banked blood was instituted in 1985. Most of the recipients of those contaminated blood products were hemophiliacs (people with a disease that prevents normal clotting of blood), who receive large numbers of transfusions.
- As of this writing, there are 11 health care workers worldwide who appear to have become infected with HIV through on-the-job contact with AIDS patients, their blood or other body fluids. The most frequent mechanism of infection among those health workers was accidental needle stick injury. In three cases, HIV-infected blood came in contact with broken skin, and in one case HIV infection followed a splash of blood to the face of a health worker who had facial acne.
- There have been no documented cases of work-related transmission of HIV to *any* EMS provider anywhere in the world.
- There have been no reported cases of HIV transmission as a consequence of performing mouth-to-mouth resuscitation or of practicing CPR on a mannikin.
- There have been no recorded cases of AIDS among people living in intimate contact with AIDS patients, except among spouses of AIDS patients who had sexual relations with the patient.

All evidence, then, points to the fact that AIDS is NOT a highly communicable disease. The only known means of transmission are through sexual contact, contaminated blood products, puncture with a contaminated needle, or across the placenta from mother to fetus.

While panic and hysteria are *not* warranted, sensible precautions *are* indicated—not just when dealing with patients known to have AIDS, but for contact with every patient; for it is impossible to determine just from taking a history or physical examination which patients are infected with the AIDS virus. Studies have shown that as many as one out of every twenty patients presenting to an urban emergency department tested positive for HIV (in patients with penetrating trauma, such as gunshot wounds, the proportion was even higher—nearly one in seven was HIV positive). For that reason, the Centers for Disease Control now recommend that blood and body-fluid precautions be consistently used for *all* patients, and those precautions are therefore referred to as "universal precautions."

> DON'T TAKE CHANCES! OBSERVE BLOOD AND BODY-FLUID PRECAUTIONS WITH *ALL* PATIENTS.

- Wear GLOVES whenever there is potential exposure to blood or other body fluids. Use heavy-duty rubber gloves for extricating accident victims or cleaning up contaminated areas. Wear surgical latex gloves for performing venipunctures, touching mucous membranes or nonintact skin, or whenever there is a possibility of exposure to blood or body fluids. Change gloves after contact with each patient. Discard used gloves immediately after use in an appropriate receptacle (e.g., plastic bag with a 'biohazard' label). Wash your hands immediately after you remove your gloves.

- Use additional barrier protection (MASK, PROTECTIVE EYEWEAR, FACE SHIELD, GOWN) during any procedure that is likely to generate splashes of blood or other body fluids.
- WASH YOUR HANDS or any other skin surfaces immediately and thoroughly if they become contaminated with blood or other body fluids.
- Handle all NEEDLES, INTRAVENOUS EQUIPMENT, and SHARP INSTRUMENTS with extreme care.
  1. *Never* recap, remove, bend, or break needles after use or manipulate them in any other way by hand.
  2. Dispose of syringes, needles, scalpel blades, and other sharp items in puncture-resistant containers, which should be kept within easy reach.
- Although saliva has *not* been implicated in HIV transmission, it is preferable for health workers to use a pocket mask (with one-way valve) or bag-valve-mask for artificial ventilation. Such devices, therefore, should always be immediately accessible—which you can ensure by always carrying a pocket mask where it was intended to be carried—in your pocket.

When the patient is known to have AIDS or is in a high-risk group (for example, a known intravenous drug user), additional routine precautions are recommended:

- Restrict pregnant EMTs from contact with known AIDS patients. While pregnancy does not increase susceptibility to AIDS, the potential consequences of HIV infection in a pregnant woman are grave, for both mother and fetus are likely to be infected. Furthermore, AIDS patients, because of their deficient immunity, often harbor other viruses, such as cytomegalovirus, that are potentially damaging to a developing fetus.
- After the transport, air out the vehicle and clean the interior thoroughly with disinfectant solution such as a 1:10 dilution of sodum hypochlorite (household bleach). Incinerate any disposable items, such as oxygen masks, that were in contact with the patient. Double-bag used linens, tag them with a biohazard label, and make sure the linens are laundered in hot water.

With commonsense precautions, like those above, there should be no danger of an EMT contracting AIDS from a patient. And there can be NO justification for an ambulance service *ever* refusing transport to a patient with AIDS. Medical professionals, by virtue of the profession they have chosen, have an obligation to care for any person who comes to them for help. Medical professionals also have a responsibility to teach the public by the example of their own behavior. The doctor, nurse, or EMT who refuses to provide his or her services to a patient with AIDS—or any patient, for that matter—abdicates that responsibility and brings discredit on the whole medical profession.

IMMUNIZATIONS

The overall immunization schedule for medical personnel is fundamentally the same as for the general public, with the addition of vaccination against hepatitis B, but it is particularly important that medical personnel make sure their immunizations are complete and up-to-date. These should include the following:

Immunizations for EMTs

- DPT (Diphtheria-Pertussis-Tetanus), tetanus booster every 10 years
- MEASLES
- MUMPS
- POLIO
- RUBELLA (German measles)
- HEPATITIS B

In addition, EMTs should have a checkup and a tuberculin test once a year.

PRECAUTIONARY MEASURES

Part of the EMT's job is to ensure that neither the ambulance personnel, the vehicle, nor the emergency equipment become sources for transmitting disease. Most of this preventive work can be accomplished through strict adherence to simple, routine procedures. In certain cases, more extensive measures are required.

ROUTINE MEASURES

The most important measures for preventing the transmission of contagious diseases are simply a matter of good personal habits. It should be an automatic and unwavering practice for the EMT to wash his or her hands thoroughly after *every* case. After transferring the patient to the care of emergency room personnel and completing any necessary records, head straight for the sink. Wash your hands with surgical scrub solution (pHisoHex or a povidone-iodine solution), and use a surgical scrub brush to get underneath the fingernails. Simply dipping your hands in a little water will not do!

WASH YOUR HANDS THOROUGHLY AFTER EVERY CALL.

As for equipment, use disposable equipment wherever possible, and dump the used equipment in a proper receptacle promptly at the end of the case. Do not carry used equipment around in the ambulance until the end of the shift. If it is disposable, dispose of it! Used linen or soiled blankets should be stashed promptly in the laundry. Equipment that is not disposable, such as the bag-valve-mask unit, should be thoroughly cleaned with soap and water followed by antiseptic solution after each use. Air the ambulance between trips, and establish a regular schedule for thorough cleaning of the ambulance interior—floor, ceiling, walls, and fixed equipment—at least once a day.

Routine Measures to Control the Spread of Disease

- WASH YOUR HANDS AFTER EVERY CALL.
- USE DISPOSABLE EQUIPMENT wherever possible, and dispose of used disposable equipment promptly.
- DISINFECT NONDISPOSABLE EQUIPMENT AFTER EACH USE.
- REMOVE LINENS AFTER EACH USE.
- AIR THE AMBULANCE AFTER EACH RUN.
- SCRUB THE AMBULANCE INTERIOR ONCE A DAY, or more often as needed.

MEASURES FOR KNOWN EXPOSURE TO COMMUNICABLE DISEASE

When it is necessary to transport a patient who has a known or suspected communicable disease, certain additional measures are recommended. These measures can be categorized according to whether they are taken before, during, or after the transport of the patient.

Before Transport

If there is advance notification that the patient has a contagious disease, the following measures should be taken prior to transport.

- FIND OUT THE NATURE OF THE ILLNESS, if known. Where possible, ambulance personnel with documented immunity should be selected for the trip (e.g., EMTs who have had chicken pox to transport a child with chicken pox).
- REMOVE ALL UNNECESSARY EQUIPMENT FROM THE VEHICLE.
- TAKE DISPOSABLE GOWNS AND MASKS for each crew member.
- MAKE UP THE STRETCHER WITH DISPOSABLE LINEN.
- TAKE PLASTIC BAGS to use later for stashing contaminated materials.

While Caring for the Patient

- DON A MASK AND GOWN before examining the patient.
- KEEP YOUR HANDS AWAY FROM YOUR FACE.

After Transferring the Patient

- PLACE IN SEPARATE PLASTIC BAGS
  1. all contaminated, disposable supplies, including protective masks and gowns worn during the call
  2. all contaminated linens and bedding
  3. all contaminated, nondisposable equipment

  Follow hospital procedures regarding disposal of bag 1. If the hospital does your laundry, leave bag 2 in the appropriate receptacle, and tag it as contaminated. Take bag 3 back to base for thorough cleaning of equipment with soap and water, followed by disinfectant solution.
- EMPTY THE AMBULANCE AND AIR IT OUT. Although airing the vehicle probably does not contribute to decontamination, it does help remove unpleasant odors. Clean and disinfect all the equipment you have removed from the vehicle. Give particular attention to respiratory equipment such as humidifiers and tubing.
- After airing, SCRUB ALL INTERIOR SURFACES OF THE AMBULANCE WITH SOAP AND WATER. THEN SCRUB AGAIN WITH A DISINFECTANT. Ninety percent isopropyl alcohol, phenolic germicide, or an alcohol-formaldehyde preparation may be used as a disinfectant.
- If you were not wearing protective garments during the call, remove all your clothing and stash it in a plastic bag until it can be laundered. Take a good, hot shower, and put on a complete change of clothes.
- WASH YOUR HANDS AGAIN WHEN YOU HAVE FINISHED CLEANING THE VEHICLE AND ITS EQUIPMENT.

Sometimes, it is not known until after the ambulance returns from a call that the patient had a contagious illness. In such instances, besides carrying out the procedures outlined above, it is important to notify any personnel who might have had contact with the patient. In addition, if another patient was transported with the infected patient, or if another patient was transported afterwards in the same vehicle (before the vehicle was disinfected), the physician of that patient should be notified.

VOCABULARY

carrier Person who harbors an infectious agent and, although not himself ill, can transmit the infection to another person.

communicable disease Disease that can be transmitted from one person to another.

communicable period Period during which an infected person is capable of transmitting his illness to someone else.

contamination Presence of harmful microorganisms on or in any person, animal, or object.

hepatitis Inflammation of the liver.

incubation period Period from infection until the appearance of the first symptoms.

jaundice Yellow coloring of the skin and sclerae.

meningitis Inflammation of the membranes covering the brain and spinal cord.

orchitis Inflammation of the testicles.

reservoir Place where germs live and multiply.

rubella Another name for German measles.

tuberculin test Skin test to determine if a person has been infected with tuberculosis.

FURTHER READING

GENERAL INFECTION CONTROL

Dettman G. Practicing infection control. *Emergency* 21(1):54, 1989.

Feiner B. Infectious diseases: Actual vs. perceived exposures. *Emerg Med Serv* 17(10):27, 1988.

LaForce FM. Immunizations, immunoprophylaxis, and chemoprophylaxis to precent selected infections. *JAMA* 257:2464, 1987.

West KH. Infection control. *Emerg Med Serv* 12(1):53, 1983.

West KH. *Infectious Disease Handbook for Emergency Care Personnel*. Philadelphia: Lippincott, 1987.

CHILDHOOD DISEASES

Centers for Disease Control. Mumps—United States, 1983–1984. *MMWR* 33(38), 1984.

Greaves, WK et al. prevention of rubella transmission in medical facilities. *JAMA* 248:861, 1982.

Howard J et al. Rubella immunization policies for health care personnel. *J Fam Pract* 17:805, 1983.

Schlech WF III et al. Bacterial meningitis in the United States, 1978 through 1981. *JAMA* 253:1749, 1985.

Strassburg MA et al. Rubella in hospital employees. *Infect Contr* 5:123, 1984.

HEPATITIS

Bader T. A protocol for needle-stick injuries. *Emerg Med* 18(2):36, 1986.

Centers for Disease Control. Recommendations of the immunization practices advisory committee update on hepatitis B prevention. *MMWR* 36(23), 1987.

Clawson JJ et al. Prevalence of antibody to hepatitis B virus surface antigen in emergency medical personnel in Salt Lake City, Utah. *Ann Emerg Med* 15:183, 1986.

Francis DP et al. The safety of the hepatitis B vaccine: Inactivation of the AIDS virus during routine vaccine manufacture. *JAMA* 256:869, 1986.

Iserson KV, Criss EA. Hepatitis B prevalence in emergency physicians. *Ann Emerg Med* 14:119, 1985.

Kunches LM. Hepatitis B exposure in emergency medical personnel: Prevalence of serologic markers and need for immunization. *Am J Med* 75:269, 1983.

Maddrey WC. Viral hepatitis today. *Emerg Med* 21(16):124, 1989.

Moss WD. Hepatitis B. *Emerg Med Serv* 12(5):48, 1983.

Pepe PE et al. Viral hepatitis risk in urban emergency medical services personnel. *Ann Emerg Med* 15:454, 1986.

Schwartz JS. Hepatitis B vaccine. *Ann Int Med* 100:149, 1984.

Snyder M. Management of health care workers remotely vaccinated for hepatitis B who sustain significant blood and body fluid exposures. *Infect Control Hosp Epidemiol* 9:462, 1988.

Valenzuela TD. Occupational exposure to hepatitis B in paramedics. *Arch Intern Med* 145:1976, 1985.

AIDS

American College of Emergency Physicians. AIDS—statement of principles and interim recommendations for emergency department personnel and prehospital care providers. *Ann Emerg Med* 17:1249, 1988.

Baker J. What is the occupational risk to emergency care providers from the human immunodeficiency virus? *Ann Emerg Med* 17:700, 1988.

Burrow GN. Caring for AIDS patients: The physician's risk and responsibility. *Canad Med Assoc J* 129:1911, 1983.

Centers for Disease Control. First 100,000 cases of acquired immunodeficiency syndrome—United States. *JAMA* 262:1453, 1989.

Centers for Disease Control. Recommendations for prevention of HIV transmission in health-care settings. *JAMA* 258:1293, 1987.

Centers for Disease Control. Update: Human immunodeficiency virus infections in health-care workers exposed to blood of infected patients. *MMWR* 32:285, 1987.

Cueva KG. The AIDS factor. *Emergency* 21(1):48, 1989.

Curran JW et al. Acquired immunodeficiency syndrome (AIDS) associated with transfusions. *N Engl J Med* 310:69, 1984.

Friedland G. AIDS and compassion. *JAMA* 259:2898, 1988.

Gerbert B et al. Why fear persists: Health care professionals and AIDS. *JAMA* 260:3481, 1988.

Hahn RA et al. Prevalence of HIV infection among intravenous drug users in the United States. *JAMA* 261:2677, 1989.

Hardy AM et al. The incidence rate of acquired immunodeficiency syndrome in selected populations. *JAMA* 253:215, 1985.

Kelen GD et al. Human immunodeficiency virus infection in emergency department patients. *JAMA* 262:516, 1989.

Landesman SH et al. The AIDS epidemic. *N Engl J Med* 31:521, 1985.

Marcus R et al. Surveillance of health care workers exposed to blood from patients infected with the human immunodeficiency virus. *N Engl J Med* 319:1118, 1988.

Nordberg M. AIDS/Infection control: Critical issues for EMS. *Emerg Med Serv* 17(10):35, 1988.

Ornato JP. Providing CPR and emergency care during the AIDS epidemic. *Emerg Med Serv* 18(4):45, 1989.

Redfield R et al. Frequent transmission of HTLV-III among spouses of patients with AIDS-related complex and AIDS. *JAMA* 253:1571, 1985.

Sande MA. Transmission of AIDS: The case against casual contagion. *N Engl J Med* 314:380, 1986.

Skeen WF. Acquired immunodeficiency syndrome and the emergency physician. *Ann Emerg Med* 14:267, 1985.

VII. ENVIRONMENTAL EMERGENCIES

"Everyone complains about the weather," said Mark Twain, "but no one does anything about it." Nearly 100 years later, people are still complaining about the weather and extremes of temperature—and are still dying on account of them. For in addition to the discomfort and inconvenience they bring, very hot or very cold environmental conditions can cause harmful and even fatal effects on the human body. In this section, we will examine the health hazards of the summer heat waves and winter freezes. We will look as well at another environmental hazard that Mark Twain did not have to worry about but that is very much a part of modern life—the hazard of radiation exposure.

29. HEAT EXPOSURE

OBJECTIVES

When one thinks of death from the heat, one tends to imagine exotic tropical or desert scenes—scores of British soldiers languishing in the "Black Hole of Calcutta" or hundreds of Moslem faithful collapsing during the pilgrimage to Mecca. In fact, however, death from the heat is not an uncommon occurrence in the United States, where an estimated 4,000 people succumb every year to the "dog days" of summer. In this chapter, we will examine the mechanisms that the body uses to protect itself from excessive heat and the types of illness that can occur when those mechanisms are overwhelmed. By the end of the chapter, the reader should be able to

1. Identify the mechanisms by which the body normally gets rid of excess heat and indicate the limitations of these mechanisms
2. Identify a patient with (a) heat cramps, (b) heat exhaustion, and (c) heat stroke, given a description of several patients with different signs and symptoms
3. Identify the correct treatment for (a) heat cramps, (b) heat exhaustion, and (c) heat stroke, given a list of possible treatments
4. List at least five measures that can be taken to minimize the risk of heat illness

HOW THE BODY EXCRETES EXCESS HEAT

The human body likes to maintain a temperature very close to 98.6°F (37°C), for it is at this temperature that the many complex enzyme systems of the body function best. In order to keep a constant temperature, however, the body must have some means of getting rid of the heat it generates in the normal course of metabolism.

The body's first response to an increase in internal temperature is to try to move the heat to the surface, where it can be more easily dissipated into the atmosphere. The way the body does this is by sending more blood to the skin surface; thus blood vessels near the surface of the body dilate to be able to hold the increased volume. This is the reason that a person who is overheated appears flushed.

Once at the body surface, the extra heat has to be shed into the atmosphere. This is accomplished through three mechanisms: convection, radiation, and conduction. CONVECTION refers to the loss of heat that takes place when moving air picks up the heat and carries it away. Convection is the principle one uses instinctively when blowing on hot food to cool it down. RADIATION occurs when heat is simply emitted from the body into the surrounding atmosphere without the help of moving air currents. A radiator used to heat a room is so named because it operates by this mechanism. CONDUCTION refers to the dissipation of heat into a solid object or a liquid

of heat stroke are changes in behavior—irritability, combativeness, signs that the patient is hallucinating—which may mislead the rescuers into thinking that the patient is "crazy" or "high" on drugs. Other victims of heat stroke may present with signs similar to those of a cerebrovascular accident (stroke). If you don't *suspect* heat stroke in such patients, treatment may be tragically delayed.

> SUSPECT HEAT STROKE AND CHECK A TEMPERATURE IN ANY PERSON BEHAVING STRANGELY IN A HOT ENVIRONMENT.

The SKIN is VERY HOT AND USUALLY DRY, reflecting the patient's VERY HIGH BODY TEMPERATURE (usually over 105°F) and lack of sweating (about 50 perent of patients *will* be sweating when first seen). Skin color is PINK OR ASHEN in Caucasians. The PULSE is RAPID, and it may be bounding or thready, depending on whether dehydration is a factor. Similarly, the blood pressure may be normal or low, again depending on upon how much, if any, fluid was lost through sweating. RESPIRATIONS are VERY RAPID, for the overheated body is burning oxygen faster than it can replace it from the atmosphere.

In the TREATMENT of heat stroke, time is critical. The brain cannot tolerate extremely high temperatures for any significant period, nor can the heart keep up with the enormous demands that very high temperatures impose upon it.

> HEAT STROKE IS A LIFE-THREATENING EMERGENCY. EVERY SECOND COUNTS!

The most important aspect of the treatment of heat stroke is to COOL THE PATIENT DOWN AS FAST AS POSSIBLE. How you go about this will depend on where you find the patient. When the patient is found in his home, it has traditionally been recommended that he be immersed in a bathtub filled with ice water to promote heat loss by conduction. There are, however, several major drawbacks to that method. To begin with it is unpleasant for the patient, who, if confused, may not be in any mood to cooperate. Furthermore, it is very awkward for the rescuers to try to manage a patient in a bathtub, especially if the patient starts to have seizures or loses consciousness. Immersion in ice water, furthermore, is apt to promote shivering, which simply increases the patient's metabolic heat production. Finally, it is very difficult to transport a patient who is in a bathtub—so transport often has to be delayed if cooling is done by conduction. For all those reasons, many experts now recommend using cooling methods that rely primarily on radiation and convection. In the home, quickly remove the patient's clothing and apply ice packs to his flanks, while massaging his neck and torso to prevent a vasoconstrictive response to the ice. Move him rapidly into the bathroom and start spraying him with *tepid* water, while fanning him constantly to promote rapid evaporation. (For that purpose, it is worthwhile for ambulances to carry a small electric fan during summer months. A standing fan can then be activated in the bathroom of the patient's home and directed at the patient as he is being sprayed with water from the shower.) Do not stop cooling procedures until the patient's rectal temperature has dropped below 103°F (39.4°C).

If the patient is found outside the home, use any means available to begin cooling him. At a construction site, for example, strip the patient to his undershorts and begin hosing him down while your partner fetches every cold pack in the ambulance. Use the cold packs to rub the victim's arms, flanks, and legs, and place ice packs in his armpits and around the groin. GET as many people to help as possible.

Once cooling has been initiated, administer OXYGEN by nasal cannula (6 liters/min). Remember, the body's need for oxygen is enormously increased when the body temperature is very high, and it is partly this increased need for oxygen that is making the heart work overtime. So give the heart a break by giving the patient the extra oxygen he needs.

As soon as you have a chance, start an INTRAVENOUS INFUSION with normal saline or Ringer's solution. The *amount* of fluid you will need to give the patient will depend on the type of heat stroke the patient is suffering. If there are signs of shock (hypotension, thready pulse), you can run the fluid in relatively quickly—about 100 to 200 ml per hour. Otherwise, keep the IV at a slow rate, to keep the vein open.

As soon as feasible, TRANSPORT the patient to the hospital. Once you are on your way to the hospital, continue rubbing the patient's body with cold packs or handfuls of ice. Do *not* cover the patient with sheets soaked in ice water, as was previously recommended in many first aid courses; covering the patient with wet sheets, in fact, impedes heat loss through evaporation. Keep close tabs on the VITAL SIGNS, especially the temperature; once the temperature falls to around 102°F (38.8°C), you can stop the ice treatments, for otherwise you might overdo it.

Management of Heat Stroke

1. COOL THE PATIENT AS FAST AS POSSIBLE: Continue cooling until body temperature falls below 103°F (39.4°C).
2. Administer OXYGEN by nasal cannula at 6 liters per minute.
3. Start an INTRAVENOUS INFUSION with normal saline or Ringer's solution; consult physician for flow rate.
4. Monitor VITAL SIGNS closely.
5. TRANSPORT to the hospital as soon as possible; continue cooling en route as necessary.

The characteristics of the various heat syndromes are summarized in Table 29-1.

PREVENTION OF HEAT ILLNESS

The heat syndromes that we have discussed in this chapter are all ENTIRELY PREVENTABLE. You and the patients you serve can get through those dog days of summer relatively unscathed by following a few commonsense guidelines:

How to Avoid Heat Illness

- ACCLIMATIZE YOURSELF to the hot weather. Limit strenuous activity or sun exposure to 15 minutes the first hot day, then add 15 minutes each day thereafter.
- WEAR LIGHT-COLORED, LOOSE-FITTING CLOTHING that deflects the sun's rays and permits adequate evaporation of sweat.
- STAY IN COOL PLACES as much as possible. AVOID SUDDEN CHANGES IN TEMPERATURE.
- PARK THE AMBULANCE IN THE SHADE.
- INCREASE YOUR DAILY INTAKE OF FLUIDS AND SALT, and increase your intake even more when you are exercising.
- REST AFTER EVERY 30 MINUTES OF EXERTION.
- BEWARE OF
  1. Temperatures over 85°F.
  2. Humidity over 60 percent.

  Avoid unnecessary exertion when those conditions are present.
- IF YOU FEEL ANY SYMPTOMS OF HEAT ILLNESS (e.g., headache, nausea, cramps in the extremities or abdomen), GET OUT OF THE HEAT AND GET MEDICAL ATTENTION.

THE HOT WEATHER KIT

It is a good idea for ambulance services to carry a special hot weather kit during those parts of the year that temperatures are apt to rise above the mid-80s°F. The kit should include a supply of towels for the EMTs (a cool, damp towel around the neck helps dissipate heat by conduction) and a portable ice

Table 29-1. *Heat Syndromes*

Characteristic	Heat Cramps	Heat Exhaustion	Heat Stroke
Predisposing factors	Strenuous work in hot place; heavy sweating with large intake of water without salt; victim usually in good physical condition	Strenuous exercise; diuretics; diarrhea or vomiting; elderly	Chronic disease; old age; alcoholism; phenothiazine or atropine drugs
Mechanism	Loss of salt	Loss of water and salt; hypovolemia	Failure of temperature-regulating system of the body
Symptoms	Painful spasms in legs and abdomen	Weakness, nausea, vomiting, dizziness, fainting	Headache, weakness, dizziness, delirium, coma
State of consciousness	Alert	May be slightly disoriented	Confused, delirious, or in coma
Body temperature	Normal	Normal or subnormal	Very high (over 105°F)
Skin	Cool, moist	Pale, cool, clammy	Usually hot, red, dry
Pulse	Normal or slightly fast	Rapid, thready	Rapid; thready in classic heat stroke, bounding in exercise-induced heat stroke
Blood pressure	Normal	Decreased	Usually normal early; hypotension in exercise-induced heat stroke
Respirations	Normal	Slightly increased	Tachypnea
Treatment	Cool environment; salted fluids by mouth; rest	Rest; cool place; IV saline	Spray and fan; oxygen; IV saline

chest, like those used for picnics. Stock the ice chest with:

- Malleable ice packs, for placement in the axillae and groin of a patient with heatstroke. You can make your own ice packs by filling rubber gloves with an alcohol/water solution (in a 1:3 ratio of rubbing alcohol to water), tying them off, and then freezing them. The alcohol will prevent them from freezing solid, so they can be molded to fit body curves.
- Gator-Ade or other salt-containing drinks, for both patients and ambulance crew. Stock a generous supply of such drinks, and imbibe them liberally throughout your shift when you are working in hot conditions.
- Frozen containers of water and bags of ice cubes, to keep everything else cold. As the ice cubes start to melt, pour some of the cold water onto the towel you're wearing around your neck.

CASE HISTORY

The patient is a 70-year-old man who was found delirious at home. The ambulance was called by a home health aide, who discovered the patient highly confused and staggering about when she came for her regular daily visit. She stated that the patient seemed all right yesterday, although he was complaining then of a headache and nausea. He is under treatment for hypertension and heart disease. He takes nitroglycerin and diuretics regularly.

The patient's apartment was extremely hot, and we found the patient dressed in winter clothes. He was delirious and completely disoriented; he did not recognize the home health aide and could not tell us his name. His skin was burning hot and dry. Pulse was 140 and slightly irregular, BP 110/60, and respirations 40 and shallow. Oral temperature was 106°F. The pupils were dilated but reactive. Neck veins were not distended. The chest was clear.

The patient was immediately stripped and immersed in a tubful of cold water, to which ice was added. His arms and legs were massaged while he was in the tub. Oxygen was administered at 6 liters per minute by nasal cannula, and on orders from Dr. Heiss, an intravenous infusion was started with normal saline at 60 ml per hour. The patient's temperature began to fall within about 5 minutes, and he was removed from the cold water after 35 minutes, when the oral temperature had reached 102.5°F. Vital signs during transport were pulse 128, BP 120/70, respirations 30, and oral temperature 102°F.

Questions to think about:

1. What risk factors for heat stroke did this patient have?
2. Did he have any warning symptoms that heat stroke might be coming on? If so, what were they?
3. Were there any environmental factors contributing to the problem? If so, what factors?
4. What signs of heat stroke was he displaying?

VOCABULARY

conduction Transfer of heat to a solid object or liquid.

convection Mechanism by which body heat is picked up and carried away by moving air currents.

radiation Emission of heat from the body into surrounding, colder air.

FURTHER READING

Birrer RB. Heat stroke: Don't wait for the classic signs. *Emerg Med* 20(12):6, 1988.

Boone WB. Management of heat stroke. *JAMA* 249:194, 1983.

Carter WA. Heat emergencies: A guide to assessment and management. *Emerg Med Serv* 9(4):29, 1980.

Clowers GH, O'Donnell TF. Heat stroke. *NEJM* 291:564, 1974.

Cummings P. Felled by the heat. *Emerg Med* 15(12):94, 1983.

Graham BS et al. Nonexertional heatstroke: Physiologic management and cooling in 14 patients. *Arch Int Med* 146:87, 1986.

Hanson PG. Exertional heat stroke in novice runners. *JAMA* 242:154, 1979.

Knochel PF. Dog days and siriasis: How to kill a football player. *JAMA* 233:513, 1975.

Kunkel DB. The ills of heat. Part I: Environmental causes. *Emerg Med* 18(14):173, 1986.

Larkin JT. Treatment of heat-related illness. *JAMA* 245:570, 1981.

Slovis C, Anderson G, Casolaro A. Survival in a heat-stroke victim with a core temperature in excess of 46.5°C. *Ann Emerg Med* 11:269, 1982.

Sprung CL. Heat stroke: Modern approach to an ancient disease. *Chest* 77:4, 1980.

Stine RJ. Heat illness. *JACEP* 8:154, 1979.

Surpure JS. Heat-related illness and the automobile. *Ann Emerg Med* 11:263, 1982.

Wettach GE, Smith DS, Stalling CE. EMS protocol for management of heat emergencies during a heat wave in an urban population. *EMT J* 5(5):328, 1981.

30. COLD EXPOSURE

OBJECTIVES

The human animal is basically a semitropical being whose body was not designed to endure prolonged exposure to extremes of cold. Being a resourceful creature, however, man has found ways to adapt to cold environments—warm clothing, home heating, sheltered transportation, and so forth. But when exposure to cold does occur, the human body has only a limited capacity to protect itself. Once this capacity is exceeded, injury and even death can occur.

Injury from the cold is chiefly a winter problem, but not exclusively so. A rafting enthusiast who falls into a swift-running stream in summer can die just as quickly from the cold (if not more so) as a hiker lost in a winter blizzard. Thus EMS personnel throughout the United States need to be familiar with the potential hazards of exposure to cold. In this chapter, we will look at the ways in which the body tries to defend itself against extremes of cold and the types of injuries produced when the body's defenses fail. By the end of this chapter, the reader should be able to

1. Identify the ways in which heat is lost from the body, given several situations of potential heat loss, and indicate how heat loss can be prevented in each instance
2. Identify the mechanisms by which the body attempts to prevent or compensate for heat loss in a cold environment
3. Identify a patient with (a) frost nip, (b) superficial frostbite, and (c) deep frostbite, given a description of several patients with various signs and symptoms, and indicate the correct management of each
4. Identify a patient with (a) moderate hypothermia and (b) severe hypothermia, given a description of several patients with various signs and symptoms, and indicate the correct treatment for each
5. Identify errors in management, given a description of cases of (a) frostbite, (b) severe hypothermia, and (c) immersion hypothermia in which incorrect measures were taken

KEEPING WARM

As we learned in the previous chapter, the human body must maintain a nearly constant core temperature in order to function properly. Even very slight changes in core temperature impair the ability to function, and large temperature variations jeopardize survival.

HOW HEAT IS LOST FROM THE BODY

When a person is placed in a cold environment, heat is lost from the body in several ways, some of which we have already discussed. First of all, heat can be lost by RADIATION; any object, including the hu-

Table 30-1. *Windchill Factors*

Wind Speed (mph)	Degrees Fahrenheit 35	30	25	20	15	10	5	0	−5	−10	−15	−20	−25	−30	Wind Description
0–5	35	30	25	20	15	10	5	0	−5	−10	−15	−20	−25	−30	Calm; no breeze
5	33	27	21	16	12	7	1	−6	−11	−15	−20	−26	−31	−35	Leaves rustle
10	21	16	9	2	−2	−9	−15	−22	−27	−31	−38	−45	−52	−58	Leaves move
15	16	11	1	−6	−11	−18	−25	−33	−40	−45	−51	−60	−65	−70	Dust raised; paper blows
20	12	3	−4	−9	−17	−24	−32	−40	−46	−52	−60	−68	−76	−81	Small branches move
25	7	0	−7	−15	−22	−29	−37	−45	−52	−58	−67	−75	−83	−89	Small trees sway
30	5	−2	−11	−18	−26	−33	−41	−49	−56	−63	−70	−78	−87	−94	Large branches move
35	3	−4	−13	−20	−27	−35	−43	−52	−60	−67	−72	−83	−90	−98	Whole trees swaying
40	1	−4	−15	−22	−29	−36	−45	−54	−62	−69	−76	−87	−94	−101	Twigs torn from trees
	VERY COLD		BITTER COLD			EXTREME COLD									

man body, that is warmer than its environment will give off heat into the surrounding air. Heat loss by radiation can occur from any part of the body, but it is most prominent above the shoulders. Indeed, on a cold day, over half the heat generated by the body can be lost through an uncovered head and neck—so your mother's dire warnings about going outside without a hat and scarf were based on sound scientific principles.

A second way that heat can be lost from the body is through CONVECTION; that is, air moving across the body surface picks up heat from the body and carries it away. Still air is a poor conductor of heat. Moving air is much more efficient, and the faster the air is moving, the faster it can remove heat from the body. For this reason, a windy, cold day is much more dangerous in terms of cold exposure than a windless day of the same temperature. Recognizing this fact, the weather bureau has developed the concept of the **windchill factor**, which measures the chilling effect of a given temperature plus a given wind speed. For instance, the chilling effect of a 30°F temperature with a 30 mile per hour wind is −2°F; that is, the net effect is just as if the temperature were actually 2 below zero on a day without any wind. The windchill factor can be determined using a standard table (Table 30-1), and it allows EMS personnel to estimate the degree of cold to which a person was exposed.

Heat can also be lost from the body by CONDUCTION, that is, by direct transfer of heat from the body to a cold liquid or solid. Water conducts heat more than 200 times faster than does air of the same temperature, so a person who falls into a cold lake, for instance, is going to cool down much more rapidly than someone standing in dry air at the same temperature. You do not have to fall into a lake to get wet, however. Clothing soaked with rain, snow, or perspiration is just as dangerous, for it will also conduct heat away from the body with great rapidity.

A fourth mechanism by which heat can be lost from the body is EVAPORATION OF MOISTURE FROM THE BODY SURFACE. Heat is required to vaporize water, and as evaporation occurs, this heat is lost from the body. Evaporative heat loss occurs, for instance, when one's clothes have become wet from sweating or from rain and then the clothing gradually dries. Wet clothes, then, are a double hazard: While they are still wet, they promote heat loss by conduction; as they dry, they cause heat loss by evaporation.

Finally, heat can be lost through RESPIRATION. When air is inhaled into the lungs, its temperature is raised to body temperature; then, when this air is exhaled, it takes the heat with it out into the atmosphere.

COLD HANDS, WARM HEART: HOW THE BODY DEFENDS AGAINST HEAT LOSS

Given all these different ways of losing heat, how does anyone ever stay warm? Fortunately, the body does have a few tricks for beating the cold, so that taking a stroll on a winter day does not have to be a fatal event. First of all, when the body is exposed to cold, it can INCREASE HEAT PRODUCTION. For one thing, the rate of metabolism goes up, with resultant production of more thermal energy. In addition, increases in muscular activity can jack up heat production considerably. Shivering, for example, can increase the body's heat production about 500 percent, while strenuous exercise can bring about increases of heat production of anywhere from 1000 to 2000 percent.

Besides increasing the amount of heat it produces, the body can also DECREASE HEAT LOSS to the environment. In order to understand how this is accomplished, one needs to think of the human body as consisting of two parts: a core and a shell. The **core** comprises the vital internal organs, such as the brain, heart, lungs, and abdominal viscera, whose temperature must be maintained nearly constant. The **shell** includes the skin, muscles, and the extremities, which can tolerate relatively wide temperature variations. The normal functioning of the human body depends critically upon a stable *core* temperature (98.6°F, or 37°C, measured orally). Even a slight drop in this core temperature—just a degree or two—slows down vital functions. Perhaps the most dangerous aspect of this general slowdown is the dulling of mental faculties; as the brain is chilled, thinking becomes sluggish, and for this reason, the victim of cold exposure is usually unaware of the danger he is in.

Because it is so crucial to maintain core temperature, the body will do so at the expense of surface temperature. This is accomplished by constricting the blood vessels to the surface of the body, thereby reducing the amount of blood flow to the body's outer layer. Heat is thus hoarded deep within the body and kept away from the skin, where it would otherwise be lost by convection, radiation, and so forth. In addition, sweating is reduced or stopped altogether. In this way, the skin and subcutaneous tissues function as a cool, dry shell that provides insulation for the vital core. The thicker the shell, the better the insulation, so fat people are relatively more protected from the cold than are skinny people.

The effects of exposure to cold on any given person will depend on the balance between the body's heat loss and heat production.

Balance Between Heat Loss and Heat Preservation

Heat Loss	*Heat Preservation*
RADIATION	INCREASED HEAT PRODUCTION
CONVECTION	Increased metabolic rate
CONDUCTION	Shivering
EVAPORATIVE COOLING	Muscular exertion
	PERIPHERAL VASOCONSTRICTION

If heat loss occurs at a faster rate than heat production, injury from the cold will occur. Such injury takes two forms: (1) local injury to an isolated part of the body and (2) generalized cooling.

LOCAL INJURIES

Most injuries from the cold are localized to the extremities or exposed parts of the body, such as the face. Local freezing injuries fall under the general heading of **frostbite**. Like burns, frostbite can be superficial or deep, depending on the intensity of the cold and the duration of exposure. The mildest form of cold injury, sometimes called "frost nip" or first-degree frostbite, usually involves exposed or poorly insulated parts of the body, such as the tips of the ears, nose, upper cheek, and the tips of the fingers or toes. Frost nip comes on slowly and generally is not painful, so the victim tends to be unaware of its occurrence unless he or she should glance into a mirror and notice an unusual whiteness of the nose, ears, and so forth. The problem is easily treated by placing a warm hand firmly over the chilled nose or ear or, when fingers are frost-nipped, by placing the fingers into the armpit. The return of warmth to the frost-nipped area is usually signalled by some redness and tingling, but tissue damage rarely occurs.

Deeper degrees of frostbite involve actual freezing of body tissues. Body cells are composed chiefly of water, and when cells are subjected to low temperatures, the water within them literally turns into ice crystals, which can damage or destroy the cells. Again, the most commonly affected areas of the body are the hands, feet, ears, and nose, all of which are distant from the warm body core and are also prone to rapid heat loss because of large surface area. There are a number of factors that *predispose* a person to develop frostbite. To begin with, the person who ventures out into the cold and wind inadequately protected against the elements is much more likely to be frostbitten than one who heeds mother's warnings and wears mittens, earmuffs, a scarf, a hat, and so forth. Secondly, anything that inferferes with peripheral circulation increases the likelihood of frostbite, for if warm blood from the body core cannot reach the body surface, the surface has no way of counteracting the external cold. There are all sorts of things that can restrict circulation to the hands, feet, and other exposed areas: tight clothing, especially tight gloves or footwear, underlying arterial disease, with narrowing of the arteries; and even the body's own defense against the cold, by which blood flow is shunted away from the periphery by vasoconstriction. General conditions such as fatigue, dehydration, or poor nutrition also render a person more susceptible to frostbite. Finally, probably the most important predisposing factor for frostbite is generalized body cooling (hypothermia), which will be discussed later in this chapter.

SUPERFICIAL FROSTBITE

Superficial, or second-degree, frostbite is by definition limited to the skin and subcutaneous tissues, like a second-degree burn. The SKIN typically appears WHITE AND WAXY. Because it is frozen, it is STIFF to palpation, but the UNDERLYING TISSUES REMAIN SOFT. Generally sensation is absent, and the patient will usually report that the area feels

NUMB. As *thawing* occurs, the injured area becomes a MOTTLED BLUE, and the patient experiences a hot, stinging sensation. Leakage of plasma from damaged capillaries leads to EDEMA in the frostbitten area, and often BLISTERS develop within a few hours after thawing. Dull or throbbing pain may persist for days or even weeks after the injury, and the injured area usually becomes extremely sensitive to any subsequent exposure to cold.

TREATMENT of superficial frostbite is somewhat different from that of deep frostbite, which we will discuss shortly, so the first step is to TRY TO DETERMINE IF YOU ARE DEALING WITH SUPERFICIAL FROSTBITE ONLY. Usually it is difficult to determine the depth of the injury when you first see it, for even a shallow frostbite injury can appear like one that is frozen solid. If the tissues beneath the skin are soft when you press down on the skin surface, the frostbite is probably superficial. If not, or if there is any doubt, treat it as deep frostbite (see next discussion).

In superficial frostbite, it is very important first to GET THE PATIENT OUT OF THE COLD. Take him indoors or into a heated ambulance, so that the body can stop hoarding its warm blood in the core and can send some of that warm blood out to the periphery, where it is needed. If an ear, nose, or foot is frostbitten, apply firm, steady pressure against the area with a warm hand. If a hand is frostbitten, have the patient insert the hand into his armpit and hold it there without moving. DO NOT RUB OR MASSAGE A FROSTBITTEN AREA, for this will only cause further damage to injured tissues.

A frostbitten area should be covered and protected from further injury. If blisters have already formed, *do not rupture them;* simply cover the blisters with dry, sterile dressings. Do *not* cover frostbitten areas with any sort of ointment, and do *not* rewarm with dry or radiant heat. Transport the patient to a medical facility for evaluation.

Management of Superficial Frostbite

- RECOGNITION: Skin may be cold and stiff, but *underlying tissues remain soft.*
- MOVE THE PATIENT TO A WARM PLACE.
- REWARM THE INJURED PART WITH BODY HEAT (warm hand on cold nose, etc.). Do NOT rewarm with dry or radiant heat.
- DO NOT RUB OR MASSAGE A FROSTBITTEN AREA.
- PROTECT FROSTBITTEN AREAS FROM FURTHER INJURY.
- COVER ANY BLISTERS WITH DRY, STERILE DRESSINGS.
- DO NOT APPLY OINTMENTS TO FROSTBITTEN SKIN.
- TRANSPORT to the hospital with the injured area elevated and protected from cold and bruising.

DEEP FROSTBITE

Deep frostbite usually involves the hands or the feet. It is a very serious injury, which, if improperly handled, can lead to amputation of part or all of a limb. A frozen extremity looks WHITE, yellow-white, or mottled blue-white, and it is HARD, COLD, and INSENSITIVE TO TOUCH. The major tissue damage occurs not from the freezing per se, but during thawing, particularly if thawing occurs gradually. When tissues thaw slowly, there is often partial refreezing of melted water, and the new ice crystals tend to be much larger than those formed during the original freeze, so they cause even greater tissue damage. As thawing occurs, the injured area becomes purple and excruciatingly painful. Gangrene may set in within a few days, requiring amputation of the injured part.

The TREATMENT of deep frostbite depends upon (1) whether the injured extremity has already been partly or completely thawed before you arrive and (2) how far the victim is from the hospital. Let us take these situations one at a time.

If the extremity is still frozen when you find the patient, it is preferable to leave it frozen until the patient reaches the hospital. Rapid rewarming is extremely difficult to carry out properly in the field. Furthermore, the thawing process is usually very painful for the patient, so it should, whenever possible, be carried out in a setting where the patient can be given strong analgesic (pain-killing) medication. For these reasons, if you are within about an hour's drive of a medical facility, LEAVE THE FROZEN EXTREMITY FROZEN, and bring the patient in. *So long as the limb is not thawed,* the patient may even walk on it if necessary. Once you get him into the ambulance, pad the injured extremity to protect the tissues from trauma, and keep it away from the heater or any other sources of dry heat. DO NOT UNDER ANY CIRCUMSTANCES RUB SNOW OR ICE ONTO THE EXTREMITY OR MASSAGE IT IN ANY WAY. Don't forget, the cells are full of ice crystals, and massaging the extremity will simply cause those ice crystals to lacerate delicate tissues. Radio ahead to the receiving hospital, so they can get a rewarming bath prepared.

If the extremity is already partially thawed or if you are several hours from the hospital, it will be necessary to carry out REWARMING in the field. To do this, you will need a water bath—a large, clean container in which the extremity can be immersed without touching the container's side or bottom. Water should be heated in a second container and then stirred into the water bath until the temperature of the bath is between 100 and 108°F (38–42°C).

The injured extremity is then gently immersed in the water bath. Keep a thermometer in the water, and when the water temperature falls below 100°F, temporarily remove the injured extremity from the bath while you add more hot water to the container. Stir the added water around and keep adding more hot water until the bath is again in the right temperature range; then reimmerse the injured extremity. THE TEMPERATURE IN THE WATER BATH MUST BE KEPT AT A CONSTANT 100 TO 108°F. Both lower and higher temperatures will cause further damage to the limb.

The rewarming procedure may require 30 to 60 minutes. It is complete when the frozen area is warm to the touch and is deep red or bluish in color (and remains red when you remove it from the bath). While rewarming is in progress, the patient should be kept warm, preferably indoors, with insulated clothing and blankets. Do not permit the patient to smoke, for nicotine causes vasoconstriction and thereby interferes with blood flow to the injured area.

Once rewarming is complete, dry the extremity VERY GENTLY with sterile dressings. Apply SOFT, STERILE DRESSINGS *lightly* over the thawed parts, being careful not to rupture any blisters. Do *not* apply any ointments to frostbitten skin. Use soft, sterile gauze or cotton to separate frostbitten fingers or toes. Transport the patient supine, with the INJURED EXTREMITY ELEVATED on soft pillows and well covered to protect it from the cold.

A word of caution: DO NOT ATTEMPT REWARMING IN THE FIELD IF THERE IS *ANY* POSSIBILITY OF REFREEZING. The potential damage from refreezing is much greater than that of remaining frozen. So if circumstances will not permit you to keep the extremity thawed out, leave it frozen.

Management of Deep Frostbite

- RECOGNITION: White, hard, cold extremity that is insensitive to touch.
- *If the extremity is still frozen and if you are within an hour's drive of the hospital:*
  1. LEAVE THE EXTREMITY FROZEN.
  2. PROTECT THE EXTREMITY FROM INJURY.
  3. TRANSPORT.
- *If the extremity is already thawing or if you are several hours from the hospital:*
  1. REWARM THE EXTREMITY IN WATER 100 to 105°F until red color returns.
  2. After rewarming, APPLY STERILE DRESSINGS TO THE THAWED AREA.
  3. ELEVATE THE INJURED EXTREMITY ON SOFT PILLOWS.
  4. PROTECT THE INJURED EXTREMITY FROM COLD AND BRUISING.
  5. TRANSPORT.
- Remember the frostbite DON'Ts:
  1. DON'T RUB SNOW ON A FROSTBITTEN PART.
  2. DON'T MASSAGE OR RUB A FROSTBITTEN AREA.
  3. DON'T REWARM WITH DRY OR RADIANT HEAT.
  4. DON'T RUPTURE BLISTERS.
  5. DON'T APPLY OINTMENTS.
  6. DON'T APPLY TIGHT BANDAGES.
  7. DON'T ALLOW A THAWED EXTREMITY TO REFREEZE.
  8. DON'T HANDLE A FROSTBITTEN EXTREMITY ROUGHLY.
  9. DON'T ALLOW THE VICTIM TO SMOKE.

The steps in managing deep and superficial frostbite are summarized in Figure 30-1.

GENERAL COOLING

General body cooling, or **hypothermia**, is more unusual than frostbite, but also much more dangerous; for if body warmth cannot be restored to the hypothermic patient promptly, death is a certainty. Temperatures need not be below freezing for hypothermic death to occur. Indeed, most cases of hypothermia occur in temperatures between 30 and 50°F. The most common victims are the elderly or chronically ill, especially those constantly exposed to cold in poorly heated homes. Alcoholics are also at great risk, for intoxication dulls their sensitivity to cold and may cause them to fall asleep in exposed areas. Alcohol, furthermore, is a vasodilator, so it undermines the body's attempts to constrict peripheral vessels and thereby form an insulating shell around the body core. Hypothermia also occurs in young, healthy individuals who are stranded outdoors in severe weather. In such individuals, poor judgment, poor survival skills, inadequate clothing and shelter, overexertion, and insufficient intake of water and carbohydrates all markedly increase the risk of suffering hypothermia, which has been called for that reason "the killer of the unprepared."

When a person is exposed to the cold, there is a predictable sequence of bodily reactions that reflect progressive fall in core temperature. At the first slight drop in core temperature, just a degree or two, the victim will usually start SHIVERING, the body's attempt to generate heat by vigorous muscular activity. As core temperature falls below 95°F (35°C), there is a general dulling of mental processes. Memory and judgment become faulty, and the speech may be slurred. At about 91°F (32.7°C), the muscles become rigid and uncoordinated, and the skin takes on a bluish tinge. The victim grows listless,

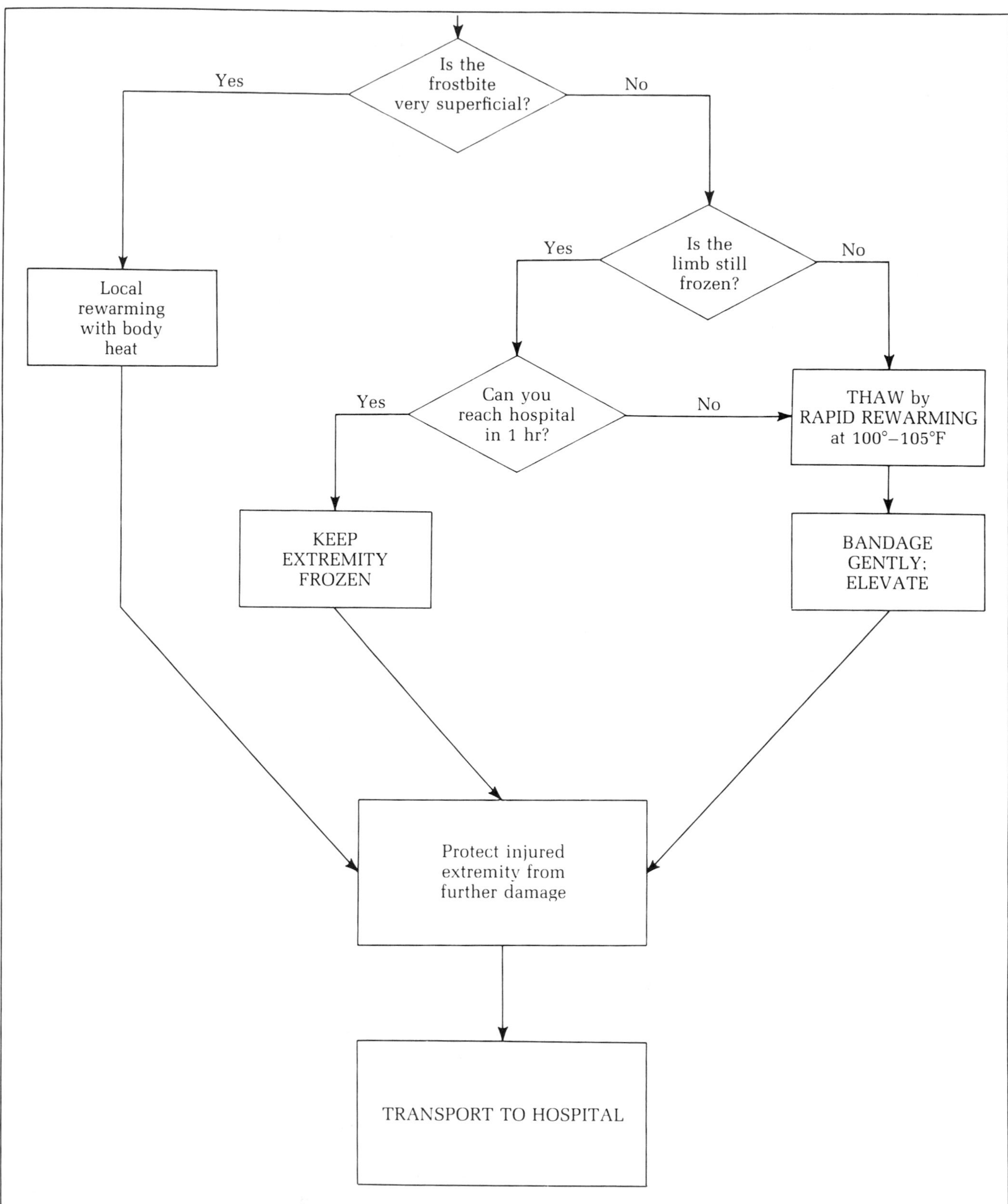

Fig. 30-1. *Management of frostbite.*

apathetic, and sleepy. By the time core temperature falls to about 86°F (30°C), the victim is stuporous. Heart rate and respirations are markedly slowed. Loss of consciousness usually occurs somewhere around a core temperature of 81°F (27.2°C), and disturbances of cardiac rhythm can develop as well. At this point, the victim typically has a glassy stare and extreme bradycardia. Below a core temperature of 78°F (25.6°C), there can be pulmonary edema. The heart becomes extremely susceptible to ventricular fibrillation, and even the slightest bump can precipitate cardiac arrest. The lower limit of survival is said to be around 74°F (23.3°C), although most patients fibrillate before their temperature falls that low. Nonetheless, one survival has been reported in a patient whose core temperature dropped to 50°F (10°C) and who had been in cardiac arrest for an hour when found. This case emphasizes the fact that a hypothermic patient should never be given up for dead, even when he or she looks convincingly like a corpse.

The sequence of events described above can develop within a few minutes when there is immersion in cold water, within an hour or two with exposure to very cold weather, or over several days in elderly or chronically ill people who have continuous exposure to moderately cold temperatures. However rapidly or slowly the hypothermia comes on, though, the underlying problem is the same: a depression in core temperature that endangers the body's vital functions. And whatever its cause, hypothermia is a dire medical emergency.

One of the keys to proper management of hypothermia is being able to recognize that hypothermia is present. This is rarely a problem if the victim is a hiker found unconscious in a snowdrift, but the elderly patient found confused and uncoordinated in a moderately cold apartment may be mistakenly assumed to have suffered a stroke or other medical illness. Thus it is very important for emergency personnel to be alert to the possibility of hypothermia in all patients found in any sort of cold environment, and a rectal temperature should always be measured in such patients.

Most standard rectal thermometers do not register below around 92°F (33.3°C), and thus the determination of *how* cold the hypothermic patient is must usually be made on the basis of the patient's signs and symptoms. This determination is important because the treatment varies according to the degree of hypothermia. For purposes of field management, victims of exposure can be divided into two categories: those with mild to moderate hypothermia and those with severe hypothermia.

MILD TO MODERATE HYPOTHERMIA (CONSCIOUS PATIENT)

A patient with mild to moderate hypothermia (rectal temperature from 94–84°F) is still CONSCIOUS, although he or she may seem indifferent and apathetic. SHIVERING may be present, and the SKIN is likely to be very PALE AND COLD TO THE TOUCH, reflecting peripheral vasoconstriction. If hypothermia developed slowly, over hours to days, there is apt as well to be an ODOR OF ACETONE ON THE BREATH, reflecting metabolic acidosis.

TREATMENT is aimed at preventing any further heat loss and rewarming the patient as rapidly as possible. To accomplish this, one must first MOVE THE PATIENT TO A PROTECTED AREA. If you cannot get the victim indoors, at least get him out of the wind, into a tent or other sheltered area. When triaging a group of exposure victims, GIVE PRIORITY TO THE THINNEST VICTIMS, for they have the least natural insulation against the cold. Entrapped victims must be protected from further cold exposure until they can be moved; use any available materials to shield them from the wind and insulate them from cold surfaces.

As soon as the victim is in a sheltered area, REPLACE ALL WET CLOTHING WITH DRY GARMENTS. Remember, moisture is a much better heat conductor than is dry cloth, and so long as the victim stays in wet clothes, rapid chilling will continue. Once the patient is in dry clothes, wrap him with any available INSULATING MATERIALS, and cover these with blankets. The patient should be kept recumbent, with insulating material beneath him, and should be covered with blankets. The arms and legs should not be placed in direct contact with the body, but rather outside the first layer of insulating material if possible. Be sure that the head and neck are covered, but leave the face free.

If medical care is not readily accessible, EXTERNAL HEAT may be provided to prevent a further drop in temperature. Hot water bottles can be placed behind the neck, in the armpits, and over the groin to promote core rewarming. Do *not* place hot water bottles or chemical heating bags over the extremities, and do *not* apply these materials in direct contact with the patient's skin, lest burns occur. Instead, wrap the heat source in a towel or similar material. If you are near a home, the best rewarming method is to put the patient in a tub of water at about 105°F (40.5°C). Out in the wilderness, shelter, insulation, and hot water bottles may be the only way to start the rewarming process.

Warm FLUIDS containing lots of SUGAR should be given by mouth, as well as any other sources of calories, such as candy bars or sugar cubes. The warm fluids probably do not, in fact, contribute very much in terms of actually raising the patient's core temperature, but warm drinks make the patient *feel* warmer and therefore more at ease. However, avoid caffeine-containing drinks, such as regular coffee, tea, or cocoa, since they are apt to have a diuretic effect, and hypothermic patients are usually already dehydrated. And DO NOT GIVE ALCOHOL, for it impairs shivering and decreases the victim's level of awareness.

BE ALERT FOR OTHER INJURIES. Frostbite is common in patients with generalized hypothermia, and the extremities should be carefully checked for local cold injury. Fractures too are apt to go unnoticed, because cold renders the patient relatively insensitive to pain. So check carefully. Treat frostbite as outlined earlier, and splint any suspected fractures before attempting to move the patient.

In transporting the patient, make sure he or she is well wrapped from head to toe in warm, insulated material, such as a sleeping bag. Bear in mind that enormous heat losses can occur from an uncovered head, so make sure the victim's head is well protected. Ideally, the patient should be enclosed in an outer wrapping of wind-resistant material as well.

Two relatively new devices show considerable promise for the field treatment of moderate hypothermia and deserve the attention of EMS personnel involved in winter search-and-rescue missions. The first is the *hydraulic sarong*, which is a thin, double-layered blanket with a network of plastic tubing running between the two layers. The blanket is wrapped around the hypothermia victim, and water heated over a camp stove is pumped through the tubing, thereby heating up the blanket and warming the victim inside. A second promising technique is the administration of *heated, humidified oxygen* to counteract respiratory heat loss from the body. Both of these techniques are still under investigation, and the EMT should keep tabs on the medical literature for further developments in this area.

SEVERE HYPOTHERMIA

A patient with severe hypothermia (rectal temperature less than 84°F) is STUPOROUS OR UNCONSCIOUS. The SKIN is ICE COLD to the touch, and the MUSCLES are RIGID. HEART SOUNDS may be INAUDIBLE, since cold tissues conduct sound very poorly, and BLOOD PRESSURE may be UNOBTAINABLE as well. The RESPIRATIONS are VERY SLOW, sometimes only 2 to 3 per minute, and PUPILS are likely to be UNREACTIVE to light.

Rewarming is vital to the survival of a patient in severe hypothermia, but it is very dangerous to attempt rewarming in the field, for slow external rewarming can lead to a condition called **rewarming shock**. This type of shock occurs if the body shell is warmed before the core, for what happens then is that blood vessels near the surface of the body start to dilate, and blood from the core floods into them. The heart is still too cold to rev up sufficiently to support the suddenly increased circulation, and it gets even colder as the blood that flooded out to the cool periphery returns to the right atrium. For this reason, ONE SHOULD NOT SPEND TIME IN THE FIELD TRYING TO REWARM SEVERELY HYPOTHERMIC PATIENTS. The victim must be brought to the hospital as rapidly as possible, with certain precautions taken en route.

To begin with, keep in mind that the severely hypothermic patient is very vulnerable to cardiac arrest from ventricular fibrillation. Thus HYPOTHERMIA VICTIMS MUST BE HANDLED VERY GENTLY, with great care taken to avoid any unnecessary jarring. If the victim's clothing is wet, it should be *cut* away, not pulled off; for undressing the patient in the normal fashion will cause too much motion. During transport, avoid sudden stops and starts, and take bumps on the road at a snail's pace.

As in any unconscious patient, the AIRWAY must be maintained, but AVOID AIRWAY ADJUNCTS, such as the oropharyngeal airway or esophageal obturator airway, for these too can induce ventricular fibrillation by excessive stimulation of the back of the throat. If BREATHING is very slow or absent altogether, you will have to ASSIST VENTILATIONS with a bag-valve-mask unit, but KEEP THE VENTILATION RATE SLOW—no more than about 5 to 10 breaths per minute—for overventilation can also trigger cardiac arrest. Administer OXYGEN, either by mask or, if you are assisting ventilations, by bag-valve-mask. If authorized to do so, start an INTRAVENOUS INFUSION with normal saline and run in about 300 ml quickly.

The real dilemma comes in assessing the C of the ABCs, for determining whether a hypothermic patient is in cardiac arrest is no easy matter. Because of the effects of cold on peripheral tissues, heart sounds may be inaudible and the pulse may not be palpable despite the fact that the patient's heart *is* still beating; so these signs are not entirely reliable. Furthermore, the pupils may be fixed and dilated despite continued cardiac function, so that sign is not helpful either. If you have a monitor with you, the problem is greatly simplified: Just hook up the monitor leads, and see what you have on the scope. If there is any kind of regular rhythm, leave the patient alone; if it is ventricular fibrillation or asystole, start CPR. Do not bother to try defibrillation, though; it will not work while the patient is hypothermic, and you are simply risking further, electric injury to the heart. Just continue CPR, and move on to the hospital.

If you do not have a monitor, you will have to make an educated guess about whether the victim's heart is still beating. Vital signs should be sought for at least a full minute before starting CPR. If there is any pulse at all, or if the patient is making any spontaneous movements, leave the victim alone, for the force of external cardiac compressions can actually cause ventricular fibrillation. *If the pulse is defi-*

Table 30-2. *Recognition and Management of Hypothermia*

Rectal Temperature	Signs and Symptoms	Field Management
Moderate hypothermia 94–84°F	CONSCIOUS, but may be apathetic, sleepy, confused, listless. Skin is PALE, COLD TO THE TOUCH. There may be an ACETONE ODOR TO THE BREATH. SHIVERING in mild cases. SUSPECT HYPOTHERMIA in any elderly or chronically ill patient found in an environment less than 50°F.	MOVE THE VICTIM TO SHELTERED AREA, OUT OF THE WIND (preferably indoors). REPLACE ALL WET CLOTHING WITH DRY GARMENTS. COVER WITH INSULATING MATERIALS AND BLANKETS. If far from a medical facility, REWARM, using a. Immersion in hot tub (105°F), or b. Hot water bottles to trunk. Give SUGAR and SWEET, HOT LIQUIDS by mouth; DO NOT GIVE ALCOHOL. WRAP PATIENT FROM HEAD TO TOE FOR TRANSPORT.
Severe hypothermia below 84°F	STUPOROUS OR COMATOSE. Skin is ICE COLD. Muscles are RIGID. PATIENT LOOKS DEAD. PUPILS DILATED, UNREACTIVE. HEART SOUNDS CANNOT BE HEARD. BLOOD PRESSURE usually UNOBTAINABLE. RESPIRATIONS 2–3/MIN. PULSE VERY DIFFICULT TO PALPATE.	DO NOT SPEND TIME IN THE FIELD TRYING TO REWARM THE VICTIM. GENTLE HANDLING! a. Cut away wet clothes; do not pull. b. Avoid jolts during transport. Maintain the AIRWAY, but DO NOT USE ADJUNCTS. ASSIST VENTILATIONS AS NEEDED, BUT SLOWLY. ADMINISTER OXYGEN. If so authorized, START AN IV with normal saline. BE CERTAIN THERE IS NO PULSE BEFORE STARTING CPR. ONCE YOU HAVE STARTED CPR, DO NOT GIVE UP! TRANSPORT the victim in slightly HEAD-DOWN POSITION.

nitely absent, start external cardiac compressions in the usual fashion.

It should be noted that the decision to start CPR must be made with due regard to the *total* rescue situation—for instance, the number of rescuers available to maintain CPR without themselves risking exhaustion and hypothermia, the terrain to be traversed, and so on.

Once you have initiated CPR, DO NOT GIVE UP, even if the patient looks very dead indeed. The same low temperatures that put the heart into fibrillation give the brain considerable protection from the effects of hypoxia, so the "magic 4 minutes" does not apply. The success or failure of CPR cannot be gauged until the patient has been rewarmed to normal body temperature, at which point defibrillation again becomes effective. Thus, when dealing with hypothermic patients, the message to remember is

> THE HYPOTHERMIC PATIENT IS NOT DEAD UNTIL HE IS REWARMED AND DEAD.

TRANSPORT the patient in a slightly HEAD-DOWN POSITION, that is, with the foot of the stretcher tilted upward about 10 degrees so that the victim's head is lower than his feet.

The recognition and management of varying degrees of hypothermia are summarized in Table 30-2.

IMMERSION HYPOTHERMIA

One specific type of hypothermia deserves separate mention, and that is the hypothermia caused by immersion in water. Immersion hypothermia is not exclusively a problem of cold climates or winter weather, for even in very warm climates, water temperatures in oceans, lakes, or swift-running rivers can fall below 70°F (21°C), and that is all that is necessary to cause significant body cooling.

The problems in immersion hypothermia are basically the same as those in any other form of hypothermia, but they develop much more rapidly. Just 15–20 minutes immersion in water less than 50°F (10°C) can be enough to bring about ventricular fibrillation and death. Furthermore, a person's instinctive behavior in water can actually hasten his own death considerably. Someone who attempts to swim, for example, will accelerate the cooling rate of his body by at least 35 percent, and conventional "drown-proofing" techniques, which put the victim's head in the water, increase the rate of heat loss by about 80 percent. This is because every movement the victim makes requires him to perfuse his cold peripheral muscles with warm core blood; this in turns cools the blood, which then returns to the core and causes a further lowering of core temperature.

For those reasons, THE VICTIM MUST BE REMOVED FROM THE WATER WITH A MINIMUM OF PHYSICAL EXERTION ON HIS PART. If at all possible, do not allow the victim to swim or to climb out of the water by himself.

After the victim has been removed from the water, his core temperature will continue to fall as cold blood from his extremities is pumped back into the core—a phenomenon termed **afterdrop**. Afterdrop seems to be partly the result of purely physical, as opposed to physiologic, phenomena, since even inanimate objects like melons will show afterdrop when fished out of cold water and subjected to external rewarming. Nonetheless, afterdrop will be increased by any maneuver that increases circulation to1the extremities, such as moving about, rubbing one's arms and legs and so on. Afterdrop is also increased if wet clothing is allowed to remain on the victim, permitting further evaporative cooling. To minimize afterdrop, then, HAVE THE PATIENT LIE AS STILL AS POSSIBLE. Do not permit him to sit, stand, or move in any way. DO NOT MASSAGE THE VICTIM'S EXTREMITIES. As soon as possible, REMOVE THE VICTIM'S WET CLOTHING, but do so with a minimum of patient movement; cut away the clothing if you have to, and replace it with dry garments. PROTECT THE VICTIM FROM THE WIND, any way you can, to prevent heat losses by convection.

All of the additional measures discussed above for general hypothermia apply to immersion hypothermia as well: gentle handling, rewarming for moderate degrees of hypothermia, and rapid evacuation to the hospital.

PREVENTION OF INJURIES DUE TO THE COLD

Many cold exposure injuries are simply the result of failure to take adequate safeguards against the elements and can be prevented with a little common sense. The EMT must know how to protect both himself or herself and the patient against heat loss in a cold environment. An understanding of the mechanisms of heat loss makes these preventive measures self-evident (Table 30-3).

Table 30-3. *Prevention of Cold Injury*

Mechanism of Body Cooling	Prevention of Heat Loss by This Mechanism
Convection	Wear insulating clothes, such as down, dacron, or foam linings Take shelter from the wind; wear windproof overgarments. Keep ears and nose covered. Wear ointment over nose, cheeks, and lips.
Conduction	Do not sit in the snow. Do not touch cold metal with bare skin. Replace wet clothing with dry clothing.
Radiation	Keep head and neck covered. Do not drink alcoholic beverages.
Evaporation	Change wet clothes immediately.
Inadequate heat production	Frequent snacks high in sugar and starch. Keep moving.
Interference with circulation	Avoid tight clothing, especially tight shoes and gloves. No cigarettes.

CASE HISTORY

The patient is a middle-aged man who was found unconscious in an alley downtown. There was no exact information about how long the patient had been there, although one bystander stated that the patient was seen in the same spot 6 hours earlier. He carried no identification. The outside temperature at the time we found the patient was 28°F.

On physical examination, the man was pale and his skin very cold to the touch. The pulse was very difficult to palpate at 44 per minute; blood pressure was unobtainable; respirations were 3 per minute. The pupils were dilated and unreactive to light. There was no evidence of head trauma. Neck veins were collapsed. Neither heart sounds nor breath sounds were audible. Both hands appeared to be frozen solid.

The patient was moved carefully to the ambulance and placed in a head-down position on the stretcher. Ventilations were assisted with a bag-valve-mask and oxygen at a rate of 8 per minute. The injured hands were elevated on pillows. Shortly after we started transport, the pulse became unobtainable, and external cardiac compressions were initiated and continued all the way to the emergency room.

Questions to think about:

1. Why were heart sounds inaudible? Did this indicate that the heart was not beating?
2. Should the EMTs have inserted an oropharyngeal airway to keep the patient's airway open? Why or why not?
3. What was the significance of the fact that the pulse became unobtainable? What might have caused this to happen?

VOCABULARY

afterdrop Continued fall in core temperature after a victim of hypothermia has been rescued from a cold environment, due to return of cold blood from the body surface to the body core.

core In reference to the human body, the part of the body comprising the heart, lungs, brain, and abdominal organs.

frostbite Freezing injury to tissues.

hypothermia Generalized cooling of the body, including the core.

rewarming shock Shock caused by sudden expansion of the circulation that follows dilation of the peripheral vessels as the body surface is rewarmed.

shell In reference to the human body, the skin, subcutaneous tissues, and extremities.

windchill factor Factor that takes into account both the temperature and wind velocity in calculating the effect of a given temperature on living organisms.

FURTHER READING

Albin N et al. Fatal accidental hypothermia and alcohol. *Alcohol* 19:13, 1984.

Avery WM. Hypothermia—the silent killer. *Emerg Med Serv* 8:26, 1979.

Bangs C. Immersion hypothermia: Preventing unnecessary deaths. *Emergency* 12(1):43, 1980.

Bangs C. Caught in the cold. *Emerg Med* 14(21):29, 1982.

Besdine RW. Accidental hypothermia—the body's energy crisis. *Geriatrics* 34:51, 1979.

Caught in cold water. *Emerg Med* 17(2):68, 1985.

Christenson C et al. Frostbite. *Am Fam Phys* 30:111, 1984.

Danzl DF et al. Multicenter hypothermia study. *Ann Emerg Med* 16:1042, 1987.

Davee TS et al. Extreme hypothermia and ventricular fibrillation. *Ann Emerg Med* 9:100, 1980.

Donner HJ. Out in the cold. *Emerg Med* 17(21):21, 1985.

Forgey WW. *Death by Exposure: Hypothermia.* Merrillville, IN: ICS Books, 1985.

Harnett RM, Pruitt JR, Sias FR. A review of the literature concerning resuscitation from hypothermia. Part I. The problem and general approaches. *Aviat Space Environ Med* 54:425, 1983.

Lathrap TG. *Hypothermia: Killer of the Unprepared.* Portland, OR: Mazamas, 1975.

Leavitt M, Podgorny G. Prehospital CPR and the pulseless hypothermic patient. *Ann Emerg Med* 13:492, 1984.

Miller JW, Danzl DF, Thomas DM. Urban accidental hypothermia: 135 cases. *Ann Emerg Med* 9:456, 1980.

Osborne L et al. Survival after prolonged cardiac arrest and accidental hypothermia. *Br Med J* 289:881, 1984.

Romet TT, Hoskin RW. Temperature and metabolic responses to inhalation and bath rewarming protocols. *Aviat Space Environ Med* 59:630, 1988.

Siebke H et al. Survival after 40 minutes submersion without cerebral sequelae. *Lancet* 1:1275, 1975.

Southwick FS, Dalglish PH. Recovery after prolonged asystolic cardiac arrest in profound hypothermia. *JAMA* 243:1250, 1980.

Stanford TM. The cold war. *Emergency* 20(11):22, 1988.

Steinman AM. Immersion hypothermia. *Emerg Med Serv* 6(4):22, 1977.

Stine RJ. Accidental hypothermia. *JACEP* 6:413, 1977.

Webb JQ. Cold to the core: Treating the hypothermic patient. *JEMS* 14(12):30, 1989.

Weyman AE, Greenbaum DM, Grace WJ. Accidental hypothermia in an alcoholic population. *Am J Med* 56:13, 1974.

White JD. Hypothermia: The Bellevue experience. *Ann Emerg Med* 11:417, 1982.

Wilkerson JA, Bangs CC, Hawyward JS. *Hypothermia, Frostbite, and Other Cold Injuries.* Seattle, WA: Mountaineers, 1986.

Working Group II. *Proceedings of the International Symposium on First Aid in Cardiopulmonary Resuscitation, Hypothermia, and Frostbite.* Geneva: LRCS. October, 1981.

Zachary L et al. Accidental hypothermia treated with rapid rewarming. *Ann Plast Surg* 9:238, 1982.

Zell SC, Kurtz KJ. Severe exposure hypothermia: A resuscitation protocol. *Ann Emerg Med* 14:339, 1985.

31. RADIATION AND HAZARDOUS MATERIALS

OBJECTIVES

Our environment is increasingly being filled up with hazardous materials. Among the hazardous materials most feared by the public are those that emit ionizing radiation. There was a time, not long ago, when we used to teach EMTs about radiation hazards mainly for the sake of completeness, for the whole matter seemed to be a rather remote problem, of theoretical interest perhaps, but not of much practical concern. The accidents at Three Mile Island in 1979 and at Chernobyl in 1986 changed all that. Those accidents created a new awareness—among the general public and medical community alike—that we live in an age where significant radiation exposure, from a variety of sources, is a constant possibility.

Radiation accidents occur infrequently, but when they do occur, they tend to provoke panic that is often out of all proportion to the dangers involved. The EMT needs to understand basic facts about radiation so that he or she can respond to a possible radiation accident without exaggerated anxiety, but with a clear and realistic concept of the risks involved. In this chapter, we will learn a bit about the nature of radiation and its effects on the human body. We shall look at some radiation accidents and see how EMS personnel can minimize the hazards—to themselves and their patients—of radiation exposure. We shall also examine some general principles of management that apply to all hazardous material incidents. By the end of this chapter, the reader should be able to

1. Identify the three principal forms of ionizing radiation and indicate the means by which a person can be shielded from each
2. List three ways by which a person can protect himself or herself from excessive exposure to a radioactive source
3. Calculate the total dose of radiation received, given the emission rate from a radioactive source and the duration of exposure
4. Indicate how alpha and beta particles can gain access to the body and list the means by which one can protect oneself from those particles
5. Identify an object or person who is radioactive, given a description of the circumstances of radiation exposure
6. Identify correct and incorrect procedures in dealing with a "dirty" radiation accident and its victims, given a list of various procedures
7. Indicate what signs and symptoms of radiation illness should be sought in persons exposed to a radiactive source
8. Identify correct and incorrect procedures for dealing with a hazardous materials ("hazmat") incident, given a list of procedures

WHAT IS RADIATION?

The word *radiation* often evokes awe and dread, conjuring up images of lethal rays that leave a trail of scorched earth and melting corpses in their wake. In fact, **radiation** simply means the transmission of energy in the form of waves or particles. Light is a form of radiation, as is sound, and neither of these forms of radiation poses any serious danger under ordinary circumstances. The kind of radiation we worry about is **ionizing radiation,** that is, radiation of certain types of particles or waves that are capable of disrupting atoms into their component charged particles (**ions**). When ionizing radiation is absorbed by living tissues, it goes banging into atoms, which are the smallest building blocks of all matter, and bumping charged particles (ions) loose from those atoms. The charged particles in turn bump into other atoms, and the process continues—like the scattering of billiard balls—until the energy of the particles is dissipated. In the process, cell structures are left in disarray.

A substance that gives off ionizing radiation is called **radioactive,** and in general there are three types of ionizing radiation that a radioactive substance can emit (Fig. 31-1). To begin with, radiation can be given off in the form of ALPHA PARTICLES. An alpha particle is actually the nucleus of an atom. It has a positive charge, and as subatomic particles go, it is rather big, heavy, and sluggish. The alpha particle has a very short range—only a few centimeters in air. It also has very little penetrating ability, and it can be stopped even by a sheet of paper. Thus alpha particles ordinarily do little damage, for they tend to be absorbed by clothing, and even if the victim is unclothed, these particles are halted by the outer layers of the skin. However, alpha particles *are* a significant hazard if they gain access to the inside of the body—through inhalation, ingestion, or an open wound.

BETA PARTICLES correspond to the electron of the atom and carry a negative charge. They are much tinier than alpha particles but also much speedier and have greater penetration. Nonetheless, beta particles can usually be stopped by heavy clothing and, like alpha particles, are dangerous mainly when they are inhaled, ingested, or delivered into an open wound.

The most penetrating and thus the most dangerous type of ionizing radiation is GAMMA RAY radiation, which is emitted from the nucleus of an atom. Gamma rays are very energetic, able to penetrate several hundred yards through the air. They pass easily through clothes and indeed through the whole body and can be stopped only by heavy lead shielding or extremely thick concrete. Gamma rays are, for all practical purposes, the same as x-rays; what makes x-rays "safe" and gamma rays dangerous is simply a

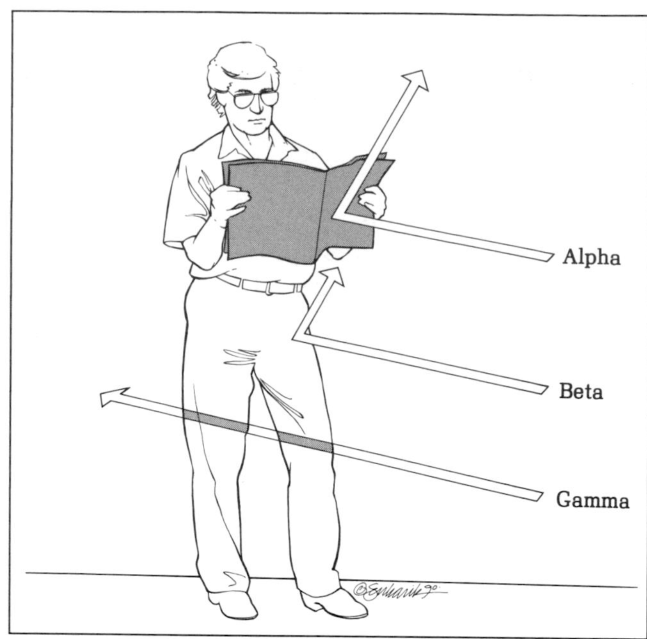

Fig. 31-1. *Types of ionizing radiation. ALPHA rays are stopped by paper. BETA rays are stopped by clothing. GAMMA rays can be stopped only by heavy shielding, such as lead.*

matter of dose. When x-rays are used for medical diagnosis, the exposure time is kept extremely brief.

Ionizing radiation—whether alpha, beta, or gamma—cannot be seen, heard, or felt. It can be detected only with special instruments, such as a Geiger counter or ionization chamber. These instruments measure the amount of ionizing radiation delivered by a radioactive source in **roentgens** (named for the man who discovered x-rays), or R, and they are usually finely calibrated to read in milliroentgens per hour (a milliroentgen is 0.001R, that is, one one-thousandth of a roentgen).

EFFECTS OF RADIATION ON THE BODY

As noted earlier, ionizing radiation attacks very tiny targets—the atoms in its path. If the atoms disrupted by ionizing radiation happen to be part of a human cell, then the structure or function of that cell may be disrupted as well, just as the function of a watch is altered if you damage one of its springs or cogs. We cannot see the changes that occur in the body's atoms or molecules after a dose of radiation, but what we *can* observe (if the radiation exposure was significant) are the effects of those molecular changes on body function. The effects may be acute, occurring within hours or days, or they may be long-term, taking years or even generations to appear. In general, the larger the dose of radiation, the more acute the effects. A person exposed to a dose of about 300 to 600 roentgens over a short period, for example, has a 50-percent chance of dying within the next month. A person exposed to about 1,000 roentgens will probably die within a couple of weeks; exposure to 2,000 roentgens can cause death within hours.

To put these doses into some kind of perspective, we need to consider the kinds of radiation exposure that a person encounters in the course of everyday life, for all of us are constantly exposed to minute amounts of radiation from cosmic rays and naturally occurring radioactive materials. The natural radiation level from cosmic rays is about 0.04R per year, or a total of about 3R in a human lifetime of 70 years. Natural radioactive substances in the soil and rock probably contribute another 3R per lifetime. Every hour of television viewing adds 0.00015R. A diagnostic medical x-ray delivers about 0.1R. Thus, when we look at radiation producing *acute* illness, we are talking about doses many thousands of times higher than that of a routine chest x-ray. Nonetheless, it should be emphasized that *any* amount of ionizing radiation, even in tiny doses delivered by cosmic rays, does some biologic harm, although that harm may not be evident for many years. We cannot do much about the radiation we receive from natural sources, but great care should be taken to avoid unnecessary exposure from other sources.

FACTORS INFLUENCING RADIATION DAMAGE

The amount of radiation damage a person suffers from a radioactive source depends on a number of factors. To begin with, there is the STRENGTH OF THE RADIATION, that is, how many roentgens per hour the source is emitting. This can be measured with a Geiger counter and should be determined, whenever possible, before entering a radiation field. Every ambulance service should have quick access to radiation monitoring equipment (which is available from Civil Defense), and EMTs should be trained in the use of a simple Geiger counter.

A second factor determining the potential severity of radiation exposure is the DURATION OF EXPOSURE. By knowing the duration of exposure and the strength of the radiation source, one can estimate the *dose* of exposure with a simple equation.

$$\text{TOTAL DOSE} = \text{dose rate (R/hr)} \times \text{exposure time}$$

What this equation says is that the longer the exposure to a radioactive substance, the bigger the dose of radiation the exposed person receives. The practical implications are clear: The exposure time of any one individual should be kept as short as possible. Say, for example, you are working near a radioactive source emitting 100R per hour (dose rate), and rescue is going to take 6 minutes, or 0.1 hour. If a single rescuer goes into the exposure zone for the whole 6 minutes, he or she will receive a radiation dose as follows:

$$\begin{aligned}\text{TOTAL DOSE} &= \text{dose rate} \times \text{exposure time}\\ &= 100\text{R/hr} \times 0.1 \text{ hour}\\ &= 10\text{R}\end{aligned}$$

But suppose there are six people on the rescue team and they divide up the work so that each of them enters the radiation zone for only 1 minute (0.017 hr) each. Then each of them will receive a dose of radiation as follows:

$$\begin{aligned}\text{TOTAL DOSE} &= \text{dose rate} \times \text{exposure time}\\ &= 100\text{R/hr} \times 0.017 \text{ hour}\\ &= 1.7\text{R}\end{aligned}$$

This is about the same exposure one would receive from a diagnostic x-ray series.

The message is clear

> KEEP EXPOSURE TIME TO A BARE MINIMUM.

Divide up the work among as many people as possible, and work as fast as you can to get yourself and the victim out of the exposure area. This will be possible only if there has been extensive practice beforehand in working in shifts, relay-race fashion.

A third factor influencing the amount of radiation damage a person sustains is the DISTANCE FROM THE RADIATION SOURCE. The exposure falls off as the inverse square of the distance, that is:

$$\text{EXPOSURE} = \frac{1}{(\text{distance})^2}$$

What this means is that if, for example, you double your distance from the radiation source, you get one-quarter the exposure; whereas if you halve the distance to the radiation source, you get four times the exposure. Let us take an example. Suppose we have a radioactive source emitting 1,000R per hour at a distance of 1 foot from the source, where the victim is lying. If we move the victim 20 feet from the source, the exposure will be reduced to 2.5R per hour ($1{,}000/20^2$). The practical significance of this relationship is very simple: THE FARTHER AWAY YOU CAN GET FROM THE RADIATION SOURCE THE BETTER, BUT MOVING EVEN A SMALL DISTANCE AWAY REDUCES THE EXPOSURE CONSIDERABLY.

SHIELDING FROM THE RADIATION SOURCE is a fourth factor that influences one's exposure and thus one's potential injury. Ordinary clothing provides adequate shielding from alpha and beta radiation. Shielding from gamma radiation requires a thick (1–2-inch) lead plate, and for this reason, it is more practical in the field to try to shield the source than to shield the rescuers. Any heavy accumulation of concrete, brick, or earth, offers some protection, and rescuers can shelter behind a thick concrete wall or embankment while making preparations to enter the exposure area.

A fifth factor that determines how much radiation damage a person will suffer is the AREA OF THE BODY THAT RECEIVES RADIATION. Radiation exposure to the whole body is much more likely to produce systemic illness than an exposure limited to one small area of the body.

Finally, radiation damage is influenced by the TYPE OF RADIATION received—alpha, beta, or gamma.

PROTECTION FROM RADIATION

Among the factors listed above, we have seen that three have practical implications for protecting oneself and one's patients from *direct* radiation exposure: TIME, DISTANCE, and SHIELDING. In addition, it is important to bear in mind that radiation can be transmitted *indirectly*, on particles of contaminated dust or smoke or in contaminated liquids. Inhalation or swallowing of such contaminated materials is extremely dangerous, for it brings the radioactive material in direct contact with internal tissues, where the ionizing radiation can wreak extensive cellular damage. Thus the EMT must take rigorous precautions in the presence of a radiation hazard to prevent accidental inhalation or ingestion of contaminated materials. This means, at the least, wearing a filtration mask. Needless to say, smoking or eating in a radiation area is strictly forbidden.

To summarize some of the general principles of protecting oneself in a radiation area:

Protection from Ionizing Radiation

- LIMIT EXPOSURE TIME TO THE MINIMUM POSSIBLE.
- PUT THE MAXIMUM DISTANCE BETWEEN YOURSELF AND THE RADIATION SOURCE.
- SHIELD THE SOURCE OR SHIELD YOURSELF.
- PROTECT YOURSELF FROM INHALING OR INGESTING CONTAMINATED MATERIALS. Do not smoke. Do not eat. Wear a filtration mask.

Before leaving the subject of protection from radiation exposure, it is important to deal with one common misconception that causes much unnecessary anxiety among EMS personnel, and that has to do with who or what is actually radioactive. We have said that a radioactive substance is one that *gives off* ionizing radiation. A PERSON OR OBJECT THAT HAS BEEN EXPOSED TO IONIZING RADIATION DOES *NOT* BECOME RADIOACTIVE, that is, does not give off radiation. If you have a chest x-ray, for instance, you receive a certain amount of radiation, but you do *not* become radioactive either during or after the exposure. Thus in a radiation accident, a person who has been exposed to even a very high dose of ionizing radiation poses no hazard to rescue personnel, and the radiation victim can be handled just as any other patient.

What does sometimes pose a problem is contamination, that is, the victim who has been sprayed with radioactive dust or smoke. We shall discuss shortly the measures that can be taken to minimize such contamination, but for our purposes here, suffice it to say that no one ever died from accidental surface contamination. Lots of people die, however, from obstructed airways, bleeding, and so forth. The message is that CONTAMINATION IS NOT A MEDICAL EMERGENCY. While decontamination should be accomplished as soon as possible, THE ABCS HAVE PRIORITY.

TYPES OF RADIATION ACCIDENTS

Radiation accidents can be categorized as "clean" accidents or "dirty" accidents. CLEAN ACCIDENTS are most likely to occur at nuclear power plants or industrial facilities where radioactive substances are routinely used. They occur when a radioactive source somehow becomes unshielded, and personnel in the vicinity are thereby exposed to radiation. By definition, a clean accident is one in which there is no contamination or in which decontamination has been carried out by radiation safety officers before you arrive. In such cases, there is no hazard to the ambulance personnel, and the exposure victims can be handled and transported as any other patients. Bear in mind that reactor sites and industrial users of radioactive materials generally have staff who are quite expert in dealing with radiation, and they will be able to provide guidance to rescue personnel. Thus, when responding to a call at a facility that routinely uses radioactive materials, follow the instructions of the plant radiation safety team.

A much more difficult problem in terms of rescue and patient care is that posed by a DIRTY ACCIDENT. The typical accident of this type is a transportation accident; and with the increasing delivery of radioactive substances by air, rail, and truck, such accidents are likely to increase. The Interstate Commerce Commission has very strict regulations regarding the packaging of radioactive materials, and radioactive shipments must carry the universal radiation symbol, a purple propellor on a yellow background (Fig. 31-2). Depite packaging precautions, however, a violent collision, especially if it results in fire or explosion, may permit release of radioactive materials, with contamination of the surrounding area.

In the next discussion, we will look at a hypothetical dirty accident and go step-by-step through the ambulance response to such a situation.

RESPONDING TO A RADIATION ACCIDENT

Let us take as our example an accident in which a truck carrying radioactive wastes collides with a car on the interstate highway, flips over, and ignites. The result is a lot of wreckage, dust, and smoke.

The response to the accident begins WHEN THE CALL COMES INTO THE DISPATCHER. One of the jobs of a dispatcher is to try to determine what, if any, hazards are present at the accident scene, and with luck the caller will report that the truck was carrying a radiation symbol. If the dispatcher is able to get such information ahead of time, he or she should (1) radio the responding ambulance to take appropriate precautions at the scene and (2) phone the proper local authorities, so that radiation safety experts can be sent to join you at the scene as soon as possible.

If the dispatcher cannot obtain any information about what the truck was carrying, your first job upon ARRIVAL AT THE SCENE will be to get a good look at the truck to check whether it carries the telltale purple and yellow symbol. Should you see that symbol, radio back to base immediately, so that the dispatcher can notify the proper authorities.

PARK THE AMBULANCE UPWIND FROM THE ACCIDENT SCENE and upstream from any liquid spills or leaks from the accident vehicle. If possible, keep the ambulance and yourselves behind some kind of SHIELDING (a heavy concrete wall, an embankment, even a big semitrailer) while you organize yourselves for the rescue process. Quickly DON PROTECTIVE CLOTHING—surgical hood, mask, shoe covers, gown or coveralls—which should ideally be available in a special Radiation Emergency Kit (Table 31-1) in the vehicle. Also clip on a dosimeter film badge, and wear it for the duration of the call. If no protective gear is available, you must adapt the clothes you are wearing to minimize contamination by alpha and beta particles carried in dust or smoke. Put on an extra layer of clothes, the more tightly woven the better, and don some kind of filtering mask. Button your shirt all the way up, and turn the collar up. Tape shirt cuffs and pant legs closed, and tape over buttonholes and other openings in your clothing through which dust might otherwise enter. Make sure to keep your head well covered, so that no hair is exposed, and protect your eyes with goggles.

A word of caution: WOMEN EMTS WHO ARE PREGNANT OR POTENTIALLY PREGNANT SHOULD STAY ON THE SIDELINES, well out of range of the radiation area. This is not male chauvinism; it is practical genetics. A developing fetus is exquisitely sensitive to the effects of radiation, and even small exposure can result in birth defects. As a matter of fact, the germ cells of both sexes (the male sperm and female ova) are also very sensitive to radiation, so the older the rescuers, the better. If you have a few 50-year-old EMTs on your squad who have no further aspirations to sire or bear children, those EMTs should be preferred to enter the radioactive area.

Once you have suited up, the first priority is to get the victim(s) out of the exposure area as rapidly as possible. Remember, your three best means of protection from a radioactive source are TIME, DISTANCE, AND SHIELDING. So you want to get in and out as fast as possible, put some distance between the victim and the radiation source, and, if possible,

Fig. 31-2. *Universal radiation symbol.*

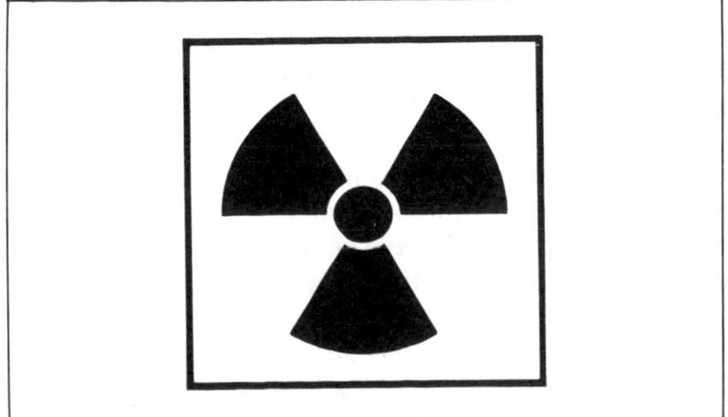

Table 31-1. *Suggested Radiation Kit for Ambulances*

Geiger-Mueller (G-M) instrument
Dosimeter badge for each EMT
5–10 heavy-duty plastic garbage bags
Packet of "radioactive" stickers to label contaminated articles
Several pairs of surgical gloves (various sizes)
Several sets of surgical hoods, gowns, and shoe covers
Filtration masks
Masking tape
Special record-keeping forms
Disaster tags

Response to ("Dirty") Radiation Accidents

1. NOTIFY LOCAL AUTHORITIES AS SOON AS A POTENTIAL RADIATION HAZARD IS DISCOVERED (e.g., upon seeing a "radioactive" symbol on a wrecked vehicle).
2. PARK THE AMBULANCE UPWIND FROM THE WRECKAGE AND UPSTREAM FROM ANY SPILLAGE.
   a. The ambulance should be at least 50 yards from any potential hazard.
   b. Where possible, put the ambulance in a SHIELDED area.
3. DON PROTECTIVE CLOTHING AND MASK.
4. APPROACH THE WRECKAGE FROM UPWIND. STAY OUT OF DUST AND SMOKE.
5. GET THE VICTIM(S) TO THE UPWIND EDGE OF THE CONTAMINATION ZONE AS FAST AS POSSIBLE.
   a. MINIMIZE THE EXPOSURE OF EACH RESCUER. Work in shifts. *Maximum* allowable exposure for one person is 100R.
   b. GET AT LEAST 20 to 30 FEET FROM THE RADIATION SOURCE.
   c. MOVE TO A SHIELDED AREA IF POSSIBLE.
6. GIVE URGENT MEDICAL CARE, AND STABILIZE THE PATIENT.
7. REMOVE THE PATIENT'S CLOTHES AND YOUR OWN PROTECTIVE GARMENTS while you are still in the control area.
8. CHECK FOR AND DOCUMENT RADIOACTIVE CONTAMINATION ON THE PATIENT'S BODY.
9. REMOVE THE PATIENT FROM THE CONTAMINATION ZONE.
10. COLLECT AND RECORD NECESSARY INFORMATION:
    a. MEDICAL: Patient's signs and symptoms (ask about NAUSEA and VOMITING).
    b. TECHNICAL: Type of radioactive material involved.
11. NOTIFY RECEIVING HOSPITAL.
12. TRANSPORT.
13. TRANSFER PATIENT TO HOSPITAL CART *OUTSIDE* HOSPITAL ENTRANCE.
14. DO NOT LEAVE THE HOSPITAL UNTIL RELEASED BY RADIATION SAFETY OFFICER, AFTER
    a. Personal decontamination.
    b. Supervised decontamination of vehicle and equipment.

Each state has a radiologic health department that can be contacted for assistance in radiation accidents, and the EMT should know how to get in touch with the state authorities. In addition, the Radiation Emergency Assistance Center/Training Site (REAC/TS) in Oak Ridge, Tennessee maintains a 24-hour "hot line" to provide telephone advice or even send a team of experts to assist at the scene. REAC/TS can be reached any hour of the day or night by calling (615) 481–1000 (Beeper 241).

HAZARDOUS MATERIALS

Up to this point, we have looked at the response to one specific type of hazardous material (hazmat) incident—that involving ionizing radiation. In fact, radiation accidents constitute only a small minority of hazmat incidents. One of the inevitable consequences of living in an industrialized world is the proliferation of hazardous materials all around us. The products of our civilization require the manufacture, transport, storage, use, and disposal of thousands of potentially toxic substances, which may be spilled or ignited at any stage between manufacture and disposal. Some 35,000 dangerous commodities are produced in the United States, and there are nearly 200 *million* shipments of hazardous materials per year in the United States. Twenty-five percent of unintentional releases of those materials occur during transport; 75 percent occur during production, storage, or use. From 1971 to 1981, more than 108,000 hazmat events occurred on U.S. highways. What all those statistics mean is one simple rule: The first thing to remember when responding to a road accident or vehicular fire, especially if a truck or train is involved, is that a hazardous material may be part of the picture.

ALWAYS CONSIDER THE POSSIBILITY OF HAZARDOUS MATERIALS WHEN RESPONDING TO A ROAD OR RAIL ACCIDENT. EVERY CARGO SHOULD BE CONSIDERED DANGEROUS UNTIL PROVED OTHERWISE.

Dealing with hazardous materials requires special training and special equipment. The EMT who plunges heedlessly forward to reach the casualties without taking careful stock of the situation is likely to become one of the casualties himself and therefore a burden to the rescue team.

DO NOT RUSH INTO A HAZMAT SCENE. STOP AND ASSESS THE SITUATION FIRST.

ESTABLISHING A HAZARD ZONE

To start with, PARK THE VEHICLE UPWIND from any potential hazardous materials spill, preferably at least 50–100 yards away, and take action at once to establish a hazard zone; that is, an area from which unauthorized persons should be excluded. One quick method for estimating the extent of the hazard zone is to use the "hazmat rule of thumb": Hold your arm out straight in front of you, with your thumb pointing upward, and center your thumb over the hazardous area (the hazardous area will include, for example, an entire overturned vehicle and the whole area over which spilled materials are visible). If your thumb does not block out the entire hazardous area from your view, you are *too close*! Move back in a direction upwind from the spill until your thumb obscures the whole area of potential hazard. That point is the border of the hazard zone. Do whatever you can to keep bystanders away from the hazard zone. And do not enter the hazard zone yourself until you have determined the identity of the hazardous material and your own capability to deal with it.

IDENTIFICATION OF THE HAZARDOUS MATERIAL

One of the most important contributions that the first ambulance on the scene can make to a hazmat response is to enable early identification of the hazardous substance involved. In the United States, trucks or trains carrying hazardous materials across state lines are required by law to follow federal regulations regarding markings on the vehicle and shipping documents.

The first thing to look for is a colored Department of Transportation placard (Fig. 31-4) on the side or back end of the vehicle (truck or railway car). The placard is a diamond-shaped sign, which is likely to be color-coded and which may contain some or all of the following:

- A pictorial representation of the hazard (for instance, a skull and crossbones to indicate poison, or a flame to indicate a flammable substance)
- A four-digit identification number, sometimes preceded by the letters "NA" (standing for North American) or "UN" (standing for United Nations). Older placards may show the name of the chemical itself (e.g., "CHLORINE") rather than an identification number.
- A single number at the bottom, which refers to the United Nations classification system (Table 31-3)

Fig. 31-4. *Sample Department of Transportation placard showing a pictorial symbol of the substance carried, a four-digit UN/NA identification number (in this case, it is the number for chlorine), and the UN hazard class number (in this case, it is the number for a gas).*

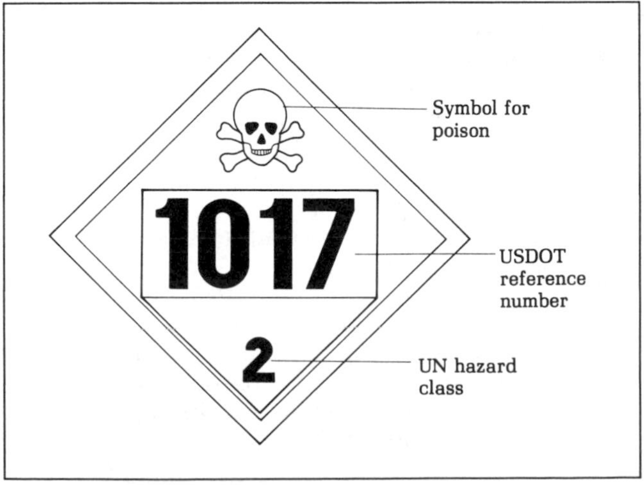

We have already mentioned that EMTs arriving first at a potential hazmat incident should not cross into the hazard zone before the hazardous material has been identified. How, then, is an EMT, who may be standing 100 yards from an overturned truck, supposed to be able to read the lettering on a placard at that distance? The answer is that your ambulance had better be equipped with BINOCULARS, or you will be out of luck. Do NOT risk personal exposure to a hazardous material in order to get close enough to read the placard on the side of a disabled truck or railway car.

Another source of information for identifying hazardous cargoes is the **bill of lading** carried in the cab of trucks or the **waybill** and **consist** carried by the conductor on trains. (The consist lists the order in which the cars are lined up in the train, and the waybill lists their contents). Those shipping documents are usually not as helpful as the placard information, since it may not be possible at first to reach the truck cab or the engine car of a train. Furthermore, shipping documents may be lost or destroyed in the course of an accident. Nonetheless, it is useful to know what to look for in such a document if you should be fortunate enough to get access to it during a hazmat incident. The waybill or bill of lading lists the name of the shipper, the company to which the product is being shipped, the four-digit UN/NA iden-

Table 31-3. *United Nations Hazardous Materials Classification Codes.*

Number	Material
1	Explosives
2	Gases
3	Flammable and combustible liquids
4	Flammable solids
5	Oxidizers and organic peroxides
6	Poisons
7	Radioactive materials
8	Corrosives

tification number, and a description of all products being transported (e.g., 10 drums gasoline, flammable liquid, 4500 lbs.

From whatever source you obtain the information, RADIO YOUR DISPATCHER at once with the four-digit identification number of the cargo. Every dispatch station should be equipped with the U.S. Department of Transportation's *Hazardous Material, The Emergency Response Handbook*; using that handbook, your dispatcher should be able to give you an initial identification of the substance involved in the incident and help you decide what to do until professional hazmat personnel reach the scene. Meanwhile, the dispatcher should control CHEMTREC (the Chemical Transportation Emergency Center in Washington, D.C.), which maintains a 24-hour toll-free hotline to provide information on handling specific hazmat incidents. The telephone numbers of CHEMTREC are (800) 424–9300 from the continental United States; 483–7616 from the Washington, D.C. area; and (202) 483–7616 from outside the continental United States (CHEMTREC will accept collect calls). The information that the dispatcher needs to furnish is as follows:

Information Needed by the CHEMTREC Communicator

- Name of caller
- Call-back number
- Shipper*
- Manufacturer's name*
- Container type
- Railcar or truck number
- Carrier's name*
- Consignee*
- Product involved, if known, or 4-digit identification number
- Location of incident
- Condition at scene, including weather
- Type of problem (e.g., spill, fire, etc.)

*Information from waybill or bill of lading.

RESCUE AND MEDICAL TREATMENT

As soon as the EMTs have enough information and professional backup to enter the hazard zone, they should remove the injured from the zone to prevent further exposure—employing whatever protective equipment is necessary under the circumstances (e.g., protective clothing, self-contained breathing apparatus). As in the case of radiation incidents, once the casualty has been removed from the hazard zone, FIRST PRIORITY GOES TO URGENT MEDICAL PROBLEMS. The usual priorities of ABC apply. If either the casualty or the EMT has come in contact with the hazardous material, then **decontamination** must also be carried out, preferably *before* transport.

Decontamination

Casualties or EMS personnel at a hazmat incident may become contaminated in a number of ways:

- Being splashed by materials during rescue operations
- Walking through puddles of hazardous liquids or across contaminated ground
- Coming in contact with gases, vapors, or particles of hazardous substances
- Touching contaminated persons or instruments

However contamination occurs, decontamination is required as soon as possible; otherwise, exposure to the hazardous material will continue and the resulting injury will become progressively more severe. When highly toxic materials are involved, decontamination may have to be carried out simultaneous with medical stabilization of the patient.

Ideally, decontamination should be conducted by trained personnel using special equipment; but that may not always be possible, especially when a critically injured patient must be moved urgently to the hospital before the decon team has arrived and deployed its gear. In decontaminating casualties, the following general principles apply:

General Principles of Decontamination

- Remove all of the victim's clothing (including shoes, socks, underwear) and place it in a sealed container, such as a plastic bag.
- Flush the skin *gently* with water for at least 15 minutes. Start at the head and work downward. Make sure that hair and body folds are thoroughly rinsed as well. Pay special attention to fingernails, underarms, groin. Then give a gentle wash with tincture of green soap and rinse again.
- If there are open wounds on the skin, wash and rinse from the wound area outward, taking care not to flush contaminants into the wound. Once the wound area is clean, cover it with an occlusive dressing or plastic wrap.
- When flushing is complete, gently dry the patient with a clean towel. Cover him with a clean sheet for transport.
- No matter how thoroughly you think you have decontaminated the casualty, be sure to notify the receiving hospital in advance that the patient may still be partially contaminated so that the hospital can implement its own hazmat protocols.

Whenever possible, it is preferable to have a separate team—EMTs who were not involved in the rescue and treatment of the casualty—transport the casualty to the hospital. In that way, the chances of bringing contaminants into the hospital are minimized, and the EMTs who did participate in rescue can, meanwhile, themselves undergo decontamination at the scene, without delaying the evacuation of the patient. All equipment, gear, and protective clothing used during the hazmat response must also undergo thorough decontamination before the rescue personnel leave the scene.

VOCABULARY

alpha particle Positively charged subatomic particle, corresponding to the nucleus of the atom, with high ionizing ability but low penetration.

beta particle Negatively charged subatomic particle, corresponding to the electron of an atom, with slightly higher penetrating ability than an alpha particle.

gamma ray Radioactive emission from the nucleus of an atom, with very high penetrating ability.

ion An atom, part of an atom, or a group of atoms that carries an electric charge.

ionizing radiation Emission of waves or particles that have the ability to disrupt atoms in their path into component ions.

radiation Transmission of energy in the form of waves or particles.

radioactive Property of emitting ionizing radiation.

roentgen (R) Unit of measurement for radiation, named for the discoverer of x-rays.

FURTHER READING

RADIATION

Beane MJ et al. Radiation primer. *EMT J* 5(4):260, 1981.

Deluca SA et al. Radiation exposure in diagnostic studies. *Am Fam Phys* 36:101, 1987.

English WE. Radioactive contamination. *Emergency* 14(1):43, 1982.

Gale RP. Immediate medical consequences of nuclear accidents: Lessons from Chernobyl. *JAMA* 258:625, 1987.

Geiger HJ. The accident at Chernobyl and the medical response. *JAMA* 256:609, 1986.

Goldstein HA. Radiation accidents and injuries. *Emerg Med* 14(15):195, 1982.

Huebner KF. Decontamination procedures and risks to health care personnel. *Bull NY Acad Med* 59:1119, 1983.

Keller PD. A clinical syndrome following exposure to atomic bomb explosions. *JAMA* 131:504, 1946.

Leonard RB, Ricks RC. Emergency department radiation accident protocol. *Ann Emerg Med* 9:462, 1980.

Lushbaugh CC, Huebner KF, Ricks RC. Medical aspects of nuclear radiation emergencies. *Emergency* 10:32, 1978.

Mettler FA. Emergency management of radiation accidents. *JACEP* 7:302, 1978.

Mettler FA, Rocco FG, Junkins RL. The role of EMTs in radiation accidents. *Emerg Med Serv* 6:22, 1977.

Miller KL, Demuth WE. Handling radiation emergencies: No need for fear. *J Emerg Nursing* 9:141, 1983.

Milroy WC. Management of irradiated and contaminated casualty victims. *Emerg Med Clin North Am* 2:667, 1984.

Richter LL et al. A systems approach to the management of radiation accidents. *Ann Emerg Med* 9:303, 1980.

Ricks RC. Radiation response. *Emergency* 21(2):28, 1989.

Solon LR. Some aspects of emergency planning for nuclear reactor accidents by New York City. *Bull NY Acad Med* 59:981, 1983.

Trott KR. Nuclear power plant disasters—health consequences and needs for subsequent medical care. *Lancet* 2:32, 1981.

HAZARDOUS MATERIALS

Bronstein A, Currance P. *Emergency Care for Hazardous Materials Exposure*. St. Louis: Mosby, 1988.

Currance PL. Staging decon operations. *Rescue* 2(4):45, 1989.

International Fire Service Training Association. Personal protective equipment for hazardous incidents. *Emerg Med Serv* 18(10):44, 1989.

Isman WE. Emergency responders at a hazardous materials incident. *JEMS* 8(2):26, 1982.

Leonard RB. Chemicals in transit: Be prepared. *Emerg Med* 14(18):17, 1984.

McKenna R. Hazardous materials incidents and the EMT. *EMT J* 5(6):400, 1981.

Staten C. Hazardous materials: The EMS response. *Emerg Med Serv* 18(10):34, 1989.

Stutz DR, Janusz SJ. *Hazardous Material Injuries: A Handbook for Pre-Hospital Care* (2nd ed.). Beltsville, MD: Bradford Communications, 1988.

U.S. Department of Health and Human Services/U.S. Department of Labor. *IOSH/OSHA Pocket Guide to Chemical Hazards*. Washington, D.C.: NIOSH, 1986.

U.S. Department of Transportation. *1987 Emergency Response Guidebook, DOT-P-5800.4*. Washington, D.C.: USDOT, 1987.

VIII. OBSTETRIC AND GYNECOLOGIC EMERGENCIES

Obstetrics is the branch of medicine that deals with the pregnant woman as she goes through the various phases of pregnancy, labor, and delivery. Gynecology deals with illnesses related to the female genital tract. In this section, we will look at emergencies in both categories: the natural and usually happy "emergency" of childbirth, the urgent medical problems that can occur during pregnancy and delivery, and some of the acute illnesses and trauma to which women are uniquely susceptible.

HOW BABIES ARE MADE

In order to understand where babies come from, one needs to know a bit about the anatomy and function of the female reproductive system. This system consists of the ovaries, fallopian tubes, uterus, and vagina (Fig. 32-1).

The OVARIES are two walnut-sized organs that sit in the right and left lower quadrants of the abdomen. The ovaries have a dual responsibility. First of all, they produce *female sex hormones*, which are released into the bloodstream and travel to various target organs throughout the body. These hormones give women their characteristic female appearance and also influence the menstrual cycle. The second job of the ovaries is to produce eggs, or **ova** (one egg is an **ovum**), and to release one ovum at regular intervals throughout a woman's reproductive life.

When an egg is released from an ovary, it travels down a special connecting duct, the FALLOPIAN TUBE, into the cavity of the womb, or UTERUS. The latter is a very muscular, pear-shaped organ that can stretch considerably when the time comes to accommodate a developing baby inside. At the distal end of the uterus is a narrow opening, called the CERVIX, which connects the uterus with the VAGINA. The cervix is the canal through which menstrual flow (and eventually a baby) passes from the womb to the outside world; it also provides for the passage of male sperm from the vagina into the uterus, for it is the muscular vagina that receives the penis during sexual intercourse. The vagina connects to the VULVA, the external female genitalia. The area between the vaginal opening and the rectum is called the PERINEUM.

THE MENSTRUAL CYCLE

Throughout a woman's reproductive years, there is a regular cycle of changes occurring in her body at approximately 1-month intervals. These phasic changes, called the menstrual cycle, start somewhere around the age of 12 (**menarche**) and cease around the age of 50 (**menopause**). Each monthly cycle begins as female hormones stimulate the lining of the uterus to thicken and form a special, highly vascular cushion, which is created just in case a fertilized egg should arrive on the scene and need a place to bed down. Approximately 2 weeks after the previous menstrual period, an egg is dispatched by one of the ovaries into the fallopian tube for the trip to the uterus. If that egg happens to meet up with a sperm whizzing up from the vagina, and if the chemistry is right, the egg will be fertilized. The fertilized egg will then start dividing and implant itself in the thickened uterine wall, and it will begin to grow—the beginning of pregnancy. If the egg is not fertilized, the uterus will shed its special lining (which is simply a layer of cells and blood) as menstrual flow, which passes out of the body through the cervix and vagina. Menstrual flow usually continues for about 5 days, following which the uterus is back at work preparing a new lining, just in case, and the whole cycle starts anew.

PREGNANCY

As noted above, if a sperm should happen to arrive on the scene on the day that the ovum starts meandering down to the uterus (about day 14 of the menstrual cycle), fertilization of the egg can occur. Once the egg is fertilized, it begins to divide and then, in

Fig. 32-1. *Female reproductive system.*

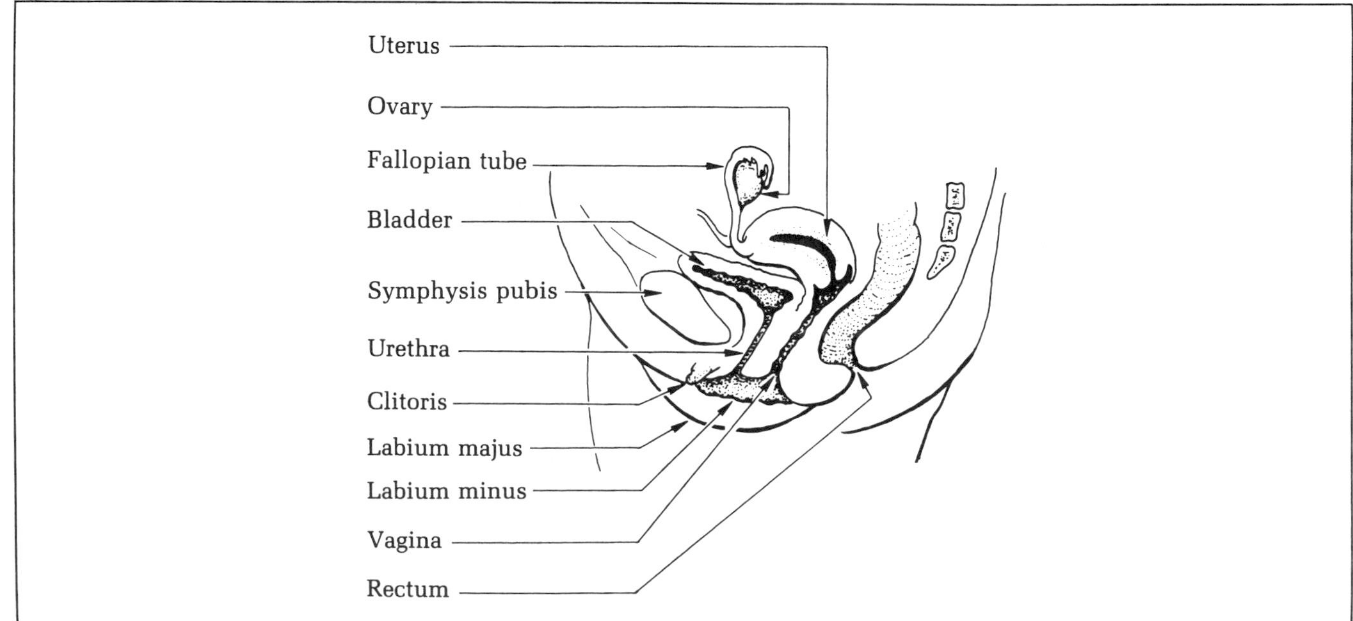

about a week, it nestles down into the thickly cushioned uterine wall to start an energetic process of cell division and growth that will culminate approximately 270 days later in the birth of a baby. Perhaps the most critical phase of that growth is the first 90 days or so of pregnancy, called the FIRST TRIMESTER. During this period, cells must begin their differentiation into specialized body tissues, a process that can be significantly disturbed if the mother is exposed to certain drugs (e.g., thalidomide), infectious illnesses (e.g., German measles), or radiation. Also during the first trimester, the specialized structures of pregnancy develop within the womb to protect and nourish the growing embryo. The embryo becomes enclosed in a special bag, called the **amniotic sac,** or "bag of waters." As the name implies, this sac contains about a liter of liquid (**amniotic fluid**) in which the developing baby paddles about. Nourishment and oxygen are provided to the embryo by a special organ of pregnancy called the **placenta,** or afterbirth, which is attached to the inside wall of the uterus. A long pipeline, the **umbilical cord,** links the fetus to the placenta and permits circulation of the blood between them.

During the SECOND TRIMESTER (the second 3 months of pregnancy), the embryo graduates into a full-fledged **fetus.** Bone structure develops, facial features appear, and hair starts to sprout from the head. The uterus expands to accommodate the enlarging fetus and becomes palpable at about the level of the mother's umbilicus. This process continues through the last 3 months of pregnancy, the THIRD TRIMESTER, during which the fetus prepares to makes its debut in the world outside the warm, protected womb. Subcutaneous fat develops to provide insulation, and the lungs mature in preparation for breathing. The uterus reaches its maximal expansion, crowding up against the mother's diaphragm.

At the end of the third trimester, when the fetus is fully mature, it is said to be at "full term," and it paddles into position to depart from mother (Fig. 32-2). Now all that remains for the baby is to make its way out of the womb and into the world. This is accomplished through a process called **labor,** in which the uterus begins a series of rhythmic contractions that increase in frequency and intensity until the baby and its placenta are ejected from the mother's body.

LABOR

Labor progresses through several well-defined stages, whose duration depends in part on whether the mother is going through her first pregnancy or whether she is already a veteran in having babies. To begin with, there is a PRODROMAL STAGE, which may go unnoticed in many cases. In this stage, the woman begins to feel a relief of pressure in her upper abdomen with a simultaneous increase of pressure in her pelvis as the baby starts its descent toward the birth canal. A plug of mucus, sometimes mixed with blood, called the **bloody show,** is expelled from the dilating cervix and discharged from the vagina. The FIRST STAGE OF LABOR begins with the onset of regular labor pains, crampy abdominal pains that radiate into the small of the back and reflect the contractions of the uterus. These early contractions come at about 5- to 15-minute intervals, and they serve to maneuver the baby into position, as well as to dilate the cervical opening through which the baby will have to make its exit. The first stage of labor lasts an average of about 12 hours in a woman having her first baby (a **primigravida**) and anywhere up to 8

Fig. 32-2. *A. Nonpregnant woman. B. Position of fetus in uterus just before birth.*

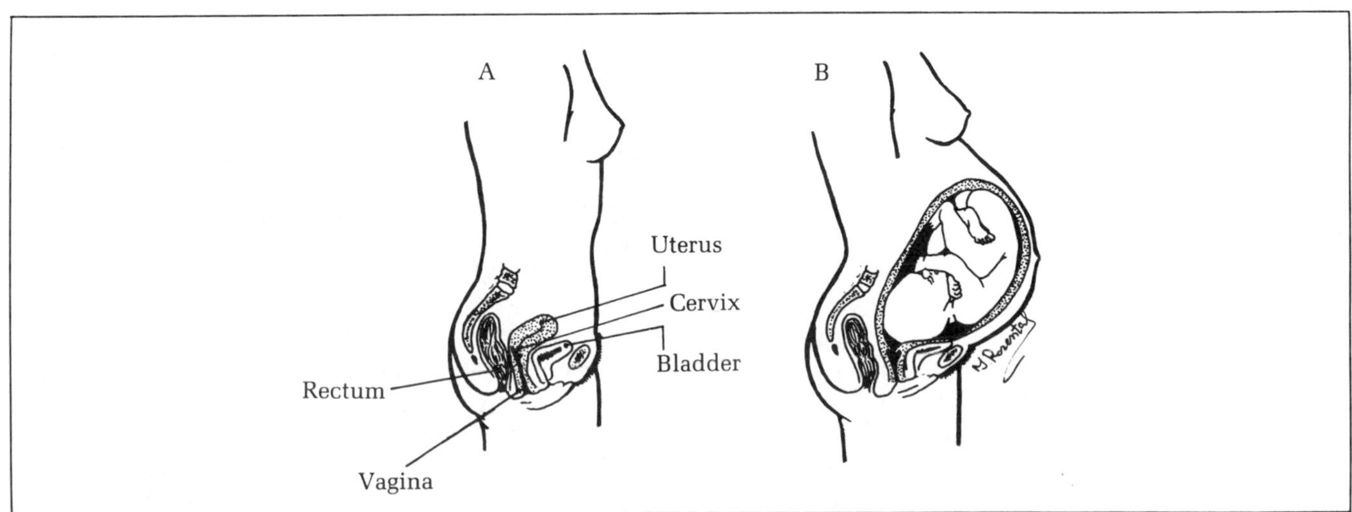

hours in a woman who has already had more than one pregnancy (a **multipara,** or "multip"). It is usually toward the end of the first stage of labor that the amniotic sac ruptures, with a dramatic gush of fluid suddenly pouring out of the vagina.

The SECOND STAGE OF LABOR begins as the baby's head enters the birth canal. The mother's pains become more intense and more frequent, now occurring 2 to 3 minutes apart. Her pulse rate increases. Sweat appears on her face. She tends to bear down with each contraction, and because of the pressure of the baby's head against her rectum, she may feel as if she has to move her bowels. The cervix meanwhile becomes fully dilated, and the **presenting part** of the baby (the part that emerges from the mother first—normally the head) begins bulging out of the vaginal opening, a process called **crowning** (Fig. 32-3). When crowning occurs, delivery is imminent. The second stage of labor is concluded when the baby is fully delivered. Altogether, the third stage of labor takes an average of about 50 minutes in a primip and about 20 minutes in a multip.

The THIRD STAGE OF LABOR, also called the placental stage, is the period from the delivery of the baby until the placenta has been fully expelled and the uterus has contracted. Uterine contraction is necessary to squeeze shut all of the tiny blood vessels left exposed when the placenta separated from the uterine wall.

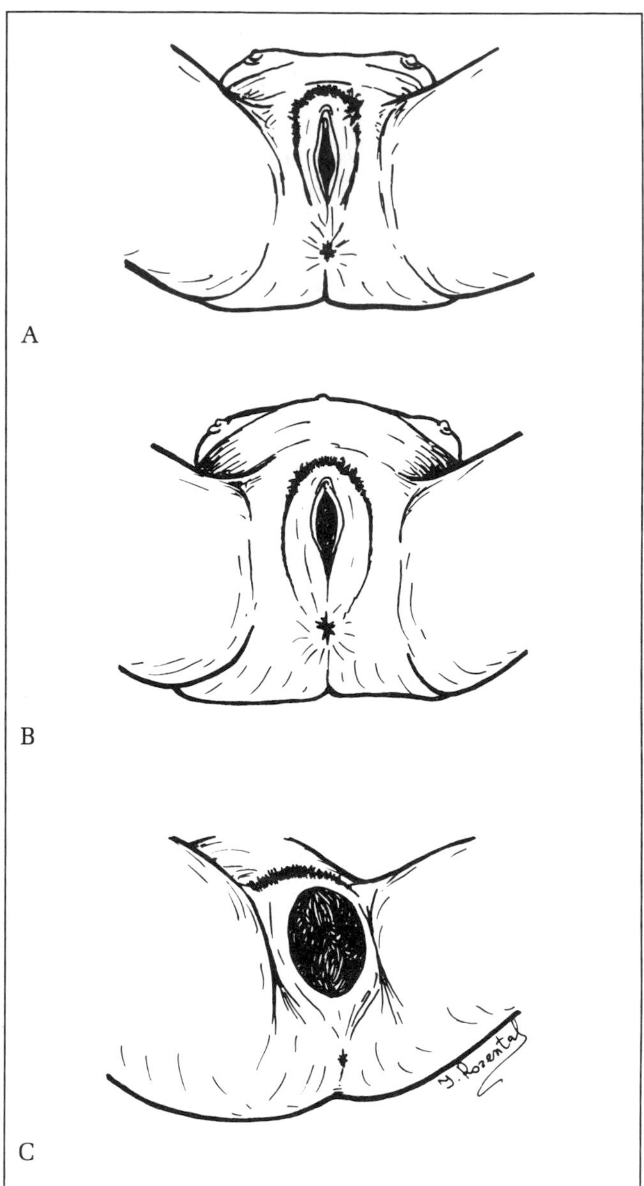

Fig. 32-3. *A. Vaginal opening in nonpregnant woman. B. Early crowning. C. Late crowning, just before delivery.*

NORMAL CHILDBIRTH

As a general rule, babies in America are born in hospitals under sterile and controlled conditions. Occasionally, however, the most carefully laid plans are thwarted by Mother Nature, and the pregnant woman finds herself in an advanced stage of labor without sufficient time to reach the hospital for delivery. On such occasions, the EMT may be called upon to assist the mother in delivering the baby. In this discussion, we will examine how the EMT can determine whether there is time to transport the mother and the steps he or she should take if it appears that delivery will not wait.

EVALUATING THE MOTHER

When an EMT is called to attend a woman in labor, the first decision he or she must make is whether there is time to transport the patient to a medical facility, which is generally the preferred environment in which to deliver a baby. Thus the EMT needs to be able to determine whether labor will continue for a while longer or whether delivery can be expected within a few minutes. To make this determination, one must ask the mother a few pertinent questions and make a quick visual examination.

To begin with, it is important to know the FREQUENCY OF THE MOTHER'S CONTRACTIONS. Labor pains that are 5 to 10 minutes apart usually indicate that you have a safe margin of time to reach the hospital; labor pains less than 2 minutes apart suggest that delivery may occur quite soon. The significance of the frequency of labor pains can be more accurately assessed by finding out WHETHER THIS IS THE WOMAN'S FIRST PREGNANCY. Remember, the second stage of labor is a much more leisurely affair in a rookie; it is the multip who is likely to go roaring through the second stage of labor, often in 15 to 20 minutes. Find out also WHETHER THE MOTHER FEELS AS THOUGH SHE HAS TO MOVE HER BOWELS. This sensation occurring during labor is a pretty good sign that the baby's head has entered the vagina, and once that happens, delivery is only minutes away.

To make sure, you need to take a look at the vaginal opening to see whether there is crowning, that is, whether the presenting part is bulging out at the entrance to the vagina. Explain to the mother what you intend to do (male EMTs should request a chaperone—the woman's husband or a female friend or relative). Have the mother lie down and remove her undergarments, and *look at*—do not touch— the vaginal opening. If you see bulging, or if the presenting part is peeking out through the vagina, you can expect delivery within a very few minutes.

The steps in determining whether delivery is imminent are summarized in Figure 32-4.

A word of caution: If the mother tells you she feels

Fig. 32-4. *Evaluating the woman in labor.*

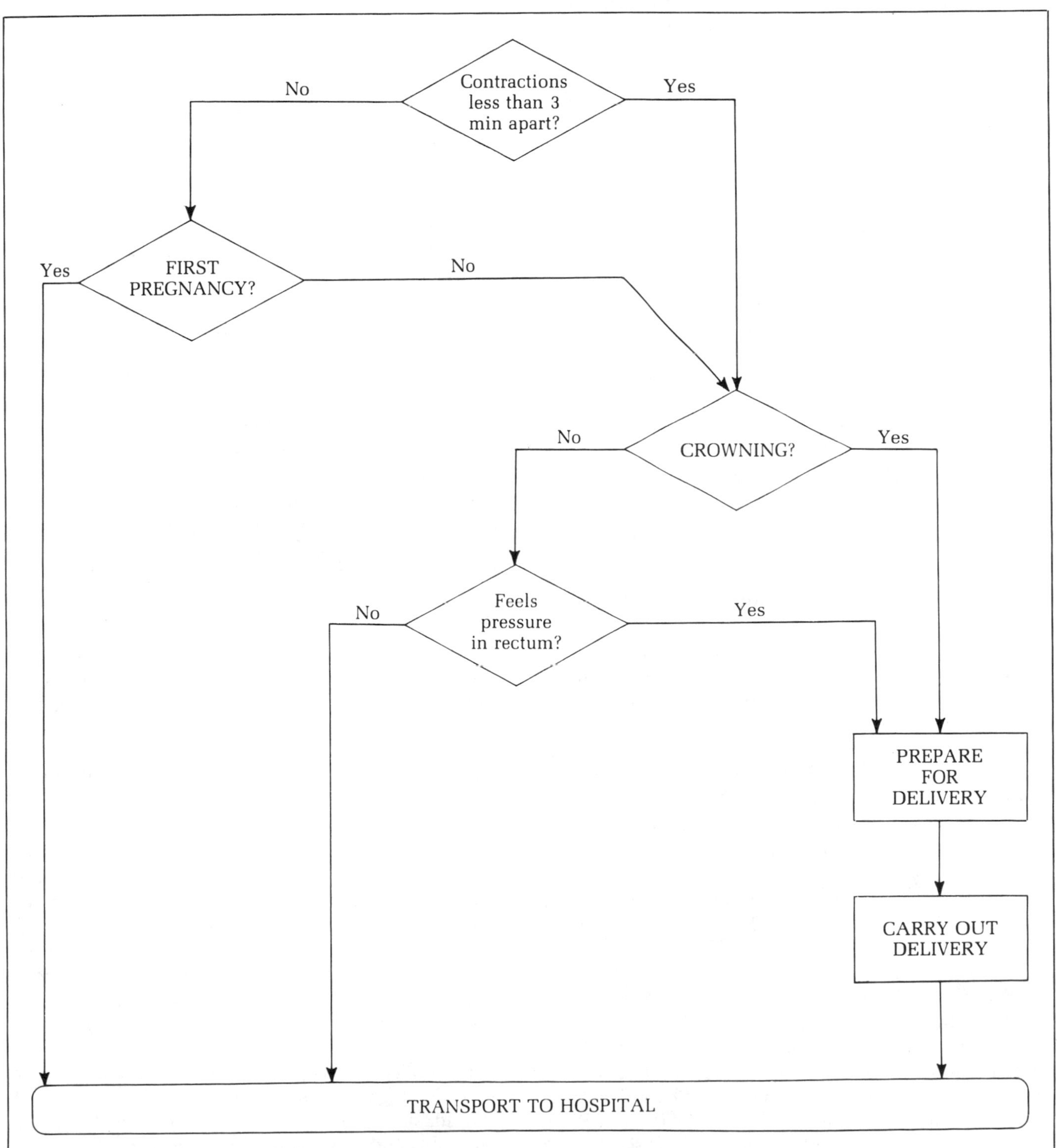

as if she has to move her bowels, DO NOT PERMIT HER TO GO TO THE TOILET, for in fact it is the baby and not her bowels that she has to move. Once delivery is imminent, furthermore, there is no way to prevent nature from taking its course, and any attempt to delay delivery will only result in harm or death to the baby and possibly to the mother as well. For that reason, NEVER ATTEMPT TO RESTRAIN OR HALT DELIVERY IN ANY WAY. Do not hold the mother's legs together. Do not have her cross her legs. It will not help. Just get yourself in gear, and start setting up pronto for the arrival of the baby.

PREPARING FOR DELIVERY

Once you have reached the conclusion that there will not be time to transport the mother to the hospital, you need to make swift but deliberate preparations to assist in the delivery of the baby. This involves preparing the scene, preparing the mother, and preparing the bystanders—all of which needs to be done more or less simultaneously. Good teamwork with your partner will be indispensable in this situation, for keep in mind that in childbirth you are dealing with *two* patients, each of whom needs special attention.

One EMT should begin at once PREPARING THE PROPER ENVIRONMENT FOR DELIVERY. If childbirth is to take place at home, the most convenient surface on which to place the mother is usually a bed. Time permitting, it is desirable to place a canvas stretcher or backboard onto the bed to facilitate moving the mother without undue handling after delivery. If delivery is to occur outside the home in a public place, it is best carried out on the wheeled ambulance stretcher, which should be positioned to ensure maximum privacy. Whether childbirth will be in bed, on a canvas stretcher, or on the wheeled stretcher, lay a clean sheet over the surface, and have the mother lie down on it—flat on her back, with knees flexed, thighs spread apart, and feet flat on the surface. The mother's buttocks should be at least 2 feet from the end of the bed, so that the baby will not be shot out onto the floor. Put a folded blanket or folded sheet beneath the mother's buttocks to elevate them 1 or 2 inches above the stretcher surface. In an automobile (yes, it happens in automobiles too), position the mother supine on the seat, with one leg flexed, resting on the seat, and the other leg hanging down to the floor.

Every ambulance should carry a STERILE OBSTETRIC KIT, whose contents are listed in Table 32-1. When the mother is positioned, this kit should be placed on a nearby table or chair, within easy reach. Open the kit, being careful not to touch anything inside, and WASH YOUR HANDS THOROUGHLY with germicidal solution. Then DON STERILE GLOVES and preferably a sterile cap and surgical

Table 32-1. *Sterile Obstetric Kit for Ambulances*

Quantity	Equipment
1 pair	Surgical scissors
4	Cord clamps
4–6	12-inch lengths of umbilical tape
4–6	Towels
2–3 pair	Surgical gloves
1	Surgical gown*
1–2	Surgical masks*
12	4 × 4-gauze sponges
12	Sanitary napkins
1	Bulb syringe
1	Baby blanket
2	Large plastic bags

*Optional.

gown as well, if these are provided in your kit. Now comes the process of DRAPING THE PATIENT. Take the first sterile towel and slip it under the mother's buttocks, taking care not to touch anything unsterile (e.g., the sheet, the mother's skin) as you do so. Lay a second sterile towel flat on the bed or stretcher between the mother's legs, just below the vaginal opening. A third sterile towel or drape should be laid across the mother's abdomen, and each thigh should be draped as well. When you finish, everything should be covered with sterile drapes except the vaginal opening.

While you have been busy getting everything properly set up at the delivery end, your partner should have been tending to the EMOTIONAL PREPARATION OF THE MOTHER AND BYSTANDERS. Remember, most women do not *plan* to have their babies at home or in a department store or at a football game, so mother is bound to be at least a little nervous and upset. Thus the EMT should comfort and reassure her. In addition, the EMT in charge of mother needs to make a quick judgment regarding the emotional state of various bystanders. Depending on who seems calmest, a female relative, friend, or the patient's husband should be asked to stay by the mother and lend emotional support; having a comforting hand to squeeze can alleviate much of the pain and anxiety of labor. Agitated bystanders should be dispatched on various errands that will keep them occupied and out of the way. Sending a panicky husband off to boil several gallons of water, for example, is often a useful maneuver; there is no need for boiling water in the delivery of a baby, but the preparation thereof keeps the father-to-be busy in the kitchen.

The EMT assigned to mother should remain *by her head* at all times, in order to turn her head to the side should she begin vomiting. An emesis basin and portable suction should be within reach.

DELIVERY
With the mother prepared and draped, the EMT who will be assisting in her delivery should take up a position just distal to her buttocks (a right-handed EMT on the woman's right, a left-handed EMT on the woman's left) and keep a close eye on the vaginal opening. The mother should be encouraged to rest between contractions; during contractions, she should be instructed to pant and avoid bearing down unless she feels she must.

WHEN THE BABY'S HEAD BEGINS TO EMERGE from the vagina, place your right hand (or if left-handed, your left hand) against the baby's head—taking care not to touch the mother's perineum—and support the head gently, with very slight pressure, to prevent the head from rocketing out of the vagina (Fig. 32-6A). Your goal in this maneuver is *not* to prevent delivery of the head, but simply to control it lest delivery be too rapid, so keep the pressure on the head *very* gentle. Usually it takes a few contractions before the head is fully delivered, and the light pressure on the baby's head may be released between contractions.

Once the head is delivered, look and feel to DETERMINE IF THE UMBILICAL CORD IS WRAPPED AROUND THE BABY'S NECK. If so, try very gently to loosen it and slip it over the baby's head, to prevent the baby from being strangled by it (Fig. 32-5). Great care must be taken not to tear the cord in the process. Should the cord be wrapped very tightly around the baby's neck, it will have to be clamped and cut: Put two sterile clamps about 2 inches apart along the cord, and use a sterile scissors to cut the cord between them. If all is well with the umbilical cord, inspect the baby's head to BE SURE THE HEAD IS NOT ENCLOSED IN THE AMNIOTIC SAC. Occasionally, the bag of waters does not break during labor, and the baby is born still enclosed inside the amniotic sac. If this occurs, use a clamp or your finger to puncture the sac, and peel it away from the baby's nose and mouth, for otherwise the infant will asphyxiate.

Fig. 32-5. *If the umbilical cord is wrapped around the baby's neck, try gently to slip the cord over its head.*

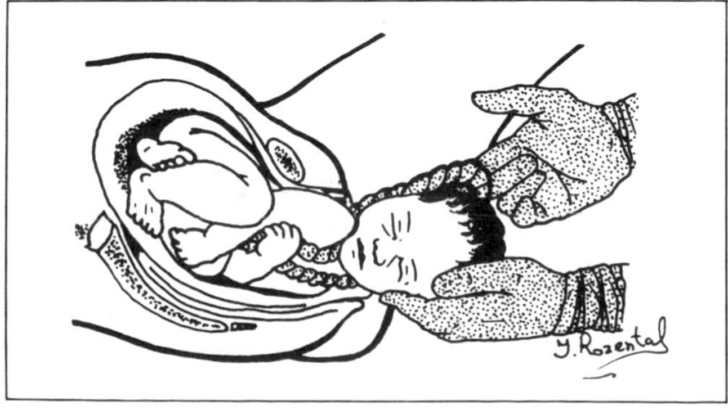

As the baby's head emerges from the vagina, it is usually facing the mother's rectum; then as the chin emerges, the head turns to face one of the mother's thighs. As the chin comes out of the vagina, slide the hand that has been controlling the baby's head beneath the head, so that the head is cradled and supported in your hand (Fig. 32-6B). With your other hand, take the BULB SYRINGE and suction the baby's mouth and nostrils. To do so correctly, squeeze the bulb *before* inserting it, *then* place the tip in the infant's mouth or nostrils, and slowly release pressure on the bulb (Fig. 32-7). Squeeze out the contents of the bulb onto a towel, then compress it again, and suction the baby's mouth and nostrils once more. This process may have to be repeated two or three times until the baby's airway is clear of mucus and amniotic fluid.

Meanwhile, as the baby's head turns to face the mother's thigh, the upper shoulder usually becomes visible in the vaginal opening. From this point on, the baby should be supported with two hands. To assist in DELIVERY OF THE UPPER SHOULDER, gently guide the head downward (Fig. 32-8). DO

Fig. 32-6. *A. Apply gentle pressure to the baby's head to prevent explosive delivery. B. Support the head as it begins to deliver.*

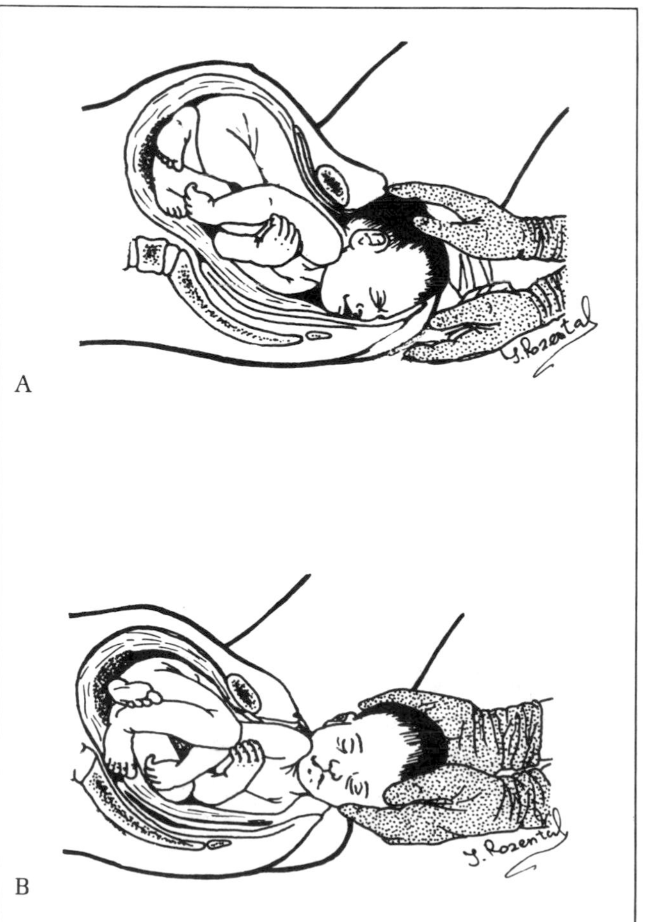

push the vaginal wall gently away from the baby's face. If you can, keep one finger in the baby's mouth to hold it open. DO NOT UNDER ANY CIRCUMSTANCES TRY TO PULL THE BABY OUT. If delivery of the head has not occurred within 2 to 3 minutes after you have established an airway, you will have to get the mother and baby to a medical facility as soon as possible. This will not be an easy task, for you must try to maintain the baby's airway at all times. That means the ride to the hospital must be exceptionally smooth, to permit you to hold the vaginal wall steadily away from the baby's face. Elevating the mother's buttocks on a pillow will be helpful in reducing the pressure of the baby's head against the birth canal.

Limb Presentation

When the presenting part is an arm or a leg (Fig. 32-14), normal delivery is impossible, and special obstetric procedures must be employed to enable a safe birth. LIMB PRESENTATION CANNOT BE MANAGED IN THE FIELD. Thus if you see an arm or leg protruding from the birth canal, TRANSPORT THE MOTHER TO THE HOSPITAL WITHOUT ANY DELAY.

PROLAPSED UMBILICAL CORD

A prolapsed umbilical cord means that the umbilical cord emerges from the vagina before the baby. Cord prolapse is a relatively unusual occurrence, but an extremely dangerous one; for as the baby descends through the birth canal, the cord will be squeezed against the pelvic wall, and the baby's supply of oxygenated blood will be shut off. To prevent asphyxiation of the baby under these circumstances, rapid measures must be taken to relieve the pressure of the baby's head against the umbilical cord.

If you see the umbilical cord protruding from the mother's vagina, have the mother lie on one side and IMMEDIATELY PLACE THE MOTHER IN A HEAD-DOWN POSITION WITH HER BUTTOCKS MUCH HIGHER THAN HER SHOULDERS. This maneuver will help keep the baby, by gravity, higher in the birth canal. Take a sterile towel from the obstetric kit, and moisten it with sterile saline. Then WRAP THE MOISTENED, STERILE TOWEL GENTLY AROUND THE PROTRUDING PORTION OF THE CORD to protect it from drying and jarring. DO NOT UNDER ANY CIRCUMSTANCES ATTEMPT TO PUSH THE CORD BACK INTO THE VAGINA. Treat it as an evisceration, and leave it where it is.

ADMINISTER OXYGEN to the mother, so that the blood that does reach the baby through the umbilical cord will be maximally oxygenated. TRANSPORT to the hospital, making sure to KEEP THE MOTHER WARM en route, with blankets as needed.

TWINS AND PREMIES

The delivery of more than one baby or the delivery of an abnormally small (premature) baby requires special measures to ensure the infant(s) the best possible start in life.

Fig. 32-14. *Limb presentations. A. Footling breech. B. Shoulder distocia with prolapse of the arm.*

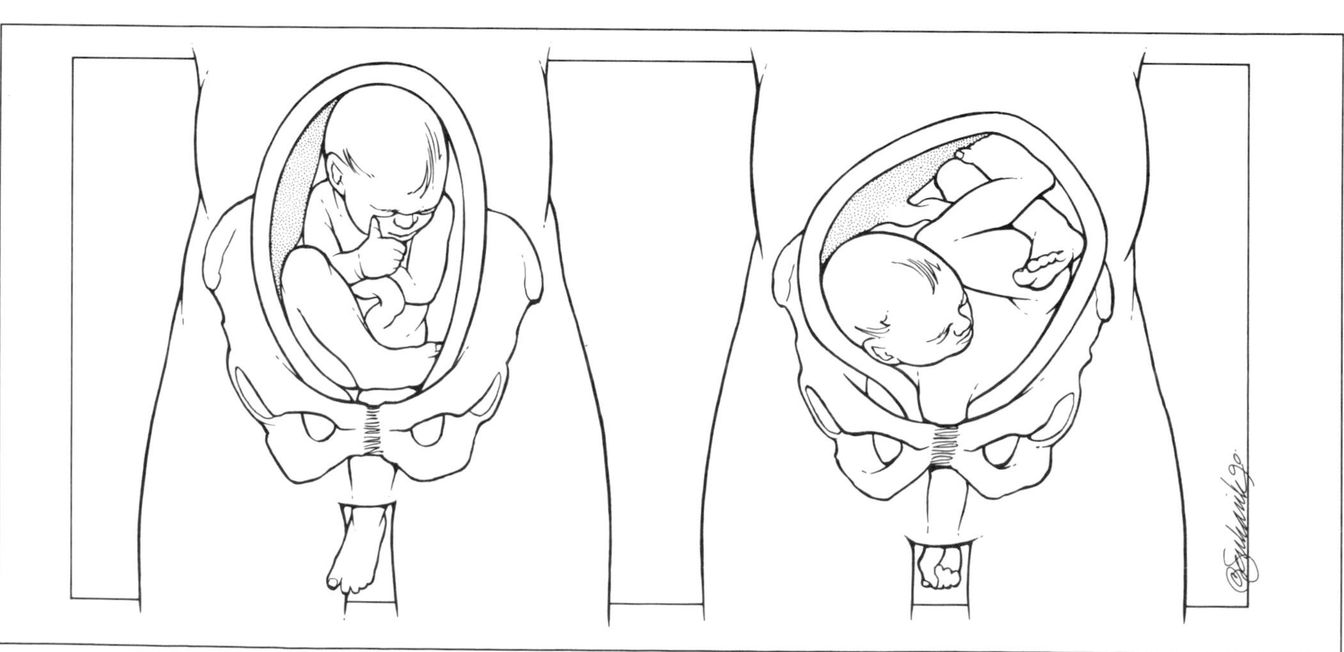

TWINS

About 1 in every 90 deliveries produces twins, so the chances of encountering a twin birth sometime in your EMT career are not all that remote. Often the mother-to-be will know in advance that she is carrying twins, having been given the news during pregnancy. Sometimes, though, the mother is not aware that she is doubly pregnant. The EMT should suspect this possibility if the woman's abdomen is unusually large or if it remains large after birth of the (first) baby.

Most twins are delivered single file, one after the other, in the same manner as single babies. When the first baby arrives, handle it as you would any other delivery. Clamp and cut the cord in the usual manner, making sure that there is no bleeding from *either* of the cut ends. Labor contractions will usually start up again within 5 to 10 minutes after the birth of the first baby, and baby number two can be expected to arrive within 30 to 45 minutes of its twin. Usually both babies are born before the first placenta is delivered. The whole process is fundamentally the same as the delivery of a single infant, except you have to do everything twice!

Twins are apt to arrive prematurely, and even if they are full term, they are often small for their age. If this is the case, they should be handled with the same special precautions given a premature infant (see below).

PREMATURE BABIES

A premature baby ("premie") is, by definition, any baby born before 8 months of pregnancy or weighing less than 2 kg (about 5½ lb). Unless you carry a scale around in the ambulance, you will usually have to make an educated guess about the baby's weight. Practice making these estimates when you do your clinical rotation through the obstetric service; guess each baby's weight, and then check your guess against the measurement on the scale. After a while, you should be able to come within about half a pound of the correct weight. Other clues to prematurity come from the history provided by the mother and the baby's general appearance. If the mother says she was not "due" for another 2 months, the baby is doubtless premature. Furthermore, premature babies *look* premature: They are skinnier, smaller, redder, and usually more wrinkled than full-term babies, and their heads seem to be way too big for their bodies.

Premies are very fragile creatures and need very special care to survive. Because their surface area is large with respect to body volume, and because there is minimal subcutaneous fat to serve as insulation, premies lose heat much faster than do full-term babies and can become hypothermic with alarming rapidity. A limited blood volume makes them exquisitely sensitive to even small amounts of bleeding, and immature immune mechanisms give premies a much greater susceptibility to infection. All of these factors must be kept in mind as one cares for the premature infant.

The first principle in caring for a premie is to KEEP THE BABY WARM. Dry the baby quickly after delivery to minimize heat loss by evaporation. Ideally, the infant should be transported in a special portable incubator, whose internal temperature and humidity can be carefully controlled. If such equipment is not available, other means will have to be found to maintain the infant's body heat. Remember, babies lose heat by the same mechanisms that big people do: radiation, convection, and so forth. So you need to insulate the baby against these types of heat loss. One of the most efficient ways of doing this is to WRAP THE BABY FROM HEAD TO TOE IN STERILE ALUMINUM FOIL, leaving only the face uncovered. Then wrape a blanket over the foil, again covering everything except the baby's face.

Just like big people, premies need an ADEQUATE AIRWAY. Check the baby's airway frequently after delivery, and use the squeeze bulb to suction out mucus from the mouth and nostrils as needed. ADMINISTER OXYGEN, but *not* in the same way you would administer it to an adult. Use a sterile towel or similar material to make a small tent above the baby's head, and pipe the oxygen flow—about 2 to 3 liters per minute—into this tent. Aim the flow toward the top of the tent, not into the baby's face.

EXAMINE THE UMBILICAL CORD CLOSELY FOR BLEEDING. Remember, premies cannot tolerate blood loss, even very tiny amounts of blood loss. So if you see any oozing at all from the cut end of the cord, apply an additional clamp or tie.

AVOID CONTAMINATION. Premies are easily infected and must be protected from exposure to potential contaminants. If at all possible, wear a surgical mask and gown when handling a premie. Do not breathe directly into its face, and keep it well away from other people, especially small children (who are always carrying some germ or other).

NOTIFY THE HOSPITAL that you are bringing in a premature baby, and tell them your estimated time of arrival. This will give the obstetric staff time to set up an incubator and make other necessary preparations to receive the infant. TRANSPORT the baby and mother expeditiously to the hospital, with close attention to the baby's airway en route.

COMPLICATIONS OF CHILDBIRTH

Complications are unusual during and after delivery, but when they do occur, the EMT must be able to spot them quickly and provide appropriate emergency management. Complications can involve the baby or the mother or both.

THE NONBREATHING BABY

Most newborn babies will start to breathe, and cry, within a few seconds after delivery, often while you are still suctioning the nose and mouth. If the newborn does not begin spontaneous breathing within about 30 seconds of delivery, or if it is born limp and seemingly without signs of life, immediate resuscitation measures will be necessary. First of all, CLEAR THE AIRWAY by suctioning the mouth and nostrils of blood and mucus, as described earlier, and place the baby on one side, with the head lower than the trunk to facilitate drainage of fluids from its mouth. STIMULATE THE BABY by flicking your index finger several times against the soles of its feet; this maneuver is often all that is required to get the baby to gasp and start breathing. If the baby remains apneic, however, you will have to begin artificial ventilation. USE MOUTH-TO-MOUTH (AND NOSE) VENTILATION ONLY: DO NOT USE ADJUNCTS, such as a bag-valve-mask or demand valve, for these will deliver too much air under too much pressure. In ventilating an infant, keep in mind a fundamental fact:

> BABIES ARE VERY LITTLE.

Thus place your mouth over the baby's nose and mouth, and give *very small breaths*—just PUFFS FROM YOUR CHEEKS (Fig. 32-15). If the infant begins breathing spontaneously after several puffs, administer oxygen—an oxygen mask held about 4 inches from the infant's face will do the trick—until the baby "pinks up" and respirations seems unlabored. If spontaneous respirations do not resume, continue artificial ventilation, and CHECK FOR A PULSE. An absent pulse signals the need to start EXTERNAL CARDIAC COMPRESSIONS. Do not forget that for babies you use only the index finger to depress the midsternum (see Chapter 7).

CPR should be continued until the baby resumes breathing on its own or is pronounced dead by a physician. Once you have started CPR, therefore, do not give up. Get set for transport, taking care to keep the baby protected with a blanket from the cold, and move on to the hospital with CPR continuing en route. The steps of resuscitation of the newborn are summarized in Figure 32-16.

There is one situation in which CPR should not be attempted in the nonbreathing newborn, and that is when it is clear that the baby died in the womb several hours or days before birth, a so-called **stillbirth.** This situation is usually not difficult to recognize, for the infant has a very unpleasant odor. In addition, the infant's head may be quite soft, and its skin is often covered with blisters. DO NOT ATTEMPT TO RESUSCITATE A STILLBORN BABY.

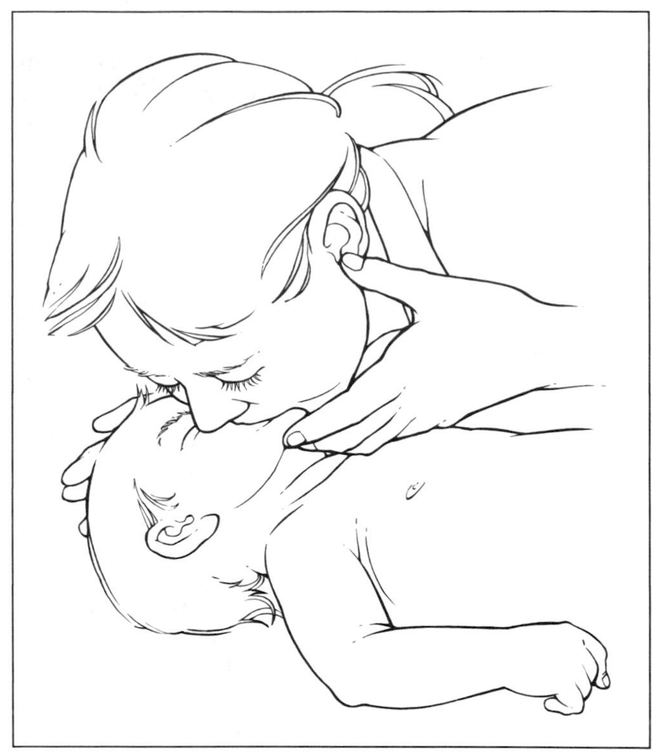

Fig. 32-15. *Artificial ventilation of the newborn. Give only small puffs from your cheeks.*

POSTPARTUM HEMORRHAGE

Postpartum hemorrhage means bleeding after delivery. As noted earlier, the mother can be expected to lose about half a unit of blood during delivery of the placenta. Such bleeding is normal and self-limited, and it is not a cause for alarm. If, however, bleeding is profuse or it does not stop shortly after the placenta has been delivered, measures must be taken to prevent the mother from going into hemorrhagic shock. The fundamental principles of treatment are the same as for any other case of impending shock, but with special consideration to the circumstances in which bleeding has occurred.

To begin with, PROTECT THE MOTHER'S AIRWAY. Vomiting is not uncommon during delivery and in shock, so you must be alert to make sure that aspiration does not occur. Be ready to turn the mother's head to the side at the first sign of vomiting, and have suction handy. ADMINISTER OXYGEN—generally 6 liters per minute by nasal cannula will be sufficient. Keep the mother in the SHOCK POSITION, that is, legs elevated, and KEEP HER WARM. Cover the vaginal opening with sanitary napkins or multitrauma pads, but DO NOT TRY TO INSERT ANY DRESSING OR PACKING INTO THE VAGINA. Use the measures described earlier to PROMOTE UTERINE CONTRACTION: massage of the uterus and putting the baby to the mother's breast. If signs of shock are already present, apply the MILITARY ANTI-SHOCK TROUSERS, and if authorized to do so, START AN INTRAVENOUS INFUSION WITH NORMAL SALINE OR RINGER'S SOLUTION.

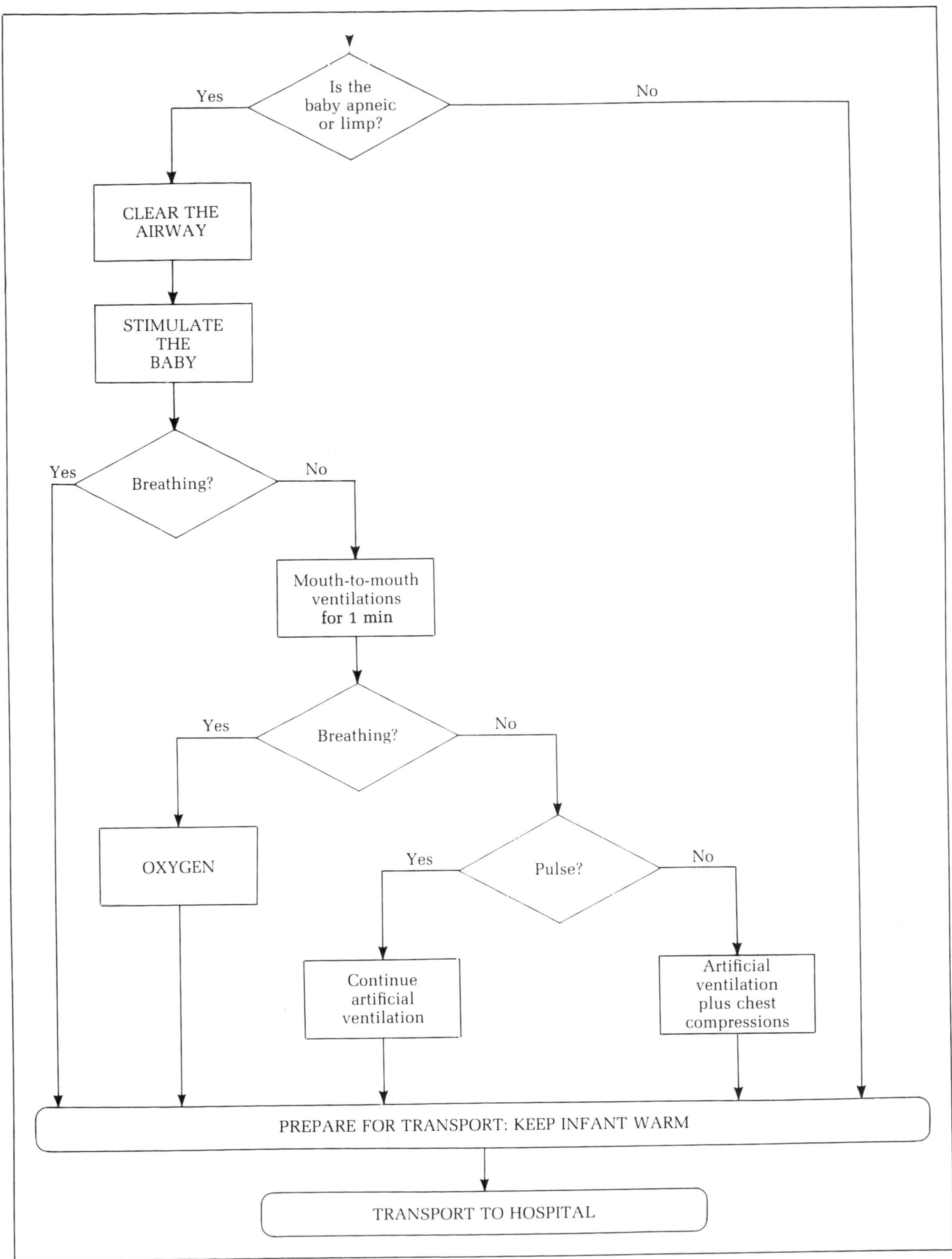

Fig. 32-16. *Resuscitation of the apneic newborn.*

to 6 months of pregnancy is said to be having a **threatened abortion**—"threatened" because it may progress to complete abortion, or the symptoms may subside, permitting the pregnancy to go to term.

The field treatment of a suspected abortion is simply reassurance and transport. Keep the woman as calm and quiet as possible, and proceed without undue haste to the hospital. High speed and sirens are not necessary and will only aggravate the situation. If the woman has passed any products of conception from her vagina (i.e., anything besides blood), collect these in a plastic bag and bring them to the hospital for examination. Be alert for the possibility of sudden, profuse hemorrhage, and monitor the vital signs frequently en route.

THIRD TRIMESTER BLEEDING

Bleeding during the last 3 months of pregnancy is always a serious matter. It may be due to any of several causes, but the two most worrisome are a premature separation of the placenta from the wall of the uterus and a malposition of the placenta such that it becomes the presenting part. In either case, exsanguinating hemorrhage can occur *within minutes.* Sometimes the bleeding is not immediately evident, for it may be confined within the uterus, and the patient presents simply with severe abdominal pain and unexplained shock. Thus the EMT must be alert to the possibility of internal bleeding whenever a woman in late pregnancy presents with signs of hypovolemia or shock.

BLEEDING IN THE THIRD TRIMESTER SHOULD ALWAYS BE REGARDED AS A CRITICAL EMERGENCY, and the woman must reach an obstetric facility as soon as possible. Keep the patient RECUMBENT, LYING ON HER SIDE. If signs of shock, such as restlessness, tachycardia, and cold, clammy skin, are already present, administer OXYGEN, and secure permission to start an INTRAVENOUS INFUSION en route to the hospital. Remember, bleeding may abruptly become very massive, so it is a good idea to have at least one large-bore intravenous line established, just in case you need to infuse a lot of fluids in a hurry. Keep the Military Anti-Shock Trousers (MAST) handy, preferably laid out on the stretcher beneath the patient, ready to be applied. If shock develops, apply and inflate the *leg sections* of the MAST.

DO NOT ATTEMPT TO EXAMINE THE PATIENT'S VAGINAL AREA, for this may precipitate exsanguinating hemorrhage. Confine your examination to a check of vital signs, and get moving to the hospital. RADIO AHEAD to the receiving hospital to let them know the nature of the case and your estimated time of arrival. In some cases, a woman with significant third trimester bleeding will have to be taken straight to the operating room, and the obstetric staff will need some lead time to get set up.

PREECLAMPSIA AND ECLAMPSIA

Eclampsia, or toxemia of pregnancy, is a condition characterized by high blood pressure, edema, and protein in the urine, and it may lead to serious complications as the pregnant woman goes into labor. Eclampsia is more common during first pregnancies, and its early signs usually become evident sometime after the twenty-fourth week of pregnancy. During this early phase, called **preeclampsia**, the woman may gain more weight than expected, as edema fluid begins to collect in her body. In addition, her blood pressure begins to creep upward. These signs are often very subtle and, unless you look for them specifically, you will probably miss them. For this reason:

> A BLOOD PRESSURE SHOULD BE RECORDED FOR EVERY PREGNANT PATIENT, REGARDLESS OF CHIEF COMPLAINT.

Normally, the blood pressure is somewhat low during the third trimester, and any blood pressure over about 130/80 should be called to the attention of the woman's physician.

Full-blown eclampsia, when present, usually occurs around the time of labor. The typical patient has massive EDEMA, which may be evident even in her face, and HYPERTENSION. She may complain of HEADACHE and sometimes of EPIGASTRIC OR RIGHT UPPER QUADRANT PAIN. Eclampsia is a very serious condition, for it is often associated with SEIZURES and COMA, and may threaten the life of both mother and baby.

If you are called to attend a pregnant woman near or at term and note any of the signs and symptoms mentioned above, immediately notify the physician at the receiving hospital of the situation. The major goal of treatment in the field is to minimize the possibility of seizures. It does not take much to precipitate a seizure in an eclamptic woman: Noise, excitement, confusion, flashing lights—any of those may trigger severe convulsions in eclampsia. Thus the first consideration in managing and transporting a woman with suspected eclampsia is to MINIMIZE ALL EXTERNAL STIMULI. Keep the woman in a quiet, darkened room until you are all set to transport. Have someone beside her at all times to provide reassurance and to protect her from injury in the event that seizures do occur. Once you are in the ambulance, transport the patient as gently and quietly as possible. NO SIRENS, NO FLASHING

LIGHTS. Keep the patient area of the ambulance darkened if possible.

Administer OXYGEN by nasal cannula, and KEEP THE PATIENT ON HER SIDE. Should seizures occur despite all your precautions, maintain the patient's airway, and protect her from injury. Keep suction close by.

SUPINE HYPOTENSIVE SYNDROME

The perceptive reader will have noticed that in all of the situations just described, and in our discussion of prolapsed umbilical cord (Chapter 32), we have stated that the pregnant woman should be transported lying on her side (preferably her left side, in order that she faces you and not the wall of the ambulance). The reason for this is a practical one. The pregnant woman in her last trimester has a large, heavy mass in her abdomen. When she lies supine, this mass—comprising the combined weight of the fetus, placenta, amniotic fluid, and uterus—tends to press down against the inferior vena cava. Compression of the vena cava in turn reduces blood return to the heart, with a consequent fall in cardiac output. The reduction in cardiac output will be even more pronounced if the woman's blood volume is in any way compromised, as in the situation of hemorrhage.

The drop in cardiac output due to pressure on the vena cava is called the supine hypotensive syndrome, for it occurs only when the pregnant woman is lying supine. The prevention and treatment are simple:

> TRANSPORT THE PREGNANT WOMAN LYING ON HER SIDE.

TRAUMA

Trauma during pregnancy is particularly worrisome because there are *two* patients involved—mother and baby—either or both of whom may sustain life-threatening injury. In general, the same priorities of treatment apply to an injured, pregnant woman as to any other victim of trauma. The AIRWAY always has first priority, and adequate OXYGENATION must be ensured at all times, for there are two lives depending on that oxygen. Inadequate BREATHING must be promptly managed with artificial ventilation, and BLEEDING should be controlled as rapidly as possible. Don't forget: The supine position will aggravate the effects of even minor blood loss, so PUT THE WOMAN ON HER SIDE as soon as it is safe to do so (i.e., after stabilization of suspected fractures). Anticipate SHOCK, and be prepared to start an intravenous infusion and apply the MAST (leg sections only) as needed.

Two important points need special emphasis. The first is that it is impossible in the field to assess potential damage to the fetus. Even when the mother appears relatively uninjured, the baby inside her may have sustained major trauma, especially in the event of a deceleration injury such as that which occurs in an automobile accident. Thus the rule to remember is:

> EVERY PREGNANT WOMAN WHO HAS BEEN INVOLVED IN AN ACCIDENT, EVEN IF HER INJURIES APPEAR MINOR, *MUST* BE EVALUATED IN THE HOSPITAL.

The second important point concerns the pregnant woman who has been critically or hopelessly injured during her third trimester. In such cases, you must always keep in mind that there are two lives involved. It may not be possible to save both lives, but sometimes the baby can be saved even when the mother cannot. What this means in practice is that you must make every effort to resuscitate a pregnant woman, even when the situation appears hopeless. Artificial ventilation with oxygen and external cardiac compressions may keep the baby alive for some time after the mother is biologically dead, and an emergency caesarian section at the hospital may then enable rescue of the infant. The message is:

> IF A PREGNANT WOMAN SUFFERS CARDIAC ARREST FROM ANY CAUSE, INITIATE CPR AND CONTINUE UNTIL YOU REACH THE HOSPITAL, EVEN IF HER CONDITION SEEMS HOPELESS.

EMERGENCIES IN THE NONPREGNANT WOMAN

The large majority of gynecologic problems, such as infections of the female genital tract and bleeding between periods, require only transport to a medical facility. We will deal here only with those emergencies that are likely to require special treatment or precautions in the field.

TRAUMA TO THE FEMALE GENITAL TRACT

The *internal* female genitalia—the ovaries, fallopian tubes, and uterus—are rarely injured because they are well protected within the pelvic girdle. Trauma massive enough to damage these organs will usually cause enormous damage to more major organs as well, and the priorities of treatment will dictate primary attention to the more life-threatening injuries. On the other hand, the *external* genitalia—the vulva, clitoris, major and minor labia, and entrance to the urethra—may suffer a variety of soft tissue injuries; and due to the rich nerve supply to the area, such injuries are apt to be very painful, even if not usually life-threatening. ABRASIONS, LACERATIONS, or AVULSIONS of the external female genitalia should be treated with STERILE MOIST COMPRESSES. If there is hemorrhage, CONTROL BLEEDING WITH LOCAL PRESSURE.

> DO NOT UNDER ANY CIRCUMSTANCES PLACE DRESSINGS INSIDE THE VAGINA.

Apply bulky dressings externally, and hold them in place with a triangular bandage fastened in the manner of a diaper.

IMPALED OBJECTS or other foreign bodies should not be removed but rather stabilized in place. BLUNT TRAUMA may cause considerable pain and swelling and should be treated with cold compresses until the patient reaches the hospital.

RAPE

Perhaps one of the most difficult emergency situations that the EMT may have to deal with is the call that comes in for a victim of sexual assault. Unfortunately this is not an uncommon emergency in our society—a rape occurs every six minutes in the United States—and it is a very complex one; for rape involves not only potential physical and psychologic injury, but also far-reaching legal ramifications.

In most cases, the victim of rape is a woman, and we will orient our discussion here to the management of female patients. It should be noted, however, that men, both heterosexual and homosexual, may also be raped, and the general principles of management outlined here are equally applicable when the victim is a man.

There are many definitions of rape, but in general rape involves attempted or actual sexual intercourse that is carried out *forcibly*, against the will of the victim. Associated physical injury is common, and even when physical damage has not been inflicted, the psychologic trauma may be enormous. As the first person on the scene, the EMT has the potential to help to alleviate that trauma or to make that trauma much worse. Perhaps nowhere else in emergency care is a calm, sympathetic, and professional attitude so important as in dealing with the victim of sexual assault.

In managing the victim of suspected rape, it is important always to bear in mind one fundamental principle:

> AN EMT IS FIRST AND FOREMOST A MEDICAL PROFESSIONAL, NOT A LAW ENFORCEMENT OFFICER.

This means that in every phase of the victim's management, your first concern should be for her physical and emotional well-being. It is *not* your primary job to collect evidence or even to notify law enforcement officials. Indeed, in some states, such as California, victims of sexual assault are given the option not to have contact with the police if they so choose. Even where police notification is mandatory, however, the victim should not be forced to make a police report prior to medical examination. Nor should you try to substitute for the police by conducting your own interrogation, for this process is very apt to make the victim feel "re-raped"; and any chance you might have had of gaining her confidence will be destroyed. If the victim *volunteers* any information about what happened to her, this information should be recorded accurately in the record, without editorial comment and preferably in the victim's own words (e.g., "The patient states, 'I was grabbed from behind by a heavy man.' "). Otherwise, confine your questions to pertinent assessment of the patient's immediate problems: Does anything hurt? Where? Does the pain radiate? Do you have any other symptoms?

EXAMINE THE VICTIM FOR INJURY THAT REQUIRES IMMEDIATE STABILIZATION. If the examination will require any disrobing of the patient—for example, in order to locate the source of bleeding from the trunk—it should preferably be conducted with another woman present. Ideally, a woman EMT should take charge of the case. DO NOT EXAMINE THE GENITALIA UNLESS THERE IS INJURY THERE THAT REQUIRES IMMEDIATE TREATMENT, for instance, profuse bleeding.

TRY WHEREVER POSSIBLE TO PRESERVE EVIDENCE. The victim should thus be *encouraged* not to change her clothes, wash, urinate, defecate, douche, gargle, or take anything by mouth. The word "encouraged" is stressed, because the victim cannot and should not be forced to follow this advice. Some rape victims feel a very strong and understandable need to wash after such an experience, as a way of cleansing themselves of the experience. They may also feel shame about appearing in the hospital in a condition they consider "dirty." You should try to explain to the victim, in a sympathetic way, the reasons why it would be best not to "clean up," but her feelings on the matter should be respected.

Bear in mind that a rape victim, like any other patient, has the right to refuse treatment and to refuse transport to the hospital, and this right should also be respected. Shame, fear, embarrassment, guilt, or any combination of these feelings may make the victim reluctant to undergo examination (and cross-examination!) at the hands of strangers. Nonetheless, should the victim refuse transport, you should make every effort to ensure that she is not simply left alone. A victim of sexual assault needs emotional support. If there is a Rape Crisis Center in your community, you should know the telephone number so that you can furnish this number to the victim. Furthermore, if at all possible, try to leave the victim in the care of a friend or relative. DO NOT ABANDON THE VICTIM OF RAPE AT THE SCENE.

In managing any case of sexual assault, and in writing up your report, always remember that RAPE IS A LEGAL DIAGNOSIS. Medical professionals in the hospital can ascertain whether *sexual intercourse* occurred; only the courts can decide whether that intercourse was actually rape. Therefore AVOID PUTTING JUDGMENTS INTO THE WRITTEN RECORD. The chief complaint is *not* "rape"; it is, "The patient states that she was raped." Remember, there is a considerable likelihood that your trip sheet will be used as evidence in court, so STICK TO THE FACTS, and make your record as accurate as possible.

In addition, take maximum care to PROTECT THE PRIVACY OF THE VICTIM. Avoid using the word "rape" when you radio in to the hospital, lest you be overheard by curious bystanders; a radio code, such as "Case R," should be established for such cases.

CASE HISTORY

The patient is an 18-year-old primigravida in her ninth month of pregnancy who called for an ambulance because she had gone into labor. She stated that her labor pains were 10 minutes apart. She complained as well of a headache and dull, steady pain in the right upper quadrant of her abdomen. She stated that she felt nauseated but had not vomited. On physical examination, she was alert and oriented. Massive edema was evident throughout her body, including the face. The pulse was 116 and regular, BP 180/110, and respirations 20. Pupils were equal and reactive to light. The remainder of the examination was unremarkable.

The patient was given 6 liters per minute of oxygen by nasal cannula and placed in the left lateral recumbent position in a darkened room while preparations were made for transport. She was then transferred to the ambulance, and transport was undertaken without lights and sirens. En route, she had a grand mal seizure, followed by vomiting. Her head was kept turned downward and her mouth was suctioned of vomitus. Vital signs were unchanged during transport, except for a transient tachycardia during the seizure.

Questions to think about:

1. What do you think is this patient's problem? What evidence do you have for your suspicion?
2. What is the normal blood pressure for an 18-year-old woman? Does the blood pressure normally get higher or lower during pregnancy?
3. Why was the patient placed in a lateral recumbent position?
4. Why were lights and sirens not used in transporting this patient to the hospital?

VOCABULARY

abortion Loss of a pregnancy before the twentieth week of gestation.

spontaneous abortion Abortion that occurs naturally; miscarriage.

threatened abortion Bleeding during the first 20 weeks of pregnancy, which may or may not lead to loss of the pregnancy.

eclampsia Syndrome of hypertension, massive edema, and protein in the urine, which may lead to seizures and coma as the pregnant woman enters labor; toxemia of pregnancy.

preeclampsia The early stage of eclampsia, marked by hypertension and protein in the urine.

rape Sexual intercourse that is inflicted forcibly on another person, against that person's will.

FURTHER READING

Agran PF et al. Fetal death in motor vehicle accidents. *Ann Emerg Med* 16:1355, 1987.

Arthur R. Postmortem cesarian section. *Am J Obstet Gynecol* 132:175, 1978.

Bocka J. OB Trauma. *JEMS* 13(10):51, 1988.

Bocka J et al. Trauma in pregnancy. *Ann Emerg Med* 17:829, 1988.

Celebrezze EM. Third trimester predelivery hemorrhage. *Emergency* 13(10):48, 1981.

Crosby WM. Traumatic injuries during pregnancy. *Clin Obstet & Gynecol* 26:902, 1983.

Cryer L et al. Crisis management: The EMT and the sexual assault victim. *EMT J* 3(4):42, 1979.

Harris BA Jr. Dealing with a difficult delivery. *Emerg Med* 16(11):22, 1984.

Hicks DJ. The patient who's been raped. *Emerg Med* 20(20):106, 1988.

Josephson GW. The male rape victim: Evaluation and treatment. *JACEP* 8:13, 1979.

Lee RV et al. Cardiopulmonary resuscitation of pregnant women. *Amer J Med* 81:311, 1986.

Muller RJ. Cesarean section in the street. *Emerg Med* 16(5):143, 1984.

Nixon RG. Third trimester obstetric complications. Part I: Antepartum hemorrhage and fetal distress. *Emerg Med Serv* 10(3):53, 1981.

Nixon RG. Third trimester obstetric complications. Part II: Eclampsia and postpartum hemorrhage. *Emerg Med Serv* 10(4):52, 1981.

Schloss B. Sexual assault. *Emergency* 11(2):47, 1979.

Seldon BS, Burke TJ. Complete maternal and fetal recovery

after prolonged cardiac arrest. *Ann Emerg Med* 17:346, 1988.

Sibai BM et al. Eclampsia: Observations from 67 recent cases. *Obstetr Gynecol* 58:609, 1981.

Tintinalli J, Hoelzer M. Clinical findings and legal resolution in sexual assault. *Ann Emerg Med* 14:447, 1984.

Tipple AL et al. Sexual assault: The problem and its management. *Minn Med* 67:433, 1984.

Whipkey R, Paris P, Stewart R. Drug use in pregnancy. *Ann Emerg Med* 13:346, 1984.

Women's woes. *Emerg Med* 14(17):26, 1982.

IX. PEDIATRIC EMERGENCIES

34. PEDIATRIC EMERGENCIES

OBJECTIVES

Pediatrics is the branch of medicine concerned with the care of children. The very fact that there *is* a special branch of medicine devoted to children indicates that children are not simply miniature adults: They have special problems that differ both qualitatively and quantitatively from those of grownups. While basic principles of emergency treatment are the same for all people (big and little), *techniques* of treatment sometimes differ in children. In this chapter, we will examine some of the special considerations in dealing with sick or injured children. We will look at the modifications necessary in fundamental techniques of emergency care and also at a few of the special emergencies to which children are particularly susceptible. By the conclusion of this chapter, the reader should be able to:

1. Describe the differences in approach to the pediatric patient as opposed to the adult patient, particularly with respect to conduct of the physical examination
2. Indicate the modifications required in (a) establishing an airway, (b) providing artificial ventilation, and (c) giving external chest compressions in an infant and small child
3. Identify a child with probable (a) croup and (b) epiglottitis, given a description of several children with various signs and symptoms, and indicate the correct prehospital treatment for each
4. Identify the correct management in the field for febrile seizures, given several treatment options
5. Identify a child with probable (a) hemorrhagic shock and (b) severe dehydration, given a description of several children with various signs and symptoms, and indicate the correct prehospital management for each
6. Identify signs suggestive of child abuse, given a list of signs, and indicate the correct management of suspected child abuse in the prehospital phase
7. Indicate the correct field management of sudden infant death syndrome

THE EPIDEMIOLOGY OF CHILDHOOD

Accidents are the leading cause of death in children over the age of 1 year. Approximately 25,000 children die from accidents in the United States each year; 100,000 are permanently maimed or crippled; and close to 2 million children are disabled for 2 weeks or longer due to injuries.

Nearly 70 percent of accidents in preschool children (and 40 percent of accidents in children of all ages) occur in or around the home. The principal causes of accidental death in children are road traffic accidents, poisoning, burns, and falls. Poisoning alone accounts for over 100,000 emergency room visits each year by children under 5, and it is estimated that nearly 1.5 million childhood poison exposures occur in the United States annually.

Childhood deaths and disability from road traffic accidents, choking, poisoning, burns, and other home accidents all have one thing in common: They are nearly all preventable.

APPROACH TO THE PEDIATRIC PATIENT

As noted above, children are not simply miniature adults. They perceive the world differently from adults; they have different fears and worries; and, depending on the child's age, there is a variable ability to communicate and understand. Furthermore, children elicit responses in the EMT different from those felt toward an adult; the sight of an injured child, for instance, is much more upsetting to the average person (be one a lay person or a medical professional) than the sight of an adult with a similar injury. For all these reasons, the emergency care of a sick or injured child is likely to be more difficult, emotionally and medically, than that of an adult, and the EMT needs to be aware of the special considerations in dealing with children.

It is a safe generalization that nearly every injured child is frightened—frightened of pain, frightened of being separated from mother, frightened of strangers (like yourself) who might have evil intentions. The EMT's behavior will often determine whether the child becomes even more frightened or whether the child is reassured and comforted.

Certain guidelines apply to the care of children in general. The principle underlying all of these guidelines is to do everything possible to gain the confidence of the child and to avoid actions that will aggravate the child's fear. The first of these guidelines is BE CALM. This is not always as easy as it sounds, for often the sick or injured child is surrounded by family or bystanders who are not calm at all, and keeping cool under such circumstances requires considerable self-discipline. If at all possible, TAKE A LITTLE EXTRA TIME TO ESTABLISH RAPPORT WITH THE CHILD. With children older than about 2 years, introduce yourself and explain your mission, bearing in mind that a child's vocabulary is not the same as that of an adult.

DO NOT SEPARATE THE CHILD FROM HIS OR HER PARENT(S), even if the parent is injured. Separation from mother is much more terrifying to a small child than injury to mother (especially if the injury can be covered once it is taken care of). Where small children are concerned, it is best to CONDUCT THE EXAMINATION WITH THE CHILD SITTING ON MOTHER'S LAP, for the physical contact with mother's body gives the child comfort and reassurance. Sit down, so that you can BE AT EYE LEVEL WITH THE CHILD, rather than towering over him. CONDUCT YOUR EXAMINATION FROM TOE TO HEAD, since most small children do not like strange people poking at their faces. DELAY THE USE OF INSTRUMENTS UNTIL THE END OF THE EXAMINATION, for children do not like these either. Meanwhile, let the child play with the stethoscope or flashlight so that he can become more familiar with it. When you do begin to use instruments, have the parent handle them insofar as possible (e.g., have mother place the bell of the stethoscope on the child's chest or hold the oxygen mask near his face). EXAMINE THE PART THAT HURTS LAST, and if any portion of the examination seems to cause the child anxiety, skip it until the end.

BE GENTLE BUT FIRM in carrying out treatment procedures. EXPLAIN IN SIMPLE LANGUAGE WHAT YOU INTEND TO DO. BE HONEST. Do not tell a child that something won't hurt if it will hurt! Try to answer the child's questions as simply as possible, and do not overwhelm him with information. Most children are not particularly interested in a detailed description of their injuries; what they want is reassurance and support. Wherever possible, ENLIST THE CHILD'S COOPERATION, as in having him hold a bandage or help with a dressing. BE FIRM. Tell the child to cooperate; do not ask him, since asking simply gives him the option to refuse! COVER BLEEDING INJURIES AS RAPIDLY AS POSSIBLE, but be sure to assure the child that his anatomy is generally intact beneath the dressing, since small children fear mutilation and loss of body parts.

In transport, again keep the child with his or her parent. If possible, allow the child to take along a favorite toy or other possession, such as a teddy bear or blanket. Try to answer his questions about what will happen in the hospital, but do not offer more detail than the child wants to hear. Keep your answers simple and honest.

There will be occasions when even the most charming EMT cannot calm the child, or when the urgency of the situation does not permit time for establishing rapport. Under such circumstances, the EMT must simply conduct the examination as swiftly and gently as possible, and take whatever measures are necessary to manage life-threatening situations.

Guidelines for Dealing with Sick or Injured Children

- BE CALM, PATIENT, GENTLE.
- BE HONEST.
- DO NOT SEPARATE THE CHILD FROM HIS OR HER PARENT(S).
- Physical Examination
    1. KEEP THE SMALL CHILD ON MOTHER'S LAP.

2. DO NOT TOWER OVER THE CHILD.
3. TOE-TO-HEAD EXAMINATION.
4. EXAMINE THE PART THAT HURTS LAST.
5. DELAY THE USE OF INSTRUMENTS UNTIL THE END OF THE EXAM.

- Treatment
  1. EXPLAIN IN SIMPLE LANGUAGE WHAT YOU INTEND TO DO.
  2. BE FIRM.
  3. TRY TO GET THE CHILD TO HELP.
  4. COVER BLEEDING INJURIES AS SOON AS POSSIBLE.

THE ABCs OF PEDIATRIC EMERGENCIES

Just as in the treatment of adults, the fundamental priorities of treating children are AIRWAY, BREATHING, and CIRCULATION. What differs in children are some of the techniques of implementing these priorities and some of the conditions that may jeopardize the ABCs.

THE AIRWAY IN CHILDREN

Establishing and maintaining an adequate airway in an infant or child is just as crucial as in an adult, and the basic technique is similar: backward tilt of the head. Bear in mind, however, that in the case of infants and small children, *extreme* hyperextension of the head may itself cause airway obstruction and therefore should be avoided. Obstruction of the upper airway by a foreign body has been discussed in detail in Chapter 5, and the student should review that section at this time. We would only reemphasize here that if the child is able to move any air past the obstruction, he should simply be given oxygen and transported rapidly to the hospital. Only if the foreign body has caused complete upper airway obstruction should the EMT attempt to remove it, in the manner outlined in Chapter 5.

In addition to obstruction caused by the tongue and foreign bodies, the child's airway may become blocked by swelling. That is particularly likely in the case of a small child: Since the airway of a small child is very narrow to begin with, it does not take much swelling to create significant airway problems. Two illnesses in particular are apt to cause narrowing of the child's upper airway: croup and epiglottitis.

Croup

Croup is a viral illness, most commonly seen in children between about 6 months and 4 years of age, that causes swelling and narrowing of the upper airway just *below the glottis* (Fig. 34-1A). It comes on gradually following a cold or other respiratory infection, and the acute attack often occurs at night. Typically, the child is relatively well during the day, with just a low-grade fever and some hoarseness, and then during the wee hours, the parents are galvanized from their beds by a very alarming, loud, BARKING NOISE ("seal bark"). The child is found lying in his crib, with pronounced STRIDOR on inhalation. If the airway is extremely narrowed, the child may show classic signs of respiratory distress: flaring of the nostrils, retractions of the intercostal and suprasternal muscles, and so forth. Restlessness and tachycardia signal the presence of hypoxia.

In treating the child with suspected croup, let him assume a POSITION OF COMFORT (usually lying down), and administer HUMIDIFIED OXYGEN. Using a cold steam vaporizer is often effective, or simply placing the child in a humid environment (e.g., a bathroom in which a steamy shower has been running) may be helpful prior to transport. Once en route to the hospital, disturb the child as little as possible, and move rapidly to the emergency room.

Epiglottitis

Epiglottitis results from bacterial infection of the epiglottis, and is potentially a very dangerous illness, for the swollen epiglottis may at any moment cause complete airway obstruction and death from asphyxia (Fig. 34-1B). Epiglottitis occurs most commonly in children slightly older than those affected by croup: the 3- to 7-year old set. It comes on very rapidly, usually in a matter of a few hours, with the swift development of HIGH FEVER and SEVERE PAIN ON SWALLOWING. Because it hurts so much to swallow, the child avoids swallowing even his own secretions, so DROOLING is prominent. Furthermore, the chid instinctively assumes a posture that keeps his airway maximally open—SITTING UPRIGHT, LEANING FORWARD, WITH THE CHIN THRUST OUTWARD—and he will strongly resist any attempt to make him lie down. SIGNS OF AIR HUNGER—restlessness, tachypnea, nasal flaring, retractions—are likely to be present, and in general the child looks very ill.

A CHILD WITH EPIGLOTTITIS IS IN GRAVE DANGER! Complete airway obstruction may occur within seconds and, if that happens, the child will die unless he is in a facility where tracheostomy can be performed immediately. Thus the most important aspect of prehospital treatment is to GET THE CHILD TO THE HOSPITAL AS FAST AS POSSIBLE. Administer HUMIDIFIED OXYGEN, and transport the child in a SITTING POSITION (he probably won't let you put him in any other position). DO NOT UNDER ANY CIRCUMSTANCES PLACE ANYTHING IN THE CHILD'S MOUTH, for this is a sure way to precipitate laryngospasm and instant, complete airway obstruction. *Do not* try to examine his throat with a tongue depressor. *Do not* use an oral thermometer. *Do not* use any kind of oropharyngeal airway. *Do not*

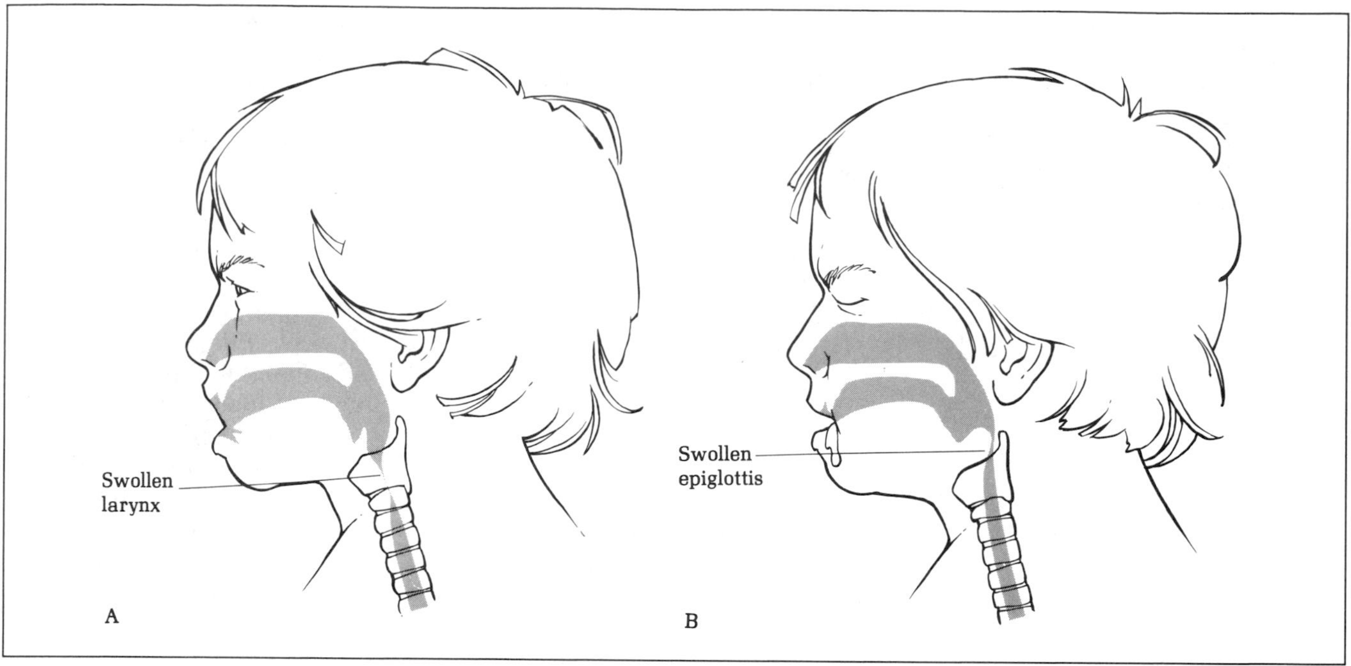

Fig. 34-1. *Illnesses that cause airway obstruction in children. A. Croup produces swelling in the larynx. B. Epiglottis produces swelling of the epiglottis.*

try to suction the mouth or throat. Just start oxygen administration, and get moving. RADIO AHEAD to the receiving hospital so that they can prepare a tracheostomy set, just in case.

BREATHING

The child who is not breathing, or not breathing adequately, needs ventilatory assistance, and in general this is best carried out by manual methods, without the use of adjuncts. Recall that for infants and small children, you cover both nose *and* mouth with your mouth for rescue breathing and that the volume of air delivered should be just enough to make the child's chest rise. Particularly in very small children, excess ventilation volumes will rapidly distend the stomach and thereby may lead to regurgitation, so take it easy. If a bag-valve-mask is used, it should be the smaller variety specially designed for pediatric use and fitted with an appropriate size pediatric mask. DO NOT USE A DEMAND VALVE ON AN INFANT OR SMALL CHILD.

CIRCULATION

The presence of a pulse may be checked at the brachial artery in an infant; in a child, the usual carotid check is adequate. Because the ventricles lie higher in the chest in infants and small children, external cardiac compressions are performed over the *midsternum*. For infants, one uses only one or two fingers to do chest compressions; for children, just the heel of one hand. The compression rate is 80 to 100 per minute, with a ventilation interposed between each 5 compressions (Fig. 34-2).

SPECIAL PROBLEMS IN CHILDREN

Most of the emergencies that may befall infants and children have been covered in other sections of this book, and the principles involved are equally applicable to children and adults, whether the problem be poisoning, anaphylaxis, drowning, fracture, or any other acute emergency. In this section, we shall deal only with those emergencies that are unique to children or that require special management in the pediatric age group.

FEBRILE SEIZURES

A *febrile seizure* is, by definition, a convulsion brought on by high fever, and approximately 2 to 5 percent of all children will have at least one such episode at some time during childhood. The peak incidence is in children between about 9 and 20 months of age, but such seizures may be seen up to the age of 5 or 6 years. In roughly 10 percent of these cases, there is a family history of similar seizures; an older brother or sister may have had the same problem, or one of the parents may have experienced such seizures during childhood. The majority of fe-

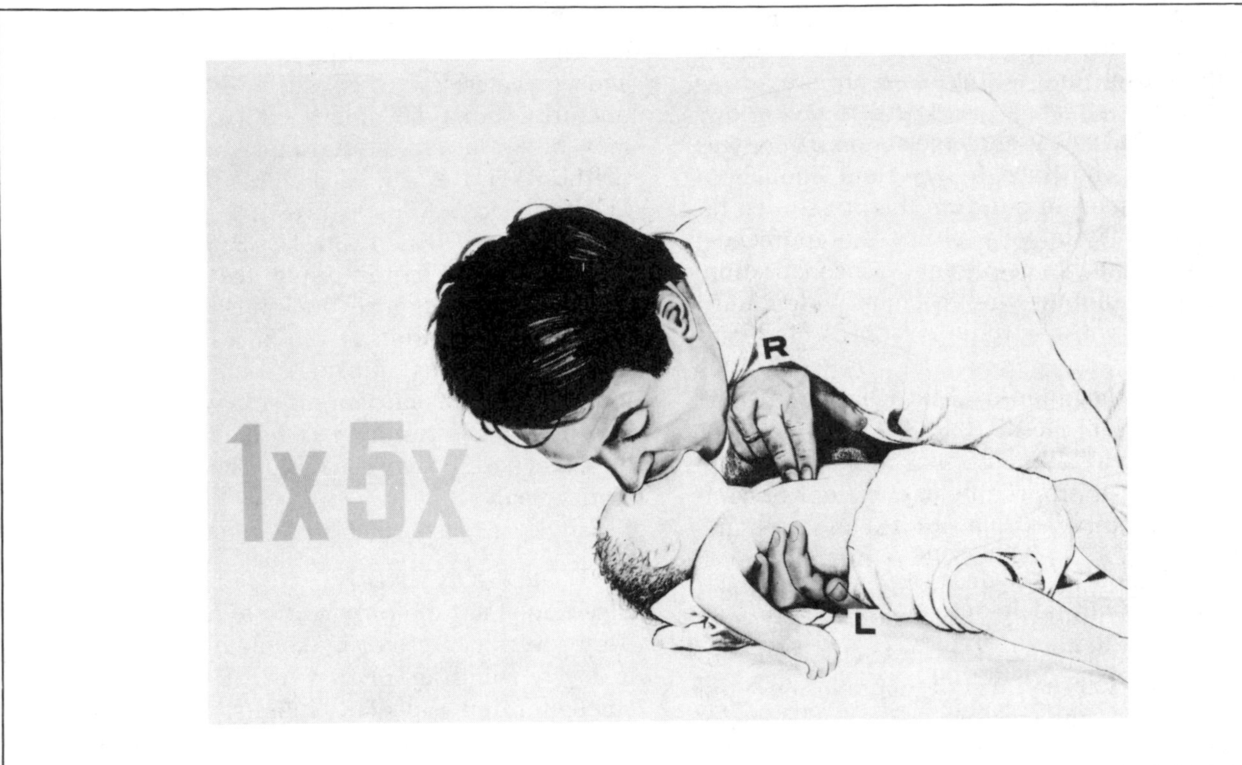

Fig. 34-2. *Resuscitation of an infant. (Reproduced courtesy Asmund Laerdal, Stavanger, Norway.)*

brile seizures are generalized, involving the whole body, and usually brief, most of them lasting less than 20 minutes. They almost always come on within the first few hours of fever, and if a seizure has not occurred in the first 24 hours of fever, it is unlikely that it will occur at all. The risk of seizures is also related to the severity of the fever: The more rapid the rise in temperature and the higher the fever, the more likely the occurrence of a convulsion. In the vast majority of cases, simple febrile seizures do not cause any permanent damage, nor do they lead to epilepsy. But because of their sudden and dramatic nature, these seizures are likely to precipitate an epidemic of panic among all concerned—parents and emergency personnel alike.

Often by the time you reach the scene, the child's seizure will have already run its course, and you will simply find him in a sleepy, post-ictal state. In this situation, you should reassure the parents and transport the child to the hospital for evaluation. If you should arrive while the child is still seizing, place him in a SEMIPRONE POSITION on a bed or other surface where he will be protected from injury. If a bite block can be easily inserted between the child's molars, go ahead and put one in; but DO NOT TRY TO FORCE A BITE BLOCK BETWEEN THE TEETH. Administer OXYGEN by nasal cannula, and keep suction handy, in the event of vomiting. Meanwhile, remove the child's clothing and try to reduce his temperature by SPONGING him WITH LUKEWARM WATER.

DO NOT USE ALCOHOL OR ICE WATER TO SPONGE A FEVERISH CHILD.

Alcohol or ice water may actually increase the child's fever by producing chills and shivering, which in turn crank up the body's rate of metabolism. So keep the water tepid, and do not let the child become chilled.

Once the seizure has either stopped or continued longer than 15 or 20 minutes, transport the child to the hospital, with close attention to his airway. Not every seizure in childhood is a febrile seizure, and only careful evaluation in the hospital will allow differentiation between a harmless febrile seizure and one associated with neurologic damage. For this reason, EVERY CHILD HAVING A SEIZURE FOR THE FIRST TIME MUST BE EXAMINED BY A PHYSICIAN.

TRAUMA IN CHILDREN

Once again, the basic principles of evaluating and treating trauma are the same in children as in adults, but the types of trauma involved and the details of treatment differ. To begin with, children have a much greater susceptibility to blunt trauma because their scanty muscle and fat tissue do not provide as much padding as an adult has. Furthermore, a low-set diaphragm and relatively large abdominal organs make injuries to the liver, spleen, and duodenum much more common in children than in adults. Internal bleeding may be very difficult to appreciate; for children are capable of extreme vasoconstriction, and thus hypotension may not become evident until the child has lost a major proportion of his blood volume.

In evaluating the injured child, then, one must be alert to EARLY SIGNS OF SHOCK. Look for APATHY AND LISTLESSNESS, as in the child who does not respond appropriately to questions or commands (or the infant who does not respond to cooing and cuddling). COLD, PALE SKIN is another important sign of probable shock, especially when the NECK VEINS AND PERIPHERAL VEINS ARE COLLAPSED. Use a tape measure to MEASURE THE ABDOMINAL GIRTH at the level of the umbilicus, and accurately record the measurement you obtain. Sometimes an increase in the circumference of the abdomen will be the first clue that there is bleeding within the abdominal cavity, so a baseline measurement should be obtained as early as possible.

Record the VITAL SIGNS, and reassess them frequently. In order to evaluate the significance of the measurements you obtain, you need to know the normal measurements for any given age; this information is summarized in Table 34-1. If you do not have a small, pediatric blood pressure cuff, you will not be able to obtain an accurate blood pressure reading, so it is probably not worth taking the time to measure the BP in those circumstances. Even if you do have a pediatric cuff, again remember that THE CHILD WILL NOT DEVELOP HYPOTENSION UNTIL HE HAS LOST A QUARTER OF HIS BLOOD VOLUME, so do not be lulled into a false sense of security just because the blood pressure is apparently normal.

Children in shock need INTRAVENOUS FLUIDS as soon as possible, usually in an initial dose of about 10 ml per pound of body weight, given as saline or Ringer's solution. If you are not authorized to start an intravenous infusion on a child, you must get the child to a medical facility fast. A pediatric MAST should be used if available. Needless to say, external bleeding should be controlled promptly, and suspected fractures, especially suspected spinal fractures, must be stabilized before the child is moved. As in adults, one must presume that ANY CHILD WITH A HEAD INJURY OR FOUND UNCONSCIOUS AFTER GENERAL INJURY HAS A CERVICAL SPINE FRACTURE UNTIL PROVED OTHERWISE. When in doubt, use a backboard.

Shock or any other severe injury calls for OXYGEN and careful attention to the airway. Children commonly vomit after injury, especially after head injury, so keep the child on his side wherever possible, and have suction handy. When there is a head injury, it is best to keep the child's head elevated about 30 degrees.

Table 34-1. *Normal Vital Signs in Children at Rest*

Age	Average BP	Pulse	Respirations
1 day–1 mo	74/40	120–150	30–70
1 mo –1 yr	85/60	115–130	20–40
2–6 yr	90/60	80–115	20–30
6–10 yr	95/62	85–100	20–25
10–18 yr	105/65	70– 75	15–20

DEHYDRATION AND HYPOVOLEMIA

Bleeding is not the only cause of shock in children. Very severe degrees of hypovolemia may occur due to fever, vomiting, or diarrhea. Keep in mind that small children, especially infants, do not have a very large fluid volume to begin with, so it does not take a great deal of vomiting or diarrhea to bring about severe dehydration, and the dehydrated child is a very sick child.

One of the most sensitive SIGNS of dehydration is progressive LETHARGY; the child becomes more and most listless and apathetic, and he does not move around. DRYNESS OF THE LIPS AND ORAL MUCOSA are almost always present in dehydration, and often the EYES APPEAR SUNKEN. In infants, the soft spot on the top of the head, THE FONTANEL, IS DEPRESSED, and the SKIN TURGOR MAY BE DECREASED; that is, if you pinch the skin, it stays pinched. URINATION BECOMES SCANTY AND INFREQUENT as the body attempts to conserve fluid; and TACHYCARDIA, with a weak, thready pulse, reflects the diminished vascular volume. An infant with these signs must be hospitalized for intravenous feeding without delay. If the child has fever, he should be sponged with lukewarm water to reduce the insensible fluid loss that fever produces; otherwise the child should be protected against undue loss of body heat and should breathe humidified oxygen en route to the hospital.

THE BATTERED CHILD

Approximately 60,000 cases of child abuse are reported in the United States each year. Perhaps as many as another half million to one million cases go unreported—a very serious figure when one considers that about 1 in 500 of these children will die from his injuries, and as many as 35 percent will suffer permanent damage. One very important fact about child abuse is that it is invariably a chronic problem: The child who is battered once is going to be battered again, often with increasing severity. What this means is that the battered child who is not identified as such on the first visit to the emergency room may arrive dead on the next visit. For this reason, it is important for all emergency care personnel to have a high index of suspicion when dealing with injured children.

What CLUES TO CHILD ABUSE should arouse one's suspicion? First of all, one should be sensitive to the BEHAVIOR OF THE PARENT(S). A mother who is DETACHED OR UNCONCERNED or does not seem to want to hold the child is worthy of note, since most parents cannot resist cuddling and comforting an injured child. It has been observed that the neglected child is often carried "like a loaf of bread," without any evidence that he is an object of special importance. The parent may be in a big hurry to leave the emergency room, even before making sure the child is safe. Be alert also to parents who give VAGUE, EVASIVE, OR CONFLICTING STORIES about the nature of the accident, especially WHEN THE DESCRIPTION OF THE ACCIDENT CANNOT ACCOUNT FOR THE OBSERVED INJURIES. A series of bruises to the back, for instance, are unlikely to have been caused by a "fall," for children tend to fall forward, not backward, and they usually sustain one bruise per fall. THE PARENT WHO HAS WAITED A LONG TIME TO BRING THE CHILD FOR TREATMENT, sometimes days or even weeks after the accident, should also arouse suspicion. A HISTORY OF RECENT VISITS TO OTHER EMERGENCY ROOMS suggests multiple episodes of abuse.

In the EXAMINATION OF THE CHILD, certain signs are highly suspicious for abuse. An abused child is apt to be withdrawn and apathetic, and does not show the usual tendency to cling to a parent for comfort. Be especially alert for the CHILD WHO DOES NOT CRY despite his injuries—another sign of fear and withdrawal. The abused child is usually a neglected child and will show SIGNS OF NEGLECT, such as diaper rash, lack of cleanliness, and poor clothing and nutrition.

Look for MULTIPLE INJURIES OF ANY KIND, especially when there are OLD BRUISES IN ADDITION TO NEW ONES. Injuries in various stages of healing indicate repeated trauma. BURNS are common in abused children, and many of these burns are very unlikely to have occurred by accident. SCALD BURNS, for example, almost always occur in a splash pattern about the shoulders and arms when accidental; a child who has been intentionally immersed in boiling water, on the other hand, will usually have a sharp line of demarcation between the burned and unburned areas of the body. MULTIPLE CIGARETTE BURNS are invariably intentional. BRUISES IN INACCESSIBLE AREAS, such as the armpits, the small of the back, or behind the knees, are very difficult to sustain accidentally, as are WELTS, STRAP MARKS, and other signs of injury inflicted by a rope, stick, or similar object.

Clues to Child Abuse: Summary

- Parental Behavior
  1. ANGER, HOSTILITY, LACK OF APPROPRIATE CONCERN
  2. VAGUE, EVASIVE, OR CONFLICTING STORIES
  3. HISTORY THAT CANNOT ACCOUNT FOR THE INJURIES OBSERVED
  4. LONG DELAY IN SEEKING TREATMENT
- The Child
  1. APATHETIC; DOES NOT CRY; DOES NOT TURN TO PARENTS FOR COMFORT
  2. APPEARS POORLY NOURISHED, POORLY CARED FOR
  3. MULTIPLE BRUISES, MULTIPLE FRACTURES
  4. OLD AND NEW INJURIES
  5. HISTORY OF SEVERAL VISITS TO DIFFERENT HOSPITALS
  6. CIGARETTE BURNS, SCALDS ON BACK, STRAP MARKS, WELTS
  7. BRUISES ON BACK, BUTTOCKS, MOUTH

What do you do when you suspect child abuse? First of all, you treat the child as you would any other injured child: Examine him carefully—indeed, very carefully—and stabilize any injuries you find. DO NOT CONFRONT THE PARENTS WITH YOUR SUSPICIONS, but maintain a calm, professional manner. In the field, your job is to deal strictly with the injuries, not to play policeman or judge.

IF YOU SUSPECT CHILD ABUSE, YOU MUST TRANSPORT THE CHILD TO THE HOSPITAL, EVEN IF THE INJURIES SEEM TRIVIAL. Remember, the next time around, the injuries may not be trivial, and hospitalization may be the only way to protect the child from another, perhaps fatal episode of abuse. When you reach the emergency department, confide your suspicions *in private* to the emergency room physician. Bear in mind that, in several states, failure of a medical or paramedical worker to report a suspected case of child abuse may lead to prosecution for criminal liability. So make sure you convey your suspicions to the responsible member of the emergency room staff. In addition, MAKE YOUR TRIP SHEET AS THOROUGH AND ACCURATE AS

POSSIBLE. Record in detail the history the parent(s) gave you, and note all of your findings on examination, including your observations at the scene (e.g., Was the home disorderly and unkempt? Was there evidence of excessive alcohol consumption at the scene?).

A special case of child abuse is that of the *sexually molested child*, and in general the same guidelines apply here as in any other case of suspected sexual assault. Examination should be kept to the minimum necessary to detect injuries that require stabilization. Do not examine the genital area unless there is obvious bleeding that requires a dressing. The child should not wash or go to the bathroom before being brought to the emergency room, and he or she should be shielded from curious bystanders.

SUDDEN INFANT DEATH SYNDROME

Every year in the United States, approximately 5,000 apparently healthy babies are tucked into their cribs at night and are found dead in their cribs the next morning. These babies are victims of the sudden infant death syndrome (SIDS), or "crib death," a condition that kills more infants between the ages of 1 month and 1 year than any other disease. The cause of crib death is unknown. Most cases occur in infants under 25 weeks old. There is a higher incidence during the colder months of the year, and there is also a higher incidence in infants of lower-income families, but wealthy families are not by any means immune to this tragedy.

There are no early warning signs of crib death, and thus there is no way to prevent it. Typically, death occurs during sleep in an apparently healthy baby, and the infant is not discovered until it is too late for successful resuscitation. It is also typical for the parents to blame themselves for the death. Because the cause of SIDS is unknown, many parents are overwhelmed with guilt and self-doubt and are tortured by the thought, "Maybe if I had done such-and-such, it wouldn't have happened."

The EMT is often the first official representative of the community to reach the scene, and he or she can therefore do a great deal of good for the family, or a great deal of harm. An accusatory attitude is entirely unjustified in this situation (or in any situation!), for it will only reinforce the family's feelings of guilt. What the family needs is support, and the best support an EMT can provide is to behave in a calm, professional manner and do all that is possible for the infant. This means starting CPR and continuing CPR all the way to the hospital, *even if you are convinced that the baby has been dead for hours*. Usually the family still clings to the hope that their baby can be saved, and it is very important for them to feel that everything medically possible was done.

THE EMT AS A HEALTH EDUCATOR

If you care about children and do not like to see injured children among your patients, you should DO SOMETHING ABOUT IT! We know a lot about the things that cause needless injury to children: medicines, toxic chemicals, matches, and flammable materials left carelessly around the house where small children can get at them; dangerous toys; failure to use child restraint devices when children are transported in motor vehicles. You know all about those things. (And you can learn more—see Further Reading for this chapter.) But many parents do not. So why not share your knowledge with the community and help prevent those injuries to children that upset you and everyone on the squad?

The time to teach child safety is NOT during the emergency call. Chances are that the parents are already feeling very guilty about whatever happened to their child. And your reciting a lecture on prevention at that juncture will only add to that guilt, for it will be seen as an accusation ("If you had been more careful, this wouldn't have happened. . .").

The time to teach child safety, then, is *before* the emergency occurs. Your squad can organize a series of seminars or perhaps mimeograph a list of safety tips for parents and distribute the list in the community. Often there is a good deal of slack time between emergency calls. Use the time creatively, for accident prevention projects.

Medicine in general (and emergency medicine in particular) is just about the only business in which we would like to have fewer customers.

What can *you* do to cut down the number of calls for emergencies in children?

VOCABULARY

crib death Term for the sudden infant death syndrome.

croup Viral disease of the upper airway that leads to partial upper airway obstruction, stridor, and a barking cough.

epiglottitis Bacterial infection of the epiglottis that may lead to abrupt, complete airway obstruction.

febrile Condition of having an elevated body temperature; feverish.

fontanel Soft spot on an infant's head, where the bones of the skull have not yet fused together.

FURTHER READING

GENERAL

Gratz RR. Children's responses to emergency department care. *Ann Emerg Med* 13:322, 1984.

Davidson L, Dierking BH. Medical emergencies in the pediatric patient: Hazardous chemical exposures. *JEMS* 14(6):74, 1989.

Holbrook PR. Prehospital care of critically ill children. *Crit Care Med* 8:537, 1980.

Jarvis DA. The unconscious child. *Emerg Med* 20(20):193, 1988.

Lipton H. Parental care. *Emergency* 21(8):43, 1989.

Oquist N. A child-proof assessment. *Emergency* 21(8):35, 1989.

Ramenofsky ML et al. EMS for pediatrics. Optimum treatment or unnecessary delay? *J Pediatr Surg* 18:498, 1983.

Reece RM. Pediatric emergencies. *Emerg Med Serv* 7:8, 1978.

Seidel JS. Emergency medical services and the pediatric patient: Are the needs being met? II. Training and equipping emergency medical services providers for pediatric emergencies. *Pediatrics* 78:808, 1986.

AIRWAY PROBLEMS

Broniatowski M. Croup. *Ear Nose Throat* 64:12, 1985.

Broniatowski M. Epiglottitis. *Ear Nose Throat* 64:22, 1985.

Denny FW et al. Croup: An 11-year study in pediatric practice. *Pediatrics* 71:871, 1983.

Dierking BH. Respiratory distress! *Emergency* 21(1):27, 1989.

Food asphyxiation in young children. *Clin Pediatr* 23:654, 1984.

Holbrook PR. On opening the airway. *Emerg Med* 14(1):137, 1982.

Lazoritz S, Saunders BS, Bason WM. Management of acute epiglottitis. *Crit Care Med* 7:285, 1979.

Rucker RW. Acute upper airway obstruction in children: Recognition and early management. *Emerg Med Serv* 9(1):45, 1980.

Tintinalli JE (Ed.) Respiratory stridor in the young child. *JACEP* 5:195, 1976.

Whitten CE. Intubating the child. *Emerg Med* 21(19):81, 1989.

CPR IN CHILDREN

Eisenberg M, Bergner L, Hallstrom A. Epidemiology of cardiac arrest and resuscitation in children. *Ann Emerg Med* 12:672, 1983.

Lewis JK et al. Outcome of pediatric resuscitation. *Ann Emerg Med* 12:297, 1983.

Ludwig S et al. Pediatric cardiopulmonary resuscitation: A review of 130 cases. *Clin Pediatr* 23:71, 1984.

Singer J. Cardiac arrests in children. *JACEP* 6:198, 1977.

Torphy DE, Minter MG, Thompson BM. Cardiopulmonary arrest and resuscitation of children. *Am J Dis Child* 138:1099, 1984.

FEVER AND FEBRILE SEIZURES

Addy DP. Cold comfort for hot children. *Br Med J* 286:1163, 1983.

El-Rahdi AS et al. Effect of fever on recurrence rate of febrile convulsions. *Arch Dis Child* 64:869, 1989.

Goldbloom RB. Sponging for fever—a second look. *Pediatric Notes* 9(19):1, 1985.

Newman J. Evaluation of sponging to reduce body temperature in febrile children. *Can Med Assoc J* 132:641, 1985.

Schmitt BD. Fever phobia: Misconceptions of parents about fever. *Am J Dis Child* 134:176, 1980.

Tomlanovich MC, Rosen P, Mendelsohn J. Simple febrile convulsions. *JACEP* 5:347, 1976.

ACCIDENTS AND TRAUMA

Agran PF, Dunkle DE, Winn DG. Motor vehicle childhood injuries caused by noncrash falls and ejections. *JAMA* 253:2530, 1985.

Baker D et al. Household electrical injuries in children: Epidemiology and identification of avoidable hazards. *AJDC* 143:59, 1989.

Berger LR et al. Promoting the use of car safety devices for infants—an intensive health education approach. *Pediatrics* 74:16, 1984.

Centers for Disease Control. Toy safety—United States, 1983. *MMWR* 33(50), 1984.

Davidson RI. Emergency care of pediatric head injuries. *Emerg Med Serv* 9(1):31, 1980.

Decker MD et al. The use and efficacy of child restraint devices. *JAMA* 252:2571, 1984.

Eichelberger M. Trauma at an early age: Penetration of a small torso. *Emerg Med* 17(3):45, 1985.

Gratz RR. Accidental injury in childhood: A literature review on pediatric trauma. *J Trauma* 19:551, 1979.

Green AR et al. Epidemiology of burns in childhood. *Burns* 10:368, 1984.

Haller JA. Trauma at an early age: A blow above the belt. *Emerg Med* 17(3):51, 1985.

Herzenberg JE et al. Emergency transport and positioning of young children who have an injury of the cervical spine: The standard backboard may be hazardous. *J Bone Joint Surg Am* 71A:15, 1989.

Huerta C, Griffith R, Joyce SM. Cervical spine stabilization in pediatric patients: Evaluation of current techniques. *Ann Emerg Med* 16:1121, 1987.

Karwacki JJ et al. Children in motor vehicles. *JAMA* 242:2848, 1979.

Ordog GJ et al. Gunshot wound in children under 10 years of age: A new epidemic. *AJDC* 142:618, 1988.

Pyper JA et al. Orthopaedic injuries in children associated with the use of off-road vehicles. *J Bone Joint Surg Am* 70:275, 1988.

Ramenofsky ML et al. Maximum survival in pediatric trauma: The ideal system. *J Trauma* 24:818, 1984.

Ramenofsky ML. Trauma at an early age: To watch an injured child. *Emerg Med* 17(3):33, 1985.

Reynolds E, Dierking B, Ramenofsky ML. Head care for kids. *Emergency* 20(9):43, 1988.

Rivara FP et al. Injuries to children younger than 1 year of age. *Pediatrics* 81:93, 1988.

Sanders RS et al. Bless the seats and the children: The physician and the legislative process. *JAMA* 252:2613, 1984.

Thompson RS et al. A case-control study of the effectiveness of bicycle safety helmets. *N Engl J Med* 320:1361, 1989.

Throckmorton K, Throckmorton DW, Knight P. Number-one killer. *Emergency* 20(5):20, 1988.

Valentine MW. Bicycle handlebar injuries in children. *Emerg Med* 20(21):37, 1988.

Wheatley J et al. Traumatic deaths in children: The importance of prevention. *Med J Australia* 150:72, 1989.

Williams A. Children killed in falls from motor vehicles. *Pediatrics* 68:576, 1981.

Ziegler MZ. Trauma at an early age: A blow below the belt. *Emerg Med* 17(3):65, 1985.

CHILD ABUSE

AAP Committee on Hospital Care. Medical necessity for the hospitalization of the abused and neglected child. *Pediatrics* 79:300, 1987.

American Medical Association, Council on Scientific Affairs. AMA diagnostic and treatment guidelines concerning child abuse and neglect. *JAMA* 254:796, 1985.

Brodeur AE. Child abuse. *Emerg Med Serv* 8(2):49, 1979.

Dunlap WC. Child abuse and the emergency medical technician. *Emerg Prod News* 8:38, 1976.

Heller RE. The epidemiology of child abuse and neglect. *Pediatr Ann* 13:745, 1984.

Hobbs J. When are burns not accidental? *Arch Dis Child* 61:357, 1986.

King J et al. Analysis of 429 fractures of 189 battered children. *J Ped Orth* 8:585, 1988.

Kottmeier PK. The intricacies of abuse. *Emerg Med* 17(3):75, 1985.

Montrey JS et al. Nonaccidental burns in child abuse. *South Med J* 78:1324, 1985.

Purdue GF et al. Child abuse by burning: An index of suspicion. *J Trauma* 28:221, 1988.

Reynolds EA, Davidson L, Dierking BH. Delivering and documenting: Care in child abuse cases. *JEMS* 14(10):71, 1989.

Robertson DM. Unusual injury? Recent injury in normal children and in children with suspected nonaccidental injury. *Br Med J* 285:1399, 1982.

Rosenberg N, Bottenfield G. Fractures in children: A sign of child abuse. *Ann Emerg Med* 11:178, 1982.

Rosenberg N et al. Prediction of child abuse in an ambulatory setting. *Pediatrics* 70:879, 1982.

Shah C, Holloway C, Valkil D. Sexual abuse of children. *Ann Emerg Med* 11:18, 1982.

Solomons G. Trauma and child abuse: The importance of the medical record. *Am J Dis Child* 134:503, 1980.

Thygerson AL. Child abuse. *Emergency* 13(10):25, 1981.

Vey PK. Child abuse: Your standard of care. *Emerg Med Serv* 13(2):89, 1984.

CRIB DEATH

Brown KR. Sudden infant death syndrome. *Emerg Med Serv* 12(5):52 and 12(6):31, 1983.

Shannon D, Kelly D. SIDS and near-SIDS. *N Engl J Med* 306:959 and 306:1022, 1982.

Strimer R, Adelson L, Oseasohn R. Epidemiologic features of 1,134 sudden, unexpected infant deaths. *JAMA* 10:1493, 1969.

SKILL EVALUATION CHECKLISTS

The following pages contain skill checklists covering the techniques of basic life support for the pediatric patient. These checklists are intended as a guide for the student in the pediatric practice of the skills described for the adult in Chapters 5, 6, and 7. These skill checklists are reprinted with the kind permission of the American Heart Association.

American Heart Association CPR and ECC Performance Sheet
One-Rescuer CPR: Infant

Name ______________________________ Date ______________

Step	Activity	Critical Performance	S	U
1. Airway	Assessment: Determine unresponsiveness.	Tap or gently shake shoulder.		
	Call for help.	Call out "Help!"		
	Position the infant.	Turn on back as unit, supporting head and neck.		
		Place on firm, hard surface.		
	Open the airway.	Use head-tilt/chin-lift maneuver to sniffing or neutral position.		
		Do not overextend the head.		
2. Breathing	Assessment: Determine breathlessness.	Maintain open airway.		
		Ear over mouth, observe chest: look, listen, feel for breathing (3–5 sec).		
	Ventilate twice.	Maintain open airway.		
		Make tight seal on infant's mouth and nose with rescuer's mouth.		
		Ventilate 2 times, 1–1.5 sec/inspiration.		
		Observe chest rise.		
		Allow deflation between breaths.		
3. Circulation	Assessment: Determine pulselessness.	Feel for brachial pulse (5–10 sec).		
		Maintain head-tilt with other hand.		
	Activate EMS system.	If someone responded to call for help, send him/her to activate EMS system.		
		Total time, Step 1—Activate EMS system: 15–35 sec.		
	Begin chest compressions.	Draw imaginary line between nipples.		
		Place 2–3 fingers on sternum, 1 finger's width below imaginary line.		
		Equal compression-relaxation.		
		Compress vertically, ½ to 1 inch.		
		Keep fingers on sternum during upstroke.		
		Complete chest relaxation on upstroke.		
		Say any helpful mnemonic.		
		Compression rate: at least 100/min (5 in 3 sec or less).		
4. Compression/ Ventilation Cycles	Do 10 cycles of 5 compressions and 1 ventilation.	Proper compression/ventilation ratio: 5 compressions to 1 slow ventilation per cycle.		
		Pause for ventilation		
		Observe chest rise: 1–1.5 sec/inspiration; 10 cycles/45 sec or less.		
5. Reassessment	Determine pulselessness. (If no pulse: Step 6.)*	Feel for brachial pulse (5 sec).		
6. Continue CPR	Ventilate once.	Ventilate 1 time.		
		Observe chest rise; 1–1.5 sec/inspiration.		
	Resume compression/ventilation cycles.	Feel for brachial pulse every few minutes.		

* If pulse is present, open airway and check for spontaneous breathing. (a) If breathing is present, maintain open airway and monitor breathing and pulse. (b) If breathing is absent, perform rescue breathing at 20 times/min and monitor pulse.

Instructor ______________________ Check: Satisfactory ________ Unsatisfactory ________

4/86

American Heart Association CPR and ECC Performance Sheet
One-Rescuer CPR: Child*

Name ______________________________ Date ______________

Step	Activity	Critical Performance	S	U
1. Airway	Assessment: Determine unresponsiveness.	Tap or gently shake shoulder.		
		Shout "Are you OK?"		
	Call for help.	Call out "Help!"		
	Position the victim.	Turn on back as unit, if necessary, supporting head and neck (4–10 sec).		
	Open the airway.	Use head-tilt/chin-lift maneuver.		
2. Breathing	Assessment: Determine breathlessness.	Maintain open airway.		
		Ear over mouth, observe chest: look, listen, feel for breathing (3–5 sec).		
	Ventilate twice.	Maintain open airway.		
		Seal mouth and nose properly.		
		Ventilate 2 times at 1–1.5 sec/inspiration.		
		Observe chest rise.		
		Allow deflation between breaths.		
3. Circulation	Assessment: Determine pulselessness.	Feel for carotid pulse on near side of victim (5–10 sec).		
		Maintain head-tilt with other hand.		
	Activate EMS system.	If someone responded to call for help, send him/her to activate EMS system.		
		Total time, Step 1—Activate EMS system: 15–35 sec.		
	Begin chest compressions.	Rescuer kneels by victim's shoulders.		
		Landmark check prior to initial hand placement.		
		Proper hand position throughout.		
		Rescuer's shoulders over victim's sternum.		
		Equal compression-relaxation.		
		Compress vertically, 1 to 1½ inches.		
		Keep hands on sternum during upstroke.		
		Complete chest relaxation on upstroke.		
		Say any helpful mnemonic.		
		Compression rate: 80–100/min (5 per 3–4 sec).		
4. Compression/ Ventilation Cycles	Do 10 cycles of 5 compressions and 1 ventilation.	Proper compression/ventilation ratio: 5 compressions to 1 slow ventilation per cycle.		
		Observe chest rise: 1–1.5 sec/inspiration (10 cycles/60–87 sec).		
5. Reassessment†	Determine pulselessness. (If no pulse: Step 6.)‡	Feel for carotid pulse (5 sec).		
6. Continue CPR	Ventilate once.	Ventilate one time.		
		Observe chest rise; 1–1.5 sec/inspiration.		
	Resume compression/ventilation cycles.	Palpate carotid pulse every few minutes.		

* If child is above age of approximately 8 years, the method for adults should be used.

† 2nd rescuer arrives to replace 1st rescuer: (a) 2nd rescuer identifies self by saying "I know CPR. Can I help?" (b) 2nd rescuer then does pulse check in Step 5 and continues with Step 6. (During practice and testing only one rescuer actually ventilates the manikin. The 2nd rescuer simulates ventilation.) (c) 1st rescuer assesses the adequacy of 2nd rescuer's CPR by observing chest rise during ventilations and by checking the pulse during chest compressions.

‡ If pulse is present, open airway and check for spontaneous breathing. (a) If breathing is present, maintain open airway and monitor breathing and pulse. (b) If breathing is absent, perform rescue breathing at 15 times/min and monitor pulse.

Instructor ______________________ Check: Satisfactory ________ Unsatisfactory ________

4/86

American Heart Association CPR and ECC Performance Sheet
Two-Rescuer CPR: Child*

Name ______________________________ Date ______________

Step	Activity	Critical Performance	S	U
1. Airway	One rescuer (ventilator): Assessment: Determines unresponsiveness.	Tap or gently shake shoulder.		
		Shout "Are you OK?"		
	Positions the victim.	Turn on back if necessary (4–10 sec).		
	Opens the airway.	Use a proper technique to open airway.		
2. Breathing	Assessment: Determine breathlessness.	Look, listen and feel (3–5 sec).		
	Ventilator ventilates twice.	Observe chest rise: 1–1.5 sec/inspiration.		
3. Circulation	Assessment: Determines pulselessness.	Feel for carotid pulse (5–10 sec).		
	States assessment results.	Say "No pulse."		
	Other rescuer (compressor): Gets into position for compressions.	Hands, shoulders in correct position.		
	Locates landmark notch.	Landmark check.		
4. Compression/ Ventilation Cycles	Compressor begins chest compressions.	Correct ratio compressions/ventilations: 5/1.		
		Compression rate: 80–100/min (5 compressions/3–4 sec).		
		Say any helpful mnemonic.		
		Stop compressing for each ventilation.		
	Ventilator ventilates after every 5th compression and checks compression effectiveness.	Ventilate 1 time (1–1.5 sec/inspiration).		
		Occasionally palpate pulse to assess compressions.		
	(Minimum of 10 cycles.)	Time for 10 cycles: 40–53 sec.		
5. Call for Switch	Compressor calls for switch when fatigued.	Give clear signal to change.		
		Compressor completes 5th compression.		
		Ventilator completes ventilation after 5th compression.		
6. Switch	Simultaneously switch:			
	Ventilator moves to chest.	Move to chest.		
		Become compressor.		
		Get into position for compressions.		
		Locate landmark notch.		
	Compressor moves to head.	Move to head.		
		Become ventilator.		
		Feel for carotid pulse (5 sec).		
		Say "No pulse."		
		Ventilate once.†		
7. Continue CPR	Resume compression/ventilation cycles.	Resume Step 4.		

* (a) If CPR is in progress with one rescuer (lay person), the entrance of the two rescuers occurs after the completion of one rescuer's cycle of 5 compressions and 1 ventilation. The EMS should be activated first. The two new rescuers start with Step 6. (b) If CPR is in progress with one professional rescuer, the entrance of a second professional rescuer is at the end of a cycle after check for pulse by first rescuer. The new cycle starts with one ventilation by the first rescuer, and the second rescuer becomes the compressor.

† During practice and testing only one rescuer actually ventilates the manikin. The other rescuer simulates ventilation.

Instructor ______________________________ Check: Satisfactory __________ Unsatisfactory __________

4/86

American Heart Association CPR and ECC Performance Sheet
Obstructed Airway: Conscious Infant*

Name ______________________ Date ______________

Step	Activity	Critical Performance	S	U
1. Assessment	Determine airway obstruction	Observe breathing difficulties.*		
2. Back Blows	Deliver 4 back blows.	Supporting head and neck with one hand, straddle infant face down, head lower than trunk, over your forearm supported on your thigh.		
		Deliver 4 back blows, forcefully, between the shoulder blades with the heel of the hand (3–5 sec).		
3. Chest Thrusts	Deliver 4 chest thrusts.	While supporting the head, sandwich infant between your hands and turn on back, with head lower than trunk.		
		Deliver 4 thrusts in the midsternal region in the same manner as external chest compressions, but at a slower rate (3–5 sec).		
4. Sequencing	Repeat sequence.	Repeat Steps 2 and 3 until either the foreign body is expelled or the infant becomes unconscious (see below).		
Infant with Obstructed Airway Becomes Unconscious (Optional Testing Sequence)				
5. Call for Help.	Call for help.	Call out "Help!" or, if others respond, activate EMS system.		
6. Foreign Body Check	Perform tongue-jaw lift. Do not perform blind finger sweep; remove foreign body only IF VISUALIZED.	Do tongue-jaw lift by placing thumb in infant's mouth over tongue. Lift tongue and jaw forward with fingers wrapped around lower jaw.		
		Remove foreign body IF VISUALIZED.		
7. Breathing Attempt	Attempt ventilation (airway is obstructed).	Open airway with head-tilt/chin-lift.		
		Seal mouth and nose properly.		
		Attempt to ventilate.		
8. Back Blows	Deliver 4 back blows.	Supporting head and neck with one hand, straddle infant face down, head lower than trunk, over your forearm supported on your thigh.		
		Deliver 4 back blows, forcefully, between the shoulder blades with the heel of the hand (3–5 sec).		
9. Chest Thrusts	Deliver 4 chest thrusts.	While supporting the head and neck, sandwich infant between your hands and turn on back, with head lower than trunk.		
		Deliver 4 thrusts in the midsternal region in the same manner as external chest compressions, but at a slower rate (3–5 sec).		
10. Foreign Body Check	Perform tongue-jaw lift, not blind finger sweep.	Do tongue-jaw lift.		
		Remove foreign body IF VISUALIZED.		
11. Breathing Attempt	Reattempt ventilation.	Open airway with head-tilt/chin-lift.		
		Seal mouth and nose properly.		
		Attempt to ventilate.		
12. Sequencing	Repeat sequence.	Repeat Steps 8–11 until successful.†		

* This procedure should be initiated in a conscious infant only if the airway obstruction is due to a witnessed or strongly suspected aspiration and if respiratory difficulty is increasing and the cough is ineffective. If the obstruction is caused by airway swelling due to infections, such as epiglottitis or croup, these procedures may be harmful; the infant should be rushed to the nearest ALS facility, allowing the infant to maintain the position of maximum comfort.

† After airway obstruction is removed, check for breathing and pulse. (a) If pulse is absent, ventilate a second time and start cycles of compressions and ventilations. (b) If pulse is present, open airway and check for spontaneous breathing. (c) If breathing is present, monitor breathing and pulse closely and maintain an open airway. (d) If breathing is absent, perform rescue breathing at 20 times/min and monitor pulse.

Instructor ______________________ Check: Satisfactory __________ Unsatisfactory __________

4/86

American Heart Association CPR and ECC Performance Sheet
Obstructed Airway: Unconscious Infant

Name ______________________ Date ______________

Step	Activity	Critical Performance	S	U
1. Assessment/ Airway	Determine unresponsiveness.	Tap or gently shake shoulder.		
	Call for help.	Call out "Help!"		
	Position the infant.	Turn on back as unit, if necessary, supporting head and neck.		
		Place on firm, hard surface.		
	Open the airway.	Use head-tilt/chin-lift maneuver to sniffing or neutral position.		
		Do not overextend the head.		
	Determine breathlessness.	Maintain open airway.		
		Ear over mouth, observe chest: look, listen, feel for breathing (3–5 sec).		
2. Breathing Attempt	Attempt ventilation (airway is obstructed).	Maintain open airway.		
		Make tight seal on mouth and nose of infant with rescuer's mouth.		
		Attempt to ventilate.		
	Reattempt ventilation (airway remains blocked).	Reposition infant's head.		
		Seal mouth and nose properly.		
		Reattempt to ventilate.		
	Activate EMS system	If someone responded to call for help, send him/her to activate EMS system.		
		Total time, Steps 1 and 2: 10–25 sec.		
3. Back Blows	Deliver 4 back blows.	Supporting head and neck with one hand, straddle infant face down, head lower than trunk, over your forearm supported on your thigh.		
		Deliver 4 back blows, forcefully, between the shoulder blades with the heel of the hand (3–5 sec).		
4. Chest Thrusts	Deliver 4 chest thrusts.	While supporting the head and neck, sandwich infant between your hands and turn on back, with head lower than trunk.		
		Deliver 4 thrusts in the midsternal region in the same manner as external chest compressions, but at a slower rate (3–5 sec).		
5. Foreign Body Check	Perform tongue-jaw lift. Do not perform blind finger sweep; remove foreign body only IF VISUALIZED.	Do tongue-jaw lift by placing thumb in infant's mouth over tongue. Lift tongue and jaw forward with fingers wrapped around lower jaw.		
		Remove foreign body IF VISUALIZED.		
6. Breathing Attempt	Reattempt ventilation.	Open airway with head-tilt/chin-lift.		
		Seal mouth and nose properly.		
		Attempt to ventilate.		
7. Sequencing	Repeat sequence.	Repeat Steps 3–6 until successful.*		

* After airway obstruction is removed, check for breathing and pulse. (a) If pulse is absent, ventilate a second time and start cycles of compressions and ventilations. (b) If pulse is present, open airway and check for spontaneous breathing. (c) If breathing is present, monitor breathing and pulse closely and maintain an open airway. (d) If breathing is absent, perform rescue breathing at 20 times/min and monitor pulse.

Instructor ______________________ Check: Satisfactory ________ Unsatisfactory ________

4/86

American Heart Association CPR and ECC Performance Sheet
Obstructed Airway: Conscious Child*

Name ______________________ Date ______________

Step	Activity	Critical Performance	S	U
1. Assessment	Determine airway obstruction.*	Ask "Are you choking?"		
		Determine if victim can cough or speak.		
2. Heimlich Maneuver	Perform abdominal thrusts (only if victim's cough is ineffective and there is increasing respiratory difficulty).	Stand behind the victim.		
		Wrap arms around victim's waist.		
		Make a fist with one hand and place the thumb side against victim's abdomen, in the midline slightly above the navel and well below the tip of the xiphoid.		
		Grasp fist with the other hand.		
		Press into the victim's abdomen with quick upward thrusts.		
		Each thrust should be distinct and delivered with the intent of relieving the airway obstruction.		
		Repeat thrusts until either the foreign body is expelled or the victim becomes unconscious (see below).		
Victim with Obstructed Airway Becomes Unconscious (Optional Testing Sequence)				
3. Additional Assessment	Position the victim.	Turn on back as unit.		
		Place face up, arms by side.		
	Call for help.	Call out "Help!" or if others respond, activate EMS system.		
4. Foreign Body Check	Perform tongue-jaw lift. Do not perform blind finger sweep; remove foreign body only IF VISUALIZED.	Keep victim's face up.		
		Use tongue-jaw lift to open mouth.		
		Look into mouth and remove foreign body IF VISUALIZED.		
5. Breathing Attempt	Attempt ventilation (airway is obstructed).	Open airway with head-tilt/chin-lift.		
		Seal mouth and nose properly.		
		Attempt to ventilate.		
6. Heimlich Maneuver	Perform abdominal thrusts.	Kneel at victim's feet if on the floor, or stand at victim's feet if on a table.		
		Place heel of one hand against victim's abdomen, in the midline slightly above navel and well below tip of xiphoid.		
		Place second hand directly on top of first hand.		
		Press into the abdomen with quick upward thrusts.		
		Perform 6–10 abdominal thrusts.		
7. Foreign Body Check	Perform tongue-jaw lift. Do not perform blind finger sweep; remove foreign body only IF VISUALIZED.	Keep victim's face up.		
		Use tongue-jaw lift to open mouth.		
		Look into mouth and remove foreign body IF VISUALIZED.		
8. Breathing Attempt	Attempt ventilation.	Open airway with head-tilt/chin-lift.		
		Seal mouth and nose properly.		
		Attempt to ventilate.		
9. Sequencing	Repeat sequence.	Repeat Steps 6–8 until successful.†		

* This procedure should be initiated in a conscious child only if the airway obstruction is due to a witnessed or strongly suspected aspiration and if respiratory difficulty is increasing and the cough is ineffective. If the obstruction is caused by airway swelling due to infection such as epiglottitis or croup, these procedures may be harmful; the child should be rushed to the nearest ALS facility, allowing the child to maintain the position of maximum comfort.

† After airway obstruction is removed, check for pulse and breathing. (a) If pulse is absent, ventilate a second time and start cycles of compressions and ventilations. (b) If pulse is present, open airway and check for spontaneous breathing. (c) If breathing is present, monitor breathing and pulse closely and maintain an open airway. (d) If breathing is absent, perform rescue breathing at 15 times/min and monitor pulse.

Instructor ______________________ Check: Satisfactory __________ Unsatisfactory __________

4/86

American Heart Association CPR and ECC Performance Sheet
Obstructed Airway: Unconscious Child

Name ______________________ Date ______________

Step	Activity	Critical Performance	S	U
1. Assessment/ Airway	Determine unresponsiveness.	Tap or gently shake shoulder.		
		Shout "Are you OK?"		
	Call for help.	Call out "Help!"		
	Position the victim.	Turn on back as unit, if necessary, supporting head and neck (4–10 sec).		
	Open the airway.	Use head-tilt/chin-lift maneuver.		
	Determine breathlessness.	Maintain open airway.		
		Ear over mouth, observe chest: look, listen, feel for breathing (3–5 sec).		
2. Breathing Attempt	Attempt ventilation (airway is obstructed).	Maintain open airway.		
		Seal mouth and nose properly.		
		Attempt to ventilate.		
	Reattempt ventilation (airway remains blocked).	Reposition victim's head.		
		Seal mouth and nose properly.		
		Reattempt to ventilate.		
	Activate EMS system.	If someone responded to call for help, send him/her to activate EMS system.		
		Total time, Steps 1 and 2: 15–35 sec.		
3. Heimlich Maneuver	Perform abdominal thrusts.	Kneel at victim's feet if on the floor, or stand at victim's feet if on a table.		
		Place heel of one hand against victim's abdomen in the midline slightly above navel and well below tip of xiphoid.		
		Place second hand directly on top of first hand.		
		Press into the abdomen with quick upward thrusts.		
		Each thrust should be distinct and delivered with the intent of relieving the airway.		
		Perform 6–10 abdominal thrusts.		
4. Foreign Body Check	Perform tongue-jaw lift. Do not perform blind finger sweep; remove foreign body only IF VISUALIZED.	Keep victim's face up.		
		Use tongue-jaw lift to open mouth.		
		Look into mouth and remove foreign body IF VISUALIZED.		
5. Breathing Attempt	Reattempt ventilation.	Open airway with head-tilt/chin-lift maneuver.		
		Seal mouth and nose properly.		
		Attempt to ventilate.		
6. Sequencing	Repeat sequence.	Repeat Steps 3–5 until successful.*		

* After airway obstruction is removed, check for pulse and breathing. (a) If pulse is absent, ventilate a second time and start cycles of compressions and ventilations. (b) If pulse is present, open airway and check for spontaneous breathing. (c) If breathing is present, monitor breathing and pulse closely and maintain an open airway. (d) If breathing is absent, perform rescue breathing at 15 times/min and monitor pulse.

Instructor ______________________ Check: Satisfactory ________ Unsatisfactory ________

4/86

X. DISTURBANCES OF BEHAVIOR

35. DISTURBANCES OF BEHAVIOR

OBJECTIVES

Everyone has feelings. Under ordinary circumstances, most people have some degree of control over their feelings. But the EMT does not deal with ordinary circumstances. If someone calls for an ambulance, it is because something out of the ordinary has occurred, usually something unpleasant or frightening or even horrifying. Under such circumstances, one can expect changes in the emotional state and behavior of just about everyone involved: the patient, bystanders, and the EMTs themselves. In this chapter, we will examine some of the reactions that are typically generated by sudden illness or injury and the ways in which an EMT can cope with these reactions. We will also look at some examples of emotionally disturbed behavior and how this behavior should be handled in the field. By the conclusion of this chapter, the reader should be able to:

1. List various emotional reactions that people commonly have to sudden illness or injury, and indicate how the EMT can deal with these reactions
2. Identify persons who should be placed under supervision at the scene of a disaster, given a description of several bystanders exhibiting various kinds of behavior
3. Identify a patient (a) at risk of suicide, (b) having an anxiety attack, and (c) displaying dangerous behavior, given a description of several patients, and indicate the correct prehospital management of each situation

NORMAL REACTIONS TO ILLNESS AND INJURY

Sudden illness or injury is a stressful event, and all of those involved in the situation—the patient, the family, bystanders, health professionals—can be expected to react in some way to the stresses of an emergency situation. It is important that EMTs have some insight into the emotional reactions involved, both in others and in themselves, in order to function effectively under trying conditions.

RESPONSES OF THE PATIENT TO ILLNESS AND INJURY

People react in different ways to being ill or injured, but there are certain common responses that one sees again and again in individuals who are suddenly stricken with pain or disability. Probably the most common response is anxiety. Such anxiety is usually a combination of REALISTIC FEARS (e.g., fear of pain, fear of permanent disability, fear of death) and also less concrete, DIFFUSE ANXIETY—a sense of having lost control over one's life. Along with these anxieties usually comes some degree of DEPRESSION, which is a normal psychologic reaction to *loss*; in the case of sudden illness or injury, the loss in question is loss of some bodily function. Many people who are injured or suddenly stricken ill will show some degree of REGRESSION as well; that is, they will behave in a less mature way than usual and become unusually dependent on others.

Another way of dealing with the stress of sudden disability is to pretend that it does not exist, a mechanism called DENIAL. The patient uses phrases like "just a little pain" to dismiss his symptoms as unimportant. Denial is especially common in previously healthy individuals with a first attack of chest pain or other serious illness. Elderly patients, on the other hand, are more apt to respond to serious illness or injury with CONFUSION. They may become partially or completely disoriented, and the presence of strangers with strange equipment only aggravates this reaction.

Probably the toughest reaction for health professionals to deal with is ANGER. It is not uncommon for people to respond to sudden illness or injury by becoming resentful of those around them, and the EMT may be bewildered when he or she becomes the object of apparently unmotivated hostility. The patient may be irritable, accusatory, or excessively demanding, and one's first impulse is to yell right back at him. Under these circumstances, it is useful to remember that the patient's anger comes from fear and pain and is not really directed at the rescue team.

RESPONSES OF THE FAMILY, FRIENDS, OR BYSTANDERS

It is not only the patient who will be reacting to the stresses of the emergency. Those at the scene with the patient are also likely to experience many of the responses already described. Furthermore, especially among family members, there are often feelings of GUILT, which are apt to translate themselves into aggressive DEMANDS FOR ACTION. Such demands may be very difficult to deal with, particularly when the family member or bystander implies that the EMT is not competent to handle the situation (e.g., "Why don't you get him to the hospital so he can be taken care of by a doctor? Why are you hanging around here? Can't you see he's hurt bad?") Such remarks can infuriate the most even-tempered of EMTs; but once again, one must keep in mind that this irritating behavior from bystanders comes from their own fear and distress.

How do you handle these reactions in patients and bystanders? First of all, you have to BE IN CONTROL OF YOUR OWN FEELINGS. Try to take a step back from the situation mentally and remind yourself, "He [or she] isn't really angry at me—just worried and scared." Remember too that the best medicine for anxiety is having someone around who seems calm and steady. Thus if you can remain cool and unflustered and can convey the feeling that the situation is under control, a great deal of the fear in people around you will be defused. That is a tall order, and no EMT is born with the ability to stay calm and unruffled in the midst of panic. Keeping "cool under fire" is something that comes with experience and with insight into one's own feelings.

RESPONSES OF THE EMT

There is nothing magical about being an EMT. EMTs are human, as are other health professionals, and consequently are subject to a variety of reactions in dealing with critically ill and injured patients. The EMT is bound to have moments of fear, anger, grief, insecurity, impatience, frustration. These feelings are natural, and there is no reason for any EMT to be ashamed of them. What is important in the field, however, is to try to keep such feelings under control. Remember that others, even those who seem hostile or critical, will be looking to you for leadership; and if you seem calm and in control of things, others will become calmer as well.

There are two reactions very common in emergency personnel that the EMT needs to guard against. The first is a tendency to become angry when family or bystanders put pressure on the EMT to rush the victim to the hospital, thus implying that the EMT is not competent to deal with the situation. The EMT who becomes angry in this situation is often the EMT who is not very secure, who secretly feels that maybe the bystanders are right in thinking that he or she cannot handle the problem. The only safeguard against such insecurity is to practice your skills to perfection and to have a very clear idea of exactly what you are and are not capable of doing. If you feel, deep down, "I can handle this," you will not be unduly upset by clamoring bystanders. And if the situation is one that you know you cannot handle, you should have no hesitation, or shame, about moving on swiftly to the hospital.

A second reaction common among emergency personnel is a feeling of irritation at patients who seem to have trivial illnesses or injuries. The EMT is trained to deal with life-threatening events, and he or she may feel it is a waste of time to be called to see a patient with a minor complaint. This feeling is *not* justified. When someone calls for an ambulance, it is because that person is in distress. It is not the function of the EMT or any other health professional to pass judgment on another person's distress. The EMT's job is to give whatever care is needed in any given case, whether it is a bandage for a scraped knee or full-scale resuscitation for cardiac arrest.

REACTIONS IN MASS CASUALTY SITUATIONS

In a situation in which many people are injured—be it a natural disaster (earthquake, flood, tornado) or a major accident (aircraft crash, explosion)—those at the scene are apt to be overwhelmed by the event. It is important for the EMT to recognize some of the common reactions to disaster, both in bystanders and in members of the rescue team, in order to help others cope with the situation and prevent a secondary disaster from mass panic.

In general, there are five basic reactions to a disaster situation. The NORMAL REACTION consists of extreme anxiety, with sweating, trembling, tachycardia, nausea, and sometimes vomiting. This is the type of reaction you are apt to see in one of your crew (the EMT who looks a bit dazed and green around the gills), and the best treatment for it is to give the person something constructive to do. Usually having a well-defined task will help the person in this state to "snap out of it" and function effectively.

Much more worrisome than this normal reaction is BLIND PANIC, in which the individual seems to have lost all reason and judgment. Panic is dangerous because it is contagious, and a person showing signs of uncontrollable panic must be isolated from other bystanders. If at all possible, find another bystander who seems reasonably calm and responsible to escort the panicky individual out of the main disaster area and to remain with that person at all times.

Another individual who needs to be removed from the disaster area is one showing signs of OVER REACTION. This person is easily identified, for he or she is talking compulsively, joking inappropriately, and running from one task to another without accomplishing anything useful. A person who is over-reacting will simply get in the way and interfere with other people who are trying to get things done.

At the other end of the spectrum is the bystander with DEPRESSION, the person who just sits numbly in one place and appears totally dazed, in what lay people call "a state of shock." Sometimes a person with a depressive reaction may be able to come out of it if given something to do; but if the individual does not respond to commands, he or she should be placed under supervision of a responsible bystander.

Finally, one occasionally sees what is called a CONVERSION REACTION among victims of mass disaster. In this reaction, the person subconsciously converts his or her anxiety into physical symptoms, such as sudden blindness or inability to move the extremities. A person having such a reaction must be triaged and treated along with other victims, according to the usual order of priorities.

The EMT should bear in mind that what people need most in a disaster situation is LEADERSHIP; and if yours is the first rescue team on the scene, it is your job to provide that leadership. Upon arriving at the scene, rescue personnel should identify themselves and take command with as much self-assurance and authority as they can muster. Frightened, dazed bystanders cannot make decisions and do not want to be given options. They should be *told* what to do, not asked. Whenever possible, ASSIGN TASKS TO BYSTANDERS, in order both to keep them occupied and to free up rescue personnel for medical activities.

PATIENTS WHO ARE EMOTIONALLY DISTURBED

So far, we have discussed reactions that occur in emotionally healthy people under stress, in the context of a critical medical emergency or mass disaster. Occasionally, however, the EMT will be called to attend a patient whose *chief complaint* is an emotional disturbance that is in some way distressing to himself or those around him. The EMT should be able to assess the general nature of such problems and to act in a manner consistent with the safety of all concerned.

IS THE PATIENT EMOTIONALLY DISTURBED?

One of the first questions the EMT needs to ask when dealing with a person whose behavior seems disturbed or "crazy" is whether that person is in fact suffering from an illness or injury that has caused the strange behavior. Recall that a DIABETIC who has taken too much insulin may behave convincingly like a paranoid, and it just takes a candy bar to restore that person to perfectly normal behavior within minutes. HEAD INJURY may also produce very bizarre behavior, as can STROKE, SEVERE INFECTION, and various metabolic disorders. Don't forget DRUGS and ALCOHOL either, which account for about half the cases of abnormal behavior seen in most emergency rooms. Never write someone off as "crazy" until you have ruled out all the other possible causes of crazy behavior; and be particularly alert for a physical cause when you get a history of a *sudden* change in the way the patient has been acting.

GENERAL GUIDELINES FOR DEALING WITH DISTURBED PATIENTS

When the EMT is called to attend an emotionally disturbed person, it is because that person's behavior is upsetting to himself or to others around him. Thus you can count on the fact that you are going to find at least one panicky person at the scene, and probably a whole group of panicky people, all of whom are expecting you to "do something." This is not an easy situation in which to work, but once again, staying calm and professional can do wonders to quiet everyone down.

In dealing with a psychiatric emergency, the EMT must BE PREPARED TO SPEND TIME WITH THE DISTURBED PATIENT. There is no place for haste in these cases, for hurrying simply conveys to the patient and bystanders that you are as nervous as they are. IDENTIFY YOURSELF CLEARLY, and arrange to TALK TO THE PATIENT ALONE. While it is often useful to have relatives or trusted friends in the room initially, after a few minutes it is usually preferable to send them into another room, where your partner can obtain their story. SIT DOWN to interview the patient; do not tower over him. BE CALM AND DIRECT. Most disturbed patients are frightened, and what frightens them most is the feeling that they are losing control of themselves. Your behavior should indicate that you have confidence in the patient's ability to maintain self-control. LET THE PATIENT TELL HIS STORY IN HIS OWN WAY. Listen quietly, and DO NOT PASS JUDGMENT. The patient has a right to his feelings, and you should respect that right. DON'T BE AFRAID OF SILENCE OR OF TEARS. Give the patient time to vent his feelings and get control of himself. Wherever possible, PROVIDE HONEST REASSURANCE; that is, show that you believe there are medical professionals who can help him with his problem. Do not, however, utter platitudes such as, "Don't worry, everything will be all right," for you will just convince the patient that you do not understand how bad the situation is. TAKE A DEFINITE PLAN OF ACTION. The patient needs to feel that something is being done, and usually will prefer to be instructed what to do rather than be confronted with too many decisions. ENCOURAGE THE PATIENT TO DO AS MUCH FOR HIMSELF AS POSSIBLE. If you are taking him to the hospital, have him gather together his own belongings. If he so chooses, let him walk to the ambulance and *sit* in the back rather than being carried on a stretcher. And in general, TREAT THE PATIENT AS SOMEONE YOU EXPECT TO GET BETTER; your confidence in him will help restore his confidence in himself. Be sure to BRING ALL THE PATIENT'S MEDICATIONS with him to the hospital, for knowledge of what pills the patient is taking will help the doctors to identify the problems for which the patient is being treated. Finally, STAY WITH THE PATIENT AT ALL TIMES, for his safety is your responsibility.

As a general rule, a patient who is seriously disturbed should be seen by a physician and evaluated for possible admission to the hospital. Problems arise when a disturbed patient refuses transport to a medical facility, for in most regions of the country, NO ONE EXCEPT A LAW ENFORCEMENT OFFICER MAY FORCIBLY RESTRAIN OR TRANSPORT A PERSON AGAINST HIS WILL. Every ambulance service should have clearly defined procedures for dealing with this situation in accordance with local statutes and good medical practice.

SPECIFIC PSYCHIATRIC EMERGENCIES

This is not a textbook of psychiatry, nor is it our purpose here to provide an encyclopedia of emotional disturbances. The aim of this section is to present a brief picture of some common psychiatric disturbances in order that the EMT may recognize these problems and deal with them appropriately in the field. Patients with psychiatric problems may present with disturbances of thinking, mood, behavior, or any combination of the three.

DEPRESSION AND SUICIDAL BEHAVIOR

The depressed person usually is not very difficult to spot, for he or she *looks* sad. A person suffering depression may be apathetic or listless, with bouts of crying, and often expresses feelings of worthlessness, pessimism, and guilt.

Depression should never be taken lightly by emergency care personnel, for it is all too often a fatal illness. The majority of successful suicides occur in depressed people, and the EMT should be alert for the danger signals suggesting suicidal intent.

Suicide is the tenth leading cause of death in the United States—taking nearly 30,000 lives a year—and it is the third leading cause of death among adolescents and young adults.

Suicide is more common in MEN, especially men who are SINGLE, WIDOWED, OR DIVORCED. More than half of all successful suicides have made a PREVIOUS SUICIDE ATTEMPT, and nearly three quarters give some CLEAR WARNING before taking their own lives.

Typically, the person who attempts or succeeds in suicide has feelings of worthlessness, hopelessness, and inability to cope with life in general. When a patient expresses such feelings, the EMT should always ask about suicidal intentions with a series of questions such as "Have you ever thought that life was not worth living? Did you ever feel you would be better off dead? Have you ever thought of harming yourself? If so, do you feel that way now? Do you have a specific plan for how you would do it?" Some health professionals are reluctant to pose those questions in the mistaken belief that they may "put ideas into the patient's head." That is not a danger. Suicide is not such an original idea that it wouldn't occur to the depressed person without someone else suggesting it. To the contrary, by broaching the subject, the EMt gives the patient a chance to talk about suicidal thoughts that may have frightened him. It is usually an enormous relief to a depressed person to be able to talk about suicidal thoughts, and sometimes just being able to talk about scary feelings makes those feelings less overwhelming.

Many patients make last-minute efforts to notify someone of their suicidal intentions. If a patient phones the ambulance service and threatens suicide, someone should stay by the phone and KEEP THE PATIENT ON THE LINE while an ambulance proceeds to the scene.

NEVER DISREGARD A SUICIDE THREAT OR GESTURE. IT IS A CRY FOR HELP—SOMETIMES THE LAST CRY FOR HELP.

Upon arrival at the scene, the EMTs should take a quick look around and discreetly remove any pills or implements with which the patient might injure himself. Be prepared to spend time talking with the patient. Encourage him to tell you about his problems. Do not be reluctant to ask him directly about his suicidal thoughts. Find out if he has ever attempted suicide before? Has he made concrete plans as to how he would kill himself? Has anyone in his family ever attempted suicide? Affirmative answers to any of these questions indicate a high risk for successful suicide, and the patient must be persuaded to be seen by a physician. DO NOT LEAVE THE SUICIDAL PATIENT ALONE, not even for a few minutes. Once you have responded to the call, the patient's safety becomes your responsibility.

Should you be called for a patient who has already attempted suicide, the patient's medical treatment has priority: The person who has slashed his wrists must have his bleeding controlled; the person who has taken a drug overdose must be managed for possible respiratory depression or other toxic problems. While carrying out urgent treatment, however, you should make every effort to establish rapport with the conscious patient, whose emotional needs should not be forgotten in the hurry to treat his physical injuries.

ACUTE ANXIETY

A person having an acute anxiety attack (panic attack) looks scared. He or she is tense and restless, often pacing, sweating, trembling. The patient may complain that his heart is pounding or that he cannot breathe. Often hyperventilation is part of the picture, with the characteristic signs and symptoms that hyperventilation produces: numbness around the mouth and in the extremities, dizziness, stabbing chest pains, carpopedal spasm.

Anxiety is like chicken pox: It is very catchy! So by the time you reach the scene, you are likely to have an epidemic of panic on your hands, with a whole horde of nervous and excited people buzzing frantically around the patient. Thus the first step in managing a patient with an acute anxiety attack is to SEPARATE THE PATIENT FROM ALL THE PANICKY PEOPLE AROUND HIM. Get the patient into a quiet room or, if no quiet room is available, into the back of the ambulance and shut the door. Identify yourself, and tell the patient in clear, confident terms that effect treatment is available for his problem. Continue to provide reassurance and support en route to the hospital.

HOSTILE AND VIOLENT BEHAVIOR

As far back as there were ambulances, ambulance personnel have always had to deal with violence or at least with the results of violence. The first ambulances were, after all, deployed to remove the wounded from the battlefield. And even in civilian practice, ambulances have always operated on the margins of violent events, picking up the casualties that violence generates. What is new in recent years, however, is the increasing tendency for ambulance personnel to become directly involved in violent incidents or even to become *targets* of violence.

The violent patient poses one of the most difficult management problems for EMS personnel. To begin with, most EMTs and paramedics see themselves as care-givers, not as "heavies," and often they find themselves unprepared—psychologically and tactically—to deal with hostile and even violent behavior. Furthermore, the encounter with a violent patient carries the constant risk that someone may get hurt—the patient himself, a bystander, the EMTs, or all of the aforementioned. The best way to try to ensure that no one does get hurt is to take preventive action—that is, to assess the potential for violence in *every* call and take steps to prevent violence.

Identifying Situations with a Potential for Violence

Preventive action starts with being psychologically prepared for a possible violent encounter, and keeping that possibility somewhere in the back of your mind in your response to *every* call. Do not rely too heavily on the information you get from your dispatcher; for example, the "old woman with a possible stroke" may have a disgruntled son with a M-16 rifle! Being psychologically prepared for violence does *not* mean becoming paranoid or treating every patient with distrust. It *does* mean developing a "nose for danger," or what has been called "survival awareness."

How do you identify potentially dangerous calls? Which scenarios, and which kinds of patients, are most likely to be associated with violence?

Risk Factors for Violence

SCENARIOS

- Any place where alcohol is being consumed (tavern, party)

- Crowd incidents
- Incidents where *violence* has already occurred (shooting, stabbing, "domestic," etc.)

DIAGNOSTIC GROUPS
- Intoxicated with alcohol
- Intoxicated with drugs (especially PCP, LSD, amphetamines, cocaine)
- Withdrawal from alcohol or drugs
- Psychosis (especially manic and paranoid types)
- Delirium from any cause (e.g., hypoglycemia, sepsis)

The risk factors listed above provide a general guideline to situations in which you need to be alert for possible violence. In any given specific case, however, the most important clues to the patient's potential for violence are found in his behavior and body language. Look for the following **warning signals:**

- POSTURE: The patient who sits tensely at the edge of his chair or grips at the armrest
- SPEECH: Loud, critical, threatening, a lot of profanity
- MOTOR ACTIVITY: Unable to sit still, paces back and forth or in circles, startles easily
- OTHER BODY LANGUAGE: Clenched fists, avoidance of eye contact, turning away when spoken to
- YOUR OWN FEELINGS: One of the most sensitive impending violence detectors is your own gut response to the patient: If your instinct tells you that you are in danger, pay attention!

Those signals should alert you to the possibility of imminent violence and should therefore trigger an almost automatic set of survival awareness actions on your part.

Management of the Violent Patient

Once you have concluded that there is a potential for violence in a situation, take the following steps:

- ASSESS THE WHOLE SITUATION. Are there factors in the surroundings that are contributing to the escalation of violence (e.g., friends who are egging the patient on)? Can those factors be removed? Is there evidence to suggest drug use, alcohol use, head injury, diabetes? Is there anyone present who can give you some background information? Did the patient's behavior come on gradually or suddenly? Does he have a history of violent behavior? Does he have any known medical problems, such as diabetes?
- OBSERVE YOUR SURROUNDINGS. Make sure you have access to an escape route. Place yourself between the patient and the door, but do not move *behind* an agitated patient. And do not turn your back on the patient, even for a moment. Make note of furniture and other potential barriers. Scan the area quickly for anything that could be used as a weapon (e.g., heavy or sharp objects) if the level of violence escalates. If a violent patient is armed with a dangerous weapon, don't try to deal with the situation yourself; back off and notify law enforcement authorities. Try to ensure that others at the scene are not endangered while you await the arrival of the police. If the patient is not armed, you may attempt to deal with him.
- MAINTAIN A SAFE DISTANCE. Moving too close to a potentially violent patient is likely to increase his anxiety level. In general, maintain a safety zone of two arm lengths; but if the patient is backing away from you, that's a sign that you're too close. Let him find a comfortable distance. Do not position yourself face-to-face with the patient but rather slightly to the side.
- TRY VERBAL RESTRAINTS FIRST. Remember, often anger and aggressive behavior are a response to illness or feelings of helplessness, and just talking to the angry person in a calm, sympathetic way may defuse some of his anger.

1. Take a moment to CONCENTRATE YOUR OWN THOUGHTS, for you will need to convey an impression of calm and self-control to the patient. You can't fake it, because the agitated patient will see right through your act.

2. IDENTIFY YOURSELVES as medical personnel who are there to try to help him. Keep your voice low—that forces the patient to stop what he is doing in order to focus on what you are saying to him.

3. Make note of his behavior, and restate your willingness to help (e.g., "You look very upset. How can we help you?")

4. ENCOURAGE THE PATIENT TO TALK about what is bothering him. *Listen* to what he says, and *show* him that you are listening by paraphrasing his words back to him ("I think I understand: Are you saying that . . .")

5. DEFINE YOUR EXPECTATIONS of the patient's behavior. Acknowledge his potential to do harm ("You could really hurt someone with that crowbar . . ."), but assure him that he will not be permitted to lose control.

6. If verbal de-escalation isn't working, BACK OFF AND GET HELP. You can simply say to the patient, "Look, I've been trying to talk with you for the past 15 minutes and we're just going in circles. So I'm going to leave you alone for a few minutes and see if you can get hold of yourself. When I come back, we'll try again to talk, but if talking still doesn't work, I'm going to have some people with me to help prevent you from hurting anyone."

- WHEN VERBAL RESTRAINT FAILS, USE PHYSICAL RESTRAINT

1. Make sure you have SUFFICIENT PERSONNEL before you attempt to overpower the patient. You will need police assistance, since in most jurisdictions it is not legal for an EMT (or anyone else) to restrain or transport a person against his will except at the express order of the police. You must, furthermore, have overwhelming force, which means a *minimum* of five trained, able-bodied people—one for each limb (a specific limb assigned in advance to each responder, so there won't be any confusion at the time action is initiated) and one for the head. Appoint one leader, who will direct the team and maintain verbal contact with the patient.

2. Sometimes the SHOW OF FORCE may in itself be sufficient to calm the patient: The mere sight of five 250-lb police officers, for example, has been known to have a remarkably tranquilizing effect on even the most belligerent patient. Don't move in on the patient right away: Give him a chance to make a graceful retreat to a nonviolent alternative behavior.

3. If the show of force is not sufficient to calm the patient, which may occur, for example, in a patient under the influence of drugs, such as PCP, you will have to move quickly to restrain the patient. First, remove any equipment or jewelry from your own person that could be used as a weapon against you (e.g., name badge, scissors worn on the belt, key chain, earrings). Make sure you have adequate restraining devices—preferably padded leather or nylon restraints—immediately available. Then, at a signal from the leader, move in *fast* from the patient's sides. Grasp him at the elbows, knees, and head and apply restraints to all four extremities. Probably the best position in which to secure him to the stretcher is supine, with his legs spread-eagled and both his arms secured to one side of the stretcher. That position will turn his head to the side, so that he won't aspirate if he should vomit.

4. Throughout the whole restraint procedure and transport, MAINTAIN VERBAL CONTACT with the patient, even if he does not appear to be paying attention to what you are saying. Once he is restrained, DO NOT REMOVE THE RESTRAINTS. Don't negotiate. Don't make deals.

5. Once restraints have been applied, CHECK THE PERIPHERAL CIRCULATION every 5 minutes to make sure the restraints are not too tight. Check the radial pulses in the arms and the dorsalis pedis pulses in the feet.

6. DOCUMENT EVERYTHING in the patient's chart—the reasons for using restraints (be specific: Give examples of the patient's behavior and the indications of his violent potential); the number of people used to subdue him; the restraining devices used; and the status of the peripheral circulation after restraints were applied.

Dealing with the After-Effects of Violence

As noted at the beginning of this section, most EMTs do not enjoy dealing with violent patients. The type of person who chooses a career in EMS is usually oriented toward rescue and care, not toward martial arts and the use of force. So the call that involves a violent patient is likely to leave the ambulance team feeling tired, angry, guilty, and just plain upset. It should, therefore, be the policy of every ambulance service to provide for a debriefing after every call that involved violence—a time when those who took part in the incident can get together and talk it over and share their feelings about what happened. EMTs who are not given such opportunities to "decompress" after tough calls are EMTs who will burn out very quickly.

VOCABULARY

conversion reaction Psychologic mechanism by which a person translates his anxiety into a physical symptom, most commonly paralysis.

regression Return to a more primitive form of behavior, as experienced by an adult who begins behaving like a child.

FURTHER READING

Bassuk EL, Fox SS, Prendergast KJ. *Behavioral Emergencies: A Field Guide for EMTs and Paramedics.* Boston: Little, Brown, 1983.

Dick T. Gloves without fingers: Using stockinette as a restraint. *JEMS* 14(12):25, 1989.

Dubin W. Evaluating and managing the violent patient. *Ann Emerg Med* 10:481, 1981.

Edwards FJ. Psychiatric emergencies, Part 1. *Emerg Med Serv* 14(3):46, 1985.

Eisenberg L. The epidemiology of suicide in adolescents. *Pediatr Ann* 13:47, 1984.

Garfinkel B, Froese A., Hood J. Suicide attempts in children or adolescents. *Am J Psychiatry* 139:1257, 1982.

Gorski, T, Carbine M. Managing the potentially violent patient. A protocol for training EMTs and paramedics. *Emerg Med Serv* 10(5):6, 1981.

Infantino JA. Controlling violent patients. *Emerg Med Serv* 13(5):23, 1984.

Jenike M. Depressed in the ER. *Emerg Med* 16(6)102, 1984.

Leisner K. Trauma: Accident or attempted suicide? *Emerg Med Serv* 18(5):30, 1989.

Makadon H, Gerson S, Ryback R. Managing the care of the difficult patient in the emergency unit. *JAMA* 252:2595, 1984.

Markush RE et al. Firearms and suicide in the United States. *Am J Pub Health* 74:123, 1984.

Patterson WM et al. Evaluation of suicidal patients: The sad persons scale. *Psychosomatics* 24:343, 1983.

Peterson L. The psychological impact of trauma: Recognition and treatment. *Am J Emerg Med* 1:102, 1983.

Rabin PL et al. Acute grief. *South Med J* 74:1468, 1981.

Roy A. Risk factors for suicide in psychiatric patients. *Arch Gen Psych* 39:1089, 1982.

Rund DA. Assessment of suicide risk. *Emerg Med Serv* 18(5):27, 1989.

Rund D. Emergency management of the difficult patient. *Emerg Med Serv* 13(3):17, 1984.

Ruple JA. Honing skills for suicide intervention. *JEMS* 15(1):149, 1990.

Schmidt TA. Evaluating and transporting patients at risk for suicide. *Emerg Med Serv* 17(8):48, 1988.

Solomon J. The suicide scenario: Rewriting the final act. *Emerg Med* 21(4):75, 1989.

Taylor C. Domestic violence: The medical response. *Emerg Med Serv* 13(5):35, 1984.

The violent patient. *Emerg Med* 15(9):26, 1983.

XI. EXTRICATION AND PATIENT HANDLING

The EMT's primary job is a medical one: that is, the provision of emergency medical care to the sick and injured. Sometimes, however, the EMT will find that before such care can be rendered, he or she must get to a patient who is trapped in a relatively inaccessible location, and every EMT should have certain basic skills in rescue procedures. When individuals specially trained in rescue and extrication are present at the scene, it is preferable that the EMT leave the disentanglement problems to the experts and concentrate his or her energies on the medical needs of the patients. Nonetheless, even when others are available to do the rescue work, the EMT must be aware of what the rescue personnel are doing and what problems they face, so that all concerned can work together effectively as a team.

In this section, we will look briefly at some of the basic techniques of gaining access to an entrapped patient, disentangling the patient from wreckage, and safely removing the patient to the ambulance. We will examine as well some methods for lifting and moving patients under various circumstances. It must be emphasized that the skills described in this section are not learned by reading about them; they are learned by doing them. Every EMT should have the opportunity to observe and practice the techniques involved under the supervision of trained rescue personnel.

36. EXTRICATION

OBJECTIVES

Extrication refers to the process by which an entrapped, injured person is approached, treated, and safely removed from the area of entrapment. There are all sorts of situations in which the victim of injury may be relatively inaccessible; he may be sealed inside an elevator, buried under the rubble of a collapsed building or mine shaft, or pinned within the wreckage of a car. Each situation poses unique dilemmas for those who must reach the patient and render care. In this chapter, we will look at the various stages of extrication, using as our model the most common extrication situation with which the EMT has to deal: extrication from a wrecked or disabled motor vehicle. By the conclusion of this chapter, the reader should be able to:

1. Identify the primary function of an EMT in a rescue situation, given a list of various functions
2. Identify the correct sequence of steps in extrication, given a list of steps in random order
3. Identify the correct *type* of tool needed for a given rescue task, given a description of the task to be performed
4. Identify the best method of gaining access to a victim in a wrecked car, given a description of the vehicle's condition and a list of various options for access
5. Indicate the priorities of treatment in managing a patient entrapped in a wrecked vehicle, given a description of the patient's injuries
6. Identify the best method of disentanglement, given a description of the nature of the patient's entrapment and a list of options for achieving disentanglement
7. Describe the method of removing an injured patient from (a) an upright vehicle and (b) a vehicle resting on its side

GENERAL PRINCIPLES OF EXTRICATION

Most of extrication is common sense, with an added bit of ingenuity. No matter what the extrication problem—be it entrapment in an overturned car or entombment beneath a pile of rubble—there are certain basic principles that apply. To begin with, it is necessary always to keep in mind that THE EMT'S FIRST AND MOST IMPORTANT RESPONSIBILITY IS TO PROVIDE PATIENT CARE. If rescue crews are not present, the EMT will have to use whatever means are available to gain access to the patient and disentangle him from the wreckage, but these tasks should never distract the EMT from the basic mission: administering care to the patient as rapidly as possible and ensuring that the patient's removal from the wreckage is carried out so as to minimize additional injury. When rescue teams *are* present, the EMT should attend to the needs of the patient while rescue activities are in progress.

A second basic principle of extrication is that if there is both an easy way and a hard way to do something, TRY THE EASIER WAY FIRST. No extra points are given for doing things the hard way. This may seem obvious, but it is remarkable how many times a rescue crew will deploy all sorts of power tools to pry and cut open a damaged car door when the opposite door is undamaged and unlocked and could be opened simply by turning the door handle.

Thirdly, extrication should be ORDERLY AND SYSTEMATIC. A systematic approach requires some planning. EMTs who come barreling out of the ambulance and begin immediately hacking away at a wrecked car are unlikely to do much good for the victim inside. Every extrication is different, and one must take a few moments to analyze the problem and determine the most efficient way to solve it—the stage that firefighters call **size-up**.

In general, once the scene has been secured, there are five stages of extrication: (1) gaining access, (2) providing urgent medical care, (3) disentangling the victim, (4) preparing for removal of the victim, and (5) removing the victim from the area of entrapment. Those stages should nearly always be carried out in the order listed. PATIENT CARE MUST ALWAYS PRECEDE REMOVAL OF THE PATIENT FROM THE WRECKAGE EXCEPT WHEN DELAY IN REMOVAL WOULD ENDANGER THE LIFE OF THE PATIENT OR RESCUER.

Finally, a good extrication is a safe extrication. ALWAYS KEEP YOUR OWN SAFETY AND THAT OF THE PATIENT UPPERMOST IN YOUR MIND. For your own safety, you should wear *leather gloves* and a *hard hat*. *Goggles* are required for cutting with power tools or breaking glass. If there is a fire danger, you should have a proper fire resistant coat. The patient too must be protected from injury that might arise during the extrication process. Hazards, such as spilled gasoline, must be attended to promptly. An unstable vehicle must be properly braced, and the patient must be shielded from flying glass or debris with a blanket or short backboard. It does precious little good to smash one's way spectacularly into a wrecked vehicle while spraying splinters of broken glass all over the patient. Safety too is a matter of common sense.

TOOLS FOR EXTRICATION

The American College of Surgeons has compiled a list of items for use in rescue that they regard as essential equipment for every ambulance (Table 36-1). In general, the tools used in extrication fall into four broad categories: disassembly tools, spreading tools, cutting tools, and pulling tools.

- DISASSEMBLY TOOLS are those used to take things apart, such as screwdrivers, wrenches, and pliers, and they tend to come in handy in all sorts of situations.

- SPREADING TOOLS are usually hydraulic, and may be either manual, such as the Porto-power, or

Table 36-1. *Essential Rescue Equipment for Ambulances**

Quantity	Item	Typical Uses
4	Triangular reflectors or battery-operated flares	To demarcate the danger zone and caution oncoming traffic
1	12-in. adjustable wrench	Disassembly
1	12-in. regular screwdriver	Disassembly
1	12-in. Phillips screwdriver	Disassembly, breaking tempered glass
1	Hacksaw with 12-in. carbide blades	Cutting through corner posts, steering wheel
1	10-in. pliers with vise grip	Breaking away covering of steering wheel
1	5-lb hammer with 15-in. handle	Making openings with cutting tools
1	Fire axe butt with 24-in. handle	Cutting roof section
1	51-in. crowbar with pinch point	Displacing and prying operations
1	Bolt cutter with 1¼-in. jaw opening and 36-in. handles	Breaking padlocks; cutting chains, fences
1	Portable power jack and spreader tool	Prying open doors, breaking seats loose
1	49-in. shovel with pointed blade	Removing debris
1	Double action tin snip (at least 8 in.)	Cutting seat belts, removing metal trim
2	Manilla ropes, each 50 ft long and ¾ in. in diameter	Stabilizing a vehicle, raising or lowering stretcher or equipment, rescue pull
1	Heavy duty hand winch (come-along) with 15-ft rated chain and grab hook	Displacing steering columns, widening door openings, pulling front seat back
4	Shoring blocks	Supporting an unstable vehicle, preventing collapse of hood when come-along is in use
1 set/EMT	Hard hat, goggles, gloves	Safety

*Adapted from the American College of Surgeons, Committee on Trauma. Essential Equipment for Ambulances. *Bull. Am. Coll. Surg.*, Sept., 1977.

power-driven, such as the Hurst or Lukas tool. Spreading tools are used to force open a door, break a car seat loose, and perform other operations that require prying one object away from another.

- CUTTING TOOLS include a variety of manually-operated devices, such as bolt cutters, hacksaws, and giant can-openers, as well as power-driven tools, such as the air chisel. As the name of the category implies, cutting tools are used for operations that require cleaving through a hard object; for instance, severing a steering wheel rim, sawing through roof-posts, or even opening up the roof of a car as one would a can of soup.

- PULLING TOOLS are exemplified by the hand winch, or "come-along," and employ a ratchet-driven drum to shorten a steel cable or chain. Pulling tools are used for displacing a steering column or pulling back a door or seat, and they are extremely versatile and useful devices.

It must be emphasized that sophisticated tools, such as the "Jaws of Life," should be used only by personnel who have been thoroughly trained in their proper operation. EVERY TOOL HAS OPERATIONAL LIMITS AND HAZARDS. The EMT should know what each of his or her tools can and cannot do and what potential dangers they create. And, once again, remember that you don't get extra points for doing things the hard way. DON'T USE THE BIG GUNS WHEN A SIMPLE TOOL WILL DO THE TRICK. Use common sense. Try the easiest approach first.

HAZARD CONTROL

Before any extrication measures may be attempted, it is necessary to secure the accident scene; that is, to eliminate hazards to the rescuers or the accident victims. The measures required to secure the accident scene will, of course, vary according to the circumstances of the accident. Such measures may include washing away spilled gasoline, controlling traffic, identifying hazardous cargoes, providing adequate lighting, or shoring up unstable vehicles. Once again, the point to remember is: EVALUATE THE SITUATION BEFORE YOU RUSH IN.

Hazard Control: Some General Principles

- All downed wires are live electric wires until proved otherwise by qualified personnel (that is, personnel from the power company). EMTs should *not* attempt to deal with downed wires.
- All traffic in the vicininty of an extrication should be shut down.
- During every vehicle extrication, there should be at least one charged fire hose manned until all patients have been removed from the vehicle to a safe place.
- Stabilize *every* disabled vehicle. Use tire chocks for vehicles that are upright.
- Do *not* try to disconnect the battery of a disabled vehicle (you may inadvertently spark an explosion).

GAINING ACCESS

The first stage of extrication is gaining access to the victim. Access needs to be as rapid as possible, with a minimum of tools and procedures. The goal of this step is simply to provide a space large enough for the EMT to reach the patient and stabilize him.

OPENING DOORS

Like every other stage of extrication, gaining access requires common sense. THE EASIEST WAY TO ENTER AN AUTOMOBILE IS THROUGH THE DOOR! Try first to open the door nearest the victim. If this door is jammed, *try all the other doors.* This may sound elementary, but, as noted earlier, many times rescuers become so engrossed with trying to open one door with all their fancy equipment that they neglect to check other doors that may be unlocked and perfectly functional.

If all the doors are locked and the victim inside is conscious, ask the victim to unlock the door. If the victim is unconscious in a locked car, a coat hanger or hacksaw blade can sometimes be used to force open the locking button on older-model cars from the outside; but this method should not be used if it cannot be carried out quickly.

If a door cannot be opened rapidly with a minimum of equipment, consider breaking a window to unlock the door from the inside. Side and rear windows of automobiles are made of tempered glass, which can be easily broken if punctured with a sharp object. A spring-loaded center punch can be used for this purpose; but if such equipment is not available, any sharp-pointed tool, such as a Phillips screwdriver, will do the job. Select a window away from the victim, and strike the glass in a lower corner, being careful not to displace it inward onto the victim. Once the glass is broken and pulled outside, reach in and unlatch the door. If the door does not open, try releasing the inside and outside door handles simultaneously. Should these maneuvers fail, another method to open the door may have to be used. This, however, will generally be time consuming, and in the meanwhile an alternative means of access should be sought.

ACCESS THROUGH A WINDOW

When quick access to the patient cannot be achieved through a door, by one of the methods just described, it may be necessary to reach the patient through a window. The fastest window access is achieved by breaking a rear or side window with a center punch. First tape the window with masking or adhesive tape to minimize dispersion of broken glass all over the interior of the vehicle. Then fire the center punch in a lower corner of the window. If shattered glass does fall within the vehicle, drop a heavy blanket or canvas tarp over it before you crawl in.

ACCESS TO AN OVERTURNED VEHICLE

A vehicle found upside-down or lying on its side presents special problems of access, for an improper approach may seriously jeopardize the safety of both victim and rescuer. To begin with, THE VEHICLE SHOULD BE STABILIZED IN THE POSITION IN WHICH IT IS FOUND. Attempts to right the vehicle may cause additional injuries to the victim(s) inside. Instead, the vehicle should be stabilized as necessary with any available materials, such as spare tires, cribbing blocks, rocks, or timber. Ropes may also be used to stabilize the vehicle in place, especially if it is in a precarious position (e.g., on a hillside). NO ATTEMPT SHOULD BE MADE TO ENTER THE VEHICLE UNTIL ITS STABILITY HAS BEEN ASSURED. If a door is open, it should be tied open to make sure that it does not slam shut at an inconvenient moment. Breaking the rear window is probably the fastest way to get in.

PROVIDING URGENT MEDICAL CARE

The whole point of gaining rapid access to the patient is to be able to initiate medical care as soon as possible. The EMT entering the vehicle should carry a blanket and a small jump kit with basic equipment such as airways, bag-valve-mask, dressings, and triangular bandages. Other equipment, such as oxygen or suction, can be handed in to the EMT as required.

Inside the wreckage, first make sure the ignition is turned off. Then the usual priorities of ABC apply. The AIRWAY must be opened, with care to avoid unnecessary motion of the patient's neck; and adequate BREATHING should be assured. This means not only providing artifical ventilation for the patient with apnea, but also checking for and closing off any sucking chest wounds. Seriously injured patients should receive OXYGEN at the earliest possible moment, and certainly oxygen administration should *not* be delayed until the patient is removed from the car. In assessing the CIRCULATION, bear in mind that effective CPR can be carried out only when the patient is supine on a hard surface; it cannot be accomplished when the patient is sitting or lying on a car seat. Thus, if a pulse is absent, the patient must be removed with all possible speed from the vehicle, even if removal means possibly aggravating other injuries. Significant BLEEDING should be controlled with direct pressure. The presence of shock or the likelihood of shock developing indicates a need to expedite disentanglement procedures in order that the patient can be placed in a supine position (preferably within the MAST garment) as rapidly as possible. If the EMT is authorized to start an intravenous infusion, every attempt should be made to do so early, even before the patient is disentangled. Shock is more easily prevented than treated.

Once the ABCs have been taken care of, OPEN WOUNDS should be dressed and FRACTURES stabilized. Manual stabilization is preferable initially, for bulky splints are nearly impossible to apply in cramped quarters and may well hinder efforts to remove the patient from the wreckage. Remember, effective splinting can be achieved by securing the injured extremity to an uninjured part of the body: A broken leg can be splinted to an uninjured leg; a broken arm can be secured to the chest with a sling and swath.

Throughout the rest of the disentanglement and removal procedures, the EMT in the car with the victim will have three main tasks:

1. MAINTAIN THE VICTIM'S AIRWAY.
2. KEEP THE VICTIM'S HEAD AND NECK STABLE, by applying a cervical collar and maintaining constant manual traction on the head (see Fig. 14-22).
3. PROTECT THE VICTIM FROM FURTHER INJURY.

These tasks require the EMT not only to keep a close eye on the patient but also to be alert to what other rescuers are doing. If the rescue team is about to knock in a window, for instance, the EMT must see to it that the patient is covered with a blanket or short backboard to shield him from possible flying glass. If the patient is conscious, the EMT should also provide reassurance, comfort, and a running explanation of what is being done.

DISENTANGLEMENT

Disentanglement is the process of removing those parts of the wrecked vehicle that are keeping the victim pinned or entrapped. The watchword of disentanglement is that you REMOVE THE VEHICLE FROM THE PATIENT, NOT THE PATIENT FROM THE VEHICLE. This is perhaps an overstatement, but it emphasizes the point that the parts of the car obstructing safe removal of the victim must be peeled away from the victim; one should never try to yank the victim loose from whatever is holding him in place. Remember a car—even a Rolls Royce—can be repaired or replaced. A human being cannot.

The first step of disentanglement is to determine what precisely is holding the victim in place. Is it the steering wheel? The dashboard? One of the pedals? Once the offending object has been identified, the next step is to decide how to remove that object in a way that will not cause further injury to the victim.

DOORS

Often the disentanglement procedure begins with an assault on the doors, for until the doors are opened or removed, it is difficult to reach the other objects causing entrapment. When vehicle doors are jammed, the rescue team should not initially spend a lot of time trying to get them open, but rather should seek access to the patient by another, quicker means, as through a window. However, once treatment is initiated, it is desirable to get one or more doors open to facilitate work inside the vehicle and provide a route for removal of the patient.

Once again, TRY THE EASIEST WAY FIRST. Double check all the doors to make sure that they do not open in the usual fashion (the EMT inside the vehicle can unlock them and release the inside latch). If that approach doesn't work, try inserting a pry bar while the inside and outside latches are held open. Should that fail, one can cut a flap of metal from around the lock and release the locking mechanism manually. Sometimes an air chisel must be used to cut the rivets holding the locking pin. A jammed door can also sometimes be opened using a Porto-power or Hydra-spreader to spread the door away from its frame until the locking pin is pulled clear of its housing. This is a time-consuming procedure. If available, a tool such as the Jaws of Life can do the same job considerably faster.

STEERING WHEEL

It is not uncommon for a victim to be pinned against the seat by the steering wheel, in which case disentanglement of the victim will require removal or retraction of the wheel. *Cutting the steering wheel* is accomplished in two steps. First, use the vise grip pliers to pull away the plastic coating on the wheel; then use a regular hacksaw or large bolt cutters to cut through the wheel ring. If this approach does not provide sufficient space for removal of the victim, it may be necessary to *pull the steering column up* so that it is out of the victim's way. The steering column is retracted by means of a come-along, wooden blocks, and chains. Using equipment, one can usually raise the wheel about 10 to 15 inches. The patient must be protected during the procedure with a heavy blanket or inverted short backboard lest he be injured by breaking glass or splintering from a plastic dashboard. A come-along must be used with great care. Improper placement of the chains may allow the steering column to slip and rebound back against the victim.

WINDSHIELD

Usually the reason for removing a windshield is to permit use of the come-along for retracting the steering column. The windshield may also have to be removed to allow more working room for the rescuers. The preferred method for removing a windshield or rear window will depend upon the way in which the window is mounted. If you can see only chrome trim around the windshield, the glass is mounted in a substance called *mastic*. If so, pry away the chrome trim and work the point of a right-angle blade behind the glass. Then draw the blade across the top and sides of the window and pry the whole windshield away in one piece. Windshields that are mounted in a U-shaped molding, called *channel*, are easier to remove. Again, first pry off the chrome trim at the top and sides of the windshield. Then jam the point of a sharp knife, like a linoleum knife, into the channel, keeping the knife blade flat against the glass. Pull the knife toward you, then down the sides of the glass. Once you've finished cutting the rubber channel, use a screwdriver to pry the glass out.

Sometimes the methods just described do not work, especially with some of the mastic-mounted windows. In that case, you may have to use a fire ax to chop through the windshield, taking proper precautions to protect the patient from flying glass.

A special problem arises when a victim is found with his head, arm, or another part of his body jammed through a broken windshield. Under these circumstances, bandaging materials should be used to pad the protruding part of the victim's body as thoroughly as possible. Once the patient is well protected, pliers can be used to break or peel back the glass in order to free the patient. Needless to say, the rescuer must wear protective gloves for such a procedure.

DASHBOARD AND PEDALS

Sometimes, particularly after head-on collisions, the patient's knees are pinned beneath the dashboard, which may impinge as well upon the pelvis. The involved part of the dashboard should be removed with a hacksaw or air chisel; once again, take care to protect the patient from injury while these tools are being deployed.

Occasionally a patient's foot will be caught between the pedals on the floor of the vehicle. If the foot is uninjured, it may be possible to free it simply by removing the victim's shoe. If, however, the foot is injured, or if removal of the shoe from an uninjured foot does not succeed in freeing the foot, the pedal will have to be forced sideways, using a Porto-power or similar device.

FRONT SEAT

When a victim is pinned in the driver's seat, he is generally wedged between the steering wheel–

dashboard combination in front and the driver's seat in back. Often the fastest way to release the patient is to move the seat backward. This in itself may provide sufficient space for removal of the patient and obviate the need for cumbersome efforts to pull back the whole steering column.

Before attempting to move the front seat in any way, you must make sure that the patient is held steady and that his feet are not entangled in the pedals or other debris. If the victim is unsupported, a sudden backward movement of the seat may cause his neck to jerk forward and his legs to be wrenched back.

Frequently it is possible to move the front seat backward simply by releasing the seat-adjustment lever and guiding the seat back along the floor tracks. If this maneuver does not work, the come-along can be passed through the rear window and attached to the car frame around the bumper, with the chain locked around the base of the seat.

ROOF

When a vehicle is lying on its side after an accident, the roof offers an excellent means of access for removing the patient. Remember, though, that the car must first be well stabilized with cribbing blocks or similar materials to prevent motion. The patient must also be forewarned that the procedure is going to be very noisy. An air chisel is then used to cut a flap in the roof, leaving the bottom edge intact; the metal is folded down toward the ground, thereby avoiding a razor edge of metal over which the patient must pass during removal from the vehicle. Roof beams can be cut with an air chisel, and then the head liner is removed with a knife.

When the car is upright, the roof may be removed to gain more working space for the rescue team. In this case, the job is most easily accomplished by cutting through the front and middle supporting posts with a hacksaw or air chisel. Once the posts are severed, a notch must be made in each side of the roof, over the back windows, and the roof is then lifted backward over the trunk.

PREPARATION FOR REMOVAL

The stage of preparation for removal is essentially a wrap-up of the previous two stages: The *patient* is stabilized to the maximum degree possible, including dressing of wounds and splinting of fractures; and an *exit route* is prepared by peeling away the last obstructing parts of the vehicle. All equipment necessary for removal, such as backboards, straps, and cravats, is assembled in proximity to the patient.

REMOVAL

The goal of this step is to get the victim out of the wreckage with an absolute minimum of movement to possibly injured parts. In general, when a car is upright, removal is most easily accomplished through a door; when the car is resting on its side, removal is better accomplished through a hole cut in the roof. Whatever the exit route, removal should be carried out in an orderly, unhurried fashion with great care taken to avoid any further injury to the patient. The technique of removing a patient from a vehicle with long and short backboards has been described in detail in Chaper 14, and the student is urged to review that material at this time.

FURTHER READING

Bailyn L. Subway and bus extrication. *Emergency* 10(4):62, 1978.

Briese GL. Elevator extrication. *EMT J* 3(3):45, 1979

Farrington JD. Extrication of victims—surgical principles. *J Trauma* 8:493, 1968.

Grant H. *Vehicle Rescue* (2nd ed.). Bowie, MD: RJ Brady, 1990.

Hatfield L. Fundamentals of extrication. *EMT J* 3(3):42, 1979.

Hazlett S. Open forum: Extrication. *Emerg Med Serv* 5:13, 1976.

Hunt DW. The ins and outs of automobile extrication. *Emerg Med Serv* 14(1):38 and 14(2):50, 1985.

Hunt D. Ten common automobile-extrication errors. *Emerg Med Serv* 18(1):15, 1989.

Jarboe T. Surviving the tensions of trench rescue. *Rescue* 2(4):55, 1989

Moore R. *Vehicle Rescue and Extrication*. St. Louis: Mosby, 1990.

Schottke DE. A systematic approach to extrication. *EMT J* 3(3):76, 1979.

Stanford TM. Rescue from the dungeon. *Emergency* 21(4):24, 1989.

Tomlinson D. Taking time to do it right. *Rescue* 2(4):22, 1989.

U.S. Department of Transportation. *Emergency Medical Technician: Crash-Victim Extrication Training Course*. Pub 5003-00164. Washington, D.C.: U.S. Government Printing Office, 1976.

37. LIFTING AND MOVING PATIENTS

OBJECTIVES

The EMT's job does not end with rendering emergency medical treatment to the patient. Once the patient has been stabilized (and, on rare occasions, even before the patient has been stabilized), he must be transferred to a stretcher and transported to the hospital. Proper techniques of lifting and carrying a patient are no less important than proper techniques of medical care, for there is great potential to do harm to the patient by lifting or carrying him incorrectly. In this chapter, we will examine methods of moving patients under emergency and nonemergency conditions, and we will describe the techniques of patient handling designed to minimize the possibility of injury to both patient and EMT. By the conclusion of this chapter, the reader should be able to:

1. Identify correct and incorrect techniques of lifting and moving a patient, given a description of several techniques
2. Identify lifting and carrying maneuvers likely to result in injury to the rescuer, given a list of various maneuvers
3. Identify situations in which a patient must be moved prior to stabilization, given a description of various situations, and indicate the best method for carrying out the move
4. Select the appropriate stretcher and means of transfer to the stretcher, given a description of a patient's condition and the setting in which he is found
5. Select the appropriate position for the patient on a stretcher, given a description of the patient's medical problem

GENERAL CONSIDERATIONS

When an EMT lifts or carries a patient, two people are at risk of injury: the patient and the EMT. Proper handling techniques are designed to minimize the risks to both as well as the unnecessary expenditure of energy by the rescue team.

PATIENT SAFETY

When a patient must be moved from one place to another, or even from one position to another, the primary consideration in selecting a method for lifting or carrying must be the safety and comfort of the patient. In later sections, we will examine various techniques of patient handling in more detail. For our purposes here, it is necessary only to mention certain general guidelines. To begin with, as a general rule, A PATIENT SHOULD NOT BE MOVED IN ANY WAY UNTIL HE OR SHE HAS BEEN FULLY STABILIZED AND IS READY FOR TRANSPORTATION TO THE HOSPITAL. As we shall see later, there are occasional exceptions to this rule; but the

EMT should know the rule and, before breaking it, should have a very good reason for doing so.

When the time does come to move a patient, PLAN AHEAD. Figure out exactly how you will lift and lower him; make sure that the stretcher is conveniently placed to minimize unnecessary manual carrying; and know precisely what exit route you will be taking. Once the patient is on the stretcher, THE PATIENT MUST BE SECURELY STRAPPED TO THE STRETCHER BEFORE IT IS LIFTED OR ROLLED. There is never any excuse for a patient falling off a stretcher, and only gross negligence can permit that to happen.

Except when going uphill or upstairs, or when loading the stretcher into the ambulance, CARRY OR WHEEL THE STRETCHER FEETFIRST: for should the stretcher accidentally bump into something, at least the patient's head will not bear the brunt of the blow. Make sure that there are SUFFICIENT STRETCHER BEARERS to carry the load comfortably, and recruit bystanders as necessary. A stretcher that is too heavy for those carrying it is a stretcher that is likely to be dropped.

NEVER RUN WITH A STRETCHER! Even in emergency evacuations from hazardous areas, there is no justification for trying to sprint away. The amount of time saved by running is negligible, and tearing off pell-mell simply increases the probability that one of the stretcher bearers will stumble and fall. A quick, orderly march (military style) will accomplish rapid evacuation and also keep the stretcher carriers moving in unison, thereby minimizing the risk of dropping the patient. Try *not* to march in step because walking in unison creates more bounce on the stretcher.

When bystanders are recruited to assist in lifting or carrying a patient, EACH ASSISTANT MUST BE INSTRUCTED FULLY AND CAREFULLY AHEAD OF TIME. The most trained and experienced people present should be situated at the most critical areas of the patient's body. Thus, for instance, in the "four-rescuer pickup" using two EMTs and two bystanders, the two EMTs should be stationed at the patient's head and chest respectively, while the bystanders are at the patient's buttocks and legs.

EMT SAFETY

An EMT consists of two sets of levers (arms and legs) linked by a central, somewhat flexible rod (the spine). Each of the lever systems attaches to the body through ball and socket joints. If force is applied suddenly to one of these joints, especially in a direction in which the joint does not normally move, a sprain, dislocation, or other injury may result. The spine, meanwhile, permits considerable forward bending, but very little backward motion. The muscles that straighten the back are much less powerful than those that move the limbs and thus are more susceptible to strain when forced to bear a heavy burden. Muscles in general do not like to remain in a state of contraction for extended periods, and they start to hurt after sustained contraction.

Improper lifting techniques may result in injury to any of these body components. Cramping of strained muscles, tearing of ligaments, dislocation of joints—any of these may occur if lifting and carrying are not done in a way that correctly deploys the body's natural system of levers. For this reason, the U.S. Department of Transportation has suggested a list of guidelines for safe lifting of patients:

Guidelines for Preventing Lifting Injuries

- KNOW YOUR PHYSICAL LIMITATIONS. Do not try to handle a load too heavy for you. When in doubt, seek assistance.
- DO NOT ATTEMPT TO LOWER A PATIENT IF YOU FEEL YOU COULD NOT LIFT HIM.
- KEEP YOURSELF BALANCED when carrying out any task requiring lifting or carrying.
- Maintain a FIRM FOOTING.
- Maintain a CONSTANT AND FIRM GRIP.
- LIFT AND LOWER BY BENDING YOUR KNEES, NOT YOUR BACK! Keep your back straight at all times. Bend your knees, and lift with one foot ahead of the other.
- WHEN CARRYING, KEEP YOUR BACK STRAIGHT. Use your shoulder and leg muscles to bear the burden, and keep your abdominal muscles tight.
- FOR PULLING, USE YOUR ARMS AND SHOULDERS, AND KEEP YOUR BACK STRAIGHT.
- CARRY OUT ALL TASKS SLOWLY, smoothly, and in unison with associates.
- MOVE YOUR BODY GRADUALLY. Avoid twisting and jerking.
- DO NOT KEEP YOUR MUSCLES CONTRACTED FOR LONG PERIODS. Rest between major exertions.
- WHENEVER POSSIBLE, SLIDE OR ROLL HEAVY OBJECTS rather than lifting them.

EMERGENCY MOVES

As noted earlier, our general rule is that a person should not be moved until he has been stabilized and fully prepared for transport. There are, however, special circumstances in which this rule may be broken, and these are circumstances in which an immediate danger either to the patient or to others is present. Fire, for example, or imminent danger of fire, necessitates removing the victim as quickly as possible. Similarly, the presence of explosives or other hazardous materials or an inability to protect the scene may require rapid evacuation of the victim. Sometimes a patient must be moved prior to stabilization because it is impossible to gain access to other, more seriously injured patients without moving him. Other times, rapid removal must be carried out in order to perform life-saving treatment, such as when one quickly moves a cardiac arrest victim to the floor or to the ground so that CPR can be performed effectively.

When an emergency move is required, there are a number of methods by which such a move can be accomplished, depending on the number of rescuers present. It should be emphasized that whenever one moves an injured patient precipitously, there is a significant danger of aggravating injury to the victim's spine. The emergency moves described here do *not* protect the patient from injury. For this reason, EMERGENCY MOVES ARE ONLY FOR EMERGENCIES! They should never be used when there is time to get the right equipment and extra assistance.

EMERGENCY ONE-RESCUER TECHNIQUES

Occasionally the EMT faces hazardous situations in which he or she must act alone to remove a patient from danger, particularly multicasualty incidents in which victims must be quickly evacuated from a smoke-filled building or from a structure in imminent danger of collapse. When smoke is involved, the EMT should wear a quick-entry mask, and the method of moving the victim should keep both victim and EMT close to the floor, where the air is better. The following moves all utilize *pulling*; and whenever a patient is pulled, EVERY EFFORT SHOULD BE MADE TO PULL THE VICTIM IN THE DIRECTION OF THE LONG AXIS OF HIS BODY, so as to minimize twisting motions of the victim's spine.

Blanket Drag

When correctly performed, the blanket drag (Fig. 37-1) is the safest and most effective one-person carry, for it provides a little support to the victim's spine and extremities, so long as the victim's head is kept close to the ground and his spine and extremities are kept in a straight line. A blanket is placed on the floor alongside the victim, with half of its width folded into pleats so that it can be slipped under the victim easily. The victim's arm on the side closer to the rescuer should then be extended over his head, and the victim is rolled toward the rescuer, onto his side, with care to keep the victim's head and body in a straight line. Once the victim is on his side, the pleated part of the blanket is pulled beneath him, and the victim is rolled gently back to a supine position. Usually it will be possible at that point to pull the pleats through and smooth out the blanket beneath the victim.

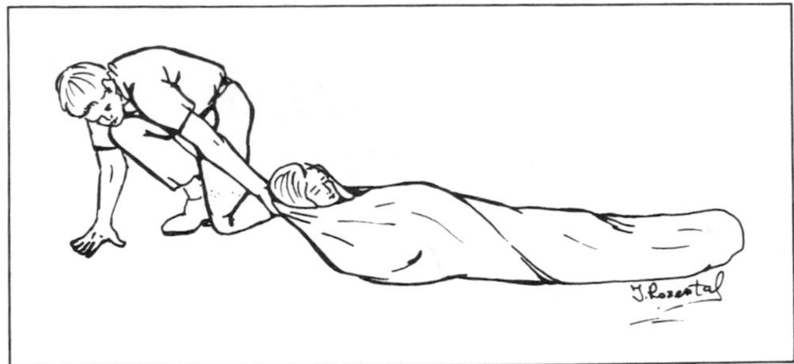

Fig. 37-1. *Blanket drag.*

When the victim is lying in the center of the blanket, place his arms across his chest, and wrap him snugly in the blanket. Then grasp the part of the blanket beneath the victim's head, and pull him to safety, keeping the head as close to the ground as possible.

If it is necessary to move the victim down a flight of stairs, you will have to pull him head-first—one of the rare occasions when this is permissible—but be sure to support his head so that it does not bump along as you go down the steps.

Clothes Drag

When a blanket is not available, the victim may be dragged by his or her clothing (Fig. 37-2). Grasp the victim's shirt behind the neck, so that the head is supported on your forearm. Once again, it is important to keep the victim's head as close to the floor as possible and to keep his head and body in a straight line. In the clothes drag, it is essential to avoid excessive constriction around the victim's neck. Should you need to drag the victim downstairs, you will have to cradle his head in your arms as you support his shoulders close to the stairs with your hands.

Fig. 37-2. *Clothes drag.*

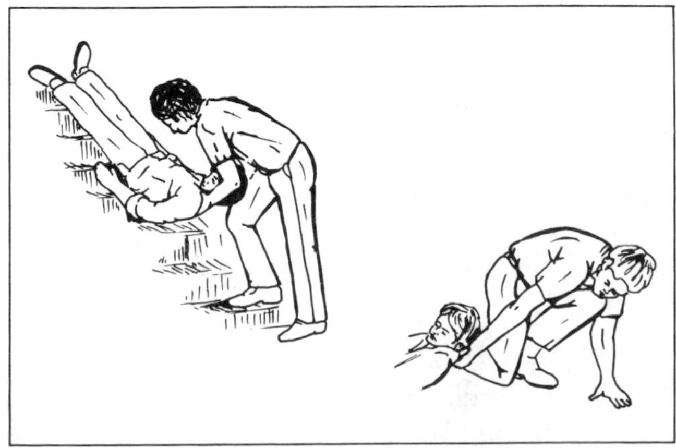

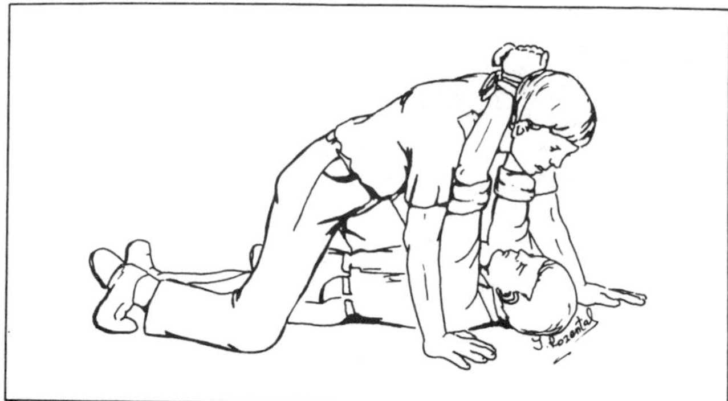

Fig. 37-3. *Fireman's drag.*

Fireman's Drag

Perhaps the most awkward and, from the point of view of patient safety, least desirable one-person carry is the fireman's drag. For this maneuver, the victim must be lying supine, with his wrists bound together with a scarf, necktie, or other material. The rescuer kneels straddling the victim, with the victim's tied hands over the rescuer's neck (Fig. 37-3). As the rescuer raises his shoulders and trunk, the victim's shoulders are lifted from the floor. The rescuer then crawls along the floor, dragging the victim with him. The fireman's drag has the disadvantages of placing considerable strain on the rescuer's neck and shoulders and leaving the victim's head unprotected and unsupported.

EMERGENCY TWO-RESCUER TECHNIQUES

When two EMTs are present, the task of evacuating a person rapidly from a hazardous area is considerably simplified, for the victim's weight may be shared between the two rescuers. As a result, the victim can usually be lifted rather than dragged, and thus the risk of injury that the victim might sustain by being pulled along the ground is reduced.

Two-Rescuer Seat Carry

To perform the seat carry, two rescuers kneel, one on each side of the patient at the level of the patient's buttocks. The patient is raised to a sitting position. If he is unconscious, his back will have to be supported; so each rescuer grips the other's arm near the shoulder to form a backrest. Then each rescuer slips his other hand beneath the victim's thigh to grasp the other rescuer's wrist, forming a seat on which to carry the victim (Fig. 37-4). When the victim is conscious and able to hold on, the rescuers may find it more comfortable to use a four-hand seat carry (Fig. 37-5).

Two-Rescuer Extremities Carry

When the rescuers must take the victim through a narrow opening, an extremities carry may be more convenient, for it allows rescuers and victim to proceed single file rather than three abreast. With one rescuer kneeling at the victim's head, the second rescuer pulls the victim into a sitting position. Using one knee to support the victim's back, the first rescuer encircles the victim's trunk with his arms while the second rescuer, crouching between the victim's legs, places his hands beneath the victim's knees. On signal from the rescuer at the head, both rescuers stand up (Fig. 37-6) and carry the victim to safety.

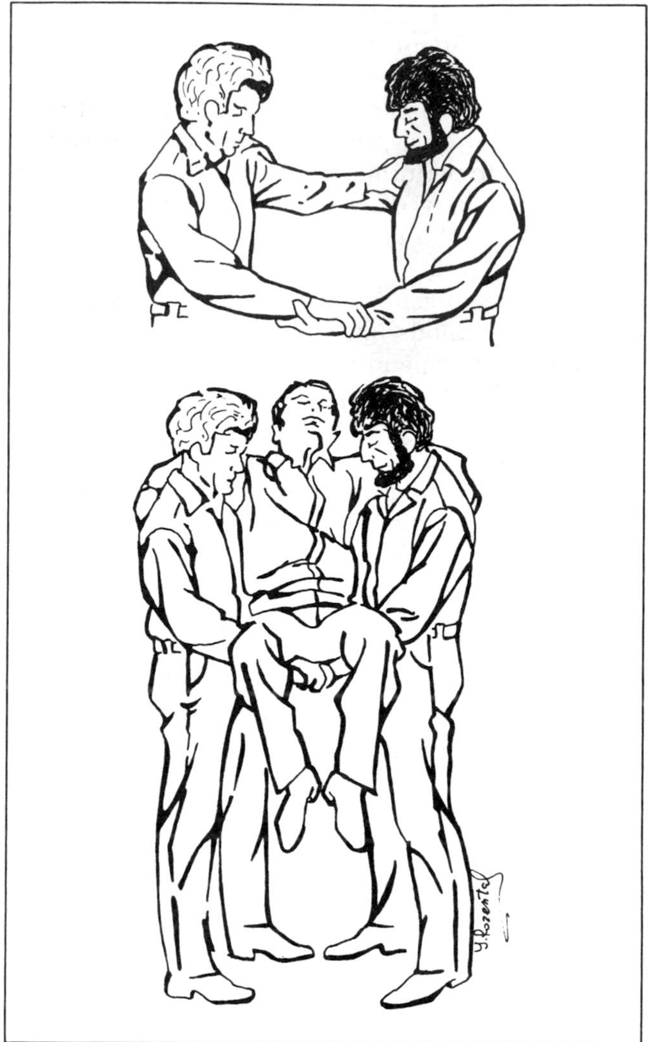

Fig. 37-4. *Two-rescuer seat carry for unconscious patient; the patient's back is supported.*

It must be emphasized again that none of the emergency moves just described, whether carried out by one or two rescuers, provides protection of the spine from further injury. The victim who is dragged or lifted hastily from a hazardous area is at great risk of suffering permanent spinal cord damage. This risk is acceptable only if there is indeed an immediate danger to the victim's life.

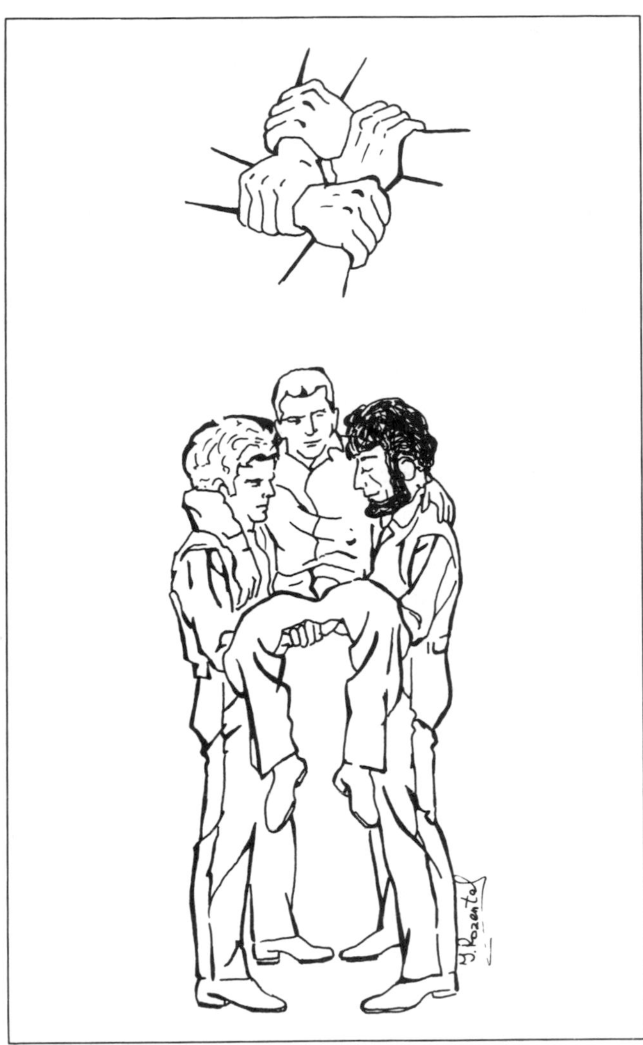

Fig. 37-5. *Two-rescuer seat carry for conscious patient, using four-hand grip to form seat.*

Fig. 37-6. *Two-rescuer extremities carry.*

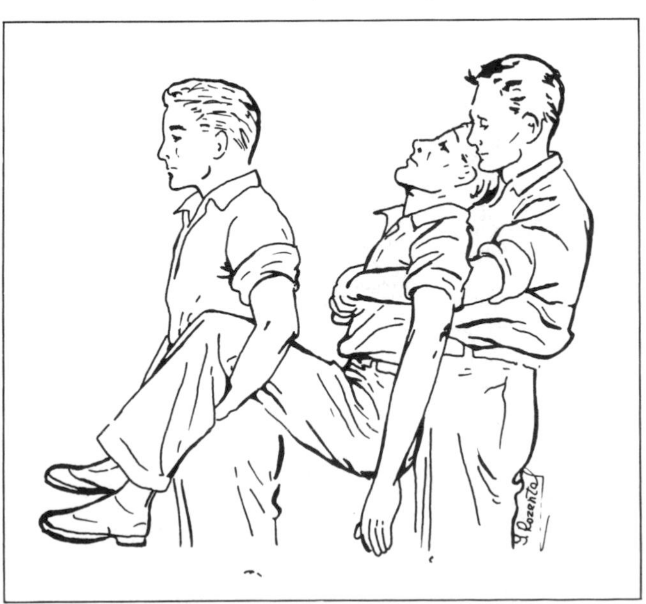

NONEMERGENCY MOVES

In the vast majority of cases, patients should be stabilized prior to being moved, lifted, or transported. This means that all injured or potentially injured parts should be immobilized as fully as possible *prior to* movement, and that injured parts must be protected from further trauma *during* movement. Every movement of the victim must be planned ahead and carried out in an orderly, unhurried fashion.

Once the victim has been immobilized, the process of moving and transporting him consists of several general steps: (1) selecting the most appropriate stretcher; (2) preparing the stretcher and accessory equipment; (3) transferring the patient to the stretcher; (4) securing the patient to the stretcher; (5) carrying the stretcher to the ambulance; (6) loading the stretcher into the ambulance; and (7) unloading the stretcher at the hospital.

TYPES OF STRETCHERS AND THEIR USES

Generally speaking, a stretcher is any device used to carry a patient—usually, but not invariably, a recumbent patient. In emergencies, stretchers may be improvised from blankets, overcoats, chairs, even fire hoses. We will confine our discussion here, however, to the types of stretchers likely to be carried in an ambulance.

Wheeled Stretchers

The wheeled stretcher is the standard ambulance cot. In its simplest and lightest form, it consists of an aluminum frame with mattress on wheels. Usually the back can be adjusted to several positions, and some versions permit the stretcher itself to be raised to various levels above the ground (Fig. 37-7A). Options are also available that enable raising the patient's knees or tilting the whole stretcher into a 10-degree head-down position, although the latter position is rarely indicated.

The wheeled stretcher is intended to be rolled rather than carried. It is most useful for moving patients over smooth, flat surfaces where there is room to maneuver. The standard wheeled stretcher is *not* easily carried up and down stairs or over difficult terrain, nor does it negotiate narrow corners very well. In many cases, therefore, it is preferable to bring the wheeled stretcher only as far as the front door, elevator, or edge of a casualty area and to carry the patient by another type of stretcher to the wheeled stretcher.

Portable Stretchers

Portable stretchers come in a wide range of designs and are intended for situations in which a wheeled stretcher cannot be readily brought to the patient. One of the most common and most versatile types of portable stretcher is the canvas pole-stretcher, or army stretcher (Fig. 37-7B). The newer models of the army stretcher fold in half and are easily stored. They are lightweight and can be suspended on wooden horses to provide a casualty station in mass disaster incidents. Their chief disadvantage is that they do not provide very much support to an injured spine. The flexible stretcher, or Reeves stretcher (Fig. 37-7C), provides somewhat more support, for the canvas is reinforced with longitudinal wooden slats. The Reeves is a good stretcher for transferring a patient from a relatively inaccessible location to the wheeled cot.

Stair Chairs

The stair chair (Fig. 37-7D) usually consists of a lightweight aluminum frame over which is stretched a nylon cover. Some portable stretchers and even wheeled stretchers can be converted to stair chairs. Whatever model is used, the stair chair is designed for carrying a patient over stairways and through narrow corridors or other confined areas. When a stair chair is not available, a standard kitchen chair can be substituted.

The stair chair is not well suited for carrying patients who must be kept in a recumbent position or for those with extensive injuries to the back or legs.

Backboards

Long backboards are primarily designed for immobilizing individuals with suspected spine injuries (see Chapter 14), but in fact they are highly versatile devices and useful in many situations in which victims must be moved supine down stairs or over difficult terrain. Long backboards are also excellent for patients with pelvic and lower extremity fractures. A backboard placed between the patient and the mattress of a standard ambulance cot provides a firm surface for performing external cardiac compressions.

Backboards come in either marine plywood or folding aluminum models. In general, the plywood backboards are superior, although they are less compact for storage.

Scoop Stretchers

The split frame, or scoop, stretcher (Fig. 37-7E) is used for immobilizing a patient with a suspected spine in-

Fig. 37-7. *Five types of stretchers commonly used in ambulances.*

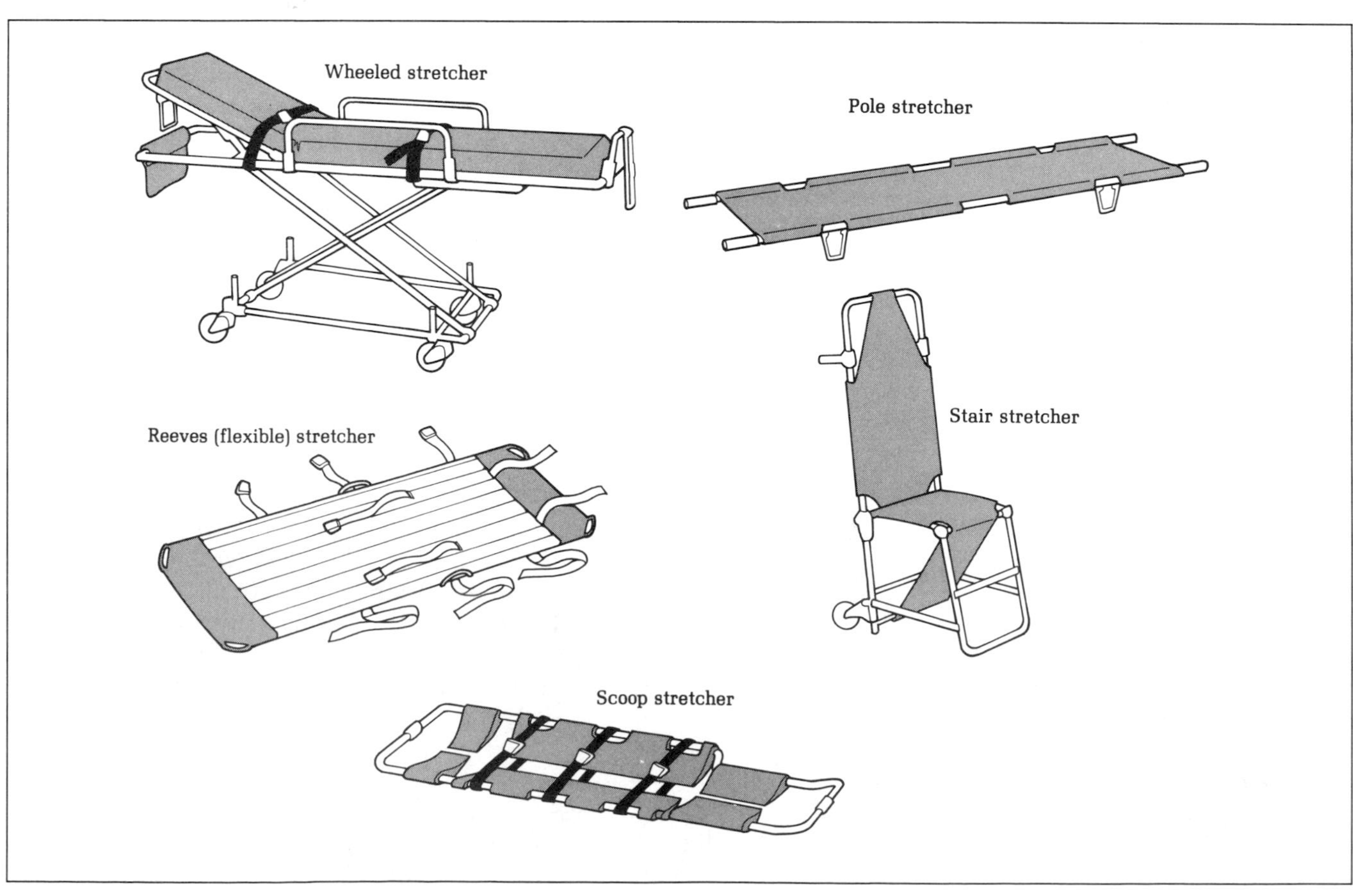

jury when one wishes to do so without moving the patient in any way. The scoop stretcher is made of aluminum and employs a scissors-type or snap-together action to enclose the patient; thus it requires that both sides of the patient be accessible, so that the two halves of the stretcher can be slid beneath the patient from each side and then locked together. Care must be taken to avoid pinching the patient or catching bits of his clothing as the stretcher halves are snapped in place.

The scoop stretcher provides excellent support and stores easily. It is readily moved through narrow passages and over difficult terrain, and it enables transfer of the patient onto an emergency room bed with a minimum of patient movement. Its use is limited chiefly by the necessity for sufficient working room. When a patient is relatively inaccessible or must be slid onto the long axis of a stretcher, a backboard is usually more convenient.

Basket Stretchers

The basket stretcher, or "Stokes basket" (Fig. 37-8), has been used for many years by the military, and is an excellent device for moving a victim over difficult terrain or lowering a victim by rope from a high place. Older models of the basket stretcher consist of a metal frame lined with chicken wire; more recent basket stretchers have a molded plastic shell attached to an aluminum frame.

To facilitate later removal of a patient from a basket stretcher, the stretcher should be lined with a blanket before the patient is placed inside. Then, when the patient must be transferred to an emergency room cart, the rescuers can simply grasp the blanket on either side of the patient and use the blanket to lift the patient from the stretcher.

Fig. 37-8. *Stokes stretcher.*

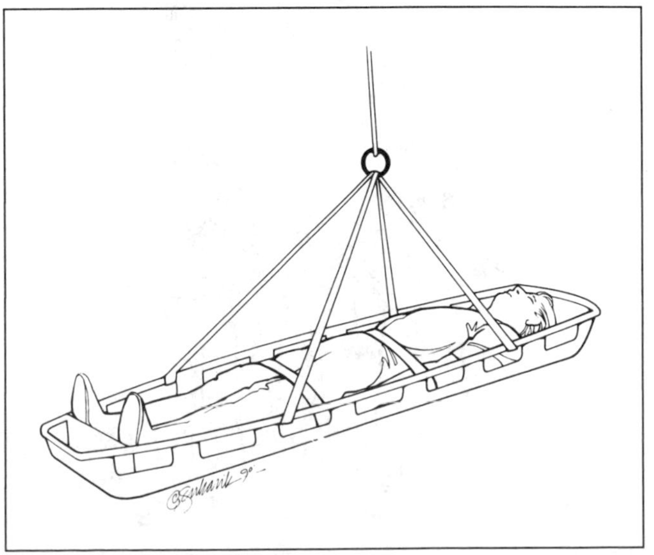

The Right Stretcher for the Job

The selection of a stretcher for a given task will depend on (1) the condition of the patient, (2) the working space around the patient, and (3) the exit route. For example, an elderly patient in bed with pneumonia can be adequately transported on a wheeled cart; but if he is on the second floor of a building with a very narrow staircase, it may be necessary to bring him downstairs on a stair chair and then transfer him to the wheeled cot at the foot of the stairs. A patient with a spine injury, on the other hand, requires immobilization on a firm stretcher, and the choice between a backboard and a scoop stretcher will be determined by the accessibility of the victim.

Some of the advantages and disadvantages of various stretchers are summarized in Table 37-1. Whatever type of stretcher is used, remember: THE PATIENT MUST BE SECURELY STRAPPED TO THE STRETCHER BEFORE BEING MOVED. Under most circumstances, it is desirable to use THREE STRAPS: one across the chest, one across the upper thighs, and one across the legs just below the knees.

LIFTING AND TRANSFERRING A PATIENT TO A STRETCHER

Most patients who require transfer to a stretcher must be moved either from ground level or from a bed. The lifting technique chosen will depend on the location of the patient, the type of stretcher being used, and the number of rescuers available to assist. A patient lying on the ground, for instance, may be slid or rolled onto a backboard, but must be lifted onto a wheeled stretcher or folded up at the hips and knees to be placed on a stair chair.

In this section, we will look briefly at some of the lifting techniques applicable to different situations. These techniques are spelled out in more detail in the Skill Evaluation Checklists at the end of the chapter.

Preparation of the Stretcher

Before a patient is moved to a stretcher, the stretcher should be fully prepared to receive him. If one is using a backboard, for example, the backboard should be lined up alongside the victim, and the straps should be in the right position to be passed beneath the backboard at the proper moment. A wheeled stretcher should be made up with clean linen, properly positioned, and its wheels locked in place. A basket stretcher shoud be lined with a blanket. The hinges on a collapsible canvas stretcher should be snapped firmly into the open position.

Transferring a Bed-Level Patient

When a patient is found in bed, it is generally easiest to transfer him directly to a wheeled cot placed at

Table 37-1. *Selection of the Right Stretcher*

Type of Stretcher	Recommended Use	Not Recommended for:
Wheeled cot	Moving patient over smooth surface	Difficult terrain, spine injury, CPR (must add backboard)
Stair chair	Carrying victim down narrow stairs or narrow passageways	Patients with severe injuries, patients who must be recumbent
Canvas stretcher (army type)	Mass casualties, rapid removal of victims	Spine injuries
Long backboard	Suspected spine injury, pelvic and lower extremity fractures, CPR, excellent all-purpose transfer stretcher	
Scoop stretcher	Suspected spine injury	Relatively inaccessible patient
Basket stretcher	Carrying victim over difficult terrain, lowering victim from a height	Spine injury (may be aggravated while placing patient on stretcher)

right angles to the bed. The simplest method of performing the transfer is usually the DIRECT CARRY, in which two EMTs stand alongside the patient. The first EMT slides one hand beneath the patient's neck to grasp the far shoulder and the other hand under the patient's back. The second EMT meanwhile slides his hands beneath the patient's hips and knees respectively. Working in unison, the two EMTs crouch slightly and lift the patient upward while at the same time rolling him toward their chests. They then step back from the bed and walk slowly to the stretcher, onto which the patient is gently lowered.

An alternative method uses a DRAW SHEET beneath the patient. The stretcher is fixed in place alongside the bed, and the two EMTs lean across the stretcher toward the bed. The first EMT grabs the head end of the sheet on which the patient is lying with one hand and supports the patient's shoulders with the other hand; the second EMT grasps the foot end of the draw sheet in one hand and supports the patient's knees with the other hand. On a signal from the head-end EMT, the patient is lifted and slid across from the bed to the stretcher. If a third person is present, he or she can help to lift and push from the other side of the bed.

When it is impossible to bring the wheeled stretcher to the vicinity of the patient's bed, it is preferable to use another stretcher as an intermediate transport device. The patient may, for example, be logrolled onto a backboard or canvas stretcher and, after being secured to that stretcher with straps, carried to a wheeled stretcher that was left at the foot of the stairs. A second transfer need be done only if the patient has to be in a sitting position; otherwise the canvas or wooden stretcher should simply be secured onto the wheeled stretcher for transport.

Transferring a Ground-Level Patient

Whenever a patient is found on the floor or the ground, the possibility of spine injury must be considered. As a general rule, one should regard such a patient as injured until proved otherwise and USE THE LOGROLL ONTO A BACKBOARD (see Chapter 14) for moving the patient. This method for moving the patient is not only the safest; it is also the simplest and the one least likely to cause injury to the rescuer. If a backboard is not available, a GROUND LIFT, using at least three rescuers, may be performed as shown in Figure 37-9.

Fig. 37-9. *Three-person ground lift.*

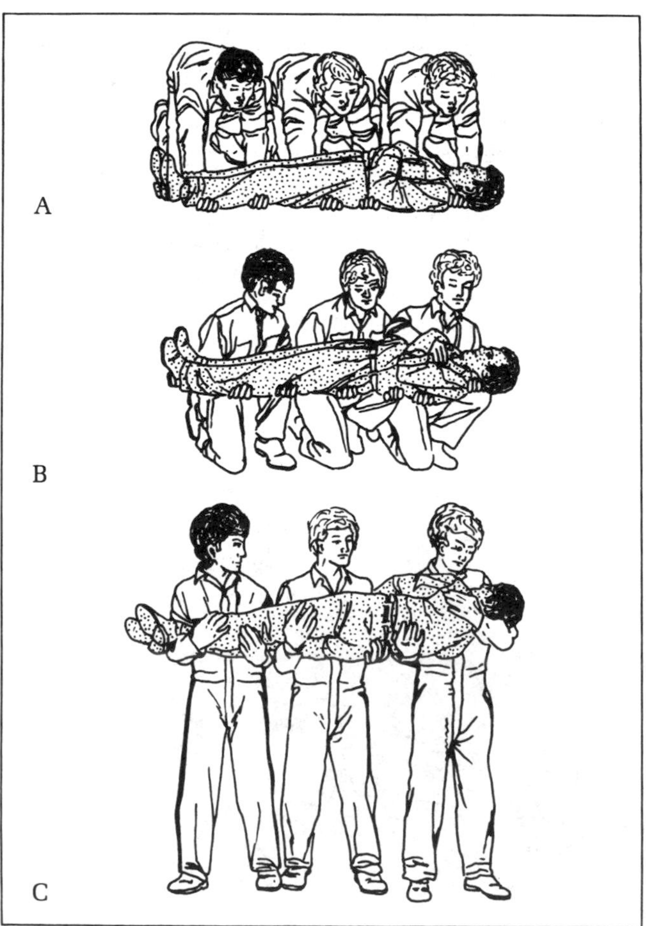

Positioning the Patient

The wheeled cot permits a variety of positions for the patient, and once the patient has been transferred to this stretcher, the appropriate position must be determined according to the patient's problem and overall condition. A patient in pulmonary edema, for example, must be transported sitting up, preferably with his legs dangling. A patient in shock, on the other hand, should be recumbent, with his legs elevated. Table 37-2 summarizes the stretcher types and positions appropriate for patients with some common conditions.

LOADING AND UNLOADING THE STRETCHER

Once the patient has been positioned comfortably on the wheeled stretcher, covered with a sheet (and blanket if necessary), and secured to the stretcher with straps, the stretcher may be moved to the ambulance. Upon reaching the ambulance, the stretcher should be positioned so that the head end is within 3 feet of the rear doors, and the stretcher should be locked in place in its lowest position. Standing on either side of the stretcher, facing one another, two EMTs crouch (with backs straight) and grasp the lower bar of the stretcher frame. With arms flexed, both rise in unison to a full standing position, thereby lifting the stretcher. The front wheels of the stretcher are lowered gently onto the floor of the vehicle, and the stretcher is rolled carefully into place, to engage the securing devices. One EMT immediately enters the patient compartment to continue care while the second EMT makes certain that the stretcher is fully locked in place.

For unloading the ambulance, the same process is carried out in reverse (see the following Skill Evaluation Checklists). In both processes, care should be taken to keep the stretcher as level as possible and to avoid sudden moves that might cause one of the EMTs to loosen his or her grip.

Table 37-2. *Stretcher Positions for Various Conditions*

Position of Patient	Condition of Patient
Flat, on backboard	Conscious patient with spine injury, pelvic fracture, lower extremity fractures
Flat, with legs elevated	Shock, fainting, CPR (with backboard beneath)
Flat, with hips elevated	Childbirth with prolapsed cord or partially delivered breech
Flat, with head elevated 10 degrees	Head injury, stroke
Lying on left side	Late pregnancy, unconscious patient (strapped to backboard if spine injury suspected)
Semisitting	Chest pain, most patients whose condition does not require another position, routine transports
Sitting upright	Dyspnea (e.g., pulmonary edema, asthma, epiglottitis)
Trendelenburg (stretcher tilted head-down)	Almost never indicated: puts pressure on diaphragm and thereby embarrasses respiration. Supine position with legs elevated is preferred in shock. Possible exception is a suspected air embolism.

FURTHER READING

Burley ME. Guidelines for the selection and use of emergency stretchers. *EMT J* 1(3):45, 1977.

Hills EA et al. Ambulance travel—head first or feet first? *Br J Clin Pract* 33:320, 1979.

Klinghoffer M. Transportation of the sick and injured. *Emerg Med Serv* 14(6):17, 1985.

Ierribilini C, Dernocoeur K. Save your back: Injury prevention for EMS providers. *JEMS* 14(10):34, 1989.

Shanaberger CJ. Don't drop the patient! *JEMS* 14(11):68, 1989.

U.S. Department of Transportation. *Emergency Medical Technician–Ambulance: Patient Handling Manual*. Pub. DOT-HS-800-504. Washington, D.C.: Government Printing Office, 1972.

SKILL EVALUATION CHECKLISTS

The following pages contain checklists for some of the skills described in this chapter. The checklists may be used as a review and as a guide for practicing the respective skills.

Performance Test
Transfer of Bed-Level Patient: Direct Carry Method

Students ______________________________ Date ______________________

____

Instructor: Place an "X" in the Fail column beside any item that is performed incorrectly, out of sequence, or omitted.

Activity	Critical Performance	Fail
Preparation of stretcher	Position stretcher perpendicular to bed: a. at side of bed nearest exit route.	
	b. head of stretcher to foot of bed, or foot of stretcher to head of bed.	
	Adjust stretcher elevation to bed-level height.	
	Unfasten safety straps from mattress.	
	Lower side rail on loading side of stretcher.	
	Lock wheels of stretcher.	
	Remove and set aside blankets and top sheet.	
	Position pillow.	
Preparation of patient	Cover patient with stretcher top sheet.	
	Remove bedding under top sheet.	
	Position patient supine with arms folded across chest, legs straight.	
Preparing to lift	Both rescuers stand between bed and stretcher facing patient.	
	R1 slides one hand beneath patient's neck to grasp far shoulder.	
	R2 slides one hand beneath patient's hip and lifts slightly.	
	R1 slides other hand under patient's back.	
	R2 slides other hand under patient's knees.	
	Together rescuers slide patient to edge of bed nearest themselves.	
	Both rescuers bend toward the patient.	
Lifting	Both rescuers crouch slightly and roll patient towards their chests: a. backs kept straight.	
	b. patient cradled in flexed arms of EMTs, resting against chests.	
	Both rescuers return simultaneously to standing position.	
Transferring the patient	Both rescuers take one step back from the bed.	
	Rescuer nearest stretcher steps backward while other rescuer steps forward until patient is parallel to stretcher.	
	Rescuers walk in unison to stretcher.	
	Both rescuers place right foot on lower bar of stretcher.	
	Both rescuers flex knees and gently lower patient to mattress.	

Activity	Critical Performance	Fail
	Rescuers slide arms from under patient's back and legs, keeping patient's head supported.	
	Head is gently lowered to pillow as supporting arm is removed.	
Positioning the patient	Instructor describes the patient's medical problem to rescuers.	
	Rescuers identify correct position for the patient.	
	Rescuers adjust stretcher to position stated.	
Preparation for moving	Patient is covered with top sheet and blanket.	
	Patient is secured to stretcher: a. one strap across chest.	
	b. one strap across upper thighs.	
	c. one strap across legs, just below knees.	
	Side rail is raised and locked in position.	
	Wheels are unlocked.	
	Stretcher is wheeled to designated location.	
Instructor ____________________		

Performance Test

Transfer of Bed-Level Patient: Draw Sheet Method

Students ______________________________ Date ______________

____

Instructor: Place an "X" in the Fail column beside any item that is performed incorrectly, out of sequence, or omitted.

Activity	Critical Performance	Fail
Preparation of patient	Cover patient with stretcher top sheet.	
	Remove patient's bedding under top sheet.	
	Loosen bottom sheet under patient to use as draw sheet.	
	Straighten bottom sheet and roll both sides in toward patient.	
	Position patient supine with arms folded on chest, legs straight.	
	Pull sheet to move patient to side of bed where stretcher will be.	
Preparation of stretcher	Adjust stretcher elevation to bed-level height.	
	Unfasten safety straps from mattress.	
	Lower side rails on both sides of stretcher.	
	Position stretcher alongside and flush with bed.	
	Lock wheels of stretcher.	
	Remove and set aside blankets.	
Moving the patient to the stretcher	Both rescuers stand beside stretcher and reach across stretcher to patient: a. first EMT stands at head end (short side) of stretcher.	
	b. second EMT stands in center of long side of stretcher.	
	Head-end EMT leans over, slides one arm under patient's head, and grasps draw sheet with free hand.	
	Foot-end EMT slides one arm under patient's knees, and grasps draw sheet with free hand.	
	Both EMTs lean against stretcher to keep it stable.	
	In unison both EMTs lift and slide patient from bed to stretcher.	
Positioning the patient	Instructor describes the patient's medical problem to rescuers.	
	Rescuers identify correct position for the patient.	
	Rescuers adjust stretcher to position selected.	
Preparation for moving	Patient is covered with a blanket.	
	Patient is secured to stretcher: a. one strap across chest.	
	b. one strap across upper thighs.	
	c. one strap across legs, just below knees.	
	Side rails are raised and locked in position.	
	Wheels are unlocked.	
	Stretcher is wheeled to designated location.	

Instructor ______________________________

Performance Test
Extremity Transfer to Stair Chair and Stair Chair Carry (Ground-Level Patient)

Students R1: ____________________ Date ____________
R2: ____________________

Instructor: Place an "X" in the Fail column beside any item that is performed incorrectly, out of sequence, or omitted.

Activity	Critical Performance	Fail
Preparation	Assemble and lock stair chair into position.	
	Place stair chair beside patient.	
	Place straps in position on stair chair and drape chair with sheet.	
	Position patient supine with legs straight.	
Raising and lifting patient	R1 kneels at patient's head.	
	R2 kneels beside patient's knees, facing R1.	
	R2 grasps patient's wrists.	
	R1 places hands beneath patient's shoulders, under armpits.	
	R2 pulls patient to sitting position as R1 assists.	
	R1 supports patient's back against one knee.	
	R1 passes arms around patient and grasps patient's wrists against patient's chest.	
	R2 slides hands beneath patient's knees.	
	Both rescuers change to crouch position.	
	Both rescuers stand in unison on signal from R1.	
	Both rescuers carry patient to chair and gently lower patient thereon.	
Positioning and securing patient	Patient is placed in center of stair chair.	
	Patient is wrapped in top sheet; blankets added as necessary.	
	Patient is secured to stair chair: a. one strap across chest.	
	b. one strap across lap.	
	c. one strap across legs.	
Chair carry	R1 stands behind chair, facing patient.	
	R1 grasps sides of backrest, near the top.	
	R1 tilts chair back.	
	R2, with back to patient, grasps chair legs: a. strong grip.	
	b. knees bent.	
	Both rescuers lift chair in unison on signal from R1.	
	Chair is kept level.	
	EMTs carry chair down a flight of stairs to wheeled stretcher.	

Activity	Critical Performance	Fail
Transfer to wheeled stretcher	On signal from R1, both rescuers set down chair stretcher.	
	Wheeled stretcher is prepared: a. placed beside and at right angles to chair stretcher.	
	b. straps unbuckled.	
	c. side rail down.	
	d. wheels locked.	
	Patient is unstrapped.	
	R1 slides hands beneath patient's armpits and encircles chest.	
	R2 slides hands beneath patient's knees.	
	On signal from R1, patient is lifted to wheeled stretcher.	
Securing patient	See skill evaluation checklist for *Transfer of Bed-Level Patient*.	

Instructor ______________________________

Performance Test
Scoop Stretcher

Students R1: ______________________ Date ______________
R2: ______________________
R3: ______________________

Instructor: Place an "X" in the Fail column beside any item that is performed incorrectly, out of sequence, or omitted.

Activity	Critical Performance	Fail
Preparation of patient	R1 holds victim's head in longitudinal traction throughout.	
	R2 applies cervical collar.	
	Victim's arms are folded across his chest.	
	Victim's wrists are tied together with cravat.	
	Victim's ankles are tied together with cravat.	
Preparation of stretcher	R2 disassembles stretcher into its two component halves.	
	R2 lines stretcher halves up on either side of patient.	
Application of stretcher	R1 continues to hold victim's head in traction.	
	R2 and R3 slide one stretcher half beneath patient.	
	R2 and R3 move to other side and slide other stretcher half beneath patient.	
	Stretcher is latched together: a. clothing is not caught in stretcher.	
	b. halves securely locked.	
	Vinyl head support properly positioned.	
Securing the patient	R1 continues traction on patient's head.	
	Patient is covered with a blanket.	
	Patient is strapped to scoop stretcher: a. one strap across chest.	
	b. one strap across upper thighs.	
	c. one strap across legs, just below knees.	
	Patient's head is secured to stretcher by cravat across forehead.	
	R1 may release traction on head.	
Moving the patient	Wheeled stretcher brought as close as possible to patient.	
	Wheeled stretcher locked.	
	Side rail lowered.	
	Straps of wheeled stretcher unbuckled.	
	Two rescuers lift stretcher by end-carry method.	
	Scoop stretcher carried level.	
	Scoop stretcher lowered gently onto wheeled stretcher.	
	Scoop stretcher secured to wheeled stretcher (by at least two straps)	
	Side rails of wheeled stretcher raised and locked.	
	Wheels unlocked.	
	Wheeled stretcher rolled to ambulance.	

Instructor ______________________________

Performance Test

Loading and Unloading a Wheeled Stretcher

Students ______________________________ Date ______________

____

Instructor: Place an "X" in the Fail column beside any item that is performed incorrectly, out of sequence, or omitted.

Activity	Critical Performance	Fail
Positioning stretcher	Roll head end of stretcher to within 3 feet of ambulance rear doors.	
	Lower stretcher to lowest position.	
	Open rear doors of ambulance and secure in open position.	
Loading stretcher	Two EMTs stand on either side of stretcher, facing one another.	
	Both EMTs crouch and grasp lower bar of stretcher frame, with: a. backs straight.	
	b. both hands (one palm up, one palm down).	
	Both EMTs flex arms and lift stretcher by standing upright on signal.	
	Stretcher is held level.	
	EMTs step sideways in unison toward ambulance door.	
	Front wheels of stretcher are placed on compartment floor.	
	Stretcher is rolled into position for securing.	
Securing to slide bar	EMTs roll head end of stretcher frame into half-ring hook.	
	EMT on left pushes spring-loaded handle of bar to open hook.	
	EMT inspects to see that stretcher is in position.	
	EMT releases bar handle so that hook catches stretcher frame.	
	EMT on right enters patient compartment.	
	EMT on left closes rear doors of ambulance.	
Unloading	EMT in patient compartment opens rear doors.	
	Rear doors are locked in open position.	
	EMTs position themselves behind ambulance, facing patient area.	
	EMT on left releases hooks from stretcher frame.	
	Both EMTs grab lower bar of stretcher with inside hand.	
	Both EMTs roll stretcher out until front wheels are near rear of compartment.	
	Both EMTs grasp lower bar of stretcher with both hands.	
	On signal, EMTs lift stretcher above ambulance floor.	
	EMTs sidestep with stretcher until it is clear of ambulance.	
	Stretcher is lowered to the ground: a. EMTs bend knees, flex arms.	
	b. backs straight.	
	c. stretcher kept level.	
	d. lowered slowly.	
	Stretcher is raised to bed-level height.	
	Stretcher is rolled feetfirst to designated location.	

Instructor ______________________________

XII. THE AMBULANCE AND THE CALL

Each day as millions of people trudge off to their offices, factories, and fields, the EMT reports to a very different place of work. For the EMT's "office" is an emergency room on wheels, and the EMT's place of work is wherever those wheels can transport the rescue team

In this section, we will look at the EMT's working environment and the mechanics of responding to a call. We shall examine the design and maintenance of the workplace: the ambulance. We shall review the equipment essential to the EMT's task. And we will look at the process by which a call is received, a response is initiated, and information about the call is communicated to those concerned. Finally, we shall examine the elements of safe emergency driving, without which even the best emergency treatment may end in tragedy for all concerned.

38. THE AMBULANCE AND ITS EQUIPMENT

OBJECTIVES

An ambulance is not just another motor vehicle. An ordinary motor vehicle has one purpose: to transport people or goods from one place to another. But an ambulance is, or should be, much more than simply a means of transportation. A modern ambulance must be an emergency room on wheels, a means of bringing immediate care *to* the sick and injured, as well as a means of bringing the sick and injured safely to a source of more definitive care. Nonetheless, when all is said and done, an ambulance—emergency room or not—is still a type of motor vehicle. Like any other motor vehicle, it can overheat, run out of gas, stall, break down, burn out a battery, have a flat tire, and suffer all the other small calamities that the internal combustion engine is heir to.

In this chapter, we shall look at this very special vehicle in detail: how it is designed, how it is equipped, how it should be maintained. By the conclusion of this chapter, the reader should be able to:

1. Identify the steps in ambulance and equipment maintenance that should be carried out (a) after each call and (b) daily
2. Indicate those items of equipment that are best stored in exterior compartments, given a list of various ambulance supplies
3. List the items desirable in a jump kit
4. Identify what items of equipment are missing, given a description of a case and an incomplete list of available equipment for caring for the patient involved
5. Locate any specified item of equipment within his or her vehicle within 15 seconds

THE AMBULANCE

Ambulances have come a long way from the horse-drawn wagons used to evacuate wounded during the Napoleonic wars. Indeed, they have come a long way even from the hearses and station wagons that constituted a majority of the ambulance vehicles in the United States just 20 years ago. Today's ambulance must meet stringent requirements for working room, equipment, and safety, as indicated in the following definition of an ambulance set down by the Committee on Ambulance Design Criteria of the U.S. Department of Transportation:

> The ambulance is defined as a vehicle for emergency care *which provides* a driver compartment and a patient compartment which can accommodate two emergency medical technicians and two litter patients so positioned that at least one patient can be given intensive life support during transit; *which carries equipment and supplies* for optimal emergency care at the scene as well as during transport, for two-way radio communication, for safeguarding personnel and patients under hazardous conditions, and for light rescue procedures; and which is *designed and constructed* to

afford maximum safety and comfort, and to avoid aggravation of the patient's condition, exposure to complications, and threat to survival.*

TYPES OF AMBULANCES

There are three basic types of ambulances that meet federal specifications. The TYPE I AMBULANCE is a conventional truck chassis to which a modular ambulance body has been added. The idea behind this kind of construction is that when the chassis wears out, the containerized patient compartment can simply be lifted off the old chassis and placed on a new chassis, thereby reducing the cost of vehicle replacement. A disadvantage of the Type I vehicle, however, is that it has no walk-through passageway between the cab and the patient compartment. The vehicle is also somewhat difficult to maneuver in high density traffic, and it consumes a considerable amount of fuel.

The TYPE II AMBULANCE, also called a standard van, is considerably less expensive than other ambulance designs and also much more maneuverable. A walk-through partition provides access from the cab to the patient area. Because it is smaller than the other two types of ambulance, it consumes less fuel, but it also has less exterior storage space. The small size also imposes engine restrictions, which in turn limit the load the vehicle can carry. Nonetheless, the Type II ambulance provides an excellent and economical vehicle and remains one of the most popular styles of ambulance throughout the United States.

The TYPE III AMBULANCE combines features of both Type I and Type II. It resembles a Type I vehicle, but the cab and body are an integral unit. Like the Type I vehicle, it offers a very spacious work area, but it also permits walk-through access between the cab and the patient compartment. It is considered to have the best ride of any type of ambulance, and it provides generous exterior storage. High cost and difficulty in servicing mechanical components are the major disadvantages of the Type III vehicle.

Any ambulance service using federal funds for vehicle procurement must comply with federal regulations for ambulance design. These regulations are spelled out in a detailed document, *Federal Ambulance Specifications KKK-A-1822B*, available from the U.S. Department of Transportation. The specifications cover all aspects of ambulance design, from electric systems and engine capacity to warning lights and vehicle color, and provide an excellent guideline even for ambulance services that are not obligated by federal funding to comply with all the regulations. Only ambulances meeting federal specifications, however, may display the Star of Life emblem (Fig. 38-1).

*From Committee on Ambulance Design Criteria, U.S. Department of Transportation, *Ambulance Design Criteria* (revised ed.). Washington, D.C.: Government Printing Office, 1974.

THE CARE AND FEEDING OF AN AMBULANCE

There is nothing more useless than an ambulance that does not run. And Murphy's Law, which states that anything that can go wrong will go wrong, predicts that if the ambulance is going to break down, it will break down during an emergency call.

An ambulance should not break down (as any good malpractice lawyer will be quick to point out!), and the risk of breakdown may be kept to an absolute minimum by a strict program of PREVENTIVE MAINTENANCE. Such a program is particularly important for an ambulance because it is a vehicle that takes a lot of punishment, that is operated by a number of different drivers, but that nonetheless must be ready to move at all times.

Preventive maintenance should be carried out systematically, according to a defined program and printed checklists. Each ambulance service will have its own maintenance schedule, based on the amount and type of use to which the vehicle is subjected. That schedule should, however, include certain tasks to be performed after each run, other tasks to be performed daily, and yet others that must be carried out at stated intervals. For instance, wherever possible, the ambulance should be *refueled* AFTER EACH RUN, for there is no telling how much fuel will be required for the next run or how many runs may have to be made consecutively before there is another chance to "gas up." The ambulance should also be aired thoroughly after every call; and expended supplies, including oxygen, should be replaced. Various mechanical components and other

Fig. 38-1. *Star of Life.*

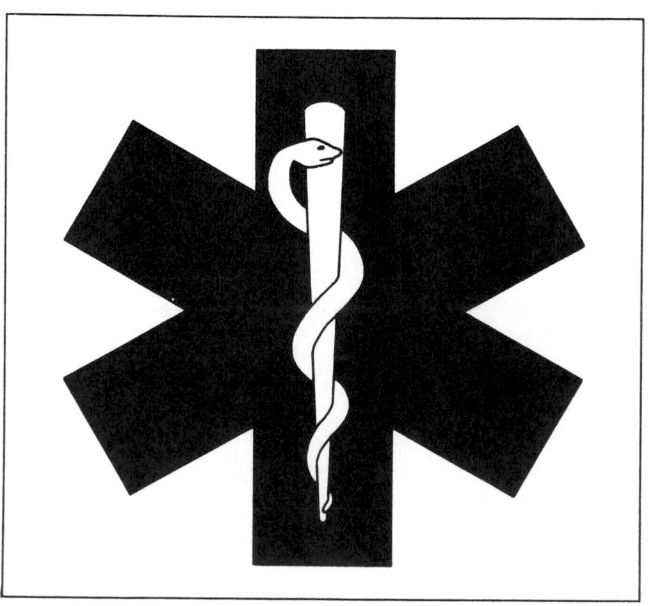

equipment need to be checked DAILY. Ambulance *tires*, for instance, take a considerable beating, often traveling over bad roads, crunching over debris, bumping into curbs. Tires, including the spare, ought to be examined daily for pressure, embedded foreign objects, and signs of wear. Under the hood, the *radiator* and *battery* need to be examined for adequate fluid levels, and the windshield washing fluid should also be refreshed as needed. *Oil levels* should be measured at the same time. All of the vehicle's *lights*, inside and out, including flashers, turn signals, and rotating beacons, should be part of the daily checklist as well. Finally, daily maintenance of the ambulance should include a thorough *scrubbing* of all interior and exterior surfaces. A dirty vehicle reflects on the attitudes and habits of its crew. EMTs take pride in their vehicles, and they know as well that a clean, shipshape ambulance increases public confidence in the service.

Beyond the daily maintenance checklist, there are other items that must be checked ON A REGULAR BASIS, such as brakes, points and plugs, transmission gauges and instruments, steering, and a variety of other mechanical components subject to wear.

Preventive Maintenance: Sample Schedule

- AFTER EACH RUN
  1. REFUEL.
  2. REPLACE expended SUPPLIES; discard trash.
  3. Check OXYGEN CYLINDERS; replace as needed.
  4. AIR the vehicle; clean the interior as needed.
- DAILY
  1. Check FLUID LEVELS in the radiator, battery, windshield washer.
  2. Check the OIL.
  3. Check TIRE PRESSURE, tread.
  4. Check all LIGHTS.
  5. Check all DOORS for proper latching.
  6. Check HEATING and VENTILATION systems.
  7. CLEAN interior and exterior thoroughly.
- AT SCHEDULED INTERVALS (e.g., every 1,000 miles)
  1. Tune up.
  2. Check brakes, clutch, transmission.
  3. Check steering.
  4. Check all instruments and gauges.
  5. Check fan belt, oil filter—replace as needed.
  6. Oil change.
  7. Replace worn windshield wipers.
  8. Rotate tires.

ESSENTIAL AMBULANCE EQUIPMENT AND SUPPLIES

What makes an ambulance an ambulance rather than just another truck is not only its special construction and design, but also the special equipment it carries. Without proper equipment, even the most resourceful EMT will be severely handicapped in trying to provide optimum care to a sick or injured person. In this section, we will look at the essential *minimum* of equipment that should be carried on every ambulance. The equipment standard presented here is based primarily on the recommendations of the American College of Surgeons and the United States Department of Transportation. These recommendations include not only medical equipment, but also equipment for transferring patients, for light rescue, and for the safety of both patients and ambulance personnel.

GENERAL CONSIDERATIONS

One of the worst moments an EMT can experience occurs when a vital piece of equipment is not present or is not functioning at a time when it is urgently needed (the second worst moment is trying to explain the incident in court!). The only way to prevent bad moments like these is to be compulsive about checking equipment and supplies. A FULL INVENTORY OF AMBULANCE EQUIPMENT SHOULD BE CARRIED OUT AT THE BEGINNING OF EACH SHIFT. This means going through the whole vehicle, *checklist* in hand, and making certain that every item, down to the last safety pin, is present and in proper working condition. Each oxygen cylinder should be checked to make certain that it has an acceptable level of pressure; the humidifier bottle should be emptied and washed with soap and water, then refilled with sterile water and reattached. Portable and fixed suction units must be tested for proper operation. All battery-operated equipment, including flashlights, should be examined for battery strength. Air splints should be checked for leaks. Any item of equipment discovered to be missing should be promptly replaced, as should soiled linens and malfunctioning equipment.

Nearly as important as what equipment you have is where you put it. Things you will need in a hurry should not be buried in the back of a remote cabinet. As far as possible, all rescue tools, backboards, splints, and other items usually needed for stabilizing the patient outside the vehicle should be in outside storage compartments. It is poor practice to have to plunge inside the patient compartment every time you need a splint or a rescue tool, for in general these items are not (or should not be) needed after the patient has been transferred into the ambulance. The storage space within the vehicle should be used mainly for supplies and equipment that may be needed in caring for the patient en route to the hospital.

Equipment and supplies are most conveniently stored in the form of special purpose KITS, such as a trauma kit or an obstetric kit, so that one does not have to grope for various odds and ends under emergency conditions. Remember, the term "search and rescue" should apply to a patient, not to ambulance gear. Kits should be of manageable size and light in weight, permitting the rescuer to grab the kit and run. Backup supplies for each kit can be stored in the vehicle. The trauma kit, for instance, need only contain a basic minimum of bandages and dressings, with additional dressing materials stored in the ambulance cabinets, in case there is not time between calls to restock the kit at the base.

In the following sections, we will look at the various kits or categories of equipment essential in a properly fitted-out ambulance.

MEDICAL EQUIPMENT AND SUPPLIES

The bulk of equipment carried in an ambulance will be used for the treatment of various medical and traumatic emergencies. Perhaps the most useful of the several kits in a well-stocked ambulance is the JUMP KIT, so named because it is the kit you grab when you jump out of the ambulance and head for the patient. The jump kit should be compact, lightweight, and easily accessible, preferably located in the cab beside the driver. A small canvas rucksack that can be slung over the shoulder is ideal. It should be a matter of reflex to TAKE THE JUMP KIT WITH YOU EVERY TIME YOU LEAVE THE AMBULANCE TO GO TO A PATIENT, regardless of the assumed nature of the call. The jump kit will contain everything you need to initiate emergency care (Table 38-1)—airways, a few dressings, a pocket mask, and so forth—and it can save several trips back to the vehicle during those early moments when time is so crucial.

A second major category of critical supplies, although a bit too cumbersome to be classified as a kit, includes all AIRWAY AND VENTILATION EQUIPMENT (Table 38-2); that is, oropharyngeal airways, bag-valve-mask unit, fixed and portable oxygen, suction apparatus, and so forth. The smaller items, such as the bag-valve-mask, airways, and suction catheters, should be stored together, again preferably in a single container or kit.

The SHOCK KIT (Table 38-3) will contain those items essential for the management of shock, namely Military Anti-Shock Trousers and intravenous infusion supplies. The shock kit can be incorporated as part of a larger WOUND KIT (Table 38-4), which contains dressings, bandages, scissors, and related materials; however, since only a few cases of soft tissue injury will actually require treatment for shock, it is generally preferable to keep the shock kit separate. For orthopedic trauma, a FRACTURE KIT (Table 38-

Table 38-1. *Sample Jump Kit*

Quantity	Equipment
3	Oropharyngeal airways, graded sizes
1	Pocket mask with oxygen inlet valve
12	4 × 4–in. gauze pads, individually wrapped
12	Povidone-iodine swabs
12	Alcohol swabs
4	Army dressings, small size
2	Army dressings, medium size
2	Multitrauma (universal) dressings
12	Triangular bandages
2	Rolls of self-adhering bandage
1	Roll of adhesive tape
12	Safety pins
1	Heavy duty scissors
1	Flashlight
2	Candy bars
1	sphymomanometer
1	stethoscope
1	pad of paper
2	ballpoint pens

Table 38-2. *Airway and Oxygen Equipment*

Quantity	Equipment
3	Oropharyngeal airways, graded sizes
3	Soft rubber nasopharyngeal airways
1	Adult size bag-valve-mask unit
1	Pediatric size bag-valve-mask unit
1	Fixed oxygen supply (3000 liter capacity) with reducing valve and spare tubing
1	Portable oxygen unit (300 liter capacity) with tubing
2	Spare portable oxygen cylinders (300 liter capacity)
6	Two-pronged nasal cannulas
6	Nonrebreathing masks
1	Installed suction unit, with spare tubing
1	Portable suction unit
6	Flexible suction catheters, graded sizes
3	Rigid, tonsil-tip (Yankauer) suction catheters
1	Bottle of clean water for rinsing suction apparatus
2	Esophageal obturator airways (where authorized)

Table 38-3. *Shock Kit*

Quantity	Equipment
1	Pair Military Anti-Shock Trousers
3	Liter bags of Ringer's solution
2	Intravenous infusion sets
6	Over-the-needle catheters, graded sizes
12	Povidone-iodine swabs
12	Alcohol swabs
2	Venous tourniquets
10	4 × 4–in. gauze pads
1	Roll adhesive tape
1	Roll self-adhering bandage
2	Small padded armboards
3	Labels for intravenous bags

Table 38-4. *Wound and Burn Kit*

Quantity	Equipment
24	4 × 4–in. sterile gauze pads (packaged in threes)
24	Band Aids
6	Medium dressings
4	Multitrauma (universal) dressings
2	Sterile burn sheets
6	Water Jel dressings, various sizes
1	Roll sterilized aluminum foil
6	Rolls self-adhering roller bandage, various widths
12	Triangular bandages
1	Roll 1-in. adhesive tape
1	Roll 3-in. adhesive tape
12	Safety pins
1	Pair heavy duty scissors

5) is necessary, including various types of splints, bandages, and chemical cold packs. Bulky splints, such as the traction splint or long board splint, will have to be stored outside the kit, but all fracture equipment should be in the same storage compartment (preferably exterior) of the vehicle. A patient with extensive fractures is likely to have injury to the spine, so a SPINAL IMMOBILIZATION KIT (Table 38-6), which includes backboard, straps, a rolled blanket, and so forth, should also be readily accessible from outside the vehicle. The short backboard, however, should be kept inside the ambulance, so that it can be handy in the event a back support is needed for CPR.

For patients, often young children, who have swallowed something dangerous, you will need a POISON KIT (Table 38-7), consisting mainly of syrup of ipecac, activated charcoal, and an emesis basin. In the happier event that you are called to participate in a delivery, a STERILE OBSTETRIC KIT (Table 38-8) will be necessary (with a backup kit in one of the cabinets, just in case the stork has a busy night).

Some basic life support ambulances carry, in addition, a locked DOCTOR'S KIT (Table 38-9), so that advanced life support equipment can be readily available in the event that a physician is present at the scene.

A given ambulance service may wish to arrange their kits differently from the way they are described here. A rescue crew may, for example, decide that their needs are better served by combining the wound kit with basic airway equipment, and so forth. There is nothing sacred about the *organization* of equipment listed here. What is important is that the equipment be complete, logically arranged, and easily accessible, and, most important of all, that you know exactly where to find it when you need it. Your daily inventories should enable you to locate any item in the vehicle within 10 to 15 seconds. If it takes longer, you should spend some more time acquainting yourself with the cabinets and special kits. In an emergency, there is no time to start searching for equipment.

Table 38-5. *Fracture Kit*

Quantity	Equipment
1	Half-ring lower extremity traction splint
1	Set air splints for upper and lower extremities
6	Padded board splints 2 splints 3 × 54 in. 2 splints 3 × 36 in. 2 splints 3 × 15 in.
20	Tongue depressors
4	Rolls self-adhering bandage
2	Rolls adhesive tape
12	triangular bandages
6	Chemical cold packs

Table 38-6. *Spinal Immobilization Kit*

Quantity	Equipment
1	Long backboard
1	Short backboard
5	3-in. × 9-ft straps with quick release buckles
3	Cervical collars, graded sizes
1	Rolled blanket, secured with cravats
12	Triangular bandages
3	Towels for padding

Table 38-7. *Poison Kit*

Quantity	Equipment
1	Bottle syrup of ipecac
2	Bottles activated charcoal
6	Paper cups
1	emesis basin
1	Liter sterile saline for irrigation
1	Contact lens remover

Table 38-8. *Sterile Obstetric Kit*

Quantity	Equipment
1	Surgical gown
2	Surgical masks
2	Pairs surgical gloves
6	Towels
1	Pair surgical scissors
4	Cord clamps
4	12-in. lengths of umbilical tape
12	4 × 4–in. gauze sponges
12	Sanitary napkins
1	Bulb syringe
1	Baby blanket
2	Large plastic bags

BASIC SUPPLIES

In addition to equipment for medical treatment, an ambulance must carry certain basic supplies for the comfort and general evaluation of the patient (Table 38-10). These supplies include blankets and linens,

Table 38-9. *Doctor's Kit*

TRACHEAL INTUBATION SET
- 1 laryngoscope handle
- 3 laryngoscope blades (2 adult, 1 pediatric)
- 10 endotracheal tubes, graded sizes
- 1 10 ml syringe
- 1 metal stylet
- 6 packets water-soluble lubricant
- 4 strips umbilical tape (24-in. lengths)
- 1 Magill forceps
- 1 hemostat

CRICOTHYROTOMY KIT
- 1 scalpel blade mounted in rubber stopper
- 2 tracheostomy tubes
- 1 sterile Kelly clamp
- 1 strip umbilical tape 24 in. long
- 6 povidone-iodine swabs

DRUG KIT

Prefilled syringes
- 4 sodium bicarbonate, 50 ml
- 2 50% dextrose, 50 ml
- 4 atropine, 1 ml (1 mg)
- 4 epinephrine, 10 ml (1 mg)
- 2 10% calcium chloride, 10 ml
- 4 lidocaine, 10 ml (100 mg)

Ampules and vials

Epinephrine	1-ml vial (1 mg/ml)
Diazepam	2-ml ampule (5 mg/ml)
Furosemide	2-ml ampule (20 mg/ml)
Aminophylline	2-ml ampule (125 mg/ml)
Hydrocortisone	4-ml vial (125 mg/ml)
Saline	

STERILE PLEURAL DECOMPRESSION SET
- 1 scalpel with assorted sterile blades
- 2 Kelly clamps
- 2 chest tubes with introducers
- 2 Heimlich valves
- 10 povidone-iodine swabs
- 10 alcohol swabs
- 10 4 × 4–in. gauze pads
- 1 roll adhesive tape

STERILE MINOR SURGICAL KIT
- 1 fine surgical scissor
- 1 needle holder
- 3 mosquito forceps
- 2 Kelly clamps
- 10 packets suture material, graded caliber
- 20 4 × 4–in. gauze pads
- 2 disposable sterile drapes

MISCELLANEOUS
- 4 Foley catheters, graded sizes
- 1 urine collecting bag
- 6 nasogastric tubes, adult and child sizes
- 1 tube sterile, water-soluble lubricant

Table 38-10. *Basic Supplies*

Quantity	Equipment
1	Stethoscope
1	Oral thermometer
1	Blood pressure gauge
1	Standard blood pressure cuff
4	Blankets
2	Pillows
2	Spare pillow cases
2	Spare sheets
4	Towels
2	Boxes disposable tissues
6	Disposable emesis basins
1	package of plastic bags
1	Package disposable drinking cups
1	Bed pan (stainless steel)
1	Urinal (stainless steel)
2	Canteens fresh drinking water
4	liters of irrigation fluid
2	Sandbags
20	Lollipops

monitoring equipment (stethoscope, thermometer, blood pressure cuff), emesis basins, and so forth. A supply of clean drinking water should be refreshed at least once daily, for you never know when you are going to get called out on a prolonged rescue mission in a place where drinking water may not be readily available. A few candy bars stashed in the jump kit can double as emergency treatment for the woozy diabetic who took too much insulin and emergency rations for the hypoglycemic EMT who did not get a chance to get dinner between calls. And don't forget the lollipops for the kids.

Table 38-11. *Stretchers and Ancillary Equipment*

Quantity	Equipment	
1	Wheeled cot	
1	Stair chair	may be combined
1	Portable stretcher	may be combined
1	Backboard set	
3	Restraining straps for each stretcher	
1	Scoop stretcher	optional
1	Basket stretcher	optional
1	Flexible (Reeves) stretcher	

STRETCHER AND ANCILLARY EQUIPMENT

Every ambulance must be equipped with several types of stretchers (Table 38-11) for carrying patients under varying circumstances. At a minimum, these should include the wheeled cot (main stretcher), long backboard, stair chair, and some type of portable stretcher. A dual purpose folding stretcher that can be laid out flat or locked into position as a stair chair is a particularly handy device when space is

Table 38-12. *Light Rescue Equipment*

Quantity	Equipment
1	12-in. adjustable wrench
1	12-in. regular screwdriver
1	12-in. Phillips screwdriver
1	Hacksaw with 12-in. carbide blades
1	Pair 10-in. pliers with vise grip
1	5-lb hammer with 15-in. handle
1	Fire axe butt with 24-in. handle
1	51-in. crowbar with pinch point
1	Bolt cutter with 1¼-in. jaw opening and 36-in. handles
1	Portable power jack and spreader tool
1	49-in. shovel with pointed blade
1	Double action tin snip (at least 8 in.)
2	Manilla ropes, each 50 ft long and ¾ in. in diameter
1	Heavy duty hand winch (come-along) with 15-foot rated chain and grab hook
4	Shoring blocks

tight. Each stretcher carried on the vehicle should be equipped with three straps for securing the patient. Wherever possible, the ambulance should be fitted with a bracket against the bulkhead to which the stair chair can be locked, enabling transport of a pulmonary edema patient in a sitting position with legs dependent.

LIGHT RESCUE EQUIPMENT

As noted in Chapter 36, every ambulance should carry a basic minimum of tools for light rescue (Table 38-12), preferably in an exterior storage compartment. Since equipment of this type acquires a good deal of grease and dirt, it should be stored separately from medical supplies.

SAFETY, LIGHTING, AND HAZARD CONTROL

An exterior storage compartment is also the best place to stash safety equipment (Table 38-13), including flares, floodlights, air masks, helmets, fire extinguishers, and the like. This category also includes the radiation hazard kit described in Chapter 31.

COMMUNICATIONS EQUIPMENT

Every ambulance should have the means by which EMTs can communicate with one another, with others at the scene, with their base, and ideally with the receiving hospital as well. To do so requires, at a

Table 38-13. *Safety, Lighting, and Hazard Control Equipment*

Quantity	Equipment
1	Set for each rescuer 1 safety helmet with chin strap 1 pair safety goggles 1 pair gloves with gauntlets 1 quick entry air mask (30-min capacity)
4	Triangular reflectors
2	Battery powered lights
2	5-lb class B:C fire extinguishers
1	Radiation hazard kit (see Chapter 31)
1	pair binoculars

minimum, a mobile two-way radio within the vehicle and a hand-held portable radio that can be carried from the vehicle to the patient. In addition, the siren should be equipped with a public address mode and amplifier to enable the rescue team to relay important information to bystanders or other rescuers in mass casualty or crowd situations.

AFTERWORD

As an EMT, you are going to be spending the majority of your time in an ambulance. That vehicle will be your transportation, your workspace, and also a large part of the image you present to the public. The life of a patient may depend on whether the ambulance is properly equipped. Your own life may depend on whether the vehicle is in good mechanical condition. You must know that ambulance inside out and treat it as a vital partner in your work.

FURTHER READING

Cameron JL et al. Bacterial contamination of ambulance oxygen humidifier water reservoirs: A potential source of pulmonary infection. *Ann Emerg Med* 15:1300, 1986.

Committee on Ambulance Design Criteria, U.S. Department of Transportation. *Ambulance Design Criteria* (revised). Washington, D.C.: Government Printing Office, 1974.

Committee on Trauma, American College of Surgeons. Essential equipment for ambulances. *Bull Amer Coll Surg* Sept., 1977.

Dahlgren BE et al. Appropriate suction device in rescue medicine. *Ann Emerg Med* 16:1362, 1987.

DeLorenzo RA, Gilmore MD. Periodic medical equipment inspection. *Emerg Med Serv* 18(8):58, 1989.

Iglewicz R et al. Elevated levels of carbon monoxide in the patient compartment of ambulances. *Am J Public Health* 74:511, 1984.

Miley MP. The infection potential of emergency medical equipment. *Emergency* 10(7):75, 1978.

Perkins Jr, White RD. Buying an ambulance. *Emergency* 11:46, 1979.

U.S. Department of Transportation. *Federal Ambulance Specifications KKK-A-1822B*. Revised, 1985.

39. DISPATCH AND COMMUNICATIONS

OBJECTIVES

There are many ways by which the EMT communicates. By dress and manner, one communicates an attitude to work. By the use of warning lights and sirens, one communicates the urgency of a call to other motorists. By words, spoken or written, one communicates information about the case to various others involved. In this chapter, we shall be concerned with the latter form of communication because it is the means by which information is transmitted all along the EMS chain. We shall examine the types of information needed at various stages of the call and the means by which that information is transmitted. By the conclusion of this chapter, the reader should be able to:

1. Identify incorrect radio transmissions, given a list of various transmissions, and rewrite them in correct form
2. Identify the meanings of commonly used ten-codes, given a list of codes
3. List the information that a dispatcher should obtain from a caller when the case is (a) a medical problem or (b) a highway accident
4. Arrange patient data in the correct sequence for transmission to the hospital, given a list of patient information in random order

SYSTEMS AND HARDWARE

When we talk about EMS communications, we are referring primarily to telephone (**landline**) and radio links among the various elements in the system (Fig. 39-1). A good EMS communications system uses a judicious combination of telephone and radio, so that neither will become overstressed by message traffic. Generally speaking, the initial link in the EMS chain—that between the person requesting help and the dispatcher—is by landline, preferably by the universal 911 emergency telephone number. Some dispatch centers in addition monitor the emergency channel 9 on Citizen's Band radio for reports of accidents or other incidents requiring an ambulance.

The second link in the communications chain—that between the dispatcher and the ambulance team—is of necessity a radio link, which permits communication with the EMTs regardless of their location. In some circumstances, the rescue team at the scene may choose to use telephone communications as well; they may, for instance, prefer to telephone their base from the patient's home in order to convey a long message or to preserve the privacy of their communications. Nonetheless, the principal link between the base or control center and the rescuers in the field is by radio.

A third essential link is that between the dispatcher and public safety units, local hospitals,

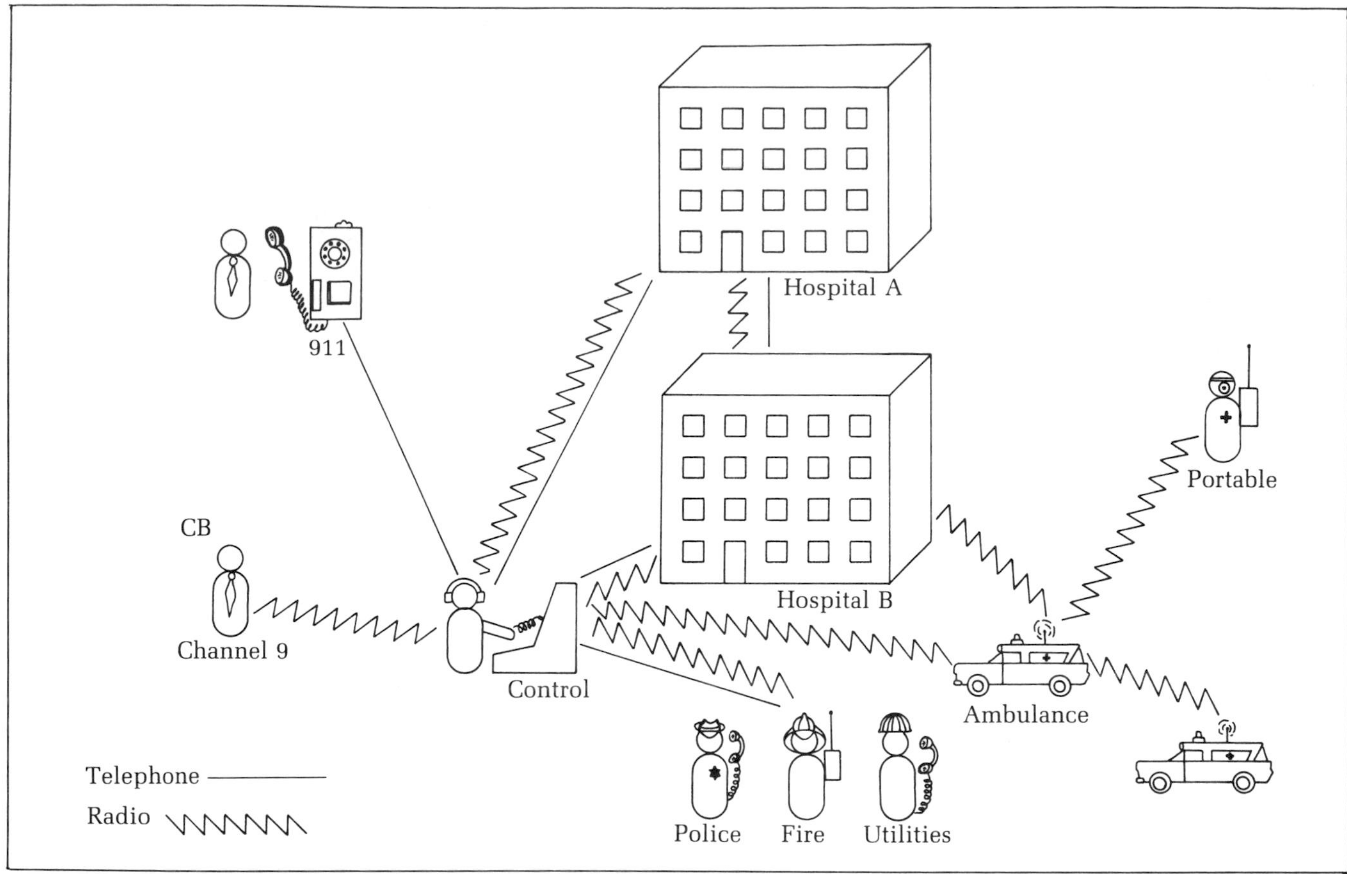

Fig. 39-1. *Sample EMS communications network.*

poison control centers, and other community agencies. For routine use, landlines are usually sufficient to maintain these connections, but radio backup is desirable for emergencies.

A fourth communications link in the EMS chain is that among rescuers in the field—from one ambulance to another, or from an EMT with a hand-held portable radio to another EMT in the vehicle. These radio links are particularly important in rescue and multiple casualty situations, in which members of the rescue team may be dispersed over a large area.

Finally, the EMS system requires a communications link between the EMT in the field and the receiving hospital. This link permits the EMT to receive advice on managing various cases from a hospital physician and also enables early notification to the hospital of incoming patients. In times of disaster, shared radio channels permit rapid interhospital communication as well and serve as a backup communication system in the event that landlines are disrupted.

RADIO EQUIPMENT

There is a wide variety of radio equipment in use today in different EMS systems, and the EMT must become familiar with the specific equipment used in his or her service. We shall deal here only with some general features that are common to most two-way radios.

As an example, let us look at one of the simpler types of two-way radios—the hand-held portable. Most hand-held portables have three control knobs. The first is an ON-OFF/VOLUME KNOB, which turns the unit on and regulates the loudness of incoming transmissions. Whenever this knob is in the "on" position, the battery is being consumed, even if the radio is silent. For this reason, the unit should be turned off whenever it is not in use, such as when you are in the ambulance and using the mobile radio.

The second knob is usually labelled SQUELCH, and its function is to suppress extraneous or interfering sounds (**noise**). In addition, most portable units now in use have a CHANNEL SELECT KNOB or keyboard that permits one to choose among two or more frequencies for transmission. **Frequency** refers to the wavelength on which one receives or transmits, and EMS services are assigned special frequencies for medical communications by the Federal Communications Commission (FCC).

In addition to these control knobs, every two-way radio has a TRANSMIT BUTTON. When the button is depressed, the receiving mode of the radio is temporarily cut off, and one can send a radio signal out through the unit. As soon as the transmit button is released, the radio becomes a receiver again, and incoming messages can be heard.

Even the smallest portable radio has some sort of ANTENNA, which extends its transmitting and receiving range. Changing the direction of the antenna or moving the radio a few feet may sometimes help overcome "dead spots" in radio reception.

In general, a portable two-way radio has a relatively small power output and therefore a relatively short range of transmission. This range can be extended by the installation of REPEATERS, which are basically small radio units that pick up the radio signal and rebroadcast it with greater power. Many EMS systems use both *fixed repeaters*, installed on towers, hills, or high buildings, and *mobile repeaters*, installed on the ambulances, to extend the range of radio communications.

Some base stations employ, in addition to telephone and radio communications, a means of combining the two, known as a TELEPHONE PATCH. Using a patch, the base can, for example, connect ("patch in") a physician phoning into the base from home with an ambulance team in radio contact from the field.

GUIDELINES FOR RADIO COMMUNICATIONS

The success or failure of a communications network depends less on the equipment than on the people using the system. The dispatcher must be able to elicit and transmit accurate information about the location and presumed problem of the patient. The EMTs must be able to convey to the hospital accurate, concise data about the patient's condition. The personnel receiving this information in the emergency room must know when to ask for additional data. In addition, all concerned must observe basic principles of courtesy, brevity, and clarity in their radio dialogues.

CLARITY OF TRANSMISSION

The purpose of communication equipment is to permit communication. This sounds obvious, and yet it is often forgotten. Simply blurting something into a microphone is not communication. In order for communication to occur, someone at the other end of the radio has to be able to hear and understand what you say. Thus the first rule of radio communications is CLARITY.

There are a number of guidelines that can help the radio user improve the clarity of a transmission. To begin with, before you begin to transmit, LISTEN TO MAKE SURE THAT THE CHANNEL IS CLEAR. If another radio transmission is in progress, wait until the parties have finished transmitting before you try to get on the air. Cutting in on someone else's transmission will only ensure that neither of you will be adequately heard.

Once the channel is quiet, PRESS THE TRANSMIT KEY FOR AT LEAST 1 SECOND BEFORE SPEAKING to ensure that the beginning of your message is not lost. GIVE THE NUMBER OR NAME OF THE UNIT BEING CALLED FIRST, then your own identification (e.g., "Mercy Hospital from Medic 3"). In this way, the unit being called is alerted immediately and will already be listening when you identify yourself, so they can reply at once, "Go ahead, Medic 3." If you call the other way around ("Medic 3 to Mercy Hospital") chances are that the recipient will not hear your identification, and time will be wasted as they try to determine who is calling them.

KEEP YOUR MOUTH CLOSE TO THE MICROPHONE, BUT NOT TOO CLOSE—about 2 to 3 inches is usually ideal. SPEAK CLEARLY AND DISTINCTLY, pronouncing each word carefully. DO NOT SHOUT, for this will simply distort the signal. SPEAK IN A NORMAL PITCH; very high-pitched or low-pitched sounds do not transmit well. DO NOT TALK WITH YOUR MOUTH FULL, for that muffles transmission, and besides you might choke. KEEP YOUR VOICE FREE OF EMOTION. You need not imitate a talking computer (a normal conversational voice is fine); just keep your voice free of panic, anger, excitement, and other feelings that can distort both your transmission and your judgment.

KEEP YOUR TRANSMISSIONS BRIEF. Air time is precious, and emergency medical frequencies are not the place for long philosophic dialogues. If you have a long message to transmit, BREAK UP THE MESSAGE INTO 30-SECOND SEGMENTS, checking at the end of each segment to determine whether it was received and understood. DO NOT WASTE AIR TIME WITH SUPERFLUOUS PHRASES, such as "be advised." Also bear in mind that courtesy is taken for granted; there is no need to use air time for social graces such as "please," "thank you," and "how nice to hear your voice."

When using a word or a name that might be misunderstood, SPELL IT OUT, using the international phonetic alphabet (Table 39-1) or a similar system. Suppose, for example, you are requesting the hospital to notify a specific doctor whose name might be mistaken for that of another doctor; you might say, "Notify Dr. Vanic. That is Dr. VICTOR-ALPHA-NOVEMBER-INDIA-CHARLIE."

When presenting numbers that might be misunderstood, TRANSMIT THE NUMBER AS A WHOLE, THEN INDIVIDUALLY. For instance, if the respirations are 15, you would say, "The respirations are fifteen, that is, one-five."

Table 39-1. *International Phonetic Alphabet*

A	ALPHA	J	JULIETTE	S	SIERRA
B	BRAVO	K	KILO	T	TANGO
C	CHARLIE	L	LIMA	U	UNIFORM
D	DELTA	M	MIKE	V	VICTOR
E	ECHO	N	NOVEMBER	W	WHISKEY
F	FOXTROT	O	OSCAR	X	X-RAY
G	GOLF	P	PAPA	Y	YANKEE
H	HOTEL	Q	QUEBEC	Z	ZEBRA
I	INDIA	R	ROMEO		

CONTENT OF TRANSMISSIONS

Radio transmission should be concise and professional in tone. Bear in mind that ANYONE MAY BE LISTENING—the medical staff of a local emergency room, the cleaning lady in another local emergency room, a twelve-year-old ambulance buff at home with his scanner. For this reason, it is essential to PROTECT THE PRIVACY OF THE PATIENT. Do not use the patient's name on the air, and do not transmit personal information. Certain types of cases, such as rape or psychiatric cases, are best identified on the air by an established code (see Codes, following).

BE IMPERSONAL. Use "we," not "I," to refer to yourself, and use proper names and titles ("Sergeant York," not "Billy") to refer to others where necessary. DO NOT TRY TO BE A COMEDIAN. There is no place for wisecracks, sarcasm, or other nonprofessional conduct on emergency medical frequencies. Similarly, DO NOT USE PROFANE LANGUAGE ON THE AIR. The penalty specified by the FCC for doing so (quite aside from the reflection on your professional character) is a fine of $10,000 or 2 years in prison or both.

USE PROFESSIONAL LANGUAGE, BUT DO NOT SHOW OFF. Once again, remember that the object of the exercise is to communicate information, not to stun your listener into awe and admiration.

AVOID WORDS THAT ARE DIFFICULT TO HEAR. The word "yes" for instance, is easily lost in transmission; use "affirmative" instead. Similarly, use "negative" instead of "no."

USE STANDARD FORMATS FOR TRANSMISSION. The patient history, for example, should always be presented in the same order. When people know what they are listening for, they are less likely to miss parts of the transmission.

When you finish transmitting, OBTAIN CONFIRMATION THAT THE TRANSMISSION WAS RECEIVED. If you do not understand any portion of the response, ask that it be repeated. IF YOU RECEIVE AN ORDER FROM A PHYSICIAN, REPEAT THE ORDER BACK TO MAKE CERTAIN THAT YOU HAVE UNDERSTOOD IT CORRECTLY.

USE EMERGENCY MEDICAL FREQUENCIES ONLY FOR EMERGENCY MEDICAL COMMUNICATIONS. If you want the dispatcher to send someone out for a corned beef sandwich on rye, telephone the base when you finish your run—do not broadcast your dinner menu over medical airways!

Table 39-2. *Common Ten-Codes*

Code	Meaning
10-1	Signal weak.
10-2	Signal good.
10-3	Stop transmitting.
10-4	O.K.
10-6	Busy; please standby unless urgent.
10-7	Out of service; unavailable for a call.
10-8	In service; available for a call.
10-9	Please repeat.
10-12	Stand by.
10-17	En route.
10-18	Urgent.
10-20	What is your location?
10-22	Disregard.
10-23	Arrived at the scene.
10-24	Completed the assignment.
10-33	Help me quick! Emergency!

CODES

Some ambulance units make extensive use of radio codes; others rely exclusively on clear English. Usually some combination of the two is preferable. Codes can significantly shorten air time, provide unambiguous information, and also enable one to transmit information that one does not wish the patient or bystanders to understand. In order for a code to be useful, however, everyone involved must know the meaning of the code words. It does not do much good to radio the hospital that you have a "Case 3, condition 2" if no one at the other end has the slightest idea what you are talking about. Thus when codes are used, they should be simple as well as standardized within a given region; a copy of the code should be posted at each radio terminal. Even in regions where radio codes are in routine use, it is advisable to dispense with all codes during mass casualty incidents. In such situations, confusion and anxiety both at the scene and in the hospitals may lead to mistakes in transmitting and receiving coded messages.

One common system of codes are the so-called ten-codes (Table 39-2). Ten codes vary somewhat among different public safety agencies, but all ten codes utilize the number 10 plus another number to indicate a given message. Numbers are used because they are brief and easily understood.

The 10-33 code deserves particular mention. When a unit gets on the air with a 10-33, or any other indication of an emergency ("May Day" or just "Help!"), all other radio users should GET OFF THE AIR. Emergency communications always have priority.

When you use ten-codes, remember that one of

Table 39-3. *Sample Medical Code*

Type of Case	Condition
1. Chest pain	1. Stable
2. Dyspnea	2. Serious
3. Coma	3. Life-threatening
4. Seizures	4. Dead
5. Cardiac arrest	
6. Other medical problem	
7. Trauma	
8. Obstetric	
9. Psychiatric	
10. Rape	

their main purposes is to speed up communications. You defeat that purpose if you stick a ten-code into a long sentence. There is no need, for instance, to say, "What is your 10-20?" Just "10-20" is sufficient. Similarly, it is a waste of time to say "10-6 for a minute." Just say "10-6."

Ten codes from 10-40 onward may be designated for special local use. For example, in your region, the various services may agree that 10-53 will mean a case of rape, or 10-76 will mean a psychiatric case. Alternatively, one may design a separate code system for medical information (Table 39-3). Using such a code, one can rapidly transmit the nature of the case to the emergency room personnel without alarming or offending the patient and without violating the patient's privacy in front of bystanders. A "Case 10, condition 1," for instance, would inform the emergency room that you are transporting a rape case in stable condition, without informing everyone at the scene of that fact. A "Case 2, condition 3" would alert the emergency room to a patient in life-threatening condition with severe dyspnea, without terrifying the patient and his family with your assessment.

Whenever such codes are used, they should be kept simple and reserved for cases in which they are really needed.

Radio jargon is best avoided, except in cases in which it is universally understood and more easily heard than the corresponding term in plain English. A few frequently used radio terms are listed below:

Frequently Used Radio Terms

affirmative	yes
copy	understand
ETA	estimated time of arrival
go ahead	proceed with your message
May Day	international distress call; help!
negative	no
spell out	please spell out phonetically a specific word
stand by	please wait

PHASES OF COMMUNICATION

Communications provide the links between the various phases of an emergency call, and each phase demands a different type of communication. In this section, we shall focus on two phases of EMS communications: (1) receipt of the call and dispatch and (2) ambulance-to-hospital communication.

THE ROLE OF THE DISPATCHER

The dispatcher is a very important person. A good dispatcher can ensure a prompt response time, prepare the rescue team for the problem they will encounter, and keep communications flowing smoothly throughout the system. An incompetent dispatcher can create havoc and fury at every level.

The job of the dispatcher may look pretty simple—just sitting for 8 hours answering the phone and talking on the radio. In fact, the dispatcher's job is not simple at all, and among the critical tasks the dispatcher must perform are the following:

1. To obtain as much information as possible about the emergency (often from an agitated, distraught caller)
2. To direct the appropriate emergency vehicle(s) to the correct address
3. To monitor and coordinate communications among everyone in the system
4. To calm the caller and, in some instances, to instruct the caller in measures that should be taken until help arrives
5. To maintain radio logs and other important records

Ideally, the dispatcher for an emergency medical service should have EMT training in addition to specialized dispatcher training because, by working as an EMT, the dispatcher learns the kind of information needed by the rescue team as well as the stresses under which they operate.

If you were dispatcher, your job would include the following responsibilities.

Receiving the Call for Help

When someone telephones an ambulance service, one must take for granted that the caller needs help, even if he is too distraught to be very clear about the nature of the problem. Whenever you are answering the phone in the dispatch center, try to put yourself in the caller's shoes. ANSWER THE PHONE PROMPTLY, within the first two or three rings, for each ring may seem like an eternity to a person who is panicky or upset. IDENTIFY YOURSELF AND YOUR AGENCY, so that the caller will know immediately that he has reached the right number. SPEAK DIRECTLY INTO THE MOUTHPIECE, AND SPEAK UP. If you mumble, the caller will not hear, and you will simply have to repeat yourself. OB-

SERVE TELEPHONE COURTESY. Be calm and professional over the phone. Tell the caller exactly what you plan to do and how soon assistance can be expected to arrive.

TAKE CHARGE OF THE CONVERSATION. Once you have identified yourself and gotten a quick idea about the caller's situation, begin asking the caller questions to which you need immediate answers. There are different systems for eliciting information; in services equipped with enhanced 911 system (E911), a lot of the information, such as phone number identification and call location, is obtained automatically through sophisticated telephone technology. Whatever system you use, you should obtain the following data within the first minute or so of the call:

1. TELEPHONE NUMBER OF THE CALLER. This information is critical, for if the call is cut off before you have obtained other necessary information (e.g., the location of the patient), you must have a way to get back to the caller. Asking for a telephone number also discourages nuisance calls.
2. LOCATION OF THE PATIENT. Get specific information, such as the street name and number, the geographic designation (e.g., East Elm or West Elm), and the name of the community. If the address is not a familiar one, get clear directions to the location, including useful landmarks.
3. NATURE OF THE CALL. Initially, one needs simply a general statement of the caller's perception of the problem; for instance, "heart attack."

With this information, you can get the ambulance underway. Ask the caller to stay on the line, and notify the appropriate unit to proceed to the scene. Tell the ambulance crew that more information will be forthcoming. Then return to the caller and find out:

4. THE SPECIFICS OF THE PATIENT'S CONDITION. Ask in particular whether the patient is conscious? breathing? bleeding? in severe pain?
5. HAZARDS AT THE SCENE. If the case involves an accident, ask specifically about fire, downed electric wires, traffic hazards, and so on.
6. Again in the case of an accident, try to get an estimate of the NUMBER OF VICTIMS and the SEVERITY OF THEIR INJURIES.

A preprinted dispatch form (see Fig. 18-2) is useful in reminding the dispatcher what questions to ask; it also provides a permanent record of the receipt and progress of the call. Whatever type of form you use, WRITE EVERYTHING DOWN. You may have a memory like a steel trap, but if you get five calls in a row, you are going to have trouble sorting them all out afterward.

Once again, have the caller stand by while you relay additional information to the responding unit. If other services are necessary (e.g., a fire company or utility service), notify the appropriate agency as well.

Once the dispatch is complete, reassure the caller that help is on the way. EXPLAIN ANY ANTICIPATED DELAYS, and where necessary give simple instructions on what to do until help arrives (e.g., hold pressure over a bleeding wound). In Seattle, Washington, a program was developed to train dispatchers how to teach CPR over the telephone in an emergency, enabling the caller to start CPR before the ambulance arrives.

Above all, keep in mind that the caller is in distress. He may be in pain or may have witnessed a terrible accident. A loved one may be in danger. Under such circumstances, the caller is likely to be agitated, perhaps irrational, and even sometimes hostile. If you respond in kind, the situation will only get worse. Your job is to try to calm the caller and to get help on the way as fast as possible. DO NOT ARGUE WITH THE CALLER; ARGUING WASTES TIME. Stay cool, keep your voice calm, and indicate by your tone that you are concerned.

Ongoing Communications with the Field

The dispatcher's job is not over when the ambulance has screeched out of the ambulance bay and the caller has hung up. From that point on, the dispatcher must monitor communications from the field and facilitate smooth coordination of the call. If extra assistance is required, it is the dispatcher's job to contact the additional units or services. If there are multiple patients or questions regarding a given hospital's readiness to receive a patient, the dispatcher must clarify the matter with the hospital(s) involved and direct the ambulance(s) to the appropriate facility. The dispatcher may also be called upon to establish a communications link between the ambulance and the hospital, or to advise an ambulance crew of changing traffic conditions. In addition, the dispatcher should record all data relating to call times, specifically:

1. Time the call was received
2. Time the ambulance left for the scene
3. Time the ambulance reached the scene
4. Time the ambulance left the scene
5. Time the ambulance arrived at the hospital
6. Time the ambulance was back in service

This information is important in evaluating the ambulance service, and it also comes in handy when responding to complaints about slow response time.

AMBULANCE-TO-HOSPITAL COMMUNICATION

The primary purpose of radio communications between the ambulance and the hospital is to provide the emergency room team with a picture of the patient that is clear enough to allow them to make appropriate preparations for the patient's arrival and ongoing care. Special equipment may have to be assembled or a particular doctor (e.g., a neurosurgeon or obstetrician) may have to be summoned. Communication with the hospital also provides the EMT with an opportunity to obtain advice on further care of the the patient en route.

When you call in to the hospital, identify your unit on each transmission. The initial report should be brief, concise, and according to the standard format that we learned in Chapter 12.

Format for Reporting Medical Information

1. Patient's AGE and SEX
2. CHIEF COMPLAINT
3. Brief, pertinent HISTORY OF THE PRESENT ILLNESS
4. Major PAST ILLNESSES
5. STATE OF CONSCIOUSNESS and DEGREE OF DISTRESS
6. VITAL SIGNS
7. PERTINENT PHYSICAL FINDINGS
8. TREATMENT GIVEN SO FAR

Information should always be reported in the above order, regardless of the order in which it was obtained.

DO NOT OFFER A DIAGNOSIS. If your report is clear and accurate, the physician should be able to reach his or her own conclusions about what is wrong with the patient. Provide additional information as requested.

If the physician gives you orders for a specific treatment, REPEAT THE ORDERS BACK FOR VERIFICATION. Question orders that are not clear. Report back when orders have been carried out, and indicate what response, if any, the patient had to the treatment in question.

Indicate your ESTIMATED TIME OF ARRIVAL, and KEEP THE HOSPITAL INFORMED OF ANY CHANGES IN THE PATIENT'S CONDITION. When you have more than one patient, number or label them (Patient A, Patient B, and so on), and report on the most critical patient(s) first.

SAMPLE TRANSMISSION

AMBULANCE: Montefiore Hospital—Unit Four.

HOSPITAL: This is Dr. Clark. Go ahead, Unit Four.

AMB: We have a 22-year-old male who was struck by a car while crossing the street. He complains of severe pain in his abdomen. He has not vomited. He did not lose consciousness. He has no known medical history. On physical exam, he is conscious and in acute distress. Pulse is 120 and thready, BP 80/50, and respirations 28 and shallow. The skin is pale, cold, and clammy. There is no external bleeding. There is no evidence of injury to the head or chest. The abdomen is bruised and rigid. Bowel sounds are absent. The left leg is slightly angulated and swollen at the midcalf. We have applied antishock trousers and a traction splint and are administering oxygen. Are there any orders?

HOSP: Unit Four—Montefiore. Start an IV with Ringer's solution, and run it wide open.

AMB: Unit Four copies: IV with Ringer's solution wide open. Stand by.

(5 min later)

AMB: Montefiore Hospital—Unit Four.

HOSP: Unit Four, go ahead.

AMB: IV is initiated. We are en route. ETA 15 minutes.

HOSP: 10–4.

(5 min later)

HOSP: Unit Four—Montefiore.

AMB: Montefiore, go ahead.

HOSP: 10–20.

AMB: Fifth and Smithfield.

HOSP: Give us another set of vitals.

AMB: 10–4. Standby.

(2 min later)

AMB: Montefiore—Unit Four.

HOSP: Unit Four, go ahead.

AMB: Pulse 100, BP 100/60, respirations 15.

HOSP: 10–9 respirations.

AMB: Respirations 15, that is, one-five. Our ETA now 5 minutes.

HOSP: Received.

(20 min later)

AMB: Medic base—Unit Four.

BASE: Unit Four, go ahead.

AMB: 10–8 at Montefiore.

BASE: Unit Four, received. KCJ976 clear.

VOCABULARY

ETA Abbreviation for estimated time of arrival.

FCC Abbreviation for Federal Communications Commission.

frequency The number of cycles per second of a radio channel, inversely related to the wavelength.

landline Communications system linked by wires, usually in reference to a telephone system.

noise Interference in a radio signal.

patch Means for connecting a telephone and a radio.

repeater Radio unit that picks up a radio signal and rebroadcasts it with greater power.

squelch Suppression of extraneous noises on a radio channel.

ten-code Radio code system using the number 10 plus another number.

FURTHER READING

Bush SG. Sending and receiving signals: The art of communications. *Emergency* 10(3):33, 1978.

Carter WB et al. Development and implementation of emergency CPR instruction via telephone. *Ann Emerg Med* 13:695, 1984.

Clawson JJ. Quality assurance: A priority for medical dispatch. *Emerg Med Serv* 18(7):53, 1989.

Dreifuss R. 911 misuse. *Emerg Med Serv* 18(7):43, 1989.

Drury CG, Schiro SG. Evaluation of an EMS communications system. *JACEP* 6:133, 1977.

Eisenberg MS et al. Emergency CPR instruction via telephone. *Am J Public Health* 75:47, 1985.

Eisenberg MS et al. Identification of cardiac arrest by emergency dispatchers. *Am J Emerg Med* 4:299, 1986.

Henke S, Orcutt L. Portable radio communications for emergency medical services. *Emerg Med Serv* 12(4):32, 1983.

Howell JE. Amateur radio: An alternative means of emergency communication. *Emerg Med Serv* 14(4):28, 1985.

Keene K. Emergency medical dispatch: The holistic approach. *Emerg Med Serv* 18(7):48, 1989.

Kulp R. Basic considerations in implementing a medical consultation radio system. *EMT J* 1(4):61, 1977.

McCorkle JE, Nagel EL, Penterman DG, Mason RA. *Basic Telecommunications for Emergency Medical Services.* Cambridge, MA: Ballinger, 1978.

Sampsel RE. Telephone-directed CPR: Does it work? *Emerg Med Serv* 18(4):49, 1989.

Slovis CM et al. A priority dispatch system for emergency medical services. *Ann Emerg Med* 14:1055, 1985.

U.S. Department of Health, Education, and Welfare. *Emergency Medical Services Communications System.* DHEW Pub. (HSM)732003. Washington, D.C.: Government Printing Office, 1972.

U.S. Department of Transportation/National Highway Traffic Safety Administration. *Communications: Guidelines for Emergency Medical Services.* DOT/HS-820214. Washington, D.C.: U.S. Government Printing Office, 1972.

Yandell DC. 911 update. *Emerg Med Serv* 18(7):36, 1989.

40. EMERGENCY DRIVING

OBJECTIVES

Approximately 26,000 emergency vehicles are involved in motor vehicle accidents each year in the United States, with a resulting 200 fatalities annually. Ambulances figure in a disproportionately high number of these accidents. In the majority of cases, the cause is excessive speed or failure of the driver to take adequate safety precautions. Proper handling of the emergency vehicle is just as important to the safety and well-being of the patient as proper medical care at the scene. In this chapter, we shall examine the principles of emergency driving. We will look at the factors that contribute to highway accidents involving emergency vehicles and the measures that may be taken to minimize these accidents. By the conclusion of this chapter, the reader should be able to:

1. Identify the situations in which speed is indicated in driving an ambulance, given a list of situations including (a) situations described by the dispatcher requiring a rapid response *to* the scene and (b) situations encountered by the ambulance crew requiring rapid transport *from* the scene
2. Identify the approximate stopping distance of an ambulance on a dry road at (a) 30 mph, (b) 40 mph, and (c) 50 mph, and list at least two factors that can increase this stopping distance
3. List three dangers in using a siren
4. Identify desirable and undesirable traits in an ambulance driver, given a list of traits
5. List at least three ways that excessive speed can be avoided on an emergency call without sacrificing an efficient response time
6. List at least five ways in which the ambulance driver can minimize the risk of an accident

WHAT CAUSES ACCIDENTS

A CAUTIONARY TALE

In April, 1989, a 32-year-old paramedic from Ohio, a veteran of 13 years of exemplary work as an EMT, responded to a report of a multi-casualty road accident. En route to the call, he approached an intersection with emergency lights flashing, sirens howling, and air horn blaring. Believing that all traffic had stopped, he entered the intersection against a red light. But suddenly a car driven by a pregnant 20-year-old woman pulled from behind a van into the intersection and right into the path of the ambulance. In the collision, the woman and her fetus were killed, and a six-year-old passenger in her car was seriously injured. Subsequently, an Ohio court convicted the paramedic of involuntary manslaughter and sentenced him to two to ten years in prison. Prior to the accident, he had never had a traffic ticket.

It is estimated that one in every ten ambulances is involved in an accident each year. An accident involving an ambulance is a very serious matter from both a professional and a legal point of view. The purpose of a modern ambulance is, after all, to enable the saving of lives and the reduction of secondary injury. When a patient suffers bodily harm because of inappropriate operation of an emergency vehicle, the crew is no less negligent than when bodily harm occurs through inadequate medical treatment. For this reason, we need to examine the causes of ambulance accidents and the means by which such accidents can be prevented.

EXCESSIVE SPEED

Probably the most frequent cause of vehicular accidents involving ambulances is operation of the ambulance at an unsafe speed. That fact inevitably leads to the question: Is high speed driving necessary *at all* for an ambulance run? To answer that question, we need to examine the two phases of the ambulance call separately: (1) travel to the scene and (2) transport of the patient to the hospital.

There is no doubt that in certain types of emergencies, such as cardiac arrest or major trauma, prompt arrival at the scene *is* important. In such cases, a significant delay in reaching the patient may mean the difference between life and death. These cases, however, constitute only a very small proportion of the calls received by most ambulance services; the remainder of the calls are not so urgent. An experienced dispatcher, with EMT training, should be able to determine with considerable accuracy the probable urgency of a given call and instruct the responding unit accordingly. The "red ball" response should be used selectively, only for those cases in which a very rapid response seems necessary or a reasonable doubt about the urgency exists. Furthermore, even when a fast response seems to be indicated, proper planning of the response (knowing where you are going and the shortest way to get there) can reduce the need for driving at very high speed.

The second phase of the call—transporting the patient to the hospital—is another matter altogether. It is very rare indeed that there is any necessity for haste in moving a patient to a medical facility. In one study of ambulance runs, it was found that less than 2 percent of all calls really required fast transport to the hospital. In most instances, high speed transport reflects the condition of the EMT, not the patient; that is, high speed is employed because the EMT is inadequately trained and lacks confidence in his or her ability to manage the patient.

The panicky EMT is not doing the patient any favors by racing off to the hospital at breakneck speed. To the contrary, a wild ride with sirens screaming may cause discomfort, fear, and even injury to the unfortunate soul on the stretcher. Many patients have reported that the most terrifying part of their illness or injury was the ambulance trip to the hospital, and it is no exaggeration to say that a patient with a heart attack may literally be "scared to death" by a precipitous ambulance ride. The patient with an acute abdomen may suffer unnecessary agony every time the ambulance takes a bump too fast. The patient with a fracture may experience severe pain with every jolt of the vehicle, for even the best splint cannot prevent *all* motion in a fractured extremity.

The attending EMT must decide in each case, according to the patient's condition, how the ambulance should be driven to the hospital and should so instruct the driver. Transport should be regarded as part of the patient's treatment and, like any other treatment, must be tailored to the particular patient's needs and condition. Thus in each case, the attending EMT must ask: IS SPEED NECESSARY?

Cases in Which Rapid Transport Is Required

- Progressive AIRWAY OBSTRUCTION (e.g., laryngeal edema, foreign body that cannot be removed)
- UNCONTROLLABLE BLEEDING
- TENSION PNEUMOTHORAX, CARDIAC TAMPONADE, or other major chest injury
- ANAPHYLACTIC SHOCK
- CARDIAC ARREST

It should be emphasized that even in the cases just listed, speed should not be so great that it interferes with ongoing treatment of the patient en route. The attending EMT who is being hurled across the ambulance every time the vehicle takes a corner cannot maintain an airway, hold pressure on a wound, provide artificial ventilation, or perform effective CPR. The driver must always take into account the requirements of those who are caring for the patient.

A little common sense is also important. It makes little sense, for instance, to dawdle at the scene and then to try to make up time by driving like a maniac to the hospital. If the call is truly a critical emergency, *do not spend unnecessary time at the scene!* Speed at the scene is a lot safer than speed on the highway.

INADEQUATE STOPPING DISTANCE

A second cause of ambulance accidents is failure to maintain a safe distance between the ambulance and the vehicle ahead; if the forward vehicle stops unexpectedly (and this happens all too often!), the ambulance traveling close on its tail does not have adequate time to stop.

The **stopping distance** of a vehicle (Table 40-1) is a

Table 40-1. *Average Stopping Distances for an Ambulance*

Speed (mph)	Stopping Distance on Dry, Level Pavement (ft)
10	18
20	52
30	100
40	170
50	280
60	425

function of both the driver and the vehicle itself. The driver element is the *reaction distance*, that is, the distance the vehicle travels from the moment the driver decides to stop until his foot hits the brake. The *braking distance* is the additional distance the vehicle then travels from the moment braking action is initiated to the moment the vehicle comes to a full stop. Together these two factors determine the stopping distance. Clearly the stopping distances listed in Table 40-1 may be influenced by the condition of the driver, the vehicle, or the road: A sleepy driver, a faulty braking system, an icy road—any of these may increase the stopping distance considerably.

INADEQUATE ATTENTION TO THE ROAD AND TRAFFIC

A third cause of accidents is failure of the driver to pay adequate attention to road conditions or traffic. Fatigue, stress, or excitement may interfere with a driver's alertness to his surroundings. Furthermore, in an ambulance, the siren may have an hypnotic effect upon an inexperienced driver, causing him or her unconsciously to increase the speed of the vehicle beyond safe limits.

Safe operation of an emergency vehicle requires total alertness both to the road itself and to other traffic, pedestrian and motorized, on the road. Changing weather conditions may cause dramatic changes in the road surface from moment to moment. During the first few minutes of a rainfall, for instance, oil rises to the road surface, and the road as a consequence may become suddenly as slippery as a sheet of ice. As the road becomes wetter, the danger of **hydroplaning** increases; that is, the ambulance wheels can literally leave the road surface and skim along on top of a layer of water, making steering impossible. A sudden drop in temperature may convert a wet road into a ribbon of ice. The driver must be constantly alert to such changes and must adjust his speed and handling of the vehicle accordingly.

Similarly the driver must be alert to what is happening on the road. He or she must be aware of the positions of other vehicles and the potential of encountering unexpected vehicles or traffic at blind intersections. Full concentration on the driving task is required.

FAILURE TO DRIVE DEFENSIVELY

Finally, ambulance accidents frequently result from the failure of the ambulance driver to operate the ambulance defensively. It is a serious mistake to assume that other motorists will behave rationally, especially when they hear a siren. Drivers of other vehicles may exhibit some very strange reactions to the approach of an ambulance. Granted, some drivers may pull over to the right as they are supposed to, but others may veer to the left or, even worse, simply come to a full stop in the middle of the street. The ambulance driver must be ready for any of these possibilities and prepared to take the necessary evasive action.

Some ambulance drivers themselves behave rather strangely behind the wheel of an emergency vehicle. An ambulance driver who would never dream of flying through a blind intersection in the family car may do exactly that with the ambulance in the mistaken belief that the siren somehow has the magic power to repel oncoming traffic. Many state statutes provide special privileges for emergency vehicles, such as proceeding through a red light. Such privileges carry risks, and they should not be invoked without a very clear necessity. A siren and flashing lights do *not* protect an ambulance from being struck by another vehicle. Only careful, attentive, defensive driving provides that protection. So remember:

> THE SIREN IS NOT MAGIC.

PRINCIPLES OF SAFE AMBULANCE OPERATION

Not every holder of a driver's license is capable of operating an ambulance on an emergency run. The EMT who secretly yearns to drive in the Indy 500, for instance, should *not* be behind the wheel of an ambulance. Nor should the driver be the crew member who is near-sighted, high-strung, or slow in his or her reactions. What qualities, then, are needed in a good ambulance driver?

First of all, an ambulance driver should be STABLE and EMOTIONALLY MATURE, able to stay cool under stress, able to control his or her frustrations rather than take them out in driving. The driver who loudly curses everyone else on the road and whose eyes glaze over every time the siren is turned on does not meet these requirements.

Secondly, the driver must be in GOOD PHYSICAL CONDITION, both in general and on any given shift. Emergency driving is stressful and demanding. As noted earlier, emergency driving requires an unusual degree of alertness and concentration. If the driver reports to work tired, upset, or taking some kind of medication that might interfere with alertness (e.g., antihistamines), a replacement driver should be assigned for that shift. A driver reporting back to work after vacation or other leave should take a warm-up run to get reacquainted with the ambulance, whose handling characteristics necessarily differ from those of the family car.

A third important quality in the driver is SENSITIVITY TO THE CONDITION OF THE PATIENT. A good ambulance driver will, for example, avoid bumpy roads when transporting a patient with an acute abdomen.

Finally, the ambulance driver must KNOW THE MAP and be thoroughly familiar with standard and alternative routes to various locations. The driver who knows the shortest way to get from point A to point B will not have to try to compensate for out-of-the-way journeys by excessive speed.

AVOIDING EXCESSIVE SPEED

A prompt ambulance response need not require breaking the speed limit. If a call is properly planned, the ambulance should be able to reach the scene swiftly without exceeding a safe rate of travel.

To begin with, it is essential for the dispatcher to TRY TO DETERMINE THE URGENCY OF THE CALL. A "possible sprained ankle" does not require a "red ball" response! To the extent possible, time should be saved off the road rather than on the road. For example, it makes little sense to sit around the base for 5 minutes to finish a cup of coffee after receiving a call, and then career out of the ambulance bay to try to make up those 5 minutes on the highway. START OUT FOR THE SCENE IMMEDIATELY UPON RECEIVING THE CALL. The cup of coffee can wait.

KNOW WHERE YOU ARE GOING AND THE QUICKEST WAY TO GET THERE. This means knowing the standard routes, the likely traffic conditions, and the possible alternative routes. CHOOSE THE PATH OF LEAST RESISTANCE, that is, the route on which you are least likely to encounter traffic jams, road construction, or other slowdowns.

USE THE SIREN SPARINGLY, and beware of its hypnotic power. Mechanical sirens in particular tend to whip the driver onward at ever-increasing speeds.

When transporting a patient to the hospital, THINK ABOUT WHETHER FAST TRANSPORT IS *REALLY* NECESSARY, THEN THINK AGAIN. Is it a critically injured patient or an insecure EMT who is being treated by the rush to the hospital? LET THE ATTENDING EMT DECIDE HOW THE VEHICLE SHOULD BE DRIVEN TO THE HOSPITAL. If the EMT in the patient compartment tells you to slow down, slow down! The EMT who is sitting beside the patient is responsible for that patient's safety and well-being, so he or she must call the shots.

SAFE DRIVING HABITS

Safe driving habits are largely a matter of common sense. If you know, for instance, that sudden braking may cause the vehicle to veer or skid, the most logical way to prevent such an occurrence is to avoid situations in which sudden braking is likely to be necessary. MAINTAIN A SAFE DISTANCE BEHIND ANOTHER VEHICLE, at least one car length for every 10 miles per hour on a dry road, two car lengths for every 10 miles per hour on a wet or icy road. Another way to ensure a safe stopping distance is by using the Two-Second Rule; that is, keep your vehicle a minimum of 2 counted seconds behind the vehicle ahead, using some reference point such as a signpost as a guide. In wet or icy weather, the Two-Second Rule becomes the Four-Second Rule.

In your standard routes, AVOID AREAS COMMONLY CONGESTED WITH TRAFFIC OR WHERE CHILDREN ARE LIKELY TO BE NUMEROUS. Driving by the local elementary school is simply looking for trouble. Playgrounds and densely populated residential areas should also be avoided wherever possible. If you must drive through a school zone, do so with *extreme* caution.

WATCH OUT AT INTERSECTIONS! The majority of ambulance accidents occur at locations where one road crosses another. *Always* slow down as you approach an intersection; do not rely on your magic siren to provide you with an invisible shield. Vary the siren tone at intersections (e.g., switch from "hi-lo" to "yelp") to try to improve audibility. Try to make eye contact with other drivers or pedestrians entering the intersection, to be certain that they have seen you. DO NOT FOLLOW ANOTHER EMERGENCY VEHICLE THROUGH AN INTERSECTION; the driver who has stopped his car to let the first emergency vehicle pass may not realize that there are two of you, and he may roll on into the intersection right after the first emergency vehicle, directly into your path. So slow down and look both ways before you go through any intersection, even when the green light is in your favor.

OBSERVE CAUTION IN TURNING AND CHANGING LANES. Signal your intentions clearly; use *both* hand signals and automatic turn signals. Do not try to pass unless you have plenty of room to do so.

On wet or icy roads, IF THE VEHICLE BEGINS TO SKID, EASE UP ON THE ACCELERATOR, but do not try to brake suddenly. Especially when hydroplaning, your object is to get the wheels back in contact with the road surface, which is best accomplished by slowing *gradually* until steering is regained.

DRIVE DEFENSIVELY. Be alert for the motorist who slows suddenly or stops altogether as he is being overtaken. Avoid passing on the right, for the driver in the left lane may suddenly remember that he is supposed to move over to the right just as you are pulling past him. Do not take anything for granted!

BUCKLE UP! In a study of ambulance accidents in Tennessee, it was found that nearly all of the serious injuries that occurred in ambulance accidents were sustained by ambulance drivers or passengers who were not wearing seat belts.

USE OF SIRENS AND WARNING DEVICES

The siren is the most over-rated and over-utilized piece of equipment on the ambulance. Improperly used, a siren is an outright danger to all occupants of the vehicle. We have already mentioned that the siren may have an hypnotic effect on the ambulance driver, impelling him unconsciously to increase the speed at which he is driving. A siren also tends to give the driver a false sense of security, creating the impression that the marvelous wailing and yelping noise alone is sufficient to clear the road magically of other vehicles. In fact, siren effectiveness is usually vastly over-estimated. A person traveling in a passenger car with the windows rolled up and the air conditioner or radio turned on may not hear the siren at all until the ambulance is practically on top of him. And at that point, a sudden blast of the siren may startle the motorist and prompt him to do something irrational, like stopping in the middle of the highway. The ambulance horn may be much more effective in these circumstances.

Meanwhile back in the passenger compartment, the siren is wreaking another kind of havoc. For the siren gives the patient two very clear messages: (1) There is something terribly wrong, and (2) the ambulance team does not feel capable of dealing with the situation. These are not the messages one wants to convey to an anxious patient. Thus the general rule is:

NEVER USE THE SIREN WHEN THERE IS A CONSCIOUS PATIENT IN THE VEHICLE.

Sirens should, on the whole, be reserved for responding *to* the call, not for the phase of transport. If very heavy traffic makes it desirable to use the siren on the way to the hospital, explain to the patient that the siren is being turned on in order to help you get through traffic, and that its use does not reflect upon his condition.

Warning lights and beacons, on the other hand, should always be lighted when the ambulance is on a call. During daylight hours, the use of headlights may also serve to alert other motorists of your advance, especially when you are overtaking another driver to whom the high-mounted emergency lights on the ambulance may not be visible.

To summarize, bear in mind the Seven Deadly Assumptions of emergency driving:

THE SEVEN DEADLY ASSUMPTIONS

1. Assumption that the other driver will see your emergency lights
2. Assumption that the other driver will hear your siren
3. Assumption that the other driver will do the right, rational thing if he does see or hear you coming
4. Assumption that the other driver understands what path you intend to take
5. Assumption that the other driver will stop at an intersection as you are coming through
6. Assumption that someone signalling a left turn will not make a right turn (or vice versa)
7. Assumption that a pedestrian will get out of your path

If you make any of these assumptions when you are driving an ambulance, sooner or later you are going to be wrong. And your being wrong may cost someone's life, so:

TAKE NOTHING FOR GRANTED WHEN YOU DRIVE AN AMBULANCE.

EMERGENCY VEHICLE OPERATIONS COURSE

Like any of the other skills discussed in this book, emergency driving is learned by doing, not reading. Every EMT entrusted with emergency ambulance operation should pass a defensive driving course and special emergency vehicle operations course (EVOC), usually available through your state department of transportation. Such programs permit the student to take the vehicle over a specially designed course in which braking, evasive maneuvers, response to skids, and other psychomotor skills may be practiced. Learning to drive the ambulance properly is no less important than learning to operate a bag-valve-mask properly.

REMEMBER, THE LIFE YOU SAVE MAY BE YOUR OWN!

VOCABULARY

hydroplaning Phenomenon that occurs on wet roads, in which a motor vehicle moves along a thin layer of water, losing contact with the road surface and thus losing steering ability.

stopping distance The distance a vehicle travels from the moment the driver decides to stop to the time the vehicle has come to a full stop.

FURTHER READING

Auerbach PS et al. An analysis of ambulance accidents in Tennessee. *JAMA* 258:1487, 1987.

Brown WA. Ambulance accidents: What to do when they occur. *Emerg Med Serv* 13(3):76, 1984.

Childs BJ, Ptacnik DJ. *Emergency Ambulance Driving*. Englewood Cliffs, NJ: Brady, 1986.

Clark JM Jr. *Emergency and High Speed Driving Techniques*. Houston: Gulf Publishing, 1976.

Cowan W. Emergency driving. *Emerg Med Serv* 5(5):72, 1976.

Davenport AF. Limited-visibility driving. *Emerg Med Serv* 14(5):39, 1985.

Elling R. Dispelling myths on ambulance accidents. *JEMS* 11(7):60, 1989.

Gentile C, McDaniel CE. Emergency vehicle operations course. *Emerg Med Serv* 7:(4):8, 1978.

Hanna JA. *Ambulance and EMS Driving*. Reston, VA: Reston, 1983.

Hanna JA. Vehicle operations in crowd situations. *Emerg Med Serv* 13(2):22, 1984.

Lewis FJ Jr. Safe operation of ambulances. *Emerg Med Serv* 4(5):51, 1975.

Morse HN. EMT law: Colliding remarks. *Emergency* 15(6):44, 1983.

Scarano S. Emergency vehicle operation. *Emergency* 10(3):22, 1978.

USEFUL REFERENCES IN EMERGENCY CARE

American Academy of Orthopedic Surgeons. *Emergency Care and Transportation of the Sick and Injured* (4th ed.). Chicago: AAOS, 1987.

Arena J. *Poisoning*. Springfield, Ill.: Thomas, 1979.

Baldwin GA. *Handbook of Pediatric Emergencies*. Boston: Little, Brown, 1989.

Barber JM, Budassi SA. *Mosby's Manual of Emergency Care*. St. Louis: Mosby, 1979.

Briese G, Schottke D. *Your First Response in the Streets*. Boston: Little, Brown, 1984.

Caroline NL. *Ambulance Calls: Review Problems in Emergency Care* (3rd ed.). Boston: Little, Brown, 1991.

Caroline NL. *Emergency Care in the Streets* (4th ed.). Boston: Little, Brown, 1991.

Caroline NL. *Life-Supporting First Aid and Resuscitation*. Geneva: League of Red Cross Societies, 1983.

Copass M, Eisenberg M. *The Paramedic Manual*. Philadelphia: Saunders, 1980.

Copass M, Eisenberg M. *EMT Defibrillation*. Westport, Conn.: Emergency Training, 1984.

Eisenberg M, Copass M. *Manual of Emergency Medical Therapeutics*. Philadelphia: Saunders, 1978.

Eisenberg M, Copass M. *Emergency Medical Therapy*. Philadelphia: Saunders, 1982.

Eisenberg M, Cummins R, Ho M. *Code Blue: Cardiac Arrest and Resuscitation*. Philadelphia: Saunders, 1987.

McNeil EL. *Airborne Care of the Ill and Injured*. New York: Springer-Verlag, 1983.

Rund DA, Rausch TS. *Triage*. St. Louis: Mosby, 1981.

Safar P, Bircher N. *Cardiopulmonary Cerebral Resuscitation* (3rd ed.). Philadelphia: Saunders, 1988.

Schwartz GR et al. (Eds.). *Principles and Practice of Emergency Medicine* (2nd ed.). Philadelphia: Saunders, 1985.

Soper RG et al. *EMT Manual*. Philadelphia: Saunders, 1984.

GLOSSARIES

GLOSSARY OF COMMON MEDICAL ROOTS

a-, an- Without
ab- Away from
ad- Toward
adeno- Gland
aer(o)- Air
alb- White
-algia Pain
ambi- On both sides
andro- Male
angio- Blood vessel
ante- Before
anti- Against
arthro- Joint
-asthenia Without strength
auto- Self

bi- Twice, two
bio- Life
blepharo- Eyelid
brachio- Arm
brady- Slow
broncho- Bronchi

cardio- Heart
carpo- Wrist
-cele Cavity, swelling
cephalo- Head
cerebro- Brain
chole- Bile, gall
chondro- Cartilage
-cide Killing of
circum- Around
contra- Against
costo- Rib
cranio- Skull
cyst- Bladder
-cyte, -cyto- Cell

dermato- Skin
diplo- Double
-dipsia Thirst, drinking
dorso- Posterior, back
-dynia Pain
dys- Abnormal, painful, difficult

-ectomy Surgical removal
-emia Blood
en- Into, within
endo- Within, innermost
entero- Intestines
epi- Upon, after, in addition to
equi- Equal
erythro- Red
-esthesia Feeling
eu- normal, good
exo- Outward
extra- Outside of, in addition to

gastro- Stomach
-genic Causing

glosso- Tongue
glyco- Sugar
-gram A written record
-graphy Visualization
gyn-, gyne-, gyneco- Woman

hem-, hema-, hemato- Blood
hemi- Half
hepato- Liver
homeo-, homo- Same
hydro- Water
hyper- Above, excess
hypo- Below, deficient
hystero- Uterus

-iasis State, condition
iatro- Physician
idio- Peculiar, self
ile- Ileum
in- Within, into, inside
infra- Beneath
inter- Between
intra- Within
irido- Iris
iso- Equal
itis Inflammation

lacto- Milk
laryngo- Larynx
leuko- White
lingua- Tongue
lipo- Fat
litho- Stone
-lysis Dissolution

macro- Large
mal- Bad, poor
mammo- Breast, mammary gland
masto- Breast
mega-, megalo-, -megaly Enlargement
melano- Black
meningo- Meninges
meno- Month
micro- Small
mono- One, single
-morphic Shape, form
myelo- Spinal cord
myo- Muscle

narco- Stupor, numbness, sleep
naso- Nose
necro- Death
neo- New
nephro- Kidney
neuro- Nerve
noct- Night

oculo- Eye
oligo- Few, little, sparse
-ology Science of
-oma Tumor, swelling
onco- Tumor
ophthalmo- Eye
orchi- Testicle
ortho- Straight, normal
-osis Disease, abnormal condition
osteo- Bone
-ostomy Surgical opening, outlet
oto- Ear
-otomy Cutting into

pan- All
para- Beside
-paresis Weakness
-pathy Disease
-penia Lack of
per- Through
peri- Around
-phagia Swallowing, eating
-phasia Speech
-philia Affinity for
phlebo- Vein
-phobia Fear
-phonia Sound, speech
photo- Light
phren- Diaphragm
pilo- Hair
-plegia Paralysis
pleuro- Pleura
-pnea Breathing
pneumo- Breath, air, lung
pod(o)- Foot
poly- Many
post- After
postero- Back
pre- Before
procto- Rectum
pseudo- False
psych- Mind
pulmo- Lung
pyelo- Pelvis of the kidney
pyo- Pus

quad-, quadri- Four

retro- Behind, backward
rhino- Nose
-rrhage, -rrhagia Excessive flow
-rrhea Profuse flow

sclero- Hard
-scopy Looking at
semi- Half
sero- Watery
-stasis Stopping, stagnation of flow
super-, supra- Above, in addition
syn- With, together

tachy- Fast
thoraco- Chest

thrombo- Clot
trans- Across, over

ultra- Beyond, excess
un- Not, reversal
uni- One
-uresis Urination
-uria Of the urine
uro- Urine, urinary organs

vaso- Vessel
ven-, veni-, veno- Vein

GLOSSARY OF TERMS USED IN THIS TEXT*

*Words in italics are defined elsewhere in this glossary.

abandonment Abrupt termination of contact with the patient without giving the patient sufficient opportunity to find another health professional to take over his medical treatment.

ABC First three steps in managing the unconscious patient: *A*irway, *B*reathing, *C*irculation.

abdomen The part of the body between the *thorax* and the *pelvis*.

abdominal thrust Maneuver in which a sharp compression is delivered over the upper abdomen in an attempt to dislodge a foreign body from the airway.

abduction Movement of a limb AWAY from the midline of the body.

abortion Loss of a pregnancy before the twentieth week of gestation.

abrasion Wound in which part of the skin surface has been rubbed or scraped away.

AC Abbreviation for alternating current.

acetabulum Depression in the pelvic bone that serves as the socket for the hip joint; formed from the junction of the *ilium*, *ischium*, and *pubis*.

acidosis Condition in which the level of acid in the body is increased above normal.

acromion Extension of the *scapula* that forms the highest point of the shoulder and articulates with the *clavicle*.

activated charcoal Substance used to adsorb ingested drugs and poisons.

acute respiratory insufficiency Any condition in which breathing is inadequate to supply oxygen to or remove carbon dioxide from the body tissues.

addiction Overwhelming involvement in the use of a drug.

adduction Movement TOWARD the midline of the body.

advanced life support Lifesaving measures that require invasive procedures—such as intravenous therapy—that may be performed only by a physician or a specially trained individual acting under a physician's supervision.

afterbirth *Placenta*.

afterdrop Continued fall in core body temperature after a victim of *hypothermia* has been rescued from a cold environment.

AIDS Acronym for acquired immunodeficiency syndrome, a viral illness that suppresses the human immune system.

air embolism Bubble of air that enters the circulation and acts as an obstruction when it becomes trapped in a blood vessel.

alcoholism *Addiction* to alcohol.

alpha particle Positively charged subatomic particle corresponding to the nucleus of an atom, with high *ionizing* ability but low penetration.

ALS Abbreviation for *advanced life support*.

alveolus Terminal air sac in the lung.

AMI Abbreviation for acute *myocardial infarction*.

amnesia Loss of memory.

amniotic fluid Liquid in which the developing *fetus* is suspended within the *amniotic sac*.

amniotic sac Membranous sac in which the developing *fetus* is enclosed; "bag of waters."
ampere Unit of electric *current.*
amputation Severing of a part of the body.
anaphylactic shock Form of *shock* that occurs as a result of a violent allergic reaction.
anesthesia Absence of feeling.
aneurysm Sac or bulge in a blood vessel due to weakening of its wall.
angina pectoris Characteristic pain from myocardial *hypoxia;* usually retrosternal; squeezing, brought on by exertion, relieved by rest.
angle of Louis Prominence on the *sternum* that lies opposite the second *intercostal space.*
anorexia Loss of appetite.
anoxia Absence of oxygen in the body tissues.
anterior Toward the front.
antibody Protein, produced in response to a specific *antigen* (foreign protein), that destroys or inactivates the antigen.
antiemetic Agent used to control or prevent vomiting.
antigen Any agent that, when taken into the body, stimulates the formation of specific, protective proteins called *antibodies.*
antivenin Serum containing *antibodies* to a specific animal venom, administered to counterattack the effects of the venom.
aorta The major artery of the body, which arises from the left *vetricle* of the heart.
apnea Absence of breathing.
appendicular skeleton The part of the skeleton comprising the shoulder girdle, upper extremity, *pelvis,* and lower extremity.
appendix Wormlike structure attached to the *cecum;* when inflamed (appendicitis), it may cause pain in the right lower quadrant.
aqueous humor Salty fluid found between the *cornea* and the *lens* of the eye.
arachnoid Middle layer of the *meninges.*
artery Vessel that carries blood AWAY from the heart.
articulation Point where two or more bones come together to form a joint.
artifact Interference in an *ECG* signal.
artificial ventilation Any means of providing air exchange to a patient who is not breathing or not breathing adequately.
assisted ventilation Use of adjunctive equipment, such as a bag-valve-mask, to increase the volume of each breath in a spontaneously breathing patient.
asystole Absence of any ventricular contractions; cardiac standstill; appears as a straight line on the *ECG.*
atelectasis Collapse of *alveoli.*
atherosclerosis Disease that causes narrowing and hardening of the coronary and cerebral arteries.
atrium Upper chamber of the right or left heart.
auscultation Listening, usually with a stethoscope, for the sounds made by internal body organs.
avulsion Injury in which part of the body is partially severed and hangs loose.
axial skeleton The part of the skeleton comprising the skull, *vertebrae,* and *thorax.*
axilla Armpit.
axillary artery Artery that supplies blood to the arm; its pulsations can be palpated in the armpit.

back blows Sharp blows delivered with the heel of the hand to the middle of the victim's back, between the shoulder blades, in an attempt to dislodge a foreign body obstructing the airway.
backboard Any of a variety of long, flat boards used to immobilize a patient with suspected spinal injury.
bandage Material used to hold a *dressing* in place.
basal skull fracture *Fracture* of the inferior part of the skull.
Battle's sign *Ecchymosis* over the *mastoid* bone; a sign of *basal skull fracture.*
beta particle Negatively charged subatomic particle, corresponding to the electron of an atom, with slightly higher penetration ability than an *alpha particle.*
bile Greenish-black fluid, secreted by the liver and concentrated in the gall bladder, that is important in the absorption of fats from the digestive tract.
biologic death Death of the organism, when irreversible brain damage has set in; also called brain death.
bladder Hollow organ of the urinary system, located in the *pelvis,* just behind the *pubic* bone, that stores urine produced by the *kidneys.*
bloody show Plug of mucus, sometimes tinged with blood, that is expelled from the *cervix* as it dilates at the beginning of *labor.*
brachial artery Artery that supplies blood to the forearm; its pulsations can be felt slightly *proximal* and *medial* to the crease of the elbow, on the *anterior* surface of the arm.
brainstem Portion of the brain, located inferior to the *cerebrum,* that controls automatic functions such as breathing and body temperature.
breech Delivery in which part of the baby's body other than the head is the *presenting part.*
bronchodilation Widening of the bronchial air passages brought about by relaxation of the muscles of the bronchial walls.
bronchospasm Violent contraction of the muscles of the bronchial walls, causing marked constriction of the *bronchi.*
bronchus One of two main branches of the *trachea,* carrying air into the lungs; plural is "bronchi."

cafe coronary Choking incident, so named because its suddenness often leads observers to mistake it for a heart attack.
calcaneus Heel bone.
callus Tissue that forms a collar joining two ends of a broken bone, gradually replaced by new bone as *fracture* healing progresses.
capillary Tiny blood vessel through which oxygen

and carbon dioxide are exchanged in the tissues of the lungs and other organs.

carbon monoxide Colorless, odorless, tasteless gas produced by incomplete combustion of organic materials; highly toxic.

carboxyhemoglobin *Hemoglobin* that is combined with *carbon monoxide* instead of oxygen.

cardiac arrest Sudden and unexpected cessation of cardiac output; for practical purposes, the cessation of pulse.

cardiac muscle Involuntary muscle, found only in the heart, that has the property of initiating its own contractions.

cardiac standstill Absence of ventricular contractions; *asystole*.

cardiogenic shock Failure of perfusion caused by damage to the pump (the heart).

cardiopulmonary resuscitation (CPR) Technique to revive a patient in *cardiac arrest* by *artificial ventilation* and *external chest compressions*.

cardiovascular collapse Form of *cardiac arrest* in which the heart continues beating but its contractions are too weak to sustain the circulation.

carina Point at which the *trachea* bifurcates into the right and left *bronchi*.

carotid Artery that supplies blood to the head and brain; its pulsations can be felt in the neck, lateral to the Adam's apple.

carpals Bones of the wrist.

carpopedal spasm Contorted position of the hand in which the fingers flex in a clawlike attitude and the thumb curls toward the palm; may be caused by *hyperventilation*.

carrier Person who habors an infectious agent and, although not himself ill, can transmit that infection to another person.

cartilage Connective tissue that lines *synovial joints* and provides structure and cushioning elsewhere in the body.

cecum First portion of the large intestine.

central nervous system (CNS) The brain and spinal cord.

cerebellum Portion of the brain, lying inferior to the *cerebrum*, that controls balance, muscle tone, and coordination of skilled movements.

cerebral embolism Free-floating blood clot that lodges in one of the arteries of the brain.

cerebral hemorrhage Bleeding into brain tissue caused by rupture of a cerebral artery.

cerebral thrombosis Obstruction of a cerebral artery by a blood clot that arises within the artery, usually in an area scarred by *atherosclerosis*.

cerebrospinal fluid (CSF) Watery fluid that bathes the brain and spinal cord.

cerebrovascular accident (CVA) Another term for *stroke*.

cerebrum Largest portion of the brain, responsible for higher functions, such as reasoning.

cervical Referring to the neck.

cervical spine First seven *vertebrae*, located in the neck.

cervix Narrow opening at the distal end of the *uterus*.

chest thrust Maneuver in which a sharp compression is delivered over the *sternum* in an attempt to dislodge a foreign body from the airway.

Cheyne-Stokes respirations Abnormal breathing pattern in which periods of *hyperpnea* are interspersed with periods of *apnea*.

chief complaint Problem for which a patient is seeking help.

chin lift Technique of opening the airway by supporting the chin in a forward position.

chronic bronchitis Form of chronic obstructive pulmonary disease characterized by excessive production of mucus, cough, and often *cyanosis*.

clavicle Collarbone.

clinical death The moment when the heart stops beating, as determined by absence of a pulse.

CNS Abbreviation for *central nervous system*.

coccyx Lowest portion of the spine; four fused *vertebrae* that constitute the tail bone.

colic Crampy pain associated with obstruction of a hollow organ.

Colles' fracture *Fracture* of the distal *radius* and *ulna*.

colon The large intestine.

coma State of unconsciousness from which a person cannot be roused, even by painful stimuli.

comatose Condition of being deeply unconscious.

comminuted fracture *Fracture* in which bone is broken into three or more pieces or in which several small cracks radiate out from the point of impact.

communicable disease Disease that can be transmitted from one person to another.

communicable period Period during which an infected person is capable of transmitting his illness to someone else.

compound fracture *Fracture* in which the bone ends are visible in or protruding from a wound.

compulsive drug use Situation in which a drug user becomes extremely preoccupied with the procurement and use of a given substance.

concussion Injury to the head causing temporary loss of function, usually of very brief duration.

conduction Transfer of heat to a liquid or solid object.

condyle Rounded projection at the end of a bone.

congestive heart failure Inadequate pumping by the heart, leading to the backup of blood behind the affected *atrium*.

conjunctiva Mucous membrane covering the *sclera* and inner surface of the eyelid.

consent Agreement, concurrence. In medicine, it usually refers to agreement by the patient to undergo some procedure.

- **implied consent** Assumed agreement to receive emergency lifesaving treatment when the patient is physically or otherwise incapable of giving knowing consent.
- **informed consent** Patient's agreement to accept

a given treatment after the nature and risks of the treatment have been fully explained to him.

contamination Presence of harmful microorganisms on or in any person, animal, or object.

controlled ventilation *Artificial ventilation* of a patient who is not breathing spontaneously.

contusion Closed injury to soft tissues; bruise.

convection Mechanism by which body heat is picked up and carried away by moving air currents.

conversion reaction Psychologic mechanism by which a person translates anxiety into a physical symptom, most commonly paralysis.

COPD Abbreviation for chronic obstructive pulmonary disease.

core In reference to the human body, that part of the body comprising the heart, lungs, brain, and abdominal organs.

cornea Clear anterior poriton of the *sclera*.

coronary arteries Vessels that carry oxygenated blood to the heart muscle.

costal arch Lower border of the ribs.

cough reflex Automatic forceful expulsion of air in response to irritation of the back of the throat.

CPR Abbreviation for *cardiopulmonary resuscitation*.

cranium Skull; the part of the head that is superior and posterior to the ears.

crib death *Sudden infant death syndrome*.

crossed-finger maneuver Technique for forcing a patient's mouth open by pushing on the lower molars with the thumb and on the upper molars with the index finger.

croup Viral disease of the upper airway in children that leads to partial upper airway obstruction, *stridor*, and a barking cough.

crowning Bulging of the *presenting part* of the baby from the mother's *vagina*.

CSF Abbreviation for *cerebrospinal fluid*.

current Flow of electric charges through a wire or other conductor.

CVA Abbreviation for *cerebrovascular accident;* a *stroke*.

cyanosis Bluish discoloration of the skin, mucous membranes, and nail beds, suggestive of inadequate oxygen in the blood.

DC Abbreviation for direct current.

decerebrate response Reaction to a painful stimulus (or sometimes to no apparent stimulus) in which all the patient's muscles go into spasm, with the legs in extreme extension.

defibrillation Use of direct current electric shock to terminate *ventricular fibrillation* and restore effective cardiac function.

delirium tremens (DTs) Potential complication of alcohol *withdrawal*, characterized by frightening hallucinations, agitation, and sometimes *cardiovascular collapse*.

demand valve Oxygen-powered resuscitator that may be triggered by the patient's inhalation.

denial Psychologic mechanism by which a person attempts to minimize or ignore serious illness.

dentures False teeth.

depressed fracture *Fracture* in which part of the skull is pushed inward toward the brain.

dermis Inner layer of the skin, containing nerves, blood vessels, glands, and hair follicles.

dextrose Form of sugar used in intravenous solutions.

diabetes mellitus Systemic disease affecting many organs, including the pancreas, whose failure to secrete *insulin* leads to an inability to utilize sugar.

diaphoresis Profuse sweating.

diaphragm Tough sheet of muscle that separates the thoracic cavity from the abdominal cavity; the principal muscle of respiration.

diastole Period of the cardiac cycle when the *ventricles* are relaxing and filling with blood.

diastolic pressure The lowest point of the blood pressure.

dislocation Displacement of a bone end from a joint.

distal Farther from the point of attachment to the body.

doral Referring to the back surface.

dorsalis pedis One of the arteries of the foot; its pulsations are palpable on the anterior surface of the foot, lateral to the tendon of the great toe.

downer Depressant drug.

down time Total time an ambulance is tied up on a call, from the time it leaves for the call until it goes back into service, ready for the next call.

dressing Material used to cover a wound.

drug dependence State in which repeated administration of a given drug is necessary to maintain a person's feeling of well-being and to prevent *withdrawal* symptoms.

DTs Abbreviation for *delirium tremens*.

duodenum First portion of the small intestine, immediately distal to the stomach.

dura mater Tough, outer layer of the *meninges*.

duty to act Legal obligation of public, and certain other, ambulance services to respond to a call for assistance in their jurisdiction.

dyspnea The sensation of being short of breath.

ecchymosis Bluish discoloration of part of the skin due to injury; a "black and blue mark."

ECG Abbreviation for *electrocardiogram*.

eclampsia Syndrome of *hypertension*, massive *edema*, and proteinuria that may lead to seizures and *coma* as the pregnant patient enters *labor;* toxemia of pregnancy.

ED Abbreviation for emergency department.

edema Swelling.

electrocardiogram Written record of the electric activity of the heart.

electrocardiograph Machine used to record the electric activity of the heart.

electrode Probe used to sense electric activity.

electrolyte Substance whose molecules dissociate into charged components when placed in water.

embolus Free-floating blood clot.

embryo Developing baby from 1 week after conception until about the end of the second month of pregnancy.

emergency medical technician Person specially trained to give basic emergency medical care at the scene of an emergency and en route to the hospital.

emphysema Form of chronic obstructive pulmonary disease characterized by destructive changes in the terminal air spaces of the lungs.

EMS Abbreviation for emergency medical services.

EMT Abbreviation for *emergency medical technician.*

entrance wound Wound at which a foreign body or electric *current* penetrates the skin to enter the body.

envenomation Process by which a venom or toxin is injected into a wound.

epidermis Outermost layer of the skin.

epidural Lying outside the *dura mater* (between the dura and the skull).

epigastrium Upper middle region of the *abdomen*, just below the *costal arches.*

epiglottis Small projection of tissue at the entrance to the *trachea* that acts as a trap door to prevent entry of foreign materials into the lower respiratory tract.

epiglottitis Bacterial infection of the *epiglottis;* may lead to abrupt, complete airway obstruction.

epilepsy Disease characterized by *seizures.*

epistaxis Nosebleed.

ER Abbreviation for emergency room.

erect Standing upright.

erythrocyte Red blood cell.

esophagus Portion of the digestive tract that lies between the throat and the stomach.

ETA Abbreviation for estimated time of arrival.

eversion Twisting of the ankle OUTWARD, so that the lateral aspect of the ankle is pressed toward the ground.

evisceration Condition in which internal organs, such as the intestines, protrude through a wound.

exhalation Passive phase of respiration, during which air is released from the lung.

exit wound Site at which a bullet, other foreign body, or electric current leaves the body.

exsanguination Bleeding to death.

extension Movement that brings the parts of a limb toward a straight condition.

external chest compressions Rhythmic pressure exerted over the *sternum* with the aim of creating an artificial circulation.

external jugular vein Principal vein draining blood from the head, sometimes visible in the neck.

external rotation Lateral turning of an extremity.

extrication Process by which an entrapped person is approached, treated, and safely removed from the area of entrapment.

fallopian tube Duct that connects the *ovary* to the *uterus.*

fasciculations Rippling movements in individual muscle bundles.

FCC Abbreviation for Federal Communications Commission.

febrile Having an elevated body temperature; feverish.

femoral artery Artery that supplies the lower extremity; its pulsations can be felt in the groin.

femur Thigh bone.

fetus Developing baby in the *uterus* after the second month of pregnancy.

fibula Smaller bone of the leg; its distal end forms the lateral *malleolus* of the ankle.

finger sweep Maneuver to clear the mouth and throat of foreign material by sweeping a finger through them.

first-degree burn Mildest form of burn, affecting only the *epidermal* layer and producing redness and swelling.

flaccidity Absence of muscle tone; limpness of the extremities.

flail chest Condition in which a segment of the chest wall flops inward during *inhalation* and bulges outward during *exhalation*, occuring when several ribs are fractured in two or more places.

flexion Act of bending a part, or the condition of being bent.

flow meter Device that controls the flow rate of oxygen from an oxygen cylinder.

fontanel Soft spot on an infant's head, where the bones of the skull have not yet fused together.

Fowler's position Position in which a patient's head is elevated 18 to 20 inches above the rest of his body (e.g., by elevating the head of the stretcher).

fracture Break in the continuity of a bone.

frenulum Fold on the lower surface of the penis; bleeds profusely if lacerated.

frequency Number of cycles per second of a radio channel, inversely related to wavelength.

frontal region Anterior region of the *cranium.*

frostbite Freezing injury to tissues.

gag reflex Automatic spasm of the airway in response to irritation of the throat.

galea Tough, inner lining of the scalp.

gall bladder Sac, located just beneath the liver, that concentrates and stores *bile.*

gamma ray *Radioactive* emission from the nucleus of an atom, has very high penetrating ability.

gauge Diameter of a needle or catheter; the higher the gauge number, the narrower the diameter of the needle.

glenoid Depression in the *scapula* that serves as the socket for shoulder joint.

glottis Opening between the *vocal cords.*

Good Samaritan law One of a variety of statutes providing limited immunity from prosecution to persons who respond voluntarily and in good faith to the aid of an injured person outside the hospital.

grand mal seizure Generalized motor *seizure.*

greenstick fracture Incomplete *fracture*, extending only part way through a bone.

hallucinogen Drug that has the capacity to stimulate hallucinations, that is, perceptions not founded on objective reality.
head tilt Maneuver to open the airway by hyperextending the head.
heart Organ located in the chest, behind the *sternum*, that pumps blood to the rest of the body.
hematemesis Vomiting blood.
hematoma Collection of blood beneath the skin, forming a lump.
hematuria Blood in the urine.
hemiparesis Weakness on one side of the body.
hemiplegia paralysis on one side of the body.
hemoglobin Pigmented protein in the red blood cell that carries oxygen and is responsible for the characteristic color of blood.
hemoptysis Coughing up blood.
hemorrhage Profuse bleeding.
hemorrhagic shock Failure of tissue perfusion caused by loss of blood.
hemothorax Presence of blood in the *pleural space*.
hepatitis Inflammation of the liver.
history of the present illness (HPI) Elaboration of the patient's *chief complaint*.
Holger Nielsen technique Method of *artificial ventilation* involving back pressure–arm lift maneuvers performed on a prone patient.
humerus The arm bone.
hydroplaning Loss of steering ability on a wet road due to suspension of the wheels on a thin film of water.
hymenoptera Class of stinging insects that includes honey bees, hornets, wasps, yellow jackets, and ants.
hypercarbia Abnormally high level of carbon dioxide in the blood, usually due to *hypoventilation*.
hyperglycemia Excess sugar in the blood.
hyperpnea Abnormally deep respirations.
hyperventilation Abnormally deep or rapid breathing that causes the level of carbon dioxide in the blood to fall below normal.
hypoglycemia Abnormally low concentration of sugar in the blood.
hypotension Low blood pressure, or deficient blood pressure.
hypothermia Generalized cooling of the body, including the *core*.
hypoventilation Breathing that is too slow or too shallow to rid the body of excess carbon dioxide.
hypovolemic shock Failure of tissue *perfusion* caused by a deficient fluid volume in the body.
hypoxia Deficiency of oxygen.
hypoxic drive Primary stimulus to breathe in some patients with *COPD*, in which a fall in the oxygen levels in the blood is the sole spur to increase respirations.

ileum Third and final section of the small intestine, joining with the large intestine at the ileocecal valve.
ilium One of two large bones that form the wings of the *pelvis*.
impacted fracture *Fracture* in which the bone ends are jammed into one another.
impaled object Foreign body that causes a puncture wound and remains embedded in the wound.
incision Wound characterized by a clean cut made with a sharp instrument, such as a knife.
incubation period Period from infection until the appearance of the first *symptoms*.
inferior Below; toward the feet.
inferior vena cava One of the two largest *veins* of the body; carries blood from the lower part of the body to the right *atrium* of the heart.
infusion Intravenous therapy with nonblood products.
inhalation Active phase of respiration during which air is drawn into the lungs.
inspection Examination of a part of the body by looking for visible signs of illness or injury.
insulin Hormone, produced in the pancreas, that regulates the level of sugar in the blood.
insulin shock State of severe *hypoglycemia* due to an excessive *insulin* dose.
intercostal muscles The muscles between the ribs, which participate in respiration.
intercostal space Space between two ribs.
internal rotation Medical turning of an extremity.
intracranial Within the skull.
intravenous line (IV) Tubing inserted within a *vein* as a means of supplying fluids or drugs directly into the bloodstream.
inversion Twisting of the ankle INWARD so that the medial aspect of the ankle is pressed toward the ground.
ion An atom, part of an atom, or a group of atoms that carries an electric charge.
ionizing radiation Transmission of energy, in the form of waves or particles, that has the ability to disrupt atoms in its path into component *ions*.
iris Circular muscle behind the *cornea* that regulates the amount of light entering the eye by constricting or enlarging the aperture at its center.
ischemia Tissue *anoxia* from diminished blood flow, usually caused by narrowing or occlusion of the artery supplying the tissue.
ischial tuberosity Most inferior and posterior portion of the *ischium*, palpable as a bump in the buttocks.
ischium One of the two bones that form the inferior portion of the pelvic ring.

jaundice Yellowish discoloration of the skin, usually due to disease of the *liver* or *gall bladder*.
jaw thrust Maneuver to open the patient's airway by pushing forward on the angles of the *mandible*.
jaw-tongue life Maneuver to open the patient's airway by inserting one's thumb in the patient's mouth, over the lower teeth, and pulling the tongue and jaw upward.
jejunum Second portion of the small intestine.
joint Place where two bones come together.

jugular notch Top border of the *sternum*.

ketoacidosis Condition that can result from uncontrolled diabetes; characterized by extreme hunger, thirst, increased urination, vomiting, and sometimes coma, with production of excessive amounts of acid and ketones in metabolism.
kidneys Paired organs located in the *retroperitoneal* space that filter the blood and produce urine.
Kussmaul breathing Respiratory pattern characteristic of diabetic *ketoacidosis*, with marked *hyperpnea* and *tachypnea*.

labor Process of uterine contractions by which the baby is expelled from the mother.
laceration Wound characterized by a ragged cut.
landline Telephone communications.
laryngectomee Person whose *larynx* has been removed surgically.
laryngectomy Surgical removal of the *larynx*.
laryngospasm Violent contractions of the muscles of the *larynx*, causing partial or complete airway obstruction.
larynx Voice box.
lateral Farther from the midline of the body.
lens Part of the eye behind the *iris* that focuses the image on the *retina*.
leukocyte White blood cell.
liability Legal obligation or responsibility.
ligament Band of fibrous tissue that connects BONE TO BONE.
linear fracture *Fracture* that appears as a single line or crack.
litigation Lawsuit.
liver Large organ in the right upper quadrant of the *abdomen* that secretes *bile*, produces many essential proteins, and performs other essential functions.
lumbar spine Part of the vertebral column in the lower back, starting just below the ribs and extending to the *pelvis*.
lungs Paired organs in the *thorax* that supply the body with oxygan and eliminate carbon dioxide.

malleolus Rounded knob on either side of the ankle; the medial malleolus is formed by the distal *tibia*, and the lateral malleolus by the distal *fibula*.
mandible Lower jaw.
march fracture Type of stress *fracture*, involving the *metacarpal* bones, caused by prolonged walking.
mastoid Bone of the skull that lies just behind the ear.
maxilla Upper jaw.
MCI Abbreviation for multiple casualty incident.
mechanism of injury Way in which an injury occurred and the forces involved in producing the injury.
medial Nearer the midline of the body.
mediastinum Space within the chest, located between the two *lungs*, that contains the *heart*, major blood vessels, *trachea*, and *esophagus*.
medulla Area in the base of the brain that controls respiration.
melanin Pigment found in varying amounts in the *epidermal* layer of the skin.
menarche Onset of menstrual function, usually around age 12.
meninges Three membranes that enclose and protect the brain.
meningitis Inflammation of the meninges, causing fever, headache, and stiff neck.
menopause Cessation of menstrual function, usually around age 50.
menstruation Cyclic uterine bleeding, occurring at about 4-week intervals in the nonpregnant woman.
mesentery Delicate tissue that carries blood vessels and nerves to and from the organs of the abdominal cavity.
metabolic acidosis Abnormal increase in the amount of organic acids in the body.
metacarpals Bones of the hand.
metatarsals Bones of the foot.
MICU Abbreviation for *mobile intensive care unit*.
midline Imaginary vertical line down the center of the anterior surface of the body.
Military Anti-Shock Trousers (MAST) Inflatable garment applied around the legs and abdomen, used in the treatment of *shock*.
mm Hg Abbreviation for millimeters of mercury, the units in which blood pressure is measured.
mobile intensive care unit Ambulance staffed by paramedics, nurses, or doctors and equipped to give *advanced life support* at the scene of an emergency and en route to the hospital.
mouth-to-mouth technique Method of *artificial ventilation* whereby air is forced into the victim's mouth from the rescuer's mouth.
mouth-to-nose technique Method of *artificial ventilation* whereby air is forced into the victim's nose from the rescuer's mouth.
mouth-to-stoma technique Method of *artificial ventilation* whereby air is forced into the *stoma* of a *laryngectomee* from the mouth of the rescuer.
multipara (multip) Woman who had had two or more pregnancies.
myocardial infarction Death of a segment of heart muscle, due to interruption of the blood supply to the area.
myocardium Heart muscle.

nasopharyngeal airway Soft rubber tube that is inserted through the nose so that its distal tip lies in the *pharynx*.
navicular One of the *carpal* bones, located just distal to the *radius*.
neck breather Person who has had a complete *laryngectomy*.
neck lift Maneuver to open the airway by lifting upward on the patient's neck.

negligence Failure to exercise the care that circumstances demand; an act of omission or commission that results in injury; carelessness.
nematocyst Stinging cell at the end of a tentacle in jellyfish, stinging corals, and similar marine animals.
neurogenic shock Failure of tissue *perfusion* caused by massive dilation of blood vessels due to failure of nervous control.
nitroglycerin Medication used by patients with *angina pectoris* for relief of chest pain; usually taken as a small, white tablet that is placed under the tongue.
noise Interference in a radio signal.
normal saline Intravenous salt solution used to replace volume.

oblique fracture *Fracture* in which the fracture line is at an angle to the shaft of the bone.
occipital region Posterior region of the *cranium*.
ohm Unit of electric resistance.
olecranon Proximal end of the *ulna* that hooks around the distal *humerus* to form the elbow.
optic nerve Nerve that extends from the back of the eye to the brain and carries signals relating to visual images.
orbit Eye socket.
orchitis Inflammation of the *testicles;* may be seen in mumps.
organophosphates Class of chemicals used in insecticides and nerve gases.
oropharyngeal airway Curved plastic device that is inserted through the mouth and passes behind the tongue, to hold the tongue away from the back of the throat.
orthopnea *Dyspnea* made worse by the *recumbent* position.
ovary Female sexual gland that produces female hormones and eggs.
ovum An egg; the plural is "ova."
oxygen Colorless, odorless gas that is essential to life and is present in the atmosphere in a concentration of 21 percent.

pallor Whiteness or paleness of the skin.
palpation Examination of part of the body by feeling for abnormal textures, contours, masses, and so forth.
palpitations Sensation of very forceful heartbeats or of the heart "skipping a beat."
pancreas Gland that secretes *insulin* and digestive enzymes.
pancreatitis Inflammation of the pancreas.
paradoxical motion Term usually applied to the movement of a *flail* segment of the chest, which is drawn inward during *inhalation* and bulges outward during *exhalation*.
paramedic Advanced level *emergency medical technician*, trained to carry out certain invasive procedures under the control of a physician.
paraplegia Paralysis of the lower extremities.
paresthesias Pins-and-needles sensations.
parietal region Posterolateral and superior region of the *cranium*.
past medical history (PMH) All of the patient's medical problems that are not directly related to the *chief complaint*.
patch Means of connecting a telephone and a two-way radio.
patella Knee cap.
pelvis Lower bony ring of the trunk.
perfusion Flow of blood through tissues.
pericardial tamponade Condition in which the *pericardium* becomes filled with blood or fluid to the extent that it compresses the heart and prevents cardiac filling.
pericardium Tough, fibrous sac that surrounds the *heart*.
perineum Skin between the *vagina* and the *rectum*.
periorbital The regionn around the eyes.
peristalsis Wavelike contractions of the muscles of hollow organs that propel the contents of the organs forward.
peritoneum Smooth layer of tissue lining the abdominal cavity.
peritonitis Inflammation of the *peritoneum*.
pertinent negative *Symptom* or *sign* that the patient DOES NOT have but might be expected to have, given his or her *chief complaint*.
phalanges Bones of the fingers or toes.
pharynx Throat.
pia mater Innermost layer of the *meninges*.
placenta Special organ of pregnancy that nourishes and oxygenates the developing *fetus*; the afterbirth.
platelet Thrombocyte; cellular element of the blood responsible for repairing leaks in blood vessels and promoting clotting.
pleura Double membrane surrounding the *lungs*.
pleural space Potential space between the two layers of the pleural membrane.
pneumothorax Air in the *pleural space*.
polydipsia Excessive intake of fluids.
polyuria Unusually frequent and profuse urination.
posterior Toward the back; behind.
posterior tibial artery One of the arteries of the foot; its pulsations can be felt posterior to the medial *malleolus* of the ankle.
postpartum After delivery of a baby.
preeclampsia Early stage of *eclampsia*, marked by hypertension and proteinuria.
premature infant Infant born before the eighth month of pregnancy or weighing less than 2 kg (5½ lb).
presenting part Part of the baby that emerges first from the mother's *vagina* during delivery.
priapism Reflex, sustained penile erection; often a sign of spinal cord injury.
primary survey Orderly, initial assessment of a patient to detect and correct immediately life-threatening conditions.
primipara (primip) Woman who has had one viable pregnancy.

prolapsed cord Situation in which the baby's *umbilical cord* protrudes from the mother's *vagina* as the *presenting part.*

prone Lying face down.

prostate Accessory sexual gland surrounding the male *urethra* as it emerges from the *bladder.*

proximal Nearer the point of attachment to the body.

pruritus Itching.

psi Abbreviation for pounds per square inch; a measurement of pressure.

pubis One of two bones that form the anterior portion of the pelvic ring.

pulmonary artery *Artery* that carries blood from the right *ventricle* of the *heart* to the lungs.

pulmonary edema Condition in which the *lungs* fill with fluid.

pulmonary vein *Vein* that carries oxygenated blood from the *lungs* to the left *atrium* of the *heart.*

pulsatile Characterized by throbbing or rhythmic motion.

pulse pressure Difference between the *systolic* and *diastolic* pressures.

P wave First component of the *ECG*, reflecting depolarization of the *atria.*

QRS complex Spiking lines on the *ECG* that follow the *P wave* and reflect depolarization of the *ventricles.*

quadrant One of the quarters into which the *abdomen* is divided by drawing imaginary perpendicular lines that intersect at the *umbilicus.*

quadriplegia Paralysis of the arms and legs.

radial artery One of the arteries to the hand; its pulsations can be felt at the wrist, just proximal to the base of the thumb.

radial nerve Nerve of the arm that controls the muscles of *extension* of the hand.

radiation (1) Emission of heat from the body into surrounding, colder air; (2) transmission of energy in the form of waves or particles.

radioactive Having the property of emitting *ionizing radiation.*

radius The larger bone of the forearm.

rales Abnomral respiratory sounds, having a crackling or bubbling quality, that indicate the presence of fluid in the *alveoli.*

rape Sexual intercourse that is forcibly inflicted on another person.

recumbent Lying down.

red blood cell Cellular component of the blood that carries oxygen; an *erythrocyte.*

reducing valve Regulator that reduces the pressure of gas inside an oxygen cylinder so that the gas emerges from the cylinder at workable pressure levels.

reduction Restoration of a broken bone to proper alignment.

regression Return to a more primitive form of behavior.

regurgitation Passive flow of gastric contents from the *stomach* into the *esophagus*, throat, and mouth.

repeater Radio unit that picks up a radio signal and rebroadcasts it with greater power.

rescue breathing Any form of *artificial ventilation* that utilizes the rescuer's exhaled air to inflate the victim's *lungs.*

reservoir Place where germs live and multiply.

respiratory arrest Cessation of breathing.

response time Total time elapsed from the moment the ambulance service receives a call for help to the moment the ambulance team reaches the patient.

resuscitation Act of reviving an unconscious person or of restoring an apparently dead person to life.

retina Layer of light-sensitive cells in the back of the eye.

retroperitoneal Referring to the area behind the *peritoneum.*

rewarming shock *Shock* due to sudden expansion of the circulation that follows dilation of peripheral vessels as a *hypothermic* patient is rewarmed.

rhonchi Abnormal respiratory sounds, having a rattling quality, that indicate the presence of mucus or other material in the *bronchi* or bronchioles.

rib One of the 12 bones forming the wall of the thoracic cavity.

Ringer's solution Intravenous salt solution used to replace volume.

risk factor Factor that increases a person's susceptibility to a given disease.

roentgen Unit of measurement for *ionizing radiation*, named for the discoverer of x-rays.

rubella German measles.

sacroiliac joint *Joint* between the *sacrum* and the *ilium.*

sacrum Portion of the vertebral column that lies inferior to the *lumbar spine* and is fused with the iliac bones of the *pelvis.*

safe residual Minimum permissible pressure in an oxygen cylinder, defined as 200 *psi.*

saliva Clear secretion from the glands of the mouth that moistens and softens food and begins the digestion of starch.

salivary glands Mucous glands of the mouth that produce *saliva.*

scapula Shoulder blade.

sciatic nerve Major nerve of the lower extremity; it runs behind the hip and down the length of the leg.

sclera Tough, white covering of the eyeball.

scrotum Sac that contains the *testes.*

sebaceous glands Glands located in the *dermis* that produce an oily substance for waterproofing the skin.

sebum Oily substance, produced by *sebaceous glands*, that gives the skin its suppleness and waterproof quality.

secondary survey Assessment of the patient undertaken to detect problems that are not immediately life-threatening but that may become more serious or life-threatening if not treated.

second-degree burn Burn involving the *epidermal* and *dermal* layers of the skin, characterized by redness and blistering.

seizure Convulsion; fit; attack of violent muscle contractions.

seminal vesicle Structure in which sperm and seminal fluid are stored prior to ejaculation.

septic shock Failure of tissue *perfusion* due to changes in the circulation that occur as a result of severe infection.

septum Dividing wall or partition, usually separating two cavities.

shell In reference to the human body, the skin, *subcutaneous* tissue, and extremities.

shock State of inadequate tissue *perfusion.*

shock position Position in which the patient is lying on his left side with his right thigh and right knee drawn up toward his waist.

sign Indication of illness or injury that the EXAMINER can see, hear, feel, smell, etc.

Silvester technique Method of *artificial ventilation* involving chest pressure—arm lift maneuvers performed on a *supine* patient.

simple fracture Closed *fracture*; fracture in which the skin is not broken.

simple pneumothorax Presence of a fixed amount of air in the *pleural space* due to a one-time leak from the *lung* surface.

skeletal muscle Voluntary muscle that is attached to bone and permits locomotion.

smooth muscle Involuntary muscle that makes up the walls of hollow organs.

snoring Noise made on inhalation when the upper airway is partially obstructed by the tongue.

sphygmomanometer Device used to measure blood pressure.

spiral fracture *Fracture*, due to twisting forces, that looks like a coil or spring on x-ray.

spleen Organ, located in the left upper *quadrant* of the *abdomen*, that is involved in the maintenace of blood cells.

splint Any device used to immobilize a part of the body.

spontaneous pneumothorax *Pneumothorax* occurring without trauma, due to rupture of a congenitally weak area of the *lung.*

sprain Injury involving the stretching or tearing of *ligaments.*

squelch Suppression of extraneous *noise* on a radio channel.

stable side position Position in which the patient is lying on his left side with his left thigh and leg flexed and his head resting on his extended left arm; NATO position.

staging area Area at a mass casualty incident in which ambulances are stationed until they are needed for evacuation of patients.

standard of care Norm for providing treatment, against which a person's performance is judged.

status asthmaticus Very severe asthmatic attack that does not respond to the usual medications; may be fatal.

status epilepticus Occurrence of two or more *seizures* without a period of full consciousness in between.

sternum Breastbone.

stillbirth Birth of a dead baby.

Stokes stretcher Basket stretcher.

stoma Hole or opening.

stomach Hollow digestive organ in the *epigastrium* that receives food material through the *esophagus.*

stopping distance Distance a vehicle travels from the moment the driver decides to stop until the vehicle comes to a full halt.

stridor High-pitched, shrill noise audible on *inhalation* when there is significant narrowing—from *edema* or spasm—of the upper airway.

stroke Sudden loss of some neurologic function, due to interruption of the blood supply to part of the brain.

subcutaneous Beneath the skin.

subcutaneous emphysema Air in the soft tissues; causes crackling when the skin is palpated; frequently accompanies large *pneumothorax.*

subdural Beneath the *dura mater.*

sucking chest wound Large, open wound of the chest wall through which air can be heard to be drawn into the chest during *inhalation.*

sudden infant death syndrome (SIDS) Sudden, unexpected death of an apparently normal infant; crib death.

superior Above; toward the head.

superior vena cava One of the two largest *veins* in the body; carries blood from the upper part of the body to the right *atrium.*

supine Lying face up.

suture Fused joint at which two or more bones of the skull come together.

symphysis pubis Point at which the two pubic bones come together.

symptom Pain, discomfort, or other abnormality that the PATIENT FEELS.

syncope Brief loss of consciousness due to temporary reduction in blood flow to the brain; fainting.

synovial joint *Joint* that permits movement of its components.

syrup of ipecac Agent used to induce vomiting.

systole Phase of the cardiac cycle in which the *ventricles* are contracting and ejecting blood.

systolic pressure High point of the blood pressure.

tachycardia Rapid heart rate.

tachypnea Rapid breathing.

tarsals Bones of the ankle.

temporal region Anterolateral region of the *cranium.*

ten-code Radio code system utilizing the number ten plus another number.

tendon Fibrous tissue that connects MUSCLE TO BONE.
tension pneumothorax *Pneumothorax* in which air collects in the *pleural space* under progressively increasing pressure.
testicle Ovoid gland, located in the *scrotum*, that produces sperm and male hormones.
testis Another word for *testicle*; plural is "testes."
tetany Sustained contraction of a muscle group.
third-degree burns Burns involving the full thickness of the skin, including the *epidermis*, *dermis*, *subcutaneous* tissue, and sometimes underlying muscle as well.
Thomas splint Splint developed by Sir Hugh Owen Thomas for applying traction to the lower extremity; half-ring splint.
thoracic spine Part of the spinal column just below the *cervical vertebrae*, comprising 12 vertebrae to which the 12 *ribs* are attached.
thorax Part of the body between the neck and the diaphragm, encased by the *ribs*; the chest.
thrombocyte *Platelet.*
thrombophlebitis Inflammation and clotting within a *vein*.
thrombus Blood clot that forms within a blood vessel and remains lodged at the point of formation.
TIA Abbreviation for *transient ischemic attack*.
tibia Larger bone of the leg; its distal end forms the medial *malleolus* of the ankle.
tolerance Progressive decrease in susceptibility to the effects of a drug after repeated doses.
tonsil tip Type of rigid suction catheter: also called Yankauer suction catheter.
tourniquet Any device applied circumferentially to a limb to impede or exclude blood flow in the limb.
toxemia *Eclampsia.*
toxin Poison produced by a living organism, such as bacteria, poisonous snakes, etc.
trachea Windpipe.
tracheal tugging Upward motion of the *trachea* on *inhalation*; a sign of respiratory distress.
traction Pulling or drawing, with the aim of bringing an injured part into a straighter condition.
transfusion Intravenous therapy with blood or blood products.
transient ischemic attack (TIA) Temporary loss of some neurologic function; often a warning sign of impending *stroke*.
transverse fracture *Fracture* perpendicular to the long axis of the bone.
traumatic asphyxia Name given to a group of clinical signs associated with severe compression injury to the chest.
triage Sorting of patients according to the seriousness of their injuries.
trimester Period of 3 months.
triple-airway maneuver Technique for opening the airway by (1) forward displacement of the *mandible*; (2) backward tilt of the head; and (3) retraction of the lower lip.
trip sheet Written record of an ambulance call.
trochanter Either of the two processes below the neck of the *femur*.
tuberculin test Skin test to determine if a person has been infected with tuberculosis.
T wave Third component of the *ECG*, reflecting the recharging phase of the *ventricles*.

ulcer Open lesion or erosion in the skin or a mucous membrane.
ulna The smaller bone of the forearm; the "funny bone."
ulnar artery One of the arteries supplying the hand; its pulsations can be felt at the wrist, on the little finger side.
umbilical cord Tube connecting the *fetus* to the *placenta*.
umbilicus Navel; belly button.
upper Stimulant drug.
ureter Tube that conducts urine from the *kidney* to the *bladder*.
urethra Tube that conducts urine from the bladder ot the outside of the body.
urticaria Hives.
uterus Pear-shaped muscular organ in a woman's lower *abdomen* that habors the developing *fetus* during pregnancy; the womb.

vagina Female genital canal.
vallecula Groove between the base of the tongue and the *epiglottis*.
vas deferens Seminal duct that conducts sperm and seminal fluid from the *testis* to the *seminal vesicle*.
vasoconstriction Narrowing of the caliber of the arteries, brought about by constriction of the muscles in the arterial walls.
vasodilation Widening of the caliber of the arteries, brought about by relaxation of the muscles in the arterial walls.
vein Vessel that carries blood TOWARD the heart.
vena cava One of the two largest *veins* in the body.
venom Poisonous substance produced by a snake, spider, etc.
ventricle Lower chamber of the right or left *heart*.
ventricular fibrillation Form of *cardiac arrest* in which the individual muscle fibers of the *heart* contract chaotically, and the heart simply quivers; appears as a wavy line on the ECG.
vertebra One of the bones making up the spinal column.
vertex Top of the head.
vitreous humor Jellylike substance within the eye, posterior to the *lens*, that gives the eye its shape.
vocal cords Paired structures in the *larynx* whose vibrations produce sound.
volar Pertaining to the palm side of the arm.
Volkmann's ischemic contractures Contracture and loss of function in the fingers and wrist due to tissue *hypoxia*; may be a complication of fractures of the *humerus* or elbow.

volt Unit of electric force.
vulva External genital organs of the female.

watt Unit of electric power (= *volts* × *amps*).
wheezes Abnormal respiratory sounds, having a whistling quality, that indicate narrowing of the lower airways.
wind-chill factor Factor that takes into account both the temperature and the wind velocity in calculating the effect of a given temperature on living organisms.

withdrawal Symptoms produced by abstinence from a drug to which one is addicted.

xiphoid process Cartilaginous lower tip of the *sternum*.

yoke Part of the *reducing valve* that connects the regulator assembly to the oxygen cylinder.

zygoma Cheek bone.

INDEX